The Oxford Handbook of Child Psychological Assessment

OXFORD LIBRARY OF PSYCHOLOGY

Editor in Chief PETER E. NATHAN

The Oxford Handbook of Child Psychological Assessment

Edited by

Donald H. Saklofske

Cecil R. Reynolds

Vicki L. Schwean

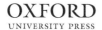

OXFORD
UNIVERSITY PRESS

OXFORD
UNIVERSITY PRESS

Oxford University Press is a department of the University of Oxford.
It furthers the University's objective of excellence in research, scholarship,
and education by publishing worldwide.

Oxford   New York
Auckland   Cape Town   Dar es Salaam   Hong Kong   Karachi
Kuala Lumpur   Madrid   Melbourne   Mexico City   Nairobi
New Delhi   Shanghai   Taipei   Toronto

With offices in
Argentina   Austria   Brazil   Chile   Czech Republic   France   Greece
Guatemala   Hungary   Italy   Japan   Poland   Portugal   Singapore
South Korea   Switzerland   Thailand   Turkey   Ukraine   Vietnam

Oxford is a registered trademark of Oxford University Press in the UK and certain other
countries.

Published in the United States of America by
Oxford University Press
198 Madison Avenue, New York, NY 10016

Library of Congress Cataloging-in-Publication Data
The Oxford handbook of child psychological assessment / edited by Donald H. Saklofske,
Cecil R. Reynolds, Vicki L. Schwean.
    p. cm.
ISBN 978–0–19–979630–4
1. Behavioral assessment of children.   2. Behavioral assessment of teenagers.   3. Psychological
tests for children.   4. Child development—Testing.   5. Psychodiagnostics.   I. Saklofske,
Donald H.   II. Reynolds, Cecil R., 1952–   III. Schwean, Vicki L.
BF722.3.O94 2013
155.4028'7—dc23
2012034712

SHORT CONTENTS

OXFORD LIBRARY OF PSYCHOLOGY

The *Oxford Library of Psychology,* a landmark series of handbooks, is published by Oxford University Press, one of the world's oldest and most highly respected publishers, with a tradition of publishing significant books in psychology. The ambitious goal of the *Oxford Library of Psychology* is nothing less than to span a vibrant, wide-ranging field and, in so doing, to fill a clear market need.

Encompassing a comprehensive set of handbooks, organized hierarchically, the *Library* incorporates volumes at different levels, each designed to meet a distinct need. At one level is a set of handbooks designed broadly to survey the major subfields of psychology; at another are numerous handbooks that cover important current focal research and scholarly areas of psychology in depth and detail. Planned as a reflection of the dynamism of psychology, the *Library* will grow and expand as psychology itself develops, thereby highlighting significant new research that will have an impact on the field. Adding to its accessibility and ease of use, the *Library* will be published in print and, later on, electronically.

The *Library* surveys psychology's principal subfields with a set of handbooks that capture the current status and future prospects of those major sub-disciplines. This initial set includes handbooks of social and personality psychology, clinical psychology, counseling psychology, school psychology, educational psychology, industrial and organizational psychology, cognitive psychology, cognitive neuroscience, methods and measurements, history, neuropsychology, personality assessment, developmental psychology, and more. Each handbook undertakes to review one of psychology's major sub-disciplines with breadth, comprehensiveness, and exemplary scholarship. In addition to these broadly-conceived volumes, the *Library* also includes a large number of handbooks designed to explore in depth more-specialized areas of scholarship and research, such as stress, health, and coping; anxiety and related disorders; cognitive development; or child and adolescent assessment. In contrast to the broad coverage of the subfield handbooks, each of these latter volumes focuses on an especially productive, more highly focused line of scholarship and research. Whether at the broadest or most specific level, however, all of the *Library* handbooks offer synthetic coverage that reviews and evaluates the relevant past and present research and anticipates research in the future. Each handbook in the *Library* includes introductory and concluding chapters written by its editor to provide a roadmap to the handbook's table of contents and to offer informed anticipations of significant future developments in that field.

An undertaking of this scope calls for handbook editors and chapter authors who are established scholars in the areas about which they write. Many of the nation's and world's most productive and best-respected psychologists have agreed to edit *Library* handbooks or write authoritative chapters in their areas of expertise.

For whom has the *Oxford Library of Psychology* been written? Because of its breadth, depth, and accessibility, the *Library* serves a diverse audience, including graduate students in psychology and their faculty mentors, scholars, researchers, and practitioners in psychology and related fields. Each will find in the *Library* the information they seek on the subfield or focal area of psychology in which they work or are interested.

Befitting its commitment to accessibility, each handbook includes a comprehensive index, as well as extensive references to help guide research. And because the *Library* was designed from its inception as an online as well as a print resource, its structure and contents will be readily and rationally searchable online. Furthermore, once the *Library* is released online, the handbooks will be regularly and thoroughly updated.

In summary, the *Oxford Library of Psychology* will grow organically to provide a thoroughly informed perspective on the field of psychology, one that reflects both psychology's dynamism and its increasing interdisciplinarity. Once it is published electronically, the *Library* is also destined to become a uniquely valuable interactive tool, with extended search and browsing capabilities. As you begin to consult this handbook, we sincerely hope you will share our enthusiasm for the more than 500-year tradition of Oxford University Press for excellence, innovation, and quality, as exemplified by the *Oxford Library of Psychology*.

Peter E. Nathan
Editor-in-Chief
Oxford Library of Psychology

ABOUT THE EDITORS

Donald H. Saklofske

Don Saklofske is a Professor, Department of Psychology, University of Western Ontario. He is editor of the Journal of Psychoeducational Assessment and Canadian Journal of School Psychology, Associate Editor of Personality and Individual Differences, and editor of the Springer Series on Human Exceptionality. Don is the current president of the International Society for the Study of Individual Differences.

Cecil R. Reynolds

A Distinguished Research Scholar at Texas A & M University, Dr. Reynolds is a Professor of Educational Psychology and a Professor of Neuroscience. He is well known for his work in psychological testing and assessment, and is the author or editor of more than 30 books, including The Handbook of School Psychology, the Encyclopedia of Special Education, and the Handbook of Psychological and Educational Assessment of Children. He also authored the widely used Test of Memory and Learning (TOMAL) and the Revised Children's Manifest Anxiety Scale. He has published a total of more than 300 scholarly works

Vicki L. Schwean

Vicki is currently Professor and Dean of Education, University of Western Ontario.

CONTRIBUTORS

Wayne Adams
Graduate Department of Clinical Psychology
George Fox University
Newberg, Oregon

Vincent C. Alfonso
Division of Psychological and Educational
   Services
Fordham University
Bronx, New York

Justin P. Allen
Department of Psychology and Research in
   Education
University of Kansas
Lawrence, Kansas

Kathleen Hague Armstrong
Department of Child and Family Studies
University of South Florida
Tampa, Florida

Tiffany L. Arrington
Department of Psychology and Research in
   Education
University of Kansas
Lawrence, Kansas

Stephen J. Bagnato
University of Pittsburgh School of
   Education
Children's Hospital of Pittsburgh
Pittsburgh, Pennsylvania

A. Lynne Beal
Private Practice
Toronto, Canada

Skylar A. Bellinger
Center for Child Health and Development
University of Kansas Medical Center
Kansas City, Kansas

Tanya Beran
Faculty of Medicine
University of Calgary
Calgary, Alberta, Canada

Jonas Bertling
Educational Testing Service
Princeton, New Jersey

Anthony Betancourt
Educational Testing Service
Princeton, New Jersey

Jeremy Burrus
Educational Testing Service
Princeton, New Jersey

Gary L. Canivez
Department of Psychology
Eastern Illinois University
Charleston, Illinois

Jenna Chin
Department of Counseling, Clinical, and
   School Psychology
University of California at Santa Barbara
Santa Barbara, California

Emma A. Climie
Faculty of Education
University of Calgary
Calgary, Alberta, Canada

Jessica Cuellar
Department of Psychology
University of North Carolina at Chapel Hill
Chapel Hill, North Carolina

Scott L. Decker
Department of Psychology
University of South Carolina
Columbia, South Carolina

Erin Dowdy
Department of Counseling, Clinical, and
   School Psychology
University of California at Santa Barbara
Santa Barbara, California

Michelle A. Drefs
Faculty of Education
University of Calgary
Calgary, Alberta, Canada

Ron Dumont
School of Psychology
Fairleigh Dickinson University
Teaneck, New Jersey

Agnieszka M. Dynda
St. John's University
Queens, New York

Tanya L. Eckert
Department of Psychology
Syracuse University
Syracuse, New York

Liesl J. Edwards
University of Kansas Medical Center
Center for Child Health and Development
Kansas City, Kansas

Stephen N. Elliott
Learning Sciences Institute
Arizona State University
Tempe, Arizona

Monica Epstein
Department of Mental Health and Law Policy
University of South Florida
Tampa, Florida

Stephen E. Finn
Center for Therapeutic Assessment
Austin, Texas

Meghann Fior
Faculty of Medicine
University of Calgary
Calgary, Alberta, Canada

Erik L. Fister
Department of Psychology and Research in
    Education
University of Kansas
Lawrence, Kansas

Dawn P. Flanagan
Department of Psychology
St. John's University
Queens, New York

James R. Flens
Private Practice
Brandon, Florida

Rex Forehand
Department of Psychology
University of Vermont
Burlington, Vermont

Craig L. Frisby
College of Education
University of Missouri
Columbia, Missouri

Mauricio A. Garcia-Barrera
Department of Psychology
University of Victoria
Victoria, British Columbia, Canada

Lauren B. Gentry
The University of Texas at Austin
Austin, Texas

Eugene Gonzalez
Educational Testing Service
Princeton, New Jersey

Jonathan W. Gould
Private Practice
Charlotte, North Carolina

Darielle Greenberg
Private Practice
Richardson, Texas

Matthew J. Grumbein
Leavenworth County Special Education
    Cooperative
Lansing USD 469
Lansing, Kansas

Ronald K. Hambleton
School of Education
University of Massachusetts Amherst
Amherst, Massachusetts

Jason Hangauer
University of South Florida
Tampa, Florida

Kimberly J. Hills
Department of Psychology
University of South Carolina
Columbia, South Carolina

Susan Homack
Private Practice
Rockwall, Texas

E. Scott Huebner
Department of Psychology
University of South Carolina
Columbia, South Carolina

Deborah J. Jones
Department of Psychology
University of North Carolina at
    Chapel Hill
Chapel Hill, North Carolina

Diana K. Joyce
University of Florida
Gainesville, Florida

R. W. Kamphaus
Department of Psychology
Georgia State University
Atlanta, Georgia

Belinda N. Kathurima
Department of Psychology and Research in
    Education
University of Kansas
Lawrence, Kansas

Alan S. Kaufman
School of Medicine
Yale University
New Haven, Connecticut.

James C. Kaufman
Learning Research Institute
California State University at
    San Bernardino
San Bernardino, California

Timothy Z. Keith
College of Education
The University of Texas at Austin
Austin, Texas

Ryan J. Kettler
Graduate School of Applied and Professional
    Psychology
Rutgers University
Piscataway, New Jersey

Sangwon Kim
Ewha Woman's University
Seoul, South Korea

H. D. Kirkpatrick
Forensic Psychologist

Eckhard Klieme
German Institute for International Educational
    Research
Frankfurt, Germany

Kathryn Kuehnle
Department of Mental Health and Law Policy
University of South Florida
Tampa, Florida

Patrick C. Kyllonen
Educational Testing Service
Princeton, New Jersey

Andrea Lee
School Psychology Program
University of North Carolina at Chapel Hill
Chapel Hill, North Carolina

Jihyun Lee
National Institute of Education
Nanyang Technological University
Singapore

Minji Kang Lee
Psychometric Methods, Educational Statistics,
    and Research Methods
University of Massachusetts Amherst
Amherst, Massachusetts

Elizabeth O. Lichtenberger
Alliant International University
San Diego, California

Petra Lietz
Australian Council for Educational Research
Melbourne, Australia

Anastasiya A. Lipnevich
Queens College
City University of New York
New York, New York

Stephen W. Loke
Department of Psychology and Research in
    Education
University of Kansas
Lawrence, Kansas

Benjamin J. Lovett
Department of Psychology
Elmira College
Elmira, New York

Patricia A. Lowe
Department of Psychology and Research in
    Education
University of Kansas
Lawrence, Kansas

Carolyn MacCann
School of Psychology
The University of Sydney
Sydney, Australia

Marisa Macy
Department of Education
Lycoming College
Williamsport, Pennsylvania

David A. Martindale
Private Practice
St. Petersburg, Florida

Nancy Mather
College of Education
University of Arizona
Tucson, Arizona

Laura G. McKee
Department of Psychology
Clark University
Worcester, Massachusetts

Brian C. McKevitt
Department of Psychology
University of Nebraska at Omaha
Omaha, Nebraska

Jennifer Minsky
Educational Testing Service
Princeton, New Jersey

William R. Moore
University of Victoria
Victoria, British Columbia, Canada

Bobby Naemi
Educational Testing Service
Princeton, New Jersey

Jeaveen M. Neaderhiser
Department of Psychology and Research in
Education
University of Kansas
Lawrence, Kansas

Christopher R. Niileksela
Department of Psychology and Research in
Education
University of Kansas
Lawrence, Kansas

Samuel O. Ortiz
Department of Psychology
St. John's University
Queens, New York

Jonathan A. Plucker
Center for Evaluation and Education Policy
Indiana University
Bloomington, Indiana

Jennifer M. Raad
Department of Psychology and Research in
Education
University of Kansas
Lawrence, Kansas

Daniel J. Reschly
Peabody College
Vanderbilt University
Nashville, Tennessee

Cecil R. Reynolds
Department of Education & Human
Development
Texas A & M University
College Station, Texas

Matthew R. Reynolds
Department of Psychology and Research in
Education
University of Kansas
Lawrence, Kansas

Cynthia A. Riccio
Department of Education and Human
Development
Texas A & M University
College Station, Texas

Richard D. Roberts
Educational Testing Service
Princeton, New Jersey

Christina M. Russell
Indiana University
Bloomington, Indiana

Donald H. Saklofske
Department of Psychology
University of Western Ontario
London, Ontario, Canada

W. Joel Schneider
Department of Psychology
Illinois State University
Normal, Illinois

Vicki L. Schwean
Faculty of Education
University of Western Ontario
London, Ontario, Canada

Jessica Oeth Schuttler
University of Kansas Medical Center
Center for Child Health and Development
Kansas City, Kansas

Jill D. Sharkey
The Gevirtz School
University of California, Santa Barbara
Santa Barbara, California

Bennett A. Shaywitz
The Yale Center of Dyslexia and Creativity
Yale University
New Haven, Connecticut

Sally E. Shaywitz
School of Medicine
Yale University
New Haven, Connecticut

Rune J. Simeonsson
School Psychology Program
University of North Carolina at Chapel Hill
Chapel Hill, North Carolina

Steven N. Sparta
UCSD Medical School
Thomas Jefferson School of Law
University of California San Diego
San Diego, California

Kathy C. Stroud
Licensed Specialist in School Psychology

Michael L. Sulkowski
University of Florida
Gainesville, Florida

H. Lee Swanson
Graduate School of Education
University of California-Riverside
Riverside, California

Hedwig Teglasi
Department of Counseling, Higher Education,
and Special Education
University of Maryland
College Park, Maryland

Deborah J. Tharinger
The University of Texas at Austin
Austin, Texas

Jennifer Twyford
University of California, Santa Barbara
Santa Barbara, California

Susan M. Unruh
Department of Counseling, Educational
Leadership, and Educational & School
Psychology
Wichita State University
Wichita, Kansas

Svenja Vieluf
German Institute for International Educational
Research
Frankfurt, Germany

John O. Willis
Senior Lecturer in Assessment
Rivier College
Peterborough, New Hampshire

Jonathan Worcester
University of South Florida
Tampa, Florida

CONTENTS

Part Four • Special and Emergent Topics in Child and Adolescent Assessment

PREFACE

Psychological assessment has paralleled the growth of psychology and its special-ties since the appearance of the famous Galton tests, the founding of psychology beginning with establishment of Wundt's laboratory, and the successful application of Binet's ability tests. Whether measuring a specific sensory process (e.g., auditory discrimination), broader psychological constructs such as personality (e.g., Big 5), or an observable behavior (e.g., frequency of motor tics) or a latent trait such as intelligence, psychologists have always espoused the importance of measuring the constructs and variables that are the domain of psychological science and using the resulting information as part of the data that can facilitate and enhance decision making in psychological practice. It is not overstating to say that measurement and assessment are the cornerstones of psychology providing the tools and techniques for gathering information to inform our understanding of human behavior.

Precision in every sense of the word is key in psychological assessment. This begins with a description and operational definition of the trait or behavior under examination derived from the theory and research necessary to add empirical sup-port. Following from this foundation is the development of scales that may include various tests (e.g., objective, self report, performance) as well as observation and interview methods to accurately measure (i.e., reliability, validity) the defined behaviors or traits. Standardizing these measures allows for even greater precision in administration, scoring, and interpretation. Data are gathered not only when the test is first published but in follow-up research that further allows for various com-parisons of the individual's responses or test scores to normative and criterion inter-pretations, including change scores whether due to maturation or 'treatment'. Thus psychological measurement addresses the fundamental questions of "how much" and within the context of assessment, contributes to the additional questions of "what and why". Measures are extensions of theory- and research- based findings such that tests developed to measure intelligence are derived from various theories that have received empirical support. In turn, the findings can be used for a variety of 'applied' purposes - to explain, predict and change behavior.

A well used phrase in the measurement/assessment area is, "the more informa-tion and the better it is, the better the decision that will be made". Psychologists have created thousands of 'tests' over the past 100 years tapping such key cognitive constructs as intelligence and memory, personality factors such as extraversion and neuroticism, and conative measures including motivation and self efficacy. As psychological knowledge expands, so does the very need to measure and assess these 'new' variables. With the emergence of contemporary models such as emo-tional intelligence and theory of mind, new measures have quickly followed. Of course it is both theory but also the development of new data analysis techniques such as structural equation modeling that has allowed us to determine how psychological constructs interact and even moderate or mediate the impact of particular factors on outcomes measures. In turn, this has enhanced the use of 'test batteries' to aid in the psychological assessment of a myriad of human 'conditions' ranging from depression and psychopathy, to learning disabilities and Attention Deficit-Hyperactivity Disorder. 'Clinical' assessment and diagnosis, necessary for determining the selection and application of the most appropriate evidence-based interventions, is grounded in the interface between a complex of key factors (both endogenous and exogenous) that can be obtained from our psychological tests and measures.

Although measurement and assessment are central to psychology, and all science-based disciplines and their resulting practices, psychological tests have been heavily criticized over the years. These criticisms not only come from other disciplines and the general public but also from psychologists themselves. For example, psychological test use has been challenged in the courts and the Response to Intevention (RTI) perspective that has gained momentum in education argues against a reliance on psychological tests for psychological and educational diagnosis. These are but two recent examples of the variability of opinion on assessment. But whether the attack comes from humanistic psychologists or radical behaviorists who might challenge the need for employing tests at all, the fact is that all psychologists engage in "assessment" through the gathering and analysis of data to aid decision making. Counseling psychologists rely heavily on 'talk' to determine a person's needs and issues whereas behaviorists are diligent in observing and measuring overt behaviors (without recourse to proposing underlying hypothetical factors) which can then be used to identify the antecedents and consequences relevant to the behavior in question. Psychoanalytically oriented psychologists may make greater use of projective techniques and free association as the 'data' for guiding their diagnosis and therapy decisions but still are engaged in the assessment process at all stages of their work with clients. These differences 'within' psychology show that assessment is not a static action but an ongoing process that starts with efforts to identify the 'issues' and continues as one observes changes related to everything from life events to therapy outcomes, including the need to reevaluate as new information comes to the fore.

The decisions that need to be made by psychologists can vary from traditional placement, selection and classification to program evaluation, early identification screening, and outcome prediction. Indeed, psychologists engage in a rather amazing array of assessments for many purposes. Psychological assessments and the measurement of various states, traits, and attributes have become valuable because in so many instances they reduce the error rates involved in predictions and decision-making. In fact, psychological assessment and the measurement process are useful only to the extent they can reduce error relative to reliance on other techniques. Determining the correct diagnosis to understand the presenting problems of a client (including the determination that there may be no pathology present), predicting who will be successful in a sales job, who will 'make it' academically in college, or whether medication has been effective in changing behavior, all require a most detailed and comprehensive assessment. In the forensic context, the extent of functional impairment in a brain injury following a motor vehicle collision, which parent a child of divorce should reside within a custody agreement, and in capital murder cases in some USA states, who is eligible for the death penalty (defendants with intellectual disability cannot be executed) are a few examples of the many predictions and decisions to which psychological test data contribute in meaningful ways.

Another traditional view is that "tests are neutral; it is what we do with them that makes them useful-useless, informative-misleading, 'good-bad', or the like. These viewpoints clearly place psychological assessment in context. Psychological tests that assess the complexities of human behavior just don't appear from nowhere, nor does their use and application automatically follow from simply administering and scoring a test. Assessment employs multimethod-multimodal techniques that rely on scientific knowledge derived from research, theoretical constructs or latent traits and models of human behavior (normal development of social behavior to models of psychiatric classification such as the DSM series). Whatever the 'methods' of assessment, there must be a demonstration of their reliability and validity. This required psychometric support is necessary to weave assessment findings into our psychological knowledge of human behavior that then may lead to prevention and intervention techniques (primary, secondary, tertiary) intended to reduce psychological challenges and promote psychological health and wellness. This process requires a high degree of clinical knowledge and professional competency regardless of one's psychological orientation. Coupled with this is an adherence to the highest professional standards and ethical guidelines.

The editors of this volume are committed to 'best practices in psychological assessment' and while psychological assessment knowledge, techniques, and applications continues to 'improve, we are reassured by a position paper published by Meyer et al (2001) American Psychologist (2001, 56, 128–165) that summarized the literature on psychological assessment. Based on an extensive review of the published literature, it was concluded that: "psychological test validity is strong and compelling, psychological test validity is comparable to medical test validity, distinct assessment methods provide unique sources of information...". It is further stated that: "...a multimethod assessment battery provides a structured means for skilled clinicians to maximize the validity of individualized assessment" and that future investigations should "focus on the role of psychologists who use tests".

A very large literature has addressed the myriad of topics of relevance to psychological assessment. There are a number of journals devoted specifically to this topic including Psychological Assessment edited by Cecil Reynolds and the Journal of Psychoeducational Assessment edited by Don Saklofske. However, the continued growth and new developments in the assessment literature requires an ongoing examination of the 'principles and practices' of central importance to psychological assessment. In particular, the psychological assessment of children and youth has undergone some of the greatest developments, and those developments are the primary focus of this book.

This volume on assessment has been organized primarily, but not exclusively, around clinical and psychoeducational assessment issues. To ensure we are on solid ground, the foundations that underlie current psychological assessment practices are revisited. For example, the mobility of people has led to major changes in the demographics of countries making cultural issues a major focus in assessment. Linked with these foundations are chapters addressing some of the fundamental principles of child assessment that particularly focus on ability, achievement, behavior and personality. Techniques and specific methods of practice can change rapidly, and we have paired such chapters where possible with the chapters (or sections within a chapter in some cases) from the two previous sections. Theory provides us with guidance in practice when techniques change, new methods are introduced, and new data are presented, as well as when we encounter new presenting issues and circumstances with patients or when asked new questions by referral sources as raised with some specific examples in the fourth section of this volume. A volume on methods that does not also focus on theory is a short-lived work. Here we hope to see theory integrated with research and practice that will enable you to read the chapters in this book, as well as future publications ,not just more profitably but critically as well.

We are especially grateful to all of our authors who wrote the informed and insightful chapters for this volume. Each is an expert who has contributed extensively to psychological assessment research and practice with children and youth and who individually and collectively have made this a book rich in content. While a number of people at Oxford University Press have had a role in this book, we are indebted to Chad Zimmerman, Sarah Harrington, and Anne Dellinger who have provided the necessary guidance and advice that has supported this book from proposal to publication. We also wish to extend our appreciation to Anitha Chellamuthu for guiding this book through the editing phases to publication.

Donald H. Saklofske
Cecil R. Reynolds
Vicki L. Schwean

PART 1

Foundations of Psychological Assessment

The Role of Theory in Psychological Assessment

Darielle Greenberg, Elizabeth O. Lichtenberger, *and* Alan S. Kaufman

Abstract

This chapter reviews the role of theory in cognitive and neuropsychological assessment from a historical perspective. Theory has been applied to both test development and test interpretation, and it provides a strong framework for valid psychological assessments. Theory-based tests of the twenty-first century such as the Kaufman Assessment Battery for Children—Second Edition (KABC-II), Stanford-Binet Intelligence Test—Fifth Edition (SB-V), Das-Naglieri Cognitive Assessment System (CAS), Woodcock Johnson Test of Cognitive Abilities—Third Edition (WJ-III), and Differential Ability Scales—Second Edition (DAS-II) are highlighted as valid and reliable testing tools. Contemporary methods of test interpretation, including the Cross Battery Assessment approach and the Planning, Attention-Arousal, Simultaneous, and Success (PASS) model of processing, are presented as valid methods of interpretation based on theory. As noted from the chapter's historical perspective, incorporating theory in an assessment helps clinicians synthesize information that is gathered from the evaluation's multiple sources, and ultimately results in more accurate interpretations and interventions.

Key Words: theory, psychological assessment, cognitive, neuropsychological, testing, Cross Battery Assessment, PASS model

For centuries, professionals have been fascinated with the functions of the human body and brain. Attempts to measure brain function, specifically cognitive abilities, date back to 2200 B.C. in China. It is believed that the emperor gave formalized tests to his officers as a way to test for fitness of duty (Kaufman, 2009). With technological advances, significant strides have been made in the area of cognitive abilities and human intelligence. However, controversy regarding the components of these abilities and how to assess them still exists (see, e.g., Flanagan & Harrison, 2012).

The purpose of this chapter is to discuss the role of theory in psychological assessment from a historical perspective. The history is rich and has had an impact on contemporary test development and interpretation. What is meant by "psychological

assessment"? Psychological assessment involves a synthesis of the information gathered from several sources, including psychological tests, family history, behavioral observations, and so forth, to understand or make statements regarding an individual's diagnosis, level of functioning, and treatment. Simply administering a test, such as the Wechsler Intelligence Scale for Children–Fourth Edition (WISC-IV; Wechsler, 2003) or even a theory-based test like the Woodcock-Johnson III (WJ III; Woodcock, McGrew, & Mather, 2001b; Woodcock, McGrew, Schrank, & Mather, 2007) or Kaufman Assessment Battery for Children–Second Edition (KABC-II; Kaufman & Kaufman, 2004a), would be considered psychological testing, and the data collected from multiple other sources in addition to this one test would round out a complete assessment. Theory has played a significant role in cognitive and neuropsychological assessments, and it is these types of assessments that are the focus of this chapter. Although we acknowledge the usefulness of theory in the development of other types of tools, such as group-administered tests, personality tests, or non-cognitive tests, our particular discussion will center around the role of theory in developing and interpreting tests of cognitive ability. The role of theory in psychological cognitive and

neuropsychological assessment is two-pronged. The first prong is the development of tests from theory, and the second is the interpretation of tests from theory.

Historical roots and landmarks

Before describing the modern role of theory in test interpretation and development, a historical review of the period from 1500 to 1970 is warranted. A timeline of historical landmarks in psychological assessment appears in Table 1.1.

Table 1.1 Timeline of Select Historical Landmarks in Psychological Assessment

2200 B.C.	Chinese emperors gave formalized tests to their officials as part of a standardized civil service testing program.
A.D. 1575	Juan Huarte published *Examen de Ingenios* (The Tryal of Wits) in which he tried to demonstrate the connection between physiology and psychology.
1799	Jean-Marc Itard worked to rehabilitate "Victor," a young wild boy found in the woods. Itard assessed differences between normal and abnormal cognitive functioning.
1644	Thomas Willis, an English physician, detailed the anatomy of the brain.
1800	Franz Gall created *phrenology*, or the idea that the prominent bumps on a person's skull determined his personality and intelligence.
1861	Pierre Broca discovered that the speech-production center of the brain was located in the ventro-posterior region of the frontal lobes (now known as "Broca's area").
1874	Carl Wernicke found that damage to the left posterior, superior temporal gyrus resulted in deficits in language comprehension. This region is now referred to as "Wernicke's area."
1837	Edouard Seguin established the first successful school for children with mental retardation.
1838	Jean Esquirol proposed that mental retardation was distinct from mental illness. He suggested that mental disabilities could be categorized into different levels.
1879	William Wundt founded the first psychological laboratory in Germany.
1884	Francis Galton theorized that intelligence was based on sensory keenness and reaction time. He set up a laboratory that used tests to measure these physical and mental abilities.
1888	James McKeen Cattell opened a testing laboratory at the University of Pennsylvania, and his work helped establish mental measurement in the United States.
1904	Charles Spearman proposed a two-factor theory of intelligence that included a general factor (g) and specific (s) factors.
1905	Albert Binet and Theodore Simon developed an intelligence test for screening school-age children.
1909	E. L. Thorndike proposed that intelligence was a cluster of three mental abilities: social, concrete, and abstract.
1917	Robert Yerkes and Lewis Terman developed the Army Alpha and Army Beta, group-administered intelligence tests.
1933	Louis Thurstone used a factor-analytic approach to study human intelligence.

(continued)

Table 1.1 (Continued)

1935	Ward Halstead established the first laboratory in America devoted to the study of brain–behavior relationships.
1939	David Wechsler published the Wechsler-Bellevue Intelligence Scale.
1949/1955	David Wechsler published the Wechsler Intelligence Scale for Children (WISC) and the Wechsler Adult Intelligence Scale (WAIS).
1959	J. P. Guilford proposed a Structure of Intellect model of intelligence.
1963	Raymond Cattell and John Horn proposed a theory of crystallized and fluid intelligence, expanding on Cattell's work in 1941.
1979	Alan Kaufman published "Intelligent Testing with the WISC-R," which launched the assessment field into merging theory into test interpretation.
1983	Alan and Nadeen Kaufman published the Kaufman Assessment Battery for Children (K-ABC).
1985	John Horn expanded the Gf-Gc model to include ten abilities.
1986	Robert L. Thorndike et al. published the Stanford-Binet—Fourth Edition, which was designed to conform to Gf-Gc theory.
1989	Richard Woodcock revised the 1977 Woodcock-Johnson Psych-Educational Battery (WJ, which was not based on theory, to develop the WJ-R, founded on 7 Broad Abilities posited by Horn's Gf-Gc theory.
1990	Colin Elliott published the Differential Ability Scale (DAS), which was based on g theory.
1993	John Carroll proposed a three-stratum theory of cognitive abilities, including general ability (level III), broad abilities (level II), and narrow abilities (level I).
1994	J. P. Das, Jack Naglieri, and John Kirby propose the Planning, Attention, Simultaneous, Successive (PASS) theory of intelligence.
1997	Kevin McGrew proposed an integrated Cattell-Horn and Carroll model of cognitive abilities, which was refined by Dawn Flanagan, Kevin McGrew, and Samuel Ortiz in 2000.
1997	Jack Naglieri and J. P. Das published the Cognitive Assessment System (CAS), which is based on the PASS theory of intelligence.
2000	Dawn Flanagan and colleagues developed the Cross-Battery approach to test interpretation.
2001	Woodcock-Johnson–3rd ed. was published, which was based on a CHC theoretical model.
2003	Stanford-Binet–5th ed. was published, which was based on a CHC theoretical model; WISC-IV was published, based on cognitive neuroscience research and theory
2004	Kaufman Assessment Battery for Children–2nd ed. was published, which was based on a dual (CHC and Luria) theoretical model.
2007	Colin Elliott published the Differential Ability Scale—Second Edition (DAS-II), which was based on CHC theory.
2008/2012	Pearson published the latest versions of Wechsler's scales, the WAIS-IV (2008) and WPPSI-IV (2012); all of Wechsler's fourth editions are based on cognitive neuroscience research and theory, especially concerning fluid reasoning, working memory, and processing speed.

Historical Antecedents Before the Nineteenth Century—Juan Huarte, Jean-Marc Itard, and Thomas Willis

Psychological assessment has its roots mainly in the nineteenth century. However, before the 1800s, there were the influential works of men such as Juan Huarte de San Juan and Jean-Marc Gaspard Itard. The sixteenth century was the beginning of the modern era, which brought about economic, political, social, and religious changes. Scientific innovations were booming. In 1575, Juan Huarte, a Spanish physician, published *Examen de Ingenios* (The Tryal of Wits) in which he tried to demonstrate the connection between physiology and psychology. This publication was considered the best-known medical treaty of its time (Ortega, 2005). Huarte believed: 1) Cognitive functions were located in the brain; 2) cognitive functions were innate; 3) human understanding was generative; 4) qualitative differences existed between humans and animals; and 5) language was a universal structure. He also theorized that language was an index of human intelligence and suggested the idea of testing to understand intelligence. Huarte's ideas greatly influenced modern psycholinguistics, organizational psychology, and psychological assessment (Ortega, 2005). Needless to say, his beliefs were revolutionary for his time.

Over two decades later, during the eighteenth century, philosophers and scholars began to question the laws, beliefs, and ideas of the aristocracy. In 1799, the work of Jean-Marc Itard drew public attention for his work with a feral young boy, "Victor," who was found in the woods. Physicians who examined Victor described him as "deaf," "retarded," "a mental defective," and "hopelessly insane and unteachable" (Ansell, 1971; Lane, 1986; Lieberman, 1982). Itard disagreed and believed that Victor's deficiencies were not the result of mental deficiency, but rather due to a lack of interaction with others. For five years, he attempted to "rehabilitate" Victor using an intense education program at the Institute of Deaf Mutes. Itard's aims were to increase his socialization, stimulation, and education. Although Itard was not successful in making Victor "normal," Victor was able to speak and read a few words and follow simple directions. Itard's program was perhaps the first of what we call today an Individualized Educational Program or Plan (IEP).

During these times, physicians were not only responsible for medically examining people like Victor, but they were also in charge of studying and explaining the relationship between brain function and behavior (known today as *neuropsychology*)

(Boake, 2008). Although not a physician, Rene Descartes, one of the greatest philosophers, was the first to note that the brain was the most vital organ in mediating behavior. He struggled with understanding and explaining the mind–body connection. After seeing an animated statue of St. Germaine, he theorized that the "flow of animal spirits" through nerves caused the body to move, which led to behaviors (Hatfield, 2007). This theory is known today as the *mechanistic* view of behavior. Descartes believed that although the body and mind interacted, they were, indeed, separate entities.

In 1664, an English physician by the name of Thomas Willis was the first to detail the anatomy of the brain. He is considered to be one of the greatest neuroanatomists of all time and the founder of clinical neuroscience (Molnar, 2004). After studying many patients and dissecting their brains, he described two types of tissue in the brain: gray and white matter. Agreeing with Descartes, he theorized that the white matter was made up of channels that dispersed the "spirits" produced by the gray matter. Willis was also convinced that the brain structures themselves influenced behavior.

Nineteenth-Century Contributions from Brain Research—Franz Gall and Pierre Paul Broca

Around the 1800s, in Austria, physician Franz Gall introduced the idea that the brain was made up of separate organs that were responsible for certain traits, such as memory and aggressiveness. He created *phrenology* or the idea that one could examine the prominent bumps on a person's skull and determine his or her personality and intelligence; a larger brain meant greater intelligence.

Although incorrect about the connection between bumps and intelligence, Gall sparked interest in the area of brain localization (or the idea that specific areas of the brain were responsible for specific functions). As advances in medicine took place, modest progress in understanding human anatomy was made. Prior beliefs had inaccurately attributed behavior to "spirits," while Gall's theories were dismissed as absurd. However, "the field was not ready for behavioral localization" (Maruish & Moses, 1997, p. 34).

After attending a conference, Pierre Paul Broca, a French physician, focused on understanding how brain damage affected people. While working in a hospital, Broca came into contact with a patient who had lost his use of speech, although he could still comprehend language. Because the patient could only say and repeat the word "tan," he became known as Tan. After Tan died in 1861, Broca performed an autopsy and found a lesion on the left side of the brain's frontal cortex. Other patients like Tan were found to have the same damaged area. From these patients, Broca postulated that the brain's left side of the frontal cortex was responsible for processing language. This region of the brain would later become known as *Broca's area*. Broca's lesion-method, which involved localization of brain function by studying the anatomy of the brain lesion, became an accepted tool for understanding the brain–behavior relationship.

Several years later, German physician Carl Wernicke suggested that not all the functions of language processing were in the area Broca described. During his work on the wards of the Allerheiligen Hospital, he found that patients who sustained damage to or had lesions on the superior posterior portion of the left hemisphere also experienced problems with language comprehension. This area was later named *Wernicke's area*. In 1874, Wernicke published a model of language organization, describing three types of language centers: 1) motor language (damage to this center produced the speech production problems described by Broca); 2) sensory language (damage to this area produced comprehension deficits); and 3) a pathway between these two centers (damage resulted in impairments in repetition) (Mariush & Moses, 1997).

Nineteenth Century Contributions from Research on Mental Deficiency—Jean Esquirol and Edouard Seguin

Along with attention to brain function localization, interest in criminals, mental illness, and mental disabilities (and the differences between them) arose. Thanks to the works of Jean-Etienne Dominique Esquirol and Edouard Sequin, mental disability was no longer associated with insanity (Aiken, 2004). Esquirol theorized that persons with mental illness actually lost their cognitive abilities. In contrast, he determined that those who were called "idiots" never developed their intellectual abilities, and he proposed several levels of mental disability (i.e., morons, idiots, etc). He also believed them to be incurable. Eduardo Sequin was a student of Itard and Esquirol. Sequin disagreed with Esquirol and believed that mental deficiencies were caused by sensory isolation or deprivation and could be mitigated with motor and tactile stimulation (Winzer, 1993). Agreeing with Itard that children with mental disabilities could learn, Sequin

expanded Itard's work into three main components: 1) motor and sensory training; 2) intellectual training; and 3) moral training. During the French Revolution, Sequin fled to the United States. He continued his work and established several schools devoted entirely to teaching children with mental retardation. Along with promoting understanding of those who had mental deficiencies, Esquirol and Sequin's work fostered a continued curiosity about intelligence and intelligence testing.

The Birth of IQ Tests in the Late 1800s— Francis Galton and James McKeen Cattell

Western society experienced many changes in culture and technology in the late 1800s. Compulsory-education laws in the United States and Europe and the rise of psychology as a quantitative science were precursors to the introduction and measurement of intelligence (Thorndike, 1997). Before the compulsory-education law, only children whose families came from higher social strata (or who were interested) attended school. The curriculum was set to meet the standards and needs of *these* students. As one can imagine, not everyone was educated. The majority of American society included people and parents who were uneducated or who were unable to speak English (due to the large number of immigrants). Giving access to public education was a way to improve literacy and assimilate immigrants. Thus, the new laws resulted in heterogeneity in the student body and a dramatic increase in student failure rates (Thorndike, 1997). Due to the astonishing failure rates, leaders believed education should not be wasted on those would not benefit, so they devised plans to "weed out" the children who were most likely to fail—intelligence testing was one method.

Along with the educational changes came the rise of psychology as a quantitative science. Gustav Fechner, Herman Ebbinghaus, Sir Francis Galton, and James McKeen Cattell were among the early forerunners who believed mental abilities could be measured (Sattler, 2008; Wasserman, 2012). While Fechner believed he had discovered "the physics of the mind," Ebbinghaus developed a way to empirically study memory and mental fatigue. In England, Sir Francis Galton believed that people were born with a blank slate and that they learned through their senses. He theorized that intelligence was based on sensory keenness and reaction time; so, people who had more acute senses were more intelligent. He developed tests to measure these physical and mental abilities and set up a laboratory in 1884, which was open to the public. In the announcement of his lab, called the Anthropometric Laboratory, he stated that one of its purposes was to serve "those who desire to be accurately measured in many ways, either to obtain timely warning of remediable faults in development, or to learn their powers" (Sattler, 2008, p. 216). However, the idea of such a laboratory was not a novel one. William Wundt is credited with the establishment of the first psychological laboratory, in Germany in 1879. Galton, with the help of his friend the mathematician Karl Pearson, was also formidable in originating the concepts of *standard deviation*, *regression to the mean*, and *correlation*. Unfortunately, his assumptions and the results of his tests were often not supported by the statistics he developed. Because of his contributions, nevertheless, Galton is often called "the father of the testing movement" (Ittenbach, Esters, & Wainer, 1997).

Galton's assistant, James McKeen Cattell, is responsible for coining the term *mental test* and for bringing Galton's ideas to the United States (Boake, 2002; Ittenbach et al., 1997; Wasserman, 2012). Cattell was interested in studying individual differences in behavior. He believed in the importance of measurement and experimentation and established his own laboratory in Pennsylvania. He developed 50 different measures to assess sensory and motor abilities, although these measures did not differ significantly from Galton's tasks. Important to the history of assessment, Cattell realized the usefulness of tests as a way to select people for training and diagnostic evaluations. As such, he attempted to bring together a battery of tests. Cattell provided us with a standard way to measure human intellectual ability rather than keeping the field of psychology as an abstract discipline (Thorndike, 1997).

The Dawn of the Twentieth Century and the Dynamic Contributions of Alfred Binet

At the end of the nineteenth century, after being publicly embarrassed for his failed work in the area of hypnosis, Frenchman Alfred Binet turned his attention to the study of intelligence. With his two daughters as his subjects, he created and played a series of short games with them. From these encounters, he theorized that intelligence involved more complex mental abilities than just the senses. Binet believed that intelligence was equated with common sense, and called intelligence "judgment…good sense…the faculty of adapting one's self to circumstances" (American Psychological Association (APA), 2004, p. 1). Binet believed that

intelligence was multifaceted and could be measured in three ways: 1) The medical method (anatomical, physiological, and pathological signs of inferior intelligence); 2) the pedagogical method (school-acquired knowledge); and 3) the psychological method (direct observations and measurements of intelligent behavior) (Foschi & Cicciola, 2006). In 1894, he devoted much of his time to researching the mental and physical differences among schoolchildren and became the director of Laboratory of Physiological Psychology in France.

By 1904, Binet was associated with a group of parents and professionals called the Free Society for the Psychological Study of the Child. This group was concerned with school failure rates. The compulsory-education laws in France impacted the government's ability (and private institutions') to provide education to all children. The result was a national system of screening exams for secondary and university education students (Schneider, 1992). The exams did not create a problem for those who advanced, but did for those considered "abnormal" due to their inability to be educated. Children who failed were deemed to belong to one of two categories: 1) Those who could not learn, and 2) those who could learn but would not do so. Those who could not learn were labeled "stupid," while the latter were referred to as "malicious." Binet's involvement with this organization led to his appointment to the French Ministry of Public Instruction, a committee created to identify "abnormal" children. With his main objective to differentiate "normal" children from the "retarded" ones, he created the "metric scale of intelligence" (Schneider, 1992, p. 114). This new approach was *not* to measure sensory or motor reaction times, but rather to measure a child's response to questions. He organized questions based on a series of increasing complexity and assumed that those who answered the more complex questions displayed higher intellectual levels. His original scale, *Measuring Scale of Intelligence*, was introduced in 1905 with the help of Victor Henri and Theodore Simon. The scale comprised 30 items measuring what he believed encompassed intelligence, such as visual coordination, naming objects in a picture, repeating a series of numbers presented orally, constructing a sentence using three given words, giving distinctions between abstract terms, etc. His test was used exclusively to determine whether children needed specialized classes. According to Binet, children who demonstrated intellectual retardation for at least two years were candidates for the classes. Along with the first

IQ test, Binet introduced the important notation of error. He realized that measuring intelligence was not completely accurate and that his tests provided only a sample of an individual's behavior. Binet's original scale and its revisions that followed (1908, 1911, and 1916) "served as both a model of form and source of content for later intelligence tests" (Boake, 2002). The Stanford-Binet Scale (1916) and its 1937 and 1960 revisions became the dominant measures of intelligence in the United States for a half-century.

The Dawn of the Twentieth Century and Charles Spearman's Theory of General Intelligence (g)

The contributions of English psychologist Charles Spearman cannot be overlooked. As a student of Wundt and influenced by Galton, Spearman was intrigued with the concept of human intelligence. While doing his research, he noted that all mental abilities were correlated to each other in some way. He concluded that scores on a mental ability test were similar—a person who performed well on one test would perform well on another (Deary, Lawn, & Bartholomew, 2008). He concluded that intelligence was a general ability that could be measured and expressed as a numerical value. Spearman believed that intelligence was made up of *general ability* or *g*, plus one or more *specific* or *s* factors, and proposed a general-factor or *g* theory. He stated:

> G means a particular quantity derived from statistical operations. Under certain conditions the score of a person at a mental test can be divided into two factors, one of which is always the same in all tests, whereas the other varies from one test to another; the former is called the general factor or G, while the other is called the specific factor. This then is what the G term means, a score-factor and nothing more.... And so the discovery has been made that G is dominant in such operations as reasoning, or learning Latin; whereas it plays a very small part indeed in such operation [sic] as distinguishing one tone from another...G is in the normal course of events determined innately; a person can no more be trained to have it in higher degree than he can be trained to be taller. (Deary et al., 2008, p. 126)

This theory was revolutionary and considered to be the first of many. In 1927, Spearman noted positive correlations (or positive manifold) among cognitive tests explained by psychometric *g* (Reynolds, 2012). When he compared children with normal ability to those with low ability, he observed that correlations were stronger in low ability groups compared to high ability groups. Spearman theorized "as a general rule the effects of psychometric g on test scores decrease as g increases, likening it to the law of diminishing returns from economics" (Reynolds, 2012, p. 3). This phenomenon has become known as Spearman's law of diminishing returns (SLODR). Along with these theories, Spearman refined the use of correlation statistics. Using factor analysis, he improved test reliability by using a correction formula to deal with the errors in his observations that obscured the "common intellective factor" (von Mayrhauser, 1992). Although his theory was criticized, Spearman's use of statistical factor analysis remains an important part of contemporary research and test development.

The Growth of the Binet and Nonverbal Tests in America in the Early Twentieth Century

Along with Binet, other individuals were studying and pursuing the measurement of intelligence. Two men, in particular, were influential pioneers—Henry Goddard and Lewis Terman. Henry Goddard is often considered the first "school psychologist" (Thorndike, 1997). In 1905, he was the director of the Vineland Training School for retarded children and was interested in their unique abilities. Although he wanted to measure the abilities of his students, no measure was available. His search led him to France, where he met Binet. Although he was skeptical, he translated the Binet-Simon scale from French to English and successfully used the scale on his students. In 1908, he introduced an adapted version of the scale, making minor revisions and incorporating standardization (2,000 American children were used). His version was used specifically to evaluate those with mental retardation. While Goddard translated and promoted the Binet-Simon scale, Lewis Terman expanded, standardized, and revised the scale. Terman was responsible for the tentative revision of the Binet-Simon scale in 1912 and the Stanford Revision and Extension of the Binet-Simon Scale in 1916. Terman is also known for renaming the *mental quotient* that Stern developed in 1914. The idea behind this *intelligence quotient* was that the use of a ratio provided a better measurement of mental retardation than the difference between two ages, because the difference did not mean the same thing at different ages (Sattler, 1992).

The beginning of World War I (WWI) initiated the need to evaluate millions of potential American soldiers for "fitness for duty." This seemed an impossible task, given the number of recruits (some of whom were immigrants) and the fact that the only measures of abilities were based on an individual administration. In 1917, Robert Yerkes and Lewis Terman led a team that developed the group-administered intelligence tests known as Army Alpha and Army Beta (Thorndike, 1997). The Army Alpha was given to the "literate" group, which covered mostly verbal abilities. Army Beta, which involved mostly nonverbal skills, was administered to the "illiterate" group or the group that performed badly on the Army Alpha. The Beta group (composed of mostly immigrants) had more difficulty performing well on the test, resulting in their rejection by the Army to serve as soldiers in WWI.

After the war, a heated debate ensued regarding the validity of the Army testing and the Stanford-Binet. Those involved were outraged about the prejudicial statements of the results of the Army testing, which claimed that individuals from different regions (North vs. South) and of ethnic minorities were inferior (Goddard was largely responsible for questionable interpretation of the test data that led to the racist claims). At the core of the debate was the nature of intelligence, a familiar controversy that began years earlier.

Twentieth-Century Opponents of Spearman's g Theory

Shortly after Spearman's theory was introduced, a debate regarding the nature of intelligence began. Critics believed that Spearman's theory was too simplistic. Thus, in 1909, Edward Lee Thorndike and his colleagues (Lay and Dean) tested the g hypothesis and concluded from their analysis, that they were almost tempted to replace Spearman's g theory by the equally extravagant theory that "there is nothing whatever common to all mental functions, or to any half of them" (R. M. Thorndike, 1997, p. 11). E. L. Thorndike believed that intelligence was a cluster of three mental abilities: 1) social (people skills); 2) concrete (dealing with things); and 3) abstract (verbal and mathematical skills) (Shepard, Fasko, & Osborne, 1999). While critics like Thorndike continued to question and denounce Spearman's theory, Spearman endlessly sparred with his critics, maintaining that his theory was sound. Although never resolved, this heated debate continued for almost 20 years.

By 1936, the Stanford-Binet was widely accepted in the United States as the standard for measuring intelligence (Roid & Barram, 2004). Finally, Spearman had "proven" his theory. But, much to his chagrin, E. L. Thorndike disagreed again. Thorndike criticized tests similar to Stanford-Binet for measuring only one aspect of intelligence; he continued to insist that intelligence was not a single construct, but much more complex.

Between 1918 and 1938, additional tests (such as Kohs' Block Design Test and the Bender Visual Motor Gestalt Test) were developed and published in response to the debate, but only a few theories (e.g., Thurstone's multiple factor analytic approach) were introduced (Thorndike, 1997). Challenging Spearman's theory, Louis Thurstone (1938) believed that intelligence was not a unitary trait and assumed that intelligence was systematically organized. Using factor analysis, he identified factors including verbal fluency, perceptual speed, inductive reasoning, numeracy, rote memory, deductive reasoning, word fluency, and space or visualization skills. He believed that each factor had equal weight in defining intelligence and labeled these factors *primary mental abilities*.

David Wechsler's Innovations in the 1930s

While many individuals were debating the Army testing issue, David Wechsler was preparing to "reinvent the wheel." Wechsler's contributions to the field of psychological assessment are unmistakable. While waiting to serve in the Army, Wechsler came in to contact with Robert Yerkes. Later, he was the assigned psychologist who administered the Army Alpha and Army Beta to recruits. As he gave the tests, he began to observe the weaknesses of these tools and was determined to use his strong clinical skills and statistical training to develop a new and improved test. Wechsler attributed the misdiagnosis of civilians as having low mental abilities to the heavy emphasis on verbal skills. He hypothesized that if civilians were evaluated on other levels, their abilities would be judged "normal." He believed:

> Intelligence is an aspect of behavior; it has to do primarily with the appropriateness, effectiveness, and the worthwhileness of what human beings do or want to do . . . it is a many-faceted entity, a complex of diverse and numerous components. . . . Intelligent behavior . . . is not itself an aspect of cognition. . . . What intelligence tests measure, what we hope they measure, is something much more important: the capacity of an individual to understand the world about him and his resourcefulness to cope with its challenges. (Wechsler, 1975, p. 135)

When he became chief psychologist at Bellevue Psychiatric Hospital in 1932, he needed a test that could be applied to his population. He stated that the Stanford-Binet scales helped in determining whether an individual had any special abilities or disabilities, but that its application was geared more toward children and adolescents than adults and that the profile interpretation was complicated and unstandardized (Boake, 2002). Creating a standardized measure, statistical in nature, for use with adults was his mission.

In 1939, after a seven-year project, Wechsler introduced his first scale—the Wechsler-Bellevue. He included many tasks from other tests, including the Army Alpha, Army Beta, Army Individual Performance Scale, and Stanford-Binet. He deemphasized previous heavy reliance on verbal skills by introducing nonverbal tasks along with verbal tasks. His selection and development of tasks was based on his belief that intelligence was part of a person's personality and comprised "qualitatively different abilities" (Sattler, 1992, p. 44). "[Wechsler's] aim was not to produce a set of brand new tests but to select, from whatever source available, such a combination of them as would best meet the requirements of an effective adult scale" (Boake, 2002, p. 397). His standardization sample included individuals ranging from seven to 59 years of age who lived in the New York area. By the 1940s, Wechsler's test had gained credibility and was widely used. Wechsler refined and revised his scales until his death in 1981. The scales continue to be modified, even today (as seen by the Wechsler Intelligence Scale for Children–Fourth Edition [WISC-IV], the Wechsler Adult Intelligence Scale–Fourth Edition [WAIS-IV]), and the Wechsler Preschool and Primary Scale of Intelligence—Fourth Edition [WPPSI-IV], although they still remain tied—to some extent—to their original scales. Unlike earlier editions of Wechsler's scales, the fourth editions are based on cognitive neuroscience research and theory, especially within the domains of fluid reasoning, working memory, and processing speed. Furthermore, Wechsler's impact on the contemporary field of assessment remains profound, particularly in transforming the field of intelligence testing psychometric measurement to clinical assessment (Kaufman, in press; Wasserman, 2012).

Mid–Twentieth-Century Contributions from Neuropsychology

While some individuals were emphasizing the concept of intelligence and how it was to be measured, others were interested in the relationship between the brain and behavior. Until the 1930s or so, the field of neuropsychology had been dominated by physicians (Boake, 2008). In 1935, Ward Halstead established the first laboratory in America devoted to the study of the brain–behavior relationship in humans. He was interested in understanding how brain damage affected cognitive, perceptual, and sensorimotor functioning. Because intelligence tests did not help quantify these deficits, he observed the daily activities of several patients and determined that their deficits were varied. Most notable were the loss of adaptive functioning and loss of flexibility of thought. Based on these observations, he compiled a battery of tests to administer in order to understand and examine the deficits. Several years later, Halstead collaborated with his former student Ralph Reitan to develop the Halstead-Reitan Battery. Reitan was responsible for researching and ultimately revising the battery. From his results, he developed indices of brain damage.

In Russia, Alexander Luria worked from a different angle. Luria developed a model of brain organization in which he theorized that brain–behavior relationship could be broken down into components he called *functional systems* (Sbordone & Saul, 2000). He believed that each area of the brain played a specific role in behavior. His theory "was acknowledged as brilliant and insightful, but was seen as forbiddingly complex and impractical for the average clinician" (Hebben & Milberg, 2009, p. 19).

Mid–Twentieth-Century Contributions from Raymond Cattell, John Horn, and J. P. Guilford

The revisions of the Wechsler-Bellevue Scale gave way to the development of additional tests and theories of intelligence between the 1940s and the 1970s. In 1941, Raymond Cattell introduced a dichotomous theory of cognitive abilities. He theorized that there were two types of intelligence—*crystallized* and *fluid* (Horn & Noll, 1997). Crystallized intelligence, Gc, involved acquired skills and knowledge based on the influences of a person's culture. In contrast, fluid intelligence, or Gf, referred to nonverbal abilities not influenced by culture.

For two decades, Cattell's theory, and theories in general, were largely overlooked. However, John Horn, a student of Cattell, was responsible for the resurgence and expansion of Cattell's theory, in 1965. Working together and utilizing Thurstone's work, Horn and Cattell theorized that crystallized and fluid intelligence also involved abilities such as visual processing (Gv), short-term memory (Gsm), long-term memory (Glr), and processing speed (Gs). In 1968, Horn added auditory processing (Ga) and refined the descriptions of other abilities (Flanagan, Ortiz, & Alfonso, 2007). The theory remains in use today as a framework for test developers and approaches to test interpretation (which is discussed later).

In 1967, J. P. Guilford's Structure of Intellect (SOI) became one of the major theories used in the field of intellectual assessment (Kaufman, 2009). Rejecting Spearman's view, Guilford believed that intelligence was composed of multiple dimensions: *operations* (general intellectual processes, such as the ability to understand, encode, and retrieve information), *contents* (how the information is perceived, such as auditory or visual) and *products* (how the information is organized, such as units and classes). This theory was innovative as it implied that there were more types of intelligence (120) than just the *g* described by Spearman. Today, the theory is utilized in the field of learning disabilities and gifted assessments. Linda Silverman, a leading expert in the field of gifted assessment, stated:

> Guilford's model was well received by educators, particularly those who decried the narrowness of some of the older conceptions of intelligence. The concept of a number of intelligences left room for everyone to be gifted in some way. But the model and the methodology have met with severe criticism within the field of psychology.... These researchers claim that there is not enough evidence to support the existence of the independent abilities Guilford has described. (Silverman, personal communication, July 8, 2008)

Theory-based tests in the twenty-first century

With an understanding of the historical landmarks, we now turn our attention to the role of theory in test development. Over the past many centuries, our fascination with human cognitive abilities has led to many dramatic developments in the measurement of, and theories related to, intellectual abilities. The links between brain and human behavior and subsequent developments linking neurological pathways and cognitive thought processes have expanded our knowledge of how best to measure human abilities. Physicians, psychologists, researchers, and legislators alike have had a role in shaping psychological assessment. Following this historical path from 2200 B.C. through the end of the twentieth century, we have learned that the field of intellectual assessment is continually evolving. We have highlighted some of the earlier theories related to the assessment of cognitive abilities, and we will now turn to the more modern theories that have shaped both test development and interpretation into the twenty-first century.

To date, the Kaufman Assessment Battery for Children–Second Edition (KABC-II; Kaufman & Kaufman, 2004a), the Stanford Binet, Fifth Edition (SB5; Roid, 2003b), the Cognitive Assessment System (CAS; Naglieri & Das, 1997a), the Woodcock Johnson–Third Edition (WJ-III; Woodcock et al., 2001b; 2007), and the Differential Ability Scales–Second Edition (DAS-II; Elliott, 2007a) are all testing tools that have been based on theory.

KAUFMAN ASSESSMENT BATTERY FOR CHILDREN—SECOND EDITION (KABC-II)

Drs. Alan and Nadeen Kaufman first introduced their Kaufman Assessment Battery for Children (K-ABC) in 1983. Their philosophy on theory and assessment was innovative and empirically based. The original K-ABC, a measure of intelligence and achievement for children aged 2½ to 12½, significantly differed from traditional tests (including the Wechsler, Woodcock-Johnson, and Stanford-Binet scales) in that it was rooted in neuropsychological theory (i.e., Luria-Das). The scales were divided in two processes: *sequential* and *simultaneous*. Those children who used sequential processing were described as solving problems in a specific, linear order, regardless of content. In contrast, children using simultaneous processing were described as solving problems in a spatial, holistic manner. This aspect of testing had not emerged until the K-ABC, even though theories of intelligence had mentioned the role of the brain. Another essential aspect of the K-ABC was its use with minority children. Cultural bias in psychological assessment has been the subject of longstanding debate among practitioners and researchers. Research had indicated that African-American children performed 15 to 16 points lower on the Wechsler scales than Caucasian children. The K-ABC significantly reduced this difference (by half) and it was said to be "culturally fair."

The KABC-II (Kaufman & Kaufman, 2004a) is used to evaluate the processing and cognitive abilities of children and adolescents aged three to 18 in a clinical, psychoeducational, or neuropsychological setting. It can be also used in conjunction with other assessment tools to identify mental retardation, intellectual giftedness, and learning disabilities. The KABC-II remains a culturally sensitive tool. Data show that Caucasians and African Americans continue to show reduced differences in global scores relative to other tests of intelligence (Kaufman et al., 2005).

The KABC-II is based on Luria's neuropsychological theory, and also uses the Cattell-Horn-Carroll (CHC) theory. The KABC-II was drastically revised from the original K-ABC. Along with subtest changes and its foundation in a dual theoretical model, the KABC-II gives the examiner the freedom to choose which of two global scores (one based on Luria theory and one based on CHC theory) is the most appropriate one for each person tested—an option that is not afforded by any other assessment tools (Kaufman, Lichtenberger, Fletcher-Janzen, & Kaufman, 2005). The choice is based on what is best suited to the child's background and reason for referral. For example, if the child is from a bilingual background, the Kaufmans suggest using the Luria Model or MPI (Mental Processing Index). In addition, if the child has or may have a learning disability in reading, they suggest using the CHC Model, which yields the Fluid Crystallized Index (FCI).

A brief review of these two theories is important to the understanding of the theory-based scales (i.e., MPI and FCI). The FCI is the global scale based on the CHC theory and measures general cognitive ability (Kaufman et al., 2005). The CHC theory is a combination of Horn-Cattell's (1968) Gf-Gc theory and Carroll's (1993) three-stratum theory (Flanagan, 2000; Schneider & McGrew, 2012). As previously mentioned, Cattell theorized that intelligence was divided into two abilities: fluid and crystallized. Crystallized intelligence or Gc involved abilities that were acquired through formal education and culture. In contrast, fluid intelligence or Gf consisted of inductive and deductive reasoning abilities that were influenced by biological and neurological factors. This theory was quite different

from the verbal–performance dichotomy used by the Wechsler tests. In 1965, Horn elaborated on the Gf-Gc theory to include the following additional cognitive abilities: visual processing (Gv), short-term memory (Gsm), long-term memory (Glr), and processing speed (Gs). In later years, he refined Gv, Gs, and Glr and added auditory processing (Ga), quantitative knowledge (Gq) and reading and writing (Grw). Horn believed that intelligence was composed of these equally weighted abilities. Figure 1.1 depicts CHC Broad Abilities classifications.

John Carroll's (1993) three-stratum theory is an extension of the Gf-Gc theory and other theories. From the results of numerous hierarchical factor-analyses based on correlational data, he theorized that intelligence or cognitive abilities have multiple levels or strata—Stratum I (narrow abilities), Stratum II (broad abilities), and Stratum III (general ability) (Kamphaus, 2008). Stratum I includes specific abilities, such as quantitative reasoning (the ability to reason inductively and deductively), listening ability (the ability to listen and comprehend), and spelling ability (the ability to spell). Stratum II involves the combinations of narrow abilities that form broader abilities, such as crystallized intelligence, fluid intelligence, quantitative knowledge, and so forth. For example, the broad ability crystallized intelligence or Gc refers to the acquired knowledge based on formal education and culture. The narrow abilities of Gc include skills such as language development, lexical knowledge, listening ability, and general (verbal) information. Finally, Stratum III encompasses general ability, or what have been labeled "general intelligence."

In contrast to the FCI, the MPI is a global scale based on Luria's model. This scale measures mental-processing ability (a child's ability to solve problems) and excludes language ability and word knowledge (Kaufman et al., 2005). As the name suggests, the Luria model is based on the work of Luria in the 1970s. Luria believed that the brain's basic functions are represented in three "blocks"—Block 1 being arousal and attention, and corresponds to

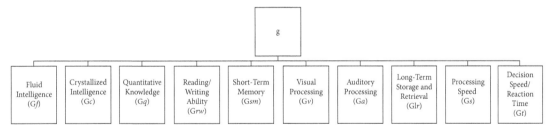

Figure 1.1 CHC Broad Abilities (Stratum II).

the reticular activating system; Block 2 being analyzing, coding, and storing information, and corresponds to the occipital, parietal, and temporal lobes; and Block 3 being executive functions, planning, and programming behavior, and corresponds to the anterior portion of the frontal lobes. Luria also believed that these "blocks" must work together in order for new material to be learned effectively. After information enters the brain, Block 2 is responsible for sending that information to Block 3. Realizing the importance of these systems, the Kaufmans included subtests measuring auditory and visual synthesis (such as requiring a child to point to a series of pictures in the correct order, corresponding to a series of words given by the examiner), as well as subtests that measure simultaneous processing that require use of Block 2 and Block 3 (such as requiring a child to point to a picture that does not go with the others around it).

The KABC-II was standardized on a sample of 3,025 children, stratified according to 2001 U.S. Census data. Reliability and validity data provide support for the psychometric properties of the test. Current literature, along with the test manual, indicates that it is a stable tool (Kaufman & Kaufman, 2004a; Kaufman et al., 2005). Internal consistency coefficients range from .69 to .97, test-retest coefficients range from .74 to .95, and validity coefficients range from .15 to .91. Like the K-ABC, the KABC-II is useful for evaluating minority children. The structure of the tool includes 18 subtests (such as copying the examiner's exact sequence of taps on the table with fist, palm, or side of the hand; assembling several blue and yellow triangles to match a picture of an abstract design; etc.) and yields one to five scales, depending on the child's age and interpretive approach used. For example, at age levels 7 to 18, ten core tasks are administered, yielding either MPI or FCI, either four scales (MPI) or five scales (FCI), and the Planning/Gf scale.

Fletcher-Janzen and Lichtenberger (2005) commented on the KABC-II's strengths and weaknesses in the areas of test development, administration and scoring, and test interpretation. In terms of test development, the KABC-II has several strengths and weaknesses. Its strengths include the following:

(1) It is based on dual theoretical models (Luria and CHC);

(2) It allows evaluators to choose the theoretical model;

(3) It evaluates a wide range of children and adolescents (ages 3–18);

(4) It allows evaluators to understand cognitive abilities in the context of academics, as it is normed with Kaufman Test of Educational Assessment–Second Edition (KTEA-II; Kaufman & Kaufman, 2004b);

(5) Its norms reflect a sample of ethnic minority responses (approximately 66%);

(6) It has ample floors and ceilings on nearly all subtests;

(7) It permits an evaluator to accept a correct response, regardless of the mode of communication (signing, writing, Spanish, etc.);

(8) The materials are well organized, sturdy, and novel; and

(9) It gives out-of-level norms for evaluating young children who might meet floors and ceilings too soon (Fletcher-Janzen & Lichtenberger, 2005).

In contrast, the KABC-II has several weaknesses in the area of test development, including the following: 1) Does not measure auditory processing (Ga) and processing speed (Gs); 2) record forms are complex; and 3) bonus points are used on three subtests, which confounds the measures (Fletcher-Janzen & Lichtenberger, 2005).

In terms of strengths of administration and scoring, the KABC-II:

(1) contains sample and teaching items that can be given in the child's native language,

(2) allows the examiner to explain items in child-specific language if the child does not understand,

(3) has short, simple instructions,

(4) has limited subjective scoring items,

(5) contains subtests that are presented in both visual and auditory forms, and

(6) has a supplemental computer scoring and interpretation software.

Weaknesses include the following: 1) Scoring on some subtests requires special attention to avoid clerical errors; 2) discontinue rules are not consistent from subtest to subtest; and 3) some children may have difficulty understanding the grammar items on Rebus (Fletcher-Janzen & Lichtenberger, 2005).

For the KABC-II, interpretation strengths are as follows:

(1) Luria and CHC models are the foundation;

(2) Use of the CHC model works well for cross-battery assessment;

(3) Interpretation is dependent on global scales and scale indexes;

(4) The interpretation system provides the evaluator with a continuous prompt to check hypotheses with other evidence;

(5) The manual provides mean MPI and FCI, scale index, and subtest scores for ethnic minority groups;

(6) Record form provides room to note basic analysis and strengths and weaknesses;

(7) Out-of-level norms are available for gifted and lower functioning children;

(8) Allows assessment of immediate and delayed memory;

(9) Allows assessment of learning and crystallized knowledge;

(10) A nonverbal index can be calculated and interpreted for children who have difficulty with oral communication (Fletcher-Janzen & Lichtenberger, 2005).

Interpretation weaknesses include: 1) the Knowledge/Gc subtests do not allow evaluators to assess expressive language, and 2) some comparisons cannot be made because of age limits on some subtests, namely "Story Completion" and "Rover" (Fletcher-Janzen & Lichtenberger, 2005).

In one study that investigated the KABC-II's consistency with the CHC theory, Matthew Reynolds and his colleagues used the standardized sample (ages 3–18) as their participant pool (Reynolds, Keith, Fine, Fisher, & Low, 2007). Multiple-sample analyses were performed. Results showed the KABC-II measures the same construct across all ages. In addition, for school-age children, the test generally matches the five CHC broad abilities it is proposed to measure. The test provides a "robust measure of g and strong measures of Gc, Gv, Glr, and Gsm, and both g and the broad abilities are important to explaining variability in subtest scores" (Reynolds et al., 2007, p. 537). However, some inconsistencies were found in Gestalt Closure, Pattern Reasoning, and Hand Movements. The subtest Gestalt Closure appeared to measure crystallized intelligence (Gc) in addition to, or perhaps instead of, visual processing (Gv). The subtest Pattern Reasoning appeared to measure visual processing (Gv) in addition to fluid reasoning (Gf). Finally, the subtest Hand Movements measures fluid reasoning (Gf) in addition to short-term memory (Gsm). In terms of clinical applications, Fletcher-Janzen and Lichtenberger (2005) report that the KABC-II is effective for individuals who are deaf or hard of hearing, autistic, have speech and language disorders, mental retardation, ADHD, and learning differences.

Sex differences in cognitive abilities in children ages 6 to 18 have been found for the KABC-II (Reynolds, Keith, Ridley, Patel, 2008). In this study, multi-group higher-order analysis of mean and covariance structures (MG-MACS) and multiple indicator-multiple cause (MIMIC) models were used on the standardization sample. Results indicated that boys showed a mean advantage in latent visual-spatial ability (Gv) at all ages and in latent crystallized ability (Gc) at ages 6 to 16. In contrast, girls scored higher on the latent, high-order g factor, at all ages, but these results were statistically significant at only ages 6 to 7 and 15 to 16.

Researchers have investigated the application of other theories as they relate to the structure of KABC-II (Reynolds, Keith, & Beretvas, 2010; Reynolds & Keith, 2007). For example, in one study, Reynolds and Keith (2007) used the standardization sample for ages 6 to 18 to confirm the presence of SLODR. Confirmatory factor analysis was performed. Results indicated that SLODR was present, and "its presence was not dependent on the hierarchical model of intelligence. Moreover, [the] findings suggest that SLODR acts on g and not on the broad abilities" (Reynolds & Keith, 2007, p. 267). In another study by Reynolds et al. (2010), a factor mixture model was performed on the standardization sample to eliminate the previous division of participants into separate groups. The results also offered support for SLODR, "most notably the g factor variance was less in high g mean classes" (Reynolds et al., 2010, p. 231). Reynolds (2012) stated that although the presence of SLODR has been detected in several batteries, its effects on "the measurement of intelligence and interpretation of test scores is less well-understood." (p. 4).

For the most up-to-date research summaries of the KABC-II, consult Reynolds et al. (2010) and Singer, Lichtenberger, Kaufman, Kaufman, and Kaufman (2012).

THE STANFORD BINET, FIFTH EDITION (SB5)

Along with the KABC-II, the Stanford Binet is another theory-based assessment tool. Its history is long, dating back to Binet and Simon in 1905. The Stanford Binet–Fifth Edition (SB5; Roid, 2003b) is based on a five-factor hierarchical cognitive model, a combination of theories developed by Carroll, Cattell, and Horn now known as the CHC model (Roid & Barram, 2004). Roid retained the theory that g comprises verbal and nonverbal abilities. The SB5 is the first intellectual battery to cover five cognitive factors: fluid reasoning, knowledge, quantitative reasoning, visual-spatial reasoning, and working memory, in both domains (verbal and nonverbal). Therefore, the SB5 yields a Full Scale IQ, Verbal IQ, Nonverbal IQ, plus the five factor indexes on each domain (Roid & Barram, 2004).

The SB5 is designed to assess an individual's general intellectual ability between the ages of three and 85 and above. It was standardized and stratified on a large sample (N = 4,800; ages 2–96) based on the 2001 U.S. Census data. Reliability and validity data provide support for the psychometric properties of the test (Roid & Barram, 2004). For example, internal consistency coefficients range from .90 to .98.

As the SB5 is a fairly new instrument, researchers need more time to explore it. However, strengths and weaknesses have emerged in terms of test development and standardization, administration and scoring, and test interpretation and application (Roid & Barram, 2004). In terms of test development and standardization, the SB5 has the following strengths: 1) Large norm sample; 2) large age range; 3) in-depth field testing and fairness reviews; 4) content-validity studies of CHC aligned factors; 5) use of item response theory; and 6) linkage with Woodcock-Johnson III Tests of Achievement (Roid & Barram, 2004). In contrast, weaknesses include: 1) it does not assess all CHC model factors; 2) it does not include many clinical and/or special group data; and 3) it correlates with only the WJ-III Achievement (Roid & Barram, 2004).

The SB5 has many strengths and weaknesses in terms of administration and scoring. Its strengths include the following:

(1) Levels are tailored to the examinee's ability;
(2) Scoring metrics are similar to other batteries;
(3) It is a child-friendly test;
(4) New Change-Sensitive Scores are used;
(5) IQ score levels have been extended on both extremes (10 to 40 and 160 to 225);
(6) Record forms are well-designed;
(7) Helpful examiner pages are included in item books; and
(8) There is an optional computer-scoring program that is easy to use (Roid & Barram, 2004).

In contrast, administration and scoring weaknesses involve the following: 1) levels may be confusing to evaluators; 2) shifting between subtests may be difficult for evaluators; 3) extended IQs are only available for Full Scale IQ; 4) nonverbal subtests do not have pure pantomime administration; 5) computer-scoring program is not included

with the kit; and 6) nonverbal knowledge may need expressive language skills (Roid & Barram, 2004).

In terms of interpretation and application, the SB5 has strengths including the following:

(1) The assessment of working memory improves diagnoses,
(2) The contrast between verbal and nonverbal subtests is useful,
(3) A comprehensive interpretive manual is included,
(4) Progress can be noted by using Change-Sensitive Scores,
(5) Early prediction of learning disabilities can be made by using Working Memory, Knowledge, and Quantitative Reasoning scores, and
(6) Extended IQs are used for assessment of giftedness and mental retardation (Roid & Barram, 2004).

The weaknesses in this area are: 1) nonverbal subtests require receptive and expressive language skills and 2) more studies of classroom application are needed (Roid & Barram, 2004).

Canivez (2008) investigated the SB5's link to theory by conducting orthogonal higher-order factor structure of the test. His participants included the three youngest age groups from the original standardization sample (N = 1,400 2–5-year-olds; 1,000 6–10-year-olds; and 1, 200 11–16-year-olds. The results of the study indicated that the SB5 "fundamentally measures general, global intelligence (Stratum III; Carroll, 1993). When examining the 10 SB5 subtest correlation matrices for the three youngest age groups, there was no evidence to suggest the presence of more than one factor as proposed by Roid.... No evidence of a five factor model was found" (Canivez, 2008, pp. 538–539).

Investigators have also looked into the effectiveness of the SB5 in assessing giftedness, autism spectrum disorders, preschool children, attention-deficit/hyperactivity disorder, autism, and working memory (e.g., Canivez, 2008; Coolican, Bryson, Zwaigenbau, 2008; Leffard, Miller, Bernstien, DeMann, Mangis, & McCoy, 2006; Lichtenberger, 2005; Minton & Pratt, 2006; Newton, McIntosh, Dixon, Williams, & Youman, 2008). Coolican and colleagues (2008) investigated the utility of the SB5 on children with autism spectrum disorders. Their participants included 63 children (12 girls, 51 boys) with a diagnosis of autism, Asperger's syndrome, and pervasive developmental disorder not otherwise specified (PDDNOS). Ninety percent of the children completed the SB5. Their results revealed a broad range of functioning;

individuals earned Full Scale IQs (FSIQs) ranging from 40 to 141. In addition, a higher percentage of children had stronger nonverbal skills than verbal skills. Minton and Pratt (2006) tested 37 students in grades two through six in Idaho. They concluded that elementary school students who were gifted or highly gifted scored significantly lower on the SB5 than on the WISC-III. This result suggests that using the two or three standard deviations from the mean as a cutoff for giftedness vs. nongiftedness was too high.

For the most up-to-date research summaries of the SB5, consult Roid and Pomplin (2012).

THE WOODCOCK JOHNSON–THIRD EDITION (WJ-III)

Although the original Woodcock Johnson was not theory-based, the Woodcock-Johnson Psycho-Educational Battery–Revised (WJ-R, Woodcock & Johnson, 1989) was grounded in Horn-Cattell theory. The latest revision, the Woodcock-Johnson III Tests of Cognitive Abilities (WJ III COG; Woodcock, Johnson, & Mather, 2001b; Woodcock et al., 2007), is based on Cattell-Horn-Carroll (CHC) theory and is designed to measure intellectual abilities of individuals from age five to 95. All three levels (stratum I, II, and III) of the CHC theory are represented on the WJ III, although the primary purpose of the test is to accurately measure broad CHC factor scores (Stratum II) (Schrank, Flanagan, Woodcock, & Mascolo, 2002). Sanders, McIntosh, Dunham, Rothlisberg, and Finch (2007) noted, "Creating tests that measured the CHC abilities allowed for analysis of within-individual variability and provided additional ipsative interpretative information" (p. 120).

The WJ III COG is divided into two major components—the standard battery and the extended battery. For the standard battery, seven cognitive factors, including comprehension-knowledge, long-term retrieval, visual-spatial thinking, auditory processing, fluid reasoning, processing speed, and short-term memory, are assessed along with the general intellectual ability. Three additional cognitive performance cluster scores can be calculated, which include verbal ability, thinking ability, and cognitive efficiency. Not all 20 tests are administered, but rather those subtests that are relevant to information the examiner seeks, as well as to the referral question. For example, the first seven subtests are administered for general intellectual ability. However, if an evaluator is wondering about an individual's short-term memory (Gsm), the two additional subtests can be administered (Schrank et al., 2002).

A useful aspect of the WJ III COG is that it has been normed with the WJ III Tests of Achievement (WJ III ACH; Woodcock, McGrew, & Mather, 2001a) so that examiners can compare cognitive and achievement abilities. The WJ III ACH consists of 22 subtests that evaluate five areas, including reading, oral language, mathematics, written language, and academic knowledge (such as science). Like the WJ III COG, the WJ III ACH is divided into a standard and extended battery. Administering nine subtests will allow for a Total Achievement score to be obtained for children age five or older. Both the WJ III COG and WJ III ACH were normatively updated in 2007, which involved a recalculation of norms for subtests and clusters (Schrank & Wendling, 2012).

The WJ III COG was standardized on a sample of 8,818 ranging from age two to 95+ and selected from more than 100 "geographically and economically diverse communities" (Schrank et al., 2002). The psychometric properties of the test indicate a stable tool (McGrew & Woodcock, 2001; Schrank et al., 2002). For the standard battery, individual test reliabilities range from .81 (Test 3: Spatial Relations) to .94 (Test 5: Concept Formation). For the extended battery, individual test reliabilities range from .74 (Test 19: Planning) to .97 (Test 18: Rapid Picture Naming). Median cluster reliability statistics range from .88 (Short-Term Memory) to .98 (General Intellectual Ability–Extended). Test-retest reliability coefficients range from .73 to .96. Convergent and discriminate validity coefficients range from .20 to .60.

The WJ III COG has several strengths and weaknesses. Its strengths include the following: 1) the battery is based on empirically strong theory of cognitive abilities; 2) interpretation of its results offers important information regarding cognitive strengths and weaknesses; 3) it is conformed with the WJ III Tests of Achievement and provides actual discrepancy norms; 4) the tool is technically stable; and 5) the materials are well made. In contrast, its weaknesses include complexity of administration and interpretation, lack of hand scoring abilities, and the need for additional research for the clinical clusters (Schrank et al., 2002).

One illustrative study that linked the WJ III COG to CHC theory was conducted by Taub and McGrew (2004), who performed confirmatory factor analysis of the battery and determined its cross-age invariance. The WJ III COG standardization sample served as the data for this study. Three sets of confirmatory factor analyses were performed. Results of the analyses provide support for the factorial invariance of the WJ COG when the 14 tests contributing to the calculation of the examinee's GIA and CHC factors scores are administered. Support is provided for the WJ III COG theoretical factor structure across five age groups (ages 6 to 90+) (Taub & McGrew, 2004, p. 72). Researchers have also looked into the effectiveness of the WJ III COG in assessing learning disabilities and attention problems (Leffard, Miller, Bernstien, DeMann, Mangis, & McCoy, 2006; Schrank et al, 2002). Schrank and his colleagues (2002) delineate several WJ III discrepancy procedures to assist in identifying specific learning disabilities, including ability-achievement, predicted achievement/achievement discrepancy, general intellectual ability/achievement discrepancy, oral language ability/achievement discrepancy, intra-ability discrepancy, intracognitive discrepancy, intra-achievement discrepancy, and intra-individual discrepancy.

Using the Woodcock-Johnson and Kaufman tests, Scott Barry Kaufman and his colleagues (2012) investigated whether cognitive g and academic achievement g are the same as the conventional g (Kaufman, Reynolds, Liu, Kaufman, & McGrew, 2012). From previous research, we know that IQ-achievement correlations are moderate to high, but that 50 to 75 percent of the variance in achievement is unaccounted for by cognitive ability. Many factors have been found to impact academics. Some of the variance is measurement error, whereas other variance is accounted for by such factors as student characteristics, school environments, and curriculum. They used two large nationally representative data sets and two independent test batteries. Second-order latent factor models and multi-group confirmatory factor analysis were used. The results indicated that COG-g and ACH-g are not the same as g. They are distinct but highly related constructs. And, importantly, Kaufman et al. (2012) gave strong support to the CHC theory-based structure of both the KABC-II and KABC-II).

For the most up-to-date research summaries of the WJ III COG and its 2007 normative update, consult S. B. Kaufman et al. (2012), Schneider and McGrew (2012), and Schrank and Wendling (2012).

THE DIFFERENTIAL ABILITY SCALES—2ND EDITION

The Differential Ability Scales (DAS; Elliott, 1990a) was developed by Colin Elliott from their predecessor, the British Ability Scales (BAS; Elliott, 1983a, 1983b), to focus on "specific abilities rather

than on 'intelligence'" (Elliott, 1997, p. 183). The second revision of the Differential Ability Scales (DAS-II; Elliott, 2007a) was designed to "address processes that often underlie children's difficulties in learning and what scientists know about neurological structures underlying these abilities" (Dumont, Willis, & Elliott, 2009, p. 5). The theoretical underpinning of the tool is not based on a single theory, but it has been connected to various neuropsychological processing models and the Cattell-Horn-Carroll theory, which has already been described above (Stavrou & Hollander, 2007).

The DAS-II is designed to evaluate children from the ages of two to 17. The test consists of 20 subtests and is divided into two overlapping age-level batteries—the Early Years (2:6–6:11) and the School Years (5:0–17:11). The Early Years battery is even further divided into a lower (2:6–3:5) and upper level (3:6–6:11). The battery yields an overall composite score labeled General Conceptual Ability (GCA), as well as several additional cluster scores, including Verbal Ability, Nonverbal Reasoning, and Spatial Ability. The Verbal Ability Cluster is a measure of crystallized intelligence or Gc, the Nonverbal Reasoning Cluster is a measure of fluid intelligence or Gf, and the Spatial Ability Cluster is a measure of visual-spatial ability or Gv. These clusters make up the core subtests. Other subtests, known as the diagnostic subtests, measure memory skills, processing speed, and school readiness.

The DAS-II was standardized and normed on 3,480 children living in the United States based on the October 2002 census. The psychometric properties of this tool indicate that it is a stable tool (Dumont, Willis, & Elliott, 2009; Stavrou & Hollander, 2007). Average internal consistency reliabilities range from .77 to .95. Test-retest reliability coefficients range from .83 to .92. In addition, the DAS-II has satisfactory concurrent validity (Dumont, Willis, & Elliott, 2009; Stavrou & Hollander, 2007). Mean overall correlation was .80.

Regarding the strengths and weaknesses of the DAS-II, the strengths include but are not limited to the following:

(1) The General Conceptual Ability Score;
(2) the Special Nonverbal Composite;
(3) ability to administer the nonverbal subtests in Spanish and American Sign Language;
(4) evaluation of differential abilities;
(5) use of Cattell-Horn-Carroll theory;
(6) fairly easy administration and scoring;
(7) child-centered;

(8) diagnostic subtests and clusters; and
(9) ability to evaluate learning differences (Dumont, Willis, & Elliott, 2009).

In contrast, weaknesses include but are not limited to the following: 1) norming that only extends to 17 years, 11 months; 2) it is a test of cognitive ability, not an IQ test; 3) it is a complex test that requires training; and 4) additional testing is required to understand the expressive language skills for younger children (Dumont, Willis, & Elliott, 2009).

Timothy Keith and colleagues have conducted confirmatory factor analyses of the DAS-II across age levels, using standardization data for ages 4–17 years, to support the CHC theoretical basis for the DAS-II for the Early Years and School-Age batteries (Keith, Low, Reynolds, Patel, & Ridley, 2010). These results confirmed the "robustness of the structure across age levels" (Elliott, 2012, p. 347).

Sex differences in cognitive abilities in children ages 5–17 have been found for the DAS-II (Keith, Reynolds, Roberts, Winter, and Austin, 2011). In this study, multi-group mean and covariance structural equation modeling was used on the standardization sample. Girls showed advantages on processing speed (*Gs*) across all ages (especially ages 8–13) and free-recall memory, a narrow ability of long term retrieval (*Glr*), for some age groups. In contrast, boys showed an advantage on visual-spatial ability (*Gv*) for most ages, ranging from less than 1 point at ages 8–10 to almost 5 points at ages 14–15. Younger girls showed an advantage on short-term memory (*Gsm*). Statistically significant sex differences were not found on latent comprehension-knowledge (*Gc*) or the latent *g* factor.

Researchers have explored the application of other theories as they relate to DAS-II, such as SLODR (Reynolds, 2012; Reynolds, Hajovsky, Niileksela, & Keith, 2011). Recently, Reynolds (2012) provided a deeper understanding of how SLODR impacts the measurement of intelligence and interpretation of test scores. The purposes of his study were: (a) to determine whether the *g* loadings of the composite scores were linear, and (b) if they were nonlinear, to demonstrate how SLODR affects the interpretation of these loadings. Using the norming sample, he performed linear and nonlinear confirmatory factor analysis. Several important contributions were made, such as (a) *Gf* was unaffected by SLODR (*Gc, Gv, Gsm*, and *Gs* decreased as *g* increased), and (b) "*g* loadings should be viewed as *g* level dependent" (p. 23).

For the most up-to-date research summaries of the DAS-II, consult Reynolds et al. (2011) and Elliott (2012).

The role of theory in contemporary test interpretation

With an understanding of the role of theory in test development, we can now shift our focus to the role of theory in contemporary test interpretation. Until recently, the importance of using theory in test interpretation had not been universally accepted or acknowledged. According to Randy Kamphaus and his colleagues (Kamphaus, Petoskey, & Morgan, 1997; Kamphaus, Winsor, Rowe, & Kim, 2012), theory was not applied to test interpretation until the late 1970s. Theory-based test interpretation has evolved significantly since the early days of Binet, who used a measuring approach. Four "waves" have been delineated in terms of the history of test interpretation: 1) Quantification of a general level; 2) clinical profile analysis; 3) psychometric profile analysis; and 4) applying theory to intelligence test interpretation (Kamphaus et al., 1997; Kamphaus et al., 2012).

The First Wave—Quantification of a General Level

Until the 1900s, identification of mental abilities was strictly medical or physical, such as "idiocy" or "imbecility." The first wave (quantification of a general level) began with Alfred Binet. As described in the previous section, in response to compulsory-education laws and increased failure rates among schoolchildren, Binet was appointed to the French Ministry of Public Instruction. His job was to develop a way to differentiate normal children from retarded ones. His 1905 *Measuring Scale of Intelligence* was created for this purpose. The interpretation was not based on a theory, but rather on two categories—whether the child was "normal" or "retarded."

By the 1920s, other descriptive terms and ranges were utilized: for example, those with IQ scores of 50 to 74 were classified as "Morons," IQ scores of 95 to 104 were described as "Average," and IQ Scores of 125 to 149 were classified as "Superior" (Levine & Marks, 1928).

Terman delineated a different classification system from Binet. His categories ranged from "Definite feeble-mindedness" to "Near genius or genius" (Davis, 1940). During World War II, Wechsler attempted to apply a description of intelligence based on statistical frequencies and distance from the mean (i.e., 50% of people who earned IQ scores of 91 to 110 were in the Average range of intelligence). Today, we continue to use a classification system, but we understand and recognize that it is only the first step to a meaningful interpretation of test results.

The Second Wave—Clinical Profile Analysis

During the mid-1940s, the use of clinical profile analysis replaced the classification system. The contribution of psychoanalytic theory to this wave is instantly recognizable, with David Rapaport, Merton Gill, and Roy Schafer being the major contributors. In 1940, Rapaport was appointed head of the Psychology and Research Departments at the famous Menninger Clinic. His interest was in understanding schizophrenia, and he did not deny that these individuals had impairments in intellectual functioning. Although Rapaport criticized the field for the lack of theory application, he justified using psychological testing in psychiatric settings (Lerner, 2007). He used a battery of tests, including the Wechsler-Bellevue Scale, Rorschach, Thematic Apperception Test, etc., and applied psychoanalytic theory to interpretation the results of each test.

Rapaport eventually collaborated with Gill and Schafer to propose a new approach (*Diagnostic Psychological Testing*) to test interpretation (Sugarman & Kanner, 2000). They believed that an IQ level had almost no diagnostic significance in their clinical work (Wiggins, Behrends, & Trobst, 2003). So they emphasized the quantitative "interrelations" among subtest scores and the qualitative aspects of individual item responses in order "to demonstrate that different types of maladjustment tend to have different distinguishing and recognizable impairments of test performance" (Wiggins et al, 2003, p. 57). Their five principles were:

(1) Every single subtest score and response was significant and representative;

(2) A comparison of the successes and failures led to further understanding of the examinee;

(3) Subtest scores were related to each other and were representative of the subject;

(4) Both the Verbal score and the Performance score was significant to the examinee's overall makeup;

(5) The data must be considered in light of other data.

The importance of scatter analysis was also described. *Scatter analysis* referred to "the relationship of any two scores or any single score to the central tendency of all the scores" (Wiggins et al., 2003, p. 58). For Rapaport and his colleagues, the Vocabulary subtest served as baseline for subtest comparisons because of its centrality and stability.

They suggested that a profile could be indicative of diagnoses such as "simple schizophrenia" or "depressives" (psychotic and neurotic). They stated, "A large percentage of schizophrenics scored relatively low on the arithmetic subtest, while they scored high on digit span. This pattern is a reversal of what is the usual pattern in neurotics, depressives, and normals" (Schafer & Rapaport, 1944, p. 280). In addition, a significant discrepancy between Digit Span Forwards and Digit Span Backwards was indicative of a psychotic process (Wiggins et al., 2003).

The Third Wave—Psychometric Profile Analysis

Access to computers and statistical software launched the third wave—"psychometric profile analysis." The major contributors of this wave included Jacob Cohen (1959), Alexander Bannatyne (1974), and Alan Kaufman (1979). Cohen (1957, 1959) conducted the first factor analyses of the Wechsler Intelligence Scale for Children (WISC; Wechsler, 1949) and the Wechsler Adult Intelligence Scale (WAIS; Wechsler, 1955). He used the standardization sample data reported in both manuals for his analyses. For the WAIS, Cohen (1957) identified *g* (general intellectual functioning) along with five Factors Scores, including Factor A (Verbal Comprehension), Factor B (Perceptual Organization), Factor C (Memory), Factor D (Picture Completion), and Factor E (Digit Symbol). His Factor Scores were obtained by averaging the subtests said to measure these abilities. Factor A was obtained by averaging scores from the Information, Comprehension, Similarities, and Vocabulary subtests. Factor B was obtained by averaging the Block Design and Object Assembly subtest scores. Finally, Factor C was obtained by averaging the Arithmetic and Digit Span subtests. Factor D and Factor E were considered "minor factors." In 1959, he analyzed the data from the WISC. His results were closely related to those obtained for the WAIS. In addition to the Verbal, Performance, and Full Scale IQs, five Factors Scores were discovered: 1) Factor A (Verbal Comprehension I); 2) Factor B (Perceptual Organization); 3) Factor C (Freedom from Distractibility); 4) Factor D (Verbal Comprehension II); and 5) Factor E (an unlabeled quasi-specific factor). Cohen indicated that Factor A seemed to involve aspects of verbal knowledge acquired by formal education, including facts (Information), verbal categorization (Similarities), and manipulation of numbers (Arithmetic). He distinguished Factor A from Factor D. Factor B required tasks on nonverbal skills, involving the interpretation and/ or organization of stimuli presented visually against a time limit. These skills included Block Design, Object Assembly, Mazes, and Picture Arrangement. Factor C involved tasks that required attention and concentration, including Digit Span, Mazes, Picture Arrangement, Object Assembly, and Arithmetic. Finally, Factor D involved the use of judgment and included Comprehension, Picture Completion, Vocabulary, and Similarities. Along with obtaining Verbal, Performance, and Full Scale IQs, Cohen delineated other Factor Scores helpful in interpreting an individual's intelligence. He also noted that his studies of the WISC and WAIS provided "insight into the process of intellectual maturation via the comparative analysis of the factorial structures for the three age groups" (Cohen, 1959, p. 285).

Like Cohen, Bannatyne (1974) offered an alternative interpretive system for the Wechsler scales. His reorganization was created in response to attempts to understand the results of the learning disabled (LD) student. The traditional Verbal, Performance, and Full Scale method did not account for the poor performances on certain subtests (i.e., Information and Vocabulary) and adequate performance on the Digit Span subtest. Bannatyne suggested analyzing these students' performances based on Spatial (ability to recognize spatial relationships and manipulate objects in space), Conceptual (ability to use general verbal language), Sequential (ability to retain visual and auditory information), and Acquired Knowledge categories (Webster & Lafayette, 1980). He proposed that a child with dyslexia would obtain a good spatial score and a poor sequencing score (Henry & Wittman, 1981). Although these categories appeared to have high reliability, inconsistent results were found among researchers (Kaufman, 1981). Kaufman noted, "One should not conclude, however, that Bannatyne's recategorizations are irrelevant to LD assessment: that would be far from the truth. Although the groupings do not facilitate differential diagnosis, they still provide a convenient framework for understanding the LD child's assets and deficits" (Kaufman, 1981, p. 522).

From Cohen's work, Kaufman (1979) constructed a systematic method for using the first three factors to interpret the scales of the Wechsler Intelligence Scale for Children–Revised (WISC-R; Wechsler, 1974). He believed:

The focus is the child, with interpretations of the WISC-R and communication of the results in the context of the child's particular background,

behaviors, and approach to the test items.... Global scores are deemphasized, flexibility and insight on the part of the examiner are demanded, and the test is perceived as a dynamic helping agent rather than as an instrument for placement, labeling.... (Kaufman, 1979)

Kaufman's approach to test interpretation was based on three premises: 1) The WISC-R subtests assess what the person has learned; 2) the subtests are examples of behavior and not comprehensive; and 3) WISC-R evaluates mental functioning under fixed experimental conditions (Kaufman, 1979). This new approach included starting with the most general and global score (Full Scale IQ) and working to the more specific levels (a single subtest) until all meaningful hypotheses about the individual were revealed. He provided case report examples as a way to illustrate his method. Kaufman was the first to merge research and theory with testing. He noted the importance of taking into consideration physical, cultural, and language factors.

The Fourth Wave—Applying Theory to Intelligence Test Interpretation

Kaufman's interpretation method launched the fourth wave of test interpretation—applying theory to intelligence testing. The best contemporary models of theoretical interpretation include the Cross-Battery Assessment approach (Flanagan, McGrew, & Ortiz, 2000) and the Planning, Attention-Arousal, Simultaneous, and Success model of processing (Naglieri & Das, 1997a). The remainder of this section will be devoted to describing these approaches.

Theory-Based Approaches in the Twenty-first Century

CROSS-BATTERY ASSESSMENT APPROACH TO INTERPRETATION

In the late 1990s, Dawn Flanagan, Kevin McGrew, and Vincent Ortiz introduced the Cross-Battery Assessment approach (XBA). They believed that the traditional "verbal" and "nonverbal" interpretative framework presented by Wechsler was ineffective in meeting the needs of contemporary theory and knowledge regarding intelligence and intelligence test batteries (Flanagan, McGrew, & Ortiz, 2000). Their review of volumes of theories and intelligence tests found that an integration of Horn-Cattell Gf-Gc theory (Horn, 1991, 1994) and the three-stratum level theory of cognitive abilities provided "the most comprehensive and empirically supported model of the structure of intelligence currently available" (Flanagan & McGrew, 1997, p. 315). They also found that no single intelligence test battery successfully operationalized the Gf-Gc theory or measured all major broad Gf-Gc abilities. This integration of theories resulted in the XBA. Flanagan and her colleagues state that the XBA "narrows the gap between practice and cognitive science" (Flanagan & McGrew, 1997, p. 314) and provides assessment professionals with a more "valid and defensible way of deriving meaning from test scores than that provided by the traditional (and largely atheoretical) Wechsler Scale approach" (Flanagan, 2000, p. 295). Furthermore, the XBA is a method of systematically analyzing broad and narrow abilities as a "cluster" rather than by individual subtests, identifies cognitive strengths and weaknesses, aids in the understanding of the relationship between cognitive and academic constructs, and provides a framework to enhance communication between professionals. They also believe that until new test batteries are developed, it is essential that professionals utilize the XBA.

The XBA is based on three pillars—contemporary CHC theory, broad CHC ability classifications, and narrow CHC ability classifications. These pillars are utilized to increase the validity of intellectual assessment and interpretation. The first pillar uses the Cattell-Horn-Carroll theory, which is the most comprehensive and empirically supported model of cognitive abilities (Flanagan & McGrew, 1997). The CHC theory was previous described.

The second pillar of XBA is the CHC broad or Stratum II classifications of cognitive and achievement tests (e.g., Gc or crystallized intelligence). Flanagan and her colleagues analyzed all subtests from the major intelligence and achievement batteries and classified them according to particular CHC broad abilities or processes. Currently, there are over 500 broad and narrow abilities classifications (Flanagan, Ortiz, & Alfonso, 2007). Having knowledge of which tests measure what abilities helps the clinician "organize tests into...clusters that contain only the measures that are *relevant* to the construct of interest" (Flanagan, Ortiz, & Alfonso, 2007, p. 23). For example, measuring short-term memory/working memory (Gsm-MW) is assessed by subtests such as Wechsler's Arithmetic, the Kaufman Assessment Battery for Children's (KABC-II's) Word Order, and the Woodcock-Johnson Third Edition's (WJ-III's) Numbers Reversed (Flanagan et al., 2007).

The third pillar of XBA is the inclusion of the CHC narrow (Stratum I) classifications of cognitive

and achievement tests according to content, format, and task demand (e.g., language development, listening ability, etc.). Flanagan and her colleagues (2007) believed that this layer is necessary to further improve assessment and interpretation validity and to ensure that underlying constructs are represented. The authors provide examples of construct representation and construct underrepresentation. They believe that the latter occurs when the assessment is "too narrow and fails to include important dimensions or facets of a construct" (Flanagan, Ortiz, & Alfonso, 2007, p. 26). An example of construct underrepresentation is the Concept Formation subtest on the Woodcock-Johnson III Tests of Cognitive Abilities (WJ III) because it measures only one narrow ability of fluid intelligence (Gf). Therefore, according to Flanagan and her colleagues, at least one other measure of Gf is needed to ensure appropriate representation of the construct. A clinician would need to use the Analysis-Synthesis test in conjunction with the Concept Formation test. In contrast, an example of construct representation is the Verbal Comprehension Index (VCI) of the Wechsler Adult Intelligence Scale–Fourth Edition (WAIS-IV; Wechsler, 2008), because this index includes Vocabulary, Similarities, and Information, all of which represent aspects of crystallized intelligence (Gc).

The guidelines, implementation, and stages of interpretation for this cross-battery approach are detailed and specific. The steps include the following:

(1) Select a primary intelligence battery;
(2) Identify the broad CHC abilities or processes measured by the primary battery;
(3) Select tests to measure the narrow CHC abilities not measured by the primary battery;
(4) Administer all tests;
(5) Enter the data into the XBA computer program;
(6) Follow the guidelines from the results of the program.

The Cross-Battery Assessment Data Management and Interpretive Assistant, a computer program, has been designed to assist the evaluator (Flanagan, Ortiz, & Alfonso, 2007). The latest resource on the clinical application of the XBA and on research studies conducted on the approach is an excellent chapter by Flanagan, Alfonso, and Ortiz (2012).

With any approach, there are strengths and weaknesses. Strengths of the cross-battery approach include its use of modern theory, improved communication among professionals, is a way to evaluate children with specific learning disabilities and cultural language differences, gives professional flexibility, and has computer-programmed assistance. The XBA affords professional flexibility. The guidelines of the approach allow evaluators to glean different types of data specific to the purpose of the evaluation. In terms of modern theory, the XBA is based on "the most empirically supported and well-validated theory of the structure of cognitive abilities/processes, namely Cattell-Horn-Carroll (CHC) theory.... By utilizing this theoretical paradigm, the XBA approach has the advantage of being current and in line with the best available scientific evidence on intelligence and cognitive abilities/ processes" (Flanagan, Ortiz, & Alfonso, 2007, p. 212). This modern theory, in turn, provides professionals with a classification system for clear, valid, and specific communication of an individual's performance similar to the *Diagnostic and Statistical Manual of Mental Disorders* (DSM) for clinicians.

Along with professional flexibility, use of modern theory, and improved communication among professionals, the XBA offers a promising system to evaluate individuals with specific learning disabilities (SLD) and those who are culturally and linguistically different (CLD) (Flanagan, Ortiz, & Alfonso, 2007). The many different definitions, measures, and interpretation approaches to learning disabilities have led to difficulties in evaluating individuals with SLD. The authors of the XBA delineate four levels (with sublevels) that must be met for a definite diagnosis of SLD, as follows:

(1) At Level I-A, a normative deficit in academic functioning is required;

(2) Level I-B, confounding factors (such as insufficient instruction, emotional disturbance, medical conditions, etc.) are considered and determined not to be the primary cause of the academic deficit(s);

(3) Level II-A, a normative deficit in a cognitive ability/process is required;

(4) Level II-B, confounding factors (such as insufficient instruction, emotional disturbance, medical conditions, etc.) are considered and determined not to be the primary cause of either the academic or the cognitive deficit(s);

(5) Level III, underachievement is demonstrated by an empirical or logical relationship between the cognitive and academic deficit(s) and by evidence of otherwise normal functioning, such as mild mental retardation;

(6) Level IV, there must be evidence of deficits in activities of daily life that require the academic skill (Flanagan, Ortiz, & Alfonso, 2007).

In addition to its strengths, the XBA has potential weaknesses, including its norm sample, complexity, time-consuming aspect, and lack of a standardization framework. First, there is no internal norm group, making the validity of the approach questionable. The XBA authors reply to and address this issue in their book *Essentials of Cross Battery Assessment* (Flanagan, Ortiz, & Alfonso, 2007). They believe that the XBA did not need a norm group since the tools used in each battery are valid. In addition, the authors suggest that examiners use assessment tools that were normed within a few years of each other, which leads to greater chances of the norming samples' being similar. A second weakness of the XBA is its complexity. This alleged weakness is seen as a strength by Flanagan and her colleagues. They believe that holding evaluators to a high standard of theory and interpretation is essential. In addition to norming issues and complexity, the XBA is seen as time-consuming. The approach requires more administration, scoring, and hypothesizing than traditional methods. Along with revisions to the approach, a computerized program has been developed to reduce the time required. Finally, when utilizing the XBA, subtests are given out of order or omitted, thus can be seen as violating standardized administration procedures.

Research on the XBA is less plentiful than the plethora of research studies on CHC theory. Researchers have been applying CHC approach to cognitive abilities for many years, and most notably, in relation to academic achievement, including reading, writing, and mathematics (e.g., Flanagan, 2000; Flanagan et al., 2012; Floyd, Keith, Taub, & McGrew, 2007; Floyd, McGrew, & Evans, 2008; Schneider & McGrew, 2012; Taub, Floyd, Keith, & McGrew, 2008). Floyd and his colleagues (2008) investigated the contributions of CHC cognitive abilities to explaining writing achievement. Their participants included the norming sample used for the WJ-III Tests of Cognitive Abilities (Woodcock, McGrew, Mather, 2001b). From a simultaneous multiple regression, the researchers were able to determine that comprehension-knowledge, processing speed, short-term memory, long-term memory, auditory processing and phonemic awareness, and fluid reasoning demonstrated moderate to strong effects on writing achievement (basic skills and written expression).

Flanagan (2000) investigated the validity of CHC approach with elementary school students. Her sample included 166 students from the Woodcock-Johnson Psycho-Educational Battery–Revised (WJ-R; Woodcock & Johnson, 1989) technical manual. These children were given the WJ-R Tests of Cognitive Ability (Extended battery) and Achievement, as well as the Wechsler Intelligence Scale for Children–Revised (WISC-R; Wechsler, 1974). Structural equation modeling was used. Findings demonstrated that the *g* factor underlying the Wechsler-based CHC cross-battery model "accounted for substantially more variance in reading achievement (25%) than the *g* factor underlying the atheoretical Verbal Comprehension-Perceptual Organization-Freedom from Distractibility (VC-PO-FD) Wechsler model" (Flanagan, 2000, p. 295). Results indicated that a Wechsler-based CHC cross-battery approach is "an effective way of ensuring valid representation of multiple cognitive abilities, especially those that have been found to affect significantly the development of reading skills" (Flanagan, 2000, p. 296).

NAGLIERI-DAS PASS APPROACH

Another contemporary and sound theory in test interpretation is the Nalieri-Das PASS approach. In the late 1970s, J. P. Das linked Luria's work to the field of intelligence by suggesting that intelligence be seen as a cognitive construct (Naglieri, 1997). According to Luria, cognitive processing occurred in three separate, but necessary units: 1) regulating of cortical tone and maintenance of attention; 2) receiving, processing, and storing of information; and 3) programming, regulating, and directing mental activity (Das, Naglieri, & Kirby, 1994). Das then described this relationship in terms of the information integration model (Das, Kirby, & Jarman, 1979). Later, Jack Naglieri and Das collaborated to develop the PASS (Planning, Attention, and Simultaneous and Successive processing) theory of cognitive processing. They believed in the importance of Luria's theory, but "focused more on the cognitive processing components rather than their specific neurological locations" (Das, Kirby, & Jarman, 1979). According to this approach, intelligence has three processes—attentional (cognitive activity), informational (simultaneous and successive), and planning.

The first process examined by the theory is attention, which is located in the brainstem and lower cortex (Kirby & Das, 1990). This process allows a person to "respond to a particular stimulus and inhibit responding to competing stimuli" (Naglieri, 1997, p. 249). The major forms of attention include arousal and selective attention. For Das and Naglieri, selective attention was of more interest than arousal, as arousal is assumed. According to the theory, *attention* refers to "specifically directed cognitive activity as well as resistance to the distraction of the competing stimuli" (Naglieri, 1997, p. 250) and is determined by both arousal and planning (Kirby & Das, 1990). Attention and arousal have been linked to task performance, which influences the informational and planning processes (Kirby & Das, 1990).

The information processes include simultaneous and successive processing, which typically operate collaboratively (Kirby & Das, 1990). The major difference is that simultaneous processing allows for "the integration of stimuli into groups where each component of the stimulus array must be interrelated to every other," and successive planning allows for "the integration of stimuli that are serial-ordered and form a chainlike progression" (Naglieri, 1997, p. 250). In essence, with successive processing, the stimuli are not interrelated; rather, each stimulus is related only to the one it follows. Information that is processed simultaneously is said to be "surveyable," because the stimuli are related and can be examined either during the activity (such as copying a design) or through recall (reproducing the design from memory) (Naglieri & Sloutsky, 1995). Simultaneous processing takes place when stimuli are perceived, remembered, or conceptualized and, thus, applied during both verbal and nonverbal tasks. Successive processing is tied to skilled movements, such as writing, because the specific skill requires a series of movements that are in a specific order (Naglieri, 1997; Naglieri & Sloutsky, 1995).

According to the theory, the planning processes use attention and information processes along with knowledge to help an individual identify and utilize the most effective solution(s) to a problem(s). This system is believed to be located in the prefrontal areas of the brain (Kirby & Das, 1990) and includes abilities such as developing a plan of action, evaluating the plan's effectiveness, impulse control, regulation of voluntary actions, and speech (Naglieri, 1997). It is the *how* of the system; how to solve problems.

The PASS processes form a "functional system that has interrelated interdependent components that are closely related to the base of knowledge, and developmental in nature and influenced by the cultural experiences of the individual" (Naglieri &

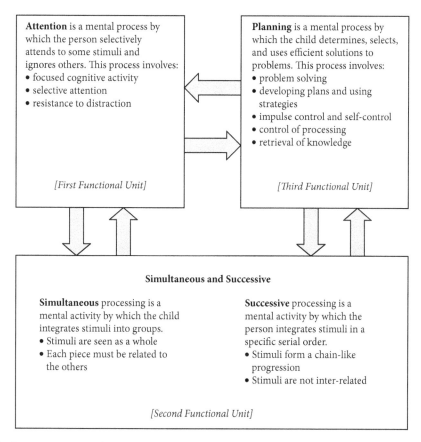

Figure 1.2 **The Cognitive Processes of PASS Theory.** The PASS processes are dynamic in nature and form an interrelated, interdependent system (as noted by the arrows in the figure).

Sloutsky, 1995, p. 14). The system is interactive; all components work together to perform nearly all of our everyday life tasks. It provides an understanding of cognitive activities (i.e., how individuals learn, think, and/or solve problems). The figure below (Fig. 1.2) describes how the system functions.

Researchers have investigated the use of the PASS theory in evaluating learning disorders, attention deficit/hyperactivity disorder, and mental retardation (e.g., Das, 2002; Kirby & Das, 1990; Kroesbergen, Van Luit, & Naglieri, 2003; Naglieri, 1997, 2001; Naglieri, Das, & Goldstein, 2012; Naglieri & Otero, 2012; Naglieri, Salter, & Edwards, 2004). Naglieri and his colleagues (2004) assessed the PASS characteristics of children with attention and reading disabilities. One hundred and eleven children were administered the Cognitive Assessment System (CAS; Naglieri & Das, 1997a). Results indicated that the children with attention disabilities scored lower on the Planning scale than children in regular education. Children with reading disabilities scored lower on the Successive scale than children in regular education and children with

attention disabilities. These children also scored lower on the Simultaneous scale than children in regular education. Das (2002) linked dyslexia with successive-processing deficits. He found that individuals with this specific reading disability make "phonological errors while reading real or made-up words or are slow in reading them (i.e., are slow decoders), or are both slow and inaccurate." (Das, 2002, pp. 31–32).

Conclusions

Psychological assessment involves a synthesis of the information gathered from several resources to understand or make statements regarding an individual's diagnosis, level of functioning or disability, and strategies for intervention or treatment. The history of assessment has its roots in many cultures, dating back to 2200 B.C. Each country focused on different aspects of understanding intelligence and developing measures to assess intelligence. Assessment abounds with many different theories, adaptations, and methods for interpretation that continue to change.

This chapter has explored the role of theory in psychological assessment, which is two-pronged—theory in test development and theory in test interpretation. Theoretically based test development and interpretation provides a strong framework for valid psychological assessments. In terms of test development, the KABC-II, SB5, CAS, WJ III COG, and DAS-II are all valid and reliable testing tools. We believe that the most valid and reliable contemporary methods of test interpretation include the Cross Battery Assessment approach (XBA; Flanagan et al., 1997; Flanagan et al., 2012) and the Planning, Attention-Arousal, Simultaneous, and Success (PASS) model of processing (Naglieri & Das, 1994; Naglieri et al., 2012). We encourage and challenge researchers and practitioners alike to continue developing tests and methods of interpretation based on theory, and to rely on the diverse theory-based instruments for the assessment of children, adolescents, and adults just as they continue rely on Wechsler's scales (Flanagan & Kaufman, 2009; Lichtenberger & Kaufman, 2013).

References

Aiken, L. R. (2004). *Assessment of intellectual functioning* (2nd ed.). New York: Springer.

Ansell, C. (1971). Wild child (*L'enfant sauvage*). *Professional Psychology*, 2(1), 95–96.

American Psychological Association. (2004). *Intelligence and achievement testing: Is the half full glass getting fuller?* Retrieved 10/10/08 from http://www.psychologymatters.org/iqtesting.html.

Bannatyne, A. (1974). Diagnosis: A note on recategorization of the WISC scaled scores. *Journal of Learning Disabilities*, 7, 272–274.

Boake, C. (2008). Clinical neuropsychology. *Professional Psychology: Research & Practice*, 39(2), 234–239.

Boake, C. (2002). From the Binet-Simon to the Wechsler-Bellevue: Tracing the history of intelligence testing. *Journal of Clinical & Experimental Neuropsychology*, 24(3), 383–405.

Canivez, G. L. (2008). Orthogonal higher order factor structure of the Stanford-Binet Intelligence Scales–5th ed., for children and adolescents. *School Psychology Quarterly*, 23(4), 533–541.

Carroll, J. B. (1993). *Human cognitive abilities: A survey of factor-analytic studies*. Cambridge, England: Cambridge University Press.

Cohen, J. (1957). A factor-analytically based rationale for the Wechsler Adult Intelligence Scale. *Journal of Consulting Psychology*, 21(6), 451–457.

Cohen, J. (1959). The factorial structure of the WISC at ages 7–6, 10–6, and 13–6. *Journal of Consulting Psychology*, 23(4), 285–299.

Coolican, J., Bryson, S. E., & Zwaigenbaum, L. (2008). Brief report: Data on the Stanford-Binet Intelligence Scales (5th ed.) in children with autism spectrum disorder. *Journal of Autistic Developmental Disorders*, 38, 190–197.

Das, J. P. (2002). A better look at intelligence. *Current Directions in Psychological Science*, 11(1), 28–33.

Das, J. P., Kirby, J. R., & Jarman, R. F. (1979). *Simultaneous and successive cognitive processes*. New York: Academic Press.

Das, J. P., Naglieri, J. A., & Kirby, J. R. (1994). *Assessment of cognitive processes: The PASS theory of intelligence*. Needham Heights, MA: Allyn & Bacon.

Davis, F. B. (1940). The interpretation of IQs derived from the 1937 revision of the Stanford-Binet Scales. *Journal of Applied Psychology*, 24(5), 595–604.

Deary, I. J., Lawn, M., & Bartholomew, D. J. (2008). Conversations between Charles Spearman, Godrey Thomson, and Edward L. Thorndike: The international examinations inquiry meetings, 1931–1938. *History of Psychology*, 11(2), 122–142.

Dumont, R., Willis, J. O., & Elliott, C. D. (2009). *Essentials of the DAS-II Assessment*. New York: Wiley.

Elliott, C. D. (1983a). *The British Ability Scales. Manual 1: Introductory handbook*. Windsor, England: NFER-Nelson.

Elliott, C. D. (1983b). *The British Ability Scales. Manual 2: Technical handbook*. Windsor, England: NFER-Nelson

Elliott, C. D. (1990a). *Differential Ability Scales*. San Antonio, TX: Psychological Corporation.

Elliott, C. D. (1997). The Differential Ability Scales. In D. P. Flanagan, J. L. Genshaft, & P. L. Harrison (Eds.), *Contemporary intellectual assessment: Theories, tests, and issues* (pp. 183–208). New York: Guilford.

Elliott, C. D. (2007a). *Differential Ability Scales, 2nd ed.: Administration and scoring manual*. San Antonio, TX: Harcourt Assessment.

Elliott, C. D. (2012). The Differential Ability Scales—Second Edition. In D. P. Flanagan & P. L. Harrison (Eds.), *Contemporary intellectual assessment: Theories, tests, and issues* (3rd ed., pp. 336–356). New York: Guilford Press.

Flanagan, D. (2000). Wechsler-based CHC cross-battery assessment and reading achievement: Strengthening the validity of interpretation drawn from Wechsler test scores. *School Psychology Quarterly*, 15(3), 295–329.

Flanagan, D. P., Alfonso, V. C., & Ortiz, S. O. (2012). The cross-battery assessment approach: An overview, historical perspective, and current directions. In D. P. Flanagan & P. L. Harrison (Eds.), *Contemporary intellectual assessment: Theories, tests, and issues* (3rd ed., pp. 459–483). New York: Guilford Press.

Flanagan, D. P. & Harrison, P. L. (Eds.) (2012). *Contemporary intellectual assessment: Theories, tests, and issues* (3rd ed.). New York: Guilford Press.

Flanagan, D. P., & Kaufman, A. S. (2009). *Essentials of WISC-IV assessment* (2nd ed.). Hoboken, NJ: Wiley.

Flanagan, D., & McGrew, K. (1997). A cross battery approach to assessing and interpreting cognitive abilities: Narrowing the gap between practice and cognitive science. In D. P. Flanagan, J. L. Genshaft, & P. L. Harrison (Eds.), *Contemporary intellectual assessment: Theories, tests, and issues* (pp. 314–325). New York: Guilford.

Flanagan, D., McGrew, K., & Ortiz, S. (2000). *The Wechsler intelligence scales and CHC theory: A contemporary approach to interpretation*. Boston: Allyn & Bacon.

Flanagan, D., Ortiz, S., & Alfonso, V. (2007). *Essentials of cross-battery assessment* (2nd ed.). New York: Wiley.

Fletcher-Janzen, E., & Lichtenberger, E. O. (2005). Strengths and weaknesses of the KABC-II. In A. S. Kaufman, E. O. Lichtenberger, E. Fletcher-Janzen, & N. L. Kaufman (Authors). *Essentials of KABC-II assessment* (pp. 168–175). Hoboken, NJ: Wiley.

Floyd, R. G., Keith, T. Z., Taub, G. E., & McGrew, K. S. (2007). Cattell-Horn-Carroll cognitive abilities and their effects on reading decoding skills: *G* has indirect effects, more specific abilities have direct effects. *School Psychology Quarterly, 22*(2), 200–233.

Floyd, R. G., McGrew, K. S., & Evans, J. J. (2008). The relative contributions of the Cattell-Horn-Carroll cognitive abilities in explaining writing achievement during childhood and adolescence. *Psychology in the Schools, 45*(2), 132–144.

Foschi, R., & Cicciola, E. (2006). Politics and naturalism in the 20th-century psychology of Alfred Binet. *History of Psychology, 9*(4), 268–289.

Hatfield, G. (2007). Did Descartes have a Jamesian theory of emotions? *Philosophical Psychology, 20*(4), 413–440.

Hebben, N., & Milberg, W. (2009). *Essentials of neuropsychological testing* (2nd ed.). Hoboken, NJ: Wiley.

Henry, S. A., & Wittman, R. D. (1981). Diagnostic implications of Bannatyne's recategorized WISC-R scores for identifying learning disabled children. *Journal of Learning Disabilities, 14*(9), 517–520.

Horn, J. L. (1991). Measurement of intellectual capabilities: A review of theory. In K. S. McGrew, J. K. Werber, & R. W. Woodcock (Eds.), *Woodcock-Johnson technical manual* (pp. 197–232). Chicago: Riverside Publishing.

Horn, J. L. (1994). Theory of fluid and crystallized intelligence. In R. J. Sternberg (Ed.), *Encyclopedia of human intelligence* (pp. 443–451). New York: Macmillan.

Horn, J. L., & Noll, J. (1997). Human cognitive capabilities: G*f*-G*c* theory. In D. P. Flanagan, J. L. Genshaft, & P. L. Harrison (Eds.), *Contemporary intellectual assessment: Theories, tests, and issues* (pp. 53–91). New York: Guilford.

Ittenbach, R. F., Esters, I. G., & Wainer, H. (1997). The history of test development. In D. P. Flanagan, J. L. Genshaft, & P. L. Harrison (Eds.), *Contemporary intellectual assessment: Theories, tests, and issues* (pp. 17–31). New York: Guilford.

Kamphaus, R. W. (2008). *Clinical assessment of child and adolescent intelligence* (2nd ed.). New York: Springer-Verlag.

Kamphaus, R. W., Petoskey, M. D., & Morgan, A. (1997). A history of intelligence test interpretation. In D. P. Flanagan, J. L. Genshaft, & P. L. Harrison (Eds.), *Contemporary intellectual assessment: Theories, tests, and issues* (pp. 32–47). New York: Guilford.

Kamphaus, R. W., Winsor, A. P., Rowe, E. W., & Kim, S. (2012). A history of intelligence test interpretation. In D. P. Flanagan & P. L. Harrison (Eds.), *Contemporary intellectual assessment: Theories, tests, and issues* (3rd ed., pp. 56–70). New York: Guilford Press.

Kaufman, A. S. (1979). *Intelligent testing with the WISC-R.* New York: John Wiley.

Kaufman, A. S. (1981). The WISC-R and learning disabilities assessment: State of the art. *Journal of Learning Disabilities, 14*(9), 520–526.

Kaufman, A. S. (2009). *IQ testing 101.* New York: Springer.

Kaufman, A. S. (in press). Biography of David Wechsler. In F. Volkmar (Ed.), *Encyclopedia of autistic spectrum disorders.* New York: Springer.

Kaufman, A. S., & Kaufman, N.L. (2004a). *Kaufman Assessment Battery for Children–2nd ed. (K-ABC-II).* Circle Pines, MN: American Guidance Service.

Kaufman, A. S., & Kaufman, N. L. (2004b). *Kaufman Test of Educational Achievement–2nd ed. (KTEA-II): Comprehensive Form.* Circle Pines, MN: American Guidance Service.

Kaufman, A. S., Lichtenberger, E. O., Fletcher-Janzen, E., & Kaufman, N. (2005). *Essentials of KABC-II Assessment.* New York: Wiley.

Kaufman, S. B., Reynolds, M. R., Liu, X., Kaufman, A. S., & McGrew, K. S. (2012). Are cognitive *g* and academic achievement *g* one and the same *g*? An exploration on the Woodcock-Johnson and Kaufman tests. *Intelligence, 40*, 123–138.

Keith, T. Z., Low, J. A., Reynolds, M. R., Patel, P. G., & Ridley, K. P. (2010). Higher-order factor structure of the Differential Abilities Scale-II: Consistency across ages 4–17. *Psychology in the Schools, 47*, 676–697.

Keith, T. Z., Reynolds, M. R., Roberts, L. G., Winter, A. L., Austin, C. A. (2011). Sex differences in latent cognitive abilities ages 5 to 17: Evidence from the Differential Ability Scales – Second Edition. *Intelligence, 39*, 389–404.

Kirby, J. R., & Das, J. P. (1990). A cognitive approach to intelligence: Attention, coding, and planning. *Canadian Psychology, 31*(3), 320–333.

Kroesbergen, E. H., Van Luit, J. E. H., & Naglieri, J. A. (2003). Mathematical learning difficulties and PASS cognitive processes. *Journal of Learning Disabilities, 36*(6), 574–582.

Lane, H. (1986). The wild boy of Aveyron and Dr. Jean-Marc Itard. *History of Psychology, 18*(1–2), 3–16.

Leffard, S. A., Miller, J. A., Bernstein, J., DeMann, J. J., Mangis, H. A., & McCoy, E. L. B. (2006). Substantive validity of working memory measures in major cognitive functioning test batteries for children. *Applied Neuropsychology, 13*(4), 230–241.

Lerner, P. M. (2007). On preserving a legacy: Psychoanalysis and psychological testing. *Psychoanalytic Psychology, 24*(4), 208–230.

Levine, A. J., & Marks, L. (1928). *Testing and intelligence and achievement.* New York: Macmillan.

Lieberman, L. M. (1982). Itard: The great problem solver. *Journal of Learning Disabilities, 15*(9), 566–568.

Lichtenberger, E. O. (2005). General measures of cognition for the preschool child. *Mental Retardation & Developmental Disabilities Research Review, 11*, 197–208.

Lichtenberger, E. O., & Kaufman, A. S. (2013). *Essentials of WAIS-IV assessment* (2nd ed.). Hoboken, NJ: Wiley.

Mariush, M. E., & Moses, J. A. (1997). *Clinical neuropsychology: Theoretical foundations for practitioners.* Hillsdale, NJ: Lawrence Erlbaum Associates.

McGrew, K. S., & Woodcock, R. W. (2001). Woodcock-Johnson III *Technical manual.* Itasca, IL: Riverside.

Minton, B. A., & Pratt, S. (2006). Gifted and highly gifted students: How do they score on the SB5? *Roeper Review, 28*(4).

Molnar, Z. (2004). Thomas Willis (1621–1675), the founder of clinical neuroscience. *Nature Reviews Neuroscience, 5*, 329–335.

Naglieri, J. A. (1997). Planning, attention, simultaneous, and successive theory and the Cognitive Assessment System: A new theory-based measure of intelligence. In D. P. Flanagan, J. L. Genshaft, & P. L. Harrison (Eds.), *Contemporary intellectual assessment: Theories, tests, and issues* (pp. 247–267). New York: Guilford.

Naglieri, J. A. (2001). Using the Cognitive Assessment System (CAS) with learning-disabled children. In A.S. Kaufman & N. L. Kaufman (Eds.), *Specific learning disabilities and difficulties in children and adolescent psychiatry* (pp. 141–177). New York: Cambridge University Press.

Naglieri, J. A., & Das, J. P. (1997a). *Cognitive assessment system.* Chicago, IL: Riverside Publishing Company.

Naglieri, J. A., Das, J. P., & Goldstein, S. (2012). Planning-Attention-Simultaneous-Successive: A cognitive-processing-based theory of intelligence. In D. P. Flanagan & P. L. Harrison (Eds.), *Contemporary intellectual assessment: Theories, tests, and issues* (3rd ed., pp. 178–194). New York: Guilford Press.

Naglieri, J. A., & Otero, T. M. (2012). The Cognitive Assessment System: From theory to practice. In D. P. Flanagan & P. L. Harrison (Eds.), *Contemporary intellectual assessment: Theories, tests, and issues* (3rd ed., pp. 376–399). New York: Guilford Press.

Naglieri, J. A., Salter, C. J., & Edwards, G. H. (2004). Using the Cognitive Assessment System (CAS) with learning-disabled children. In A. S. Kaufman and N. L. Kaufman (Eds.), *Specific learning disabilities and difficulties in children and adolescents: Psychological assessment and evaluation* (pp. 141–177). Cambridge, England: Cambridge University Press.

Naglieri, J. A., & Sloutsky, V. M. (1995). Reinventing intelligence: The PASS theory of cognitive functioning. *The General Psychologist, 31*(1), 11–17.

Newton, J. H., McIntosh, D. E., Dixon, F., Williams, T., & Youman, E. (2008). Assessing giftedness in children: Comparing the accuracy of three shortened measures of intelligence to the Stanford-Binet Intelligence Scales, 5th ed. *Psychology in the Schools, 45*(6), 523–536.

Ortega, J. V. (2005). Juan Huarte de San Juan in Cartesian and modern psycholinguistics: An encounter with Noam Chomsky. *Psicothema, 17*(3), 436–440.

Reynolds, M. R. (2012). Interpreting the *g* loadings of intelligence test composite scores in light of Spearman's law of diminishing returns. Manuscript accepted for publication in *School Psychology Quarterly*.

Reynolds, M. R., & Keith, T. Z. (2007). Spearman's law of diminishing returns in hierarchical models of intelligence for children and adolescents. *Intelligence, 35*, 267–281.

Reynolds, M. R., Keith, T. Z., & Beretvas, N. (2010). Use of factor mixture modeling to capture Spearman's law of diminishing returns. *Intelligence, 38*, 231–214.

Reynolds, M. R., Keith, T. Z., Fine, J. G., Fisher, M. E., & Low, J. A. (2007). Confirmatory factor structure of the Kaufman Assessment Battery for Children–2nd ed.: Consistency with Cattell-Horn-Carroll theory. *School Psychology Quarterly, 22*(4), 511–539.

Reynolds, M. R., Keith, T. Z., Ridley, K. P., & Patel, P. G. (2008). Sex differences in latent general and broad cognitive abilities for children and youth: Evidence for higher-order MG-MACS and MIMIC models. *Intelligence, 36*, 236–260,

Roid, G. H. (2003b). *Stanford-Binet Intelligence Scales–5th ed.*. Itasca, IL: Riverside Publishing.

Roid, G. H., & Barram, R. A. (2004). *Essentials of Stanford-Binet Intelligence Scales (SB5) assessment*. New York: Wiley.

Roid, G. H., & Pomplun, M. (2012). The Stanford-Binet Intelligence Scales, Fifth Edition. In D. P. Flanagan & P. L. Harrison (Eds.), *Contemporary intellectual assessment: Theories, tests, and issues* (3rd ed., pp. 249–268). New York: Guilford Press.

Sanders, S., McIntosh, D. E., Dunham, M., Rothlisberg, B. B., & Finch, H. (2007). Joint confirmatory factor analysis of the Differential Ability Scales and the Woodcock-Johnson Tests of Cognitive Abilities–3rd ed. *Psychology in the Schools, 44*(2), 119–138.

Sattler, J. M. (1992). Historical survey and theories of intelligence. In J. M. Sattler, *Assessment of children: Revised and updated 3rd ed.* (pp. 37–60). San Diego: Jerome M. Sattler, Publisher.

Sattler, J. M. (2008). *Assessment of children: Cognitive foundations (5th ed.)*. San Diego: Jerome M. Sattler, Publisher.

Sbordone, R. T., & Saul, R. E. (2000). *Neuropsychology for health care professionals and attorneys: 2nd ed.*. CRC Press.

Schafer, R., & Rapaport, D. (1944). The scatter: In diagnostic intelligence testing. *A Quarterly for Psychodiagnostic & Allied Studies, 12*, 275–284.

Schneider, W. (1992). After Binet: French intelligence testing, 1900–1950. *Journal of the History of the Behavioral Sciences, 28*, 111–132.

Schneider, W. J., & McGrew, K. S. (2012). The Cattell-Horn-Carroll model of intelligence. In D. P. Flanagan & P. L. Harrison (Eds.), *Contemporary intellectual assessment: Theories, tests, and issues* (3rd ed., pp. 99–144). New York: Guilford Press.

Schrank, F. A., Flanagan, D. P., Woodcock, R. W., & Mascolo, J. T. (2002). *Essentials of WJ III Cognitive Abilities Assessment*. New York: Wiley.

Schrank, F. A., & Wendling, B. J. (2012). The Woodcock-Johnson III Normative update. In D. P. Flanagan & P. L. Harrison (Eds.), *Contemporary intellectual assessment: Theories, tests, and issues* (3rd ed., pp. 297–335). New York: Guilford Press.

Shepard, R., Fasko, D., & Osborne, F. (1999). Intrapersonal intelligence: Affective factors in thinking. *Education, 119*, 663.

Singer, J. K., Lichtenberger, E. O., Kaufman, J. C., Kaufman, A. S., & Kaufman, N. L. (2012). The Kaufman Assessment Battery for Children—Second Edition (KABC-II) and the Kaufman Test of Educational Achievement—Second Edition (KTEA-II). In D. P. Flanagan & P. L. Harrison (Eds.), Contemporary intellectual assessment: Theories, tests, and issues (3rd ed., pp. 269–296). New York: Guilford.

Sugarman, A., & Kanner, K. (2000). The contribution of psychoanalytic theory to psychological testing. *Psychoanalytic Psychology, 17*(1), 3–23.

Stavrou, E., & Hollander, N. L. (2007). Differential Ability Scales–2nd ed. (DAS-II). *The School Psychologist, Fall*, 120–124.

Taub, G. E., Floyd, R. G., Keith, T. Z., & McGrew, K. S. (2008). Effects of general and broad cognitive abilities on mathematics achievement. *School Psychology Quarterly, 23*(2), 187–198.

Taub, G. E., & McGrew, K. S. (2004). A confirmatory factor analysis of Cattell-Horn-Carroll theory and cross-age invariance of the Woodcock-Johnson Tests of Cognitive Abilities III. *School Psychology Quarterly, 19*(1), 72–87.

Thorndike, R. M. (1997). The early history of intelligence testing. In D. P. Flanagan, J. L. Genshaft, & P. L. Harrison (Eds.), *Contemporary intellectual assessment: Theories, tests, and issues* (pp. 3–16). New York: Guilford.

Thurstone, L. L. (1938). *Primary mental abilities*. Chicago: University of Chicago Press.

Von Mayrhauser, R. T. (1992). The mental testing community and validity: A prehistory. *American Psychologist 47*(2), 244–253.

Wasserman, J. D. (2012). A history of intelligence assessment: The unfinished tapestry. In D. P. Flanagan & P. L. Harrison (Eds.), *Contemporary intellectual assessment: Theories, tests, and issues* (3rd ed., pp. 3–70). New York: Guilford Press.

Webster, R. E., & Lafayette, A. D. (1980). Distinguishing among three subgroups of handicapped students using Bannatyne's recategorization. *The Journal of Educational Research, 73*(4), 237–240.

Wechsler, D. (1949). *Wechsler Intelligence Scale for Children*. San Antonio, TX: Psychological Corporation.

Wechsler, D. (1955). *Wechsler Adult Intelligence Scale*. San Antonio, TX: Psychological Corporation.

Wechsler, D. (1974). *Wechsler Intelligence Scale for Children—Revised*. San Antonio, TX: Psychological Corporation.

Wechsler, D. (1975). Intelligence defined and undefined: A relativistic approach. *American Psychologist*, 135–139.

Wechsler, D. (2003). *Wechsler Intelligence Scale for Children – 4th ed.*. San Antonio, TX: Psychological Corporation.

Wechsler, D. (2008). *Wechsler Adult Intelligence Scale–4th ed.*. San Antonio, TX: Psychological Corporation.

Wechsler, D. (2012). *Wechsler Preschool and Primary Scale of Intelligence – 4th ed.*. San Antonio, TX: Pearson.

Wiggins, J. S., Behrends, R. S., Trost, K. K. (2003). *Paradigms of personality assessment*. Guilford Press.

Winzer, M. (1993). *History of special education: From isolation to integration*. Washington, DC: Gallaudet University Press.

Woodcock, R. W., & Johnson, M. B. (1989). *Woodcock-Johnson Tests of Cognitive Ability—Revised*. Chicago: Riverside.

Woodcock, R. W., McGrew, K. S., & Mather, N. (2001a). *Woodcock-Johnson III Tests of Achievement*. Itasca, IL: Riverside.

Woodcock, R. W., McGrew, K. S., & Mather, N. (2001b). *Woodcock-Johnson III Tests of Cognitive Abilities*. Itasca, IL: Riverside.

Woodcock, R. W., McGrew, K. S., Schrank, F. A., & Mather, N. (2007). *Woodcock-Johnson III Normative Update*. Rolling Meadows, IL: Riverside.

Testing: The Measurement and Assessment Link

Scott L. Decker

Abstract

This chapter broadly reviews measurement theory, scale development, testing, and assessment. The chapter is divided into two broad areas to represent distinct phases of testing involving test development and test application. A model is provided to illustrate the integrated role of testing with measurement and assessment components. Theories of measurement are reviewed with the use of the Item Response Theory, not only for the purpose of objective measurement, but as a basic model to analyze how personal attributes interact with test stimuli. Interpretive phases of tests within an assessment process are described, which include decision-making, prescriptive action, and social outcomes.

Key Words: psychological testing, measurement, item response theory, decision-making

Introduction

Measurement theory, scale development, testing, and assessment are all important contributors to test development and and test application. Despite the detailed research in each of these areas, there are few models which focus on the integration and inter-relationship across these components. The model described in this chapter is used to illustrate the integrated role of testing with measurement and assessment components. Furthermore, measure-ment theories are discussed to illustrate the impor-tance of objective in the analysis of how personal attributes interact with test stimuli. Extensions of the model to the interpretive phases of tests within an assessment process are also described.

The chapter is divided into two conceptual sections: (a) pre-application or development stage of testing, and (b) the application stage of testing. During the test development stage, theory and measurement are used for the purpose of understanding the test (i.e., developing construct validity). During the applica-tion stage, the test is used to understand the object it was designed to measure. The purpose of dividing the chapter into these two sections is to provide a better integration of the numerous components in assess-ment, which include aspects of theory, measurement, measurement models, testing, decision-making, diagnosis, and prescriptive action. Additionally, these two sections coincide with contemporary categories of validity (Embretson, 1983). These concepts form a layer of interconnected concepts. For example, test-ing depends on measurement, which includes scal-ing, which in turn depends on the theoretical basis of a construct. *Assessment* is the integration of mul-tiple sources of information for the purpose of mak-ing a judgement that leads to a prescriptive action. A *test*, or testing, is a device used to measure behavior which provides information in the assessment pro-cess. Measurement theory provides a critical founda-tion for constructing tests as measurement tools. Test interpretation is a part of a decision-making process in which some action, such as an intervention, is to be implemented. Interventions influence outcomes which are evaluated by social goals and values.

Fundamental Issues in Testing

Psychology is replete with conceptual ideas of the inner workings of mental phenomena and postulated causes of behavior. Lacking, however, is the objective measurement of many of these theories and constructs. As a result, paradigms in psychology wax and wane. Often, the constructs of one theory rename the constructs of another theory. Few theories, however, provide objective measures by which to test the theoretical propositions of the theory. Stated differently, few objective measures exist to test the theoretical propositions of most psychological theories. As such, measurement has been described as the "Achilles' heel" of psychological research (Pedhazur & Schmelkin, 1991).

Like in psychology in general, there is disagreement within the specific area of psychological measurement. Measurement models differ in Classical Test Theory from Item Response Theory (to be addressed later). Debate on the role of measurement scale of a test to permissible use of statistical procedures has raged for almost half a century (J. Stevens, 1996). As an additional confounding influence, different researchers use different terminology to describe similar aspects of testing. Terms such as "assessment instruments" are used, although some view assessment and testing as very different. Are "instruments" and "tests" equivalent? Similarly, the definition of "measurement model" and "measurement scale" are used interchangeably.

An additional difficulty in discussing testing, measurement, or assessment is that all of these topics are interrelated. This leads to an extraordinary complexity involved with each of these topics. As a possible consequence, these topics are often extensively written about, but in isolation and disconnected from the other topics. Similarly, many standard assessment textbooks provide adequate coverage on each of these topics but often do not provide an integration of the different components. Often, extensive psychometric evidence for the tests is provided, but applications of the test are dismissed and the test user is left to figure out how to appropriately apply the test, using "clinical judgement" (Kamphaus & Campbell, 2006; Sattler, 2001). Because the ultimate application for test usage has been left unspecified, this may have partially contributed to a growing dissatisfaction with the use of norm-referenced testing. As a result, context-based methods of testing that attempt to more directly link assessment from a specific context (e.g., functional behavior analysis, curriculum-based assessment, portfolio assessment) have grown in popularity, although they have substantially less psychometric rigor.

Foundations of Testing: Measurement

The foundation of testing is measurement. One important historical root of measurement in the behavioral sciences can be traced to Krantz, Luce, Suppes, and Tversky's (1971) *Foundations of Measurement*. The three-volume set provided the basis for what has become known as the *representational theory of measurement* (Krantz, Luce, Suppes, & Tversky, 1971). In representational theory, measurement involves understanding an empirical observation that can be recoded in terms of mathematical structures (Luce & Suppes, 2001). Simplifying, "measurement" includes an object of measurement or the measurement of an object attribute. Object attributes, presumed to vary across different objects, can be coded, or represented, with different numerical values. The initial coding of empirical phenomena with numerals is qualitative. The abstraction of the phenomenon into numerals that are used as numbers in a number system that has quantitative properties is the basis of measurement. Significant debate in this fundamental step has long been a characteristic in the history of measurement. Using physical sciences as a model and reserving measurement for what we now would consider interval and ratio scales, Campbell (1920) insisted that all measurement must satisfy certain properties such as concatenation or additivity. Because psychological measurement rarely demonstrated such properties, Campbell concluded psychology could not be considered a science (Campbell, 1920).

This influenced the development of formal definitions of scaling. Stevens's definition of measurement as "the assignment of numbers to aspects of objects or events according to one or another rule or convention" is perhaps the most popular definition of measurement (Stevens, 1968, p. 850). Stevens's scaling is the assignment of numbers to a sample of behavior along a dimension characterized by some unit of metric. Stevens suggested four types of metrics that continue to be popular: *nominal, ordinal, interval,* and *ratio* (Stevens, 1946). Given their ubiquity in psychology, they will only be discussed briefly. *Nominal* amounts to naming or classify objects or persons into one or more categories. In nominal measurement of attributes, an attribute is either present or not. *Ordinal* involves the detection of an attribution and the rank ordering of the attribution. That is, object can be rank ordered (high to low) by the number assignment to the attribute. *Interval* measurement entails not only rank ordering but the "amount" or quantity of difference, with constant or equal amounts between number assignments. Finally, *ratio* includes interval properties but also includes a true "zero" point for the absence of the attribute. Weight and height are two examples of ratio measures, and the widespread use of these measures and being ratio is not coincidental. For a more exhaustive review, see Pedhazur and Schmelkin, 1991.

Various aspects of these early conceptual models of measurement in behavioral science have continued to be debated for over half a century (Gaito, 1980; Guttman, 1977; Lord, 1946; Michell, 1986). However, Stevens's influence on the definition of measurement can clearly be seen in modern conceptualizations of measurement. Townsend and Ashby (1984) described measurement as a process of assigning numbers to objects in such a way that interesting qualitative empirical relations among the objects are reflected in the numbers as well as in the properties of the number system (Townsend & Ashby, 1984), or similarly to objects of measurement (Reynolds, 1986). Additionally, many modern approaches have sided with Stevens by including classification (nominal) and ranking (ordinal) as types of measurement (Pedhazur & Schmelkin, 1991).

Furthermore, various other methods of measurement have been described, but most capture concepts similar to those described in the Representational Theory of Measurement. For example, some have made a distinction between a *natural variable* and a *scaled variable* (Krantz et al., 1971). A natural variable is a variable that is defined by using the actual objects of interest that does not depend on abstract symbols such as numbers, on which scaled variables do depend (Reckase, 2000). Natural variables are directly observable from the objects of interest, whereas scaled variables are not. Natural variables can be conceptualized as detectable from direct observation and are discrete in that the observed event can be classified or be distinguished from other events or the absence of the event. For example, an observable event must be detected such that a determination of whether it is present/absent, or yes/no, can be made, or different gradations can be determined. Scaled variables are a conversion of these observable events into a metric of measurement by some rule. The scaled variable can be a raw score or a raw score corrected for a subject's developmental age.

Applications of Psychometric Models in Measurement

Psychological theory describes the attributes of the object of measurement, the different values an attribute may have, and a causative explanation for differences in values across objects. Often in psychology the object of measurement is a person. The attributes that are of interest are behavior and mental processes that influence behavior. The attributes that are measured are dictated by theory. Similarly, the types of prompts or questions used in testing are dictated by theory. Different theories have different types of emphasis for different attributes. A *construct* is defined as the concept or characteristic that a test is designed to measure. Because constructs are unobservable, different lines of valid evidence are needed to provide information relevant to a specific interpretation of test scores. Furthermore, validity is generally the degree to which evidence and theory support the interpretation of test scores and is considered the most fundamental factor in evaluating a test (American Educational Research Association (AERA), American Psychological Association (APA), & National Council on Measurement in Education (NCME), 1999).

Measurement theory provides only an abstraction of attributes, whereas theory describes attributes in detail. Additionally, measurement describes the process of quantifying attribute values but does not describe what values should be quantified. The meaning of the number may differ by the type of number used to represent the attribute. For example, people share physical attributes (e.g., height, weight) but differ in the values of these attributes (100 lbs, 200 lbs).

Scale is a term used to describe the transformation of behavioral performance, typically in response to questions, into numbers and how to present the questions in order to get the best measurement. Formally, *scale* is the set of rules that are used to assign a number to an attribute (Thorndike, 2005). A familiar scale of measurement for the attribute of length in physical objects is the assignment of inches (the basic measurement unit) from a ruler or tape measure. Another common metric is temperature, which may use either Fahrenheit or Celsius measurement units.

Scaling in behavioral measurement is "messier" than in the physical sciences, or, one might say, it involves a larger degree of error. Scaling in psychology typically involves the assignment of numbers to behavioral responses. The behavioral responses are typically from predetermined stimuli with set rules for assigning numbers. Examples of such scaling are eliciting responses that can be scored as correct or incorrect, and adding the number of correct responses to get an overall score for a set of items. Scaling may also involve a set of rules to transform the raw score into another measurement scale, such as normative score (percentile, standard, or normalized).

In scaling behavioral measurements, there are different frames of references, or measurement models, that can be used. The two main paradigms are *random sampling theory* and *item response theory* (Suen, 1990), although this is sometimes referred to as *classical test theory* or *item response theory* (Embretson & Reise, 2000). Random sampling theory, which involves both classical test theory and generalizability theory, is based on a true score model. The premise is in any testing situation no person can be exposed to all the possible items within a construct domain. Therefore, the limited sample of items provides an *observed score,* which is viewed as an approximation to a *true score.* These psychometric models essentially address the problem of how to generalize from a sample to a larger population. Classical test theory has been the dominate paradigm until recently. Classic test theory has numerous limitations. Some of the most important involve estimating item difficulties, sample-dependent statistics, single reliability estimates, and problems in comparing scores across similar tests.

Due to these and other limitations in classical test theory, item response theory (IRT) has become the most frequently used psychometric paradigm, especially in test development. IRT is a type of latent trait model that presumes a unitary dimension to describe the attribute that is being measured. A benefit to IRT models is that the model scales behavioral responses based on the joint interaction of a person's ability with the item difficulty (Figure 2.1). The basic idea is that when a person's ability is greater than the item difficulty, then the person has a higher probability

of correctly answering the item. Conversely, when the item difficulty is greater than the person's ability, the person should incorrectly answer the item. When the item difficulty and the person's ability are equally matched, there is a 50/50 chance of getting the item correct. This basic relationship is modeled with a logistical curve (Figure 2.2).

Model-based measurement in IRT is fundamentally different from classical test theory. Similar to the measurement of physical objects, one does not need to invent a new "ruler" for every object investigated. Instead, the ruler or tape measure is used as an existing model. Item response models work on a similar premise. Although IRT models differ in the number of parameters used in the model, only the Rasch (one-parameter) model will be described here. There are also two- and three-parameter models that include parameters for item discrimination and guessing. These models are not presented, because they are extensions of the basic Rasch model, and some have argued the adding these additional parameters compromises aspects of objective measurement (Wright & Stone, 1979). The Rasch model describes the outcome of a person's ability interacting with a stimulus (item) with some difficulty that results in a binary outcome, such as pass/fail, correct/incorrect, etc. The underlying model is a logistics curve that models success and failure based on a person's ability and an item's difficulty. Unlike in classical test theory, the values for the item difficulties are not sample-dependent, just as the units of measurement do not change on a ruler based on the object being measured. The probabilistic outcome is a function of the difference in the person's ability (B) and the difficulty of the item (D). Rasch (1960) described the specific ordinal relationship to describe probabilities of a test simply as "a person having a greater ability than

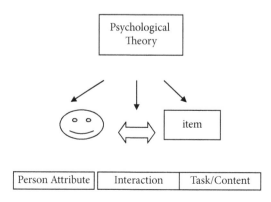

Figure 2.1 Schematic of theory in specifying person by task interaction.

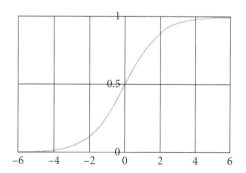

Figure 2.2 Logistical curve of ability with probability of response.

another person should have the greater probability of solving any item of the type in question (p. 117). Formally, when B = D, the probability of a correct response is 50/50. When B > D, the probability of a correct response increases from .5, and decreases when B < D. Formally, the probability of a correct answer is given in the following equation:

$$P(x = 1) = e^{(B-D)}/1 + e^{(B-D)}$$

where e is the natural log function (2.7183) which is raised to the difference in the person's ability (B) and the item difficulty (D). The resulting units of measurement are described as *logits*, which are typically set to the arbitrary value of 0 as the mean. Suppose someone with a logit ability of 3 completed a spelling item that was calibrated to have a difficulty of 1. Using equation 1, the probability of correctly answering the item can be determined as:

$$P(1) = 2.7182^{(3-1)} / 1 + 2.7182^{(3-1)} = .88$$

Similarly, if a person with a logit ability of 3 interacted with an item calibrated with a difficulty of 4, obviously, the probability of success would be much less than in the previous example; and more specifically:

$$P(1) = 2.7182^{(3-4)} / 2.7182^{(3-4)} = .27$$

The relationship of different ability–difficulty differences can be viewed in Table 2.1. Object measurement is the repetition of a measuring unit and describes a constancy in measurement not dependent on the sample or measurement instrument. Notice from Table 2.1, the probability of success is the same for the same differences in measurement

Table 2.1 Probability Outcomes Based on Person Ability and Item Difficulty

B-D	P(x = 1)
3.0	.95
2.0	.88
1.0	.73
0.0	.50
−1.0	.27
−2.0	.12
−3.0	.05

regardless of the value of the measurement. For example, there is a probability of .73 regardless of whether the person's ability/item difference is 3-2, or 2-1, or -1-(-2).

Although conjoint measurement, which enables equal interval scaling (Stevens, 1946), technically includes Weak Order, Independence, Double Cancellation, Solvability, and Archimedean Condition (Kyngdon, 2008), the Rasch model's fulfillment of these properties, or approximate fulfillment, has led many to conclude it is the only measurement model in psychology that provides interval scaling (Andrich, 1988; Bond & Fox, 2001; Embretson, 1999; Embretson & Reise, 2000; Woodcock, McGrew, & Mather, 2001; Wright & Stone, 1979). Some disagree with these claims since there is still difficulty in verifying the equal interval nature of the actual underlying psychological or causal process of behavioral responses (Kyngdon, 2008). Additionally, some have argued IRT metrics are still arbitrary until observed scores, no matter the form, are mapped onto meaningful behaviors (Blanton & Jaccard, 2006). Regardless, such probabilistic features that are not sample-dependent represent a substantial improvement in psychometric measurement from that of its historic predecessor, classical test theory (Embretson, 2006).

This transformation of test values that provide indicators of behavior to a measurement scale is the quintessential distinction in testing as the "use of an instrument" from testing as "measurement." The degree to which a test adequately "measures" a construct, rather than provides an arbitrary representation, is directly related to the degree to which valid inferences can be made on the change in amount of a construct. Thus, the issue of understanding the measured representation of psychological constructs is not just a technical issue relevant for quantitative psychologists, but is the foundation in which all concepts in psychology that involve constructs, which is the nearly the whole of psychology. In practice, items calibrated with the Rasch model are selected to have different difficulties that adequately cover the range of ability. The scale with selected items is then used for practical applications.

Psychological measurement, which involves both psychological theory and measurement, will continue to evolve. As demonstrated by measurement models, psychology will always involve the analysis of a person–item interaction, where the item may be an item or some other contextual variable identified or derived by psychological theory. Although far from perfect, the foundations of measurement with representational theory of measurement and the application of measurement models as used in IRT probably represent the pinnacle, or near pinnacle, of measurement in the behavioral sciences. It is difficult to imagine what new purely measurement developments could occur that would fundamentally change psychological measurement beyond that provided by IRT models.

Testing

Keeping the complex nature of measurement in mind, testing can now be more directly addressed. A *test* is an evaluative device used to sample an examinee's behavior in a specified domain that is scored using a standardized process (AERA et al., 1999). The objective of testing is to describe a characteristic of a subject as a numerical score to represent the quantity of the characteristic (Suen, 1990). Objects of measurement are psychological constructs. When used in assessment, tests are used to obtain information and reduce uncertainty (McFall & Townsend, 1998).

Although a test can be simply defined as a device for scoring behavior, the intricacies in this process are complex. A test is the assembly of stimuli that elicit behavioral responses from a test taker in which behavioral responses are numerically coded. The stimuli are typically calibrated, or ordered by difficulty, to form a scale that measures an attribute of an object (i.e., personal characteristic). The selection of the test stimuli or content is theoretically based. Additionally, a test provides information on the status of an attribute by recording some observable event or behavior. Linking recorded observations from the test to a measurement unit is an aspect of scaling.

Testing, as a component of psychological assessment, typically provides a measurement of a person's attribute (i.e., mental process). Multiple tests are used to measure different attributes to provide a comprehensive assessment to assist in the assessment decision-making process.

Behavioral responses are scaled by recording behaviors, usually with a predetermined response format, representative of the construct. Constructs have a dimension; that is, higher or lower amounts of a construct. The dimension represents the range of values to describe individual differences in attribute values across different objects. Objects are multidimensional (i.e., multi-characteristics) but are typically measured by unidimensional tests. Different attribute levels, as indicated by score values, are then examined or correlated with other attribute values

from different constructs as well as with important outcomes or events. For example, intelligence tests measure intelligence by combining multiple subtests measuring some theoretical attribute of intelligence. Scores are corrected for age-related variance and converted to a scale of a mean of 100 and a standard deviation of 15. The differences in levels of intelligence across different people result in a distribution, typically normal or Gaussian, across the measurement scale. Correlational methods can investigate the relationship of variations in intelligence with variations in other variables such as personality and academic achievement. The question as to whether intelligence can be represented by a single variable, and the nature of that single variable, is not an issue of measurement. Rather, this is an issue of theory and validity. Similarly, the accuracy and stability of assigning numbers to represent differences in attributes is an issue of reliability, which influences measurement but is not measurement.

Testing in Assessment

At the time of writing this chapter, the Supreme Court of the United States made a decision in which testing was at the center of the lawsuit. In the *Ricci v. DeStefano* case (decision made in June, 2009), 20 firefighters sued the city of New Haven, Connecticut, alleging that they were discriminated against. Firefighters promotions were determined based on a test, but the test scores resulted in perceived disproportionate number of promotions of white firefighters. As a result, the test was declared invalid, and the results were discarded for fear of a lawsuit by the non-white firefighters. However, discarding the result of the test was also viewed as discrimination—against the white firefighters (and one Hispanic firefighter), and resulted in a lawsuit. Ultimately, the Supreme Court ruled that the city should not have thrown out the exam, arguing that by doing so, the city was using race as a criterion for promotion, which violated Title VII of Civil Rights Act of 1964, in which employment decisions cannot be made based on race.

The point of mentioning this Supreme Court case is not to state an opinion on the verdict or address the issue of test bias (see Reynolds, Lowe, & Saenz, 1999, for more on test bias). The point here is to simply illustrate the complex and numerous layers of meaning involved in testing, which extends beyond just a device for measuring. Tests are always developed and administered for some purpose. The purpose is usually driven by some social need (e.g., promotion, intervention, or classification).

In each situation, judgement is required based on a decision-making process. The judgement then results in some action that satisfies the social need. Furthermore, social benefit, or perceptions of social benefit, may influence not just assessment but test development. In the New Haven firefighters' case, the city officials were required to make a judgement, first on test scores and then on the permissible use of test scores, which influenced social outcomes. As such, judgement and decision-making, as well as the resulting actions and the outcomes of those actions, are important components in assessment and provide an important link between theory, measurement, testing, assessment, and social outcomes.

Figure 2.3 depicts the integrative influence in the relationship between testing, measurement and assessment. As the role of theory, measurement, measurement scale, and assessment have been discussed previously in this chapter, the remainder of the chapter will cover *judgement, prescriptive action,* and *social outcome*. Although clinical judgement research is readily available, the process of translating a judgement into some action is not. Often, the action taken is more contextually derived and is difficult to determine in the abstract. Similarly, social outcomes are important but rely upon some action, which in turn relies upon judgement and assessment. In most treatment utility paradigms, assessment and decision-making are taken for granted and not represented in the models. Often such research demonstrates the utility of a behavioral intervention using a single-subject design and concludes that the change in baseline during the intervention did not require any sophisticated cognitive or personality tests. Not included, but important within an applied context, is "why," or the justification, an intervention was deemed to be needed and "why" the particular intervention was chosen. Such processes in behavioral research have remained covert mental processes of the experimenters.

Figure 2.3 represents a cyclical process that suggests that the major components of measurement, testing, and assessment are interrelated. Testing, in development or application, is interconnected to theory, measurement, and social values and consequences.

Not intended to be a unitary model of construct validity, the present model intended to (1) emphasize the sequential relationship of key stages in the application of tests in an assessment process, and (2) to emphasize the interrelatedness of these key stages. The Nomological Network (Messick, 1995) model consists of distributed but connected

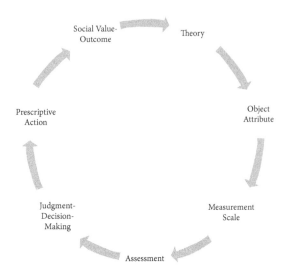

Figure 2.3 Sequential cycle of measurement, testing, and assessment.

nodes. Although this is accurate, it may not capture the sequential nature of the assessment process nor the sequential process of measurement or decision-making and how they are interconnected. Theory guides scale development, which influences which measures are used in a particular assessment. Similarly, judgements are the result of an assessment process and lead to an action that is "theoretically" believed to have a desirable social outcome; thus social value and theory are connected. Thus, the end of the chain of reasoning in testing loops back to the beginning in that it influences the actual design of the test. This is also partially idealized. For example, test development typically starts and ends with the accuracy in measuring a construct. As suggested by Figure 2.3, test development may also benefit by starting with (1) what is the social value of measuring a particular attribute, (2) what action or intervention can be taken based on information about an attribute, or (3) how can decisions be made based on a measurement of an attribute. Here, test development begins with the end in mind.

Assessment

Assessment is a broader term than *testing* that involves the integration of test information with other sources of information (AERA et al., 1999). Assessment is a framework for constructing a unified meaning from various sources of information. Assessment goes beyond test scores and involves a multi-step and multidimensional evaluation of an individual.

Assessment marks the point at which a test, constructed via the methodology previously presented, is used as a tool of investigation rather than being the focus of the investigation. Assessment is:

> concerned with the clinician who takes a variety of test scores, generally obtained from multiple test methods, and considers the data in the context of history, referral information, and observed behavior to understand the person being evaluated, to answer the referral questions, and then to communicate findings to the patient, his or her significant others, and referral sources. (Meyer et al., 2001, p. 143)

Because contextualized decision-making is required, assessment is not a completely objective process. As Matarazzo (1990) described in his APA presidential speech, assessment is "a highly complex operation that involves extracting diagnostic meaning from an individual's personal history and objectively recorded tests scores…it is the activity of a licensed professional, an artisan familiar with the accumulated findings of his or her young science…." (p. 1000).

Assessment is often described in multiple stages. Sattler (2008) described assessment as an 11-step process that includes collecting data from multiple sources that include both formal testing procedures as well as observations, and clinical judgement. McFall and Townsend (1998) described assessment as consisting of eight layers that integrated various aspects involved in assessment. Layer 1 consisted of postulates, which were assumptions, beliefs, or values. Layer 2 was a formal theoretical model. Layer 3 was described as referents or observable instantiations, Layer 4 was instrument methods; followed by Layer 5 of measurement model; Layer 6, data reduction; Layer 7, data analysis; and Layer 8, interpretation and inference. A loop connects Layer 8 with Layer 2 to demonstrate the influence of inferences on the questions that gave rise to the assessment process (McFall & Townsend, 1998). According to McFall and Townsend (1998) the purpose of assessment was one of obtaining information and reducing uncertainty.

Most models of assessment generally describe the process of transforming test data into usable information as part of "test interpretation." Sattler notes that test interpretation is the most challenging step in the assessment process, and it involves integrating assessment data, making judgements, and exploring implications (Sattler, 2008). Interpretation of test scores to provide meaningful information is central in the assessment process. Blanton and Jaccard

(2006) indicated meaning from test scores "must be established through research that links specific scores to the observable events that are relevant to the underlying psychological dimension of interest" (Blanton & Jaccard, 2006, p. 33). Similarly, scaled scores are believed to aid interpretation by indicating how a given score compares to those of other test takers (AERA et al., 1999). Procedural, objective, algorithmic methods for deriving "meaning" from test scores are generally not recommended because of the complexities involved with assessment, which include linking validity studies to a contextual purpose.

Interpretation of test scores is connected to the validity evidence for a test. According to the Standards, "Test scores ideally are interpreted in light of the available normative data, the psychometric properties of the test, the temporal stability of the constructs being measured, and the effect of moderator variables and demographic characteristics" (AERA) et al., 1999, p. 121). Tests are valid to the degree in which evidence supports inferences from the test. The evidence to support inferences is based on validity evidence; thus test validity is central to test interpretation. *Validity* refers to the degree that evidence and theory support the interpretations of test scores (AERA et al., 1999).

Models of test validity have evolved over time to more accurately represent the nuances of process involved in the application of tests in assessment. Traditional validity research amounted to obtaining evidence that the test was measuring what it was suppose to measure (Campbell & Fiske, 1959). Here, construct validity was the central focus and obtained primarily by evidence of a test's correlation with other tests with a similar label, and no, or lower, correlations with tests having a different label. Construct validity has been traditionally viewed as empirically established after the test was constructed (Cronback & Meehl, 1955). The "meaning" of test scores was determined by their relation with other variables, which formed what was termed a "nomological network." Similarly, the nomological network model of validity attempted to expand construct validity to incorporate other aspects of the assessment process (Cronbach & Meehl, 1955). This view was criticized at its inception as confusing "meaning" with "significance" (Bechtoldt, 1959). Over time, the validity concept has become "encrusted with additional meanings" and is likely to require revisions (Schwager, 1991).

Additionally, nomological networks have been difficult to define (Cronbach, 1988). Embretson (1985)

attempted to provide clarification by distinguishing construct representation from nomothetic span. *Construct representation* involves evidence to understand the processes, strategies, and knowledge that persons use to respond to test items and how these behaviors are represented by test scores. *Nomothetic span* is the evidence to support how individual differences as represented by test scores are related to external variables and the utility of those relationships. Different researchers promote different types of validity and use different terminology. For example, *nomological span* (Embretson, 1983) is synonymous with *external validity* (Cook & Campbell, 1979), which in turn is referred to as a *nomological network* (Messick, 1995), which creates additional problems for relating validity evidence to test interpretation.

Such criteria attempt to bridge the gap in assessment between using tests in data collection and making inferences leading to judgement with tests. Additionally, such criteria imply published validity on a test will make the connection for the clinician. Unfortunately, published research on most psychological tests does not provide such guidance.

In an attempt to focus less on the mechanical issues of construct validity, Messick (1980) has attempted to better address the connection between test "interpretation" and the social consequences of tests. Messick unification is described in the following diagram:

Other researchers have begun to de-emphasize construct validity, which has traditionally been viewed as the core pillar of assessment, and placed more emphasis on the social consequences aspect. The focus on social outcomes as the credentialing criteria of usefulness has been termed *treatment utility*. Treatment utility is "the degree to which assessment is shown to contribute to beneficial treatment outcome" (Hayes, Nelson, & Jarrett, 1987, p. 963). This functional approach would argue the only utility of testing is the degree to which it is associated with change in some valued social outcome. This

approach places "treatment validity" at the core of validity (Fuchs, Fuchs, & Speece, 2002) and has led some to suggest norm-referenced tests should be discontinued due to a lack of treatment validity (Gresham, 2002; Reschly & Grimes, 2002).

Contemporary models of validity are therefore fragmentary. Integrating these different points of view has been difficult. The social consequences, such as treatment benefit, should be more highly weighted than in traditional models. However, sole focus on social outcomes creates numerous problems (Decker, 2008; Reynolds, 1986). As Messick (1980) states,

> What matters is not only whether the social consequences of test interpretation and use are positive or negative, but how the consequences came about and what determined them. In particular, it is not that adverse social consequences of test use render the use invalid but, rather, that adverse social consequences should not be attributable to any source of test invalidity, such as construct under-representation or construct-irrelevant variance. (p. 748)

In Figure 2.3, processes are represented as beginning in assessment, judgement, prescriptive action, and social outcome. In support of treatment utility theories, much can be gained by first asking, "What is the benefit?" However, in support of construct theories, even social benefit involves "theory"; how the benefit came about is important, not just whether or not the benefit occurred, and some form of decision-making that informs prescriptive action is part of all interventions.

Attributes exist in individuals as finite, discrete properties but are measured as continuous variables labeled as constructs. Test interpretation involves numerous scores on continuous scales. However, the social value of assessment is one of deriving a discrete judgement. Thus, assessment requires the judgement of discrete probabilities from continuous scales to map to some prescriptive outcome. Currently, the categorical interpretation of test scores is arbitrarily given by dividing the normal distribution curve into ordinal categories (e.g., below average, average, above average). Indeed, qualitative outcomes appear to be the most informative to patients (depressed, not depressed) and may provide a linkage from test scores to real-world outcomes.

Table 2.2 Messick's View of the Interaction of Test Interpretation with Prescriptive Action and Social Outcome Variables

	Test Interpretation	Test Use
Evidential basis	Construct validity (CV)	CV + relevance/utility (R/U)
Consequential basis	CV + value implications (VI)	CV + R/U + VI + social consequences

Adapted from Messick, 1980.

Judgement and Decision-Making

The complexities of making judgements from assessment data are vast due not only to all the issues in measurement theory, the theory of the construct being measured, and situational factors during testing, but also due to how these factors impact, or are impacted by, the contextual issues involved in applied assessment applications, which include social consequences. This gets to the interrelatedness of these different concepts. Unfortunately, the complexity increases as it is at this point that interpretation is defined by cognitive events of the clinician and thus a large number of new variables become influential. The role of clinical interpretation as part of the assessment process is perhaps the most important link in the chain (McFall & Townsend, 1998). However, it is also mostly described in qualitative terms such as "integrative," "holistic," "comprehensive," and "synthesis." Granted, this is due in part to the vast complexities involved that do not readily lend themselves to statistical modeling. Additionally, contemporary models of validity do not specify how clinicians should make evaluative decisions based on a certain context. Yet, evaluative clinical decisions are the primary mechanism that leads to prescriptive action and in turn to outcome. As a result, such processes are unaccounted for and remain implicit and ambiguous, or are determined to be irrelevant.

Perhaps part of the reason why "interpretation" and validity are often not specified or specified in multiple ways is because of the complexity and challenges involved. Part of the challenge is that validity research, often conducted under controlled conditions, may not always be relevant for the contextual issues in applied practice. Additionally, clinical decision-making is intimately a part of the assessment process, and different types of validity are prioritized based on the decision-making demands of researchers or clinicians (Kazdin, 2003). One validates, not a test, but an interpretation of data arising from a specified procedure (Cronbach, 1971). Recall that test validity is in part determined by evidence suggesting the test is measuring what it is "intended" to measure. However, "intentions" change based on contextual situations. A test can be perfectly valid and reliable but have no link or implication for real-world processes that are relevant to a clinical situation.

The primary confounding problem that has historically plagued assessment is the lack of integration between the different components involved in measurement and assessment within an applied context, such as treatment. Historically, psychological or cognitive measures have been developed to fit a particular theory, and evidence is provided to validate a test as a measure of a theory. Traditionally, the outcome of testing was interpretation. The actual applications of how many practitioners would be using the instrument to make decisions has been of secondary value. True, test developers cannot anticipate all the possible uses for a particular test. However, these tests are then used by practitioners, and it is left up to the practitioner to know how to apply the test to assist him in making a decision in a specific context.

A review of research on clinical judgement is beyond the scope of this chapter (for a review see Garb, 1998; Garb & Schramke, 1996). In this chapter, two descriptions of cognitive phenomena in test interpretation will be discussed. Based on social-psychological research beginning with Solomon Asch in the 1940s, social psychologists have extensively researched how individuals develop overall impressions or judgements based on the accumulation of data (Lewicka, 1997). Lewicka (1988) distinguished between "diagnostic" and "prospective" processes, which have also been termed "categorical" versus "piecemeal" or top-down/bottom-up (Fiske & Pavelchak, 1986). Diagnostic inferences involve inferring a category membership based on specific features of an object (attribute→category); whereas prospective inference infers features of an object based on its category membership (category→attribute). Diagnostic inferences are bottom-up and data-driven; whereas prospective inferences are top-down and theory-driven. Essentially, observations are categorized to form concepts. Concepts in turn help us understand observations. In assessment, clinician judgement is influenced by the degree to which observations and concepts are used. When a concept is formed prior to data collection and not supported by data collection but maintained in prescriptive action, this is called *bias*.

During testing, clients are provided scores on various dimensions that represent attributes derived from theoretical constructs. In assessment, clinicians use scores on dimensions in supporting both diagnostic and prospective judgements that justify prescriptive actions in a social context. The whole foundation of clinician judgement resulting in social benefit rests on the mechanics of measurement, beginning with the assignment of a number to an attribute of a person.

It is important for clinicians to be aware of the type of decision that is required in an assessment process. This involves thinking through the referral question and clearly stating the problem, determining possible outcomes of an assessment, and determining how outcomes will be prioritized based on assessment data. This provides an important connection between clinical judgement and prescriptive action that leads to social outcomes. Structuring assessment judgement outcomes is helpful in this process.

Although psychological assessments can be used for numerous goals (e.g., measure client attribute; determine disability, strengths, and weakness, etc.), we will limit the scope here to classification. Classification systems establish rules for placing individuals within a specific class and provide a means of investigating correlates of class membership, such as treatment outcomes (Sattler, 2001). In an assessment context where the clinician is asked to provide a diagnostic judgement, the judgement can be one of meter reading (Blanton & Jaccard, 2006), will be used to specify an interpretive statement made by the clinician that is a direct translation of a test score to another scaled frame of reference. For example, norm-referenced tests have charts indicating qualitative labels of, for example, "above average," "average," "below average." "Inferred" interpretation is inferential. It involves direct interpretations of a test in which but goes beyond the test data. Diagnostic judgements—disability classification, for example—use numerous sources of data, none of which would directly lead to a clinical judgement.

As a simple example, suppose a clinician is asked to determine whether a person has a disorder or not (criterion classification), based on one data point that provides a positive or negative indicator. This interaction can be modeled in a classification matrix. Data can accurately classify individuals by suggesting

they have the condition, when they do, or they do not have the condition, when they do not. The other outcomes could be that the data incorrectly indicate the person either has or does not have the condition when the converse is true. Notice this example is simplistic in that psychological test data rarely provide a binary outcome of disorder/no disorder. Additionally, there are complexities involved in determining true criterion status. (Interested readers may consult the following sources for more detailed aspects of this process: Elwood, 1993; Franklin & Krueger, 2003; Gigerenzer, 2002.) However, the example is intentionally simplified for demonstration.

In such a scenario, a classification matrix describing the hypothetical outcomes of the test may be useful. Although such a matrix is frequently found in many assessment textbooks, such information is rarely reported for standardized commercial instruments used by psychologists (Elwood, 1993). There are several challenges to the use of such tables in practice. One problem, the *base rate problem*, has long been recognized and results from most of the clinical conditions' having a low prevalence rate (Meehl & Rosen, 1955). In such conditions, positive predictive values almost always suggest classifying an individual as not having the disorder despite test data.

One means of overcoming this limitation is to use Bayesian methods (Franklin & Krueger, 2003). Bayes's method is useful because it starts with the base rate probabilities of outcomes (disorder prevalence), then revises the probabilities based on new information.

As an example, Figure 2.4 shows the base rate probability for different diagnostic judgements that may be made when using assessments in schools. The overwhelmingly most likely categorical decision to be made from a random evaluation of any child in school is "normal." Thus, any information suggesting a different category would have to be overwhelmingly informative to overcome this large base rate. Unfortunately, no such information exists. Fortunately, Bayes's theorem provides a method to resolve this issue.

Bayes's theory is a method of revising probabilities based on data. As a simple example, suppose the base rate of classifications for a group of disabilities frequently made in children are as shown in Figure 2.4. Furthermore, suppose the probability of classification for each of the disabilities is related to IQ differentially. For example, the probability of not having a clinical condition is linearly associated with IQ. Children with learning disabilities on average may have an average or slightly below-average IQ, as do children with ADHD. Children with mild mental

Table 2.3 Decision-Making Matrix for Determining Judgement and Test Correspondence

Criterion Classification

Test Results

	+	−
+	A	B
−	C	D
	A + C	B + D

A = Sensitivity (A/A + C)
B = False positive
C = False negative
D = Specificity (D/B + D)
Positive predictive power = A/A + B
Negative predictive power = D/C + D

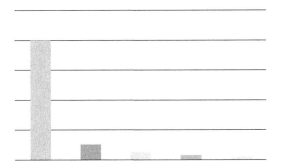

Figure 2.4 Initial probability for categorical judgements based on base rates.

retardation (MMR) have lower IQs and by definition, typically two standard deviations. Children with pervasive developmental disorders like autism may have on average low IQs, but children within this classification may also have large standard deviations.

Suppose that, during the assessment process, an IQ score was obtained and resulted in a score of 75. Further suppose that the probability of being normal given an IQ of 73 was .20, and the probability of not being normal given an IQ of 73 was .80. That is, 80% of children with an IQ of 73 are found to have some clinical condition and are judged "not normal" or "developmentally atypical." However, there is about a 20% chance of finding children who test this low on an IQ test but do not exhibit any atypical developmental features or any other impairment. What is the value in changing the probabilities of determining a child is normal based on this information?

Bayes's theorem states that the probability of having a condition (C) given the data (D) is equal to the probability of the data given that the hypothesis is true (sensitivity), multiplied by the base rate, then divided by a normalizing factor that includes test specificity. Here the values are:

P(D|C) = .20 (probability of getting 73 given normal, sensitivity)

P(C) = .80 (base rate of normal)

P(D|~C) = .80 (probability of getting test score given NOT normal, specificity)

P(C|D) = P(D|C)*P(C) / P(D|C) * P(C) + P(D| not C)*(1–P(C)

If these numbers are entered into Bayesian formula, then the probability of being normal goes from .80 (base rate) to:

P(C|D) = .20* .80 / .20* .80 + .80*(1– .80)
P(C|D) = .50

Suppose further that it was known that the probability of having MMR, given a test score of 73, was .80 and a specificity .20. That is, 80% of children with an IQ of 73 may also be shown to have low adaptive behavior, family history of MMR, very severe academic deficits that progressively drop by grade, etc. How would this information change the likelihood of MMR?

Using the same procedure as before, only changing the base rate to 3% (prevalence of MMR), the new probability is .11. Disregarding the effect of the other classification, the new graph revised where the probability of "normal" goes from .80 to .50 and the probability of MMR goes from .03 to .11 (Figure 2.5).

Now, additional information, such as "adaptive behavior," which has its own sensitivity and specificity with normal and MMR, can be added to further change the likelihood of different categories. Similarly, background information such as gender, ethnicity, or age, could be added to influence the results (see Franklin & Krueger, 2003, for more complex examples using Baysian networks). Eventually, multiple sources of information can be "integrated" to inform a categorical judgement. This procedure directly addresses the base rate problem as well as other problems that have plagued clinical inference (McFall & Treat, 1999). The base rate problem is overcome by the accumulation of highly sensitive and specific information. Additionally, it is proposed that this process "simulates" what good clinicians do when they "integrate" or "holistically" appraise test data within the assessment process. Additional implications will be discussed at the end of the chapter.

Prescriptive Action

The purpose of clarifying classification decisions is not just to provide a better "label," but rather to reduce the uncertainty of options in classification schemes, which in turn provides ready access to research on interventions (Kamphaus, Reynolds, & Imperato-McCammon, 1999). That is, classification or diagnosis supports prescriptive actions. Tests

Figure 2.5 Probability revision given IQ scores.

are used in assessment to provide information that reduces uncertainty in decision-making, which leads to a judgement, which in turn leads to a prescriptive action.

The term *prescriptive action* is used here to represent the fact that assessment is not conducted for the purpose of getting scores on tests. Judgements and conclusions by themselves are useless unless such judgements guide future actions. The term *treatment* is not used but, rather, is considered a type of prescriptive action. Not all prescriptive actions must be physical acts; they can also be "states of knowledge." A clinician may do an assessment and make a judgement that a patient's memory is impaired, it has decreased over time, and this decline indicates dementia. In some cases the prescriptive action may be to inform client so the client can make necessary arrangements. In other cases it may be a referral for medication, assisted living, etc. As such, the term *prescriptive action* is used to indicate the actions that were taken, or belief states that were changed, as a result of the assessment judgement. Prescriptive action is a mediator between assessment and social outcome. Additionally, assessment for the purpose of writing reports that includes recommendations does not fully specify that recommendations are prescriptive actions, although often only indirectly related to assessment data. The results of assessment, and the interpretive process, should provide evidence to increase or decrease the probability of different hypotheses, which in turn lead to different prescriptive actions. As such, the pinnacle, or goal, of assessment is not test interpretation. The results of assessment, and the interpretive process, should test hypotheses that lead to different actions. The link between test interpretation, decision-making, prescriptive action, and outcome is rarely formulated as a unified model because often there is a high degree of contextual dependence in applied contexts. Neuropsychologists may conduct assessments to determine whether someone has suffered a brain injury, the nature of the injury, and the extent of functional loss. The type of judgement made depends on the prescriptive action, or purpose of the assessment. Suggesting a specialized intervention to remediate a cognitive processing weakness is of little value when the original purpose of the assessment was to determine whether the client is competent to stand trial! It is important that the prescribed action, judgement, and assessment process be in alignment. Although the contextual dependence of prescriptive action limits its specification because it may differ by context (and there are numerous contexts), it may still be specified in the abstract.

Figure 2.3 and the specification of judgement and prescriptive action as precursors to social outcome may help clarify some substantial problems in contemporary assessment literature. The problem is how to determine the utility of psychological assessment. Figure 2.3 also makes it clear that the utility of test in an assessment process cannot be directly determined by social outcome or benefit that results or does not result from the assessment. Assessment is several steps removed from beneficial client outcomes. Rather, the utility of tests depends on how they are used in a context to inform judgements that lead to different actions or outcomes.

Interventions are a type of prescriptive action that includes intentional manipulations to cause a change of some attribute or indicator in an intended direction. One difficulty in treatment is selecting an intervention from among numerous possible interventions. In school-based practice, numerous children having difficulty reading are prescribed phonological interventions, which are supported by research. Unfortunately, many of these children do not improve because they do not have problems in phonological processing, which a 10-minute test in phonological processing would have suggested. A child may do poorly in reading instruction, perhaps due to social-emotional problems like depression. Such a child may show improvement in reading skills as a result of reading intervention, although the underlying problem of depression remains and may affect future academic behavior. In such situations, what would be the value of administering a test that would have clarified the attributes of a child and would have in turn led to a better prescriptive action? Currently, there is no metric for determining this value. Similarly, there is no metric for reducing uncertainty in determining the underlying problem or selecting the appropriate intervention. Testing reduces the uncertainty in these possibilities. The use of testing to reduce the possibilities of error in defining the underlying problem of a child is not included in behavioral studies of treatment validity. Such studies often "assume" that a child's status is known (e.g., depression, reading problems, etc.) and then asks how would giving a test reduce depression or improve reading (see Fletcher, Lyon, Fuchs, & Barnes, 2007, as an example in reading). Testing provides information about the attributes of an individual that contributes to decision-making within an assessment process, which in turn contributes to interventions that influence outcomes.

Other factors also impact decisions, as do the actual prescriptive actions taken that are more causally related to treatment outcomes. The problem here is analogous to that of measurement. There is a construct with natural attributes, and one must assign labels to it in order to study it. Namely, the process involved in clinical decision-making, prescriptive action, and social outcome must be pre-specified and structured as data. Testing provides information when test results reduce the uncertainty in decision-making possibilities. Testing need not reduce the probability of one category to certainty (p = 1.0) to be informative, but rather just change the distribution of possibilities (see previous example). Additionally, the process of "judgement" and "prescriptive action" need not be simply grouped under an umbrella of "interpretation" and assumed to be impenetrable to analysis. Measurement theory suggests a solution. Clarify the underlying attributes through theory, label them, and investigate.

Social Outcome

Of course, like judgements, prescriptive actions are not selected in a vacuum but rather linked to social utility. That is, a prescriptive action is selected because it is judged or predicted to result in some benefit. Traditionally, this has been framed as *consequential validity*, but as a line of validity evidence rather than, as indicated here, as a more central element of assessment. The reason why such social goals or outcome variables need greater representation in test development is because such goals provide feedback on how to construct the decision-making model. The decision-making model informs the type of validity evidence needed for a test, which in turn influences how a test is constructed, as demonstrated in the previous example of maximizing information value for decision-making thresholds.

Demonstrating how psychological assessment services provide utility in psychological outcomes has been a defining characteristic of contemporary psychological practice. Influenced by managed health care, evidence-based practice has focused on "outcomes" by which to evaluate psychological services (Maruish, 1994). Effectiveness in providing services is determined by the degree to which specified outcomes are obtained. The influence of this philosophy is vast, and an outcomes orientation has influenced everything in psychology, from standards in training, to insurance reimbursement from third-party payments.

The use of psychological tests has not escaped this scrutiny. Interestingly, there are conflicting opinions on the utility of assessment in impacting treatment outcomes. Some have suggested that assessment is of little to no value (Hayes et al., 1987), which is supported by many researchers with a behavioral orientation (Gresham & Witt, 1997; Reschly & Gresham, 1989). Similarly, some have suggested that outcomes should be the core aspect of test validity (Fuchs et al., 2002). Others have presented cogent arguments on the limitations of such an approach (Cone, 1989; Decker, 2008). Additionally, meta-analysis of more than 125 studies led to the conclusion that there is strong evidence for psychological test validity, that psychological test validity is comparable to that of many medical tests, assessment instruments provide unique information, and clinician decision-making is enhanced by the results of psychological tests (Meyer et al., 2001).

The misunderstanding inherent in approaches that dismiss the utility of psychological testing comes from a lack of specification in the application of psychological services. Namely, the role of decision-making is neglected. Administering Block Design from the Wechsler tests will not cause a desired outcome. However, results of such a test may provide information within the assessment process that requires clinician decisions to inform some course of action. Similarly, testing helps us record change as a result of intervention. Although traditional single-subject design methods are used, psychometric methods may also apply to interventions. The termed *intervention psychometrics* has been used to describe the application of psychometric theory to intervention methods (Decker, 2008).

Despite the inherent benefits in the focus on outcomes, there are some drawbacks. Perhaps the two most important are the two most general. First, the sole focus on any one thing inevitably leads to a neglect of other concepts. Second, singularity of focus often causes an oversimplification that creates a model unable to match the complexities of practical applications. Outcomes are important but perhaps no more so than methodologies determining service needs, adequate measurement representation of person-need, and adequate representation of the type of services matched to needs. Such measurement is needed if it can ever be determined that a particular configuration of matching needs to services through a diagnostic process creates a benefit beyond that which could be obtained through no diagnostic process or random matching.

An additional issue must be mentioned in the process of integrating data with social values. Similar to descriptions of assessment as top-down/bottom-up, or diagnostic/prescriptive, there are problems with describing assessment as driven by social values as a top-down process in assessment. Historic social examples have shown the push of social values is not always just. The dichotomy of data as indicators of reality and social values as interpretive mechanisms has historically been a core theme to describe the relationship between science and religion. Science, as an attempt to describe the world as accurately as possible, and religion, as a prescriptive approach to how the world should be guided, have been at odds many times. Other examples can be given, but my guess is the reader gets the idea. Test validation, as such, may not be described as a methodical process involving reliability coefficients but may better been viewed as a "belief management" technique: that is, evidence is provided to support beliefs (i.e., clinical inferences), which in turn justify actions. *Validity* is a method of determining the degree of which beliefs concerning constructs can be "believed." However, given the current status of validity research, there is yet a procedure in which the quantification of beliefs can be attained. How much, or how many lines, of validity evidence are needed before one's action is selected over another? How are beliefs and actions to be connected? What if two contradictory belief systems are both supported by different lines of validity evidence? The Bayesian approach to hypothesis testing (previously presented) may serve as one technique to more explicitly represent clinician decision-making, which in turn helps make explicit the value of assessment. Currently, nothing in the current system of test validity exists to resolve these issues.

Figure 2.3 makes explicit judgement is linked to prescriptive action which is linked to social goals, which in turn are linked to theory. Table 2.4 provides different judgement, prescriptive action, and outcomes for different assessment contexts. Although it is difficult to define all possible values

for each stage, it is possible to provide broad indictors for each stage of assessment.

Here the emphasis is on pre-specification of possible events at each stage. The events listed for these stages in Table 2.4 are simplified to the point of being irrelevant for the listed assessment applications, but more specific and sophisticated classification schemes exist for each of the areas (see Wodrich & Schmitt, 2006, for an example of school-based classification). Such models provide direct linkage of assessment to actions that may be taken as a result of testing. For example, an educator may solely be interested in identifying children who are at risk for reading problems. This implies a binary decision-making outcome ("at –risk" or "not at –risk"). The test used to make such a decision need not be a comprehensive measure that measures the entire range of reading capability. Rather, such a test need only maximize information at the decision-making threshold for making a decision as to whether a child is at risk or not at risk.

Conclusion

This chapter broadly reviewed measurement theory, scale development, testing, and assessment. The chapter was divided into two broad areas to represent distinct phases of testing involving test development and test application. The integrated role of testing with measurement and assessment components was demonstrated. Theories of measurement are reviewed with the use of the Item Response Theory, not only for the purpose of objective measurement but as a basic model to analyze how personal attributes interact with test stimuli. Interpretive phases of tests within an assessment process are described, which include decision-making, prescriptive action, and social outcomes. This

Table 2.4 Linking assessment and outcomes through judgment and actions

Assessment Purpose	Judgement	Prescriptive Action	Outcome
Disability	Disability present Disability absent	Not eligible Eligible	Educational modification
Forensic (competence to stand trial)	Competent Incompetent	Stand trial Do not stand trial	Social justice
Risk	At risk Not at risk	Protect No protection	Safety
Neuropsychological	Brain injury No brain injury	Remediation/ accommodation	Life adjustment
Intervention	Determine problem	Intervene on problem	Improvement

extension is based ambiguous concepts inherent in contemporary test theory. The interconnected "network" of concepts in testing contributes to the complexity of understanding testing, but nonetheless is necessary. Testing depends on measurement, which in turn depends on the theoretical basis of a construct. Assessment depends on testing, or typically, multiple tests for interpretation. Interpretation is a sub-part of a decision-making process in which some action, such as an intervention, is to be implemented. Interventions influence outcomes, which are evaluated by social goals and values.

Perhaps due to the complexities involved with testing, numerous misunderstandings have occurred that result not only in controversy in research but in misapplication of tests in society. Furthermore, the historic difficulties of not clarifying "interpretive" issues in testing have led to variations in the application of psychological testing, with some of the variability extending into the misapplication of practice. One need only look at the historic use of IQ measures as an example. Despite the fact the measures of intelligence are perhaps the greatest successful application of psychology, the negative connotations that surround lower IQ have created a negative impression on society, and it is doubtful that the term *IQ* will become vindicated. Additionally, the disconnection between how a test is developed and how it is used has led to criticisms involving the treatment utility of tests. This issue was indirectly addressed in this chapter by providing a clarification of why practitioners perceive the value of tests but that value is not captured in research studies. The value of assessment in treatment is not a result of assessments directly causing a change in functional status. Rather, tests used in assessment reduce uncertainty in the decision-making process, which leads to prescriptive action that causes change in social outcomes. This provides an explanation for why assessments have not been adequately tested within a treatment validity paradigm, but evidence is still required to demonstrate the decision-making utility of assessment for particular applications. A Bayesian model is reviewed as a demonstration of how this may be accomplished.

The purpose of reviewing the Rasch model in detail was to demonstrate how qualitative data can be quantified and converted to a unit of measurement. Similarly, most diagnostic classification schemes, although categorical, can be placed along a dimensional continuum (e.g., symptom severity, number of symptoms). Additionally, the value of social outcomes can be rank ordered. Most would agree that full recovery or return to normal parameters of functioning is a more desired outcome for a client than simply being informed of the diagnosis, which in turn is more valuable than not knowing what the problem is at all. Providing a unitary metric of social outcomes to monitor treatment progress may be useful.

Messick, in a review of different perspectives of construct theory, concluded with:

> The use of constructs to develop intuitive systems of meaning for observed relationships appears to be a fruitful heuristic if buttressed by convergent and discriminant evidence to validate the interpretation of test scores as measures of constructs and to validate observed relationships as reflective of meaningful connections in the nomological system (p. 587).

The model presented here for integrating testing with measurement and assessment may similarly be viewed as a "fruitful heuristic" in clarifying the utility of psychological assessment.

Future Directions

There are several future implications for research and practice based on the model presented in this chapter. Test construction may benefit from more focus and clarification of the social outcomes specified by the theory that guides test development. Similarly, clarification of the information value of a test is needed, as well as increased focus on the theoretical analysis of the resulting decision-making. That is, what service is to be provided and what is its benefit.

Another implication is that the assessment field needs to develop better metrics of "information." Such metrics exist but are not a part of mainstream psychometrics. The study of information was most formally begun by Claude Shannon (Shannon, 1948). The intended applications of the study of information were in the digital transmission of communication channels. Numerous attempts have been made to apply information theory to topics in psychology, with only a few successes (Luce, 2003). In contemporary research, its most important applications have come from statistics. For purposes of this chapter, the importance of information is that information can be formally measured. Central to its conceptualization is the statistical probability of an event to determine the likelihood of an actual event. Essentially, information theory quantifies statistically rare events as more informative. Entropy is maximized when a system of variables is completely random. As events become more orderly, entropy decreases.

Finally, another future implication of the model presented here is to provide "scale" value to prescriptive action and social outcomes. Just as measurement requires a representation of an attribute, unified models of assessment need better representations of judgement, prescriptive actions, and social outcomes. Representing attributes of these stages would enhance the investigation of how these processes are involved in assessment and would make clear how they contribute to social outcomes. Until such processes are made explicit, they will continually be viewed as a "black box" and either held in high esteem by some or disregarded by others.

Future Directions

1. How could commercial test developers assist clinicians who would want to use Bayesian models of diagnostic decision-making?

2. Is it possible to develop an abstract clinician decision-making model that fits most situations in which psychological tests are used?

3. How could it be determined that a more context-specific decision-making model is better than a general, all-purpose decision-making model?

4. What are the different values that the variable "social benefit" may take?

Acknowledgment

The author would like to thank Dr. Catherina Chang for reviewing this chapter.

References

AERA, APA, & NCME. (1999). *Standards for educational and psychological testing.* Washington, DC: American Educational Research Association.

Andrich, D. (1988). *Rasch models for measurement.* Newbury Park, CA: Sage.

Bechtoldt, H. (1959). Construct validity: A critique. *American Psychologist, 14,* 619–629.

Blanton, H., & Jaccard, J. (2006). Arbitrary metrics in psychology. *American Psychologist, 61,* 27–41.

Bond, T. G., & Fox, C. M. (2001). *Applying the Rasch model: Fundamental measurement in the human sciences.* Mahwah, NJ: Lawrence Erlbaum Associates.

Campbell, D. T., & Fiske, S. T. (1959). Convergent and discriminant validation by the multitrait-multimethod matrix. *Psychological Bulletin, 56,* 81–105.

Campbell, N. R. (1920). *Physics, the elements.* Cambridge, UK: Cambridge University Press.

Cone, J. D. (1989). Is there utility for treatment utility? *American Psychologist, 44*(9), pp. 1241–1242.

Cook, T. D., & Campbell, D. T. (1979). *Quasi-experimentation: Design and analysis issues for field settings.* Chicago: Rand McNally.

Cronbach, L. (1988). Five perspectives on validity argument. In H. Wainer & H. I. Braun (Eds.), *Test validity.* Hillsdale, NJ: Erlbaum.

Cronbach, L. J. (1971). Test validation. In R. L. Thorndike (Ed.), *Educational measurement* (2nd ed.). Washington, DC: American Council on Education.

Cronbach, L. J., & Meehl, P. E. (1955). Construct validity in psychological tests. *Psychological Bulletin, 52,* 281–302.

Decker, S. L. (2008). Intervention psychometrics: Using norm-referenced methods for treatment planning and monitoring. *Assessment for Effective Interventions, 34*(1), 52–61.

Elwood, R. (1993). Clinical discrimination and neuropsychological data. *The Clinical Neuropsychologist, 7*(2), 224–233.

Embretson, S. E. (1983). Construct validity: Construct representation versus nomothetic span. *Psychological Bulletin, 93,* 179–186.

Embretson, S. E. (1985). Multicomponent latent trait models for test design. *Test design: developments in psychology and psychometrics, 195–218.*

Embretson, S. E. (1999). *New rules of measurement: What every psychologist and educator should know.* Mahwah: NJ: Lawrence Erlbaum Associates.

Embretson, S. E. (2006). The continued search for nonarbitrary metrics. *American Psychologist, 61*(1), 50–55.

Embretson, S. E., & Reise, S. P. (2000). *Item response theory for psychologists.* Mahwah, NJ: Lawrence Erlbaum Associates.

Fiske, S. T., & Pavelchak, M. (1986). Category-based versus piecemeal-based affective responses: Development in schema-triggered affect. In R. M. Sorrentino & E. T. Higgins (Eds.), *Handbook of motivation cognition: Foundations of social behavior* (Vol. 1; pp. 167–202). New York: Guilford Press.

Fletcher, J. M., Lyon, R. G., Fuchs, L. S., & Barnes, M. A. (2007). *Learning disabilities: From identification to intervention.* New York: The Guilford Press.

Franklin, R. D., & Krueger, J. (2003). Bayesian inference and belief networks. In R. D. Franklin (Ed.), *Prediction in forensic and neuropsychology: Sound statistical practices* (pp. 65–87). Mahwah, NJ: Lawrence Erlbaum Associates, Publishers.

Fuchs, L. S., Fuchs, D., & Speece, D. L. (2002). Treatment validity as a unifying construct for identifying learning disabilities. *Learning Disability Quarterly, 25,* 33–45.

Gaito, J. (1980). Measurement scales and statistics: Resurgence of an old misconception. *Psychological Bulletin, 87*(3), 564–567.

Garb, H. N. (1998). *Studying the clinician: Judgement research and psychological assessment.* Washington, DC: American Psychological Association.

Garb, H. N., & Schramke, C. J. (1996). Judgement research and neuropsychological assessment: A narrative review and meta-analysis. *Psychological Bulletin, 120*(1), 140–153.

Gigerenzer, G. (2002). *Calculated risks: How to know when numbers deceive you.* New York: Simon & Schuster.

Gresham, F. M. (2002). Responsiveness to intervention: An alternative approach to the identification of learning disabilities. In R. Bradley, L. Danielson, & D. P. Hallahan (Eds.), *Identification of learning disabilities: Research to practice* (pp. 467–519). Mahwah, NJ: Lawrence Erlbaum.

Gresham, F. M., & Witt, J. C. (1997). Utility of intelligence tests for treatment planning, classification, and placement decisions: Recent empirical findings and future directions. *School Psychology Quarterly, 12*(3), 249–267.

Guttman, L. (1977). What is not what in statistics. *The Statistician, 26,* 81–107.

Hayes, S. C., Nelson, R. O., & Jarrett, R. B. (1987). The treatment utility of assessment: A functional approach to evaluating assessment quality. *American Psychologist, 42,* 963–974.

Kamphaus, R. W., & Campbell, J. M. (2006). *Psychodiagnostic assessment of children: Dimensional and categorical approaches.* Hoboken, NJ: John Wiley & Sons.

Kamphaus, R. W., Reynolds, C. R., & Imperato-McCammon, C. (1999). Roles of diagnosis and classification in school psychology. In C. R. Reynolds & T. B. Gutkin (Eds.), *The handbook of school psychology* (3rd ed.; pp. 292–306). Hoboken, NJ, US: John Wiley & Sons Inc.

Kazdin, A. E. (2003). *Research design in clinical psychology.* Boston: Allyn & Bacon.

Krantz, D. H., Luce, R. D., Suppes, P., & Tversky, A. (1971). *Foundations of measurement: Vol. 1: Additive and polynomial representations.* New York: Academic Press.

Kyngdon, A. (2008). The Rasch model from the perspective of the representational theory of measurement. *Theory & Psychology, 18*(1), 89–109.

Lewicka, M. (1988). On objective and subjective anchoring of cognitive acts: How behavioral valence modifies reasoning schemata. In: W. J. Baker, L. P. Mos, H. V. Rappard, & H. J. Stamm (Eds.), *Recent trends in theoretical psychology.* New York: Springer-Verlag, 285–301.

Lewicka, M. (1997). Is hate wiser than love? Cognitive and emotional utilities in decision making. In R. Ranyard, W. R. Crozier & O. Svenson (Eds.), *Decision making: Cognitive models and explanations* (pp. 90–108). New York: Routledge.

Lord, F. (1946). On the statistical treatment of football numbers. *American Psychologist, 8*(750–751).

Luce, D. (2003). Whatever happened to information theory in psychology? *Review of General Psychology, 7*(2), 183–188.

Luce, R. D., & Suppes, P. (2001). Representational measurement theory. In J. Wixted & H. Pashler (Eds.), *The Stevens handbook of experimental psychology* (3rd ed.; Vol. 4; pp. 1–41). Hoboken: John Wiley & Sons.

Maruish, M. E. (1994). Introduction. In M. E. Maruish (Ed.), *The use of psychological testing for treatment planning and outcome assessment* (pp. 3–21.). Hillsdale, NJ: Lawrence Erlbaum Associates.

McFall, R. M., & Townsend, J. T. (1998). Foundations of psychological assessment: Implications for cognitive assessment in clinical science. *Psychological Assessment, 10*(4), 316–330.

McFall, R. M., & Treat, T. A. (1999). Quantifying the information value of clinical assessments with signal detection theory. *Annual Review of Psychology, 50*, 215–241.

Meehl, P. E., & Rosen, A. (1955). Antecedents probability and the efficiency of psychometric signs, patterns, or cutting scores. *Psychological Bulletin, 52*, 194–216.

Messick, S. (1980). Test validity and the ethics of assessment. *American psychologist, 35*(11), 1012.

Messick, S. (1995). Validity of psychological assessment: Validation of inferences from person's responses and performances as scientific inquiry into score meaning. *American Psychologist, 50*, 741–749.

Meyer, G. J., Finn, S. E., Eyde, L. D., Kay, G. G., Moreland, K. L., Dies, R. R., . . . & Read, G. M. (2001). Psychological testing and psychological assessment: A review of evidence and issues. *American psychologist, 56*(2), 128.

Michell, J. (1986). Measurement scales and statistics: A class of paradigms. *Psychological Bulletin, 100*(3), 398–407.

Pedhazur, E. J., & Schmelkin, L. P. (1991). *Measurement, design, and analysis.* Hillsdale, NJ: Lawrence Erlbaum Associates.

Rasch, G. (1960). Studies in mathematical psychology: I. Probabilistic models for some intelligence and attainment tests. Oxford, England: Nielsen & Lydiche.

Reckase, M. D. (2000). Scaling techniques. In G. Goldstein & M. Hersen (Eds.), *Handbook of psychological assessment* (3rd ed.; pp. 43–64). Oxford, England: Elsevier Science Ltd.

Reschly, D., & Grimes, J. (2002). Best practices in intellectual assessment. In A. Thomas & J. Grimes (Eds.), *Best practices in school psychology* (Vol. 4; pp. 763–773). Washington, DC: National Association of School Psychologists.

Reschly, D. J., & Gresham, F. M. (1989). Current neuropsychological diagnosis of learning problems: A leap of faith. In *Handbook of clinical neuropsychology* (pp. 503–519). New York: Plenum.

Reynolds, C. R. (1986). Measurement and assessment of childhood exceptionality. In I. B. Weiner, R. T. Brown, & C. R. Reynolds (Eds.), *Wiley series on personality processes. Psychological perspectives on childhood exceptionality: A handbook* (pp. 65–87). New York: Wiley-Interscience.

Reynolds, C. R., Lowe, P. A., & Saenz, A. L. (1999). The problem of bias in psychological assessment. In C. R. Reynolds & T. B. Gutkin (Eds.), *The handbook of school psychology* (3rd ed.; pp. 549–546.). New York: Wiley.

Sattler, J. M. (2001). *Assessment of children: Cognitive applications* (4th ed.). San Diego: Jerome M. Sattler, Publisher.

Sattler, J. M. (2008). *Assessment of children: Cognitive foundations.* San Diego: Jerome M. Sattler, Publisher.

Schwager, K. W. (1991). The representational theory of measurement: An assessment. *Psychological Bulletin, 110*(3), 618–626.

Shannon, C. E. (1948). A mathematical theory of communication. *Bell Systems Technical Journal, 27*, 379–423.

Stevens, J. (1996). *Applied multivariate statistics for the social sciences* (3rd ed.). Mahwah, NJ: Lawrence Erlbaum Associates.

Stevens, S. S. (1946). On the theory of scales of measurement. *Science, 103*, 677–680.

Stevens, S. S. (1968). Measurement, statistics, and the schemapiric view. *Science, 161*, 849–856.

Suen, H. K. (1990). *Principles of test theories.* Hillsdale, NJ: Lawrence Erlbaum Associates.

Thorndike, R. M. (2005). *Measurement and evaluation in psychology and education* (7th ed.). Upper Saddle River, NJ: Prentice Hall.

Townsend, J. T., & Ashby, F. G. (1984). Measurement scales and statistics: The misconception misconceived. *Psychological Bulletin, 96*, 394–401.

Wodrich, D. L., & Schmitt, A. J. (2006). *Patterns of learning disabilities.* New York: The Guilford Press.

Woodcock, R. W., McGrew, K. S., & Mather, N. (2001). *Woodcock-Johnson III.* Itasca: Riverside Publishing.

Wright, B. D., & Stone, M. H. (1979). *Best test design.* Chicago: MESA Press.

Measurement and Statistical Issues in Child Assessment Research

Matthew R. Reynolds *and* Timothy Z. Keith

Abstract

This chapter focuses on measurement and statistical issues in child psychological assessment research. Topics with worked examples include multiple regression, confirmatory factor analysis, the Schmid-Leiman transformation, measurement invariance, and MIMIC models. Comparisons are made between simultaneous and sequential regression, higher-order and hierarchical factor models, and multiple-group mean and covariance structure analysis and MIMIC models. The chapter also discusses issues such as dealing with missing data, formative versus reflective measurement, and categorical versus continuous latent variables.

Key Words: hierarchical models, measurement invariance, higher-order confirmatory factor analysis, MIMIC models, multiple regression

Introduction

Research in psychological assessment permeates the practice of psychology. Psychological assessment relies on psychological measurement research, which in turn relies on psychological theory. Psychological assessment research itself is a broad topic. Here we will skip statistical and measurement basics because these topics are well explicated elsewhere (e.g., McDonald, 1999). The chapter will begin with a discussion of multiple regression, an increasingly popular method that is not always well understood. Following multiple regression, a variety of topics such as dealing with missing data, confirmatory factor analysis, and measurement invariance will be reviewed. Worked examples will be provided for some of them.

Some of the issues discussed in this chapter may be considered advanced, though they have been around for a few decades. Modern computing, however, makes for easy implementation of these procedures. In fact, we believe some of these advances should be part of standard practice in psychological assessment research. It is our intention to keep the presentation style as non-technical as possible with the goal of raising awareness; applied examples will demonstrate interesting and important questions that may be asked and answered using these methods. The references provide much more technical detail and should be consulted by readers who are interested in learning more. A theme of this chapter is that researchers should design research that is consistent with theory, and use methods to critically test those theories. To do so, it is essential to have good theories to draw from, and to have tools useful to test them. We believe the topics covered in this chapter include some of those tools.

Multiple Regression

Most readers will be familiar with multiple regression, a popular analytical tool that allows researchers to answer questions about the effects of presumed causes on presumed effects. Two popular approaches, simultaneous and sequential regression, will be compared and contrasted in an example.

The two approaches are sometimes either treated as entirely different methodologies or are applied rigidly according to a cookbook set of rules. In the example it will be demonstrated that the statistical processes underlying the approaches are not different, and that the differences between the two are often found in interpretation only. Understanding the similarities and differences of the two approaches is useful so that the appropriate approach can be applied to specific research questions.

Data from the Early Childhood Longitudinal Study–Kindergarten (ECLS-K), a large-scale, publicly available dataset, were used in this example. Four variables were used to explain the science achievement of fifth-grade students: sex of the student (Sex, dummy coded so that boys = 0 and girls = 1), first-grade reading ability (Prior Reading), self-perceived competence in all academic areas (Perceived Competence), and teacher ratings of children's approach to learning (Learning Approach), which includes behavior such as attention and organization skills. The ECLS-K includes these variables among a multitude of others.[1] The sample for this example included 1,027 children.

There are three common approaches to multiple regression: simultaneous, sequential, and stepwise. Stepwise regression will not be illustrated here. The method is used only for predictive purposes, not explanatory (we will discuss these two purposes in more detail later on), and we do not encourage its use. There are numerous reasons that this atheoretical approach should be avoided, including the fact that it capitalizes on chance findings due to random sampling fluctuations and because it does not require a researcher to think (see Keith, 2006; Thompson, 1995).

Simultaneous Regression

Simultaneous regression (also known as *standard multiple regression* or *forced-entry multiple regression*) is commonly used in explanatory research. Simultaneous regression produces estimates of the direct (unique) effect of the explanatory variables on the outcome variable. Specifically, correlations among the explanatory variables are accounted for so that the unique effects of the explanatory variables are estimated after the effects of the other variables have been removed. The method is useful for comparing the relative influences of variables on a single outcome variable of interest. All of the explanatory variables are entered or "forced" into the regression equation simultaneously. It is typical that R^2 (i.e., the proportion of the outcome variance explained by the optimal linear combination of predictors) and standardized (β) and unstandardized regression (b) coefficients are interpreted in simultaneous regression.

In this example, Science Achievement was regressed on Sex, Learning Approach, Prior Reading, and Perceived Competence. The linear combination of these variables explained 37% of the variation in Science Achievement (R^2 = .37, F [4, 1022] = 149.03, p < .01). When the other variables were held constant, Sex (b = –3.98, β = –.21, p < .001), Learning Approach (b = 2.47, β = .17, p < .001), and Prior Reading (b = .54, β = .52, p < .001) each had statistically significant effects on Science Achievement. The effect of Perceived Competence (b = .19, β = .01, p = .61) was not statistically significant when the other variables were statistically controlled. A qualitative comparison of the standardized effects shows that Prior Reading (β = .52) was the most important influence on subsequent Science Achievement.

Sequential Regression

In sequential regression, the explanatory variables are not forced into the equation at once; rather, they are entered sequentially in what are often referred to as *blocks* (this type of regression is also often referred to as *hierarchical regression*). The order of entry has important interpretative implications and should be based on a researcher's knowledge or beliefs about causal order. In this example, Sex was entered in the first block, Prior Reading was entered in the second block, and Learning Approach and Perceived Competence were entered simultaneously in the third block.

Sex was entered in the first block because it has time precedence over the other explanatory variables. For example, reading ability in the first grade does not explain a child's sex, but a child's sex may have important implications for first-grade reading ability. Perhaps one could *predict* a child's sex by including first-grade reading in a prediction equation, but the interest here is in *explanation*. Moreover, the prediction of a child's sex based on reading ability is uninteresting and does not make sense.

In block two, Prior Reading was entered. Prior reading is likely to influence fifth-grade science achievement because students who are better at reading will read more and build their stored knowledge base. It may also affect perceived academic competence and learning approaches in fifth grade, which are developed from prior experiences. Learning Approach and Perceived Competence were entered together in the third and final block, based on the belief that both of the variables combined add to the explanation of Science Achievement. They were entered last because lack of organizational skills and inattentiveness probably interfere with learning. Moreover, perceived academic competence is a general construct, most likely acquired over years of schooling, and thus this perceived competence should influence engagement and performance in specific academic areas like science.

Proper entry is critical in sequential regression, so it is worth considering further. It is plausible that how much a student knows in science influences teacher ratings of that student's approach to learning. If a student lacks knowledge in science, then that student may appear inattentive and unorganized in science class. The ratings are based on general academics, however, and not science, so the original order makes sense. The important point is that researchers must carefully consider order of entry and must also be prepared to defend their decisions (and defend them much more rigorously, within a theoretical framework, than we have done here).

Given this emphasis on the order of entry in sequential regression, our decision to enter Learning Approach and Perceived Competence together in one block may seem curious. Such a decision may suggest that the researchers are unsure of the proper causal sequence of the variables, or alternatively, that they believe that the variables assess related, overlapping constructs, and are interested in the effect of that overarching construct. Researchers should examine these kinds of decisions, or non-decisions, because they have important interpretative consequences. Finally, researchers should be prepared to defend their reasoning for including variables and omitting potential common causes in a regression. That is what solid research is about, and the omission of important common causes renders interpretation of the regression coefficients invalid.

For the sequential regression, Sex was entered into the equation first. ΔR^2 was used to determine if there was a statistically significant improvement in the proportion of variance explained in Science Achievement after Sex was included. ΔR^2 (.016) was statistically significant (F [1, 1025] = 17.09, $p < .01$). Sex improves the explanation of Science Achievement above that of having no explanatory variables in the equation. Although ΔR^2 is most commonly interpreted in sequential regression, some researchers also interpret the coefficient associated with each variable as it is added to the equation. For the current example, these are $b = -2.44$

and $\beta = -.13$, and the b suggests that, on average, girls score 2.44 points lower on the Science test than do boys (the negative coefficient means that girls, coded 1, score lower than boys, coded 0). *If variables are entered in the proper order, these coefficients represent the total effect of Sex on Science Achievement,* and this effect is different from the direct effect of Sex obtained from the simultaneous results. (We will return to this issue later.)

Second, Prior Reading was added to the equation, resulting in a statistically significant ΔR^2 = .32 (F [1, 1024] = 506.10, $p < .01$). Explanation of Science Achievement was improved beyond the proportion of variance explained by Sex alone. The effect of Prior Reading ($b = .60$, $\beta = .57$) was large. This effect represents the *total* effect of prior Reading on Fifth-Grade Science Achievement, both directly and possibly indirectly through the soon to be added variables Learning Approach and Perceived Competence. Someone unaware of what the regression coefficients in sequential regression represent might be confused by the coefficients related to Sex produced at this step. The coefficients for Sex have changed ($b = -3.31$, $\beta = -.17$). Does this mean that Sex is more important than it was previously? We will address this issue in more detail below.

Last, Learning Approach and Perceived Competence were added as a block, resulting in a $\Delta R^2 = .028$ (F [2, 1022] = 22.27 $p < .01$) that was statistically significant. The addition of these two variables, in combination, improves the explanation of individual differences in Science Achievement. Regression coefficients estimated for Sex ($b = -3.98$, $\beta = -.21$, $p < .001$), Prior Reading ($b = .54$, $\beta = .52$, $p < .001$), Learning Approach ($b = 2.47$, $\beta = .17$, $p < .001$), and Perceived Competence ($b = .19$, $\beta = .01$, $p = .61$) in this step were identical to those obtained in the simultaneous regression. We now have several sets of coefficients that could be interpreted from the sequential regression. If we are interested in interpreting the effects, which are appropriate, and which should we interpret? Perhaps this interpretation is best explained by comparing the results with the results from the simultaneous regression.

Simultaneous and Sequential Regression: A Comparison

Path diagrams will be used to help compare simultaneous and sequential regression. A path model of the simultaneous regression is shown in Figure 3.1. In the diagram, the rectangles represent observed variables; the arrows, or paths,

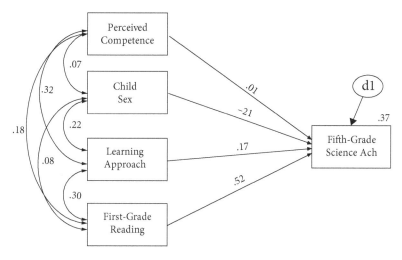

Figure 3.1 Simultaneous Regression in Path Form.

show a directed relation between the variables; the double-headed arrows represent a non-directive relation (i.e., correlation); and the oval represents a disturbance, commonly referred to as a *residual variance* in regression. In structural equation modeling, ovals typically represent latent, or unmeasured, variables. In this example, the oval represents all influences on the corresponding measured variables other than those shown in the model; these influences are not measured or modeled, and may include measurement error, nonlinear effects, random unknown influences, and all other unknown influences on the outcome (Arbuckle & Wothke, 1999; Bollen, 2002).

In the simultaneous regression shown in Figure 3.1, the explanatory variables correlate with each other, and each explanatory variable has a path connecting it directly to the outcome (Science Achievement), representing the presumed effect of these variables on science achievement. These effects are direct. Because the interrelations among the variables are controlled (by allowing them to correlate), these effects are also referred to as *unique effects*. Whatever is not explained by the linear effects of the explanatory variables is captured in the disturbance.

Compare this path model to the sequential regression path models shown in the left side of Figure 3.2. In the sequential regression there are three steps corresponding to what happened at each block of variable entry. Sex is entered first (Figure 3.2, Block 1), Prior Reading second (Figure 3.2, Block 2), and Learning Approach and Perceived Competence third (Figure 3.2, Block 3). An obvious difference between simultaneous (Figure 3.1) and sequential regression (on the left in Figure 3.2) is that some

of the non-directed arrows are now directed. The variables on the left side of Figure 3.2 show an order from left to right, and that ordering reflects the causal assumptions made in the sequential regression and justified, albeit rather weakly, earlier in this chapter.

Figure 3.2 shows two types of path models, with the disturbances not included. The models on the left illustrate the causal reasoning underlying our sequential regression coefficients. The path models on the right demonstrate the coefficients associated with each step that are produced in the output. Although most analyses using sequential regression focus on R^2 and ΔR^2 interpretations, we will focus on the interpretation of coefficients from the regression because these effects are often confused. Note, however, that the R^2 values are the same regardless of whether the example on the left or right is used (these values are shown on the top right of the Science Achievement outcome variable in each Figure). It is instructive to uncover what is happening during a sequential regression, and this becomes clear with a focus on the coefficients estimated at each block.

Starting on the left in Figure 3.2, Block 1 shows Science Achievement regressed on Sex. The regression coefficient ($\beta = -.13$) is interpreted as the total effect of Sex on Science Achievement (generally, we would interpret the unstandardized coefficient when focusing on a dummy variable, but the standardized coefficients are used in subsequent blocks, and so will be used in this first block. See Keith, 2006, for guidelines for interpreting standardized versus unstandardized coefficients, and Table 3.1 for the unstandardized coefficients).

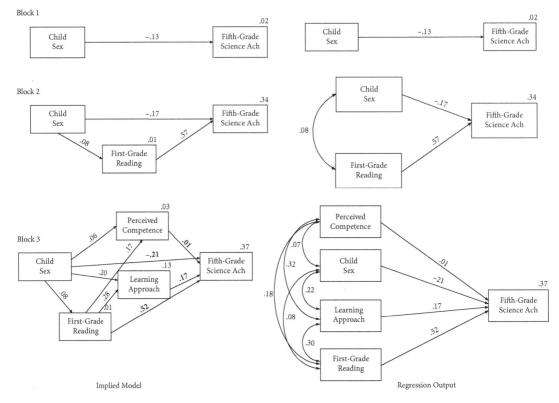

Figure 3.2 Sequential Regression Comparison in Path Forms.

In Block 2, Prior Reading was added. Shown in the second model on the left, Sex had a direct effect on Science Achievement and on Prior Reading, and thus through Prior Reading, an *indirect* effect on Science Achievement. On the right hand side of Figure 3.2 in Block 2 is the model that was *actually* run in Block 2, and the regression coefficients produced in the computer output. It may look like a simultaneous regression, and indeed it is, but with only two predictors. The standardized effect ($\beta = -.13$) associated with Sex in Block 1 was different from the standardized coefficient ($\beta = -.17$) in Block 2. The total effect from Block 1 ($\beta = -.13$) is now split into the direct effect ($\beta = -.17$) and the indirect effect, with the indirect effect equalling the path from Sex to Prior Reading times the path from Prior Reading to Science Achievement ($.08 \times .57 \approx .04$). The indirect

Table 3.1 Comparison of Direct Effects from Simultaneous Regression and Total Effects from Sequential Regression

Variable	Direct effects obtained in simultaneous regression		Total effects obtained in sequential regression	
	$b(SE_b)$	β	$b(SE_b)$	β
Sex	−3.98(.49)	−.21	−2.44(.59)[a]	−.13
Prior Reading	.54(.03)	.52	.60(.03)[b]	.57
Learning Approach	2.47(.40)	.17	2.47(.40)[c]	.17
Perceived Competence	.19(.38)	.01	.19(.38)[c]	.01

Note: [a] From Block 1; [b] From Block 2; [c] From Block 3. Note that the effects for Learning Approach and Perceived Competence are the same across models because these variables were entered in the last block of the sequential regression.

effect is not calculated in the regression output, but this indirect effect is easily obtained by subtracting the direct effect (–.17) in Block 2 from the total effect (–.13) in Block 1 = .04. To answer the question posed earlier, the apparent effect of Sex does increase from the first to the second model because part of the *total* effect of Sex is explained by Prior Reading, and in this case, the indirect effect is positive, while the direct effect is negative. That is, girls have higher prior reading scores. The effect of Prior Reading on Science Achievement is also estimated (i.e., β = .57). If the causal order is correct, this effect represents the total effect of Prior Reading on Science Achievement. In Table 3.1, the direct effects interpreted in a simultaneous regression and total effects from the sequential regression are shown for comparison.

Last, Perceived Competence and Learning Approach were entered. On the left in Figure 3.2, Block 3, the estimates actually produced in the regression output in Block 3 are bolded. The estimates are identical to the direct effects obtained in a simultaneous regression. And of course a simultaneous regression is exactly what is shown on the right in Block 3. Calculations could be used to estimate the indirect effects. But if a researcher was really interested in all of these effects, this procedure can easily be performed in a structural equation modeling (SEM) program so that the direct, indirect, and total effects are all calculated (and statistical significance can be tested). The model in the SEM program would probably be specified to match the model in the left of Figure 3.2, Block 3.

We hope this illustration allowed the reader to make some mental connections between the two approaches. Why go through the trouble of illustrating these similarities and differences? First, many researchers are interested in the *unique* effects of variables on some outcome. That is, researchers are often interested in the effect of the explanatory variable of interest on the outcome, *controlling for other variables* in the model. They often use sequential regression and estimate the unique effect by adding the variable in the last block. It should be clear now, however, that these effects are easily captured in either simultaneous or sequential regression. The multiple blocks in a sequential regression are not required if this is the interest, even though sequential regression is often used by researchers for this purpose. Second, if researchers have a causal ordering in mind and they want to use sequential regression, it is important that they understand the nature of the coefficients they are

interpreting. In fact, drawing out a path diagram as shown on the left of Figure 3.2 would be beneficial so it is clear what types of effects are obtained. We urge both users and consumers of sequential regression research to routinely draw the models underlying their and others' regressions. Of course, if one is capable of drawing a model, it may be easier to simply analyze the model via a structural equation modeling program!

Summary of Multiple Regression

Keith (2006) outlined additional similarities and differences between the two regression approaches, and a few will be mentioned here. There are many similarities, and even the differences are not necessarily true differences, but rather are differences in rigidly applied conventional interpretations. Note however that ΔR^2 is generally used as a test of statistical significance and interpreted in sequential regression.[2] It is common, however, to see regression coefficients also reported and interpreted in sequential regression. R^2 and the statistical significance of the regression coefficients are generally interpreted in simultaneous regressions. R^2 in simultaneous regression is identical to the R^2 obtained in the final step in sequential regression when all of the explanatory variables are included. When coefficients are interpreted, however, it should be noted that sequential regression is focused on total effects, and simultaneous regression is focused on direct effects. Simultaneous regression also allows comparisons of the relative (direct) effects using standardized coefficients, and can typically be used to answer questions researchers use sequential regression to answer. And lastly, sequential regression might be considered when testing for moderators or for curves in the regression plane, but only if the researcher is interested in an overall test of an interaction effect or several interaction effects in a block. (This issue will be discussed more in the section on moderation.)

Simultaneous and sequential regression may be used for either explanation or prediction. In explanation, the regression coefficients represent the effects of the presumed causes on the outcome variable of interest, given the adequacy of the model. Prediction equations can also be obtained so that optimal linear combinations of variables can be used to predict an outcome. In our experience, most researchers are interested in explanation even though they may pretend that they are only interested in prediction. One typical scenario (and we encourage the reader to do a quick literature search to find a multitude of examples) is for authors to discuss prediction in the introduction and results, and then switch to explanation when the findings are discussed. This is the research version of a bait and switch! The researcher may not even know that a switch has taken place, but any time a researcher makes a statement along the lines of "this research suggests that increases in variable x would lead to increases in variable y," he or she has made an explanatory interpretation. Researchers should ask themselves whether the purpose of their research is *really* prediction or whether it is really explanation before they begin the process (Keith, 2006). To thine own self be true!

Lastly, although we have yet to note *explicitly* that researchers should use the method to match the purpose of their research, we are doing so here. *A priori* conceptual models are associated with structural equation modeling, but it should be obvious that such models are similarly important in regression. Therefore, researchers need to decide what type of regression, or combination of regressions, will be most consistent with their theoretical models.

Mediation

There are plenty of excellent sources on mediation, so this introduction will be brief (Mackinnon, 2008; Shrout & Bulger, 2002; see also Kristopher Preacher's website: www.quantpsy.org). Mediation occurs when a variable that is between the presumed cause and outcome partially or fully explains the effect of the presumed cause on the outcome. A test of mediation is generally considered a test of the indirect effect of one variable through another variable. Although sequential regression may be used to get an idea about or sometimes test mediation, tests of mediation are probably better off performed in structural equation modeling programs. The study of mediating variables is important because these variables provide an understanding of change mechanisms; for example, an understanding of how treatment effects arise. They are especially interesting because they help explain how outcomes come about.

Moderation

Multiple regression may be used to test for interaction effects, or what is commonly referred to as *moderation*. Moderation is commonly tested via sequential regression. In child assessment research, moderation is often used to test predictive bias or invariance. For example, do scores from a reading fluency measure predict reading comprehension equally well for boys and girls (see Kranzler, Miller, & Jordan, 1999)? That is, does sex moderate the relation between reading fluency and reading comprehension? To test for an interaction using multiple regression (i.e., moderated multiple regression), first, a new variable is created as the cross-product of the two variables of interest (e.g., sex multiplied reading fluency scores). Centering any continuous variables prior to creating the cross product is also often used to improve interpretation (Aiken & West, 1991; Keith, 2006), so for example the reading fluency scores would be centered. Next, the main effects (e.g., sex and reading fluency scores centered) are entered in the first block; the cross-product (sex times reading fluency scores centered) is entered in the second block. This cross-product, or interaction term, is added to determine if the interaction term adds unique information to the explanation of the outcome variable. If it adds to the explanation, then it may be said that the effect of one variable (reading fluency) on the outcome (reading comprehension) *depends* on or is moderated by the other variable (sex). Especially with a single cross-product, this analysis could also be performed in simultaneous regression, with the statistical significance of the unstandardized coefficient used as a test of significance for the cross product. The use of sequential regression, however, allows an omnibus test for multiple cross products or the calculation of an effect size (viz., ΔR^2) for the interaction term (Turrisi &Jaccard, 2003, p. 86). See Keith (2006) for more examples of using regression to test for moderation.

Missing Data

Missing data are a perennial concern for researchers. Advances in statistical theory in recent years, along with excellent and accessible reviews of missing data assumptions and techniques, have substantially improved our knowledge of how to handle missing data (e.g., Graham, 2009; Schafer & Graham, 2002; Wothke, 2000). In fact, rather than just *dealing* with missing data, implementing planned "missingness" into research designs may be a cost-effective, efficient method of collecting data (McArdle, 1994). We will provide a brief explanation of missing data assumptions and techniques, but we encourage the reader to refer to some of the excellent sources for more in-depth and informed coverage (Enders, 2010; Graham, 2009; Schafer & Graham, 2002; Wothke, 2000).

There are three general mechanisms assumed to underlie missing data: Missing Completely at Random (MCAR), Missing at Random (MAR), and Missing Not at Random (MNAR; Little & Rubin, 1987; Rubin, 1976). MCAR requires the assumption that missing data do not differ from those that are non-missing. Say a researcher was interested in studying the effects of IQ and motivation on achievement. After the data were collected, the researcher noticed that scores from the motivation variable were missing for several cases. If data were MCAR, then the missingness of motivation cases was unrelated to motivation scores themselves, as well as to the IQ and achievement scores. The MCAR assumption is required for researchers to use the common deletion methods of handling missing data (i.e., pairwise and listwise deletion). If the assumption is met, then the biggest concern about deleting cases should be a loss of statistical power. If the assumption is not met, then parameter estimates, such as means and regression coefficients, and standard errors of those coefficients, may be inaccurate.

MAR, the second assumption, implies data are missing at random. Indications of why data are missing, however, may be found in the other variables included in the dataset. For example, if motivation scores were missing, the missingness can at least be explained partially by IQ scores, achievement scores, or both. That is, it may be that higher-achieving individuals were more likely to answer the motivation questions. If data are MAR, modern methods such as maximum likelihood estimation and multiple imputation may be used to obtain unbiased estimates. When data are MAR, but the deletion methods are used in analysis, parameter estimates are likely to be biased in that they over- or underestimate the population values, and this bias will probably to be difficult to detect.

The third possibility is that data are missing not at random, or MNAR. This type of missingness presents a problem. The missing values depend on something not measured in the dataset, and the reasons for their absence are unknown or unmeasured.

Knowledge of these three underlying mechanisms provides a framework from which a researcher can work. The good news is that it is typical for the mechanism to be at least somewhat understood. Moreover, when a researcher errs in making the assumption of MAR (when MNAR is really the case), the effects on the estimates in the model may be minimal (Graham, Hofer, Donaldson, MacKinnon, & Schafer, 1997).[3] Finally, even if MCAR is assumed by the researcher, the methods discussed below are better to use than the outdated deletion and mean substitution methods because all of the cases can be used in the analysis.

Outdated Methods

Listwise deletion, pairwise deletion, and mean substitution are examples of commonly used, but outdated methods. Deletion methods are a simple way of handling missing data because cases are simply dropped from the analysis. Deletion, however, results in fewer participants and will result in biased estimates if the MCAR assumption is not met. Mean substitution, like it implies, involves substituting a mean for missing scores, and is a simple, outdated, and potentially hazardous approach to handling missing data. Although all cases are included in the analysis when mean substitution is used, this procedure should be avoided because it produces biased estimates. Because the same value (the mean) is substituted repeatedly for the missing values of that variable, the variance will be reduced, as will the relation of that variable with the other variables in the model (Wothke, 2000). Other outdated methods include regression-based and hot deck imputations, but these approaches also suffer from limitations. Rather than discussing these methods further, we recommend the application of modern methods and will focus on those (Schafer & Graham, 2002).

Modern Methods

There are a few modern model–based approaches to deal with missing data, including the expectation maximization algorithm (which uses a maximum likelihood approach) and multiple-group structural equation modeling, but here we will discuss two popular and relatively easy-to-implement methods: maximum likelihood (ML) and multiple imputation (MI). These model-based methods require the less stringent MAR assumption compared to the outdated methods that require MCAR.

ML is the first model-based method. Space precludes a detailed description of the procedure, but a few important points can be made (see Wothke, 2000). First, ML estimation does not impute individual values; rather, the parameter estimates are obtained from using all of the available information in the observed data. Second, in large-sample statistical theory it is well known that ML produces consistent estimates that reflect the population values when data are multivariate normal. Third, ML estimation (with missing data) is available in structural equation modeling (SEM) software, and its implementation does not require additional work for the researcher. In fact, multiple regression models can be analyzed in SEM programs, making it easy to implement ML methods when data are missing. Last, and perhaps most important, ML results in similar or, more likely, more consistent and less-biased estimates than those obtained after performing deletion and mean imputation; these differences may be dramatic when the data are MAR (Wothke, 2000).

Multiple imputation (MI) is another model-based method. Like ML, the statistical theory of MI is established. In MI, rather than imputing one value for each missing value in the dataset, a set of values representing plausible values is imputed for each missing datum, creating several new datasets with different sets of these new plausible values. Analyses are conducted on each dataset, like they would be with a complete dataset, and the results are pooled. Valid statistical inferences can thus be made, as the results incorporate the uncertainty due to the missing data (Graham, 2009). Like ML, MI generally assumes multivariate normal data, although it seems to also handle multivariate non-normal data fairly well. Given a large sample size, the estimates from ML or MI should be similar. Many statistical programs now include programs for dealing with MI, making it fairly simple to implement.

Researchers should recognize that missing data are not something to be ignored, but something that should be dealt with thoughtfully. Trying to understand the mechanisms that underlie missingness can assist in a better understanding of the data that are available as well as those missing. MI and ML are two fairly simple ways to deal with missing data, even when large amounts of data are missing. Given the relative ease of implementation, these methods should be considered the standard since they outperform outdated procedures, allowing researchers to use all of their data.

Factor Analysis

Factor analysis is an invaluable tool for understanding latent constructs and evaluating validity, and is commonly used to evaluate psychological assessment (measurement) instruments. The purpose of factor analysis is to uncover latent psychological attributes that account for correlations among observed variables. Quite simply, factor analysis is useful for understanding whether an instrument measures what it is supposed to measure. Although commonplace and useful in assessment research, factor analysis and other complex methods cannot make up for lack of relevant theory, common sense,

knowledge-base, and carefulness of a researcher. Factor analysis may be misused and abused, intentionally or unintentionally.

The two main types of factor analysis are confirmatory (CFA) and exploratory (EFA) factor analysis. We will focus on CFA in this chapter, with only a few comments on EFA. EFA is older, growing out of Spearman's early twentieth-century explorations of the nature of intelligence (Spearman, 1927). With EFA, researchers choose the method (e.g., principal factors, maximum likelihood), the criteria for selecting factors (e.g., eigenvalues greater than one, *a priori* knowledge), the criteria for meaningful loadings, and the rotation method, and then interpret the results. Each step requires judgement, and multiple factor solutions are often examined. If done well—by researchers who are careful in developing the measures, and who apply combinations of criteria, use good judgement, and have knowledge of the relevant literature—EFA can be an invaluable tool in uncovering latent variables that explain relations among observed variables. But, EFA may also be abused. It is not unusual to see researchers put little thought into the theory that guides measurement; gather data; use inflexible criteria for factor extraction and rotation; and interpret their findings as if they were revealed truth. The judgement required to be good at EFA is a feature, not a design flaw! For more information about EFA, readers should refer to other, excellent sources (e.g., Preacher & MacCallum, 2003; Wolfle, 1940).

One other topic worth mentioning concerning EFA is the distinction between factor analysis and principal components analysis (PCA). A component obtained in a PCA is different from a factor obtained in a factor analysis. A component is a composite variable. Factors are latent variables. Most psychological attributes are conceptualized as latent variables, not composites, and these attributes should be invariant across the different instruments designed to measure them. One of the long-standing critiques of PCA is that the components (i.e., composites) are not psychologically meaningful (Wolfle, 1940). Factor analysis is thus the appropriate tool to use in latent variable research, not PCA.

Second, the procedures are used for different purposes. PCA, a descriptive procedure, was developed for data reduction and to maximize the variance explained in observed variables. Factor analysis, a model-based procedure, was designed to uncover psychologically meaningful latent variables that explain the correlations among observed variables. Factor analysis thus analyzes the common variance, separating it from the unique variance. Unique and common variances are not separated in PCA. These distinctions have not stopped researchers from substituting PCA for factor analysis. As some have noted, perhaps this is because even some popular statistical programs do not differentiate the two (see Borsboom, 2006, for a discussion). Although space precludes further discussion of this issue, there are other excellent treatments of the topic (e.g., Preacher & MacCallum, 2003; Widaman, 2007; Wolfle, 1940). For a demonstration of potential different findings related to the use of PCA—and outdated missing data methods—in applied research, see Keith, Reynolds, Patel, and Ridley (2008).

Confirmatory Factor Analysis

CFA requires a researcher to specify the number of factors and the pattern of zero and free factor loadings *a priori*. CFA is commonly used in psychological assessment research to address questions related the measurement of psychological constructs and construct validity. We will work through an example to demonstrate the usefulness of CFA in establishing construct validity in an individually administered intelligence test. Throughout the example, we will describe and deal with various issues that may arise when conducting CFA.

During the last 20 years there has been a shift in the development of intelligence measurement instruments; many developers now rely on underlying theory during the developmental phase. The shift represents a major advancement that has not only informed measurement, but has likewise informed research and theory (Keith & Reynolds, 2010). The most popular theory, or perhaps better described as a *taxonomy*, underlying the development of these instruments is the Cattell-Horn-Carroll (CHC) theory of intelligence (McGrew, 2009), a theory that combines Cattell-Horn's Gf-Gc theory (Horn & Noll, 1997) and John Carroll's three-stratum theory (Carroll, 1993).

The Kaufman Assessment Battery for Children–II (KABC-II; Kaufman & Kaufman, 2004) is an example of a popular measure of child and adolescent intelligence in which theory was used during the developmental phase. In fact, the KABC-II may be interpreted using either CHC theory or Luria's information processing theory. In our CFA examples, we will use the norming data from the KABC-II to evaluate the measurement structure of the test. The CFA models will be consistent with the scoring structure using the CHC theory interpretation only. The scoring structure for the KABC-II battery includes index scores for five CHC broad

abilities and a general ability referred to as the Fluid-Crystallized Index (FCI), as well as a few tests to supplement the broad ability indexes. The five broad CHC index scores include Gc (Knowledge), Gv (Visual Processing), Gf (Fluid Reasoning), Glr (Long-Term Retrieval), and Gsm (Short-Term Memory). Gc is measured with three subtests, Gv with four, Gf with two, Glr with four, and Gsm with three. We should note that the standard battery has fewer subtests, and some subtests were included as supplemental tests. The supplemental tests were used in our CFA to maximize the information available.

The data used in this example were age-standardized scores obtained from adolescents who ranged in age from 15 to 18. The sample included 578 participants. There were missing values for a few of the cases. The MCAR assumption was tenable. Rather than deleting cases, however, we chose to include *all* of the cases in the analyses using ML in Amos (Arbuckle, 2006) to handle missing data. Untimed scores were substituted for timed scores because in previous research the timed scoring procedure has been shown to introduce construct-irrelevant variance (Reynolds, Keith, Fine, Fisher, & Low, 2007). First-order and higher-order CFA models were estimated, and these are described below.

FIRST-ORDER MODELS
Specification

A first-order CFA model with five factors representing the five broad-ability factor indexes is shown in Figure 3.3. Essentially, we are interested in answering this question: Does the hypothesized latent structure underlying the observed data match the KABC-II measurement (scoring) structure? We address this question empirically by explicitly matching our factor model to the five broad-ability indexes. In Figure 3.3, the ovals represent latent variables; rectangles represent the observed variables; directed arrows represent directed effects; and nondirected arrows represent correlations/covariances.

Each factor is indicated only by the specific subtests that make up that broad index (Figure 3.3). Relevant theory (Jensen, 1998) and the use of an overall test score would also suggest that the factors should be correlated; therefore, the first-order model allows for intercorrelations among the factors rather than specifying them as independent of each other. The Glr measurements each included a delayed recall version of the original test. The residual variances associated with the first measurement and corresponding delayed measurement were specified to correlate freely (e.g., Rebus with Rebus

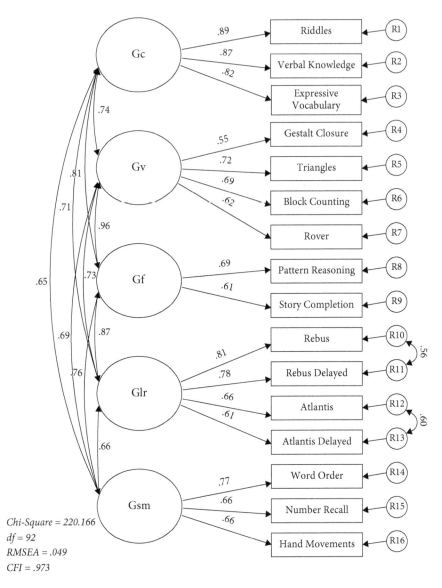

Chi-Square = 220.166
df = 92
RMSEA = .049
CFI = .973

Figure 3.3 KABC-II First-Order Factor Structure with Standardized Loadings.

Delayed). These correlated specific factors represent overlap between the tests above and beyond what is explained by the G*lr* factor. Although our input model is not presented, the residual variance paths and one loading per factor were fixed to one so that the scales were properly set and the model was properly identified.

Model Evaluation

Indexes have been developed to assist researchers in evaluating fit. (More detailed explanation of these indexes is given elsewhere [e.g., Marsh, Hau, & Grayson, 2005].) For this example, model fit was evaluated with the root mean square error of approximation (RMSEA; Steiger & Lind, 1980)

and comparative fit index (CFI; Bentler, 1990), with values below .05 and above .95 indicating good fit, respectively. In addition, chi-squared (χ^2) was used to evaluate the fit of single models, and change in chi-squared ($\Delta\chi^2$) was used to evaluate competing nested models (i.e., models that can be derived by constraining additional parameters in a model). Chi-squared demonstrates excessive power to detect model misfit in large sample sizes, but, in general, the lower the χ^2 value relative to *df*, the better.

Results

The fit indexes for this measurement model indicated model fit was acceptable: χ^2 (92) = 220.17, RMSEA = .05, CFI = .97. The model with standardized factor loadings is shown in Figure 3.3. The factor loadings were all substantial.[4] Like the directed paths in path analysis, one can interpret these loadings as regression coefficients. For example, the .88 standardized effect of Gc on Riddles suggests that a one standard deviation increase in latent Gc would result in a .88 standard deviation increase in a Riddles score.

The results support the interpretation of the broad-ability indexes on the KABC-II. It is not uncommon, however, for some subtests to measure more than one latent broad ability. Such subtests are often described as being *factorially complex* (McDonald, 1999). For example, to perform well on complex memory tasks requiring multiple steps, a person may employ a novel cognitive strategy to reduce the memory load, therefore reducing the memory requirement for successful performance. Novel problem–solving ability is associated with Gf, and working memory and Gf typically correlate strongly. The Hand Movements subtest on the KABC-II is an example of test that requires relatively complex memory; it is thus plausible that people high in Gf could reduce the memory load of the task via their novel problem–solving abilities. To test this hypothesis, we loosened the strict assumption that all subtests measure only one factor and allowed Hand Movements to indicate Gf and Gsm, or "cross-load." This model fit the data well: χ^2 (91) = 180.81, RMSEA = .04, CFI = .98. Moreover, the improvement in model fit was statistically significant, as indicated by $\Delta\chi^2$ (1) = 39.36, p < .01. When allowed to load on both factors, Hand Movements had a standardized loading of .40 on the Gf factor and .30 on the Gsm factor.

There are a few salient points related to this finding. First, Hand Movements is a supplemental test and not part of the standard battery. Perhaps the authors were not confident enough that this indicator reflected Gsm, and it was not included in the standard battery for this reason. Therefore, the finding does not invalidate the measurement of Gsm using the broad index. Second, the finding provides some initial evidence that Hand Movements may measure more than Gsm, or that it is factorially complex. Third, when such *post hoc* modifications are made, there are always increased risks for sample-specific findings that may or may not be important.

Resolving what latent cognitive abilities Hand Movements measures will be left up to future research. One excellent method that could be used to investigate further what it measures is cross-battery factor analysis (CB-FA); that is, a factor analysis of Hand Movements with Gsm and Gf tests from other intelligence batteries. Cross-battery factor analyses (and cross-battery confirmatory factor analysis, CB-CFA, in particular) across measurement instruments is an extremely useful method used to understand what tests measure (Keith & Reynolds, 2010, 2012). On a related note, it is not uncommon to see researchers factor analyze only the standard tests in a battery, even when both standard and supplemental tests are available; or, alternatively, to conduct two analyses, one including all tests and one including only those from the standard battery. We generally discourage this approach. Except under rare circumstances (e.g., a poorly designed or theoretically murky test), more measures will generally lead to a deeper understanding of the underlying constructs. In the present example, Hand Movements may be less desirable because it is factorially complex, but its inclusion, and its theoretically predictable cross-loading, also supports the validity of the underlying constructs. That is, Hand Movements can be understood as requiring novel reasoning as well as short-term memory. The fact that it shows substantial cross-loadings on two such factors supports those factors as indeed representing Gf and Gsm, respectively. The alternative, analyzing fewer measures, has the potential to mislead; when fewer tests are analyzed, factors are more likely to represent narrower abilities, and are more likely not to appear at all. When understanding the constructs underlying the test is the purpose, more is almost always better.

HIGHER-ORDER MODELS
Specification

In addition to the five CHC broad abilities, the KABC-II provides an index of a general mental ability, the FCI index. The next step is to match the analytic model (technically now a structural model because the covariance among the first-order factors were structured) with the overall scoring structure of the test. We consider the higher-order model, such as the one shown in Figure 3.4, the most appropriate. Typically, general intelligence (g) is considered to influence performance on all measures of cognitive ability. The nature of g cannot be understood by surface characteristics of the items or tests designed to measure it, however, as tests that look completely different on the surface often have similar loadings on a g factor (Jensen, 1998). Instead, g is conceptualized at a higher level of abstraction than the broad abilities, which *are* typically defined by surface characteristics of the measurement instruments. Therefore, we believe that the higher-order model most accurately

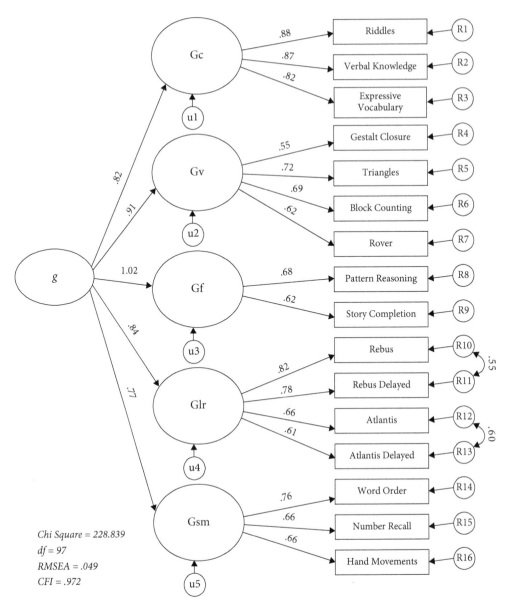

Figure 3.4 KABC-II Second-Order Factor Structure with Standardized Loadings.

mirrors current conceptions of human cognitive abilities (see Carroll, 1993; Jensen, 1998).

There are a few interesting things to note about the higher-order model shown in Figure 3.4. First, the second-order factor, *g*, in part, accounts for the covariance among the first-order factors. This conceptualization provides a more restricted and parsimonious account of the data than does the first-order model. In the higher-order model, there are five loadings on the *g* factor, while in the first-order model there were 10 correlations among the factors. Second, the *g* factor is indicated by the five latent variables and not the observed variables. It is a latent variable indicated by latent variables; *g* is at a higher order of

abstraction. In addition, *g* is considered to be more general than the broad abilities because it influences performance on all tests, albeit indirectly through those broad abilities. There are no "direct" effects of *g* on the subtests. The effect of *g* is completely mediated by the broad ability factors. Direct effects may be included,[5] but the representation in Figure 3.4 is both parsimonious and theoretically consistent with contemporary theory (Carroll, 1993; Jensen, 1998). Last, in Figure 3.4, notice the ovals, labeled with "u's," with arrows directed at the first-order factors. These uniquenesses, or disturbances, represent the variance left unexplained by *g*. These disturbances are interesting because they represent the unique aspects of the broad abilities. That is, they represent unique variance only, not unique (or specific) and error variance, as do the residuals for the subtests. They reference the first-order factors, and the factors are perfectly reliable (cleansed of error), unlike the subtests.

Results

The higher-order model fit well: χ^2 (97) = 228.83, RMSEA = .05, CFI = .97. The fit of the model along with relevant theory would indicate that the higher-order model was a plausible model for these data. However, there was also an oddity in the standardized factor loadings: The factor loading of Gf on g was 1.02 (Figure 3.4). How can a standardized loading be greater than one? It is possible, like in regression (Jöreskog, 1999), although such a result is almost always worth investigating further. Although not shown in Figure 3.4, in addition to the loading of 1.02, the unique variance (u3) for Gf was not statistically significantly different from zero. These two pieces of information suggest that Gf and g may not be statistically distinguishable, or that they are correlated perfectly. Interestingly, some have posited that Gf and g are identical (Gustafsson, 1984). An identical Gf and g is a theoretical question, however, because perfectly correlated variables need not be identical constructs. Nonetheless, by fixing the Gf unique variance (u3) to zero, rerunning the model, and then evaluating whether the model fit worse based on $\Delta\chi^2$, the *statistical* equivalence of the two variables in this sample could be tested. We ran such an analysis. The model with the u3 fixed to zero fit the data well: χ^2 (98) = 229.27, RMSEA = .05, CFI = .97. The $\Delta\chi^2$ (1) was 0.44 (p = .51), and was not statistically significant, suggesting that Gf and g are *statistically* equivalent, a finding not uncommon for higher-order analyses of intelligence data (Keith & Reynolds, 2012).

Higher-Order Models and the Schmid-Leiman Transformation

As already noted, in the higher-order model shown in Figure 3.4, g only affected the subtests indirectly, via the first-order factors. Said differently, the broad abilities completely mediate the effect of g on the subtests. Thus it is possible to calculate the total effect of g on each of the subtests in order to get some sense of the loading of each subtest (indirectly) on g. It would also be possible to compare this loading on g to the subtest's loadings on the broad abilities to get some sense of the relative effect of g versus the broad ability. The factor loadings of each subtest on its broad ability and on g are shown

Table 3.2 KABC-II Loadings on the First-Order Factors (see Figure 3.4 for the First-Order Factor Names) and the Second-Order g Factor. The final column shows the residualized first-order factor loadings, with the effect of g removed.

Subtest	First-Order	g	Residualized First-Order
Riddles	.885	.728	.503
Verbal Knowledge	.868	.714	.494
Expressive Vocabulary	.824	.677	.469
Gestalt Closure	.555	.504	.232
Triangles	.724	.658	.303
Block Counting	.685	.622	.288
Rover	.617	.560	.258
Pattern Reasoning	.693	.693	.000
Story Completion	.627	.627	.000
Rebus	.817	.688	.440
Rebus Delayed	.783	.660	.421
Atlantis	.657	.554	.352
Atlantis Delayed	.610	.514	.328
Word Order	.764	.590	.486
Number Recall	.656	.507	.417
Hand Movements	.662	.511	.421

in Table 3.2. This may feel like cheating in some sense of the word, however, because for both loadings the effect of the broad abilities on the subtests is used. So, for example, the loading of Word Order on Gsm is .76, whereas the loading of Word Order on g is .76 × .77 = .59. Given that all of g loadings go through the first-order factors, these loadings are constrained by the loading of the first-order factor on g.

If the double use of the first-order loadings makes you feel uncomfortable, an alternative would be to ask: What is the residual effect of the broad abilities after g is taken into account? One way to calculate these residual effects is to square the g loadings (to obtain the variance accounted for by g) and subtract these from the R^2 for each subtest (a statistic available in any SEM program). The resulting value would represent the variance explained uniquely by the broad abilities, after accounting for the variance explained by g. The square root of that

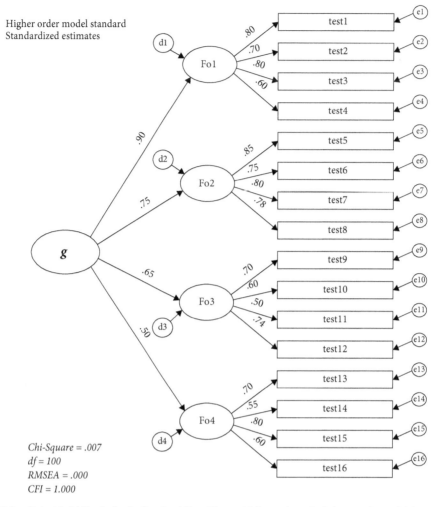

Figure 3.5 Higher-Order Model Results for the Simulated Data. The model fits nearly perfectly because the model shown was used to generate the data.

unique variance would then represent the unique loading of each subtest on the broad abilities after *g* is taken into account. These values are also shown in Table 3.2 in the last column on the right.

To further illustrate these and subsequent points, we will switch to simulated data. Figure 3.5 shows a straightforward factor model of 16 tests measuring four first-order factors and *g*, a higher-order factor. The model and the data are designed to be consistent with findings from analyses of intelligence test data. (The model fits these data perfectly, or nearly perfectly, because the model shown was used to simulate a matrix, which was then used in the analysis.) The first factor (Fo1) is most similar to *g*, and there is variability among the tests in how well they measure each broad ability. Figure 3.5 shows the loadings of each test on the broad abilities, and the first

column of numbers in Table 3.3 shows the loadings of each test on *g*. The second column of numbers in Table 3.3 shows the residualized loading of each test on the corresponding broad ability, or the unique effect of each broad ability on their subtest indicators, after accounting for *g*.

Discussion of the unique effect of the broad abilities suggests another way to calculate these effects. Figure 3.6 shows a slight variation of the higher-order model. In the initial figure, the disturbances of the first-order factors were scaled by constraining the path from the disturbance to the factor to 1.0 (what Kline, 2011, calls "unit loading identification" [ULI]). In Figure 3.6, an alternative method was used to scale the disturbances: The variances of the disturbances were set to 1, and the paths from the disturbances to the factors were estimated (unit variance identification, or UVI). With

Table 3.3 Loadings on the Higher-Order g Factor Versus the Residualized First-Order Factor Loadings, Calculated with Two Methods, for the Simulated Data

	g	First Order $\sqrt{R^2 - g^2}$	First Order $ul \times fol$
Test 1	.720	.349	.349
Test 2	.630	.305	.305
Test 3	.720	.349	.349
Test 4	.540	.262	.262
Test 5	.638	.562	.562
Test 6	.563	.496	.496
Test 7	.600	.529	.529
Test 8	.585	.516	.516
Test 9	.455	.532	.532
Test 10	.390	.456	.456
Test 11	.325	.380	.380
Test 12	.481	.562	.562
Test 13	.350	.606	.606
Test 14	.275	.476	.476
Test 15	.400	.693	.693
Test 16	.300	.520	.520

Note: First-order loadings represent the first-order factor effect on the test, with effects of g removed and calculated with two different methods (see text for explanation).

this specification, it is possible to calculate the indirect effects from the disturbances (the *unique variances* of the first-order factors) to the tests. So, for example, the effect of d4 on test 16 is .866 x .600 = .5196, or .520. Again, this is the unique effect of the first-order factor, with the effect of g removed. These values are shown in the final column of Table 3.3; they are the same as those shown in the previous column.

This calculation of the unique, or residualized, effects of the first-order factors, after accounting for the second-order factor, is analogous to the common Schmid-Leiman procedure in exploratory factor analysis. Table 3.4 shows the Schmid-Leiman transformation for these same data. The solution is based on an exploratory principal factors analysis of the simulated data used for

Figures 3.5 and 3.6 (and Table 3.4), with extraction and promax rotation of four factors. As can be seen by comparing Table 3.4 with Table 3.3, the estimates from this exploratory analysis are quite close to those from the confirmatory analysis. (It should be noted that the ordering of factors was changed; that is, what is labeled as "Factor 1" in the table actually came out as "Factor 2" in the EFA). Again, the table comparisons show that residualizing the first-order factor loadings from a higher-order model is methodologically equivalent to a Schmid-Leiman transformation.

Several points are worth mentioning about these procedures. First, they go by a variety of names. Here we have referred to this as a *residualization of the first-order factor loadings*, accounting for the second. Others may refer to this as an *orthogonalization* (e.g., Watkins, Wilson, Kotz, Carbone, & Babula, 2006) because the first-order factors have been made *orthogonal* (uncorrelated with) the second-order factor. This concept is well illustrated in Figure 3.6, where the unique factors are uncorrelated with the second-order g factor. It would also be correct to refer to these loadings as the g *loadings* and the unique effects of the first-order factors. Some writers may simply refer to these as *first* and *second-order factor loadings*, apparently not recognizing that the first-order loadings are with g statistically controlled.

EFFECTS VERSUS PROPORTION OF EXPLAINED VARIANCE

Readers may wonder why we focused on factor loadings rather than variances. After all, one method used to calculate the factor loadings did so by converting the g loadings to variances. We believe the focus on factor loadings rather than variances is appropriate for several reasons. First, factor loadings are the original metric. They are readily interpretable as effects; that is, the effect of g, or the broad abilities, on the tests. Second, the focus on factor loadings also makes this procedure easily interpretable as a Schmid-Leiman transformation. Finally, because variances focus on the original metric squared, they provide misleading estimates of the relative importance of the factors (Darlington, 1990; Keith, 2006, Chap. 5).

TOTAL VERSUS UNIQUE EFFECTS

A final point concerning this residualization is the reminder that the tables show the loadings of g, and the loadings of the first-order factors *with g controlled*, or the total effect of g and the unique

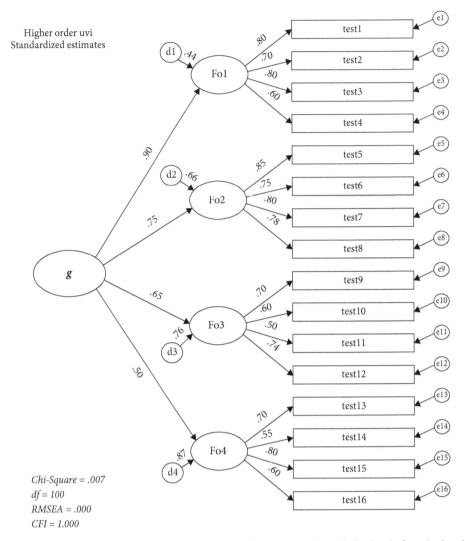

Chi-Square = .007
df = 100
RMSEA = .000
CFI = 1.000

Figure 3.6 Higher-Order Model Estimated Using Unit Variance Identification. Note the standardized paths from the disturbances to the first-order factors.

effect of the first-order factors. As such, the technique gives interpretive predominance to *g*, essentially a tacit, Spearman-like notion that *g* is most important. There is nothing wrong with this interpretation as long as researchers and readers understand it. Readers who believe that first-order factors should be given interpretive predominance (a Thurstone-like notion) could reasonably argue for the opposite of this procedure: the interpretation of the first-order factor loadings versus the unique effect of *g*, *while controlling for the first-order factors.* Because the strict higher-order model has *g* affecting the subtests only through the broad abilities, for this approach the first-order factor loadings (i.e., the "First-Order" in Table 3.2) represent the effect of the broad abilities on the subtests, but the effect of *g* on the subtests would all be equal to zero

(because there are no direct effects of *g* on the broad abilities)! Thus we recommend reporting results of this transformation, but also reporting the original, un-residualized, first-order factor loadings.

An Alternative to the Higher-Order Hierarchical Model

The higher-order model is the most common method of estimating both broad (e.g., Gf, Gc) and general (*g*) abilities in the same model. Another type of hierarchical model is often referred to as the *nested-factors* or *bi-factor model.* In this type of hierarchical model, the general and broad factors are at the same level; an example using the simulated model is shown in Figure 3.7. Note that methodologists have used different names to refer to such models. The higher-order model is sometimes called

Table 3.4 Schmid-Leiman Solution for the Simulated Data. The loadings are based on an exploratory principal factors analysis with promax rotation of four factors. The first-order loadings represent the effect of the first-order factor on the test, with the effects of *g* removed.

	g	Fo1	Fo2	Fo3	Fo4
Test 1	.712	.012	.366	.002	.005
Test 2	.623	.011	.320	.002	.005
Test 3	.712	.012	.366	.002	.005
Test 4	.533	.009	.274	.002	.005
Test 5	.633	.567	.005	.000	.002
Test 6	.559	.501	.004	.001	.002
Test 7	.597	.534	.005	.001	.002
Test 8	.581	.520	.005	.001	.002
Test 9	.454	.001	.002	.000	.532
Test 10	.390	.001	.002	.000	.456
Test 11	.325	.001	.002	.000	.380
Test 12	.481	.003	.002	.000	.562
Test 13	.352	.000	.000	.606	.000
Test 14	.276	.000	.000	.476	.000
Test 15	.402	.001	.001	.691	.000
Test 16	.302	.001	.000	.519	.001

a *hierarchical model* (e.g., Gustafsson & Balke, 1993; Mulaik & Quartetti, 1997), and the nested-factors model is often referred to as the *bi-factor*, or simply the *hierarchical*, model (McDonald, 1999). Here we refer to models such as those in Figures 3.5–3.6 as *higher-order models*, and those in Figure 3.7 as *hierarchical models*.

Conceptually, it may appear that this hierarchical approach provides a more direct approach to residualization than the Schmid-Leiman transformation shown in Tables 3.3 and 3.4. And this expectation appears confirmed by the values shown in Figure 3.7. The fit of the model is the same as it was for the higher-order model, and the loadings of the tests on *g* are identical to those shown in Table 3.3 (the symbol *G* is sometimes used to symbolize this factor because it is now a first-order, rather than a second-order, factor; Reynolds & Keith, 2007). Most importantly, the loadings of the tests on Fo1 through Fo4 are the same as the residualized

loadings for these factors in the higher-order model (Table 3.3).

It would seem, then, that a hierarchical model provides a simpler method for producing a Schmid-Leiman residualization. But this is not always the case. In fact, the only reason the two methods produced the same results is because a higher-order model was used to create the data in the first place. Note that, in Figure 3.5, the only way the second-order *g* factor can affect the tests is via the first-order factors. As a result, there are proportionality constraints on the residualized first-order factor loadings, by factor. So, for example, the first-order factor loading divided by the second-order factor loading is approximately .485 for the first four tests (which are on factor Fo1), .881 for tests 5–8 (on Factor Fo2), and so on.

Figure 3.8 shows a hierarchical model using a different set of simulated data. For this model, the hierarchical model shown was used to create the simulated data. Note that although the *g* loadings are similar to those shown for previous models, the loadings for Fo1 through Fo4 are different. More importantly, there are no proportionality constraints for this model.

Figure 3.9 and Table 3.5 show the results a higher-order solution for this same data. Note that, for this solution, there is no longer a nearly perfect fit of the model to the data. Note also the difference in factor loadings for the hierarchical solution versus the higher-order solution (Table 3.5). Finally, note the proportionality constraints for the first-order/*g* factor loadings for the higher-order solution, and the lack of those constraints for the hierarchical factor loadings. The higher-order model requires these constraints because the only way that *g* can affect the tests is indirectly, via the first-order factors.

What do these differences mean for the estimation of hierarchical models? Several points are worth noting. First, this comparison makes it obvious that the higher-order model is a more constrained version of the hierarchical model. Said differently, all higher-order models are hierarchical models, but not all hierarchical models are higher-order models. Relatedly, if a higher-order process created the data, a higher-order model and a hierarchical model will fit the data equally well. In contrast, if a hierarchical process (without proportionality constraints) created the data, then a hierarchical model will fit the data better than a higher-order model. Thus, in some sense, a comparison of a hierarchical model with a higher-order model is a test of which process created the data, and whether *g* affects first-order latent factors, or subtests directly.

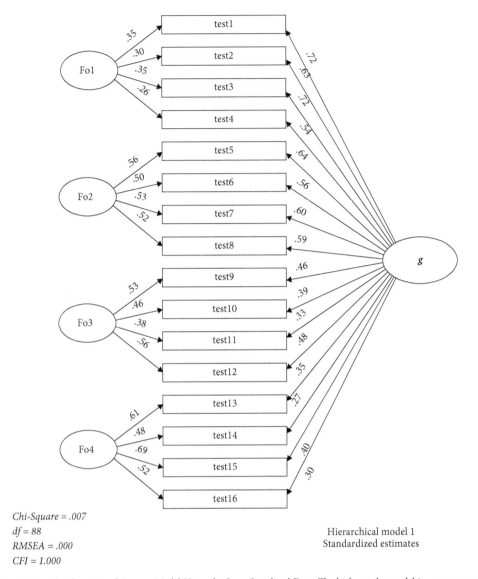

Chi-Square = .007
df = 88
RMSEA = .000
CFI = 1.000

Hierarchical model 1
Standardized estimates

Figure 3.7 A Hierarchical, or Nested Factors, Model Using the Same Simulated Data. The higher-order model is a more constrained version of this model.

Another way of saying this is that a comparison of the models tests the proportionality constraints required by the higher-order model (for further discussion of these issues, see Mulaik & Quartetti, 1997; or Yung, Thissen, & McLeod, 1999).[6]

This discussion would seem to suggest that one should prefer hierarchical models to higher-order models. After all, they will fit the data at least as well, and often better. But the entire process of modeling involves placing theoretically derived constraints on data, so we should not simply choose one model because it will have a higher probability of fitting well. As preached repeatedly in this chapter, theory must drive modeling, and must drive analysis. In

the area of intelligence, we believe that higher-order models are theoretically more defensible, more consistent with relevant intelligence theory (e.g., Jensen, 1998), than are less constrained hierarchical models.

Measurement Invariance

Psychological-assessment researchers often develop new instruments under the assumption that differences in the underlying psychological attributes produce individual differences in the observed test scores. It is typically implicitly assumed that the measurement of the latent attributes underlying those scores operate the same

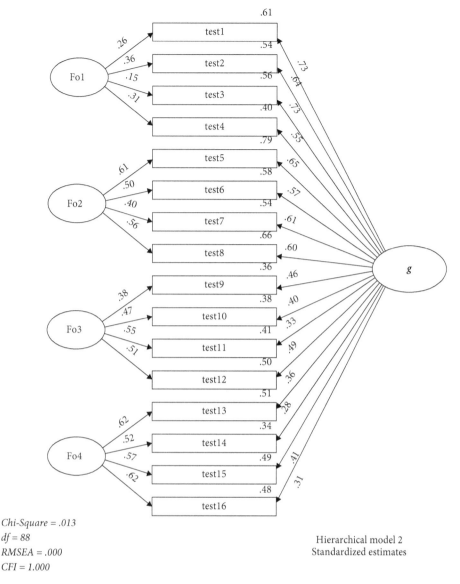

Figure 3.8 A Hierarchical Model Using a Second Simulated Data Set. This model was used to generate the data.

way across different groups of people (e.g., males and females). Nonetheless, it is important that this assumption be explicit and tested empirically. One of the more important advancements in measurement, and one that is particularly germane to psychological-assessment research, is the development of a set of factor analytic procedures to assess for measurement invariance (Meredith, 1993). Here we will discuss the assessment of measurement invariance using factor analysis.

Measurement invariance is the assumption that observed scores should be identical in individuals who have identical values of a latent trait (Meredith, 1993). That is, a measurement is unbiased. For

example, if males and females are administered a measure of intelligence, their scores should depend only on their latent intellectual ability, not on their sex. Measurement invariance is extremely important in test development and in research involving group comparisons (e.g., sex, culture, treatment/control groups) of psychological attributes and test bias. We will discuss this concept in detail via a worked example of how to establish measurement invariance at the subtest level in an individually administered measure of intelligence. We will use multiple-group confirmatory factor analysis, or what is commonly referred to as *multiple-group, mean and covariance structure* analysis (MG-MACS).

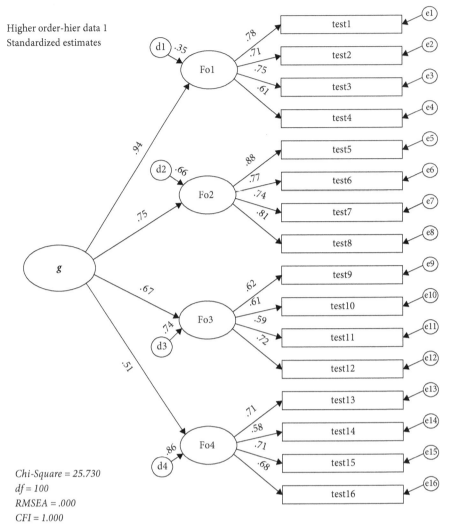

Higher order-hier data 1
Standardized estimates

Chi-Square = 25.730
df = 100
RMSEA = .000
CFI = 1.000

Figure 3.9 A Higher-Order Model for the Second Simulated Data Set. This model does not fit the data as well, because the model that created the data did not have the first-order and *g* factors proportionality constraints hidden within the higher-order model.

Age-standardized scores from the norming sample of the KABC-II (Kaufman & Kaufman, 2004) were used in the following example. Data from children and adolescents ages six to 18 were collapsed across the age range (1,189 females and 1,186 males). Previous research has demonstrated age invariance for the KABC-II, so collapsing across different age levels was deemed acceptable (Reynolds et al., 2007).

MG-MACS was used to test for measurement invariance across sex by adding parameter constraints sequentially in a set of multi-group models, moving from unconstrained to more constrained models. In multi-group models, factor models are estimated for more than one group (e.g., one for males and one for females). After the models are established, different sets of parameter constraints are added sequentially across groups, making the

overall model more restricted and parsimonious. For example, the factor loading of Word Order on the *Gsm* factor can be fixed to be the same for males and females. Including these various parameter constraints allows for tests of measurement invariance as well as substantive hypotheses relating to group differences in the latent attributes. The first-order factor model used in our CFA (Figure 3.3) example was used as our CFA model within each group in this example. Although a first-order model was used here, the MG-MACS approach can be extended to higher-order factor models to test various hypotheses about group differences in the second-order factor in addition to the first-order factors (see Reynolds, Keith, Ridley, & Patel, 2008 for examples with these same KABC-II data).

Table 3.5 Comparison of a Hierarchical versus a Higher-Order Solution for the Second Simulated Data Set. These data were simulated via a hierarchical model.

	Hierarchical Model		Higher-Order Model	
	g	First-Order	g	First-Order
Test 1	.734	.257	.732	.277
Test 2	.642	.363	.666	.252
Test 3	.734	.155	.704	.267
Test 4	.550	.310	.574	.217
Test 5	.651	.605	.664	.580
Test 6	.574	.504	.576	.504
Test 7	.612	.404	.554	.484
Test 8	.596	.555	.612	.535
Test 9	.464	.381	.412	.458
Test 10	.398	.466	.406	.452
Test 11	.331	.552	.396	.440
Test 12	.490	.509	.480	.534
Test 13	.357	.619	.362	.615
Test 14	.280	.516	.296	.503
Test 15	.408	.568	.360	.612
Test 16	.306	.619	.343	.583

RMSEA, CFI, and $\Delta\chi^2$ were used to evaluate fit. Changes in these values when constraints are added across models may indicate non-invariance, and that the hypothesis of the parameter equivalence across groups is not tenable. ΔCFI has been recommended by some (Cheung & Rensvold, 2002), but also may be considered too liberal of a criterion by others. Here, $\Delta\chi^2$ was used also to evaluate competing nested models, although some may consider this too conservative of a criterion. For the measurement invariance analyses, we used a more liberal cutoff of $p < .001$ for $\Delta\chi^2$ due to model complexity and the number of parameter constraints, but for tests of substantive hypotheses (typically involving fewer parameter constraints) a less conservative p-value was used. These are the types of decisions researchers may have to make during the course of a study. It is also possible, and likely best practice, to present the results of several criteria and discuss any discrepant findings.

Factorial Invariance Models

Configural, factor loading (also known as *metric* or *weak factorial invariance*), measurement intercept (*scalar* or *strong factorial invariance*), and subtest residual (*strict factorial invariance*) invariance models were tested, in that order, to test for measurement invariance (Meredith, 1993). Strict factorial invariance is most consistent with the definition of measurement invariance. We also applied invariance constraints to factor variances and covariances, and compared latent factor means across sex: these are tests of differences in the nature of the latent cognitive abilities for males and females, and not related to measurement invariance.

The order of invariance models may differ depending on the preference of the researcher. Researchers may begin with the most constrained model and release constraints; other researchers may choose to test for invariance of the covariance structure before introducing the mean structure;

and others may have different preferences regarding model identification. Our experience suggests that the conclusions drawn from the analyses will generally be quite similar either way, provided the analysis was conducted thoughtfully. We started with less constrained models and moved sequentially to more constrained models; that is, more of the model parameter estimates were fixed to be equal across sex. As we moved to more constrained models, the invariance constraints applied in previous model remained, unless noted otherwise.

CONFIGURAL INVARIANCE

The first step was to establish the factor structure for males and females, or configural invariance (with an example setup in Amos shown in Figure 3.10). The factor structure is identical to the CFA model used in our original KABC-II example.

In the configural model in Figure 3.10, the reference indicator for each factor has a fixed loading of one to properly scale the factors. The factor means are fixed to zero for each group, and the observed means of the subtests are estimated freely within each group. The number of factors and the pattern of factor loadings are the same for each group. All of the parameters estimated in a single group are estimated freely within each group in this configural model. This model is analogous to running independent confirmatory factor models for males and females, and then combining the information.

This multi-group model was estimated. The model fit information indicates acceptable fit (χ^2 [184] = 654.00, CFI = .97; Corrected RMSEA = .05). Note that the df for this model is different from the previous first-order CFA example (184 df versus 92 df). In a multi-group model, parameters unconstrained across groups are estimated within each group. The χ^2 value and df for this configural model are thus identical (within errors of rounding) to the values we would obtain for males and females if we ran CFAs separately for them, and subsequently summed the χ^2 and df from those two models (i.e., Males = χ^2 [92] = 318.7, Females = χ^2 [92] = 335.3).

In many SEM programs, including Amos, the RMSEA needs to be corrected when using multi-group analysis. When the models were run independently, the RMSEA = .046 for Males and .047 for Females. If we ran a model on the full sample without differentiating male and female groups, the RMSEA = .047. Because the groups are considered independent, the RMSEA is expected to be similar to the RMSEA obtained in the full sample. In the configural model, however, the uncorrected RMSEA

= .033. To account for multiple groups we applied a correction recommended by Steiger (1998): The RMSEA of .033 was multiplied by the square root of two (because there are two groups). The corrected RMSEA = .047 is what would be expected.

Based on the fit indexes and what is known about the KABC-II, the factor configuration across groups appeared acceptable, and thus we proceeded with invariance tests. Unacceptable results would pose some problems. The model would need to be reevaluated. An acceptable model for both groups should be established before proceeding to the following invariance steps.

FACTOR LOADING INVARIANCE

The step that typically follows configural invariance is invariance of the factor loadings, sometimes referred to as *metric* or *weak factorial invariance* (Meredith, 1993; Widaman & Reise, 1997). The factor loadings represent the link from theoretical to empirical worlds (Nesselroade & Thompson, 1995). And to test for invariance of the factor loadings, all of the corresponding (unstandardized) factor loadings were constrained to be equal across groups (see Figure 3.11). Factor loading invariance is a necessary but not sufficient condition for establishing measurement invariance (Meredith, 1993). As shown in Table 3.6 ("Factor Loadings"), the fit of the model is acceptable ($\Delta\chi^2$ [195] = 675.99, p = .02) when compared to the fit of the configural invariance model. The decrement in fit was not substantial, especially considering the large sample size and sensitivity of χ^2 to sample size. Using a $p < .001$ criterion, the $\Delta\chi^2$ did not fit significantly worse than the configural model (p = .02). As a result, factor loading (or weak factorial) invariance is tenable.

If factor loading invariance is established, then group comparisons related to the first-order factor variances and covariances may be made. In a structural equation model, if factor loading invariance is established, one can then compare effects (paths from one latent variable to another) across groups. If the interest of the researcher is in comparing means in a CFA or SEM, however, then intercept invariance needs to be established as well. If factor loading invariance is not established, the subtests are not measuring the factors in the same way for males and females (although sometimes a researcher may establish partial invariance if only a few of the loadings were non-invariant). Without factor loading invariance, making comparisons between the groups based on the observed scores or the latent factors would be like comparing apples and oranges.

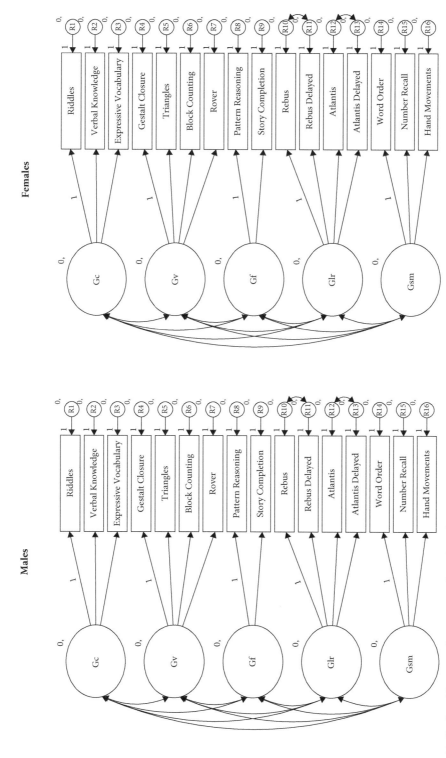

Figure 3.10 Configural Invariance Setup in Amos for Males and Females.

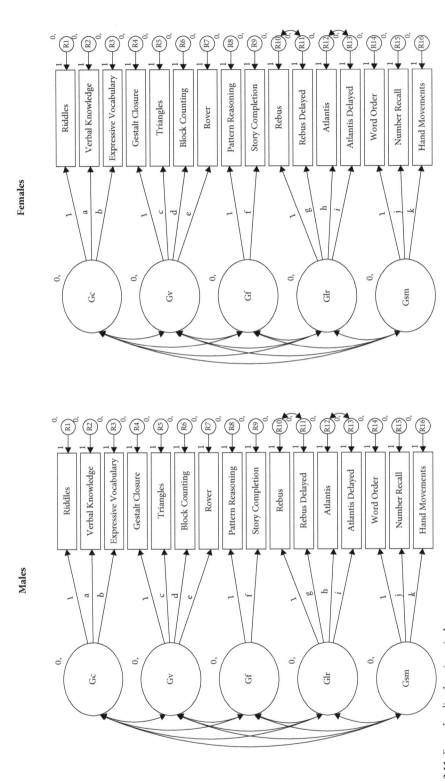

Figure 3.11 Factor Loading Invariance in Amos.

Table 3.6 Tests of Factorial Invariance

First-Order Model	χ^2	df	$\Delta\chi^2$	Δdf	p	CFI	RMSEA
Factorial Invariance							
Configural	654.01	184				0.97	0.05
Factor Loadings	675.99	195	21.98	11	0.02	0.97	0.05
Intercepts	720.05	206	44.06	11	<0.01	0.97	0.05
Subtest Residuals	748.20	222	28.15	16	0.03	0.97	0.05
Latent Variable Comparisons							
Factor Variances	754.70	227	6.50	5	0.26	0.97	0.04
Factor Covariances	771.80	237	17.10	10	0.07	0.97	0.05

Note: Compare each model with previous model.

INTERCEPT INVARIANCE

In this step, we explicitly tested the structure of the observed means as well by adding equality constraints on all of the corresponding measurement intercepts, in addition to the constraints from the previous model. This test, however, requires a few other adjustments to properly identify the model. In the configural model, the latent factor means were fixed to be zero, identical across groups, while the observed means (intercepts) were freely estimated within each group.[7] In this intercept invariance model, the first-order factor means for females remained fixed to zero; the factor means for males, however, were freed. Because the measurement intercepts were constrained to be equal, the latent factor mean estimates for males now represent latent mean differences from females.

Many readers are familiar with modeling covariance structures (e.g., factor loadings, factor variances and covariances) when conducting factor analysis, but are not familiar with modeling the means. By constraining the intercepts to be equal, and only allowing for observed score mean differences to pass through the factor, we are testing whether differences in the factor means can account for the difference in the observed means of the subtests. That is, are the observed differences in means on the various subtests a result of differences in the latent means? Alternatively, if a subtest intercept differs between groups (when between-group differences are allowed in the factor means), then the factor cannot completely explain the mean difference on that subtest between groups. For example, if on the KABC-II we allowed males and females to differ in their latent means on the G*sm* factor and found there was a significant intercept difference in the Word Order subtest, we would conclude that any mean difference on the latent G*sm* factor cannot account completely for the mean difference found on the Word Order subtest. The implication is that males and females scores do not differ on Word Order because of G*sm* only (what the test is supposed to measure), but because of something else. For example, it might reflect a difference in something specifically related to that subtest or something else that is not being considered or measured. The consequences of such a difference would be that the Word Order subtest displays uniform bias (i.e., one group scores lower on the subtest for reasons other than the differences in the latent factor), and if factor or observed means are being compared, and Word Order scores are included, then mean differences in the factor may not reflect differences in G*sm*. If there is an interest in comparing males and females on observed or factor means from the KABC-II, intercept (i.e., strong factorial) invariance must be established (Meredith, 1993). Of course, we do not know yet whether or not there are differences; this hypothesis needs to be tested formally within our model.

The results of the addition of the intercept constraints are shown in Table 3.6 ("Intercepts Model"). The change in the *df* between the factor loading and intercept model was 11 (16 subtest intercepts constrained equal, minus the 5 factor means freed for males). If a very strict interpretation were used (i.e., $\Delta\chi^2$), the addition of constraints resulted in a fit that differed significantly from zero. The other fit indexes did not indicate worse fit. Regardless, it is worth investigating further.

One might ask whether the degradation of fit was the result of a specific subtest or a combination of several. It was due primarily to one: Block Counting was a source of local misfit. The observed score sex difference in Block Counting cannot be accounted for by the latent mean difference in Gv. Put differently, there is something specific about Block Counting that the Gv factor difference cannot account for. In this situation, we have a few other indicators of Gv, so we could free the constraint on the measurement intercepts for Block Counting and still make comparisons on the latent Gv mean. We will address this issue in more detail later in a brief discussion of partial invariance. For now, because this was not an example of gross non-invariance, we assume that intercept invariance was met to a satisfactory degree. Mean differences in the subtests can be accounted for by mean differences in the broad ability factors.

Reaching this level of strong factorial invariance is important because latent mean differences can now be compared. In addition, cross-group comparisons of composite (summed) test scores assume this level of invariance (intercepts and loadings are invariant).

RESIDUAL INVARIANCE

The last model used to test for measurement invariance was residual invariance; in addition to the previous constraints, the sixteen corresponding measurement residuals were also constrained to be equal across groups. If residual invariance (strict factorial invariance) is established, then group differences in the factor means and variances account fully for all group differences in subtest scores. If residual invariance is not met, the constraints for the specific residual variance may be removed, and factor means may still be compared. This type of invariance is consistent with measurement invariance because group differences in observed means and variances would only be attributed to group differences in the latent variables. Note though that group comparisons on factor or observed means may be made if either strong or strict factorial invariance is achieved.

The model fit did not degrade significantly (See Table 3.6, "Subtest Residuals"). Scores on the KABC-II test are unbiased when comparing males and females and strict factorial invariance is tenable. This means that researchers interested in group differences on the KABC-II may make defensible group comparisons of latent variables, and that practitioners may be confident that scores obtained for individuals when using the KABC-II do not depend on the sex of the child. This type of information is extremely important to applied psychologists, and from an applied-psychology perspective, the study could end here. Researchers,

however, may be interested in sex differences related to the five broad cognitive abilities.

Latent Broad-Ability Comparisons

Measurement invariance was established via tests of factorial invariance. When assessing for measurement invariance, the latent means, latent variances, and latent covariances are allowed to differ across groups. Questions related to group differences in these parameters are unrelated to measurement invariance. Although differences in the broad abilities should not be compared if invariance was not established (although partial invariance may be used), a researcher may still be interested in trying to explain why it could not be established. There may even be examples of situations where one would expect non-invariance; for example, if a researcher expected two groups to differ on one specific subtest because it included questions that only one group would be able to answer because the questions were specific to the culture of that group.

Here, however, because measurement invariance was established, we also investigated whether there were sex differences in the latent broad abilities. Latent mean differences were estimated in both the intercept and residual invariance models, and because strict factorial invariance was established, either model could be used to test for differences in the broad abilities, although the residual variances model is the more parsimonious model.

LATENT MEANS

Sex differences in latent means using MG-MACS are typically evaluated with two methods. One method is to constrain the latent means to be equal and refer to the $\Delta\chi^2$ to determine whether the addition of the constraint resulted in a degradation of fit. If there is a significant degradation in fit, the groups demonstrate a mean difference on the latent broad ability(s). The second method is to locate the statistical significance tests for males' latent means in the output of either the measurement intercept or residual invariance model. The females' latent means were fixed to zero, so if the males' latent means were statistically significantly different from zero, they are significantly different from females. Negative means indicate higher means for females; positive means indicate higher means for males. The output from both intercept and residual variance invariance models indicated that five of the broad ability mean differences were statistically significant. Females showed an advantage in Gf (−.22), Glr (−.35), and Gsm (−.22). Males showed an advantage in Gv (.47) and Gc (.25). The conclusions regarding the latent means were the same using either approach ($\Delta\chi^2$ or significance tests). And although the magnitude of these latent mean differences may be unclear from an interpretative standpoint, they can be converted back to the original IQ score metric. See Reynolds et al. (2008) for further analysis in studying these differences when a higher-order general factor is included.

LATENT VARIANCES AND COVARIANCES

Researchers may also be interested in substantive questions about the variances and covariances across groups, although the interpretation of these differences is more ambiguous than those of the means. First, the corresponding factor variances were constrained to be equal. The degradation in model fit was not statistically significant ($\Delta\chi^2$ [5] = 6.50, p = .31). Males and females draw upon the same range of broad abilities. Because the factor variances were invariant, we next tested whether the covariances were significantly different. Applying these constraints did not result in a statistically significant degradation in fit ($\Delta\chi^2$ [10] = 17.10, p = .07). The broad abilities are equally related across sex. Note that if the variances of the broad abilities were significantly different across groups, we would have not tested for differences in the covariances. Note also that these findings also suggest invariance in loadings and unique variances for a higher-order model, since these would be estimated from the first-order variances and covariances.

MIMIC Models

Researchers may be familiar with a group of models referred to as *multiple-indicator multiple-cause* models (Jöreskog & Goldberger, 1975; Muthén, 1989). These are models in which latent variables, which are indicated by observed measures, also have variables (e.g., Sex) as causes. Like the MG-MACS models, these models may be used to test for group (mean) differences in latent factors and may also be used to test for intercept invariance. We will limit our discussion of MIMIC models to a comparison with MG-MACS models, and how to use this method to test for intercept invariance and group differences in the first-order factors. The first-order factor model from the KABC-II will be used.

One assumption of MIMIC models, which is tested with MG-MACS models, is that the variance-covariance matrix is invariant across groups (Kano, 2001), or even more explicitly, all of the model parameters related to the variance-covariance matrix are invariant across groups: factor loadings, residual variances, factor variances, and covariances. Hence, the observed KABC-II data for males and females would be assumed to arise from a common covariance matrix. Given that this assumption is met, MIMIC models may also be used to test for mean differences in the factors. The results we obtain should be the same as the latent mean differences found in the MG-MACS example.

See Figure 3.12 for a visual representation of the model. The common factors, which are regressed on Sex (dummy coded so females = 0 and males = 1), now have disturbances associated with them. These disturbance variables represented the variance in the factors not explained by Sex. The unstandardized estimates shown on the paths from Sex to the broad factors represent latent mean differences between males and females. Negative values are in favor of females, positive values in favor of males. These estimated values are identical to the latent mean differences obtained in the MG-MACS approach. Because the assumption of a common variance-covariance matrix was met (or more specifically, a common covariance structure as the latent variances, latent covariances, unstandardized factor loadings, and residual variances were equal in the MG-MACS tests), the results should be identical, and they were.

We hope we have highlighted some of the differences in assumptions related to MIMIC and MG-MACS models. Awareness of assumptions underlying the two approaches is always useful for gaining an appreciation and understanding of techniques. MG-MACS models are more flexible in that all of the assumptions may be tested explicitly. Some might consider MIMIC approaches easier to implement, especially for those who are more inclined to use regression-type methods. Nevertheless, assumptions must be met before groups are compared, and MG-MACs are more explicit in testing these assumptions. Lastly, it is also possible to combine the two types into hybrid models that allow for very interesting comparisons of latent variables (Keith et al., 2008; Lubke, Dolan, Kelderman, & Mellenbergh, 2003; Marsh, Tracey, & Craven, 2006).

Partial Intercept Invariance with MIMIC and MG-MACS

MIMIC models require the assumption that two groups share a common covariance matrix (Kano, 2001). If that assumption is met, MIMIC models may also be used to test for intercept invariance by including directs effect from the group (e.g., Sex) to

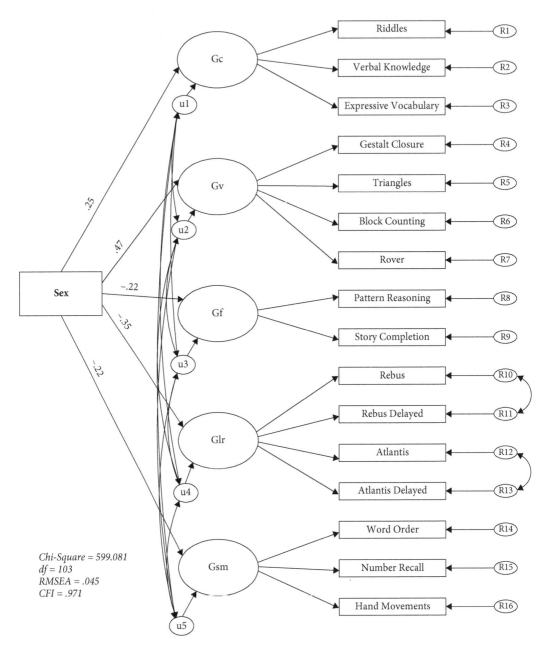

Figure 3.12 MIMIC Model for Sex Differences in First-Order Factor Means in the KABC Latent Broad Abilities. Unstandardized estimates are shown with positive effects indicating a male advantage and negative effects indicating a female advantage.

the observed indicator. To illustrate, we return to the MG-MACS and MIMIC models with the KABC-II data. In the MG-MACS example, we could have concluded that sex differences in Gv could not account for observed mean differences in Block Counting (if a strict interpretation of $\Delta\chi^2$ was used). Based on that conclusion, the invariance constraint on the measurement intercept associated with the Block Counting test could have been removed, and this model could have been used to test for latent

mean differences with partial measurement invariance for Gv (Byrne, Shavelson, & Muthén, 1989). Given that there are several indicators of Gv, this would be considered acceptable. Intercept invariance can also be tested using MIMIC models. In Figure 3.13, notice a direct effect from the Sex variable to the observed indicator Block Counting, in addition to the effects from Sex to the factors. The direct effect from Sex to Block Counting is statistically significant. Beyond the Gv factor difference,

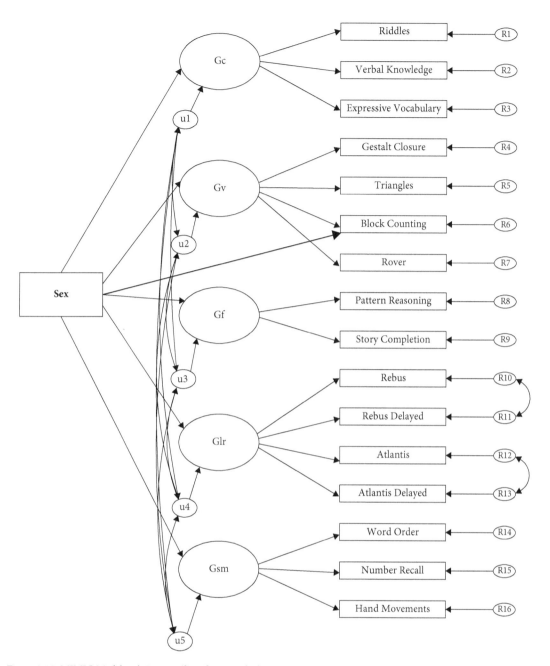

Figure 3.13 MIMIC Model with Direct Effect of Sex on Block Counting.

there is a sex difference between males and females on Block Counting. Again, the mean sex difference on this subtest cannot be accounted for fully by differences in the factor. Or, for those who are familiar with item response theory terminology, the Block Counting test acts differentially across sex (i.e., uniform bias). Allowing for the direct effect from Sex to Block Counting corresponds to freeing the equality constraints on the Block Counting intercept in the MG-MACS analysis.

This illustration should also bring something else to mind: mediation. *Mediation* refers to the effect of one variable explained via another. It should be clear from the MIMIC model diagram shown in Figure 3.13 that the Gv factor partially mediates sex differences in the observed Gv variables. The Gsm, Glr, Gf, and Gc factors, however, fully mediate the effects of sex on observed differences in the subtests. Or, to put it differently, with intercept invariance, differences in the latent factor means should *fully mediate* differences in the observed scores related to that factor.

Variables and Their Measurement

An essential part of solid assessment research is that researchers think critically about how their observed data arise. Fancy statistical techniques will not save one from sloppy thinking; even complex statistical analyses cannot make a silk purse from a sow's ear. This section introduces several additional important issues a researcher should think about before developing measurement instruments, and before analyzing and interpreting scores from those instruments. Attention to these issues should improve the quality of research because they force researchers to think carefully about what they are trying to measure, how the measurements come about, and which type of variable to include in an analysis.

Categorical versus Continuous Latent Variables

Almost all variables in psychology are considered to be *latent* variables. For example, social anxiety is a construct that cannot be observed, but differences in latent social anxiety should produce differences in how individuals respond to questions designed to measure that latent construct. If social anxiety is hypothesized as a latent variable, then researchers might be interested in whether latent social anxiety is either a category (type) or a dimension (continuous). Those who believe that anxiety is a type or categorical latent variable would say that a person either has social anxiety or doesn't, whereas those who ascribe to a continuous definition would say that the severity of anxiety depends on where along the latent social anxiety dimension a person is located (see Meehl, 2006, for more discussion). This distinction has both practical implications for the design of measurement instruments and theoretical implications related to understanding important psychological phenomena. Moreover, the distinction is important because a researcher would then need to be clear whether the latent anxiety variable in their model is a categorical or a continuous latent variable. Briefly, we will discuss a few points related to distinctions between categorical (type) and continuous (dimensions) latent variables.

The first point is that observed scores do not inform the nature of the latent variable. That is, continuous or categorical observed variables do not inform us whether latent variables are continuous or categorical. For example, in one type of continuous latent variable model, the common factor model, the latent variable may be indicated by continuous or categorical variables. Alternatively, in the latent class model (where a class is a latent categorical variable), the latent class variable is indicated by categorical observed variables; but in yet another categorical latent variable model, the latent profile model, the latent variable is indicated by continuous variables.

Second, it can be shown that a common factor model (continuous) is very difficult to distinguish from a latent profile (categorical) model (Bartholomew, 1987). And although some analytic techniques may assist us in distinguishing between categorical versus continuous latent variables empirically, the distinction is typically based on theory, not statistics. Researchers should therefore think carefully about whether the latent variable underlying the observed data is one of a continuum or category. From a measurement perspective, the measurement model designed for a continuous construct is used to develop scales where ultimately a score is obtained in an attempt to estimate the rank order of where a person is located along the latent dimension. Alternatively, a measurement model used with a latent categorical structure would be developed with the goal of classifying individuals in the appropriate group (e.g., anorexic versus non-anorexic). Latent class variables are variables used typically to represent *qualitatively* different groups of people.[8]

Finally, there are interesting developments in factor analysis and item response theory that allow for the use of both categorical and continuous latent variables (e.g., Lubke & Muthén, 2005). These models will provide opportunity for many interesting applications. Certainly it would also be exciting to see similar developments in psychological theory. Perhaps advances in these methods will provide researchers with more clarity for theory development, or more developed theories in some areas of psychological will continue to drive the development of new methods to test them.

Reflective versus Formative Measurement

Issues related to reflective and formative measurement have been generating considerable interest recently (see Bollen, 2007; Edwards & Bagozzi, 2000; Howell, Breivik, & Wilcox, 2007). Assessment researchers should be aware of this distinction because it is important to the measurement of constructs in research. Perhaps the distinction between the two types is most easily demonstrated

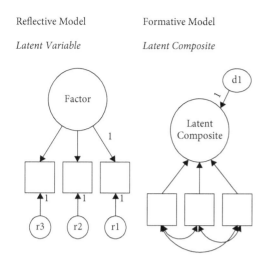

Reflective Model   Formative Model

Latent Variable   *Latent Composite*

Figure 3.14 Reflective and Formative Latent Variable Measurement.

via the direction of path arrows. In reflective measurement, the causal direction flows from the latent variable to the indicators (effect indicators) (see Figure 3.14). In formative measurement, the causal direction flows from the indicators (causal indicators) to the latent composite variable.

Reflective models are most commonly used in psychology. Factor analysis and internal reliability estimates assume a reflective model (Bollen & Lennox, 1991). In reflective measurement, it is assumed that equally reliable indicators are interchangeable, which is not the case with formative indicators. Most, if not almost all, variables in psychology are conceptualized as latent variables measured via reflective or "effect" indicators. Nevertheless, a decision to use a reflective model should not be automatic; theoretical justification is required.

In reflective models, the latent variable is the common cause of the interrelations among the indicators (e.g., a confirmatory factor model). For example, visual-spatial ability affects performance on all tests that require some aspect of visual-spatial manipulation. Differences in visual spatial ability produce individual differences in the observed scores on visual-spatial tests. The factor model on the left of Figure 3.14 is a model representing reflective measurement. The unique and error variance are removed at the indicator level and captured in the residual variance. The latent variable causes, or is reflected in, the indicators. An increase in the level of the factor will correspond to higher scores on each of the indicators.

The model on the right of Figure 3.14 represents a formative latent variable, or a latent "composite."

An example of such a formative variable might be overall time spent reading.[9] Someone might read magazines, books, articles online, or the backs of cereal boxes. If a person increases the time spent reading books, overall time spent reading increases, but it says nothing about time spent reading the backs of cereal boxes. That is, increased reading time does not imply that reading across the different areas will increase. In formative measurement, the constructs are caused or formed by the correlated measures. The disturbance variable captures whatever is not explained the indicators. In Figure 3.14, the model on the right is statistically under-identified, meaning that if the model were analyzed it would not converge, and unique estimates could not be obtained. These types of models typically need to be evaluated within a structural equation model where there is some type of external criteria. As a result, the interpretation of the latent composite also typically depends on other variable(s). The constructs or interpretations of these constructs will likely change depending on the indicators or dependent variables included in the model.

Our purpose here was to introduce these terms and reiterate the importance of clearly defining measurement prior to research. Most, if not all, psychological attributes will be measured reflectively; nevertheless, this is not a given, and researchers need to think critically about measurement. Interested readers should consult several additional, excellent sources on this topic (e.g., Bollen, 2007; Bollen & Lennox, 1991; Edwards & Bagozzi, 2000; Howell, Breivik, & Wilcox, 2007; MacCallum & Browne, 1993).

Composite versus Latent Variables

Examples of reflective latent variables and formatively measured latent composites were discussed in the previous section. Here we discuss a related issue: the decision to study latent variables versus composite variables (e.g., variables used in our multiple regression analysis).

It is important to note that when we refer to "composite variables" here, we are not referring to "latent variables." The diagram shown in Figure 3.15 will help clarify the distinction. The difference between this Figure 3.15 and the formatively measured latent variable (Figure 3.14, on the right) is that a disturbance term has been removed, and rather than use an oval to represent the variable, a rectangle was used. The composite variable, therefore, represents a linear composite of observed indicators. The model is similar to a principal component model

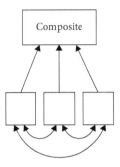

Figure 3.15 Observed Linear Composite Variable.

where measurement error and unique variance are captured in the component itself. Earlier, PCA was discussed as an unacceptable method of studying latent variables, and here it should be clear that a principal component is a *composite* variable, a variable where error and other unique or unaccounted influences are not removed.

When analyzing data, researchers often study their variables of interest indirectly via the substitution of composite variables rather than studying them directly through latent variables. Composite variables are caused by their indicators, or measured formatively, analogous to the latent "composite" variables. Composites include measurement error and invalidity. Aggregated items, components from principal component analysis, and extracted factor scores that have been summed are all examples of composite variables. Composite variables are not latent variables. Composites may provide ideas about the latent variables the researcher are really interested in, but the composite itself is not equivalent to the latent variable (Bollen & Lennox, 1991). For example, multiple regression is performed with multiple composite variables used as explanatory variables and as an outcome variable, each providing hints of latent variables. Because composites are used, however, the estimates of coefficients obtained from multiple regression analysis are inconsistent, and a researcher does not know whether they are biased upward or downward, or even if they are biased at all (Bollen, 1989, pp. 166–167). Most assessment researchers are interested in studying and measuring latent variables. Well-conceived latent variables are consistent with the theoretical constructs, and thus measurement and analytical models should reflect theoretical models. Child-assessment research should therefore be focused on the study of latent variables, because latent variables underlie what is observed.

Other Issues

There is a host of issues we did not discuss in this chapter. Psychometrics and statistics is a dynamic field, and this chapter could only deal with a limited number of issues, and even with those we encourage readers to refer to our sources for more detailed descriptions. A couple of other issues deserve at least a mention because they are so common.

Test Bias

Test bias was addressed partially in the section on moderation and in the section on measurement invariance using MG-MACS and MIMIC models. Measurement invariance is extremely important in making sure differences in the latent traits are reflected in test scores, and not group membership. But there are other means used to evaluate bias, especially with regard to external criterion, often referred to as *prediction invariance*. It is likely that assessment researchers are more familiar with prediction invariance, as it has been used more often in applied assessment research and is of particular importance for selection into important programs. As discussed, prediction invariance (or bias) is often evaluated with moderated multiple regression models using one variable to predict a criterion across groups. The regression slope and intercepts should not differ across groups for prediction invariance to be tenable (or if tested in a multi-group path model in a SEM program, the residual variances may also be tested for equality across groups). Readers may wish to refer to other sources for a more detailed discussion on test bias (e.g., Reynolds & Lowe, 2009) and the seemingly surprising but common incompatibility of measurement invariance and predictive invariance (Borsboom, Romeijn, & Wicherts, 2008; Millsap, 2007).

Regression to the Mean

Given that two variables (e.g., pretest–post-test scores; scores from two different measures) are not perfectly correlated, the rank order of individual's scores will differ across measurements, with extreme scores more likely to be closer to the mean. This regression to the mean is a statistical fact. Those who are rank ordered at the top or bottom will tend to be replaced, or scores that are furthest from the mean on one variable will tend not to be as extreme on the other variable. A correlation coefficient represents the amount of nonregression toward the mean: the closer to +/–1, the less regression toward the mean (Campbell & Kenny, 1999). The most important implication from regression to the mean is that substantive meaning should not be given to these changes in rank ordering. Campbell and Kenny (1999) provided an excellent treatment on this topic: it should be required reading for anyone who is interested in treatment or program evaluation.

Conclusion

We have covered a variety of measurement and statistical issues and examples in this chapter. Although some of our examples (e.g., higher-order models; MIMIC models) are considered structural equation models, we have not formally discussed structural equation modeling in this chapter. There are numerous resources available on structural equation modeling ranging from complex to simple (Bollen, 1989; Keith, 2006); obviously, with our focus on latent variables, we see structural equation modeling as vital tool in psychological assessment research. For example, complex structural equation modeling could be applied to better match various multi-method assessment approaches. We also believe one key to future research is that important measurement issues be worked out before structural equation modeling is used. As we stated in the beginning, psychological assessment is contingent on measurement, which is contingent on theoretically important psychological attributes. Psychological assessment research should involve each of these aspects.

Acknowledgments

We are grateful to Alan Kaufman and Mark Daniel for access to the KABC-II data. We also thank Randy Floyd for providing assistance with the Schmid-Leiman section and Matthew Irvin for comments on an early version of this chapter. We are solely responsible for any errors or opinions expressed in this article.

Correspondence may be addressed to: Matthew R. Reynolds, University of Kansas, Psychology and Research in Education, Joseph R. Pearson Hall, 1122 W Campus Rd., Lawrence, Kansas 66045-3101; Fax: 785-864-3820, email: mreynolds@ku.edu.

Notes

1. The ECLS-K also includes sampling weights and strata variables (geographic and public versus private schools), but these were not included in this analysis. For ease of exposition, we took a random sample consisting of 10% of the total cases and only included the cases with complete data. We will address better methods to deal with missing data later.

2. Semipartial (or part) correlations, equal to the square root of ΔR^2, may also be used to test unique effects and may be a better measure of the importance of an effect than is ΔR^2. See Darlington (1990) and Keith (2006) for further discussion.

3. We make this statement cautiously and do not advocate that researchers just assume the MAR and run their analysis. Thinking critically about the data and running sensitivity analyses are recommended. See Graham and colleagues (1997) and Graham (2009) for a more detailed discussion.

4. Weak loadings do not necessarily indicate that anything is wrong with the model, because the goal is to explain the correlations among tests, not maximize the variance explained.

5. There is a limited number of direct effects that may be included. For each group of tests indicating a first-order factor, unless other model constraints are applied, one direct effect would need to be omitted, or fixed to zero, for proper model identification.

6. It is possible to have hybrid-type models, in which g affects tests both directly and via first-order factors; such models will quickly result in problems with identification, however. Hierarchical models are often difficult to estimate, and, in our experience, start values are often needed to make the models work. Note that the hierarchical models shown here have uncorrelated factors, a common constraint. Such constraints also require a minimum of three tests per factor, however, or empirical under-identification will result. Hence, it is not uncommon to find constraints on the hierarchical model that do not necessarily make sense theoretically.

7. Given that this step requires both the fixing and the freeing of parameter constraints, it may appear that this model is not nested with the previous model. That is not the case. We could have identified the original multi-group model by fixing each factor's reference variable intercept to be zero across groups and freeing the constraint that the latent factor means equal zero. The factor means would have represented the mean of the reference variable subtest (i.e., the mean of Riddles). These differences in model identification do not make a difference in the outcome, but this alternative method of model identification would have more clearly demonstrated the nested nature of these models.

8. Latent classes may also represent mixture components, where each class represents a distinct distribution which may not have psychological meaning. The discussion is outside of the scope of this chapter (see Dolan & van der Maas, 1998; and Lubke & Spies, 2007, for a discussion).

9. We will use the term *latent composite variable*. Some reserve the term *latent variable* for reflective measurement only (e.g., MacCallum & Browne, 1993). And of course, one could also argue that enjoyment of reading is an internal characteristic that affects the amount one reads across settings. In that case, Reading Time (or enjoyment) would be better modeled as a reflective, i.e., traditional, latent variable.

References

Aiken, L. S., & West, S. G. (1991). *Multiple regression: Testing and interpreting interactions*. Thousand Oaks, CA: Sage.

Arbuckle, J. L. (2006). *Amos (Version 7.0)*. Chicago: SPSS.

Arbuckle, J. L., & Wothke, W. (1999). *Amos 4.0 user's guide*. Chicago: SPSS.

Bartholomew, D. J. (1987). *Latent variable models and factor analysis*. London: Charles Griffin & Co., Ltd.

Bentler, P. M. (1990). Comparative fit indexes in structural models. *Psychological Bulletin, 107*, 238–246.

Bollen, K. A. (1989). *Structural equations with latent variables*. New York: Wiley.

Bollen, K. A. (2002). Latent variables in psychology and the social sciences. *Annual Review of Psychology, 53,* 605–634.

Bollen, K. A. (2007). Interpretational confounding is due to misspecification, not to type of indicator: Comment on Howell, Breivik, and Wilcox (2007). *Psychological Methods, 12,* 219–228.

Bollen, K. A., & Lennox, R. (1991). Conventional wisdom on measurement: A structural equation perspective. *Psychological Bulletin, 110,* 305–314.

Borsboom, D. (2006). The attack of the psychometricians. *Psychometrika, 71,* 425–440.

Borsboom, D., Romeijn, J.-W., & Wicherts, J. M. (2008). Measurement invariance versus selection invariance: Is fair selection possible? *Psychological Methods, 13,* 75–98.

Byrne, B. M., Shavelson, R. J., & Muthén, B. (1989). Testing for the equivalence of factor covariance and mean structures: The issue of partial measurement invariance. *Psychological Bulletin, 105,* 456–466.

Campbell, D. T., & Kenny, D. A. (1999). *A primer on regression artifacts.* New York: Guilford.

Carroll, J. B. (1993). *Human cognitive abilities: A survey of factor-analytic studies.* New York: Cambridge University Press.

Cheung, G. W., & Rensvold, R. B. (2002). Evaluating goodness-of-fit indexes for testing measurement invariance. *Structural Equation Modeling, 9,* 233–255.

Darlington, R. B. (1990). *Regression and linear models.* New York: McGraw-Hill.

Dolan, C. V., & van der Maas, H. L. J. (1998). Fitting multivariate normal finite mixtures subject to structural equation modeling. *Psychometrika, 63,* 227–253.

Edwards, J. R., & Bagozzi, R. P. (2000). On the nature and direction of relationships between constructs and measures. *Psychological Methods, 5,* 155.

Enders, C. K. (2010). *Applied missing data analysis.* New York: Guilford.

Graham, J. W. (2009). Missing data analysis: Making it work in the real world. *Annual Review of Psychology, 60,* 549–576.

Graham, J. W., Hofer, S. M., Donaldson, S. I., MacKinnon, D. P., & Schafer, J. L. (1997). Analysis with missing data in prevention research. In K. Bryant, M. Windle, & S. West (Eds.), *The science of prevention: Methodological advances from alcohol and substance abuse research* (pp. 325–366). Washington, DC: American Psychological Association.

Gustafsson, J.-E. (1984). A unifying model for the structure of intellectual abilities. *Intelligence, 8,* 179–203.

Gustafsson, J.-E., & Balke, G. (1993). General and specific abilities as predictors of school achievement. *Multivariate Behavioral Research, 28,* 407–434.

Horn, J. L., & Noll, J. (1997). Human cognitive capabilities: Gf-Gc theory. In D. P. Flanagan, J. L. Genshaft, & P. L. Harrison (Eds.), *Contemporary intellectual assessment: Theories, tests and issues* (pp. 53–91). New York: Guilford.

Howell, R. D., Breivik, E., & Wilcox, J. B. (2007). Reconsidering formative measurement. *Psychological Methods, 12,* 205.

Jensen, A. R. (1998). *The g factor.* Westport, CT: Prager.

Jöreskog, K. (1999). *How large can a standardized coefficient be?* Retrieved October 15, 2008, from http://www.ssicentral.com/lisrel/advancedtopics.html.

Jöreskog, K. G., & Goldberger, A. S. (1975). Estimation of a model with multiple indicators and multiple causes of a single latent variable. *Journal of the American Statistical Association, 70,* 631–639.

Kano, Y. (2001). Structural equation modeling for experimental data. In R. Cudeck, S. d. Toit, & D. Sörbom (Eds.), *Structural equation modeling: Present and future. Festschrift in honor of Karl Jöreskog* (pp. 381–402). Lincolnwood, IL: Scientific Software International.

Kaufman, A. S., & Kaufman, N. L. (2004). *Kaufman Assessment Battery for Children Second Edition: Technical manual.* Circle Pines, MN: American Guidance Service.

Keith, T. Z. (2006). *Multiple regression and beyond.* Boston, MA: Allyn and Bacon.

Keith, T. Z., & Reynolds, M. R. (2010). Cattell-Horn-Carroll abilities and cognitive tests: What we've learned from 20 years of research. *Psychology in the Schools, 47,* 635–650.

Keith, T. Z., & Reynolds, M. R. (2012). Using confirmatory factor analysis to aid in understanding the constructs measured by intelligence tests. In D. P. Flanagan, & P. L. Harrison (Eds.), *Contemporary intellectual assessment: Theories, tests, and issues* (3rd ed., pp. 758–799). New York: Guilford.

Keith, T. Z., Reynolds, M. R., Patel, P. G., & Ridley, K. P. (2008). Sex differences in latent cognitive abilities ages 6 to 59: Evidence from the Woodcock Johnson III tests of cognitive abilities. *Intelligence, 36,* 502–525.

Kline, R. (2011). *Principle and practice of structural equation modeling* (3rd ed.). New York: Guilford.

Kranzler, J. H., Miller, M. D., & Jordan, L. (1999). An examination of racial/ethnic and gender bias on curriculum-based measurement of reading. *School Psychology Quarterly, 14,* 327–342.

Little, R. J., & Rubin, D. B. (1987). *Statistical analysis with missing data.* New York: Wiley.

Lubke, G. H., Dolan, C. V., Kelderman, H., & Mellenbergh, G. J. (2003). On the relationship between sources of within- and between-group differences and measurement invariance in the common factor model. *Intelligence, 31,* 543–566.

Lubke, G., & Muthén, B. O. (2005). Investigation population heterogeneity with factor mixture models. *Psychological Methods, 10,* 21–39.

Lubke, G. H., & Spies, J. R. (2007). Choosing a "correct" factor mixture model: Power, limitations, and graphical data exploration. In G. R. Hancock & K. M. Samuelsen (Eds.), *Advances in latent variable mixture models* (pp. 343–362). Charlotte, NC: Information Age.

MacCallum, R. C., & Browne, M. W. (1993). The use of causal indicators in covariance structure models: Some practical issues. *Psychological Bulletin, 114,* 533–541.

Marsh, H. W., Hau, K., & Grayson, D. (2005). Goodness of fit in structural equation modeling. In A. Maydeu-Olivares & J. J. McArdle (Eds.), *Contemporary psychometrics: A festschrift for Roderick P. McDonald* (pp. 275–340). Mahwah, NJ: Erlbaum.

Marsh, H. W., Tracey, D. K., & Craven, R. G. (2006). Multidimensional self-concept structure for preadolescents with mild intellectual disabilities: A hybrid multigroup-mimic approach to factorial invariance and latent mean differences. *Educational and Psychological Measurement, 66,* 795–818.

McArdle, J. J. (1994). Structural factor analysis experiments with incomplete data. *Multivariate Behavioral Research, 29,* 409–454.

McDonald, R. P. (1999). *Test theory: A unified treatment.* Mahwah, NJ: Erlbaum.

McGrew, K. M. (2009). CHC theory and the human cognitive abilities project: Standing on the shoulders of the giants of psychometric intelligence research. *Intelligence, 37,* 1–10.

MacKinnon, D. P. (2008). *Introduction to statistical mediation analysis*. New York: Erlbaum.

Meehl, P. (2006). *A Paul Meehl reader: Essays on the practice of scientific psychology*. Mahwah, NJ: Erlbaum.

Meredith, W. (1993). Measurement invariance, factor analysis, and factorial invariance. *Psychometrika 58*, 525–543.

Millsap, R. E. (2007). Invariance in measurement and prediction revisited. *Psychometrika, 72*, 461–473.

Mulaik, S. A., & Quartetti, D. A. (1997). First-order or higher-order general factor? *Structural Equation Modeling, 4*, 193–211

Muthén, B. O. (1989). Latent variable modeling in heterogeneous populations. *Psychometrika, 54*, 557–585.

Nesselroade, J. R., & Thompson, W. W. (1995). Selection and related threats to group comparisons: An example comparing factorial structures of higher and lower ability groups. *Psychological Bulletin, 117*, 271–284.

Preacher, K. J., & MacCallum, R. C. (2003). Repairing Tom Swift's electric factor analysis machine. *Understanding Statistics, 2*, 13–43.

Reynolds, C. R., & Lowe, P. A. (2009). The problem of bias in psychological assessment. In T. B. Gutkin & C. R. Reynolds (Eds.), *The handbook of school psychology* (4th ed., 332–374). Hoboken, NJ: Wiley.

Reynolds, M. R., & Keith, T. Z. (2007). Spearman's law of diminishing returns in hierarchical models of intelligence for children and adolescents. *Intelligence, 35*, 267–281.

Reynolds, M. R., Keith, T. Z., Fine, J. G., Fisher, M. F., & Low, J. A. (2007). Confirmatory factor analysis of the Kaufman Assessment Battery for Children–2nd ed.: Consistency with Cattell-Horn-Carroll theory. *School Psychology Quarterly, 22*, 511–539.

Reynolds, M. R., Keith, T. Z., Patel, P. G., & Ridley, K. P. (2008). Sex differences in latent general and broad cognitive abilities for children and youth: Evidence from higher-order MG-MACS and MIMIC models. *Intelligence, 36*, 236–260.

Rubin, D. B. (1976). Inference and missing data. *Biometrika, 63*, 581–592.

Schafer, J. L., & Graham, J. W. (2002). Missing data: Our view of the state of the art. *Psychological Methods, 7*, 147–177.

Shrout, P. E., & Bolger, N. (2002). Mediation in experimental and nonexperimental studies: New procedures and recommendations. *Psychological Methods, 7*, 422–445.

Spearman, C. (1927). *The abilities of man: Their nature and measurement*. Caldwell, NJ: Blackburn Press.

Steiger, J. H. (1998). A note on multiple sample extensions of the RMSEA fit index. *Structural Equation Modeling: A Multidisciplinary Journal, 5*, 411–419.

Steiger, J. H., & Lind, J. (1980, June). *Statistically based tests for the number of common factors*. Paper presented at the annual meeting of the Psychometric Society, Iowa City, IA.

Thompson, B. (1995). Stepwise regression and stepwise discriminant analysis need not apply here: A guidelines editorial. *Educational and Psychological Measurement, 55*, 525–534.

Turrisi, R., & Jaccard, J. (2003). *Interaction effects in multiple regression* (Vol. 72). Thousand Oaks, CA: Sage.

Watkins, M. W., Wilson, S. M., Kotz, K. M., Carbone, M. C., & Babula, T. (2006). Factor structure of the Wechsler Intelligence Scale for Children–4th Edition among referred students. *Educational and Psychological Measurement, 66*, 975–983.

Widaman, K. F. (2007). Common factors versus components: Principals and principles, errors, and misconceptions. In R. Cudeck & R. C. MacCallum (Eds.), *Factor analysis at 100: Historical developments and future directions* (pp. 177–203). Mahwah, NJ: Erlbaum.

Widaman, K. F., & Reise, S. P. (1997). Exploring the measurement invariance of psychological instruments: Applications in the substance use domain. In K. J. Bryant, & M. Windle (Eds.), *The science of prevention: Methodological advances from alcohol and substance abuse research* (pp. 281–324). Washington, DC: American Psychological Association.

Wolfle, D. (1940). *Factor analysis to 1940*. Chicago: The University of Chicago Press.

Wothke, W. (2000). Longitudinal and multi-group modeling with missing data. In T. D. Little, K. U. Schnabel, & J. Baumert (Eds.), *Modeling longitudinal and multiple group data: Practical issues, applied approaches, and specific examples* (pp. 219–240). Hillsdale, NJ: Erlbaum.

Yung, Y.-F., Thissen, D., & McLeod, L. D. (1999). On the relationship between the higher-order factor model and the hierarchical factor model. *Psychometrika, 64*, 113–128.

Psychometric Versus Actuarial Interpretation of Intelligence and Related Aptitude Batteries

Gary L. Canivez

Abstract

Interpretation of intelligence tests involves making various inferences about the individual based on their performance. Because there are many different scores within intelligence tests reflecting different levels (Full Scale, factors, subtests) and there are many different comparisons provided in test manuals and the extant literature, there is a multitude of possible inferences. This chapter is concerned with reviewing the various available scores and comparisons with suggested interpretations and a review of the empirical investigations of their psychometric fitness (reliability, validity, utility). Differentiation of psychometric interpretation versus actuarial interpretation methods is presented, as well as a review of research related to each. Most intelligence test interpretation methods are considered psychometric in nature, and most lack sufficient reliability, validity, or utility for individual clinical use; improvements in the clinical assessment of intelligence may result from greater development and use of actuarial approaches.

Key Words: intelligence test interpretation, reliability, validity, utility, actuarial decision-making, clinical decision-making

Introduction

Interpretation of intelligence tests involves drawing inferences about an individual based on scores obtained on a particular test. Because contemporary intelligence tests provide many different types of scores, there is a variety of inferences that could be made about any individual. Furthermore, various intelligence tests are constructed to reflect different theories of intelligence or cognitive abilities, and interpretations may also be based on the particular theory upon which the test is based. While a test may be created to reflect a particular theory, clinicians may also apply alternate or competing theories in the interpretation of test scores. Legitimate inferences about an individual from various intelligence test scores or procedures, however, must *each* be supported by reliability, validity, and utility research on the various scores, comparisons, and their uses.

Standards for Educational and Psychological Testing (American Educational Research Association, American Psychological Association, and the National Council on Measurement in Education [AERA, APA, NCME], 1999) provides numerous guidelines for considering the reliability and validity of test scores that should be applied to intelligence test scores. Such guidelines apply to test authors and publishers, but ultimately it is the test user who must decide which test scores, comparisons, and procedures possess sufficient evidence of reliability and validity to report and interpret. Test scores that do not possess adequate reliability, validity, and utility will lead the test user to make inaccurate and inappropriate inferences about the individual when interpreting those test scores and comparisons. Such inaccurate and inappropriate inferences may well lead to recommendations for classification, diagnosis, or treatment that may also be wrong. Weiner (1989) cogently noted that in order to practice in an ethical manner, psychologists must "(a) know what their tests can do and (b) act accordingly" (p. 829). Numerous ethical standards also concern the use of tests and measurement procedures in clinical practice (APA, 2010; National Association of School Psychologists [NASP], 2010).

Interpretation of intelligence tests may involve description of the individual's performance, prediction of the individual's performance in related areas such as classroom learning or performance on academic achievement tests, classification or diagnosis of the individual, and informing or recommending treatments. Each of these "interpretations" requires empirical support for appropriate use. With respect to individual test scores, it has been argued that if a score is to be used for individual decisions or clinical decision-making, reliability indices should meet or exceed .85 (Hills, 1981) or .90 (Aiken, 2000; Guilford & Fruchter, 1978; Nunnally & Bernstein, 1994; Ponterotto & Ruckdeschel, 2007; Salvia & Ysseldyke, 1988, 2001). Specific inferences about the individual are tied more to the various estimates of the validity of test scores and their diagnostic utility; however, scores that lack sufficient reliability cannot be valid or of diagnostic utility. It is within this framework that psychometric and actuarial intelligence test interpretations are examined.

History of IQ Test Interpretations

Kamphaus, Winsor, Rowe, and Kim (2005) provided a useful description of the history of intelligence test interpretation. The earliest application of intelligence test interpretation was associated with a classification of the individual's test score (and thus the individual) according to descriptive terms based on the overall test score and prediction of school functioning. The earliest classification systems contained descriptive terms (viz., "idiots," "imbeciles," "morons"; Levine & Marks, 1928) that are considered pejorative by today's standards. Each intelligence test presently published also contains descriptive classifications for test score ranges, and these are frequently the first "interpretation" made. Kamphaus et al. also noted that present-day descriptive terms typically reflect some aspect of score deviation from the average range, but each test contains somewhat different descriptors and may include different score ranges. While the earliest intelligence tests provided one overall test score (i.e., IQ), present-day intelligence tests contain numerous scores reflecting different levels of the test. Such scores include an overall, omnibus Full Scale score; several factor-based scores or indexes; subtest scores; ipsative or deviation scores derived from comparing subtest or factor scores to the individual's overall mean score; and theoretically or logically combined subtest composite scores.

Kamphaus et al. (2005, p. 26) referred to a "second wave" of test interpretation proposed by Rapaport, Gil, and Schafer (1945–1946) that ushered in an approach to intelligence test interpretation still in use by many today. The approach advocated by Rapaport et al. was that of going beyond the overall, omnibus Full Scale IQ and examining the shape of the subtest profile to provide a description of subtest highs and lows for the individual. These strengths and weaknesses were presumed to reflect some aspect of psychopathology as well as consideration for intervention. Wechsler's examination (1944) of differences between verbal and performance scales as well as subtest profile shape and deviations was also included in this second wave and reflected Wechsler's clinical approach to test interpretation. This is in contrast to Wechsler's note that subtests are merely different practical estimates for measuring general intelligence.

Criticism of these early interpretation methods on empirically based psychometric grounds led to what Kamphaus et al. (2005) referred to as the "third wave," wherein application of psychological measurement methods was used to evaluate various intelligence test scores and interpretation methods. Cohen's investigation (1959) of the factor structure of the Wechsler Intelligence Scale for Children (WISC; Wechsler, 1949) was one of the first of its kind and provided an empirical means for identifying subtest association to factors or dimensions underlying the WISC. While Wechsler assigned WISC subtests to the verbal or performance scale based on subtest content, Cohen's factor analysis empirically assigned subtests to factors based on their shared variance, and resulted in the three-factor structure (Verbal Comprehension, Perceptual Organization, and Freedom from Distractability) of the WISC. Cohen was critical of WISC subtest scores based on the high levels of shared variance and low subtest specificity (non-error variance unique to the subtest). Subsequently, this three-factor structure was frequently replicated with other samples and Cohen's WISC factor names were retained in both the second (WISC-R; Wechsler, 1974) and third editions of the WISC (WISC-III; Wechsler, 1991). Kaufman (1979) provided a means for calculating scores for the three factors to provide more factorially pure scores than the VIQ and PIQ.

Kaufman's significant influence on intelligence test interpretation is reflected in the hierarchical and sequential process of interpretation and subtest analyses (Kaufman, 1979, 1994; Kaufman & Lichtenberger, 2000, 2006) frequently taught in graduate programs and used by practitioners (Alfonso, Oakland, LaRocca, & Spanakos, 2000; Groth-Marnat, 1997; Kaufman, 1994; Pfeiffer, Reddy, Kletzel, Schmelzer, & Boyer, 2000). Levels of test interpretation were ordered from the most reliable and valid scores (Full Scale IQ and composite scores) to the least reliable and valid scores (single subtest scores). Kaufman's approach continued the clinical interpretation method of unique profile shape (subtest strengths and weaknesses) much like that of Rapaport et al. (1945–1946), but his profile interpretation method of comparing an individual's subtest scores to their own overall mean performance was through the identification of statistically significant strengths and weaknesses and consideration of base rates. This ipsative approach examines intraindividual differences and is an *ideographic* interpretation approach, in contrast to the *nomothetic* interpretation approach (normative comparisons) provided by the standard scores of intelligence tests. Sattler (1982, 1988, 1992, 2001, 2008) and Sattler and Ryan (2009) also provided for similar intelligence test interpretations based on a sequential order from the global score to subtest comparisons.

Reliability and validity research highlighting major problems with ipsative comparisons and profile interpretations (discussed in detail later in this chapter) led to what Kamphaus et al. (2005) referred to as the "fourth wave" where intelligence theory was applied to intelligence test construction and interpretations. The earliest intelligence tests were seemingly constructed from a pragmatic perspective and some would say atheoretical. Thorndike (1990, p. 226) noted Alfred Binet was "theoretically agnostic" with regard to the Binet-Simon scale. Zachary (1990) noted David Wechsler's minimal explication of theory in constructing the original Wechsler-Bellevue (WB) scales in 1939. However, as several have pointed out, when constructing and modifying his tests, Wechsler used Spearman's (1904, 1927) theory of general intelligence (*g*) and was also influenced by other contemporary intelligence theories (Saklofske, 2008; Tulsky et al., 2003; Zhu & Weiss, 2005). Wechsler's definition of *intelligence* (i.e., "global capacity"; Wechsler, 1939, p. 229) also reflected Spearman's *g*.

Contemporary intelligence tests are now greatly influenced by theories of intelligence or models of intelligence measurement in their construction and interpretation. Presently, one of the most influential models of intellectual measurement is that of Carroll (1993, 1995, 1997a, 2003), which proposes that intelligence tests measure various intellectual abilities that are hierarchically ordered. Carroll's (1993, 2003) three-stratum theory of cognitive abilities proposes some 50–60 narrow abilities (Stratum I) at the bottom (subtests), 8–10 broad-ability factors (Stratum II) in the middle (first-order factors), and the general ("g") ability factor (Stratum III) at the top (second-order factor) and reflected by the overall FSIQ or global IQ. Many contemporary intelligence tests are constructed to reflect Carroll's model of intelligence measurement either explicitly or implicitly. The American Psychological Association task force study of intelligence (Neisser et al., 1996) noted that the hierarchical nature of intelligence measurement was the most widely accepted view, and this still appears to be true.

Another theoretical perspective of intelligence measurement closely related to, and preceding that of Carrol, is the Gf-Gc theory of Cattell and Horn (Cattell, 1943; Horn, 1988, 1991; Horn & Cattell, 1966; Horn & Noll, 1997). Cattell and Horn's Gf-Gc theory describes aspects of reasoning abilities that allow the individual to solve novel problems (*fluid intelligence* [Gf]) and abilities acquired through the individual's exposure to aspects of their culture such as language and educational experiences (*crystallized intelligence* [Gc]). Extension of Gf-Gc theory by Horn (1991) and Horn and Noll (1997) is similar to that of Carroll with some 8–9 or more broad dimensions but does not include higher-order *g*, arguing there was insufficient construct validity evidence for singular *g*.

Cattell-Horn-Carroll (CHC) theory is an approach wherein researchers melded the work of Cattell and Horn with that of Carroll (Evans, Floyd, McGrew, & Leforgee, 2001; Flanagan, 2000; McGrew, 2005), but this is an odd combination, given that Carroll provided evidence for higher-order *g* while Horn argued that singular *g* did not exist and was a statistical artifact. Carroll's model, Cattell and Horn's model, or the combined CHC model are often cited as theoretical foundations or influences in present versions of intelligence tests such as the Wechsler Intelligence Scale for Children–Fourth Edition (WISC-IV: Wechsler, 2003), Wechsler Adult Intelligence Scale–Fourth Edition (WAIS-IV: Wechsler, 2008a), Stanford-Binet

Intelligence Scales–Fifth Edition (SB-5: Roid, 2003a), Differential Ability Scales–Second Edition (DAS-II: Elliott, 2007a), Wide Range Intelligence Test (WRIT: Glutting, Adams, & Sheslow, 2000a), Reynolds Intellectual Assessment Scales (RIAS: Reynolds & Kamphaus, 2003), Kaufman Adolescent and Adult Intelligence Test (KAIT: Kaufman & Kaufman, 1993), and Kaufman Assessment Battery for Children–Second Edition (KABC-II: Kaufman & Kaufman, 2004a).

Luria's neuropsychological theory was the foundation for the development of the Kaufman Assessment Battery for Children (K-ABC; Kaufman & Kaufman, 1983) and later, the development of the Planning, Attention, Simultaneous, Successive (PASS) theory (Das, Naglieri, & Kirby, 1994) which is the foundation for the Cognitive Assessment System (CAS: Naglieri & Das, 1997a). While the KABC-II is linked to and can be interpreted according to CHC theory, it is also linked to and can be interpreted according to Luria's theory through its dual theoretical foundation (Kaufman & Kaufman, 2004a). CAS interpretation follows the PASS theory and is related to Luria's three functional units of the brain (Naglieri, 1997; Naglieri & Das, 1990, 1997b).

Kamphaus et al. (2005) noted that, in practice, clinicians frequently interpret not only the overall Full Scale/Composite intelligence test score, which is an estimate of Spearman's g (Spearman 1904, 1927) and the apex of Carroll's hierarchy (1993), but also interpret factor-based scores *and* ability profiles produced from subtest strengths and weaknesses. These subtest profile-interpretation systems (Flanagan & Kaufman, 2004; Kaufman, 1994; Kaufman & Lichtenberger, 2000; Sattler, 2001, 2008; Sattler & Ryan, 2009) are exceedingly popular in psychology training and clinical practice (Alfonso et al., 2000; Groth-Marnat, 1997; Kaufman, 1994; Pfeiffer et al., 2000).

Despite their popularity, clinicians *must* confront the issue of whether there is sufficient empirical support for *all* these interpretation methods and the resulting inferences. While many test publishers, test authors, workshop presenters, and textbook authors present all the above methods for interpreting intelligence tests and argue for their utility, it is the test user who must decide which methods have adequate reliability, validity, and utility for clinical application and making inferences and decisions about the individual they assess. By interpreting all such scores, the clinician is adding (or replacing) interpretations beyond the overall Full Scale score

and thus, knowledge of such score interpretation improvement *beyond* the overall IQ score is imperative (Brody, 1985). Furthermore, interpretation of scores at every level of the test ignores the fact that scores at the subtest and factor level are themselves correlated and *not* independent, representing mixtures of g and subtest variance (Carroll, 1993). These and other critically important interpretation issues are further explicated throughout this chapter.

Psychometric Interpretation Methods

Descriptions of intelligence test interpretation methods from stage one through stage four (Kamphaus et al., 2005) are ostensibly *psychometric* interpretation methods. Interpretations based on psychometric grounds are interpretations based on various scores provided by the intelligence test as well as derived scores or comparisons of different scores. These scores can be used in descriptive (level of performance), predictive (estimate of performance on related variable), and classificatory (assignment to diagnostic group) ways. Clinicians use test scores and analysis information as well as test session observations, background information, interview information, etc., and make a clinical decision, judgement, or inference regarding the individual. Such decisions might be considered *clinical* decisions rather than *actuarial* (statistical) decisions because it is the clinician's *judgement* of meaning of the score(s) that guides the interpretation (decision) rather than strict adherence to a statistically based (formula) interpretation (decision) (Meehl, 1954, 1957; Meehl & Rosen, 1955).

Intelligence test scores are (or can be) associated with a hierarchical model similar to Carroll's (1993, 2003) Stratum III (omnibus, Full Scale score), Stratum II (factor-based scores), or Stratum I (subtest scores). These scores are standardized scores and reflect comparison to the normative group appropriate for the individual. Interpretations from the standardized scores are nomothetic and allow for understanding how the individual performed relative to others their age in the population. Other derived scores such as ipsative factor score comparison, pairwise factor score comparisons, ipsative subtest comparisons, and pairwise subtest comparisons are rooted in the clinical intelligence test interpretation approaches articulated by Rapaport et al. (1945–1946), Kaufman (1979, 1994), Kaufman and Lichtenberger (2000, 2006), Sattler (1982, 1988, 1992, 2001, 2008), and Sattler and Ryan (2009) and are ideographic. These are comparisons of the individual to himself or herself. Another means by which clinicians may interpret scores from intelligence tests is the combination of various subtest scores into composite scores based on some logical or theoretical connection (Kaufman, 1994; Kaufman and Lichtenberger, 2000, 2006; Sattler, 2001, 2008; Sattler & Ryan, 2009).

Finally, some have argued that no single intelligence test adequately measures all of Carroll's (1993, 2003) Stratum II dimensions, or Horn and Noll's (1997) Gf–Gc factors, and in order to better assess these broad intelligence dimensions, subtests from different intelligence tests should be combined in what is referred to as "cross-battery assessment" (Flanagan & McGrew, 1997; Flanagan & Ortiz, 2001; Flanagan, Ortiz, & Alfonso, 2008; McGrew & Flanagan, 1998). Cross-battery assessment is rooted in the aforementioned CHC theory. Such cross-battery assessment is proposed to better account for an individual's varied broad abilities (Stratum II) in cognitive assessment; which in turn is used to understand their educational difficulties, provide better differential diagnosis, and guide interventions. While the cross-battery assessment approach attempts to improve assessment of cognitive abilities and has intuitive appeal, there are numerous substantial psychometric problems cogently pointed out by Glutting, Watkins, and Youngstrom (2003), which have yet to be adequately empirically addressed. Other issues noted later in this chapter also have implications for such interpretations. Thus, individual clinical use of such cross-battery interpretation methods is not recommended.

Examination of psychometric interpretation methods proceeds in order of the hierarchy and structure of intelligence tests (Carroll, 1993, 1995; Neisser et al., 1996). This order also parallels the psychometric interpretation procedures recommended by Kaufman (Flannagan & Kaufman, 2004; Kaufman, 1994; Kaufman & Lichtenberger, 2002, 2006) and Sattler (Sattler, 2008; Sattler & Ryan, 2009) as well as contemporary intelligence test authors through their test technical and interpretation manuals.

Global IQ Score Interpretation/Stratum III

The first level of intelligence test interpretation involves the reporting and description of the overall, omnibus, global, or Full Scale score; which is measured or estimated by two or more subtests within the scale. Full Scale scores represent an estimate of g or Spearman's general intelligence factor (Spearman, 1904, 1927), which is the apex of Carroll's (1993, 1995) hierarchical model. Substantial evidence for interpretation of global Full Scale scores (g estimates) exists (Gottfredson, 2002, 2008; Jensen, 1998; Kubiszyn et al., 2000; Lubinski, 2000; Lubinski & Humphreys, 1997; Neisser et al., 1996).

Interpretation of Full Scale scores typically begins with a presentation and description of the standard score, percentile rank, and confidence interval (obtained score or estimated true score) for the standard score to account for measurement error, consistent with *Standards for Educational and Psychological Testing* (AERA, APA, NCME, 1999). Classification of the Full Scale score within a descriptive category (or range of descriptive categories around the confidence interval) reflecting some deviation from average is also frequently made (i.e., average, above average, significantly below average). These normative descriptors are intended to provide an illustration of how the individual performed relative to others their age. This is necessary given the interval level measurement such standardized scores represent.

Another aspect of interpretation of the Full Scale score is an inference as to what to expect from the individual in regard to their acquisition of academic skills (i.e., academic achievement). The predictive validity of intelligence test Full Scale scores is well documented (Bracken & Walker, 1997; Brody, 2002; Brown, Reynolds, & Whitaker, 1999; Flanagan, Andrews & Genshaft, 1997; Gottfredson, 2008, Konold & Canivez, 2010; Naglieri & Bornstein, 2003) and intelligence is a construct that precedes and influences the development of academic achievement because as Jensen (1998) noted "school learning itself is g-demanding" (p. 279). Watkins, Lei, and Canivez (2007) also demonstrated that verbal and perceptual measures of intelligence (WISC-III) predicted future academic achievement in reading and mathematics but reading and mathematics *did not* predict future measured intelligence, thus supporting Jensen's position of the temporal precedence and influence of intelligence on academic achievement.

Full Scale scores are also used in making classification or diagnostic decisions regarding psychopathology, disability, and giftedness. Classification or diagnosis of mental retardation (MR)/intellectual disability (ID) requires by definition "significantly subaverage general intellectual functioning" (Public Law 108–446 [IDEIA]; U. S. Department of Education, 2006, p. 46756) or "significantly subaverage intellectual functioning" (APA, 2000, p. 49). It is generally agreed that a score 2 *SD* below the population mean would satisfy this criterion. Historically, the operational definition for classifying specific learning disability (SLD), according to IDEA prior to IDEIA 2004, involved first a severe discrepancy between predicted academic achievement given a certain level of intelligence and actual academic achievement. This criterion was concerned with the *unexpectedly* low achievement associated with the concept of learning disability (Reynolds, 1984). While federal law no longer mandates the use of the severe discrepancy criterion, states may allow local school districts to continue using this criterion in SLD classification (IDEIA 2004) and predicted (expected) achievement is based on a person's general intellectual ability. DSM-IV-TR (APA, 2000) specifies individually measured achievement from a standardized test that "is substantially below that expected given the person's chronological age, measured intelligence, and age-appropriate education" (p. 53, p. 54, p. 56) for classification of its SLD type disorders (viz., Reading Disorder, Mathematics Disorder, Disorder of Written Expression, respectively). Assessment for intellectual giftedness also has implications for intelligence testing and it is generally thought that a Full Scale intelligence test score 2*SD* above the population mean would satisfy the criterion of significantly above average intelligence.

GLOBAL SCORE PSYCHOMETRIC SUPPORT

Psychometric support for Full Scale IQ, or related omnibus scores, is strong and includes the highest internal consistency estimates, short-term temporal stability, long-term temporal stability, and predictive validity coefficients (Bracken & McCallum, 1998b; Canivez & Watkins, 1998; Elliott, 2007b; Glutting, Adams, & Sheslow, 2000b; Kaufman & Kaufman, 1983, 1993, 2004a, 2004b; Naglieri & Das, 1997b; The Psychological Corporation, 1999; Reynolds & Kamphaus, 2003; Roid, 2003b; Wechsler, 2002a, 2002b, 2003, 2008b; Wechsler & Naglieri, 2006; Woodcock, McGrew, & Mather, 2001). In studies of long-term temporal stability of WISC-III IQ scores, the Full Scale IQ possessed the highest stability coefficient of all scores available and this also held across a variety of demographic variables (sex, age, race/ethnicity, disability) (Canivez & Watkins, 1998, 1999, 2001). Similar results were also reported by Krohn and Lamp (1999) for the K-ABC and Stanford-Binet Intelligence Scale: Fourth Edition (SB:FE: Thorndike, Hagen, & Sattler, 1986). These are expected findings according to true score theory, and reflect the power of aggregate scores that contain less error variance. Assessing temporal stability

is important as it addresses one of the major sources of error variance in intelligence tests not addressed by the internal consistency estimate (Hanna, Bradley, & Holen, 1981). Hanna et al. also noted the importance of assessing intelligence test measurement error related to scoring and administration errors.

IQ tests have a rich history of accounting for meaningful levels of academic achievement variance (Brody, 2002; Naglieri & Bornstein, 2003), with average IQ-achievement correlations near .55 across age groups (Neisser et al., 1996; Brody, 2002). Thorndike (1986) also noted approximately 85% to 90% of predictable criterion variable variance is accounted for by a single general score. Among co-normed intelligence and achievement tests it is quite common to observe concurrent IQ-achievement correlations near .70. It is often said that the most important application of intelligence tests is their ability to forecast student achievement (Brown, Reynolds, & Whitaker, 1999; Weiss & Prifitera, 1995) and the prediction of school performance with intelligence tests has been a primary use since the creation of the first Binet-Simon Scale of Intelligence (Binet & Simon, 1905).

Broad Factor/Verbal-Nonverbal Score Interpretation/Stratum II

VERBAL VS. NONVERBAL ASSESSMENT

Recognition of literacy issues affecting standardized intelligence testing was noted in the early 1900s and influenced the creation and use of the Army Alpha (verbal) and Army Beta (nonverbal) tests (Thorndike, 1997), with Yoakum and Yerkes (1920) noting the use of Army Beta for recruits who failed Army Alpha to prevent "injustice by reason of relative unfamiliarity with English" (p. 19). Wechsler (1939) also recognized the need to assess intellectual abilities through both verbal *and* nonverbal (performance) means. The selection and aggregation of subtests into composite scores were originally based on subtest task requirements, and, Wechsler noted, "the subtests are different measures of intelligence, not measures of different kinds of intelligence" (1958, p. 64). For Wechsler, verbal and performance measures were not different types of intelligence, but rather different ways to measure it. Verbal and performance measures relate to Carroll's (1993) Stratum II dimensions, which he referred to as "flavors" of g. Authors of contemporary *nonverbal* intelligence tests note that it is the method of assessment that is nonverbal rather than the cognitive process involved in solving the tasks (Bracken &

McCallum, 1998a, 1998b; Naglieri, 2003a, 2003b; Wechsler & Naglieri, 2006). Naglieri wrote, "the term *nonverbal* refers to the content of the test, not a type of ability" (2003a, p. 2). Thus, the content or demands of subtests and composites may differ but they still measure general intelligence. Spearman referred to this as the "indifference of the indicator" (1927, p. 197).

For individuals who have hearing impairments or are deaf, have receptive or expressive language deficits, or are from ethnic minority groups with limited English proficiency; nonverbal assessment of intellectual abilities is particularly useful (Bracken & McCallum, 1998b; Naglieri, 2003a). This is primarily because the verbal (English) methods would likely underestimate the intellectual abilities of such individuals. But there are other clinical groups for whom differences between verbal and nonverbal (performance) estimates have been reported or hypothesized. These include individuals with traumatic brain injury, bilingualism, autistic disorder, Asperger's disorder, and delinquents or psychopaths. Most intelligence test technical manuals (i.e., WPPSI-III, WISC-IV, WAIS-IV, KAIT, UNIT, KABC-II, DAS-II) typically provide clinical group and matched normal group comparisons in test performance that sometimes illustrate similar verbal–nonverbal differences but frequently contain small samples that are intended to be only preliminary investigations.

VERBAL–NONVERBAL (VIQ-PIQ/VCI-PRI) COMPARISONS

Kaufman and Lichtenberger (2006) devoted two chapters to VIQ and PIQ differences as they related to neuropsychology (brain functioning or injury) and clinical research and use. Many of the studies were of adults and with WB or WAIS data, but some studies were with children and adolescents and WISC data. Their review of more than 50 studies and approximately 2,700 patients who had unilateral brain damage generally supported the PIQ > VIQ for left-hemisphere lesions and VIQ > PIQ for right-hemisphere lesions on the WB, WAIS, and WAIS-R, but there was greater consistency for the right-hemisphere lesion groups. Variables that appeared to have possible moderating effects included age, sex, race or ethnicity, and educational attainment. Group difference studies are not sufficient for individual diagnostic use of such signs, and Kaufman and Lichtenberger noted calls by Matarazzo and colleagues (Bornstein & Matarazzo, 1982, 1984; Matarazzo, 1972; Matarazzo &

Herman, 1984) for due caution for such individual use of VIQ-PIQ differences by attending to base rates in the population. Furthermore, it is one thing to assess an individual with known brain injury and lesion, observe VIQ-PIQ differences of a large magnitude, and infer the likely cause for the VIQ-PIQ difference to the brain damage; but in the absence of brain injury or lesion, to infer such from VIQ-PIQ differences is a much riskier proposition.

Such inferential problems from test scores or other "signs" in psychology have been pointed out at least as far back as 1955 (Meehl & Rosen, 1955) and are also articulated by others (Lilienfeld, Wood, & Garb, 2000; McFall 2005; Swets, Dawes, & Monahan, 2000; Watkins, 2009; Watkins, Glutting, & Youngstrom, 2005) as it relates to the Reverend Thomas Bayes' (1702–1761) theorem of conditional probabilities and base rates. Leonard and Hsu (1999) and Nickerson (2004) provide excellent descriptions of Bayes' theorem (Bayes, 1763) and its implications and applications. One feature of diagnostic tests often highlighted is *sensitivity*, which indicates the probability of obtaining a positive test result, given that the person has the target disorder. However, in diagnostic use of a test, a clinician is much more interested in *positive predictive power*, or the probability of a person's having the target disorder, given a positive test result. A similar contrast is that of *specificity*, which indicates the probability of obtaining a negative test result, given that the person *does not* have the target disorder; and *negative predictive power*, the more important indicator of the probability of a person's not having the target disorder, given a negative test result. With respect to low base rates, it is difficult for tests to improve accuracy in individual cases (Lilienfeld et al., 2006; McFall, 2005; Meehl, 2001; Meehl & Rosen, 1955).

In the case of VIQ-PIQ differences and inferences regarding brain injury and function, inverse probabilities suggest that there may well be a much greater proportion of individuals with brain injury and lesions who show VIQ-PIQ differences (sensitivity) than individuals with VIQ-PIQ differences who also have brain injury and lesions (positive predictive power). Neuropsychologists are also probably more likely to see patients referred for evaluations who have brain damage and observed VIQ-PIQ (VCI-PRI) discrepancies; and while those who have brain damage are more likely to show VIQ-PIQ (VCI-PRI) discrepancies, neuropsychologists may overestimate the value of these VIQ-PIQ (VCI-PRI) differences because they are not likely to see those with VIQ-PIQ (VCI-PRI) discrepancies who do not have brain damage.

Review and summary of research provided by Kaufman and Lichtenberger (2006) regarding PIQ > VIQ for delinquents or "psychopaths" indicated that some distinct group difference studies found such differences as suggested by Wechsler (1944, 1958), but results overall were reportedly mixed. Kaufman and Lichtenberger noted that use of this PIQ > VIQ "sign" as recommended by Wechsler should not be used for individual diagnosis due to a lack of empirical support. Inconsistency of PIQ > VIQ findings for individuals with autistic disorder was also noted, in addition to small effect sizes, and thus determined to be of no diagnostic clinical use (Kaufman & Lichtenberger). More recently, a large Swedish study of individuals with Asperger's disorder, autism, or pervasive developmental disorder–not otherwise specified (PDD-NOS), based on DSM-IV criteria (American Psychiatric Association, 1994), found profile level (overall IQ) differentiated Asperger's from autism and PDD-NOS, but scatter and shape of profiles were small (Zander & Dahlgren, 2010). Within the autism group, a mean VCI-POI difference of 9 points (*SD* = 20.5) in favor of POI was observed and represented a medium effect size, but Zander and Dahlgren also noted individual profiles were too variable for individual diagnostic use of the Swedish version of the WISC-III (Wechsler, 1999) in differentiating among PDD diagnoses.

Cronbach (1990), however, noted problems with interpreting difference scores due to their low reliability. VIQ-PIQ difference scores, for example, have been shown to have poor temporal stability (too low for individual clinical use) and thus likely of questionable utility (Canivez & Watkins, 1998, 1999, 2001; Cassidy, 1997). The inference from significant VIQ-PIQ differences is that the individual has stronger cognitive skills in one area than the other, as well as giving rise to speculation as to the implications of the difference. However, if the difference score is not sufficiently reliable, it cannot be valid or of diagnostic value. Also, what such an analysis and inference ignores is the fact that VIQ and PIQ scores are not independent and such inferences from them are obscured by shared variance.

While Canivez, Neitzel, and Martin (2005) did not examine VIQ-PIQ differences in their study on relationships between the WISC-III, KBIT, Adjustment Scales for Children and Adolescents (ASCA: McDermott, Marston, & Stott, 1993), and academic achievement; with a sample (*N* = 207) of various students (non-disabled, learning disability,

mental retardation/intellectual disability, and emotional disability); additional VIQ-PIQ analyses of this dataset were conducted for this chapter. Correlations between VIQ-PIQ discrepancies and all ASCA syndromes (core and supplementary) and global adjustment scales ranged from –.004 to .056 (*p* >.05) and ranged from –.003 to .099 (*p* >.05) with measures of academic achievement. Furthermore, there were no significant differences in VIQ-PIQ discrepancies between the four diagnostic groups. Glutting, Youngstrom, Oakland, and Watkins (1996) also examined relations between WISC-III scores and ASCA (and other measures) and found low WISC-III IQ and index score correlations ranging from –.27 to .18 (M_r = –.04) across all ASCA syndromes and global adjustment scales.

While some research may indicate distinct group differences with respect to VIQ > PIQ or PIQ > VIQ, this is necessary but not sufficient for individual diagnostic utility, and until such diagnostic utility is demonstrated in differentiating individuals within these groups, clinicians should not assume that a VIQ/VCI and PIQ/POI/PRI difference is an indicator, marker, or sign for that diagnostic group. Study of distinct clinical groups may well reflect the problem of inverse probabilities where members of a distinct group may likely demonstrate VIQ-PIQ "signs" (sensitivity), but those who demonstrate VIQ-PIQ "signs" may not necessarily be members of that distinct clinical group (positive predictive power). Kaufman and Lichtenberger (2006) noted that, "when evaluating V–P differences for individuals instead of groups, extreme caution must be exercised" (p. 316). In the absence of diagnostic utility research affirming the diagnostic utility of scores for individual diagnostic purposes (especially their positive predictive power), interpretation of those scores should probably be curtailed.

FACTOR/BROAD-ABILITY SCORE COMPARISONS

Beginning with the WISC-IV, revised Wechsler scales no longer provide VIQ and PIQ scores and now only report factor index scores as Stratum II abilities, as they are more factorially pure indexes of latent abilities. Like Full Scale scores, interpretation of factor or broad-ability scores typically first involves a presentation and description of the standard score, percentile rank, and confidence interval (obtained score or estimated true score) for each standard score to account for measurement error (AERA, APA, NCME, 1999). Classification of factor or broad-ability scores within a descriptive category (or range of descriptive categories around the confidence interval) reflecting some deviation from average is also frequently made (i.e., "average," "below average," "significantly above average"). Like Full Scale scores, these normative descriptors are intended to provide an illustration of how the individual performed relative to others their age and are a function of the interval level measurement the standardized scores represent.

Because there are multiple factor or broad-ability scores, test authors and publishers provide in their respective manuals procedures for comparing these scores to each other. Tables of critical values of difference scores as well as base rates for differences are presented in test manuals and provide clinicians a convenient way to determine which factor or broad-ability scores differ and how rare such a difference was in the standardization sample. Like VIQ-PIQ differences, the inference from significant differences between factor or broad-ability scores is that the individual has stronger cognitive skills in one area than the other and there is speculation as to the implications of these strengths and weaknesses. Factor or broad difference scores that are not sufficiently reliable cannot be valid or of value. Like the VIQ and PIQ scores, factor or broad area scores are not independent and inferences from them are also obscured by shared variance.

FACTOR/BROAD-ABILITY PSYCHOMETRIC SUPPORT

Psychometrically, factor scores or broad-ability scores typically have internal consistency estimates, short-term stability estimates, and predictive validity coefficients that are generally lower than the Full Scale score but higher than individual subtest scores (Bracken & McCallum, 1998b; Elliott, 2007b; Glutting, Adams, & Sheslow, 2000b; Kaufman & Kaufman, 1983, 1993, 2004a, 2004b; Naglieri & Das, 1997b; The Psychological Corporation, 1999; Reynolds & Kamphaus, 2003; Roid, 2003b; Wechsler, 1997, 2002a, 2002b, 2003, 2008b; Wechsler & Naglieri, 2006; Woodcock et al., 2001). This is expected, as true score theory predicts that scores with more items and subtests will have less error variance and thus greater reliability and true score variance. This also means that factor scores or broad-ability scores typically include more error variance than the Full Scale score. However, some factor scores or broad-ability scores have better reliability estimates than others, partly related to the number of subtests (and items) that comprise the factor-based score. In long-term stability studies of the WISC-III (Canivez & Watkins, 1998, 1999,

2001) for example, it was found that across the total sample and across age, sex, race or ethnicity, and disability groups that the VCI, POI, FDI, and PSI scores had lower stability coefficients than the FSIQ but more importantly, only the VCI and POI scores showed long-term temporal stability coefficients close to being high enough for individual interpretation or decision-making ($r \geq .85$; Hills, 1981; $r \geq .90$; Aiken, 2000; Guilford & Fruchter, 1978; Nunnally & Bernstein, 1994; Ponterotto & Ruckdeschel, 2007; Salvia & Ysseldyke, 1988, 2001). The FDI and PSI score stability coefficients were too low (too unstable) for individual clinical use. Similar results were also obtained by Krohn and Lamp (1999) for the K-ABC and SB:FE.

FACTORIAL/STRUCTURAL VALIDITY

While some factor-based scores might possess acceptable reliability coefficients (internal consistency, short-term stability, long-term stability) and reliability is a foundation for possible score validity, validity is ultimately more important. Also, "validity is always *specific to some particular use or interpretation*" (Linn & Gronlund, 1995, p. 49). Investigations of the internal or structural validity of intelligence tests is often conducted via factor analyses (exploratory [EFA] *and* confirmatory [CFA]), but recently, some intelligence test authors and publishers (Elliott, 2007b; Roid, 2003b, Wechsler, 2008b; McGrew & Woodcock, 2001) opted to report only results from CFA. This is in contrast to previous practice (and some current practice) wherein both EFA *and* CFA results were both reported (Bracken & McCallum, 1998b; Elliott, 1990; Glutting et al., 2000b; Kaufman & Kaufman, 1993; Naglieri & Das, 1997b; Wechsler, 1991, 2002a, 2002b; Wechsler & Naglieri, 2006). Gorsuch (1983) noted the complimentary nature of EFA and CFA, suggesting that greater confidence in the internal structure of a test is obtained when EFA and CFA are in agreement. As noted by Frazier and Youngstrom (2007), there is good cause for concern regarding the disagreement between the number of latent factors reported in contemporary intelligence tests based only on CFA procedures (or the most liberal EFA factor-extraction criteria) and the number of factors suggested with EFA procedures using the most psychometrically sound methods for determining the correct number of factors to extract and retain. For example, DiStefano and Dombrowski (2006) and Canivez (2008) provided markedly different results for the SB-5 than the CFA results presented in its technical manual (Roid, 2003b).

Another EFA approach to investigate the internal structure of intelligence tests is the Schmid and Leiman (1957) procedure, which was recommended by Carroll (1993, 1995, 1997a, 2003); McClain (1996); Gustafsson and Snow (1997); Carretta and Ree (2001); Ree, Carretta, and Green (2003); and Thompson (2004). Because the narrow abilities (subtests) and broad abilities (factors) are themselves correlated, subtest performance on cognitive abilities tests reflect combinations or mixtures of both first-order *and* second-order factors. Carroll argued that variance from the second-order factor should be extracted first to residualize the first-order factors, leaving them orthogonal to each other and the second-order factor. Thus, variability associated with the higher-order factor is accounted for prior to interpreting variability in the lower-order factors. In this way, it is possible to see how the reliable test variance is partitioned to higher- and lower-order dimensions. However, almost no test manuals provide these analyses for practitioners to review.

When the Schmid and Leiman (1957) procedure has been used with contemporary intelligence tests, the higher-order factor (g) accounted for the largest portion of variance, and considerably smaller portions of variance remained at the lower-order (factors) level (Bracken & McCallum, 1998b; Canivez, 2008, 2011; Canivez, Konold, Collins, & Wilson, 2009; Canivez & Watkins, 2010a, 2010b; Domrowski & Watkins, in press; Dombrowski, Watkins, & Brogan, 2009; Nelson & Canivez, 2012; Nelson, Canivez, Lindstrom, & Hatt, 2007; Watkins, 2006; Watkins, Wilson, Kotz, Carbone, & Babula, 2006). This is one reason the primary (if not exclusive) interpretation should be at the Full Scale score level. Clinicians *should be* provided such information about the portions of test variance captured at the different levels of the test in test manuals to facilitate decisions about the importance of the different dimensions and what should be interpreted. Unfortunately, this information is absent from most contemporary intelligence test technical manuals. However, decisions about the validity and interpretation of intelligence tests cannot be sufficiently answered or resolved using only structural validity or internal structure perspective (EFA or CFA) (Canivez et al., 2009; Carroll, 1997b; Kline, 1994; Lubinski & Dawis, 1992).

FACTOR/BROAD-ABILITY INCREMENTAL VALIDITY

When considering intelligence test validity and interpretation across multiple levels and scores from a test, it is critical to consider the *external* validity investigations such as predictive validity and incremental validity of lower-level scores beyond that of higher-level scores (Haynes & Lench, 2003; Hunsley, 2003; Hunsley & Meyer, 2003). In this way the relative importance of factor scores versus the global Full Scale score may be assessed. However, *validity* should not be confused with *diagnostic utility* (Meehl, 1959; Mullins-Sweatt & Widiger, 2009; Wiggins, 1988), as the latter is concerned with the application of test score interpretation to the individual. It follows that construct validity and criterion-related validity, Cronbach and Meehl (1955) preferred construct validity, are a prerequisite without which utility is not possible.

A major aspect of intelligence test use is its utility in assisting in the diagnosis or classification of an individual (e.g., MR, SLD, GT). Examination of the diagnostic or predictive utility is also a prerequisite for the ethical use of test scores (Dawes, 2005). Ultimately, the greatest utility would be the ability of a test or set of variables to accurately determine the likelihood of treatment response under specified conditions (i.e., treatment validity). However, prediction is, in and of itself, important, regardless of treatment utility (Glutting, Watkins, & Youngstrom, 2003) and is frequently investigated.

The importance of incremental validity investigations in general, and in the case of multilevel intelligence test interpretation in particular, is based on an important scientific principle articulated by William of Ockham (alt. "Occam"): the law of parsimony (Occam's razor), which states "what can be explained by fewer principles is needlessly explained by more" Jones, 1952, p. 620). Thus, science favors a less complex explanation over a more complex explanation for phenomena. In the case of intelligence test interpretation, the Full Scale score, an estimate of g, is a more parsimonious index than the lower-level factor or broad-ability scores (and subtest scores) and satisfies the law of parsimony. Intelligence test Full Scale scores demonstrate substantial criterion-related validity (Neisser et al., 1996; Carroll, 1993; Gottfredson, 1997, 2008, 2009; Jensen, 1998; Lubinski, 2000; Lubinski & Humphreys, 1997), so in order for the factor scores to be relevant, they must demonstrate *meaningful* predictive validity *beyond* that afforded by the Full Scale score.

Besides describing performance on factor-based scores or broad-ability scores, clinicians are often instructed to consider predictive utility and explanation of performance in academic achievement areas reflecting the higher- and lower-order factor scores.

For example, if significant differences between factor scores exist, or if factor scores deviate from the individual's mean factor performance, that variability among factor scores suggests to some that the FSIQ is not interpretable and that the clinician must examine and interpret the examinee's unique pattern of performance on the factors or broad abilities (Flanagan & Kaufman, 2004; Hale & Fiorello, 2004; Kaufman, 1994; Kaufman & Lichtenberger, 2002, 2006; Lezak, 1995; Sattler, 2008; Sattler & Ryan, 2009; Weiss, Saklofske, & Prifitera, 2003; Wolber & Carne, 2002). Others (Gridley & Roid, 1998; Hale & Fiorello, 2004; Hildebrand & Ledbetter, 2001) have suggested that under these conditions the FSIQ would not be a valid predictor of the individual's academic achievement. Even when there are no differences among factor scores, interpretation of the factor scores may still be done. Those promoting the clinical approach to test interpretation of factor index variability often argue that, while the deviations might not be appropriate for diagnosis, the ability patterns (strengths and weaknesses) could be helpful for instructional strategies, interventions, or treatments or provide hypotheses about the individual (Flanagan & Kaufman, 2004; Kaufman, 1994; Kaufman & Lichtenberger, 2002, 2006; Sattler, 2008; Sattler & Ryan, 2009).

Whether or not such factor score differences provide useful indications for treatment, accommodations, or hypothesis-generation will, in part, be based upon their incremental validity. A primary use of intelligence tests is to predict or account for academic achievement, and if the index scores are to be of practical clinical utility, they must account for meaningful portions of achievement variance *beyond* that provided by the Full Scale score (Haynes & Lench, 2003; Hunsley & Meyer, 2003). This is a necessary, but not sufficient, condition for clinical utility and use with *individuals*. In considering incremental validity, there are two approaches that are often taken and are highly dependent upon the nature of the question being asked and the level of analysis.

In their innovative and highly influential article "Distinctions Without a Difference:...," Glutting, Watkins, Konold, and McDermott (2006) thoroughly examined the validity of observed scores *and* latent factors from the WISC-IV in estimating reading and mathematics performance on the WIAT-II using the WISC-IV—WIAT-II standardization linking sample. Both approaches are important and legitimate methods, but they answer different questions and use different statistical procedures. If one is interested in testing theory and *explaining* latent achievement constructs from latent intelligence constructs, then the use of structural equation modeling (SEM) is an appropriate statistical method (Glutting et al., 2006). However, because the latent constructs are not directly observable, *and* latent construct scores are difficult to calculate and not readily available, there are no direct practical clinical applications (Oh, Glutting, Watkins, Youngstrom, & McDermott, 2004). If one is interested in clinical application of test scores in *predicting* academic achievement from intelligence test scores, hierarchical multiple regression analysis (HMRA) is an appropriate statistical method (Glutting et al. 2006) and may be the most common statistical method in incremental validity (McFall, 2005). HMRA techniques utilize the observed IQ and factor scores that psychologists have available to them. Unlike the perfectly reliable latent constructs in SEM, in clinical assessment and interpretation for individuals, psychologists *must* use observed scores from tests, and those scores contain measurement error.

Glutting et al. (2006) demonstrated that the WISC-IV FSIQ predicted substantial portions of variance in reading and mathematics scores on the WIAT-II, but the four factor index scores (VCI, PRI, WMI, PSI) did not contribute additional meaningful prediction beyond the FSIQ. Other studies of incremental predictive validity before and after Glutting et al. (2006) provided similar results (Canivez, 2011; Freberg, Vandiver, Watkins, & Canivez, 2008; Glutting, Youngstrom, Ward, Ward, & Hale, 1997; Kahana, Youngstrom, & Glutting, 2002; Ryan, Kreiner, & Burton, 2002; Watkins, Glutting, & Lei, 2007; Youngstrom, Kogos, & Glutting, 1999). Glutting et al. concluded that their results were very like "previous epidemiological studies from both the United States and Europe that showed specific cognitive abilities add little or nothing to prediction beyond the contribution made by *g* (Jencks et al., 1979; Ree, Earles, & Treachout, 1994; Salgado, Anderson, Moscoso, Bertua, & de Fruyt, 2003; Schmidt & Hunter, 1998; Thorndike, 1986)" (2006, p. 110).

Furthermore, in their SEM analyses, Glutting et al. (2006) found only the higher-order *g* and the VC latent construct offered significant *explanations* of reading and mathematics constructs (PR, WM, and PS constructs provided no increases in explanation). Similar SEM findings were also reportedly obtained with the Woodcock-Johnson Revised Tests of Achievement (WJ-R; Woodcock & Johnson, 1989) (Keith, 1999; McGrew, Keith, Flanagan,

& Vanderwood, 1997) and with the WISC-III (Wechsler, 1991; Oh et al., 2004). Kuusinen and Leskinen (1988) and Gustafsson and Balke (1993) reportedly reached similar conclusions with other measures of ability and achievement (Glutting et al., 2006).

Why the factor scores failed to add incremental predictive validity over and above the FSIQ may relate to the earlier discussion of hierarchical EFA where the lower-order factors accounted for substantially smaller portions of reliable variance (Canivez, 2008, 2011; Canivez & Watkins, 2010a, 2010b; Nelson & Canivez, 2012; Nelson et al., 2007; Watkins, 2006; Watkins et al., 2006). If test authors and publishers are interested in improving the incremental predictive validity of cognitive tests, it may be necessary to (a) increase the number of subtests estimating the factor scores to capture more variance, and/or (b) construct cognitive subtests that contain less *g* variance (and more Stratum II or broad-ability variance). However, at present, empirical results continue to corroborate the overwhelming majority of the reliable criterion variable variance is predicted by the single Full Scale intelligence test score (Thorndike, 1986).

Multiple regression analysis research with the WJ-III cognitive clusters predicting reading (Evans, Floyd, McGrew, & Leforgee, 2001) and writing (Floyd, McGrew, & Evans, 2008) found some clusters were more important than others. However, these were not *hierarchical* multiple regression analyses first accounting for *g* and then accounting for cluster score improvement in predicting academic achievement. Thus, the incremental validity of clusters beyond *g* was not investigated. Other recent WJ-III research used SEM procedures to examine direct vs. indirect *explanations* of *g* with direct vs. indirect *explanations* of broad-ability dimensions in areas of reading decoding (Floyd, Keith, Taub, & McGrew, 2007) and mathematics achievement (Taub, Floyd, Keith, & McGrew, 2008). Both studies noted the WJ-III influences of *g* were large but indirect through the broad-ability dimensions. However, as Floyd et al. noted, the WJ-III has a problem regarding possible criterion contamination that could inflate the predictive power of some broad-ability dimensions. Determining direct vs. indirect influences of general intelligence is further complicated and unresolved due to issues of singularity, multicollinearity, and reported Heywood cases in SEM of the J-III in the Floyd et al. study (i.e., Gf–g, Glr–g, Gsm–g [three-stratum model] and Gf–g [two-stratum model]; paths at 1.0). Another

important issue remains, despite these authors' arguments for practitioner use of SEM results in informing test interpretation. Glutting et al. (2006) pointed out,

> We previously demonstrated the following: (a) The constructs from SEM rank children differently than observed scores, and children's relative position on factor-based constructs (e.g., VC) can be radically different than their standing on corresponding observed factor scores (the VCI); (b) construct scores are not readily available to psychologists; and (c) although it is possible to estimate construct scores, the calculations are difficult and laborious (cf. Oh et al., 2004, for an example). Therefore, one of the most important findings here is that psychologists cannot directly apply results from SEM. (p. 111)

Thus, SEM results provide theoretical *explanations* for relationships between the cognitive and achievement variables, but this does not mean that there is direct application in the prediction of achievement performance from the cognitive test scores. Thus, the incremental predictive validity of factor or broad-ability scores for clinical use is very much in doubt.

Perhaps the most extreme view regarding the clinical value of the FSIQ is that of Hale, Fiorello, and colleagues (Fiorello, Hale, Holdnack, Kavanagh, Terrell, & Long, 2007; Fiorello, Hale, McGrath, Ryan, & Quinn, 2001; Hale & Fiorello, 2004; Hale, Fiorello, Bertin, & Sherman, 2003; Hale, Fiorello, Kavanagh, Holdnack, & Aloe, 2007; Hale, Fiorello, Kavanagh, Hoeppner, & Gaither, 2001), who proclaimed the invalidity of the FSIQ in predicting academic achievement when significant intracognitive variability (factor or subtest scatter or variation) was observed. They argued that practitioners should "never interpret the global IQ score if there is significant scatter or score variability" (Hale & Fiorello, 2001, p. 132).

The approach that Hale, Fiorello, and colleagues used to render such a recommendation is that of regression commonality analysis of global and factor-index scores from the WISC-III (Wechsler, 1991), and achievement scores from the Wechsler Individual Achievement Test (WIAT; Wechsler, 1992). Another method (later deemed inappropriate) was their entering factor or broad-ability scores into the first block of hierarchical multiple regression and entering the Full Scale score in the second block to test how much incremental validity there is in the Full Scale score over and above the lower-order factor or broad-ability scores. This approach was criticized by Glutting et al. (2006), who wrote that while it had "intuitive appeal," and was "employed on occasion (Hale, Fiorello, Kavanagh, Hoeppner, & Gaither, 2001)" (p. 106), such use violates the law of parsimony such that psychologists would favor a more complex accounting for predictive validity rather than the less complex predictor (g) when the many factors at best only account for marginally more achievement variance.

A special issue of the journal *Applied Neuropsychology* further addressed these issues and the merits and conclusions of the approach of Hale, Fiorello, and colleagues (Reynolds, 2007). Fiorello et al. (2007) applied regression commonality analysis to WISC-IV factor index scores obtained from the 228 participants previously diagnosed with learning disability (LD), attention deficit–hyperactivity disorder (ADHD) and traumatic brain injury (TBI) from the special-groups data reported in the WISC-IV Technical Manual (Wechsler, 2003b). However, they only included participants with FSIQ scores between 80 and 120 "to ensure extreme scores did not affect study results" (Fiorello et al., 2007, p. 5). Primary conclusions of their results were that the WISC-IV FSIQ is not appropriate for interpretation for these groups (those with intracognitive variability) due to small, shared variance of the four index scores; and individual idiographic interpretation is appropriate based on sizable unique variance components.

The manuscript of Fiorello et al. (2007) was provided to several statistics and psychological measurement experts for critique and comment who provided very different assessments and conclusions. Dana and Dawes (2007); Faust (2007); and Watkins, Glutting, and Lei (2007) pointed out numerous methodological errors as well as empirical evidence arguing against the Hale, Fiorello, et al. use of regression commonality analysis. Hale et al. (2007) provided a rejoinder to address the critiques but appeared to only restate their original position rather than rebut the critiques and data presented (Dana & Dawes, 2007; Faust, 2007; Watkins et al., 2007). Daniel (2007) also provided a critique of Fiorello et al. and used a simulation study to demonstrate that high levels of index-score scatter *did not* affect the FSIQ predictive validity. Schneider (2008), quite dissatisfied with the Hale et al. (2007) rejoinder indicating they did not recognize the flaws in their analyses, provided yet another critique of the Hale, Fiorello, and colleagues' application of regression commonality analysis. Daniel (2009) also provided evidence that WISC-IV subtest or factor score

variability does not invalidate the FSIQ in predicting WIAT-II performance, as he showed in comparisons of high- and low-variability groups. In an investigation of the predictive validity of the DAS general conceptual ability index (GCA; Elliott, 1990) when significant and unusual scatter was observed, Kotz, Watkins, and McDermott (2008) found no significant differences in predicting academic achievement by the GCA across groups showing significant *and* clinically unusual differences between factors.

In summary, while factor or broad-ability scores may possess higher reliability estimates than subtest scores, and some have acceptable reliability estimates to support individual decision-making, the validity research does not provide strong enough support for their interpretations in many instances. Furthermore, this discussion was concerned with the issue of statistical incremental validity, not clinical incremental validity, which Lilienfeld, Wood, and Garb (2006) noted could negatively affect decisions based on the "dilution effect," whereby "presenting participants with accurate but nondiagnostic information… often results in less accurate judgments" (p. 11), as reported by Nisbett, Zukier, and Lemley (1981). Unless stronger support is provided for their incremental validity, clinicians should restrain their clinical interpretations to the Full Scale score in most, if not all, instances.

Subtest-Based Score Interpretation/Stratum I

Interpretation of intelligence test subtest scores is most frequently conducted through examination of subtest deviations from the individual's average subtest performance through ipsative comparisons, an ideographic procedure. As noted by Rapaport et al. (1945–1946), the examination of subtest highs and lows (strengths and weaknesses) for an individual was to provide the clinician with valuable information about the individual that could assist in diagnosis and treatment. Zeidner (2001) recommended the use of cognitive strengths and weaknesses derived from the WISC-III as the basis for psychoeducational recommendations. As with other test scores, investigation of reliability and validity of subtest scores is a requirement for determining their utility and thus interpretability.

SUBTEST PSYCHOMETRIC SUPPORT

While Full Scale scores (and some factor or broad-ability scores) demonstrate uniformly high estimates of reliability and validity, the same cannot be said for subtest scores. Great variability exists within and between various intelligence tests as to the magnitude of their subtest reliability estimates. Invariably, intelligence test subtests typically have lower internal consistency estimates than composite scores (Bracken & McCallum, 1998b; Elliott, 2007b; Glutting et al., 2000b; Kaufman & Kaufman, 1983, 1993, 2004a, 2004b; Naglieri & Das, 1997b; Psychological Corporation, 1999; Reynolds & Kamphaus, 2003; Roid, 2003b; Wechsler, 2002, 2003, 2008b; Wechsler & Naglieri, 2006; Woodcock et al., 2001). Importantly, internal consistency estimates provide the highest estimates of intelligence subtest reliability because they do not consider important sources of error such as temporal stability, scoring errors, or administration errors (Hanna et al., 1981). In examining the long-term stability of WISC-III scores, Canivez and Watkins (1998) found the stability coefficients for subtests ranged from .55 to .75; thus, none showed acceptable stability for individual clinical decision-making. Considering more stringent criteria for reliability estimates for individual clinical interpretation (Aiken, 2000; Hills, 1981; Guilford & Fruchter, 1978; Nunnally & Bernstein, 1994; Ponterotto & Ruckdeschel, 2007; Salvia & Ysseldyke, 1988, 2001), many (most) intelligence test subtests are inadequate. For the subtests with reliability coefficients (internal consistency, short-term stability, long-term stability) that meet or exceed minimum standards, it is also necessary to know how much subtest specificity exists (reliable subtest variance *unique* to that subtest). More importantly, subtest score *validity*, particularly incremental validity, must be empirically supported, or their measurement may simply be redundant.

IPSATIVE SUBTEST COMPARISONS

While interpretation of individual subtest scores in isolation is not very common, the use of intricate subtest interpretation systems (Kaufman, 1994; Kaufman & Lichtenberger, 2000, 2006; Sattler, 2001, 2008; Sattler & Ryan, 2009) is very popular, both in psychology graduate training and in clinical practice (Alfonso et al., 2000; Groth-Marnat, 1997; Kaufman, 1994; Pfeiffer et al., 2000). The argument is that if there is substantial scatter or variability among the subtests, then an IQ score (or factor score) "represents a summary of diverse abilities and does not represent a unitary entity" (Kaufman & Lichtenberger, 2000, p. 424). The specific patterns of subtest scores presumably invalidate global intelligence indices (Groth-Marnat, 1997), and subtest scores and subtest composites become the principal

focus of test interpretation. Subtests that are significantly higher or lower than the child's own average (i.e., ipsative comparisons) are deemed strengths or weaknesses; and while some authors (Kaufman & Lichtenberger, 2000; Sattler, 2008; Sattler & Ryan, 2009) point out that such ipsative or subtest comparisons are not diagnostic, they simultaneously claim that such strengths and weaknesses allow the psychologist to formulate hypotheses concerning the underlying problems and implications for the individual. Such hypotheses are then to be examined with other data sources and used for recommending educational or psychological treatment.

If these hypotheses are to be of use, they must be based on scores or results that have acceptable reliability, otherwise one may be formulating hypotheses about characteristics or possible interventions with essentially random indicators. Furthermore, "Any long-term recommendations as to a strategy for teaching a student would need to be based on aptitudes that are likely to remain stable for months, if not years" (Cronbach & Snow, 1977, p. 161). If suggestions regarding differential teaching styles, curricular materials, interventions, and learning environments (Kaufman, 1994; Kaufman & Lichtenberger, 2000; Sattler, 2008; Sattler & Ryan, 2009) are made based on subtest interpretive methods, then investigation of the reliability and validity of such subtest interpretive methods is imperative.

IPSATIVE SUBTEST COMPARISON PSYCHOMETRIC SUPPORT

Watkins (2003) provided a comprehensive and thorough review of the literature regarding intelligence test subtest analyses and noted the overwhelming shortcomings and failures of subtest analyses to reliably and validly inform psychological practice. The temporal stability of WISC-R's (Wechsler, 1974) cognitive strengths and weaknesses was examined by McDermott, Fantuzzo, Glutting, Watkins, and Baggaley (1992), who found that classification stability of the relative cognitive strengths and weaknesses identified by subtest elevations and depressions was near chance levels. Livingston, Jennings, Reynolds, and Gray (2003) also found the multivariate stability of WISC-R subtest profiles across a three-year retest interval too low for clinical use. Watkins and Canivez (2004), in examining WISC-III subtest ipsative strengths and weaknesses and numerous subtest composites across a three-year retest interval, found agreement, on average, at chance levels. Furthermore, *none* of the 66 subtest composites reached the minimum level of agreement necessary for clinical use (Cicchetti, 1994). Given the poor reliability of ipsative and subtest composite scores, that such scores or profiles would be valid and diagnostically useful is highly unlikely.

Review of the literature on subtest analysis validity and utility (Watkins, 2003; Watkins, Glutting, & Youngstrom, 2005) showed that subtest scores, patterns, and analyses were unable to adequately identify global neurocognitive or neuropsychological deficits presumably related to learning disability (Watkins, 1996), nor were they related to or valid for diagnosis of learning disabilities (Daley & Nagle, 1996; Glutting, McGrath, Kamphaus, & McDermott, 1992; Hale & Raymond, 1981; Hale & Saxe, 1983; Kahana et al., 2002; Kavale & Forness, 1984; Kline, Snyder, Guilmette, & Castellanos, 1992; Livingston et al., 2003; Maller & McDermott, 1997; Mayes, Calhoun, & Crowell, 1998; McDermott & Glutting, 1997; McDermott, Goldberg, Watkins, Stanley, & Glutting, 2006; McGrew & Knopik, 1996; Mueller, Dennis, & Short, 1986; Ree & Carretta, 1997; Smith & Watkins, 2004; Thorndike, 1986; Ward, Ward, Hatt, Young, & Mollner, 1995; Watkins, 1999, 2000, 2003, 2005; Watkins & Glutting, 2000; Watkins & Kush, 1994; Watkins, Kush, & Glutting, 1997a, 1997b; Watkins, Kush, & Schaefer, 2002; Watkins & Worrell, 2000). Furthermore, subtest analyses were not valid in the classification of behavioral, social, or emotional problems (Beebe, Pfiffner, & McBurnett, 2000; Campbell & McCord, 1996, 1999; Dumont, Farr, Willis, & Whelley, 1998; Glutting et al., 1992; Glutting et al., 1998; Lipsitz, Dworkin, & Erlenmeyer-Kimling, 1993; McDermott & Glutting, 1997; Piedmont, Sokolove, & Fleming, 1989; Reinecke, Beebe, & Stein, 1999; Riccio, Cohen, Hall, & Ross, 1997; Rispens et al., 1997; Teeter & Korducki, 1998).

Kaufman (1994) argued that an individual's cognitive pattern "becomes reliable by virtue of its cross-validation" (p. 31) if it is supported by other clinical information and observations. In Kaufman's system, clinicians are thought of as detectives attempting to make sense out of profiles and searching for clues to the individual's strengths and weaknesses within the test and also by supplemental test information (Kaufman & Lichtenberger, 2006). Dawes (1994), however, noted the difficulty (impossibility) of combining different types (and amounts) of information in clinical decision-making, but asserted that the suggestion that unreliable cognitive subtest scores or patterns become valid for the individual when informally and subjectively integrated with a complex mixture of other assessment data simply is not consistent with the empirical literature (Dawes, Faust, & Meehl, 1989). Psychologists are particularly vulnerable to errors in clinical decision-making precisely in situations such as this (Davidow & Levinson, 1993; Faust, 1986, 1990; Watkins, 2003, 2009). Thus, as Faust (1990) noted, the "common belief in the capacity to perform complex configural analysis and data integration might thus be appropriately described as a shared professional myth" (p. 478). Kaufman and Lichtenberger (2006) noted, "The validity that comes from group data may never be available for the individual profile approach that we advocate" (p. 413).

Watkins and Canivez (2004) concluded as follows:

(a) Recommendations based on unreliable ipsative subtest comparisons or subtest composites must also be unreliable;

(b) Intelligence subtest analysis procedures that lack reliability or agreement across time cannot be valid;

(c) Most students will exhibit several relative cognitive strengths and weaknesses, so their presence should not be interpreted as unusual or pathognomonic;

(d) The fact that several strengths and weaknesses will typically be observed makes it more likely that errors will result from inferring pathology from them; and

(e) Using an essentially random component (i.e., the subtest profile or subtest composite) and then searching for corroborating information, is likely to decrease the accuracy of clinical decision-making.

Meehl and Rosen (1955) noted such impacts in judgement accuracy when attempting to detect low-prevalence strengths or weaknesses. For an elaborative description of the many types of diagnostic decision-making and clinical judgment errors and how clinicians can avoid them, the reader is directed to Watkins (2009), Garb (2005), and Garb and Boyle (2003).

Despite all this negative empirical research, test authors and publishers continue to describe ipsative subtest analysis procedures in test manuals (Bracken & McCallum, 1998b; Elliott, 2007b; Glutting et al., 2000b; Kaufman & Kaufman, 1983, 1993, 2004a, 2004b; Naglieri & Das, 1997b; Reynolds & Kamphaus, 2003; Roid, 2003b; Wechsler, 2002, 2003, 2008b; Wechsler & Naglieri, 2006). Some test authors, however, have attempted to minimize their use of ipsative sub-test comparisons because of their awareness of the lack of empirical support (Glutting et al., 2000b; Reynolds & Kamphaus, 2003). Textbook authors also continue to describe and promote ipsative and subtest composite interpretations (Flanagan & Kaufman, 2004; Kaufman & Lichtenberger, 2000, 2006; Sattler, 2008; Sattler & Ryan, 2009). Continued presentation of such procedures perpetuates the decades-long shared professional myth that such analyses, in the hands of the trained and skilled clinician, provide important clues in understanding the individual examinee. Lilienfeld et al. (2006) presented several reasons why questionable psychological tests remain popular, and two in particular appear to be operating in the domain of ipsative comparisons and profile analyses in intelligence tests. They referred to the belief in special expertise and intuition in combining test scores and other information to render valid interpretations from invalid scores as "the Alchemist's Fantasy," and the influence of "Clinical Tradition and Educational Inertia" also seems to perpetuate these practices. Macmann and Barnett (1997) may well be correct in their characterization of these ipsative subtest interpretations as the "myth of the master detective" (p. 197).

Psychometric Interpretation Conclusion

Each of the psychometric interpretation methods discussed above requires the psychologist to consider the scores and render an inference or decision about the individual based on their judgment. Elliott (2007b) wrote, "Profile interpretation is clinical rather than statistical; suggestive rather than definitive; and concerned with hypothesis generation" (p. 93). However, as Dawes (1994) pointed out, "*The accuracy of the judgment of professional psychologists and other mental health workers is limited, however, by the accuracy of the techniques they employ*" (p. 107). While there is abundant research support for the clinical interpretation of omnibus, Full Scale intelligence test scores, such is not the case for clinical interpretation of factor scores; and especially subtest scores, profiles, or patterns. Clinical interpretation of intelligence test subtests is essentially the interpretation of scores that have too much error for individual use and will lead to significant errors in formulating hypotheses as well as in diagnosis and treatment recommendations. Even factor-based or broad-ability scores are questionable when their incremental predictive validity estimates are unremarkable, as previously illustrated.

At present, ample evidence for clinical interpretation of Full Scale scores from intelligence tests exists and should be the primary, if not exclusive, interpretation focus. For those promoting subtest and factor score or broad-ability score interpretations, it is incumbent on them to provide strong empirical evidence for their interpretation procedures, particularly their utility in the correct prediction of diagnostic groups or disorders, and more importantly, differential treatment (McFall, 1991, 2000). At present, such evidence does not exist.

Actuarial Interpretation Methods

Actuarial test interpretation involves a statistically based decision regarding an individual based on scores from one or more measures (one or more variables). Data could include test scores from standardized tests, but also could include ratings, interview information, and historical information. The statistical combination of available data (i.e., logistic regression, discriminant function analysis, multiple regression, etc.) optimizes the prediction. These statistical procedures are able to differentially weight variables in predictions, and only the variables that have significant contribution to prediction are retained and used. Such complex combinations of variables are something clinicians simply are unable to do (Dawes et al., 1989; Faust, 1990). Decisions one might be interested in making about an individual include classification of the individual's profile (i.e., "Which empirically based profile does the individual's profile most resemble; or is it unique?"), diagnostic or classification decisions (i.e., differential diagnosis), or determining the probability of success for a given treatment (i.e., given this individual's characteristics, treatment x is expected to produce some likely response). It is sometimes argued that, in order to make an actuarial interpretation of an intelligence test, one must have access to formulae or data that have been developed and (hopefully) cross-validated on a new sample to provide a comparison of an individual's test score(s). Such methods require available outcome data by which one may derive algorithms for comparison.

Over 50 years ago, Paul Meehl set in motion a debate on actuarial prediction (decision making) by seeking answers to questions about the relationship between clinical and actuarial (statistical) prediction in his seminal book, *Clinical versus statistical prediction: A theoretical analysis and review of the evidence* (Meehl, 1954). His self-proclaimed "wicked book" (Meehl, 1979, p. 564) or "disturbing little book" (Meehl, 1986, p. 370) reviewed and examined the clinical decision-making (prediction) abilities of clinicians versus actuarial/statistical formula–based predictions. Meehl's conclusion was that the actuarial approach was superior and should be used more frequently. Since that time, there have been numerous studies comparing clinical (informal or impressionistic) and actuarial (formal, mechanical, algorithmic) predictive methods, and it has been fairly consistently shown that the actuarial method is as accurate or more accurate than clinical methods (Dawes, Faust, & Meehl, 1989; Grove & Meehl, 1996; Grove, Zald, Lebow, Snitz, & Nelson, 2000). While 8 of the 136 studies in the Grove et al. (2000) meta-analysis showed superiority of the clinical method, 7 of the 8 benefitted from *more* information via clinical interview not made available to the actuarial method. While most studies in the Grove et al. meta-analysis found a statistical equivalence between the clinical and actuarial methods, it has been argued that in the event of a tie, there should be preference for the actuarial method, because once developed it is less expensive in time and money, less laborious, and allows for consistent application in a dispassionate manner (Dawes et al., 1989; Meehl, 1954).

Why might an actuarial/statistical/mechanical method of prediction be superior? The answer appears to be, in part, its consistent application. All one need do is correctly enter the appropriate scores or data into the formula, and the formula calculates the prediction consistently. It has been reported numerous times that humans (expert clinicians included) are susceptible to numerous errors in judgement, including confirmation bias, overconfidence, fundamental attribution error, misperception of regression, representativeness, insensitivity to prior probabilities or base rates, misperception about chance (i.e., illusory correlations, conjunction fallacy, inverse probabilities, insensitivity to sample size [law of small numbers], pseudodiagnosticity), and hindsight bias (Garb, 1997, 1998; Kahneman, Slovic, & Tversky, 1982; Meehl & Rosen, 1955; Tversky & Kahneman, 1974; Watkins, 2009). McDermott (1981) also noted problems such as the inconsistent application of diagnostic criteria (decision rules), inconsistent weighting of diagnostic cues, and inconsistent decision-making processes (strategies or sequences) among school psychologists. However, entering data into formulae in a consistent manner allows the algorithm or calculations to be applied consistently and resulting decisions from them to be applied consistently as well. Another important aspect of actuarial or statistical

superiority rests in the variables included in the formula. Statistical methods of multiple regression, logistic regression, and discriminant function analysis are able to differentially and optimally weight variables to provide the most accurate predictions of the criterion variable, and this provides another advantage over that of a clinician (Grove & Meehl, 1996). It is for these and other reasons that Grove and Meehl argued that actuarial methods should be widely applied and false arguments against it should be rejected.

Research on actuarial interpretations of intelligence tests is quite sparse. Literature searches crossing key terms such as *intelligence test, psychometric intelligence, interpretation, actuarial, statistical, classification, diagnosis,* or *prediction* produced no empirical research applied to actuarial intelligence test interpretation. There are, however, some applications and approximations worth examining.

Statistical/Actuarial Approaches: Classification of Intelligence Test Profiles

Intelligence test subtest (or factor score) profile analysis as systematized by Kaufman (Kaufman, 1979, 1994a; Kaufman & Lichtenberger, 2000) and Sattler (1982, 1988, 1992, 2001, 2009; Sattler & Ryan, 2009) is an ideographic method that uses the individual's mean performance as the basis for comparing subtest (or factor) scores, and determination of strengths or weaknesses is based on significant deviation from that mean. As previously reviewed, these ipsative approaches are neither reliable nor valid in distinguishing clinical group memberships. However, another approach to examining subtest profiles in tests is a *normative* method whereby characteristic profiles are identified through procedures such as cluster analysis (Hale, 1981; McDermott, 1998; Ward, 1963).

Several methods of cluster analysis are available and involve examining individuals' scores on a test and grouping similarly scoring individuals into mutually exclusive groups or clusters with a minimal loss of information. McDermott (1998) developed a three-stage hierarchical clustering method, *Multistage Euclidean Grouping* (MEG), which incorporated recommended cluster analysis techniques such as application of Ward's (1963) method (e.g., Konold, Glutting, McDermott, Kush, & Watkins, 1999), combining hierarchical and nonhierarchical clustering algorithms, and included built-in replications (Milligan & Hirtle, 2003). Once clusters are identified, they are then examined for characteristics (internal and external) that deviate from other clusters' in order to describe distinguishing characteristics. Clusters may differ in proportions of demographic characteristics such as sex, race or ethnicity, and socioeconomic status (SES), as well as performance or scores on other measures (achievement, learning behaviors, personality, psychopathology). When an individual's test scores are compared to the various profiles defined by the clusters, their profile might be assigned to a particular cluster based on similarity, or perhaps the individual has scores that reflect similarity to no other profile, in which case the profile is deemed unique.

A number of intelligence tests have been examined through cluster analysis in order to determine what profiles exist from a normative perspective. Cronbach and Gleser (1953) noted that profiles are defined by three characteristics (a) level/elevation (i.e., average performance), (b) shape/pattern (i.e., highs and lows or peaks and valleys), and (c) scatter/variability (i.e., range of scores); and profile shape/pattern is determined after removing the level and scatter information. Tests such as the WPPSI, WISC-R, WISC-III, WAIS-R, DAS, UNIT, KABC, and McCarthy Scales of Children's Abilities (MSCA; McCarthy, 1972) have had their standardization samples subjected to cluster analysis and resulting normative profiles described (Donders, 1996; Glutting, & McDermott, 1990a, 1990b; Glutting, McDermott, & Konold, 1997; Glutting, McGrath, Kamphaus, & McDermott, 1992; Holland & McDermott, 1996; Konold et al., 1999; McDermott, Glutting, Jones, & Noonan, 1989; McDermott, Glutting, Jones, Watkins, & Kush, 1989; Schinka & Vanderploeg, 1997; Wilhoit & McCallum, 2002). In all of these examples, the primary distinguishing feature appears to be that of profile level/elevation, which is a reflection of overall ability (g). The next distinguishing characteristic of normative profiles appears to be shape/pattern, which often is reflected by broad differences between the test's verbal/crystallized and nonverbal/fluid/visual tasks.

What a normative typology based on cluster analysis affords is a means by which an individual's profile may be *empirically* compared and classified and in a manner that does not discard reliable test variance like the ipsative subtest profile method does (Jensen, 1992; McDermott et al., 1992). Also, group similarity coefficient statistics, such as $r_{p(k)}$ (Tatsuoka, 1974, p. 31; Tatsuoka & Lohnes, 1988, pp. 377–378) or D^2 (Cronbach & Gleser, 1953; Osgood & Suci, 1952), provided an index of similarity to the normative profile types that account for all three profile characteristics. If, for example, none of the normative core profile type comparisons produces an $r_{p(k)}$ value > .40 (Konold et al., 1999; McDermott, Glutting, Jones, Watkins, et al., 1989; McDermott, Glutting, Jones, & Noonan, 1989), then the individual's profile was classified as unique or atypical. Another method of profile comparison is based on Euclidian distance or generalized distance theory (D^2) (Osgood & Suci, 1952), and although somewhat less precise, it is easier to calculate and apply and thus more convenient.

These nonlinear multivariate profile analysis methods are better than clinically based ipsative methods in that they simultaneously consider both linear and nonlinear characteristics of the profile, simultaneously examine multiple subtest scores, and empirically determine similarity (or uniqueness) to the normative core profiles from a nationally representative sample. However, like other test scores, profile similarity or classification must also demonstrate acceptable reliability, validity, and utility.

CLUSTER COMPARISON PSYCHOMETRIC SUPPORT

While normative core profiles have been (or can be) developed for intelligence tests, the measurement properties of the profiles need to be investigated, as well as the measurement properties of individuals' profiles. It was earlier shown that ipsative subtest profiles (strengths and weaknesses) and subtest composite scores were not stable across time and therefore could not be (and were not) valid.

Short-term stability of profile classifications has yielded fairly consistent results for the MSCA (general κ_m =.728; Glutting & McDermott, 1990a), K-ABC (general κ_m =.497; Glutting et al., 1992), and DAS (general κ_m =.541; Holland & McDermott, 1996). Partial κ_m coefficients were also found to be statistically significant for MSCA core profiles (Glutting & McDermott, 1990a) as well as for K-ABC core profiles and a group of unusual K-ABC profiles (Glutting et al., 1992). WPPSI profile short-term stability was lower (general κ_m =.216; Glutting & McDermott, 1990b).

While short-term stability for empirically based profiles was moderate, Livingston et al. (2003) found that empirically derived subtest profiles did not possess acceptable long-term stability; however, they did not evaluate profile stability by comparison to the core taxonomy. Borsuk, Watkins, and Canivez (2006) explored the long-term stability of WISC-III cluster membership based on nonlinear multivariate profile analysis for 585 students across a mean retest interval of 2.82 years. Individual profiles at Time 1 and Time 2 were classified according to the normative core WISC-III profiles (Konold et al., 1999) using D^2 (Cronbach & Gleser, 1953; Osgood & Suci, 1952) and the critical D^2 value of 98 established by Konold et al. Agreement for all profile types across time (κ_m =.39, p <.0029; Fleiss, 1971) and partial κ_m coefficients for each individual profile (.26 to .51) indicated that cluster membership based on nonlinear multivariate profile analysis was generally not sufficiently stable over a three-year period showing generally poor agreement (Cicchetti, 1994). Profiles 6 and 8 showed fair and statistically significant stability necessary to justify future validity research (Cicchetti, 1994). Although it appears that several intelligence test profile–type memberships possess some degree of short-term stability, long-term stability results for the WISC-III (Borsuk et al., 2006) were generally poor. As such, even the empirically based WISC-III subtest profile-type memberships were not suitable for making educational decisions about students. Thus, at this point, both nonlinear multivariate *and* clinical (ipsative) approaches to profile analysis lack empirical support for contribution to individual diagnosis or educational decision-making.

If empirically derived profiles were at some point found to be reliable, they then must also provide incremental validity over and above general intelligence scores *and* must assist in diagnostic utility for clinical use. However, like ipsative subtest interpretive methods, normative approaches to subtest interpretation have inadequate empirical support in their diagnostic utility (Glutting et al., 1992; Glutting, McDermott, Konold, Snelbaker, & Watkins, 1998; McDermott et al., 1992), and it is appropriate to heed the recommendation, even for normatively based profiles, to "just say no" (McDermott, Fantuzzo, & Glutting, 1990) to all subtest analyses and interpretations in clinical practice.

Statistical/Actuarial Approaches to Classification and Diagnosis

Ultimately, actuarial (statistical) classification and diagnosis should include co-normed measures assessing relevant domains (intelligence, academic achievement, adaptive behavior, personality, learning behaviors, psychopathology) and include large, demographically representative standardization samples. This would allow the generation of multivariate statistical comparisons and enable empirical classification and differential diagnosis. With a demographically representative sample, base-rate

estimates for the population would be available for empirically delineated and defined pathologies. This, however, is not yet available.

One group of instruments that is an approximation is the Adjustment Scales for Children and Adolescents (ASCA; McDermott, Marston, & Stott, 1993), the Learning Behaviors Scale (LBS; McDermott, Green, Francis, & Stott, 1999), and the DAS (Elliott, 1990). In the nationally representative standardization of ASCA by The Psychological Corporation, 1,260 of the 1,400 youths in the ASCA standardization sample were also administered the DAS, and 1,252 had teacher ratings on the LBS. In the cluster analysis of the ASCA (McDermott, 1993, 1994; McDermott & Weiss, 1995) 22 distinct profiles (14 major types, 8 clinical subtypes) were identified based on the six ASCA core syndromes. Following identification of distinct profiles, McDermott and Weiss were able to describe the characteristics of cluster profile types according to features that differed significantly from other profile types on demographic variables (age, sex, SES, race/ethnicity), cognitive abilities (general conceptual, verbal, nonverbal), academic achievement (word reading, numerical skills, spelling), and ability–achievement discrepancies. Using generalized distance scores (D^2), an individual's core syndrome profile is classified as most similar to one of the 22 normative profiles producing the lowest D^2 value and characteristics of the profile likely related to the youth in question. While this application is not directed at intelligence per se, a similar procedure could provide greater understanding and empirically based classification. This co-normed set of tests also allowed McDermott et al. (2006) to examine aspects of intelligence, processing speed, classroom learning behaviors, problem behaviors, and demographic variables in identifying differential risk of learning disabilities from an epidemiological perspective. Important differences were identified in differential risk and classification depending on some of these variables as well as the method of determining learning disability (low achievement vs. ability–achievement discrepancy).

SYSTEMS ACTUARIAL CLASSIFICATION

Recognizing the problem of the lack of consistency or agreement among (and within) diagnosticians in child clinical psychology and school psychology diagnostic decision-making, McDermott (1980) developed a multidimensional system for the actuarial differential diagnosis of children with disabilities. This multidimensional actuarial classification

(MAC) was the forerunner of the McDermott Multidimensional Assessment of Children program (M-MAC; McDermott & Watkins, 1985). Implicit in this process is the notion that there must be reliable application of diagnostic criteria and consideration of multivariate analyses. Without reliability in clinical decision-making, there can be no validity. The M-MAC was generations ahead of its time in terms of both technology and comprehensive actuarial classification. Sadly, nothing like it even exists today!

M-MAC (and its predecessor MAC) applied a classification system that considered both abnormal *and* normal development and provided classifications based, in part, on objective measures of intelligence, academic achievement, adaptive behavior, and psychopathology; recognizing that variations within and between these would provide for differential classification or diagnosis. Because the diagnostic decision rules and mathematical comparisons are applied consistently, the classifications across similar or identical cases are reliable. This is a necessary first step for any method of diagnosis. With respect to intelligence test interpretation, M-MAC provided differential diagnosis for mental retardation (e.g., both intelligence *and* adaptive behavior measures were at least two standard deviations below the mean) and learning disabilities (e.g., IQ–achievement discrepancy, consideration of significant and rare achievement problems, and absence of mental retardation, sensory impairment, etc.). Prevalence rates were also applied and increased the validity of classifications (Glutting, 1986a). M-MAC also provided for the development of recommended intervention programs (1,111 specific behavioral objectives in reading, math, learning, and/or adaptive skills) to address the previously identified diagnostic needs of the child (Glutting, 1986b).

Evaluation of MAC (McDermott, 1980; McDermott & Hale, 1982) with a sample of 73 youths referred to an outpatient clinic resulted in agreement across areas (mental retardation, specific learning disability, behavioral/emotional disorder, communication/perceptual, reading problem, mathematics problem) 86% beyond chance when MAC results were compared to experts'. Agreement between two experts for cases averaged 76.5% beyond chance, but experts were not significantly in agreement for classifications of learning disability or mathematics problems. Agreement for MAC (expert applied vs. novice applied) across disorders was perfect! Thus, as observed elsewhere (Dawes, Faust, & Meehl, 1989; Grove & Meehl, 1996;

Grove et al., 2000), actuarial interpretations by MAC were generally better than those of experts. Actuarial classification or diagnosis by programs like MAC or M-MAC provide advantages of basing diagnostic decisions on data (i.e., test scores) that are standardized and normed on representative samples, mathematical comparisons of scores from different tests, and statistical decision rules and application of diagnostic criteria are applied consistently and in accordance with diagnostic standards established by governmental agencies or professional organizations.

Actuarial Interpretation Conclusion

Research regarding the benefits of actuarial methods for classification and diagnosis has been available for some time, yet clinical application in interpretation of intelligence and other tests has generally failed to capitalize on this. Actuarial interpretation affords systematic and reliable application and ability for multivariate consideration of variables that affect reliable and valid differential diagnosis. Where the M-MAC program from the 1980s required numerous 5.25" floppy disks to be swapped during computations, the technological advances in computer processing power and storage capacity would allow the complex algorithms to be run on today's handheld computers and smart phones. Better clinical practice and more ethical practice would be afforded by actuarial and empirical applications in intelligence test interpretation.

A final note regarding actuarial methods is necessary concerning their limits (Dawes et al., 1989). An actuarial method is only as good as the measures included for predictions and the available outcomes. Research and evaluation of the actuarial algorithms and accuracy of decisions is necessary in order to continually improve. Quality control and revision based on theory development and research are most certainly necessary as the field advances. Also, actuarial methods should not be considered infallible, as there will always be errors in diagnostic decision-making and within psychology, and because there appear to be no biological or positive markers for disorders, we never really know with certainty whether or not individuals have a particular disorder. As such, clinicians must cope with the reality of practicing with uncertainty.

General Conclusion

Interpretation of intelligence tests requires careful consideration of the empirical support for their reliability, validity, and utility. At present there appear to be no specific actuarial systems of intelligence test interpretation leading to prediction or differential diagnosis. Available research, considered in its entirety, suggests that most, if not all, interpretation should be based on the overall, or omnibus score (FSIQ). This is not to say that cognitive or intellectual abilities are only one thing (*g*), but at present our ability to measure more than general intellectual abilities is less than adequate when considering important uses such as in prediction of academic achievement and diagnostic decision-making. The inadequacies of lower-level scores beyond the Full Scale score will lead to greater errors in diagnostic decision-making and treatment recommendations. This research has been available for decades, yet numerous test authors and publishers, textbook authors, and university trainers of clinicians continue to perpetuate the clinical interpretation method and the shared professional myth of the utility of subtest and other interpretations and often ignore this research altogether. It is hoped that a new generation of psychologists will heed the empirical evidence and advice of those who have repeatedly called for abandonment of subtest interpretations. It is time to follow Weiner's (1989) sage advice that effective psychodiagnosticians:

(a) know what their tests can do and (b) act accordingly. Knowing what one's test can do—that is, what psychological functions they describe accurately, what diagnostic conclusions can be inferred from them with what degree of certainty, and what kinds of behavior they can be expected to predict—is the measure of a psychodiagnostician's competence. Acting accordingly—that is, expressing only opinions that are consonant with the current status of validity data—is the measure of his or her ethicality. (p. 829)

However, in clinical assessment, intelligence is but one domain to be considered, and any consideration of multiple domains simultaneously requires multivariate analyses that tax human information processing and clinical judgement. Tests covering many important domains (intelligence, achievement, personality, psychopathology, adaptive behavior, learning behaviors) simultaneously normed on representative population samples would help us improve differential diagnosis and better understand psychopathology base rates, and allow for actuarial interpretation for individual examinees. In the absence of such an ambitious venture, perhaps one day soon a systems-actuarial interpretation program like M-MAC will be created to account for the multivariate measurement of psychopathologies, of which intelligence is one part, to improve the clinical decision-making process when questions of intelligence confront the clinician. Such a method would at least assure that diagnostic criteria would be consistently applied. Only then will there be the possibility of valid classification and diagnosis.

Author Note

Gary L. Canivez is Professor of Psychology at Eastern Illinois University, principally involved in training school psychologists. His research interests include applied psychometric investigations of the reliability, validity, and utility of intelligence, achievement, and psychopathology measures; and investigations of test bias.

The author would like to thank Drs. Marley W. Watkins, W. Joel Schneider, Scott O. Lilienfeld, and Peter V. W. Hartmann for extremely helpful critiques, comments, and suggestions concerning earlier versions of this chapter.

Correspondence regarding this manuscript should be addressed to Gary L. Canivez, Ph.D., Department of Psychology, 600 Lincoln Avenue, Charleston, Illinois 61920-3099. Dr. Canivez may also be contacted via email at glcanivez@eiu.edu, glcanivez@gmail.com, or the World Wide Web at http://www.ux1.eiu.edu/~glcanivez.

References

Aiken, L. R. (2000). *Psychological testing and assessment* (10th ed.). Needham Heights, MA: Allyn & Bacon.

Alfonso, V. C., Oakland, T. D., LaRocca, R., & Spanakos, A. (2000). The course on individual cognitive assessment. *School Psychology Review, 29,* 52–64.

American Educational Research Association, American Psychological Association, & National Council on Measurement in Education. (1999). *Standards for educational and psychological testing.* Washington, DC: American Educational Research Association.

American Psychiatric Association. (1994). *Diagnostic and statistical manual of mental disorders* (4th ed.). Washington, DC: APA.

American Psychiatric Association. (2000). *Diagnostic and statistical manual of mental disorders* (4th ed., text rev.). Washington, DC: APA.

American Psychological Association. (2002, 2010 Amendments). *Ethical principles of psychologists and code of conduct.* Washington, DC: APA.

Bayes, T. (1763). An essay towards solving a problem in the doctrine of chances. *Philosophical Transactions of the Royal Society, 53,* 370–18. (Reprinted in G. A. Barnard [1958], *Studies in the history of probability and statistics.*) *Biometrika, 45,* 293–315.

Beebe, D. W., Pfiffner, L. J., & McBurnett, K. (2000). Evaluation of the validity of the Wechsler Intelligence Scale for Children–Third Edition comprehension and picture arrangement subtests as measures of social intelligence. *Psychological Assessment, 12,* 97–101.

Binet, A., & Simon, T. (1905). Methodes nouvelle pour le diagnostic du niveau intellectual des anormaux [New methods for the diangnosis of the intellectual level of subnormals]. *L'Annee Psychologique, 11,* 1991–244.

Bornstein, R. A., & Matarazzo, J. D. (1982). Wechsler VIQ versus PIQ differences in cerebral dysfunction: A literature review with emphasis on sex differences. *Journal of Clinical Neuropsychology, 4,* 319–334.

Bornstein, R. A., & Matarazzo, J. D. (1984). Relationship of sex and the effects of unilateral lesions on the Wechsler intelligence scales: Further considerations. *Journal of Nervous and Mental Disease, 172,* 707–710.

Borsuk, E. R., Watkins, M. W., & Canivez, G. L. (2006). Long-term stability of membership in a WISC-III subtest core profile taxonomy. *Journal of Psychoeducational Assessment, 24,* 52–68.

Bracken, B. A., & McCallum, R. S. (1998a). *Universal Nonverbal Intelligence Test.* Itasca, IL: Riverside Publishing.

Bracken, B. A., & McCallum, R. S. (1998b). *Universal Nonverbal Intelligence Test: Examiners manual.* Itasca, IL: Riverside Publishing.

Bracken, B. A., & Walker, K. C. (1997). The utility of intelligence tests for preschool children. In D. P. Flanagan, J. L. Genshaft, & P. L. Harrison (Eds.), *Contemporary intellectual assessment: Theories, tests, and issues* (pp. 484–502). New York: The Guilford Press.

Brody, N. (1985). The validity of tests of intelligence. In B. Wolman (Ed.), *Handbook of intelligence* (pp. 353–389). New York: Wiley.

Brody, N. (2002). *g* and the one–many problem: Is one enough? In *The nature of intelligence* (Novartis Foundation Symposium 233) (pp. 122–135). New York: Wiley.

Brown, R. T., Reynolds, C. R., & Whitaker, J. S. (1999). Bias in mental testing since bias in mental testing. *School Psychology Quarterly, 14,* 208–238.

Campbell, J. M., & McCord, D. M. (1996). The WAIS-R comprehension and picture arrangement subtests as measures of social intelligence: Testing traditional interpretations. *Journal of Psychoeducational Assessment, 14,* 240–249.

Campbell, J. M., & McCord, D. M. (1999). Measuring social competence with the Wechsler picture arrangement and comprehension subtests. *Assessment, 6,* 215–223.

Canivez, G. L. (2008). Orthogonal higher-order factor structure of the Stanford-Binet Intelligence Scales for children and adolescents. *School Psychology Quarterly, 23,* 533–541.

Canivez, G. L. (2011). Hierarchical factor structure of the Cognitive Assessment System: Variance partitions from the Schmid-Leiman (1957) procedure. *School Psychology Quarterly, 26,* 305–317.

Canivez, G. L. (2011, August). *Interpretation of cognitive assessment system scores: Considering incremental validity of PASS scores in predicting achievement.* Paper presented at the 2011 Annual Convention of the American Psychological Association, Washington, DC.

Canivez, G. L., Konold, T. R., Collins, J. M., & Wilson, G. (2009). Construct validity of the Wechsler Abbreviated Scale of Intelligence and Wide Range Intelligence Test: Convergent and structural validity. *School Psychology Quarterly, 24,* 252–265.

Canivez, G. L., Neitzel, R., & Martin, B. E. (2005). Construct validity of the Kaufman Brief Intelligence Test, Wechsler Intelligence Scale for Children–Third Edition, and Adjustment Scales for Children and Adolescents. *Journal of Psychoeducational Assessment, 23,* 15–34.

Canivez, G. L., & Watkins, M. W. (1998). Long term stability of the Wechsler Intelligence Scale for Children–Third Edition. *Psychological Assessment, 10,* 285–291.

Canivez, G. L. & Watkins, M. W. (1999). Long term stability of the Wechsler Intelligence Scale for Children–Third Edition among demographic subgroups: Gender, race, and age. *Journal of Psychoeducational Assessment, 17,* 300–313.

Canivez, G. L., & Watkins, M. W. (2001). Long term stability of the Wechsler Intelligence Scale for Children–Third Edition among students with disabilities. *School Psychology Review, 30,* 438–453.

Canivez, G. L., & Watkins, M. W. (2010a). Investigation of the factor structure of the Wechsler Adult Intelligence Scale–Fourth Edition (WAIS-IV): Exploratory and higher-order factor analyses. *Psychological Assessment, 22,* 827–836.

Canivez, G. L., & Watkins, M. W. (2010b). Exploratory and higher-order factor analyses the Wechsler Adult Intelligence Scale–Fourth Edition (WAIS-IV) adolescent subsample. *School Psychology Quarterly, 25,* 223–235.

Carretta, T. R., & Ree, J. J. (2001). Pitfalls of ability research. *International Journal of Selection and Assessment, 9,* 325–335.

Cassidy, L. C, (1997). *The stability of WISC-III scores: For whom are triennial reevaluations necessary?* Unpublished doctoral dissertation, Kingston, RI: University of Rhode Island.

Carroll, J. B. (1993). *Human cognitive abilities: A survey of factor analytic studies.* New York: Cambridge University Press.

Carroll, J. B. (1995). On methodology in the study of cognitive abilities. *Multivariate Behavioral Research, 30,* 429–452.

Carroll, J. B. (1997a). The three-stratum theory of cognitive abilities. In D. P. Flanagan, J. L. Genshaft, & P. L. Harrison (Eds.), *Contemporary intellectual assessment: Theories, tests, and issues* (pp. 183–208). New York: Guilford.

Carroll, J. B. (1997b). Theoretical and technical issues in identifying a factor of general intelligence. In B. Devlin, S. E. Fienberg, D. P. Resnick, & K. Roeder (Eds.), *Intelligence, genes, and success: Scientists respond to the bell curve* (pp. 125–156). New York: Springer-Verlag.

Carroll, J. B. (2003). The higher-stratum structure of cognitive abilities: Current evidence supports *g* and about ten broad factors. In H. Nyborg (Ed.), *The scientific study of general intelligence: Tribute to Arthur R. Jensen* (pp. 5–21). New York: Pergamon Press.

Cattell, R. B. (1943). The measurement of adult intelligence. *Psychological Bulletin, 40,* 153–193.

Cicchetti, D. V. (1994). Guidelines, criteria, and rules of thumb for evaluating normed and standardized assessment instruments in psychology. *Psychological Assessment, 6,* 284–290.

Cohen, J. (1959). The factorial structure of the WISC at ages 7–6, 10–6, and 13–6. *Journal of Consulting Psychology, 23,* 285–299.

Cronbach, L. J. (1990). *Essentials of psychological testing* (5th ed.). Boston: Addison–Wesley.

Cronbach, L. J., & Gleser, G. C. (1953). Assessing similarity between profiles. *Psychological Bulletin, 50,* 456–473.

Cronbach, L. J., & Meehl, P. E. (1955). Construct validity in psychological tests. *Psychological Bulletin, 52,* 281–302.

Cronbach, L. J., & Snow, R. E. (1977). *Aptitudes and instructional methods: A handbook for research on interactions.* New York: Irvington Publishers.

Daley, C. E., & Nagle, R. J. (1996). Relevance of WISC-III indicators for assessment of learning disabilities. *Journal of Psychoeducational Assessment, 14,* 320–333.

Dana J., & Dawes, R. M. (2007). Comment on Fiorello et al., "Interpreting intelligence test results for children with disabilities: Is global intelligence relevant?" *Applied Neuropsychology*, *14*, 21–25.

Daniel, M. H. (2007). "Scatter" and the construct validity of FSIQ: Comment on Fiorello et al. (2007). *Applied Neuropsychology*, *14*, 291–295.

Daniel, M. H. (2009, August). *Subtest variability and the validity of WISC–IV composite scores.* Paper presented at the 2009 annual convention of the American Psychological Association, Toronto, ON, CA.

Davidow, J., & Levinson, E. M. (1993). Heuristic principles and cognitive bias in decision making: Implications for assessment in school psychology. *Psychology in the Schools*, *30*, 351–361.

Dawes, R. M. (1994). *House of cards: Psychology and psychotherapy built on myth.* New York: The Free Press.

Dawes, R. M. (2005). The ethical implications of Paul Meehl's work on comparing clinical versus actuarial prediction methods. *Journal of Clinical Psychology*, *61*, 1245–1255.

Dawes, R. M., Faust, D., & Meehl, P. E. (1989). Clinical versus actuarial judgment. *Science*, *243*, 1668–1674.

Das, J. P., Naglieri, J. A., & Kirby, J. R. (1994). *Assessment of cognitive processes: The PASS theory of intelligence.* Boston: Allyn & Bacon.

DiStefano, C., & Dombrowski, S. C. (2006). Investigating the theoretical structure of the Stanford-Binet–Fifth Edition. *Journal of Psychoeducational Assessment*, *24*, 123–136.

Dombrowski, S. C., & Watkins, M. W. (in press). Exploratory and higher order factor analysis of the WJ-III full test battery: A school aged analysis. *Psychological Assessment.*

Dombrowski, S. C., Watkins, M. W., & Brogan, M. J. (2009). An exploratory investigation of the factor structure of the Reynolds Intellectual Assessment Scales (RIAS). *Journal of Psychoeducational Assessment*, *27*, 494–507.

Donders, J. (1996). Cluster subtypes in the WISC-III standardization sample: Analysis of factor index scores. *Psychological Assessment*, *8*, 312–318.

Dumont, R., Farr, L. P., Willis, J. O., & Whelley, P. (1998). 30-second interval performance on the coding subtest of the WISC-III: Further evidence of WISC folklore? *Psychology in the Schools*, *35*, 111–117.

Elliott, C. D. (1990). *Differential Ability Scales.* San Antonio, TX: The Psychological Corporation.

Elliott, C. D. (2007a). *Differential Ability Scales–2nd edition.* San Antonio, TX: The Psychological Corporation.

Elliott, C. D. (2007b). *Differential Ability Scales–2nd edition: Introductory and technical handbook.* San Antonio, TX: The Psychological Corporation.

Evans, J. J., Floyd, R. G., McGrew, K. S., & Leforgee, M. H. (2001). The relations between measures of Cattell-Horn-Carroll (CHC) cognitive abilities and reading achievement during childhood and adolescence. *School Psychology Review*, *31*, 246–262.

Faust, D. (1986). Research on human judgment and its application to clinical practice. *Professional Psychology: Research and Practice*, *17*, 420–430.

Faust, D. (1990). Data integration in legal evaluations: Can clinicians deliver on their premises? *Behavioral Sciences and the Law*, *7*, 469–483.

Faust, D. (2007). Some global and specific thoughts about some global and specific issues. *Applied Neuropsychology*, *14*, 26–36.

Fiorello, C. A., Hale, J. B., Holdnack, J. A., Kavanagh, J. A., Terrell, J., & Long, L. (2007). Interpreting intelligence test results for children with disabilities: Is global intelligence relevant? *Applied Neuropsychology*, *14*, 2–12.

Fiorello, C. A., Hale, J. B., McGrath, M., Ryan, K., & Quinn, S. (2001). IQ interpretation for children with flat and variable test profiles. *Learning and Individual Differences*, *13*, 115–125.

Flanagan, D. P. (2000). Wechsler-based CHC cross-battery assessment and reading achievement: Strengthening the validity of interpretations drawn from Wechsler test scores. *School Psychology Quarterly*, *15*, 295–329.

Flanagan, D. P., Andrews, T. J., & Genshaft, J. L. (1997). The functional utility of intelligence tests with special education populations. In D. P. Flanagan, J. L. Genshaft, & P. L. Harrison (Eds.), *Contemporary intellectual assessment: Theories, tests, and issues* (pp. 457–483). New York: The Guilford Press.

Flanagan, D. P., & Kaufman, A. S. (2004). *Essentials of WISC–IV assessment.* Hoboken, NJ: Wiley.

Flanagan, D. P., & McGrew, K. S. (1997). A cross-battery approach to assessing and interpreting cognitive abilities: Narrowing the gap between practice and cognitive science. In D. P. Flanagan, J. L. Genshaft, & P. L. Harrison (Eds.), *Contemporary intellectual assessment: Theories, tests, and issues* (pp. 314–325). New York: Guilford.

Flanagan, D. P., & Ortiz, S. O. (2001). *Essentials of cross-battery assessment.* New York: Wiley.

Flanagan, D. P., Ortiz, S. O., & Alfonso, V. C. (2008). *Essentials of cross-battery assessment* (2nd ed.). New York: Wiley.

Fleiss, J. L. (1971). Measuring nominal scale agreement among many raters. *Psychological Bulletin*, *76*, 378–382.

Floyd, R. G., Keith, T. Z., Taub, G. E., & McGrew, K. S. (2007). Cattell-Horn-Carroll cognitive abilities and their effects on reading decoding skills: g has indirect effects, more specific abilities have direct effects. *School Psychology Quarterly*, *22*, 200–233.

Floyd, R. G., McGrew, K. S., & Evans, J. J. (2008). The relative contributions of the Cattell-Horn-Carroll cognitive abilities in explaining writing achievement during childhood and adolescence. *Psychology in the Schools*, *45*, 132–144.

Frazier, T. W., & Youngstrom, E. A. (2007). Historical increase in the number of factors measured by commercial tests of cognitive ability: Are we overfactoring? *Intelligence*, *35*, 169–182.

Freberg, M. E., Vandiver, B. J., Watkins, M. W., & Canivez, G. L. (2008). Significant factor score variability and the validity of the WISC-III Full Scale IQ in predicting later academic achievement. *Applied Neuropsychology*, *15*, 131–139.

Garb, H. N. (1997). Race bias, social class bias, and gender bias in clinical judgment. *Clinical Psychology: Science and Practice*, *4*, 99–120.

Garb, H. N. (1998). *Studying the clinician: Judgment research and psychological assessment.* Washington, DC: American Psychological Association.

Garb, H. N. (2005). Clinical judgment and decision making. *Annual Review of Clinical Psychology*, *1*, 67–89.

Garb, H. N., & Boyle, P. A. (2003). Understanding why some clinicians use pseudoscientific methods: Findings from research on clinical judgment. In S. O. Lilienfeld, S. J. Lynn, & J. M. Lohr (Eds.), *Science and pseudoscience in clinical psychology* (pp. 17–38). New York: Guilford.

Glutting, J. J. (1986a). The McDermott Multidimensional Assessment of Children: Applications to the classification of childhood exceptionality. *Journal of Learning Disabilities, 19,* 331–335.

Glutting, J. J. (1986b). The McDermott Multidimensional Assessment of Children: Contribution to the development of individualized education programs. *Journal of Special Education, 20,* 431–445.

Glutting, J. J., Adams, W., & Sheslow, D. (2000a). *Wide Range Intelligence Test.* Wilmington, DE: Wide Range, Inc.

Glutting, J. J., Adams, W., & Sheslow, D. (2000b). *Wide Range Intelligence Test: Manual.* Wilmington, DE: Wide Range, Inc.

Glutting, J. J., & McDermott, P. A. (1990a). Score structures and applications of core profile types in the McCarthy Scales standardization sample. *Journal of Special Education, 24,* 212–233.

Glutting, J. J., & McDermott, P. A. (1990b). Patterns and prevalence of core profile types in the WPPSI standardization sample. *School Psychology Review, 19,* 471–491.

Glutting, J. J., McDermott, P. A., & Konold, T. R. (1997). Ontology, structure, and diagnostic benefits of a normative subtest taxonomy from the WISC-III standardization sample. In D. P. Flanagan, J. L. Genshaft, & P.L. Harrison (Eds.), *Contemporary intellectual assessment: Theories, tests, and issues* (pp. 349–372). New York: Guilford.

Glutting, J. J., McDermott, P. A., Konold, T. R., Snelbaker, A. J., & Watkins, M. W. (1998). More ups and downs of subtest analysis: Criterion validity of the DAS with an unselected cohort. *School Psychology Review, 27,* 599–612.

Glutting, J. J., McGrath, E. A., Kamphaus, R. W., & McDermott, P. A. (1992). Taxonomy and validity of subtest profiles on the Kaufman Assessment Battery for Children. *Journal of Special Education, 26,* 85–115.

Glutting, J. J., Watkins, M. W., Konold, T. R., & McDermott, P. A. (2006). Distinctions without a difference: The utility of observed versus latent factors from the WISC-IV in estimating reading and math achievement on the WIAI-II. *Journal of Special Education, 40,* 103–114.

Glutting, J. J., Watkins, M. W., & Youngstrom, E. A. (2003). Multifactored and cross-battery assessments: Are they worth the effort? In C. R. Reynolds & R. W. Kamphaus (Eds.), *Handbook of psychological and educational assessment of children: Intelligence, aptitude, and achievement* (2nd ed., pp. 343–374). New York: Guilford.

Glutting, J. J., Youngstrom, E. A., Oakland, T., & Watkins, M. W. (1996). Situational specificity and generality of test behaviors for samples of normal and referred children. *School Psychology Review, 25,* 94–107.

Glutting, J. J., Youngstrom, E. A., Ward, T., Ward, S., & Hale, R. L. (1997). Incremental efficacy of WISC-III factor scores in predicting achievement: What do they tell us? *Psychological Assessment, 9,* 295–301.

Gorsuch, R. L. (1983). *Factor analysis* (2nd ed.). Hillsdale, NJ: Erlbaum.

Gottfredson, L. S. (1997). Intelligence and social policy. *Intelligence, 24,* 288–320.

Gottfredson, L. S. (2002). Where and why g matters: Not a mystery. *Human Performance, 15,* 25–46.

Gottfredson, L. S. (2008). Of what value is intelligence? In A. Prifitera, D. Saklofske, & L. G. Weiss (Eds.), *WISC-IV clinical assessment and intervention* (2nd ed., pp. 545–564). Amsterdam: Elsevier.

Gottfredson, L. S. (2009). Logical fallacies used to dismiss the evidence on intelligence testing. In R. P. Phelps (Ed.), *Correcting fallacies about educational and psychological testing* (pp. 11–65). Washington, DC: American Psychological Association.

Groth-Marnat, G. (1997). *Handbook of psychological assessment* (3rd ed.). NY: Wiley.

Gridley, B. E., & Roid, G. H. (1998). The use of the WISC-III with achievement tests. In A. Prifitera & D. Saklofske (Eds.), *WISC-III clinical use and interpretation* (pp. 249–288). New York: Academic Press.

Grove, W. M., Meehl, P. E. (1996). Comparative efficiency of informal (subjective, impressionistic) and formal (mechanical, algorithmic) prediction procedures: The clinical-statistical controversy. *Psychology, Public Policy, & Law, 2,* 293–323.

Grove, W. M., Zald, D. H., Lebow, B. S., Snitz, B. E., & Nelson, C. (2000). Clinical versus mechanical prediction: A meta-analysis. *Psychological Assessment, 12,* 19–30.

Guilford, J. P., & Fruchter, B. (1978). *Fundamental statistics in psychology and education* (6th ed.). New York: McGraw-Hill.

Gustafsson, J.-E., & Balke, G. (1993). General and specific abilities as predictors of school achievement. *Multivariate Behavioral Research, 28,* 407–434.

Gustafsson, J.-E., & Snow, R. E. (1997). Ability profiles. In R. F. Dillon (Ed.), *Handbook on testing* (pp. 107–135). Westport, CT: Greenwood Press.

Hale, J. B., & Fiorello, C. A. (2001). Beyond the academic rhetoric of "g": Intelligence testing guidelines for practitioners. *The School Psychologist, 55,* 113–139.

Hale, J. B., & Fiorello, C. A. (2004). *School neuropsychology: A practitioner's handbook.* New York: Guilford.

Hale, J. B., Fiorello, C. A., Bertin, M., & Sherman, R. (2003). Predicting math competency through neuropsychological interpretation of WISC-III variance components. *Journal of Psychoeducational Assessment, 21,* 358–380.

Hale, J. B., Fiorello, C. A., Kavanagh, J. A., Holdnack, J. A., & Aloe, A. M. (2007). Is the demise of IQ interpretation justified? A response to special issue authors. *Applied Neuropsychology, 14,* 37–51.

Hale, J. B., Fiorello, C. A., Kavanagh, J. A., Hoeppner, J. B., & Gaither, R. A. (2001). WISC-II predictors of academic achievement for children with learning disabilities: Are global and factor scores comparable? *School Psychology Quarterly, 16,* 31–55.

Hale, R. L. (1981). Cluster analysis in school psychology: An example. *Journal of School Psychology, 19,* 51–56.

Hale, R. L., & Raymond, M. R. (1981). Wechsler Intelligence Scale for Children–Revised patterns of strengths and weaknesses as predictors of the intelligence achievement relationship. *Diagnostique, 7,* 35–42.

Hale, R. L., & Saxe, J. E. (1983). Profile analysis of the Wechsler Intelligence Scale for Children–Revised. *Journal of Psychoeducational Assessment, 1,* 155–162.

Hanna, G. S., Bradley, F. O., & Holen, M. C. (1981). Estimating major sources of measurement error in individual intelligence scales: Taking our heads out of the sand. *Journal of School Psychology, 19,* 370–376.

Haynes, S. N., & Lench, H. C. (2003). Incremental validity of new clinical assessment measures. *Psychological Assessment, 15,* 456–466.

Hildebrand, D. K., & Ledbetter, M. F. (2001). Assessing children's intelligence and memory: The Wechsler Intelligence Scale for Children–Third Edition and the Children's Memory Scale. In J. J. W. Andrews, D. H. Saklofske, & H. L. Janzen (Eds.), *Handbook of psychoeducational assessment: Ability, achievement, and behavior in children* (pp. 13–32). New York: Academic Press.

Hills, J. R. (1981). *Measurement and evaluation in the classroom* (2nd ed.). Columbus, OH: Merrill.

Holland, A. M., & McDermott, P. A. (1996). Discovering core profile types in the school-age standardization sample of the Differential Ability Scales. *Journal of Psychoeducational Assessment, 14*, 131–146.

Horn, J. L. (1988). Thinking about human abilities. In R. Nesselroade & R. B. Cattell (Eds.), *Handbook of multivariate experimental psychology* (2nd ed., pp. 645–685). New York: Plenum Press.

Horn, J. L. (1991). Measurement of intellectual capabilities: A review of theory. In K. S. McGrew, J. K. Werder, & R. W. Woodcock, *WJ-R technical manual* (pp. 197–232). Chicago: Riverside.

Horn, J. L., & Cattell, R. B. (1966). Refinement and test of the theory of fluid and crystallized general intelligences. *Journal of Educational Psychology, 57*, 253–270.

Horn, J. L., & Noll, J. (1997). Human cognitive capabilities: Gf-Gc theory. In D. P. Flanagan, J. L. Genshaft, & P. L. Harrison (Eds.), *Contemporary intellectual assessment: Theories, tests, and issues* (pp. 53–91). New York: Guilford.

Hunsley, J. (2003). Introduction to the special section on incremental validity and utility in clinical assessment. *Psychological Assessment, 15*, 443–445.

Hunsley, J., & Meyer, G. J. (2003). The incremental validity of psychological testing and assessment: Conceptual, methodological, and statistical issues. *Psychological Assessment, 15*, 446–455.

Jencks, C., Bartlett, S., Corcoran, M., Crouse, J., Eaglesfield, D., Jackson, G., et al. (1979). *Who gets ahead? The determinants of economic success in America*. New York: Basic Books.

Jensen, A. R. (1992). Commentary: Vehicles of *g. Psychological Science, 3*, 275–278.

Jensen, A. R. (1998). *The g factor: The science of mental ability*. Westport, CT: Praeger.

Jones, W. T. (1952). *A history of Western philosophy*. New York: Harcourt, Brace.

Kahana, S. Y., Youngstrom, E. A., & Glutting, J. J. (2002). Factor and subtest discrepancies on the Differential Abilities Scale: Examining prevalence and validity in predicting academic achievement. *Assessment, 9*, 82–93.

Kahneman, D., Slovic, P., & Tversky, A. (1982). *Judgement under uncertainty: Heuristics and biases*. Cambridge: Cambridge University Press.

Kamphaus, R. W., Winsor, A. P., Rowe, E. W., & Kim, S. (2005). A history of intelligence test interpretation. In D. P. Flanagan and P. L. Harrison (Eds.), *Contemporary intellectual assessment: Theories, tests, and issues* (2nd ed., pp. 23–38). New York: Guilford.

Kaufman, A. S. (1979). *Intelligent testing with the WISC-R*. New York: Wiley-Interscience.

Kaufman, A. S. (1994). *Intelligent testing with the WISC-III*. New York: Wiley.

Kaufman, A. S., & Kaufman, N. L. (1983). *Kaufman Assessment Battery for Children*. Circle Pines, MN: American Guidance Service.

Kaufman, A. S., & Kaufman, N. L. (1993). *Kaufman Adolescent and Adult Intelligence Test*. Circle Pines, MN: American Guidance Service.

Kaufman, A. S., & Kaufman, N. L. (2004a). *Kaufman Assessment Battery for Children–Second Edition*. Circle Pines, MN: AGS Publishing.

Kaufman, A. S., & Kaufman, N. L. (2004b). *Kaufman Brief Intelligence Test–Second Edition*. Circle Pines, MN: AGS Publishing.

Kaufman, A. S., & Lichtenberger, E. O. (2000). *Essentials of WISC-III and WPPSI-R assessment*. New York: Wiley.

Kaufman, A. S., & Lichtenberger, E. O. (2006). *Assessing adolescent and adult intelligence* (3rd ed.). Hoboken, NJ: Wiley.

Kavale, K. A., & Forness, S. R. (1984). A meta-analysis of the validity of Wechsler Scale profiles and recategorizations: Patterns or parodies? *Learning Disability Quarterly, 7*, 136–156.

Keith, T. Z. (1999). Effects of general and specific abilities on student achievement: Similarities and differences across ethnic groups. *School Psychology Quarterly, 14*, 239–262.

Kline, P. (1994). *An easy guide to factor analysis*. London: Routledge.

Kline, R. B., Snyder, J., Guilmette, S., & Castellanos, M. (1992). Relative usefulness of elevation, variability, and shape information from WISC-R, K-ABC, and Fourth Edition Stanford Binet profiles in predicting achievement. *Psychological Assessment, 4*, 426–432.

Konold, T. R., & Canivez, G. L. (2010). Differential relationships among WISC-IV and WIAT-II scales: An evaluation of potentially moderating child demographics. *Educational and Psychological Measurement, 70*, 613–627.

Konold, T. R., Glutting, J. J., McDermott, P. A., Kush, J. C., & Watkins, M. W. (1999). Structure and diagnostic benefits of a normative subtest taxonomy developed from the WISC-III standardization sample. *Journal of School Psychology, 37*, 29–48.

Kotz, K. M., Watkins, M. W., & McDermott, P. A. (2008). Validity of the General Conceptual Ability score from the Differential Ability Scales as a function of significant and rare interfactor variability. *School Psychology Review, 37*, 261–278.

Krohn, E. J., & Lamp, R. E. (1999). Stability of the SB:FE and K-ABC for young children from low-income families: A 5-year longitudinal study. *Journal of School Psychology, 37*, 315–332.

Kubiszyn, T. W., Meyer, G. J., Finn, S. E., Eyde, L. D., Kay, G. G., Moreland, K. L., et al. (2000). Empirical support for psychological assessment in clinical health care settings. *Professional Psychology: Research and Practice, 31*, 119–130.

Kuusinen, J., & Leskinen, E. (1988). Latent structure analysis of longitudinal data on relations between intellectual abilities and school achievements. *Multivariate Behavioral Research, 23*, 103–118.

Leonard, T., & Hsu, J. S. J. (1999). *Bayesian methods: An analysis for statisticians and interdisciplinary researchers*. Cambridge, UK: Cambridge University Press.

Levine, A. J., & Marks, L. (1928). *Testing intelligence and achievement*. New York: Macmillan.

Lezak, M. D. (1995). *Neuropsychological assessment* (3rd ed.). New York: Oxford University Press.

Linn, R. L., & Gronlund, N. E. (1995). *Measurement and assessment in teaching*. Englewood Cliffs, NJ: Prentice-Hall.

Lilienfeld, S. O., Wood, J. M., & Garb, H. N. (2000). The scientific status of projective techniques. *Psychological Science in the Public Interest, 1*, 27–66.

Lilienfeld, S. O., Wood, J. M., & Garb, H. N. (2006). Why questionable psychological tests remain popular. *The Scientific Review of Alternative Medicine, 10*, 6–15.

Lipsitz, J. D., Dworkin, R. H., & Erlenmeyer-Kimling, L. (1993). Wechsler comprehension and picture arrangement subtests and social adjustment. *Psychological Assessment, 5*, 430–437.

Livingston, R. B., Jennings, E., Reynolds, C. R., & Gray, R. M. (2003). Multivariate analyses of the profile stability of intelligence tests: High for IQs, low to very low for subtest analyses. *Archives of Clinical Neuropsychology, 18*, 487–507.

Lubinski, D. (2000). Scientific and social significance of assessing individual differences: "Sinking shafts at a few critical points." *Annual Review of Psychology, 51*, 405–444.

Lubinski, D., & Dawis, R. V. (1992). Aptitudes, skills, and proficiencies. In M. D. Dunnette & L. M. Hough (Eds.), *Handbook of industrial and organizational psychology* (2nd ed., Vol. 3, pp. 1–59). Palo Alto, CA: Consulting Psychology Press.

Lubinski, D., & Humphreys, L. G. (1997). Incorporating general intelligence into epidemiology and the social sciences. *Intelligence, 24*, 159–201.

Macmann, G. M., & Barnett, D. W. (1997). Myth of the master detective: Reliability of interpretations for Kaufman's "intelligent testing" approach to the WISC-III. *School Psychology Quarterly, 12*, 197–234.

Maller, S. J., & McDermott, P. A. (1997). WAIS-R profile analysis for college students with learning disabilities. *School Psychology Review, 26*, 575–585.

Matarazzo, J. D. (1972). *Wechsler's measurement and appraisal of adult intelligence* (5th ed.). Oxford, UK: Williams & Wilkins.

Matarazzo, J. D., & Herman, D. O. (1984). Base rate data for the WAIS-R: Test-retest stability and VIQ-PIQ differences. *Journal of Clinical Neuropsychology, 6*, 351–366.

Mayes, S. D., Calhoun, S. L., & Crowell, E. W. (1998). WISC-III profiles for children with and without learning disabilities. *Psychology in the Schools, 35*, 309–316.

McCarthy, D. (1972). *McCarthy Scales of Children's Abilities*. San Antonio, TX: Psychological Corporation.

McClain, A. L. (1996). Hierarchical analytic methods that yield different perspectives on dynamics: Aids to interpretation. *Advances in Social Science Methodology, 4*, 229–240.

McDermott, P. A. (1980). A computerized system for the classification of developmental, learning, and adjustment disorders in school children. *Educational and Psychological Measurement, 40*, 761–768.

McDermott, P. A. (1981). Sources of error in psychoeducational diagnosis of children. *Journal of School Psychology, 19*, 31–44.

McDermott, P. A. (1993). National standardization of uniform multisituational measures of child and adolescent behavior pathology. *Psychological Assessment, 5*, 413–424.

McDermott, P. A. (1994). *National profiles in youth psychopathology: Manual of adjustment scales for children and adolescents*. Philadelphia, PA: Edumetric and Clinical Science.

McDermott, P. A. (1998). MEG: Megacluster analytic strategy for multistage hierarchical grouping with relocations and replications. *Educational and Psychological Measurement, 58*, 677–686.

McDermott, P. A., Fantuzzo, J. W., & Glutting, J. J. (1990). Just say no to subtest analysis: A critique on Wechsler theory and practice. *Journal of Psychoeducational Assessment, 8*, 290–302.

McDermott, P. A., Fantuzzo, J. W., Glutting, J. J., Watkins, M. W., & Baggaley, A. R. (1992). Illusions of meaning in the ipsative assessment of children's ability. *The Journal of Special Education, 25*, 504–526.

McDermott, P. A., & Glutting, J. J. (1997). Informing stylistic learning behavior, disposition, and achievement through ability subtests—Or, more illusions of meaning? *School Psychology Review, 26*, 163–176.

McDermott, P. A., Glutting, J. J., Jones, J. N., & Noonan, J. V. (1989). Typology and prevailing composition of core profile types in the WAIS-R standardization sample. *Psychological Assessment, 1*, 118–125.

McDermott, P. A., Glutting, J. J., Jones, J. N., Watkins, M. W., & Kush, J. C. (1989). Identification and membership of core profile types in the WISC-R national standardization sample. *Psychological Assessment, 1*, 292–299.

McDermott, P. A., Goldberg, M. M., Watkins, M. W., Stanley, J. L., & Glutting, J. J. (2006). A nationwide epidemiological modeling study of learning disabilities: Risk, protection, and unintended impact. *Journal of Learning Disabilities, 39*, 230–251.

McDermott, P. A., Green, L. F., Francis, J. M., & Stott, D. H. (1999). *Learning Behaviors Scale*. Philadelphia, PA: Edumetric and Clinical Science.

McDermott, P. A., & Hale, R. L. (1982). Validation of a systems-actuarial computer process for multidimensional classification of child psychopathology. *Journal of Clinical Psychology, 38*, 477–486.

McDermott, P. A., Marston, N. C., & Stott, D. H. (1993). *Adjustment Scales for Children and Adolescents*. Philadelphia, PA: Edumetric and Clinical Science.

McDermott, P. A., & Watkins, M. W. (1985). *Microcomputer systems manual for McDermott Multidimensional Assessment of Children*. New York: The Psychological Corporation.

McDermott, P. A., & Weiss, R. V. (1995). A normative typology of healthy, subclinical, and clinical behavior styles among American children and adolescents. *Psychological Assessment, 7*, 162–170.

McFall, R. M. (1991). Manifesto for a science of clinical psychology. *The Clinical Psychologist, 44*, 75–88.

McFall, R. M. (2000). Elaborate reflections on a simple manifesto. *Applied and Preventive Psychology, 9*, 5–21.

McFall, R. M. (2005). Theory and utility—key themes in evidence-based assessment: Comment on the special section. *Psychological Assessment, 17*, 312–323.

McGrew, K. S. (1997). Analysis of the major intelligence batteries according to a proposed comprehensive Gf-Gc framework. In D. P. Flanagan, J. L. Genshaft, & P. L. Harrison (Eds.), *Contemporary intellectual assessment: Theories, tests, and issues* (pp. 151–179). New York: Guilford.

McGrew, K. S. (2005). The Cattell-Horn-Carroll theory of cognitive abilities: Past, present, and future. In D. P. Flanagan and P. L. Harrison (Eds.), *Contemporary intellectual assessment: Theories, tests, and issues* (2nd ed, pp. 136–181.). New York: Guilford.

McGrew, K. S., & Flanagan, D. P. (1998). *The Intelligence Test Desk Reference (ITDR): Gf-Gc cross-battery assessment*. Boston: Allyn & Bacon.

McGrew, K. S., Keith, T. Z., Flanagan, D. P., & Vanderwood, M. (1997). Beyond g: The impact of Gf-Gc specific cognitive ability research on the future use and interpretation of intelligence tests in the schools. *School Psychology Review, 26*, 189–201.

McGrew, K. S., & Knopik, S. N. (1996). The relationship between intra-cognitive scatter on the Woodcock-Johnson Psycho-Educational Battery–Revised and school achievement. *Journal of School Psychology, 34*, 351–364.

McGrew, K. S., & Woodcock, R. W. (2001). *Technical manual. Woodcock-Johnson III*. Itasca, IL: Riverside Publishing.

Meehl, P. E. (1954). *Clinical versus statistical prediction: A theoretical analysis and review of the evidence*. Minneapolis, MN: University of Minnesota Press.

Meehl, P. E. (1957). When shall we use our heads instead of the formula? *Journal of Counseling Psychology, 4*, 268–273.

Meehl, P. E. (1959). Some ruminations on the validation of clinical procedures. *Canadian Journal of Psychology, 13*, 102–128.

Meehl, P. E. (1979). A funny thing happened to us on the way to latent entities. *Journal of Personality Assessment, 43*, 564–581.

Meehl, P. E. (1986). Causes and effects of my disturbing little book. *Journal of Personality Assessment, 50*, 370–375.

Meehl, P. E. (2001). Comorbidity and taxometrics. *Clinical Psychology: Science and Practice, 8*, 507–519.

Meehl, P. E., & Rosen, A. (1955). Antecedent probability and the efficiency of psychometric signs, patterns, or cutting scores. *Psychological Bulletin, 52*, 194–216.

Milligan, G. W., & Hirtle, S. C. (2003). Clustering and classification methods. In J. A. Schinka, & W. F. Velicer, J. A. (Eds.), *Handbook of psychology: Research methods in psychology*, Vol. 2 (pp. 165–186). Hoboken, NJ: Wiley.

Mueller, H. H., Dennis, S. S., & Short, R. H. (1986). A meta-exploration of WISC-R factor score profiles as a function of diagnosis and intellectual level. *Canadian Journal of School Psychology, 2*, 21–43.

Mullins-Sweatt, S. N., & Widiger, T. A. (2009). Clinical utility and DSM-V. *Psychological Assessment, 21*, 302–312.

Naglieri, J. A. (1997). Planning, attention, simultaneous, and successive theory and the Cognitive Assessment System: A new theory-based measure of intelligence. In D. P. Flanagan, J. L. Genshaft, & P. L. Harrison (Eds.), *Contemporary intellectual assessment: Theories, tests, and issues* (pp. 247–267). New York: Guilford.

Naglieri, J. A. (2003a). *Naglieri nonverbal ability test–Individual administration*. San Antonio, TX: Harcourt Assessment.

Naglieri, J. A. (2003b). Naglieri nonverbal ability tests: NNAT and MAT-EF. In R. S. McCallum (Ed.), *Handbook of nonverbal assessment* (pp. 175–190). New York: Kluwer.

Naglieri, J. A., & Bornstein, B. T. (2003). Intelligence and achievement: Just how correlated are they? *Journal of Psychoeducational Assessment, 21*, 244–260.

Naglieri, J. A., & Das, J. P. (1990). Planning, attention, simultaneous, and successive (PASS) cognitive processes as a model for intelligence. *Journal of Psychoeducational Assessment, 8*, 303–337.

Naglieri, J. A., & Das, J. P. (1997a). *Cognitive Assessment System*. Itasca, IL: Riverside Publishing.

Naglieri, J. A., & Das, J. P. (1997b). *Cognitive Assessment System: Interpretive handbook*. Itasca, IL: Riverside Publishing.

National Association of School Psychologists. (2010). *Principles of professional ethics*. Bethesda, MD: NASP.

Neisser, U., Boodoo, G., Bouchard, Jr. T. J., Boykin, A. W., Brody, N., Ceci, S. J., et al. (1996). Intelligence: Knowns and unknowns. *American Psychologist, 51*, 77–101.

Nelson, J. M., & Canivez, G. L. (2012). Examination of the structural, convergent, and incremental validity of the Reynolds Intellectual Assessment Scales (RIAS) with a clinical sample. *Psychological Assessment, 24*, 129–140.

Nelson, J. M., Canivez, G. L, Lindstrom, W., & Hatt, C. (2007). Higher-order exploratory factor analysis of the Reynolds Intellectual Assessment Scales with a referred sample. *Journal of School Psychology, 45*, 439–456.

Nickerson, R. S. (2004). *Cognition and chance: The psychology of probabilistic reasoning*. Mahwah, NJ: Erlbaum.

Nisbett, R. E., Zukier, H., & Lemley, R. E. (1981). The dilution effect: Nondiagnostic information weakens the implications of diagnostic information. *Cognitive Psychology, 12*, 248–277.

Nunnally, J. D., & Bernstein, I. H. (1994). *Psychometric theory* (3rd ed.). New York: McGraw-Hill.

Oh, H. J., Glutting, J. J., Watkins, M. W., Youngstrom, E. A., & McDermott, P. A. (2004). Correct interpretation of latent versus observed abilities: Implications from structural equation modeling applied to the WISC-III and WIAT linking sample. *Journal of Special Education, 38*, 159–173.

Osgood, C. E., & Suci, G. J. (1952). A measure of relation determined by both mean differences and profile information. *Psychological Bulletin, 49*, 251–262.

Piedmont, R. L., Sokolove, R. L., & Fleming, M. Z. (1989). An examination of some diagnostic strategies involving the Wechsler intelligence scales. *Psychological Assessment, 1*, 181–185.

Pfeiffer, S. I., Reddy, L. A., Kletzel, J. E., Schmelzer, E. R., & Boyer, L. M. (2000). The practitioner's view of IQ testing and profile analysis. *School Psychology Quarterly, 15*, 376–385.

Ponterotto, J. G., & Ruckdeschel, D. E. (2007). An overview of coefficient alpha and a reliability matrix for estimating adequacy of internal consistency coefficients with psychological research measures. *Perceptual and Motor Skills, 105*, 997–1014.

The Psychological Corporation (1999). *Wechsler Abbreviated Scale of Intelligence*. San Antonio, TX: Psychological Corporation.

Public Law (P.L.) 108–446. Individuals with Disabilities Education Improvement Act of 2004 (IDEIA). (20 U.S.C. 1400 et seq.). 34 CFR Parts 300 and 301. Assistance to States for the education of children with disabilities and preschool grants for children with disabilities; Final Rule. *Federal Register, 71* (156), 46540–46845.

Rapaport, D., Gil, M. M., & Schafer, R. (1945–1946). *Diagnostic psychological testing* (2 vols.). Chicago: Year Book Medical.

Ree, M. J., & Carretta, T. R. (1997). What makes an aptitude test valid? In R. F. Dillon (Ed.), *Handbook on testing* (pp. 65–81). Westport, CT: Greenwood Press.

Ree, M. J., Carretta, T. R., & Green, M. T. (2003). The ubiquitous role of g in training. In H. Nyborg (Ed.), *The scientific study of general intelligence: Tribute to Arthur R. Jensen* (pp. 262–274). New York: Pergamon Press.

Ree, M. J., Earles, J. A., & Treachout, M. S. (1994). Predicting job performance: Not much more than g. *The Journal of Applied Psychology, 79*, 518–524.

Reinecke, M. A. Beebe, D. W., & Stein, M. A. (1999). The third factor of the WISC-III: It's (probably) not freedom from distractibility. *Journal of the American Academy of Child and Adolescent Psychiatry, 38*, 322–328.

Reynolds, C. R. (1984). Critical measurement issues in assessment of learning disabilities. *Journal of Special Education, 18*, 451–476.

Reynolds, C. R. (2007). Subtest level profile analysis of intelligence tests: Editor's remarks and introduction. *Applied Neuropsychology, 14*, 1.

Reynolds, C. R., & Kamphaus, R. W. (2003). *Reynolds Intellectual Assessment Scales*. Lutz, FL: Psychological Assessment Resources.

Riccio, C. A., Cohen, M. J., Hall, J., & Ross, C. M. (1997). The third and fourth factors of the WISC-III: What they don't measure. *Journal of Psychological Assessment, 15,* 27–39.

Rispens, J., Swaab, H., van den Oord, E. J. C. G., Cohen-Kettenis, P., van Engeland, H., & van Yperen, T. (1997). WISC profiles in child psychiatric diagnosis: Sense or nonsense? *Journal of the American Academy of Child and Adolescent Psychiatry, 36,* 1587–1594.

Roid, G. H. (2003a). *Stanford-Binet Intelligence Scales–Fifth Edition.* Itasca, IL: Riverside Publishing.

Roid, G. H. (2003b). *Stanford-Binet Intelligence Scales–Fifth Edition: Technical manual.* Itasca, IL: Riverside Publishing.

Ryan, J. J., Kreiner, D. S., & Burton, D. B. (2002). Does high scatter affect the predictive validity of WAIS-III IQs? *Applied Neuropsychology, 9,* 173–178.

Salgado, J. F., Anderson, N., Moscoso, S., Bertua, C., & de Fruyt, F. (2003). International validity generalization of GMA and cognitive abilities: A European community meta-analysis. *Personnel Psychology, 56,* 573–605.

Salvia, J., & Ysseldyke, J. E. (1988). *Assessment in special and remedial education* (4th ed.). Boston: Houghton Mifflin.

Salvia, J., & Ysseldyke, J. E. (2001). *Assessment* (8th ed.). Boston: Houghton Mifflin.

Saklofske, D. H. (2008). Forward. In D. Wechsler (Author), *Wechsler Adult Intelligence Scale–Fourth Edition.* San Antonio, TX: Pearson.

Sattler, J. M. (1982). *Assessment of children's intelligence and special abilities* (2nd ed.). Boston: Allyn & Bacon.

Sattler, J. M. (1988). *Assessment of children* (3rd ed.). San Diego, CA: Author.

Sattler, J. M. (1992). *Assessment of children* (3rd ed., revised and updated). San Diego, CA: Author.

Sattler, J. M. (2001). *Assessment of children: Cognitive applications* (4th ed.). San Diego, CA: Author.

Sattler, J. M. (2008). *Assessment of children: Cognitive applications* (5th ed.). San Diego, CA: Author.

Sattler, J. M. & Ryan, J. J. (2009). *Assessment with the WAIS-IV.* San Diego, CA: Author.

Schinka, J. A., & Vanderploeg, R. D. (1997). Profile clusters in the WAIS-R standardization sample. *Journal of the International Neuropsychological Society, 3,* 120–127.

Schmid, J., & Leiman, J. M. (1957). The development of hierarchical factor solutions. *Psychometrika, 22,* 53–61.

Schmidt, F. L., & Hunter, J. E. (1998). The validity and utility of selection methods in personnel psychology: Practical and theoretical implications of 85 years of research findings. *Psychological Bulletin, 124,* 262–274.

Schneider, J. (2008). Playing statistical Ouija board with commonality analysis (and other errors). *Applied Neuropsychology, 15,* 44–53.

Smith, C. B., & Watkins, M. W. (2004). Diagnostic utility of the Bannatyne WISC-III pattern. *Learning Disabilities Research and Practice, 19,* 49–56.

Spearman, C. (1904). General intelligence, objectively determined and measured. *American Journal of Psychology, 15,* 201–293.

Spearman, C. (1927). *The abilities of man.* New York: Macmillan.

Swets, J. A., Dawes, R. M., & Monahan, J. (2000). Psychological science can improve diagnostic decisions. *Psychological Science in the Public Interest, 1,* 1–26.

Tatsuoka, M. M. (1974). *Classification procedures: Profile similarity.* Champaign, IL: Institute for Personality and Ability Testing.

Tatsuoka, M. M., & Lohnes, P. R. (1988). *Multivariate analysis* (2nd ed.). New York: Macmillan.

Taub, G. E., Keith, T. Z., Floyd, R. G., & McGrew, K. S. (2008). Effects of general and broad cognitive abilities on mathematics achievement. *School Psychology Quarterly, 23,* 187–198.

Teeter, P. A., & Korducki, R. (1998). Assessment of emotionally disturbed children with the WISC-III. In A. Prifitera & D. H. Saklofske (Eds.), *WISC-III clinical use and interpretation: Scientist-practitioner perspectives* (pp. 119–138). New York: Academic Press.

Thompson, B. (2004). *Exploratory and confirmatory factor analysis: Understanding concepts and applications.* Washington, DC: American Psychological Association.

Thorndike, R. L. (1986). The role of general ability in prediction. *Journal of Vocational Behavior, 29,* 332–339.

Thorndike, R. L., Hagen, E. P., & Sattler, J. M. (1986). *Technical manual, Stanford-Binet Intelligence Scale: 4th edition.* Chicago, IL: Riverside.

Thorndike, R. M. (1990). Origins of intelligence and its measurement. *Journal of Psychoeducational Assessment, 8,* 223–230.

Thorndike, R. M. (1997). The early history of intelligence testing. In D. P. Flanagan, J. L. Genshaft, & P. L. Harrison (Eds.), *Contemporary intellectual assessment: Theories, tests, and issues.* New York: Guilford.

Tulsky, D. S., Saklofske, D. H., Chelune, G. J., Heaton, R. K., Ivnik, R. J., Bornstein, R., et al. (2003). *Clinical interpretation of the WAIS-III and WMS-III.* San Diego, CA: Academic Press.

Tversky, A., & Kahneman, D. (1974). Judgment under uncertainty: Heuristics and biases. *Science, 185,* 1124–1131.

Ward, J. J., Jr. (1963). Hierarchical grouping to optimize an objective function. *American Statistical Association Journal, 58,* 236–244.

Ward, S. B., Ward, T. B., Hatt, C. V., Young, D. L., & Mollner, N. R. (1995). The incidence and utility of the ACID, SCIDS, and SCAD profiles in a referred population. *Psychology in the Schools, 12,* 267–276.

Watkins, M. W. (1996). Diagnostic utility of the WISC-III developmental index as a predictor of learning disabilities. *Journal of Learning Disabilities, 29,* 305–312.

Watkins, M. W. (1999). Diagnostic utility of WISC-III subtest variability among students with learning disabilities. *Canadian Journal of School Psychology, 15,* 11–20.

Watkins, M. W. (2000). Cognitive profile analysis: A shared professional myth. *School Psychology Quarterly, 15,* 465–479.

Watkins, M. W. (2003). IQ subtest analysis: Clinical acumen or clinical illusion? *The Scientific Review of Mental Health Practice, 2,* 118–141.

Watkins, M. W. (2005). Diagnostic validity of Wechsler subtest scatter. *Learning Disabilities: A Contemporary Journal, 3,* 20–29.

Watkins, M. W. (2006). Orthogonal higher-order structure of the WISC-IV. *Psychological Assessment, 18,* 123–125.

Watkins, M. W. (2009). Errors in diagnostic decision making and clinical judgment. In T. B. Gutkin & C. R. Reynolds (Eds.), *Handbook of school psychology* (4th ed., pp. 210–229). Hoboken, NJ: Wiley.

Watkins, M. W., & Canivez, G. L. (2004). Temporal stability of WISC-III subtest composite strengths and weaknesses. *Psychological Assessment, 16,* 133–138.

Watkins, M. W., Lei, P., & Canivez, G. L. (2007). Psychometric intelligence and achievement: A cross-lagged panel analysis. *Intelligence, 35,* 59–68.

Watkins, M. W., & Glutting, J. J. (2000). Incremental validity of the WISC-III profile elevation, scatter, and shape information for predicting reading and math achievement. *Psychological Assessment, 12*, 402–408.

Watkins, M. W., Glutting, J. J., & Lei, P.-W. (2007). Validity of the full-scale IQ when there is significant variability among WISC-III and WISC-IV factor scores. *Applied Neuropsychology, 14*, 13–20.

Watkins, M. W., Glutting, J. J., & Youngstrom, E. A. (2005). Issues in subtest profile analysis. In D. P. Flanagan and P. L. Harrison (Eds.), *Contemporary intellectual assessment: Theories, tests, and issues* (2nd ed, pp. 251–268). New York: Guilford.

Watkins, M. W., & Kush, J. C. (1994). Wechsler subtest analysis: The right way, the wrong way, or no way? *School Psychology Review, 23*, 638–649.

Watkins, M. W., Kush, J. C., & Glutting, J. J. (1997a). Discriminant and predictive validity of the WISC-III ACID profile among children with learning disabilities. *Psychology in the Schools, 34*, 309–319.

Watkins, M. W., Kush, J. C., & Glutting, J. J. (1997b). Prevalence and diagnostic utility of the WISC-III SCAD profile among children with disabilities. *School Psychology Quarterly, 12*, 235–248.

Watkins, M. W., Kush, J. C., & Schaefer, B. A. (2002). Diagnostic utility of the learning disability index. *Journal of Learning Disabilities, 35*, 98–103.

Watkins, M. W., Wilson, S. M., Kotz, K. M., Carbone, M. C., & Babula, T. (2006). Factor structure of the Wechsler Intelligence Scale for Children–Fourth Edition among referred students. *Educational and Psychological Measurement, 66*, 975–983.

Watkins, M. W., & Worrell, F. C. (2000). Diagnostic utility of the number of WISC-III subtests deviating from mean performance among students with learning disabilities. *Psychology in the Schools, 37*, 303–309.

Wechsler, E. (1939). *The measurement of adult intelligence.* Baltimore, MD: Williams & Wilkins.

Wechsler, D. (1944). *The measurement of adult intelligence* (3rd ed.). Baltimore, MD: Williams & Wilkins.

Wechsler, D. (1949). *Wechsler Intelligence Scale for Children.* New York: Psychological Corporation.

Wechsler, D. (1958). *The measurement and appraisal of adult intelligence* (4th ed.). Baltimore, MD: Williams & Wilkins.

Wechsler, D. (1974). *Wechsler Intelligence Scale for Children–Revised.* New York: Psychological Corporation.

Wechsler, D. (1991). *Wechsler Intelligence Scale for Children–3rd Edition.* San Antonio, TX: Psychological Corporation.

Wechsler, D. (1992). *Wechsler Individual Achievement Test.* San Antonio, TX: Psychological Corporation.

Wechsler, D. (1997). *Wechsler Adult Intelligence Scale–3rd Edition.* San Antonio, TX: Psychological Corporation.

Wechsler, D. (1999). *The Wechsler Intelligence Scale for Children—3rd Edition (Swedish version).* Stockholm, Sweden: Psykologiförlaget.

Wechsler, D. (2002a). *WAIS-III/WMS-III technical manual, updated.* San Antonio, TX: Psychological Corporation.

Wechsler, D. (2002b). *Wechsler Preschool and Primary Scale of Intelligence–3rd Edition.* San Antonio, TX: Psychological Corporation.

Wechsler, D. (2003). *Wechsler Intelligence Scale for Children–4th Edition.* San Antonio, TX: Psychological Corporation.

Wechsler, D. (2008a). *Wechsler Adult Intelligence Scale–4th Edition.* San Antonio, TX: Pearson.

Wechsler, D. (2008b). *Wechsler Adult Intelligence Scale–4th Edition: Technical and interpretive manual.* San Antonio, TX: Pearson.

Wechsler, D., & Naglieri, J. A. (2006). *Wechsler Nonverbal Scale of Ability.* San Antonio, TX: The Psychological Corporation.

Weiner, I. B. (1989). On competence and ethicality in psychodiagnostic assessment. *Journal of Personality Assessment, 53*, 827–831.

Weiss, L. G., & Prifitera, A. (1995). An evaluation of differential prediction of WIAT achievement scores from WISC-III FSIQ across ethnic and gender groups. *Journal of School Psychology, 33*, 297–304.

Weiss, L. G., Saklofski, D. H., & Prifitera, A. (2003). Clinical interpretation of the Wechsler Intelligence Scale for Children–Third Edition (WISC-III) Index scores. In C. R. Reynolds & R. W. Kamphaus (Eds.), *Handbook of psychological and educational assessment of children: Intelligence, aptitude, and achievement* (2nd ed., pp. 115–146). New York: Guilford Press.

Wiggins, J. S. (1988). *Personality and prediction: Principles of personality assessment.* Malabar, FL: Krieger Publishing Company.

Wilhoit, B. E., & McCallum, R. S. (2002). Profile analysis of the Universal Nonverbal Intelligence Test standardization sample. *School Psychology Review, 31*, 263–281.

Wolber, G. J., & Carne, W. F. (2002). *Writing psychological reports: A guide for clinicians* (2nd ed.). Sarasota, FL: Professional Resources Press.

Woodcock, R. W., & Johnson, M. B. (1989). *Woodcock-Johnson–Revised Tests of Achievement.* Itasca, IL: Riverside Publishing.

Woodcock, R. W., McGrew, K. S., & Mather, N. (2001). *Woodcock-Johnson III Tests of Cognitive Abilities.* Itasca, IL: Riverside Publishing.

Yoakum, C. S., & Yerkes, R. M. (1920). *Army mental tests.* New York: Henry Holt & Company.

Youngstrom, E. A., Kogos, J. L., & Glutting, J. J. (1999). Incremental efficacy of Differential Ability Scales factor scores in predicting individual achievement criteria. *School Psychology Quarterly, 14*, 26–39.

Zachary, R. A. (1990). Wechsler's intelligence scales: Theoretical and practical considerations. *Journal of Psychoeducational Assessment, 8*, 276–289.

Zander, E., & Dahlgren, S. O. (2010). WISC-III Index Score profiles of 520 Swedish children with pervasive developmental disorders. *Psychological Assessment, 22*, 213–222.

Zeidner, M. (2001). Invited foreword and introduction. In J. J. W. Andrews, D. H. Saklofske, & H. L. Janzen (Eds.), *Handbook of psychoeducational assessment: Ability, achievement, and behavior in children.* New York: Academic Press.

Zhu, J., & Weiss, L. (2005). The Wechsler scales. In D. P. Flanagan and P. L. Harrison (Eds.), *Contemporary intellectual assessment: Theories, tests, and issues* (2nd ed., pp. 297–324). New York: Guilford.

The Scientific Status of Projective Techniques as Performance Measures of Personality

Hedwig Teglasi

Abstract

"Psychological constructs" are phenomena that are not seen directly but exert influence on individuals' responses to the real world and to items on tests. Constructs such as "intelligence" or "motivation" are valued because they organize otherwise piecemeal observations. Science aims to understand real-world phenomena through systematic observations and iterative refinement of constructs about how observations "go together." Measurement *per se* is not science but a tool to observe phenomena. The "scientific status" of an instrument rests on its construct validity, meaning that the construct in question causes variation in responses to real-world conditions and to test items. Insofar as variation in projective test responses are caused by constructs' capturing phenomena that matter in the lives of individuals, projective techniques are legitimate tools for science and practice. Shortcomings of clinical instruments are rooted in some combination of insufficient understanding of the target phenomenon (need to improve theory), flawed conceptualization of causal relations of the phenomenon to variations in scores on the test (need to improve measures), improper selection of real-world criteria (need to improve match between predictor and predicted constructs), or unreliability of the measure (need to improve psychometric properties).

Key Words: psychological constructs, scientific status, projective techniques, personality, psychometrics, assessment

Prelude

Critics of projective techniques have assumed incorrectly that self-report and projective tests of the same variable measure the same phenomenon and hence are interchangeable. Pitting one assessment procedure against another is misguided in light of research documenting that questionnaire and projective methods provide distinct and complementary information about phenomena. "When truth is evident, it is impossible for parties and factions to rise. There never has been a dispute as to whether there is daylight at noon" (Francis Marie Arouet de Voltaire, [1694–1778], *Philosophical Dictionary*, 1764).

The complexities of human behavior cannot be captured by a single method of assessment. Therefore, questions of scientific status and of the practicality of

a given instrument are linked to the larger issue of how well a clinical assessment battery captures the influences of various relevant phenomena. It has been said that "The aim of science is to seek the simplest explanation of complex facts. We are apt to fall into the error of thinking that the facts are simple because simplicity is the goal of our quest. The guiding motto in the life of every natural philosopher should be 'seek simplicity and distrust it'" (Alfred North Whitehead [1861–1947] English mathematician and philosopher, *Concepts of Nature*, 1920, p. 163).

As researchers in various psychology subfields have backed away from language loaded with excess meaning, particularly those introduced in the context of psychodynamic theory, they have substituted newer terms for similar phenomena (e.g., *implicit memory* for *unconscious memory*; *person schema* for *object representation*; *cognitive avoidance* for *repression*; *pre-attentive processing* for *preconscious processing*; *defensive attribution* for *ego defense*; and *central executive* for *ego*; see Bornstein, 2005). In this chapter, use of the term "performance measure of personality" as synonymous with "projective technique" is not meant to signal repudiation of its conceptual foundations in the "projective hypothesis." Indeed, "most of the change we think we see in life is due to truths being in and out of favor" (Robert Frost, "The Black Cottage," *North of Boston*, 1914).

The original tenets of the "projective hypothesis" are well supported by current theory and empirical evidence. However, proponents of projective techniques have expressed dissatisfaction with the term *projective* for two basic reasons. First, the central insights of the "projective hypothesis" have been incorporated into current research and theory across multiple psychology subfields (Teglasi, 1998), and terminology such as *personality performance measure* acknowledges this broader conceptual and empirical base. Second, terms that dichotomize personality tests as "projective" versus "objective" are problematic because of the untenable implications that "objectivity" is inherent in questionnaire measures but missing from projective tests, and that the two sources of information are equivalent and interchangeable (Meyer & Kurtz, 2006).

Introduction

The issue of scientific status, posed in the title of this chapter in reference to projective techniques, applies equally to all measurement. Professionals are accountable for selecting clinical assessment tools with consideration of their strengths and limitations for intended uses. Psychological measurement is not science but a tool that serves science as well as practice.[1] A measure's utility for applied purposes and its scientific merit are intertwined in that both depend on how well the instrument captures a phenomenon that exists in the real world.

Phenomena of interest to scientists come in two varieties: those that are amenable to being directly observed or sensed (such as temperature, latency of a response, or duration of a specific behavior) and those that are known indirectly from observed patterns (such as intelligence, personality, psychopathology, emotional reactivity, or motivation). The amount of gasoline in a car's tank, though estimated by the meter inside the cabin, may be glimpsed directly, whereas psychological phenomena such as "intelligence" are invisible.[2] Just like the gasoline in the tank,

these psychological phenomena, called *constructs*, are assumed to exert their influences on what happens in the real world even when there are no instruments to measure them (e.g., a broken fuel gauge). A series of behaviors may be explained in reference to a construct such as a person's intelligence or motivation. Similarly to scientific theories, constructs are valued because they lend coherence to otherwise piecemeal observations. Measures are useful to the extent that they give a faithful account of the construct to which they refer, provided that the construct itself is sufficiently understood to organize observations in the real world. Phenomena and measures are distinct, and acknowledging shortcomings of a particular instrument does not mean that the phenomenon is irrelevant. The idea of "construct validity" is what ties measurement to science and what makes a test valuable for practice.

The scientific quest to understand a phenomenon is akin to the proverbial story of the blind men exploring different parts of the elephant. The explorers agree that the elephant exists as an entity but, based on limited observations, each comes to his own conclusion about the nature of the *whole* elephant. Reliance on a single observer (or measure) to define the elephant (or a construct, such as "intelligence") may lead to the elevation of a part to the status of the whole; whereas arguments among the various observers ("the elephant is hard"—tusk; "it is very soft"—the ear; "it is like a rope"—the tail) or low convergence among different measures of a construct has the potential to yield glimpses of the whole: that is, unless the voice of one observer or one measurement approach drowns out the others. Clinical assessment tools measuring a construct in different ways may provide different perspectives on the whole, promoting differentiation and integration of constructs, whereas exclusive reliance on a single mode of measurement may add detail to a limited conception.

If data about a construct accumulate with the use of a single measurement approach, the version of the construct associated with that measure may become accepted by the scientific community but may not adequately capture the phenomenon as it exists in nature. If, on the other hand, different measures lead to different conclusions about the construct, scientists, like the blind men exploring the elephant, may argue about which version is correct. Attempts to chart unknown (or partially known) territory require ongoing revisions of working hypotheses about what the landscape looks like. Keeping in mind that essential features may yet be elusive, scientific criticism should aim not only to improve measures but also to refine constructs.

Construct Validity and Practical Utility

The idea of "construct validity" is predicated on the assumption that the construct being measured refers to an actual phenomenon, such as intelligence, that causes variation in real-world responses and to responses on test items (see Borsboom, Mellenbergh, & van Heerden, 2003, 2004). The phenomenon (intelligence) is assumed to exist apart from the ways that it is measured (intelligence tests), thereby allowing researchers to take a dual focus, one to refine the construct itself and the other to improve its measures. The task of psychological science is to delineate the constructs accounting for observed regularities in the real world and to devise measures that faithfully capture those constructs. Prediction from a test to a real-life criterion is a function of the constructs influencing variation in both.[3]

Current understanding of construct validity was foreshadowed in the works of Cronbach and Meehl (1955), who argued that demonstration of construct validity depends on a "nomological network" of lawful relations among entities. However, documenting lawful networks of relations among measures of constructs involves complex considerations, including precise understandings of constructs, theory of the relations among constructs, assumptions about the linkages of measures with constructs, and psychometric properties of the measures. The primary evidence bearing on "construct validity" comes from knowledge of the causal influences exerted by the construct on item responses and not directly from a measure's psychometric properties or correlations with other measures (see Borsboom et al., 2003, 2004; Smith, 2005).

A commonly used validation procedure, the "multi-trait–multi-method (MTMM)" matrix became a fashionable way to tease apart sources of variance attributable to measurement methods versus constructs (Campbell & Fiske, 1959). Support for a construct entails patterns showing higher correlations among different measures of the same construct (*convergent* validity) and lower correlations among similar measures of different constructs (*discriminant* validity). Although providing important information, examining the pattern of convergences and divergences does not settle the core issue of validity, the existence of an attribute that influences responses in the real world, and its causal impact on test responses. Evidence of construct validity, or lack thereof, is not provided by tables of correlations but by substantive psychological theory. Refinement of theory occurs through increasing differentiation of constructs that refer to real-life phenomena.

For instance, the construct of aggression has been unpacked into its various *forms* (overt and relational) and *functions* (proactive and reactive; see Card & Little, 2006) and into components that are *implicit,* influenced by mental sets operating largely outside of awareness, and *explicit,* influenced by values directly attributed to the self (Winter, John, Stewart, Klohnen, & Duncan, 1998**).** Correlations among undifferentiated measures of aggression or predictions from test scores to external criteria without considering relevant distinctions are not sufficient to inform construct validity.

A measure's construct validity enables its practical utility. By definition, drawing valid conclusions from tests is possible only if the intended phenomenon causes variation in responses on test items and in real-life conditions. Since the same constructs are assumed to underlie variation in responses to the predictor (test score) and to the predicted (real-life) variables, construct validity applies equally to both (Messick, 1989). This emphasis on construct validity places equal value on prediction and explanation as fundamental to establishing the utility of conclusions based on test scores. The essence of construct validity is the mapping of constructs as causal mechanisms explaining variation in responding to items on measures and to real-life circumstances.

Incremental Construct Validity

The property of *incremental validity* is ascribed to an instrument if it adds information to other measures in the battery by raising the overall correlation with the criterion (Mayer, 2003; Mischel, 1968). Viewed as a practical matter, incremental validity answers the question of whether a psychologist should or should not include a particular test in a set of measures (Wood, Garb, Lilienfeld, & Nezworski, 2002; Wood, Nezworski, Lilienfeld, & Garb, 2003). However, from the perspective of construct validity, what contributes incrementally to variance in a criterion is the addition of constructs, not measures. Some measures may encompass multiple constructs, whereas others may represent a single narrow construct. Therefore, in the conduct of psychological evaluations, what should be justified is the inclusion of each construct as optimally measured. If measures stand in for constructs, it does not seem logical to think of measures as predictors of other measures. A new term, *incremental construct validity,* is needed to capture the idea that constructs, not measures predict criteria, and that several constructs may contribute to complex and multiply determined criteria.

The foundation of *incremental construct validity* is the *construct validity* of conclusions derived from each measure. *Incremental construct validity* means that the *construct*, as measured by a particular test (with construct validity), contributes to variation in a predicted criterion beyond other constructs as variously measured. In his account of incremental validity in the assessment of adult psychopathology, Garb (2003) focused on the measures without reference to construct validity. Taking a box score approach toward the prediction of specific diagnoses, Garb came to the general conclusion that findings were more encouraging for the use of interviews, personality inventories, and brief self-ratings than for projective techniques. However, from the perspective of *incremental construct validity*, it would be necessary to identify the multiple constructs influencing the criterion, including constructs that play moderating or mediating roles, as well as the impact of method variance. Since adult diagnoses are often based on self-report interviews, constructs measured with similar techniques, such as interviews or questionnaires may share more variance. The demonstration of incremental construct validity requires careful consideration of the constructs and measures involved both in the predictors and criteria. If primacy were given to incremental construct validity, the practical issue of which tests should be selected would depend on answers to two questions: Which constructs are pertinent to a criterion, and what are the best available measures of those constructs (as predictors and as criteria)?

Conceptual Distinctions Relevant to Projective Techniques

The scientific community judges whether or not a phenomenon is worthy of study and whether its measures meet professional standards. Provided that a psychological phenomenon such as *projection* is accepted by (some) members of the scientific community, the measures based on the construct are met with an open mind. Among various scientific communities in psychology, constructs resembling projection masquerade under different names even as the term remains controversial. The development of models across different research traditions to explain phenomena similar to projection, regardless of terminology, may be considered a form of "replication" strengthening the construct. Within the field of projective assessment, the construct of projection has various meanings because they refer to different real-world phenomena, and various

understandings of the term *projection* signal the need for conceptual distinctions that may be informed by findings across psychology subfields.

Different Conceptions of Projection

A fundamental assumption of all projective assessment methods, the "projective hypothesis" posits that stimuli from the environment are perceived and organized by the individual's specific needs, motives, feelings, perceptual sets, and cognitive structures, and that, in large part, this process occurs automatically and outside of awareness (Frank, 1939; 1948). The influences of preexisting mental sets or schemas on the interpretation of ongoing encounters are ubiquitous, applying to both adaptive and maladaptive modes of processing information. However, some use the term *projection* to refer to faulty information-processing due to mental sets and defense mechanisms that distort reality.

Restricting the concept of projection to faulty information-processing has led to questioning whether or not certain responses to stimuli such as the Rorschach cards are products of projection. Those who view projection as limited to percepts that are idiosyncratic (such as distortions or elaborations) do not consider normative perceptions and classifications of stimuli as involving projection. Exner (1991) explained that the Rorschach Inkblot Method (RIM) is not a projective device because responses are more influenced by stimulus properties, and less by projection. Similarly, reasoning that well-defined stimuli do not elicit projection, the authors Roberts and Gruber (2005) changed the name of the *Roberts Apperception Test for Children* (one of a number of offshoots of the Thematic Apperception Test) to *Roberts-2*, deliberately omitting the word "apperception," which means "attributing an interpretation to perception." They asserted that this storytelling measure is not and never has been a projective test because the stimuli are not ambiguous but represent clearly recognized, everyday situations.

Given that projection is about the influence of preexisting mental sets or schemas on current information processing, the "pull" of the stimulus is a key consideration. The aim of projective techniques is not to measure free-floating thoughts without context, but to gauge how individuals use their schemas to negotiate the performance demands set by the stimuli and instructions of a particular task. The ambiguity of the stimulus to be identified or interpreted is an important source of individuality in responding to personality performance measures. However, restricting projection as pertinent only to ambiguous stimuli does not account for idiosyncratic responses to well-defined stimuli or for individualistic elaborations of commonly given responses. Rorschach cards with easily recognizable blot contours are more likely to elicit certain percepts with high frequency, but such "popular" responses to a blot area may involve embellishment (such as attributing movement) not readily explained by the stimulus. Apart from the nature of the stimuli, potential sources of ambiguity in the Rorschach task include the instructions, the extent to which the responses are open-ended, and the obscurity of performance expectations to respondents (no single correct solution and no awareness of scoring criteria). Presentation of an inkblot with instructions to tell the examiner "what might this be" leaves it up to the individual to decide how many responses to give and whether to focus on the whole blot or the parts. Similarly, well-defined scenes on the *Roberts-2* may elicit story themes consistent with the "popular pull," but a conventional interpretation is only a starting point, with many aspects of the unfolding narrative bearing the imprint of individuality.

Restricting projection to responses shaped by distorted mental structures is difficult because this view of projection does not fully capture the well-accepted phenomenon that prior knowledge influences all aspects of current information-processing. To clarify the workings of the projective hypothesis, it is necessary to differentiate among different types of schemas and the conditions to which they apply in the contexts of assessment and real life.

Constructs Supporting Projective Techniques Across Psychology Subfields

Two well-documented conceptual distinctions clarify the contribution of projective methods to clinical assessment. One distinction is between what persons report and what persons actually experience. The other distinction is between how persons function under relatively well-defined and ill-defined performance conditions. Table 5.1 describes three types of measures: (a) performance tasks presenting conditions that are *maximal* (more well-defined, such as IQ and achievement tests); (b) performance tasks presenting conditions that are *typical* (less well-defined, such as personality performance tasks such as storytelling); and, (c) questionnaires and interviews to elicit self-report.

WHAT PERSONS REPORT AND WHAT THEY ACTUALLY EXPERIENCE

Personality constructs come in two varieties, paralleling two modes of thought used by individuals to process information about themselves, others, and the world (Epstein, 1994; Fazio, 1990; Greenwald, Banaji, Rudman, Farnham, Nosek, & Mellott, 2002; Wilson, Lindsey, & Schooler, 2000): *explicit* (i.e., controlled or conscious) and *implicit* (i.e., automatic or non-conscious). Explicit and implicit constructs change and develop through different routes, the former by social influence and the latter by the individual's synthesis of lived experience (McClelland et al., 1989; Teglasi & Epstein, 1998). Implicit personality develops on the basis of affective experience and authentic encounters, whereas explicit personality is grounded in social values, encompassing what persons think they *should* want to do or believe based on what is important to their identity and promoted by social values (e.g., Burton, Lydon, D'Alessandro, & Koestner, 2006). *Explicit* personality constructs are active in situations that are salient for that construct, due to structures and incentives and are measured with self-report. *Implicit* personality constructs manifest in settings that allow individuals to make choices that are based on preferences and are measured with performance tasks.

Measures of explicit personality, provided by self-report, tend to correlate only modestly with measures of implicit personality, provided by projective techniques, and predict behaviors under different conditions (see Bornstein, 2002; James & Mazerolle, 2002; Kihlstrom, 1999; McClelland et al., 1989; Spangler, 1992). For instance, explicit achievement motivation (self-reported) fosters engagement in motive-relevant actions in the presence of situational prompts, whereas implicit achievement motivation (derived from TAT stories) directs individuals to engage in such behaviors spontaneously (see review, Spangler, 1992).

This duality of implicit and explicit personality as measured respectively with performance tasks and self-report corresponds considerably with two modes of information processing: one that is automatic, operating outside of awareness, and another, which is effortful and subject to awareness (for reviews, see Evans, 2008; Lieberman, 2007). The emphasis of the projective hypothesis on information processing without awareness is in tune with current views of the "unconscious" as qualities of the mind, not in immediate awareness, that influence conscious thought and behavior (James, 1998;

Table 5.1 Self Report and Performance Measures

	Self Report/Other Report	Performance Measure Typical	Performance Measure Maximal
Other terms	direct, explicit, objective, report-based	implicit, indirect, projective, performance-based	ability, intelligence, achievement
Basic assumptions	What is reported is accessible to introspection but may or may not be willingly disclosed	What is revealed operates outside of awareness, not necessarily amenable to introspection or to self-report	Responses demonstrate ability in a certain domain (crystallized or fluid, general or specific)
Instructions and stimuli set task demands	Instructions restrict variation in responses to differing degrees (forced-choice or open-ended)	Instructions expand variations in responses (less structure). Stimuli are complex or ambiguous, allowing individuals to select the focus of attention and to define the task	Instructions restrict variation in responses (more structure)
Responses	Responses may be constrained by options (true/false, Likert scales, multiple-choice) or be open-ended (interviews)	Responses are open-ended as to detail and organization, with leeway for individualistic approaches	Responses are guided by the instructions, and information for problem solution is provided
Strengths	Predict relevant criteria, efficient to administer and score	Predict relevant criteria, less subject to faking, not reliant on insight or on willingness to disclose information, reveal what is outside of awareness and give information about the process of thinking	Predict relevant criteria, clear guidelines for scoring
Limitations	Susceptible to self-presentation bias, limitation of self knowledge and reluctance to share information. Respondent may misinterpret items, and answers do not tell about the basis of the response. More predictive when settings are structured to increase salience of self presentation	Labor-intensive administrative and coding procedures, more predictive of performance and adjustment when tasks and settings are less structured	More predictive of performance and adjustment when settings and tasks are more structured
Criteria for judging responses	Responses to questionnaires are judged in relation to norms	Responses are judged by multiple criteria in the absence of a single correct solution; extensive norms may or may not be available	Responses are judged by a single criterion of correctness in line with norms

Uleman, 2005). The powerful role of unconscious information-processing on perception, thought, behavior, and motivation has been convincingly documented (Bargh & Morsella, 2008; Duckworth, Bargh, Garcia, & Chaiken, 2002). The central insights of the projective hypothesis are at the core of contemporary social cognitive theory, which posits that cognitive interpretations are important drivers of behavior and that prior conceptions inform

real-time information processing, often automatically, without deliberate effort.

Individuals bring to their day-to-day encounters both automatic and effortful modes of information processing, along with implicit and explicit components of their personality. However, individuals are not able to report on the implicit cognitive and affective processes that operate outside of awareness (Nisbett & Wilson, 1977), and, when given response options, may succumb to the desire to present themselves in a particular light (Cronbach, 1990; Edwards, 1957). What individuals report may also be influenced by cues about expected responses (as conveyed by *demand characteristics*, Orne, 1962). The fewer cues provided about response expectations, the more difficult it is to manage impressions (see Teglasi, 1993). Social desirability scales (e.g., Crowne & Marlowe, 1960; Paulhus, 1998; Stöber, 2001) aim to tease apart the contribution of wanting to present the self in a favorable light from the phenomenon the scale intends to assess. Yet, attempts to control for social desirability may not increase construct validity (Borkenau & Ostendorf, 1992; McCrae & Costa, 1983) because socially desirable responding may arise from processes that occur with self awareness through intentional *impression management,* or without awareness through *self-deception,* due to introspective limits (Paulhus, 1984). Self-report sheds light on explicit versions of constructs, being restricted by limits of awareness and the subjects' willingness to disclose information (Greenwald et al., 2002). Discrepancies between implicit and explicit measures of personality may be due to conflicts between two views of the self, not necessarily attributable to conscious impression management. For assessment, the challenge is to comprehend various ways of understanding the self, including the desire to make a certain impression.

HOW PERSONS PERFORM UNDER WELL-DEFINED AND ILL-DEFINED CONDITIONS

The performance context is relevant to the assessment of a wide range of psychological constructs. As analogues of real-life settings, the nature of performance tasks, whether tests of ability or of personality, is relevant to the phenomenon being assessed.

Performance tasks vary along a continuum of *maximal* and *typical* conditions. Maximal performance conditions provide clear-cut problems that have a limited number of correct solutions, whereas typical conditions require individuals to identify the problem and to formulate responses that maximize individual discretion (see Table 5.2; Sackett, Zedeck, & Fogli, 1988; Sackett, 2007).

Standard IQ tests, intended to assess the *ability* to solve well-defined (with clearly correct solutions) rather than ill-defined (with many potential solutions) problems (Pretz, Naples, & Sternberg, 2003), provide maximal performance conditions. On the other hand, problem-solving in ambiguous conditions involves both the *ability* to reason and the disposition to do so, including the *sensitivity* to recognize the moments that call for reasoning and the *inclination* to invest the necessary energy (Perkins & Ritchhart, 2004). This distinction between tests of personality and tests of ability is inherent in the *method* of measurement and not in the *content* domain. For instance, social skills may be assessed as *ability* under conditions of *maximal* performance by asking individuals to role play or to select responses to a contrived problem. However, such procedures shed little light on the *personality,* which orchestrates when and how the individual would use that ability under *typical* conditions.

The distinction between maximal and typical performance measures is important because it corresponds to differences in real-life conditions. Performance in an assessment context predicts outcomes in real-life settings, provided that both make similar functional demands. Consider two forms of sustained attention that are salient under different conditions, *contingency-shaped attention* and *goal-directed persistence* (see Barkley, 1997). Contingent attention is driven by novelty, incentives,

Table 5.2 Typical and Maximal Conditions of Performance

Typical Conditions	Maximal Conditions
Person is not aware of being observed or evaluated; is not likely to exert unusual effort.	Person perceives the task to be important and puts forth heightened level of effort and attention
Person is not aware of performance criteria and there are multiple correct solutions, hence the task pulls for characteristic ways of responding	Expectations and performance criteria are not equivocal as there is a limited range of correct responses
Person's responses are monitored over extended time or require competencies that are consolidated over time through concerted effort, enabling performance of complex tasks that reflect a history of more typical exertions	Observations of the person's responses are restricted to a short time span, which allows for an uncharacteristic spurt of effort that cannot be sustained

or presence of supervision (external sources of attention regulation), whereas goal-directed persistence is active when the individual pursues tasks or a course of action independently of immediate feedback or ongoing reinforcement (internal sources of attention regulation). Contingency-shaped attention, directed by immediate situational pulls, seems to align with maximal performance conditions and explicit motives, whereas goal-directed persistence, absent incentives or cues, seems to align with typical performance conditions and with the operation of implicit motives.

The maximal–typical distinction applies equally to social interactions and to task performance. Routine social encounters such as ordering a meal in a restaurant require the use of a highly scripted schema representing clear rules as to what is expected, whereas more ambiguous social encounters, such as being teased by a peer, require the synthesis of multiple schemas to consider the context, the peer's intention, one's own immediate or longer term purposes, potential responses, and so forth. Ambiguous social encounters call on the individual to discern the meaning of changing cues, to infer the existence of a problem or conflict and to determine whether and how to respond. Likewise, in daily life, individuals face tasks on continua that range from being clearly delineated (guiding what to do as well as how and when to do it) to being relatively undefined (providing limited cues that point to what information is important to consider or how to prioritize aspects of a complex task).

Projective Hypothesis and Types of Schemas

Consistent with the projective hypothesis, the schema is the basic mental unit that guides day-to-day information processing, allowing interpretation of the current situation to be informed by what has been learned previously. Prior knowledge shapes subsequent perception and conception in virtually every context, but this all-encompassing formulation of the operation of schemas and of the projective hypothesis is unpacked by making distinctions among different types of schemas and among the conditions in which they are relevant.

Implicit and Explicit Schemas

All schemas are outgrowths of the capacity of human beings to detect, process, and use information about co-variations of stimuli and events in their surroundings (such as a change in contingencies), often without deliberate effort or conscious awareness (Lewicki, Hill, & Czyzewska, 1992). Schemas differ from behavioral skills or factual knowledge in that the schema is a structure, organizing facts and ideas that influence the use of skills and knowledge. Schemas serve as templates for information processing by providing categories to encode information, pointing to what is relevant, filling in what is missing, and connecting ideas. Schemas come in explicit and implicit versions, influencing processing of information through the two modes discussed earlier: a) *automatic, implicit,* and *outside of awareness* and b) *effortful, explicit,* and *amenable to awareness.*

Public and Personal Schemas

As summarized in Figure 5.1, *public schemas* comprise shared knowledge structures *or* collective perceptions, and *personal schemas* encompass individual knowledge structures or perceptions. In some situations, both public and personal schemas apply. *Public* schemas capture the regularities of the external world and are therefore amenable to proof by logic, evidence, or social consensus. There are two types of public schemas that are subject to different types of proof: *logical* schemas, such as mathematical formulas or scientific principles; and *social* schemas, or scripts for what happens in routine situations. Logical schemas, describing observed relationships among facts or ideas (such as the formula for calculating the circumference of a circle; the layout of an airport) are maintained or changed through critical analysis, logical proof, or direct evidence. *Social schemas* or *scripts* organize regularities in routine events (how to order a meal in a restaurant; what happens when visiting the dentist), are widely

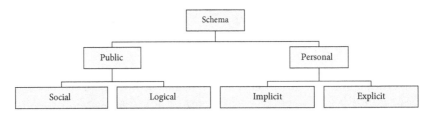

Figure 5.1 Public and Personal Schemas.

held in a culture, and are maintained or changed by consensus, not necessarily logic. The perceived co-variations of external events may remain tacit or implicit (Dowd & Courchaine, 2002; Lewicki, Czyzeswka, & Hill, 1997), playing an important role in recognition of the often-unstated rules that govern the regularities in the milieu. Social skills programs that focus on increasing children's social awareness or prosocial behavioral repertoire in well-defined conditions address public social schemas.

Personal schemas coordinate the inner and outer worlds. Explicit and implicit personal schemas apply respectively to assessment with self report and personality performance measures. *Implicit personal schemas* are outgrowths of experiences, incorporating ideas about sources of emotions such as distress or about efficacy to regulate uncomfortable states, to cope with challenges, or to attain desired outcomes. *Explicit personal schemas* are mental models about the self, including motives that a person endorses (self-attributes) on the basis of social values (wanting to be a good student) but not necessarily supported by patterns of regularities in actual experience (enjoying the activities relevant to being a good student). Explicit personal schemas are active in situations structured to provide cues or incentives (reminders, supervision, or clear expectations) salient for a given schema. In contrast, implicit personal schemas operate as the default, often without awareness, in situations that are ambiguous (resembling those of personality performance measures).

As individuals notice patterns in the external world such as links between actions and outcomes as well as regularities in their emotional states in relation to the stream of external events, they form expectations about what actions can or cannot bring about desired effects. A history of faulty information-processing reinforces incomplete or distorted mental sets or schemas that bias subsequent information processing, thereby maintaining vicious cycles. Although qualities of implicit personal schemas (measured by stories ascribed to TAT pictures) such as their accuracy, organization, and complexity, are linked to temperament (Bassan-Diamond, Teglasi, & Schmidt, 1995; Lohr, Teglasi, & French, 2004), once developed, these qualities take on a life of their own with relevance to adjustment, mental health (Lohr et al., 2004), and reading comprehension (Blankman, Teglasi, & Lawser, 2002).

Personality performance measures present standard tasks but allow leeway for individuality in the interpretation of the stimuli and in the organization of the response. To the extent that the stimuli are not amenable to interpretation by public schemas, individualistic schemas come into play. However, individuals may impose personal schemas on structured stimuli or social scripts on ambiguous stimuli. Assessment clarifies the qualities of the schemas that help or hinder understanding of and responding to relevant real-world contexts, both well-defined and ill-defined.

Schema-based interventions (e.g., Riso, du Toit, Stein, & Young, 2007) are designed to address maladaptive schema-driven information processing due to faulty (distorted, simplified, or incomplete) personal or social schemas or to difficulty balancing among various implicit and explicit schemas. Schema-based interventions may harness effortful processing to bring automatic tendencies to awareness and to reconcile conflicts between implicit and explicit personal schemas. However, to fully address gaps or distortions of information processing promoted by implicit personal schemas, interventions need to account for influences contributing to schema development and continued maintenance (such as temperamentally rooted problems regulating attention or emotion; Teglasi & Epstein, 1998). Otherwise, cognitive therapeutic interventions may produce changes in explicit personality without altering implicit processes or structures (Dowd, 2006).

Projective Techniques/Personality Performance Measures
Description of Projective Techniques

All projective tests present a task with standard elements, but they vary in their specific stimuli, instructions, leeway for responding, and system for interpreting the responses (see Figure 5.2, below; Rabin, 1981; Lindzey, 1961; Teglasi, 1993). Projective techniques highlight the imprint of individuality by incorporating various degrees of ambiguity into performance conditions that allow many potentially correct solutions.

STIMULI

Stimuli that are easily recognized in a culture constrain interpretations because they are explained by public schemas. Ambiguous stimuli permit alternative perceptions and interpretations, allowing for assessment of schemas that come to mind as the default in conditions of uncertainty. There are different perspectives on the degree of ambiguity that is ideal for personality assessment. Some researchers favor high ambiguity (e.g., Frank, 1939) but

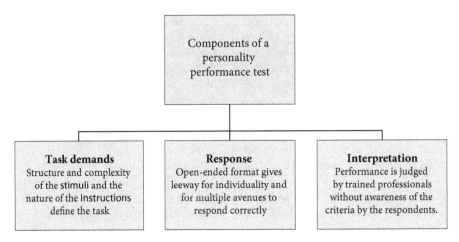

Figure 5.2 Components of a Personality Performance Test.

others prefer medium ambiguity (e.g., Murstein, 1965; Kaplan, 1967). Still others maintain that lack of ambiguity is best (Epstein, 1966). The optimal degree of ambiguity in the stimulus may depend on the purposes of the test. As the stimulus pull becomes weaker, the imprint of implicit personal schemas becomes increasingly influential. Yet, if information processing is seriously impaired, the individual may misinterpret even highly structured stimuli.

INSTRUCTIONS

Instructions for eliciting responses and procedures to query or encourage responses also pertain to the nature of the task as structured or ambiguous. Some personality performance tasks, such as human figure drawings, do not present stimuli at all, and ambiguity is a function of the instructions and obscurity of standards by which performance is to be judged. For instance, the request to "draw a person" is more structured when followed by the instruction to draw the "best person you can and not a stick figure." The Rorschach instruction "What might this be?" minimizes cues about how to approach the task.

RESPONSES

Regardless of the degree of ambiguity of stimuli and instructions, personality performance tasks that call for open-ended responses expand avenues for individuality in the production and organization of ideas. Stimulus cards that present highly structured scenes to elicit stories may constrain the themes but still allow a great deal of variation in the development of narratives, including the detail and coherence of ideas.

INTERPRETATION

Insofar as respondents are unaware of the interpretive criteria, the task demands are equivocal. The same set of open-ended responses may be interpreted in various ways, and the nature of the coding system and the expertise of the interpreter are relevant to what a given projective test actually measures. Even though personality performance measures do not specify a single correct solution, responses are not expected to be random but to be in tune with the task demands set by the stimuli and instructions. In the absence of single "correct" solutions, complex coding systems have been developed to ascertain the meaning of the responses, and it is necessary to document construct validity for each set of stimuli, instructions, and interpretive procedures (see Jenkins, 2008; Teglasi, 2010; Teglasi & Locraft, 2008).

Contribution of Projective Techniques/ Personality Performance Measures

Conceptual distinctions reviewed earlier between implicit and explicit personality constructs and between maximal and typical performance conditions are crucial for the status of "personality" as a scientific construct. In his textbook on personality and assessment, Mischel (1968) reviewed findings about the relationship between personality trait measures and relevant behavioral outcomes, reporting weak correlations (rarely exceeding .30), which led to his questioning the viability of personality as a construct. The transactional position (e.g., Magnusson & Endler, 1977) stressed the idea that behaviors are not only a function of factors within the *person* but also of the *situation* to which the person is responding. One of the strongest moderators of the link between personality traits and behavior is the extent to which the situation is governed by rules and normative expectations for appropriate behavior, as opposed to the expected responses being obscure (see Snyder & Ickes' [1985] distinction between strong and weak situations). Analogously, tests with well-defined performance conditions assess ability constructs, whereas those with ill-defined performance conditions measure personality constructs.

A framework for organizing psychological constructs in terms of transaction with environments is central to the assessment enterprise. Individuals bring implicit and explicit version of constructs to social and non-social domains and use both automatic and effortful modes of information processing in typical and maximal learning and performance conditions. Implicit and explicit versions of personality constructs cannot be averaged together, because they operate in different contexts. Therefore, theoretical formulations are needed to guide their integration. One suggestion is the *channeling hypothesis* (Winter, Stewart, Klohnen, & Duncan, 1998), which states that explicit self-beliefs channel how a motive is expressed. Consider an individual whose implicit inclination to be aggressive is at odds with his self-definition (shown in Figure 5.3; and see Frost, Ko, & James, 2007). To resolve this disparity and maintain a favorable self-view, the individual may engage in reasoning to justify his hostile acts and, depending on the norms of the setting, may express aggression openly or through indirect channels.

Compromises between implicit and explicit inclinations that are not socially sanctioned, such as aggression, may differ in nature from compromises among socially promoted motives such as achievement. Consider a fifth-grade student (with above-average intelligence) who is explicitly motivated to be a good student basing her sense of identity on getting good grades (see Figure 5.4). However, her low implicit motivation plays out in her day-to-day experience of becoming bored and frustrated, avoiding work in the absence of incentives. She puts forth more effort when the task is clear and supported by immediate feedback, such as when her parents supervise her homework. Recently, however, as expectations that she will work more independently have increased, so has her frustration and task incompletion. As seen in Figure 5.4, when explicit achievement motivation is not supported by implicit motivation (interest), the individual processes information more superficially and sets goals that emphasize performance (gain approval, grades) over mastery (understanding the material; see Moller & Elliot, 2006). Cumulatively, superficial information processing takes its toll on the development of mastery.

What do personality performance measures contribute to understanding transactions between persons and environments? They provide unique information to enable understanding of each of three vantage points on transactions between persons and situations: (a) internal dynamics; (b) situation-specific dynamics; and (c) developmental dynamics (see Teglasi, Newman, & Nebbergall, 2012).

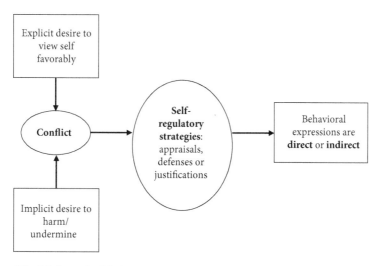

Figure 5.3 Implicit and Explicit Aggression Motives.

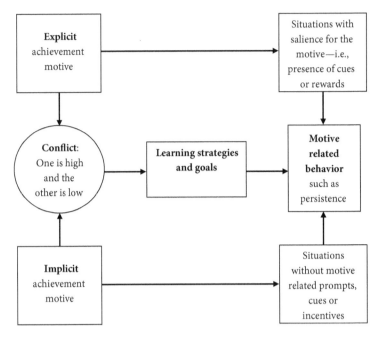

Figure 5.4 Implicit and Explicit Achievement Motives.

INTERNAL DYNAMICS

The whole person is understood as *the context* in which various psychological constructs (implicit and explicit) and mental processes (effortful and automatic modes of attention, self-regulation) converge to influence responses in a particular setting. Compromises among intra-individual factors and joint influences of various reciprocally interactive attributes (such as attentional and emotional self-regulation) are understood by obtaining information from various sources, including personality performance measures.

SITUATION-SPECIFIC DYNAMICS

Transactions between individuals and their external worlds are situation-specific, making it necessary to understand persons *in context*. Psychological constructs characterizing persons (schemas, executive functions) play out differently in settings (both in the assessment and real-world contexts) that vary on a continuum of typical and maximal conditions. Accordingly, responses to performance tests and to real-life challenges, as well as reports of various informants (peers, teachers, supervisors), are viewed in reference to applicable performance conditions (e.g., informant rating in a familiar, highly structured setting).

DEVELOPMENTAL DYNAMICS

Schemas play a pivotal role in developmental dynamics as they are products of *prior*

contexts and influence exchanges in current settings. Situation-specific responses are not directly pulled by current conditions but are informed by schemas. As individuals discern regularities in their transactions with certain contexts, they form mental sets housing knowledge about self, others, and the world that inform their subsequent appraisals, emotions, and behaviors in those contexts. To learn from experience, the individual must incorporate new categories into preexisting schemas by recognizing when the current repertoire is not adequate to understand or respond to the situation. Personality performance measures are used to assess implicit personal schemas and clarify the processes by which existing mental sets are adapted to impose meaning on ill-defined stimuli and to organize ideas (Teglasi, 2010).

The administration of measures that reveal implicit and explicit versions of targeted constructs in typical and maximal conditions, social and non-social, allow for case conceptualizations that are systematically organized around these elements to understand persons *as* context, *in* context, and *of* prior contexts (see Teglasi, Simcox, & Kim, 2007; Teglasi et al., ,2012).

Scientific Status of Projective Techniques

The provocative title of one critique, "The Scientific Status of Projective Techniques" (Lilienfeld, Wood, & Garb, 2000), incorrectly implies that the evidence presented, in the form of box scores of hits and misses of hypothesized correlations, speaks to the issue of the scientific merit of this class of instruments. Reviews of the empirical evidence regarding the use of projective or other clinical assessment techniques have the potential to advance research and practice, provided that they address construct validity, the core elements of which are (see Smith, 2005): theory development, hypothesis specification, research design, empirical evaluation, and implications of data for theory. The scientific rigor of a review of empirical findings should be judged by how well it accounts for each of these elements of the construct validation process.

1. Theory

Does the review recognize the theoretical grounding of the assessment tool in question, including recent advances in theory and implications for use of the measure? Lilienfield and colleagues (2000) treated projective techniques as if they were alternatives to self-report methods (Hughes, Gacono, & Owen, 2007), basing their largely negative conclusions on a mere caricature of the projective rationale (Hibbard, 2003). They dismiss construct validity as being independent of practical utility, asserting that . . . "an index derived from a projective technique may possess construct validity without being useful for predictive purposes in real world settings" (p. 28). By sidestepping the issue of construct validity, Lilienfield and colleagues give up the opportunity to contribute to theory development.

2. Informative hypotheses

Does the review differentiate between studies that pose informative tests of hypotheses from those that do not? It is incumbent on reviewers to flag studies that do not pose adequate tests of hypotheses and to raise questions about the relationship of the construct to both the predictor (measure) and the predicted (criterion). As Hibbard points out, Lilienfield and colleagues do not distinguish between studies designed to validate aspects of the measures from those aiming to explore relations among variables.

3. Sound research design

Does the review provide an accurate and comprehensive treatment of the extant literature by including the relevant studies and judging their adequacy to test the hypotheses and to rule out alternative explanations? Credibility of the conclusions drawn from a review of the evidence bearing on the value of a clinical measure depends on the inclusion and scrutiny of the research design of individual studies. The review of Lilienfield and colleagues provided a tally of findings that do or do not support the use of projective tests for the purpose of diagnosis without sufficient scrutiny of the quality of the research design and, as noted by Hibbard (2003), they included studies using the measure in ways that do not resemble their use by clinicians.

4. Explanation of the degree to which observations confirm hypotheses

Does the review provide possible explanations for patterns in the data within and across studies, explaining correspondences or disparities between observations and hypotheses? A tally of positive and negative correlations (zero order and multiple) does not substitute for a conceptual accounting of patterns of findings such as given by Spangler (1992), who highlighted different patterns of external correlates associated with self-reported and performance (TAT) measures of achievement motivation.

5. Ongoing revisions of both theory and measures

Does the critique treat empirical data in ways that are relevant to advancing theory? With respect to Lilienfield and colleagues' 2000 review, Hibbard (2003) points out numerous flaws, including their ignoring of longstanding and contemporary arguments (or simple extensions thereof) relevant to the scientific consideration of reliability, incompletely or inaccurately reporting data published in the time frame of the review, and excluding or misreporting relevant validity studies. Apart from the aggregation of multiple errors noted by Hibbard, a major shortcoming of the review is its failure to address issues of construct validity, which limits its usefulness in informing practice, research, and theory.

Conclusion

Comprehensive reviews of the evidence about projective (or any other) clinical instruments (personality performance tests) appropriately raise questions about the psychometric properties and utility of instruments for certain purposes. However, the scientific status of an instrument can only be addressed by reviews that scrutinize the accumulated evidence to answer the two interrelated questions: How well does the instrument measure the target phenomenon, and how well does that phenomenon explain responses in real-world contexts? Together, these two questions address the issues of construct validity and scientific status. The phenomena on which projective devices are based are robust, having received support across multiple psychology subfields. Theory-grounded reviews that distinguish between measures of implicit and explicit personality constructs (e.g., Spangler, 1992; Winter et al., 1998) support the scientific merit of the distinction as capturing unique phenomena that are measured with different techniques, develop via different routes, and have different relations with external correlates. Accordingly, policy and ethics guidelines regarding the clinical use of psychological tests must be mindful of the implications of relevant distinctions within a single construct for generalizing from test responses to functioning in real world contexts. Moreover, testing guidelines should extend beyond a focus on the *construct validity* of single instruments to consider *case validity*, which rests with the selection and the synthesis of the measures to be included in a given protocol (*case validity*; Teglasi et al., 2012).

Notes

1. *Science* is defined in *Webster's Dictionary* as (a) "knowledge or a system of knowledge covering general truths or the operation of general laws, especially as obtained and tested through scientific methods"; and as (b) "a system or method reconciling practical ends with scientific laws."

2. Techniques such as brain imaging show activation of neural networks during mental processes.

3. Not all measures claim to assess a construct, and the relationship between a construct and its measure is not necessarily causal. In such cases, the idea of construct validity does not apply (see Borsboom et al., 2004).

References

Bargh, J. A., & Morsella, E. (2008). The unconscious mind. *Perspectives on Psychological Science, 3*, 73–79.

Barkley, R. A. (1997). Behavioral inhibition, sustained attention, and executive functions: Constructing a unified theory of ADHD. *Psychological Bulletin, 121*, 65–94.

Bassan-Diamond, L., Teglasi, H., & Schmitt, P. (1995). Temperament and a story telling measure of self-regulation, *Journal of Research in Personality, 29*, 109–120.

Blankman, C., Teglasi, H.(co-first authors), & Lawser, M. (2002). Thematic apperception, narrative schemas, and literacy. *Journal of Psychoeducational Assessment, 20*, 268–289.

Boorsboom, D., Mellenbergh, G. J., & van Heerden, J. (2004), The concept of validity. *Psychological Review, 111*, 1061–1071.

Borsboom, D., Mellenbergh, G. J., & and Jaap van Heerden, J. (2003). The theoretical status of latent variables. *Psychological Review, 110*, 203–219

Borkenau, P., & Ostendorf, F. (1992). Social desirability scales as moderator and suppressor variables. *European Journal of Personality, 6*, 199–214.

Bornstein, R. F. (2005). Reconnecting psychoanalysis to mainstream psychology: Opportunities and challenges. *Psychoanalytic Psychology, 22*, 323–340.

Bornstein, R. F. (2002). A process dissociation approach to objective-projective test score interrelationships. *Journal of Personality Assessment, 78*, 47–68.

Burton, K., Lydon, J., Alessandro, D., & Koestner, R. (2006). The differential effects of intrinsic and identified motivation on well-being and performance: Prospective, experimental, and implicit approaches to self-determination theory. *Journal of Personality and Social Psychology, 91*(4), 750–762.

Campbell, D. T., & Fiske, D. W. (1959). Convergent and discriminant validation by the multitrait-multimethod matrix. *Psychological Bulletin, 56*, 81–105.

Card, N. A., & Little, T. D. (2006). Proactive and reactive aggression in childhood and adolescence: A meta-analysis of differential relations with psychosocial adjustment. *International Journal of Behavioral Development, 30*, 466–480.

Cronbach, L. J. (1990). *Essentials of psychological testing* (5th ed.). New York: Harper/Collins.

Cronbach, L. J., & Meehl, P. E. (1955). Construct validity in psychological tests. *Psychological Bulletin, 52*, 281–302.

Crowne, D. P., & Marlowe, D. (1960). A new scale of social desirability independent of psychopathology. *Journal of Consulting Psychology, 24*, 349–354.

Dowd, E. T. (2006). What changes in cognitive therapy? The role of tacit knowledge structures. *Journal of Cognitive and Behavioral Psychotherapies, 6*, 21–29.

Dowd, E. T., & Courchaine, K. E. (2002). Implicit learning, tacit knowledge, and implications for stasis and change in cognitive psychotherapy. In R. L. Leahy & E. T. Dowd (Eds.), *Clinical advances in cognitive psychotherapy* (pp. 325–344). New York: Springer.

Duckworth, K. L., Bargh, J. A., Garcia, M., & Chaiken, S. (2002). The automatic evaluation of novel stimuli. *Psychological Science, 13*, 513–519.

Edwards, A. L. (1957). *The social desirability variable in personality assessment and research.* New York: Dryden.

Epstein, S. (1966). Some considerations on the nature of ambiguity and the use of stimulus dimensions in projective techniques. *Journal of Consulting Psychology, 30*, 183–192.

Epstein, S. (1994). Integration of the cognitive and psychodynamic unconscious. *American Psychologist, 49*, 709–724.

Evans, J. (2008). Dual processing accounts of reasoning, judgment, and social cognition. *Annual Review of Psychology, 59*, 255–278.

Exner, J. E. (1991). *The Rorschach: A comprehensive system: Vol. 2. Interpretation* (2nd ed.). New York: Wiley.

Fazio, R. H. (1990). Multiple processes by which attitudes guide behavior: The MODE model as an integrative framework. In M. P. Zanna (Ed.), *Advances in experimental social psychology* (Vol. 23, pp. 75–109). New York: Academic Press.

Frank, L. D. (1939). Projective methods for the study of personality. *Journal of Psychology, 8*, 389–413.

Frank, L. D. (1948). *Projective Methods.* Springfield, IL: Thomas.

Frost, B. C., Ko, C. E., & James, L. R. (2007). Implicit and explicit personality: A test of a channeling hypothesis for aggressive behavior. *Journal of Applied Psychology, 92*, 1299–1319.

Garb, H. N. (2003). *What's wrong with the Rorschach?* San Francisco: Jossey-Bass.

Greenwald, A. G., Banaji, M. R., Rudman, L. A., Farnham, S. D., Nosek, B. A., & Mellott, D. S. (2002). A unified theory of implicit attitudes, stereotypes, self-esteem, and self-concept. *Psychological Review, 109*(1), 3–25.

Hibbard, S., 2003. A critique of Lilienfeld et al.'s (2000) "The Scientific Status of Projective Techniques." *Journal of Personality Assessment, 80*, 260–271.

Hughes, T. L., Gacono, C. B., & Owen, P. F. (2007). Current status of Rorschach assessment: Implications for school the school psychologist. *Psychology in the Schools, 44*, 281–291.

James, L. R. (1998). Measurement of personality via conditional reasoning. *Organizational Research Methods, 1*, 131–163.

James, L. R., & Mazerolle, M. D. (2002). *Personality in work organizations.* Thousand Oaks, CA: Sage Publications.

Jenkins, S. R. (2008). Teaching how to learn reliable scoring. In S. R. Jenkins (Ed.), *A handbook of clinical scoring systems for thematic apperceptive techniques* (pp. 39–66). New York: Erlbaum.

Kaplan, M. F. (1967). The effect of cue relevance, ambiguity, and self-reported hostility on tat responses. *Journal of Projective Techniques & Personality Assessment, 31*(6), 45–50.

Kihlstrom, J. F. (1999). The psychological unconscious. In L. R. Pervin & O. John (Eds.), *Handbook of personality* (2nd ed.; pp. 424–442). New York: Guilford.

Lewicki, P., Czyzewska, M., & Hill, T. (1997). Cognitive mechanisms for acquiring "experience": The dissociation between conscious and nonconscious cognition. In J. D. Cohen and J. W. Schooler (Eds.), *Scientific approaches to the question of consciousness (Carnegie Mellon symposium on consciousness)* (pp. 161–177). Hillsdale, NJ: Erlbaum.

Lewicki, P., Hill, T., & Czyzewska, M. (1992). Nonconscious acquisition of information. *American Psychologist, 47*, 796–801.

Lilienfeld, S. O., Wood, J. M., & Garb. H. N. (2000). The scientific status of projective techniques. *Psychological Science in the Public Interest, 1*, 27–66.

Lindzey, Gardner. 1961. *Projective techniques and cross-cultural research.* New York: Appleton-Century-Crofts.

Lieberman, M. D. (2007). Social cognitive neuroscience: A review of core processes. *Annual Review of Psychology, 58*, 259–289.

Lohr, L., Teglasi, H., & French, M. (2004). Schemas and temperament as risk factors for emotional disability, *Personality and Individual Differences, 36*, 1637–1654.

Magnusson, D., & Endler, N. S. (1977). Interactional psychology: Present status and future prospects. In D. Magnusson & N. S. Endler (Eds.), *Personality at the crossroads: Current issues in interactional psychology.* Hillsdale, NJ: Lawrence Erlbaum Associates.

Mayer, J. D. (2003). Structural divisions of personality and the classification of traits. *Review of General Psychology, 7*, 381–401.

McClelland, D. C., Koestner, R., & Weinberger, J. (1989). How do self-attributed and implicit motives differ? *Psychological Review, 96*, 690–702.

McCrae R. R., & Costa P. T. (1983). Social desirability scales: More substance than style. *Journal of Consulting and Clinical Psychology, 51*, 882–888.

Messick, S. (1989). Validity. In R. L. Linn (Ed.), *Educational measurement* (3rd ed.; pp. 13–103). New York: MacMillan.

Meyer, G. J., & Kurtz, J. E. (2006). Advancing personality assessment terminology: Time to retire "objective" and "projective" as personality test descriptors. *Journal of Personality Assessment, 87*, 223–225.

Mischel, W. (1968). *Personality and assessment.* New York: Wiley.

Moller, A. C., & Elliot, A. J. (2006). The 2 x 2 achievement goal framework: An overview of empirical research. In A. V. Mitel (Ed.), *Focus on educational psychology research* (pp. 307–326). New York: Nova Science Publishers.

Murstein, B. I. (1965). The stimulus. In B. Murstein (Ed.), *Handbook of projective techniques.* New York: Basic Books.

Nisbett, R., & Wilson, T. (1977). Telling more than we can know: Verbal reports on mental processes. *Psychological Review, 84*, 231–259.

Orne, M. T. (1962). On the social psychology of the psychological experiment: With particular reference to demand characteristics and their implications. *American Psychologist, 17*, 776–783.

Paulhus, D. L. (1984). Two-component models of socially desirable responding. *Journal of Personality and Social Psychology, 46*, 598–609.

Paulhus, D. L. (1998). Interpersonal adaptiveness of trait self-enhancement: A mixed blessing? *Journal of Personality and Social Psychology, 74*, 1197–1208.

Perkins, D. N., & Ritchhart, R. (2004). When is good thinking? In D. Y. Dai & R. J. Sternberg (Eds.), *Motivation, emotion, and cognition: Integrative perspectives on intellectual functioning and development* (pp. 351–384). Mahwah, NJ: Erlbaum.

Pretz, J. E., Naples, A. J., & Sternberg, R. J. (2003). Recognizing, defining, and representing problems. In J. E. Davidson & R. J. Sternberg (Eds.), *The psychology of problem solving* (pp. 3–30). New York: Cambridge University Press.

Rabin, A. I. (1981). Projective methods: A historical introduction. In A. I. Rabin (Ed.), *Assessment with projective techniques* (pp. 1–22). New York: Springer.

Riso, L. P., du Toit, P. L., Stein, D. J., & Young, J. E. (2007). *Cognitive schemas and core beliefs in psychological problems: A scientist-practitioners guide.* Washington DC: American Psychological Association.

Roberts, G. E., & Gruber, C. (2005). *Roberts-2.* Los Angeles: Western Psychological Services.

Sackett, P. R., Zedeck, S., & Fogli, L. (1988). Relations between measures of typical and maximum job performance, *Journal of Applied Psychology, 73*, 482–486.

Sackett, P. R. (2007). Revisiting the origins of the typical-maximum performance distinction, *Human Performance, 20*, 179–185.

Smith, G. T. (2005). On construct validity: Issues of method and measurement. *Psychological Assessment, 17*, 396–408.

Snyder, M., & Ickes, W. (1985). Personality and social behavior. In G. Lindzey & E. Aronson (Eds.), *Handbook of social psychology* (3rd ed.). New York: Random House.

Spangler, W. D. (1992). Validity of questionnaire and TAT measures of need for achievement. *Psychological Bulletin, 112*, 140–154.

Stöber, J. (2001). The Social Desirability Scale-17 (SDS-17): Convergent validity, discriminant validity with age. *European Journal of Psychological Assessment, 17*, 222–232.

Teglasi, H. (1993). *Clinical use of story telling: Emphasizing the TAT with children and adolescents.* Boston: Allyn & Bacon.

Teglasi, H. (1998). Assessment of schema and problem-solving strategies with projective techniques. In M. Hersen & A. Bellack (Series Eds.) & C. Reynolds (Vol. Ed.), *Comprehensive clinical psychology: Vol. 4. Assessment* (pp. 459–499). London: Elsevier Science Press.

Teglasi, H. (2010). *Essentials of TAT and other storytelling assessments* (2nd ed.). New York: Wiley.

Teglasi, H., & Epstein, S. (1998). Temperament and personality theory: The perspective of cognitive-experiential self-theory. *School Psychology Review, 27*, 534–550.

Teglasi, H., Locraft, C., & Felgenhauer, K. (2008). Empathy: schemas and social information processing, In S. Jenkins (Ed.), *A handbook of clinical scoring systems for thematic apperceptive techniques* (pp. 573–605). Mahwah, NJ: Lawrence Erlbaum Associates.

Teglasi, H., Nebbergall, A., & Newman, D., (2012). Construct validity and case validity in assessment. *Psychological Assessment, 24*, 464–475.

Teglasi, H., Simcox, A., & Kim, N. Y. (2007). Personality constructs and measures. *Psychology in the Schools, 44*, 215–228.

Uleman, J. S. (2005). On the inherent ambiguity of traits and other mental concepts. In B. F. Malle & S. D. Hodges (Eds.), *Other minds: How humans bridge the divide between self and others* (pp. 253–267). New York: Guilford Publications.

Whitehead, A. N. (1920). *The concept of nature*. Cambridge: Cambridge University Press.

Wilson, T. D., Lindsey, S., & Schooler, T. (2000). A model of dual attitudes. *Psychological Review, 107*, 101–126.

Winter, D. G., John, O. P., Stewart, A. J., Klohnen, E. C., & Duncan, L. E. (1998). Traits and motives: Toward an integration of two traditions in personality research. *Psychological Review, 105*(2), 230–250.

Wood, J. M., Garb, H. N., Lilienfeld, S. O., & Nezworski, M. T. (2002). Clinical assessment of personality. *Annual Review of Psychology, 53*, 519–543.

Wood, J. M., Nezworski, M. T., Lilienfeld, S. O., & Garb, H. N. (2003). *What's wrong with the Rorschach? Science confronts the controversial inkblot test*. New York: Jossey-Bass.

Large-Scale Group Score Assessments: Past, Present, and Future

Bobby Naemi, Eugene Gonzalez, Jonas Bertling, Anthony Betancourt,
Jeremy Burrus, Patrick C. Kyllonen, Jennifer Minsky, Petra Lietz, Eckhard Klieme,
Svenja Vieluf, Jihyun Lee, *and* Richard D. Roberts

Abstract

The influence of large-scale group score assessments on research, policy, and practice in education has increased dramatically over the past few decades. The goal of this chapter is to provide an overview of the value and scope of this program of research. The chapter begins by providing an overview of the history of large-scale assessment. Next, it focuses on current research and development surrounding the National Assessment of Educational Progress (NAEP, a government-mandated assessment in the United States) and the Programme for International Student Assessment (PISA, a large-scale survey and assessment commission by the Organisation for Economic Co-operation and Development, OECD). We also briefly review other landmark large-scale group score assessments. Throughout, we highlight the growing use of noncognitive variables in these assessments. The chapter concludes with a discussion of some of the topics and approaches likely to guide future directions in this domain.

Key Words: large-scale group score assessment, international assessment, noncognitive assessment, NAEP, PISA

Introduction

Large-scale assessments, in the broadest sense, are defined as surveys of knowledge, skills, or behaviors in a given domain, usually with an attempt to describe a population of interest. They typically involve sampling (a) knowledge and skills using a comprehensive theoretical framework, (b) a relatively large number of items or tasks to cover the domain, and (c) relatively large samples of people representative of the population of interest. Results tend to be reported and aggregated at the group level, which is why "group score" is sometimes added to the description. To avoid overburdening the people surveyed, large-scale assessments often make use of multiple-matrix sampling designs, which allow them to survey smaller subsets of participants with a fewer number of items. Through the use of these methods, large-scale group score assessments produce reliable scores for groups at the expense of reliable scores for individuals.

Large-scale assessments are administered nationally or internationally. The classic example of a national large-scale assessment is the U.S. National Assessment of Educational Progress (NAEP). NAEP has been administered to samples of students within the United States since the 1960s, and covers a wide range of school-based subjects, such as mathematics, science, reading, writing, history, civics, and so forth. NAEP is usually administered at the fourth, eighth, and twelfth grades, which means, by default, it is concerned with different age groups at different levels of schooling. Note that the United States is not alone in administering national assessments, though it is relatively unparalleled in terms of its scope and frequency. For example, between 1995 and 2006, 22 countries in Sub-Saharan Africa alone administered one form or another of a national assessment (see United Nations Educational, Scientific and Cultural Organization [UNESCO], 2007). Table 6.1 provides a listing of countries across the globe (by regions given in the aforementioned report) that have administered one form or another of a national assessment over this time period.

International large-scale assessments are no less prevalent. Major surveys include the Trends in International Mathematics and Science Study (TIMSS; see Mullis, Martin, & Foy, 2008), the Progress in International Reading Literacy Study (PIRLS; see Mullis, Martin, Kennedy, & Foy, 2007), the Programme for International Student Assessment (PISA; see OECD, 2010a), and the International Civic and Citizenship Education Study (ICCS; see Schulz, Ainley, Fraillon, Kerr, & Losito, 2010). There also assessments of a regional nature, such as those sponsored by UNESCO in Latin America and Southern Africa, and those covering out-of-school populations such as the International Adult Literacy Study (IALS; see Kirsch, 2001), and the Programme

for International Assessment of Adult Competencies (PIAAC; see PIAAC Literacy Expert Group, 2009).

The use of these large-scale international assessments to measure educational processes and outcomes has become more and more prominent over the past few decades. In particular, the ubiquity of country rankings and cross-national comparisons, often heavily discussed in the media, serve as a testament to the perceived importance of the indicators and outcomes measured by these assessments. For example, PISA, conducted by the Organisation for Economic Co-operation and Development (OECD) grew from 43 participating countries in 2000 to 67 participating educational systems in 2012. This growth also applies to other large-scale international assessments operated by the International Association for the Evaluation of Education Achievement (IEA). TIMSS, for example, grew from 40 eighth-grade educational systems in 1995 to 56 in 2007, while PIRLS grew from 35 participating systems in 2001 to a projected participation of 55 in 2011. Current projections suggest that TIMSS and

Table 6.1 Countries That Have Administered National Assessments Between 1995 and 2006 (United Nations Educational, Scientific and Cultural Organization, 2007)

Sub-Saharan Africa

Burkina Faso, Central African Republic, Eritrea, Ethiopia, Gambia, Ghana, Guinea, Kenya, Lesotho, Malawi, Madagascar, Mauritius, Mozambique, Namibia, Niger, Nigeria, Seychelles, Senegal, South Africa, Swaziland, Uganda, Zambia

Arab States

Algeria, Djibouti, Egypt, Jordan, Kuwait, Lebanon, Mauritania, Morocco, Oman, Qatar, Saudi Arabia, United Arab Emirates

East Asia and the Pacific, and South and West Asia

Australia, Bangladesh, Cambodia, Cook Islands, Fiji, India, Indonesia, Japan, Lao PDR, Malaysia, Maldives, Myanmar, New Zealand, Pakistan, Philippines, Republic of Korea, Samoa, Singapore, Solomon Islands, Thailand, Tonga, Tuvalu, Vanuatu, Viet Nam

Latin America and the Caribbean

Anguilla, Argentina, Bahamas, Belize, Bolivia, Brazil, Chile, Colombia, Costa Rica, Cuba, Dominican Republic, Ecuador, El Salvador, Guatemala, Guyana, Haiti, Honduras, Jamaica, Mexico, Nicaragua, Panama, Paraguay, Peru, Saint Kitts and Nevis, Uruguay, Venezuela

Central and Eastern Europe and Central Asia

Albania, Azerbaijan, Bulgaria, Croatia, Estonia, Georgia, Hungary, Lithuania, Mongolia, Montenegro, Poland, Romania, Serbia, Slovakia, The former Yugoslav Republic of Macedonia, Turkey

Western Europe and North America

Belgium, Canada, Denmark, Finland, France, Germany, Iceland, Ireland, Israel, Italy, Luxembourg, Malta, Netherlands, Norway, Portugal, Spain, Sweden, Switzerland, United States, United Kingdom (England, Scotland, Wales)

PIRLS will be administered to a combined set of 85 educational systems in 2011. Further support for the increase in the use of large-scale assessment data comes from Rutkowski, Gonzalez, Joncas, and von Davier (2010), who reported an increase in research interest in these large-scale assessments through a search of the Wilson Education Full Text database. Findings demonstrated a growth in published research involving TIMSS, PIRLS, or PISA from 340 articles between 1995 and 1999 to 851 articles between 2005 and 2009. Clearly, the prevalence of international large-scale assessment is on the rise. The goal of this chapter is to give the reader the flavor of these large-scale assessments, while simultaneously outlining important issues these studies address that can benefit educational research, policy, and practice.

The data gathered by large-scale international assessments represents an enormously valuable source of information on a host of issues and topics relevant to educational research and policy, data that can be difficult or impossible to gather in smaller, within-country contexts. Performance results in many cases are reported as a series of scores, with the goal of providing information about how students are performing at a given threshold or score category (Ercikan, 2006). These score reports have led to increasingly high stakes for many large-scale assessments as accountability measures.

The chapter begins with a brief history of large-scale international assessment, which has a colorful and vibrant past. Next, we focus on one particular national large-scale assessment, with a long history: NAEP. We then discuss a small selection of these programs, including their current status and general features. Space simply precludes covering all of the programs that have been conducted, as attested by the list of assessment programs identified in Table 6.1, as well as Table 6.2, which highlights major studies and large-scale student assessment administrations since 1961. We conclude with a discussion of where large-scale group score assessment research might head in the future.

The Past: A History of Large-Scale Group Score Assessment

The end of the Second World War and the associated reconstruction of economic and educational systems were accompanied by an unprecedented expansion of education. This expansion extended across all levels, from early childhood education through universities and institutes for adult education (Connell, 1980). This growth, among other things, led to the development of educational research as a major field of scholarly inquiry.

Origins

In 1946, the constitution of the United Nations Educational, Scientific and Cultural Organization (UNESCO) was ratified by 20 countries with the aim of integrating educational, scientific, and cultural activities across countries and cultures in the quest for world peace. In 1952, a group of scholars met at the UNESCO Institute for Education in Hamburg, Germany, in what might nowadays be called a think-tank. The goal of this group was to consider how information might be obtained more systematically in terms of educational processes and outcomes across the world, beyond the national studies that had been undertaken in some countries up to that time. Specifically, the aim of the group was to obtain this information and determine what educational systems could learn from each other (UNESCO, 2010).

Against this background, the IEA was founded in 1958 with the goal of studying the process of education across the world. As one of its first activities, the Pilot Project was undertaken from 1959–1961 in twelve education systems (i.e., Belgium, England, Germany, Finland, France, Israel, Poland, Scotland, Sweden, Switzerland, the United States, and then-Yugoslavia) to examine the feasibility of a cross-national study of educational achievement. The project assessed achievement in the areas of reading comprehension, mathematics, science, geography, and non-verbal ability from samples of about 1,000 13-year-old students in each country. This particular age group had been chosen because, at that time, this was the oldest age group for which nearly the whole cohort was still at school in the participating countries. The Pilot Project showed, for the first time, that it was possible to conduct an international assessment study on a relatively large scale, despite major challenges in terms of logistics and translation (Foshay, Thorndike, Hotyat, Pidgeon, & Walker, 1962).

The Pilot Project was followed by a study in 1964 of mathematics achievement levels of 13-year-olds and students at the pre-university year (Husén, 1967). The study design improved in that probability samples of the two target populations were drawn to enable proper population estimates and the estimation of sampling error. Again, twelve countries (i.e., Australia, Belgium, England, Germany, Finland, France, Israel, Japan, the Netherlands, Scotland, Sweden, and the United States) participated, with

Table 6.2 Characteristics of Major Large-Scale Group Score Student Assessments Conducted Since 1961

Year	Study	RD	Conducted By	Constructs Measured	Pop/Age (years)	Intl	# Count
1961	Twelve-Country Study	No	International Association for the Evaluation of Educational Achievement (IEA) / UNESCO Institute in Hamburg	Math; reading; geography; science; non-verbal ability	13	Yes	12
1964	First International Mathematics Study (FIMS)	No	IEA	Math	13; 17–18	Yes	12
1968	The Equality of Educational Opportunity Study (EEOS) "Coleman Study"	No	United States Department of Health, Education, and Welfare	Verbal skills; nonverbal associations; reading comprehension; math	* 6; 8; 11; 17	No	1 (USA)
1969	National Assessment of Educational Progress (NAEP)	Yes	National Center for Education Statistics (NCES)	Math; reading; science; writing; arts; civics; economics; geography; U.S. history	* 9; 13; 17	No	1 (USA)
1971	Reading Comprehension	No	IEA	Reading comprehension; speed of reading; word knowledge	* 10; 14; 17	Yes	14
1971	Literature Education	No	IEA	Literature	* 14; 17	Yes	9
1971	French as a Foreign Language	No	IEA	French: reading; listening; writing; speaking	* 14; 17	Yes	8
1971	First International Science Study (FISS)	No	IEA	Biology; chemistry; physics	* 10; 14; 17	Yes	18
1971	English as a Foreign Language	No	IEA	English: reading; listening; writing; speaking	*14; 17–18	Yes	9

Year	Study	RD	Conducted By	Constructs Measured	Pop/Age (years)	Intl	# Count
1971	NAEP	Yes	NCES	Math; reading; science; writing; arts; civics; economics; geography; U.S. history	* 9; 13; 17	No	1 (USA)
1971	Civics Education	No	IEA	Civics education	10; 14; 17	Yes	10
1979	Second International Mathematics Study (SIMS)	No	IEA	Arithmetic; algebra; geometry; measurement; statistics	13; 17	Yes	18
1980–1985	Classroom Environment Study	Yes	IEA	Science; math; history	* 10–13	Yes	9
1983–1988	Written Composition	No	IEA	Written composition	*10; 16; 18	Yes	14
1984	Second International Science Study (SISS)	No	IEA	Science	10; 14; 17	Yes	23
1987	International Assessment of Educational Progress (IAEP)	Yes	Educational Testing Service (ETS)	Math; science	9; 13	Yes	20
1987–1993	Computer in Education Study (CompEd)	No	IEA	Use of computers in schools	10; 13; 17–18	Yes	23
1990–1992	Trial State Assessment	No	NCES	Math	13	No	1 (USA)
1991	Reading Literacy Study	No	IEA	Reading	9; 14	Yes	31
1991	International Assessment of Educational Progress (IAEP)	Yes	ETS	Math; science; geography; performance assessment	9; 13	Yes	20
Year	Study	RD	Conducted By	Constructs Measured	Pop/Age (years)	Intl	# Count
1994	Pre-Primary Project (PPP)	Yes	IEA	Cognitive and language development; family background; teachers' characteristics; structural features of settings; children's experiences	4 (and tested again at 7)	Yes	10
1995	Third International Mathematics and Science Study (TIMSS)	Yes	IEA	Math; science	* 8; 9; 12; 13	Yes	40

(continued)

Table 6.2 (Continued)

Year	Study	RD	Conducted By	Constructs Measured	Pop/Age (years)	Intl	# Count
1995	TIMSS Advanced (TIMSS-a)	Yes	IEA	Advanced math; physics; math; science literacy	*17–18	Yes	22
1995	Language Education Study (LES)	No	IEA	English; French; German; Spanish	*16; 18	Yes	25
1995	Southern and Eastern Africa Consortium for Monitoring Educational Quality (SACMEQ)	Yes	SACMEQ; UNESCO International Institute for Educational Planning (IIEP).	Reading; math	*11	Yes	7
1997	Laboratorio Latinoamericano para la Evaluacion de la Calidad Educativa (LLECE)	No	UNESCO's Regional Bureau for Education in Latin America and the Caribbean	Math; language	*8; 9	Yes	13
1999	Third International Mathematics and Science Study—Repeat (TIMSS-R)	Yes	IEA	Math; science	*13	Yes	38
1999	Civic Education (CivED)	No	IEA	Civic and citizenship education	*14; 16–19	Yes	28
Year	Study	RD	Conducted By	Constructs Measured	Pop/Age (years)	Intl	# Count
2000	Programme for International Student Assessment (PISA)	Yes	OCED	Math; science; reading	15	Yes	48
2000	SACMEQ	Yes	SACMEQ; UNESCO IIEP	Reading; math	*11	Yes	14
2001	Progress in International Reading Literacy (PIRLS)	Yes	IEA	Reading	*9	Yes	35
2001	Progress in International Reading Literacy (PIRLS TRENDS study)	No	IEA	Reading	9	Yes	9
2003	PISA	Yes	OCED	Math; science; reading; problem solving	15	Yes	41

Year	Study	RD	Conducted By	Constructs Measured	Pop/Age (years)	Intl	# Count
2003	TIMSS	Yes	IEA	Math; science	*9; 13	Yes	49
2003	Trial Urban District Assessment (TUDA)	Yes	NCES	Math; reading; science	*9; 13	No	1 (USA)
2006	PISA	Yes	OCED	Math; science; reading	15	Yes	57
2006	PIRLS	Yes	IEA	Reading	*9	Yes	40
2007	TIMSS	Yes	IEA	Math; science	*9; 13	Yes	52
2007	Segundo Estudio Regional Comparativo y Explicativo (SERCE)	No	UNESCO's Regional Bureau for Education in Latin America and the Caribbean	Math; science; language	*8; 11	Yes	16
2007	SACMEQ	Yes	SACMEQ; UNESCO IIEP	Reading; math	*11	Yes	14
2008	TIMSS-a	yes	IEA	Math; physics	*17–18	Yes	10
2009	PISA	Yes	OCED	Math; science; reading	15	Yes	65
2009	International Civic and Citizenship Education Study (ICCS)	No	IEA	Civic and citizenship education	*13	Yes	38
Year	**Study**	**RD**	**Conducted By**	**Constructs Measured**	**Pop/Age (years)**	**Intl**	**# Count**
2010–2013	Latin America Laboratory for Assessment in the Quality of Education (Third Regional Explanatory and Comparative Study, TERCE)	No	UNESCO's Regional Bureau for Education in Latin America and the Caribbean	Reading; writing; arithmetic; practical competencies	Students; Teachers	Yes	11
2011	European Indicator of Language Competence	No	European Council	Reading; listening; speaking; writing	15	Yes	16

Note. Abbreviations for columns: Year (Year), Study Name (Study), Repeated Design (RD), Organization, Conducted By (Conducted By), Constructs and Subjects Measured (Constructs Measured), Population and Age (Pop/Age), International Study (Intl), Number of Countries (# count). Asterisk (*) indicates that only grade-level information was provided and an approximate age was given for the students' grade level.

the project involving over 133,000 students from 5,400 schools. In addition to achievement data, background information was collected from these students as well as from 13,000 teachers and 5,400 principals by way of questionnaires. Analyses were aimed at testing specific hypotheses in four main areas: (a) the effects of school organization on mathematics achievement, (b) curriculum and instruction, (c) support for education, and (d) the relationships of socio-economic and geographic factors with mathematical achievement.

Around this time period, the United States Department of Health, Education, and Welfare commissioned the Equality of Educational Opportunity Study (EEOS), more commonly known as the "Coleman Study" (Coleman, 1968). The study grew out of efforts to address social policy issues relating to ethnicity, religion, and national origin prompted by the Civil Rights Act of 1964. As part of the survey, students from five grade levels (first, third, sixth, ninth, and twelfth grades) completed questionnaires assessing demographic and background variables, attitudes towards learning, education and career goals, and racial attitudes, alongside tests of verbal ability, reading comprehension, nonverbal associations, and mathematics. In addition, principals and teachers completed questionnaires examining education and teaching experience, salary, academic discipline, verbal facility, and racial attitudes. The study proved to be a landmark effort in linking national social policy goals to large-scale surveys and assessments.

Both the Pilot Project and the Coleman Study represented examples of how meaningful analyses could be undertaken with comparable data from large-scale assessments of school-aged children. For the Pilot Project in particular, two additional developments took place. First, the theoretical foundations to guide these assessments were further developed. Second, the scope of the assessments was extended to cover a wider range of school subjects.

The theoretical developments involved the consideration of a number of models. These included a general model for cross-national comparisons in education, which started with the environment and the economy, which then gave rise to a demand for human resources and curriculum development (Dahlöf, 1967). These demands were translated into objectives, and finances were used to fund processes that resulted in educational attainment. Based on this schema, a comprehensive model of educational processes was put forward by Super (1967). This model started with the social and cultural capital

that was evident in inputs categorized as financial conditions, production conditions, and human conditions. Processes followed that covered educational structure, equipment, agents, curricula, and instructional methods. These were modeled to lead to outputs in the form of performance in terms of knowledge, skills, attitudes, educational levels, and competencies, which, in turn, were utilized in the contexts of employment, community, and family. These contexts were identified as being reflective of national development in terms of human, economic, and political development.

Several additional models highlighted other important aspects thought to have an impact on performance in large-scale group score assessments. For example, the model of selectivity and retentivity argued that differences in countries' performance in mathematics were a consequence of the number and type of students retained in a cohort (Walker, 1967). Carroll's (1963) model of school learning specified the relationships between aptitude, perseverance, opportunity to learn, ability to understand instruction, and quality of instruction and their impact on student performance. In addition, the model put forward by Rosier and Keeves (1991) underlined the importance of the intended, implemented, and achieved curriculum in describing and understanding student performance.

Large-Scale Assessment Research: The Second Wave

The Six-Subject Survey was the second major development in large-scale group score assessment research. Specifically, it extended the content coverage of large-scale cross-national assessments in schools and enabled the testing of the conceptual models described above. Conducted between 1970 and 1971, the Six-Subject Survey assessed performance in science (Comber & Keeves, 1973), reading comprehension (Thorndike, 1973), literature (Purves, 1973), French as a foreign language (Carroll, 1975), English as a foreign language (Lewis & Massad, 1975), and civic education (Torney, Oppenheim, & Farnen, 1976). The Six-Subject Survey also increased coverage as far as geography and economic development were concerned in comparison to past assessments. A total of 23 different education systems participated across the six subjects, although not all systems participated in each subject area (Peaker, 1975).

Led by the IEA, conceptual and content development came together during this period, based on extended content area coverage and improved test design. For example, Carroll's model was tested using data from the French as a Foreign Language study, while the curriculum model was examined using data from the First and Second IEA Science Studies (Comber & Keeves, 1973; Postlethwaite & Wiley, 1992), as well as the Second International Mathematics Study (Robitaille & Garden, 1989).

Over the next two decades, IEA conducted the following studies: the Second International Mathematics Study (Robitaille & Garden, 1989); the Second International Science Study (Keeves, 1992); the Reading Literacy Study 1990–91 (Elley, 1994); the Third International Mathematics and Science Study (Beaton, Martin, Mullis, Gonzalez, Kelly, & Smith, 1996; Beaton, Mullis, Martin, Gonzalez, Kelly, & Smith, 1996); and the Third International Mathematics and Science Study Repeat (or TIMSS-R) in 1999 (Martin et al., 2000; Mullis et al., 2000). The IEA also extended to new areas of interest as they arose (e.g., Computers in Education [Pelgrum & Plomp, 1993]; Written Composition [Purves, 1992]; and the Pre-Primary Project [Olmsted & Weikart, 1994]).

Each of these large-scale assessments also had new design elements that resulted in fresh insights. For example, TIMSS-R 1999 allowed for the comparison of different age cohorts between the first wave of data collection in 1995 and the second wave of data collection in 1999 (as students progressed from Grades 4 to 8). Often these studies were prompted by important policy issues. Take again the TIMSS. The background for these studies began in the late 1980s, when the U.S. government decided to set a goal that, by the year 2000, the nation would be number one in educating students. A series of reforms were thus put into place in the late 1980s and early 1990s. The results for the United States in 1995 indicated a relatively good performance for the fourth graders, but showed that American eighth graders lagged behind their peers from around the world. TIMSS-R in 1999 was designed, among other reasons, to investigate whether the cohort of fourth graders in 1995, once they reached the eighth grade, would still hold on to their relatively high results compared to the rest of the countries. Researchers hypothesized that in 1995, the reforms from the 1980s and 1990s may have resulted in favorable results among fourth graders, but might not have yet reached the older cohort of students. The results did not support this hypothesis: American eighth graders were still lagging behind their peers in 1999. Similarly, the Pre-Primary Project (Olmstedt & Weikart, 1994)

enabled the nine education systems that participated in Phases 1 and 2 to examine how the quality of life of preschool children in various care and education environments influenced these children's development, as participants were first assessed at age four with a follow-up at age seven.

Large-Scale International Assessment Research: Towards the Current Major Programs

Out of these earlier studies, the two current main large-scale assessments conducted by the IEA emerged. These are the Trends in International Mathematics and Science Study (TIMSS) and the Progress in International Reading Literacy Study (PIRLS). TIMSS has been conducted every four years since 1995 and assesses the mathematics and science achievement of a representative sample of students in Grades 4 and 8. Twelfth graders were assessed in 1995 and in 2008. At the time of writing, fifty-eight fourth grade education systems and 59 eighth grade education systems were participating in the current form of the assessment (i.e., TIMSS 2011). Data collection for PIRLS, which is conducted every five years, also occurred in 2011. The target population for PIRLS is the grade level that represents four years of schooling in the 53 participating education systems, providing that the mean age at the time of testing is at least 9.5 years.

TIMSS designs the studies based on the intended curriculum (what is supposed to be taught), the implemented curriculum (what is actually taught), and the achieved curriculum (what students have actually learned). PIRLS focuses on the achievement of young children (between 9 and 10 years) and the experiences that they have at home and school in learning to read. In the PIRLS framework, *reading literacy* is defined as "the ability to understand and use written language forms required by society and/or valued by the individual" (Mullis et al., 2011, p. 11) Options for young readers include reading to learn, reading for enjoyment, or reading to participate in various communities of readers. The choice of age for PIRLS is based on the general understanding that, at that age, students have made the transition from learning to read to reading to learn.

In 2012, the Organization for Economic Cooperation and Development (OECD) will have conducted the fifth cycle of its Programme for International Student Assessment (PISA), which began in 2000 and is undertaken every three years. PISA regularly assesses three domains: reading literacy, mathematics literacy, and science literacy. Each cycle, one of these domains is tested in greater depth to allow for greater coverage in every third cycle or every nine years. In addition to these domains, PISA occasionally assesses other aspects considered important, such as problem-solving (in 2003 and in 2012) or financial literacy (in 2012). In addition to the cognitive assessments, PISA includes background questionnaires for students, parents, and schools that provide a rich database on attitudes and behaviors of 15-year olds (e.g., mathematics motivation, self-concept, or enjoyment of reading) as important performance predictors and noncognitive outcomes of education.

Unlike TIMSS and PIRLS, which are studies developed and based largely on an analysis of what is taught across the participating countries, PISA assesses students' literacy in the three subject areas mentioned above. In other words, the guiding principle in the PISA test design is to assess the extent to which students have acquired reading, mathematics, and science literacy skills deemed necessary to be fully functioning citizens. "Fully functioning citizens" are defined here as individuals who will be able to constructively contribute to the economies in which they are educated (in OECD countries, e.g.; OECD, 2010a). A more detailed review of constructs assessed in PISA appears below. Because its goal is to measure whether students have the skills necessary to be fully functioning citizens, PISA focuses on 15-year-old students. This is the age group that in most OECD countries is considered the year prior to being able to join the workforce. These students are also generally found to be towards the end of compulsory education in OECD countries.

There are 67 participating systems in PISA 2012, 34 of which are OECD member countries. PISA assessments produce a large array of technical reports. For example, in the 2009 cycle, six volumes were produced, each focusing on a specific issue: students' literacy (OECD, 2010a), equity of educational opportunities (OECD, 2010b), characteristics of successful students (OECD, 2010c) characteristics of successful schools (OECD, 2010d), changes in reading performance from 2000 to 2009 (OECD, 2010e), and digital reading (OECD, 2011).

Large-Scale National Assessments: The History of NAEP

The preceding review concerned itself mainly with international large-scale assessments. National assessments, as we suggested earlier, have a long and colorful history as well, though providing an exhaustive history of all such programs might well fill a book (or two). To ensure some historical coverage of these programs, we focus on the National Assessment for Educational Progress (NAEP), the large-scale assessment regularly conducted in the United States, which is something of a flagship for this approach.

NAEP has been measuring student progress since 1964 and has become the "Nation's Report Card." The development of NAEP was spearheaded by Francis Keppel, the U.S. Commissioner of Education from 1962 to 1966, with the goal of obtaining empirical evidence concerning the condition of American schools in order to report on the progress of students for the U.S. Office of Education. Planning for the development of such an assessment program sprang from two conferences and the establishment of an Exploratory Committee on Assessing the Progress of Education (ECAPE), all funded by the Carnegie Corporation (Jones, 1996).

The idea for the assessment was initially conceptualized by psychologist Ralph Tyler, who thought it necessary to measure what students know and how they compare to their age cohort (Carr, Dogan, Tirre, & Walton, 2007). The main goal was to examine changes in student performance over time. Tyler conceived that the assessment should: (a) test general knowledge; (b) not discriminate among individuals; (c) provide a more accurate measure of the least, average, and most educated individuals in society; (d) include adults; and (e) be administered to individuals of certain ages (Greenbaum, Garet, & Solomon, 1975). Furthermore, Tyler emphasized the importance of considering the outcomes of the assessment, including the potential that the assessment could become part of the standards for curricula. Another expectation was that student data should be assessed at the state and local levels. This suggestion was met, however, with criticism. Various educational institutions became concerned that the results of the assessment would be used to make improper comparisons (Vinovskis, 1998). Thus, it was initially decided that reporting would be done on the basis of the four regions of the United States.

Tyler, along with ECAPE and a technical advisory committee (including members such as Lee Cronbach and John Tukey) proposed possible content areas to be assessed and developed, sampling guidelines, as well as procedures for scoring, data analysis, and reporting (Jones, 1996). The following content areas were chosen based on their correspondence to school curricula: reading, mathematics, writing, literature, science, social studies, citizenship, art, music, and career and occupational development. The initial plan was to assess two of these areas per year, in five-year cycles, for all U.S. residents, including those of ages 9, 13, and 17, as well as young adults (26- to 36-year-olds; Vinovskis, 1998).

The ideas put forth by Tyler and the various committees were generally kept intact, although some amendments and refinements were made. The first national assessments were conducted in 1969. During this year, the administration and management of student assessments came under the jurisdiction of the Education Commission of the States (ECS), which was composed of various states. ECS then created a Project Policy Board to oversee operations, and the project was then renamed the National Assessment of Educational Progress (Vinovskis, 1998). Funding for NAEP primarily came from the Carnegie Foundation and received some support from the federal government. By 1972, funding was exclusively provided by the federal government.

The first administration of NAEP occurred in 1969, at about the same time as the International Association for the Evaluation of Educational Achievement began conducting international large-scale assessment studies. In its first administration, NAEP assessed science, writing, and citizenship content areas for students aged 9, 13, and 17, out-of-school 17 year-olds, as well as adults aged 16 to 35. The second administration in 1971 assessed the same age groups in reading and literature content areas. Reports of student performance emphasized the individual items, about half of which were printed in the report along with their p values, however, an overall summary of results was not supplied (Linn, 2001). In 1982, the Educational Testing Service (ETS) won the NAEP contract, and significant changes were made. Documentation for the new design of NAEP was disseminated in a report by Messick, Beaton, and Lord (1983). The report encompassed an overview of the conceptual framework along with rationalizations for the new design that focused on improving the relevance of NAEP to educational policy by addressing performance standards and school effectiveness. An additional focus was on technical innovations, such as sampling by grade and age, which allowed for direct links to other state and local assessments, as well as school practices. Sampling by grade was based on the idea that age alone would not necessarily capture the

relevant populations of interest to inform schools and policy makers. Furthermore, the adoption of item-response theory and plausible values methodology allowed for the reporting of average scaled performance for groups of students and improved measurement. Around this time, it also became possible to track the trends of the different assessments and especially those that had common items (Linn, 2001).

In 1988, the National Assessment Governing Board (NAGB) was established for the purpose of independently providing policy guidance to NAEP (Jones, 1996). NAGB was given responsibility for selecting the subject areas to be assessed, as well as the frameworks that provide information concerning the content of each of the assessments (Linn, 2001). That same year, Congress allowed states to receive state-level NAEP results if they participated in the Trial State Assessment (TSA) during the 1990 and 1992 NAEP administrations. New programs subsequently emerged (e.g., Trial Urban District Assessment [TUDA], which began in 2003 and assesses samples of students from across the nation's largest cities).

Currently, state-level participation in NAEP is mandatory for reading and mathematics in the fourth and eighth grade; however, it is voluntary for states to participate in other NAEP subjects and grades (NAGB, 2010). The day-to-day operations associated with NAEP are exceedingly complex. The responsibility for the overall project is the National Center for Education Statistics (NCES) in the U.S. Department of Education. As mentioned earlier, NAGB continues to set the policy and develop the assessment specifications. The actual assessments are presently administered with the help of nine contractors, who are variously involved in sampling, item development, test delivery and production, psychometrics, and reporting.

Current State of the Art in Large-Scale Group Score Assessments

Over the past 60 years, large-scale group score assessments in school education, whether international (e.g., PISA, TIMSS and PIRLS) or national (e.g., NAEP), have come a long way, such that a wealth of data is now available for use by researchers to inform practitioners and policy makers in education. The remainder of this chapter provides a more detailed overview of constructs measured and items used by NAEP and PISA, which serve as exemplars of national and international large-scale assessments, respectively. In addition, we highlight three other major large-scale assessments mentioned in the overview; specifically, TIMSS, PIRLS, and ICCS. Note this is a very small subset of large-scale group score assessments as our preceding review suggests, though these five assessments do represent those having some of the greatest impact on research and public policy.

The National Assessment of Educational Progress (NAEP)

The National Assessment of Educational Progress assesses and reports on students' knowledge of academic subjects, including mathematics, reading, geography, writing, civics, economics, U.S. history, science, and the arts. A few additional subject areas are also currently in development, including foreign language, world history, and technology and engineering literacy. Subjects are assessed at grades 4, 8, and 12, and reporting is done on an aggregate national level, with the exception of mathematics, reading, science, and writing, which are also reported at the state level. State assessments began in 1990 (Linn, 2001), but by law, results cannot be reported for individuals or schools (Beaton & Zwick, 1992).

The main NAEP assessments are also augmented by long-term-trend NAEP assessments. Although both main and long-term-trend NAEP assessments examine the content areas of mathematics and reading, there are four differences that do not allow for a direct comparison between them:

(1) *Frequency*. Long-term-trend NAEP is measured every four years, while main NAEP assessments are measured every two years.

(2) *Content*. Long-term-trend NAEP has remained almost unchanged, while main NAEP frameworks are updated around every decade.

(3) *Sample*. Long-term-trend students are chosen based on age (9, 13, and 17 years), while main NAEP students are selected by grade (4, 8, and 12).

(4) *Results*. Long-term-trend NAEP reports results on a national level using scale scores and performance levels in order to see how student performance has changed over time. Main NAEP reports results using scale scores and achievement levels.

COGNITIVE ASSESSMENT

Each NAEP cognitive assessment is built around an organizing framework, which is the blueprint that guides the development of the assessment instrument and determines the content to be assessed (NAEP, 2010). Developing a framework generally involves the following components: (i) widespread participation and reviews by educators and state education officials; (ii) reviews by steering committees whose members represent policymakers, practitioners, and members of the general public; (iii) involvement of subject supervisors from education agencies; (iv) public hearings; and (v) reviews by scholars in the field, including staff in the National Center for Education Statistics (NCES), and by a policy advisory panel (NAEP, 2010). NAEP has developed frameworks for a variety of subjects, including: arts; civics; economics; foreign language; geography; mathematics; reading; science; U.S. history; and writing (NAEP, 2010).

As the content and nature of the NAEP assessments evolve to match instructional practice and the latest research, the ability of the assessment to measure changes over time is reduced. While short-term trends can be measured in many of the NAEP subjects (e.g., mathematics, reading), the most reliable instruments of change over time are the NAEP long-term-trend assessments (Rampey, Dion, & Donahue, 2009).

The NAEP long-term-trend assessments in reading and mathematics were administered throughout the U.S. in 2007 and 2008 to samples of students aged 9, 13, and 17 years. Because the long-term-trend program uses substantially the same assessments decade after decade, it has been possible to chart educational progress since 1971 in reading and 1973 in mathematics (Rampey et al., 2009). Overall, the national trend in reading showed gains in average scores at all three ages since 2004. Average reading scores for 9- and 13-year-olds increased in 2008 compared to 1971, but the reading score for 17-year-olds was not significantly different (Rampey et al., 2009). In mathematics, average scores for 9- and 13-year-olds increased since 2004, while the average score for 17-year-olds did not change significantly. Average scores were 24 points higher than in 1973 for 9-year-olds and 15 points higher for 13-year-olds. The average mathematics score for 17-year-olds was not significantly different from that in 1973 (Rampey et al., 2009).

In terms of achievement gaps, most racial/ethnic score gaps were narrowed compared to that observed with the first assessment. While the reading score gaps between White and Black students at all three ages showed no significant change from 2004 to 2008, the gaps did narrow in 2008 compared to 1971. White–Hispanic gaps in reading scores also showed no significant change from 2004 to 2008 but were smaller in 2008 than in 1975 at ages 9 and 17 years. Across all three age groups, neither the White–Black nor White–Hispanic gaps in mathematics changed significantly from 2004 to 2008, but both were smaller in 2008 than in 1973 (Rampey et al., 2009).

In addition to achievement scores, results indicated higher percentages of 13- and 17-year-olds enrolled in advanced mathematics in 2008 than in past years (Rampey et al., 2009). Taking higher-level mathematics courses was generally associated with higher scores on the 2008 mathematics assessment at ages 13 and 17. For example, 13-year-olds who were enrolled in algebra classes scored higher on average than those enrolled in pre-algebra or regular mathematics. The percentages of 13-year-olds who reported taking pre-algebra or algebra in 2008 were higher than the percentages in 1986. The percentage of 17-year-olds who reported they had taken pre-calculus or calculus was higher in 2008 than in 1978, as was the percentage who had taken second-year algebra or trigonometry (Rampey et al., 2009).

NONCOGNITIVE INDICATORS AND OUTCOMES

In addition to the subject-specific cognitive items, NAEP also administers a series of background questions, which collect information from students, teachers, and school administrators about background variables (including several noncognitive factors) that are related to student achievement (National Assessment of Educational Progress, 2011a). Gathering this information serves, in part, to fulfill reporting requirements of federal legislation. Specifically, under the No Child Left Behind Act (No Child Left Behind Act of 2001, 2008), NAEP is required to collect information on and report achievement results disaggregated by the following variables: gender, race, ethnicity, socioeconomic status (SES), disability status, and English language learner (ELL) status. In addition to fulfilling federal requirements, information from the background items also serves to give context to NAEP results and allow researchers to track factors associated with academic achievement (National Assessment of Educational Progress, 2011b).

While some differences exist in the way that each type of background questionnaire is developed, there are shared principles that underlie the forms given to student, teacher, and school. First, the Governing Board provides initial guidance on what is developed, and the Governing Board has multiple opportunities to review and provide input. Additionally, all background questionnaires share a development process that seeks to reduce burden on respondents and ensures data quality while continuing to meet the needs of the NAEP program (NAEP, 2011b).

There are three types of noncognitive data collected in the background questionnaires: (1) student reporting categories (or demographics), (2) contextual/policy information, and (3) subject-specific information (NAEP, 2011b). With regard to general student reporting categories, since the first NAEP assessment in 1969, achievement results have always been disaggregated by subgroups of the population (i.e., as previously noted, gender, race, ethnicity, socioeconomic status, disability status, and English language learner status [NAEP, 2011b]). In addition to the required reporting categories, NAEP also collects information about factors presumed to be associated with academic performance, including homework habits, the language spoken in the home, and the quantity of reading materials in the home (National Assessment of Educational Progress, 2011c).

Contextual and policy information items primarily focus on students' educational settings and experiences, and collect information about students' attendance (days absent), family discourse (talking about school at home), reading load (pages read per day), and exposure to English in the home (NAEP, 2011c). There are also items that ask about students' effort on the assessment, and the difficulty and importance of the assessment. Answers on the questionnaires provide information on how aspects of education and educational resources are distributed among different groups. Policy-related questions are reserved for the teacher and school questionnaires. These items collect data on basic characteristics of the school, the student body, and teachers, including factors such as: grade span of school, school enrollment, expenditures per pupil, student/teacher ratios, teacher background and training, qualifications, and classroom organization (NAEP, 2011b). Together, these school, teacher, and student level variables provide a basic context for understanding achievement.

The subject-specific items in NAEP are focused and limited. These items cover three categories of information: (1) time spent studying the subject; (2) instructional experiences in the subject; and (3) motivation and perceptions about the subject and the assessment (NAEP, 2011c).

Programme for International Student Assessment

As mentioned above, the Programme for International Student Assessment (PISA) assesses three domains in each three-year cycle: reading, mathematics, and science. Questionnaires are provided to students (15-year-olds), schools, and (in some, but not all countries) parents. For the 2012 cycle, a greater effort was made to expand the scope and depth of the assessment to incorporate both innovative new item types and constructs that have not been typically measured in past PISA cycles, yet were included in other international studies. An overview of these constructs is discussed below.

A central goal of PISA is to collect and report on indicators of student achievement. These include student performance (literacy, or more generally, life skills), noncognitive outcomes (such as student motivation and well-being), educational careers, context variables (such as the students' cultural, ethnic and socioeconomic backgrounds) and, finally, process characteristics at the school and system levels (including evaluation and accountability policies, student selection and allocation, parental involvement, staff cooperation, and opportunities to learn). PISA also provides indicators that cover relationships between these factors (e.g., the so-called social gradient, which measures the strength of the relationship between socioeconomic status and performance, or the relationship between educational resources and outcomes).

PISA defines *literacy* as the capacity of students to use texts of various kinds, mathematical tools, and science-based reasoning as they encounter, interpret, and solve problems and make decisions in real-life situations. PISA also attempts to measure broader cognitive skills, such as strategies for learning and thinking and problem-solving competency. A central tenet of PISA is that success in school—and in life—depends on being committed, sharing values and beliefs, respecting and understanding others, being motivated to learn and to collaborate, and being able to regulate one's own learning behavior. These constructs can be perceived as prerequisites of cognitive learning, but may also themselves be judged as goals of education, as the OECD project Defining and Selecting Key Competencies (DeSeCo) has elaborated (Rychen & Salganik, 2003). Therefore, PISA addresses noncognitive outcomes like attitudes, beliefs, motivation, aspirations, and learning-related behavior (e.g., self-regulation, strategies, and invested time). Another important noncognitive outcome, truancy, has received increased attention as an important (negative) indicator of student's use of learning opportunities, which is also predictive of school drop-out and deviant behavior (Kearney, 2008; Lee & Burkam, 2003). In summary, PISA represents a rich and wide source of data for a host of potential research questions, bringing together both cognitive and noncognitive indicators and outcomes at multiple levels in a single large-scale assessment.

Progress in International Reading Literacy Study (PIRLS)

The Progress in International Reading Literacy Study (PIRLS) is an international comparative study of the reading literacy of young students coordinated by the IEA. PIRLS examines the reading achievement and reading behaviors and attitudes of students in the grade where most nine-year-old students can be found (which is the equivalent of fourth grade for the United States and most participating countries).

In addition to measuring achievement, PIRLS collects information about students' attitudes towards reading and their reading habits. Furthermore, parent, teacher, and school principal questionnaires gather information about students' home and school experiences in developing reading literacy, while curriculum questionnaires provide information about national context such as reading goals and curricula.

Results from the 2006 administration of PIRLS show that countries can make progress in improving children's academic achievement (Mullis et al., 2007). Most of the highest-achieving countries in 2006 showed significant improvement since 2001, including the three top-performing countries. The results also show that girls have had higher reading achievement than boys in all countries since 2001. The difference was substantial in many countries, raising concerns about the educational prospects of so many low-achieving boys during their adolescent years and beyond (Mullis et al., 2007).

Additionally, the questionnaires revealed that only about half the students across the countries assessed in 2006 agreed that they enjoyed reading and appreciated books, reflecting a troubling downward trend since 2001. Moreover, fewer students in 2006 reported reading for fun. Almost one-third hardly ever read for fun (twice monthly at most) (Mullis et al., 2007). However, PIRLS 2006 reinforces on a worldwide basis the well-established finding that children from homes fostering literacy become better readers. Students had higher reading achievement when they were from homes where their parents enjoyed reading and read frequently, books were in abundance, and students were engaged in literacy activities—from alphabet blocks to word games—from an early age (Mullis et al., 2007).

Trends in International Mathematics and Science Study (TIMSS)

The Trends in International Mathematics and Science Study (TIMSS) provides data on the mathematics and science achievement of U.S. fourth- and eighth-grade students compared to that of students in other countries. Designed to align broadly with mathematics and science curricula in the participating countries, TIMSS examines the degree to which students have learned mathematics and social concepts and skills likely to have been taught in school. TIMSS assessments emphasize questions and tasks that offer better insight into the analytical, problem-solving, and inquiry skills and capabilities of students. In addition, students, teachers, and school principals in each participating country are asked to complete questionnaires concerning the context for learning mathematics and science, so as to provide a resource for interpreting the achievement results and to track changes in instructional practices.

Results from the 2007 administration of TIMSS show that fourth graders, in both mathematics and science, showed improvement rather than decline in more countries (Mullis et al., 2008). Steady improvement since the first TIMSS in 1995 was seen in a range of countries. However, this pattern is less pronounced at the eighth grade level. Although close to a dozen countries showed improvements, most countries either showed little change or declined. At the fourth and eighth grade levels, the differences in achievement between boys and girls were negligible in mathematics and science for over a third of the countries sampled. In the remaining countries, girls had higher achievement scores than boys, especially in mathematics (Mullis et al., 2008). In addition, a key noncognitive finding was that at both grade levels, high achievement in both math and science was associated with positive attitudes toward these subjects, high levels of self-confidence in learning mathematics and science, and high values placed on these subjects as important to future success (Mullis et al., 2008).

International Civic and Citizenship Education Study (ICCS)

The International Civic and Citizenship Education Study (ICCS) examines how young people undertake their citizen roles in their respective countries. The study is based on a previous pioneering IEA study known as The Civic Education Study (CIVED), which was carried out from the year 1999 to 2000 in 28 countries. Similar to TIMSS, the ICCS targets students who are determined to be in their eighth year of schooling; for most countries, this represents the eighth grade, with a minimum mean student age of 13.5 years.

ICCS includes cognitive tests designed to examine knowledge, competencies, and conceptual understanding of civic and citizenship education. The assessment also includes noncognitive background questionnaires that collect information concerning student dispositions, activities, attitudes, and behaviors relating to civics and citizenship. Similarly, questionnaires for teachers and schools examine information about teaching and class management practices, school governance, climate, and other background variables. In order to address important culture-specific issues associated with each country sample, a National Context Survey is also used to assess the political, cultural, and educational contexts associated with civic and citizenship education in each country. To this end, regional modules are also used to examine and account for region-specific issues for groups of countries, with existing regional modules focusing on Latin America, Europe, and Asia.

Initial results from the 2009 administration of ICCS in 38 countries, based on 140,000 Grade 8 students, 62,000 teachers, and 5,300 school principals, provide a bounty of information on citizenship and civic education in an international context. Specific findings point to differing approaches in each country towards delivering civics and citizenship education. In addition, results demonstrated that, on average, a substantial proportion of students performed below minimum proficiency levels on a scale of civic knowledge (Schulz et al., 2010). Background questions also provided interesting results. For example, female students demonstrated significantly more civic knowledge than male students in most countries. In general, factors such as school experiences, having an open or receptive climate for classroom discussion, and socioeconomic status were all shown to be important contributors to civic and citizenship education. Overall, this assessment contributes a more nuanced and richer understanding of the role of citizenship and civic education in issues of importance for educational reform.

The Future of Large-Scale Group Score Assessments

Large-scale or group score assessments have the potential to answer important research questions of great value to researchers, practitioners, and policy-makers. In light of lessons learned from each of these assessments, we offer the following overall considerations for future large-scale educational assessment research. These questions need to be answered with a certain degree of consensus amongst participating countries, and to make these guidelines more concrete, we will use an assessment of critical thinking as a running example.

Policy Relevance and Interest

• The issues identified should be relevant to policy concerns in many countries. Do policy-makers around the world care if their students can think critically? How is critical thinking related to the performance of a country in terms of important educational, political, and economical indicators?

• There should be public interest in the particular issue. Do the citizens of many countries care if their students can think critically?

• The information obtained should be of value in understanding, and taking steps to improve, student performance and other outcomes. Will an assessment of critical thinking ultimately lead to improved academic and economic performance within countries?

• The issue should be related to a construct in which trends over time are of importance. Do we care if critical thinking skills improve from year to year? Do we expect students to become better at critical thinking as a function of their education?

• International comparisons should relate to important policy issues. If it is found that students from some countries tend to be more critical thinkers than others, will that lead to the implementation of policy designed to improve critical thinking in the lower performing countries?

Appropriateness for an International Assessment

• The issue should be one that can be addressed cross-culturally and should have a similar meaning across countries. If students from different countries achieve the same score on critical thinking, does that mean they are equivalent in critical thinking skills? Would we expect these students to produce responses that are equivalent

to critical thinking problems? These questions are reflective of concerns relating to Differential Item Functioning (DIF; see Magis, Beland, Tuerlinckx, & De Boeck, 2010), which can appear when test items are highly culturally complex. Test items with high cultural complexity require large amounts of specific culturally shared knowledge that is not part of the construct that should be measured. As such, items developed for international assessments should avoid relying on any specific culturally shared knowledge.

• The assessments used to measure these constructs should be reliable and valid. Do large-scale assessments of critical thinking measure the construct consistently? Can they predict important outcomes such as academic and economic output?

Technical Feasibility

• It should be technically feasible to address the issue within the context of the assessment design. Is it possible to design assessments of critical thinking for large-scale assessments?

• The time and cost associated with developing the assessments used to measure these constructs should be reasonable. Are assessments of critical thinking so complex that building them becomes prohibitively expensive?

• Researchers should consider whether there are less expensive ways to collect the information. Are there cheaper ways to assess critical thinking in a large-scale fashion? Is there some existing database already available that can be integrated into the existing assessment?

Given these constraints and guidelines, large-scale assessment research has the potential to contribute greatly to a base of scientific knowledge. There are also many examples where large-scale assessment results have been used to change educational systems and influence the direction of educational policy around the globe (see Dossey & Lindquist, 2002; Robitaille, Beaton, & Plomp, 2000; Wiseman, 2010). For instance, the term *Pisa-Schock* was coined to refer to a large and long-lasting discussion in the German political world after the results of the first PISA study showed poor student performance in Germany, which led to a wide-ranging reform agenda (Ertl, 2006). Specific outcomes included giving far greater attention to educational topics in politics and policy discussions, the introduction of national educational standards, and the formation of new curriculum development processes, which resulted in concrete changes in testing in German schools and universities.

Similarly, the reaction to recently falling PISA scores in Japan was also dubbed "PISA shock" by the Japanese media, and it has led to a number of specific educational policy changes (Foster, 2010). These changes come in the context of a previous 10-year program of "pressure-free education" that was designed to encourage more application of knowledge and less rote memorization. Faced with criticism for PISA results indicating Japanese students were falling behind rival nations, Japanese education administrators ordered a number of changes, such as adding 1,200 pages to elementary school textbooks and adding one to two hours of school for most students. These changes are themselves facing both praise and criticism as a potential regression to the stricter, rote-memorization methods that "pressure-free education" was designed to discourage.

The German and Japanese reactions to the results from PISA were notable, but certainly not unique. To demonstrate a flavor for political and policy reactions to large-scale assessment research results from a wider spectrum, see Table 6.3 for a select number of quotes from leading figures in the United States and across the globe.

Large-scale group score assessments such as PISA have clearly had an impact, both at the level of political and educational leadership, and school policy. Along these lines, and based on the advances and accomplishments made through existing studies and frameworks, we see the future of large-scale assessment research following a number of potentially fruitful paths. In particular, we highlight several approaching areas of innovation.

Computer-Based Assessment

Computerized (or electronic methods) represent the most obvious area for new and unique

Table 6.3 Selected Reactions to PISA 2009 Results from World Leaders and Governments

Quote	Leader	Nation	In response to	Source
"For me, it's a massive wake-up call…have we ever been satisfied as Americans being average in anything? Is that our aspiration? Our goal should be absolutely to lead the world in education.…I know skeptics will want to argue with the results, but we consider them to be accurate and reliable, and we have to see them as a challenge to get better.…the United States came in 23rd or 24th in most subjects. We can quibble, or we can face the brutal truth that we're being out-educated."	Arne Duncan, Secretary of the Department of Education	United States of America	Poor U.S. ranking in PISA 2009 results	(Anderson, 2010)
"Fifty years later, our generation's Sputnik moment is back.…As it stands right now, America is in danger of falling behind."	Barack Obama, President	United States of America	Poor U.S. ranking in PISA 2009 results	(Dillon, 2010).
"Since 2000, Finnish reading skills have decreased somewhat.…Ten years ago, one in five youths said they did not read for pleasure. Now that figure is one in three, and 50% for boys."	Henna Virkkunen, Minister of Education	Finland	Finland dropping from first place in PISA 2009 results	BBC, 2010)
"[Mexico] not only achieved but surpassed the goals we had set ourselves [in reading comprehension and math]."	Felipe Calderon, President	Mexico	Improved ranking in PISA 2009 results	(Oppenheimer, 2010).

approaches to large-scale group score assessment. Computer-based approaches can provide benefits in two different ways: 1) better or more efficient assessments of skills that are already widely measured, and 2) assessment of newer skills that are currently difficult or impossible to measure with paper-and-pencil approaches.

Adaptive approaches that are calibrated to a student's level of knowledge or competence are an example of how computer-based assessments can be designed to provide both more accurate measurement and a more stimulating and targeted method of measurement than traditional paper-and-pencil multiple-choice assessments that require a simple linear approach. The stimulation in this sense can come from students' ability to answer questions through a more interactive method that is based on their moment-to-moment responses.

Additional advantages of computer-based approaches to assessment include the potential to use multimedia stimuli and unique item formats; a lack of a need to store, distribute, or print test materials; the possibility of scrambling item sequences to improve security, and the potential to provide immediate results or feedback to students. An additional important benefit of computer-based assessment is its ability to capture item response-time data, which can both inform item development and serve as an important validity check. Sheuermann and Björnsson (2009) offer a more detailed discussion of these advantages, but even a brief overview is enough to demonstrate that the future of large-scale assessment research is almost inextricably tied to advances afforded by computer-based testing. Even though there are disadvantages to this approach, such as the potential for students to experience computer anxiety, and the questionable economic or practical utility of using computer-based testing across the globe (e.g., in rural areas), the potential advantages remain compelling. One approach in particular provides an advantage in promoting greater stimulation or engagement from students than do traditional paper-and-pencil methods: by the use of computer-based simulations.

Simulations

Simulations have the potential to better contextualize skills by providing real-life situations with which students can interact. In this way, the competencies or skills being assessed can be examined to give us a richer and more complete picture than typical Likert-type or multiple-choice questions.

For example, recent work at the Educational Testing Service involved the use of video-based situational judgement tests where students were asked to judge the effectiveness or ineffectiveness of specific behaviors observed in videotaped school and workplace scenarios. The contextualized scenarios provided a simulation-based method of assessment that was engaging and shown to predict achievement outcomes (Roberts et al., 2011). We believe such simulation-based approaches have promise for promoting engagement and connecting the constructs measured in large-scale studies to relatable real-life scenarios for students. Advances in simulation approaches will lead not only to better measurement, but also to better prediction of important outcomes for large-scale group score assessments.

Collaboration and Exploration

A final future area of innovation relates to the idea of collaborative or connective large-scale assessment research. Given modern technological capacities that have made collaboration and the dissemination of information more feasible than at any moment in history, we see the future of large-scale assessment research as involving further collaboration and cooperation. Along these lines, organizations and countries could ideally work together to develop concurrent assessments that complement rather than duplicate efforts, forming frameworks that allow the exploration of distinct but still vital research questions.

For example, researchers are currently exploring how NAEP data can be "cross-walked" with U.S. Census data in order to form a richer and more coherent picture of the measured constructs. These efforts specifically involve providing a more complete operationalization of socio-economic status than is currently provided by the NAEP questionnaire. Future collaborations along this line can allow for data sets to complement one another, and communicating in this way can provide a great benefit for analysis and conceptualization of important antecedents of student achievement.

NAEP also provides a specific tool that we see as representing an emblematic and extremely promising direction for the use and dissemination of large-scale assessment data: the NAEP Data Explorer (NDE). The NDE is a freely available online tool that allows for researchers to generate customized tables and graphics based on data from past NAEP administrations. Users can conduct regression analyses, compare variables, examine trends, and otherwise freely analyze and explore the data sets in both a versatile and user-friendly way. In terms of both accessibility and transparency, we see this tool as a promising way for researchers to collaborate and more easily disseminate results from large-scale assessments, which should lead to further innovations and progress in the field of large-scale group score assessment research.

Conclusion

The work being done in large-scale assessment studies is vital and groundbreaking, and although the chapter highlights the current innovations in the use of selected noncognitive predictors and outcomes, the authors suggest that the potential for further expansion of the outcome space in the field of international large-scale assessment research is great. The growth of noncognitive variables represents a promising avenue for future research, as evidenced by the use of such measures in PISA and NAEP. A growing consensus on the value of such measures and outcomes has formed, not just in the fields of psychology and education, but also through the work of economists such as Lindqvist and Vestman (2011), who found that noncognitive skills measured at age 18 predicted labor market outcomes such as wages and employment status for 30+-year-olds. In fact, noncognitive predictors outperformed cognitive predictors of these outcomes by as much as a factor of three, providing further evidence that such constructs can no longer be ignored in future large-scale assessment research.

Overall, we believe that the use of sound conceptual and methodological frameworks and an expanded set of cognitive and noncognitive predictors and outcomes can allow international large-scale assessment studies to be improved for the future. In this chapter, we have attempted, albeit in a limited amount of space, to present at least a broad overview of the past, present, and future of large-scale group score assessments. From the landmark studies of 1955, to the modern research of today, we hope that we have outlined how the work in NAEP, TIMSS, PISA, PIRLS and a host of additional assessments has contributed immensely to our knowledge of student performance across the globe. As we have argued, the results of large-scale assessment research has had an impact on schools and children from Washington to Hong Kong, and by understanding the history of this work, we will be able to better prepare a plan for future research that will benefit both science and practice.

Author Note

All statements expressed in this chapter are the author's and do not reflect the official opinions or policies of the various testing programs, countries, or authors' host affiliations. Correspondence concerning this article should be directed to Bobby Naemi, email: bnaemi@ets.org.

References

Anderson, N. (2010, Dec. 7). International test score data show U.S. firmly mid-pack. *The Washington Post*. Retrieved from http://www.washingtonpost.com/wp-dyn/content/article/2010/12/07/AR2010120701178.html?sid=ST2010120701251.

BBC (2010, Dec.). Finland loses top spot to Asians. BBC Europe. Retrieved from http://www.bbc.co.uk/news/world-europe-11939566.

Beaton, A. E., Martin, M. O., Mullis, I. V. A., Gonzalez, E. J., Kelly, D. L., & Smith, T. A. (1996). *Science achievement in the middle school years: IEA's Third International Mathematics and Science Study*. Chestnut Hill, MA: Center for the Study of Testing, Evaluation, and Educational Policy, Boston College.

Beaton, A. E., Mullis, I. V. A., Martin, M. O., Gonzalez, E. J., Kelly, D. L., & Smith, T. A. (1996). *Mathematics achievement in the middle school years: IEA's Third International Mathematics and Science Study*. Chestnut Hill, MA: Center for the Study of Testing, Evaluation, and Educational Policy, Boston College.

Beaton, A. E., & Zwick, R. (1992). Overview of the National Assessment of Educational Progress. *Journal of Educational Statistics*, *17*, 95–109.

Carr, P., Dogan, E., Tirre, W., & Walton, E. (2007). Large-scale indicator assessments: What every educational policymaker should know. *Yearbook of the National Society for the Study of Education*, *106*, 321–339.

Carroll, J. B. (1963). A model of school learning. *Teachers College Record, 64* (8), 723–733.

Carroll, J. B. (1975). *The teaching of French as a foreign language in eight countries*. Stockholm: Almqvist and Wiksell; and New York: John Wiley.

Coleman, J. S. (1968). Equality of educational opportunity. *Equity & Excellence in Education, 6* (5), 19–28.

Comber, L. C., & Keeves, J. P. (1973). *Science education in nineteen countries*. Stockholm: Almqvist and Wiksell.

Connell, W. F. (1980) *A history of education in the twentieth-century world*. New York: Teachers College Press.

Dahlöff, U. (1967). Relevance and fitness analysis in comparative education. In D. E. Super (Ed.), *Towards a cross-national model of educational achievement in a national economy*. New York: Teachers College, Columbia University.

Dillon, S. (2010, Dec. 7). Top test scores from Shanghai stun educators. *The New York Times*, p. A1.

Dossey, J. A., & Lindquist, M. M. (2002). The impact of TIMSS on the mathematics standards movement in the United States. In D. F. Robitaille & A. E. Beaton (Eds.), *Secondary analysis of the TIMSS data* (pp. 63–79). Netherlands: Springer Netherlands.

Elley, W. B. (Ed.). (1994). *The IEA study of reading literacy: Achievement and instruction in thirty-two school systems*. Oxford, UK: Pergamon Press.

Ercikan, K. (2006). Developments in assessment of student learning and achievement. In P. A. Alexander and P. H. Winne (Eds.), *Handbook of educational psychology (2nd ed.)*. New York: Lawrence Erlbaum Associates.

Ertl, H. (2006). Educational standards and the changing discourse on education: The reception and consequences of the PISA study in Germany. *Oxford Review of Education, 32*, 619–634.

Foshay, A. W., Thorndike, R. L., Hotyat, F., Pidgeon, D. A., & Walker, D. A. (1962). *Educational achievements of thirteen-year-olds in twelve countries*. Hamburg: UNESCO Institute for Education.

Foster, M. (2010). Japan fattens textbooks to reverse sliding rank. *USA Today*. Retrieved from: http://www.usatoday.com/news/education/2010-09-06-japan-thicker-textbooks_N.htm.

Greenbaum, W., Garet, M. S., & Solomon, E. (1975). *Measuring educational progress*. New York: McGraw-Hill.

Husén, T. (Ed.). (1967) *International study of achievement in mathematics*. Stockholm: Almqvist and Wiksell.

Jones, L. V. (1996). A history of the National Assessment of Educational Progress and some questions about its future. *Educational Researcher, 25*, 15–22.

Kearney, C. A. (2008). Helping school refusing children and their parents: A guide for school-based professionals. New York: Oxford University Press.

Keeves, J. P. (Ed.) (1992) *The IEA Study of Science III: Changes in science education and achievement: 1970 to 1984*. Oxford, UK: Pergamon Press.

Kirsch, I. (2001). *The International Adult Literacy Survey (IALS): Understanding what was measured (Research Report 01–25)*. Retrieved from: http://www.ets.org/Media/Research/pdf/RR-01-25-Kirsch.pdf.

Lee, V. E., & Burkam, D. T. (2003). Dropping out of high school: The role of school organization and structure. *American Educational Research Journal, 2*, 353–393.

Lindqvist, E., & Vestman, R. (2011). The labor market returns to cognitive and noncognitive ability: Evidence from the Swedish Enlistment. *American Economic Journal: Applied Economics, 3*, 101–128.

Lewis, E. G., & Massad, C. E. (1975). *The teaching of English as a foreign language in ten countries*. Stockholm: Almqvist and Wiksell.

Linn, R. L. (2001). *The influence of external evaluations on the National Assessment of Educational Progress* (CSE Technical Report 548). CRESST: University of Colorado at Boulder.

Magis, D., Beland, S., Tuerlinckx, F., & De Boeck, P. (2010). A general framework and an R package for the detection of dichotomous differential item functioning. *Behavioral Research Methods, 42*, 847–862.

Martin, M. O., Mullis, I. V.A ., Gonzalez, E. J., Gregory, K. D., Smith, T. A., Chrostowski, S. J., Garden, R. A, & O'Connor, K. M. (2000). TIMSS 1999 *International Science Report. Findings from IEA's repeat of the Third International Mathematics and Science Study at the eighth grade*. Chestnut Hill, MA: Boston College. Available at: http://timssandpirls.bc.edu/timss1999i/science_achievement_report.html; last accessed April 20, 2011.

Messick, S., Beaton, A., & Lord, F. (1983). *National Assessment of Educational Progress reconsidered: A new design for a new era* (Report 83-10). Princeton, NJ: Educational Testing Service.

Mullis, I.V.S ., Martin, M. O., & Foy, P. (2008). *TIMSS 2007 International Mathematics Report. Findings from IEA's Trends in International Mathematics and Science Study at the fourth and eighth grades*. Chestnut Hill, MA: IEA TIMSS & PIRLS International Study Center.

Mullis, I. V. S ., Martin, M. O., Gonzalez, E. J., Gregory, K. D., Garden, R. A., O'Connor, K. M., et al. (2000). TIMSS 1999 *International Mathematics Report. Findings from IEA's repeat of the Third International Mathematics and Science Study at the eighth grade*. Chestnut Hill, MA: Boston College. Available at: http://timssandpirls.bc.edu/timss1999i/pdf/T99i_Math_All.pdf; last accessed April 20, 2011.

Mullis, I. V. S., Martin, M. O., Kennedy, A. M., & Foy, P. (2007). *IEA's Progress in International Reading Literacy Study in primary school in 40 Countries*. Chestnut Hill, MA: TIMSS & PIRLS International Study Center, Boston College.

Mullis, I. V. S., Martin, M. O., Kennedy, A. M., & Trong, K. L. (2011). *PIRLS 2011 assessment framework*. Chestnut Hill, MA: TIMSS & PIRLS International Study Center.

National Assessment of Educational Progress (2010). *NAEP Frameworks*. Retrieved from: http://nces.ed.gov/nationsreportcard/frameworks.asp.

National Assessment of Educational Progress. (2011a). *NAEP instruments*. Retrieved from: http://nces.ed.gov/nationsreportcard/tdw/instruments/.

National Assessment of Educational Progress. (2011b). *Non-cognitive items and questionnaires*. Retrieved from: http://nces.ed.gov/nationsreportcard/tdw/instruments/noncog.asp.

National Assessment of Educational Progress. (2011c). *Non-cognitive items in student booklets*. Retrieved from: http://nces.ed.gov/nationsreportcard/tdw/instruments/noncog_student.asp.

No Child Left Behind Act of 2001, 20 U.S.C. § 6319 (2008).

OECD (2010a). *Volume I, what students know and can do: Student performance in reading, mathematics and science*. Paris: Organization for Economic Cooperation and Development.

OECD (2010b). *Volume II, Overcoming social background: Equity in learning opportunities and outcomes*. Paris: Organization for Economic Cooperation and Development.

OECD (2010c). *Volume III, Learning to learn: Student engagement, strategies and practices*. Paris: Organization for Economic Cooperation and Development.

OECD (2010d). *Volume IV, What makes a school successful? Resources, policies and practices*. Paris: Organization for Economic Cooperation and Development.

OECD (2010e). *Volume V, Learning trends: Changes in student performance since 2000*. Paris: Organization for Economic Cooperation and Development.

OECD (2011). *Volume VI, Students online: Reading and using digital information*. Paris: Organization for Economic Cooperation and Development.

Olmsted, P. P., & Weikart, D. P. (1994). *Families speak: Early care and education in 11 countries*. Ypsilanti, MI: High/Scope Press.

Oppenheimer, A. (2010, Dec. 28). Commentary: PISA results are a wake-up call for Argentina's education system. *The Miami Herald*. Retrieved from http://www.mcclatchydc.com/2010/12/18/v-print/105399/commentary-pisa-results-are-a.html.

Peaker, G. F. (1975). *An empirical study of education in twenty-one countries: A technical report*. Stockholm: Almqvist and Wiksell; and New York: John Wiley.

Pelgrum, W. J., & Plomp, T. (Ed.). (1993). *The IEA study of computers in education: Implementation of an innovation in 21 education systems*. Oxford, UK: Pergamon Press.

PIAAC Literacy Expert Group. (2009). *PIAAC Literacy: A conceptual framework* (OECD Education Working Paper No. 34). Retrieved from http://www.oecd.org/

officialdocuments/displaydocumentpdf?cote=edu/wkp(2009)13&doclanguage=en.

Postlethwaite, T. N., & Wiley, D. E. (1992). *The IEA Study of Science II: Science achievement in twenty-three countries.* Oxford, UK: Pergamon Press.

Purves, A. C. (1973). *Literature education in ten countries.* Stockholm: Almqvist and Wiksell.

Purves, A. C. (Ed.). (1992). *The IEA Study of Written Composition II: Education and performance in fourteen countries.* Oxford, UK: Pergamon Press.

Rampey, B. D., Dion, G. S., & Donahue, P. L. (2009). *NAEP 2008 trends in academic progress* (NCES 2009–479). Washington, DC: National Center for Education Statistics, Institute of Education Sciences, U.S. Department of Education.

Roberts, R. D., Betancourt, A. C., Burrus, J., Holtzman, S., Libbrecht, N., MacCann, C., et al. (2011). *Multimedia assessment of emotional abilities: Development and validation.* Army Research Institute Report Series. Arlington, VA: ARI.

Robitaille, D. F., Beaton, A. E., & Plomp, T. (Eds.). (2000). *The impact of TIMSS on the teaching and learning of mathematics and science.* San Francisco, CA: Pacific Educational.

Robitaille, D. F., & Garden. R.A. (Eds.). (1989). *The IEA Study of Mathematics II: Context and outcomes of school mathematics.* Oxford, UK: Pergamon Press.

Rosier, M. J., & Keeves, J. P. (eds.) (1991). *The IEA study of Science I: Science education and curricula in twenty three countries.* Oxford, UK: Pergamon Press.

Rutkowski, L., Gonzalez, E., Joncas, M., & von Davier, M. (2010). International large-scale assessment data: Issues in secondary analysis and reporting. *Educational Researcher, 39,* 142–151.

Rychen, D. S., & Salganik, L. H. (Eds.). (2003). *Key competencies for a successful life and a well-functioning society.* Göttingen, Germany: Hogrefe & Huber.

Schulz, W., Ainley, J., Fraillon, J., Kerr, D., & Losito, B. (2010). *ICCS 2009 International Report: Civic knowledge, attitudes and engagement among lower secondary school students in thirty-eight countries.* Amsterdam: IEA.

Sheuermann, F., & Björnsson, J. (Eds.). (2009). The transition to computer-based assessment: New approaches to skills assessment and implications for large-scale testing. Luxembourg: European Communities.

Super, D. E. (Ed.). (1967). *Towards a cross-national model of educational achievement in a national economy.* New York: Teachers College, Columbia University.

The National Assessment Governing Board (2010). *20th anniversary conference proceedings: NAEP and the progress of education in America.* Washington, DC: National Assessment Governing Board.

Thorndike, R. L. (1973). *Reading comprehension education in fifteen countries: An empirical study.* Stockholm: Almqvist and Wiksell; and New York: John Wiley.

Torney, J. V., Oppenheim, A. N., & Farnen, R. N. (1976). *Civic education in ten countries.* Stockholm: Almqvist and Wiksell.

United Nations Educational, Scientific and Cultural Organization. (2007). Education for all global monitoring report 2008: Education for all by 2015 will we make it? Retrieved from: http://unesdoc.unesco.org/images/0015/001548/154820e.pdf.

United Nations Educational, Scientific and Cultural Organization. (2010). Activity Review 2009. Retrieved from: http://unesdoc.unesco.org/images/0018/001882/188290E.pdf.

Vinovskis, M. A. (1998). *Overseeing the nation's report card: The creation and evolution of the National Assessment Governing Board (NAGB).* Paper prepared for the National Assessment Governing Board.

Walker, D. A. (1967). Mathematical achievement and school retentivity. In T. Husén, *International study of achievement in mathematics* (pp. 116–135).

Wiseman, A. W. (Ed.). (2010). *The impact of international achievement studies on national education policymaking.* Bingley, England: Emerald Group Publishing Limited.

Testing, Assessment, and Cultural Variation: Challenges in Evaluating Knowledge Claims

Craig L. Frisby

Abstract

The academic and psychometric literature is filled with many competing knowledge claims related to the confidence with which cognitive and personality tests can be selected, administered, and interpreted with test-takers from culturally diverse groups. There are three broad sources of knowledge claims that can inform consumers about the appropriateness of test usage with individuals from culturally different examinees: (1) conclusions drawn from high-quality empirical research, (2) claims and criticisms embedded in sociopolitical ideologies and crusades, and (3) ethical and legal professional testing standards. Major claims from each of these sources are identified and summarized, followed by an analysis of the compatibility and conflict between information emanating from these knowledge sources.

Key Words: cognitive and personality testing, assessment, legal and ethical test standards, cultural groups, test bias

There is no shortage of resources purporting to raise awareness among professionals concerning how the design, administration, and interpretation of psychological tests may need to be altered in light of ethnic, racial, or language subpopulation differences both within and between countries (e.g., Grigorenko, 2009; Hambleton & Li, 2005; Kaufman, 2005; Reynolds & Lowe, 2009; Suzuki & Ponterotto, 2008; Valencia & Suzuki, 2001).

Most writing on this topic begins with the implicit assumption that test usage, scoring, and administration with culturally diverse groups is fraught with certain dangers, which need to be understood in order for test users to use tests fairly. What is rarely discussed are the sources of the knowledge claims from which test users derive their information; their credibility, and how these sources may sometimes reinforce or contradict each other.

The purpose of this chapter is twofold. First, the essential characteristics of three sources for

knowledge claims about the development, administration, and interpretation of psychological tests for "culturally diverse" groups will be discussed. No knowledge source exists in a vacuum, but rather influences, and is influenced by, other sources. Second, the interrelationships between these three sources for psychological test knowledge claims (as these relate to test use with culturally diverse groups) are discussed. The chapter ends with concluding thoughts and suggestions for professionals who use psychological tests.

Sources for Knowledge Claims About Psychological Tests and Culturally Diverse Groups

Knowledge claims about the use of psychological tests with culturally diverse groups arise from three primary sources: (1) converging conclusions drawn from high-quality empirical research, (2) tenets embedded within sociopolitical ideologies, and

(3) ethical and legal professional standards related to the use and interpretation of tests and assessments with individuals from culturally diverse groups.

Conclusions from High-Quality Empirical Research

When investigators are described as engaging in "high-quality" empirical research, this means that a body of techniques, referred to collectively as the *scientific method*, is used to investigate naturally occurring phenomena, test hypotheses, acquire new knowledge, correct misconceptions or inaccuracies in existing knowledge bases, and integrate disparate pockets of previous or existing knowledge (Maxim, 1999). Research is labeled as "scientific" when evidence (data) is measurable and observable; clearly articulated hypotheses are formulated and subsequently tested using a wide variety of experimental designs and the statistical analysis of data. Parallel to this process, well-supported hypotheses (independently investigated) coalesce to form *theories*—which, in turn, guide the formulation of new hypotheses and the collection and statistical analysis of new data. Good theories enable predictions to be made, which in turn help researchers interpret their research findings within a meaningful context. Scientific research is contrasted with "unscientific" methods for formulating knowledge claims, which include (but are not limited to) appeals to authority, popular opinion, ideological biases, custom and tradition, or wishful thinking (Ruggiero, 2001).

Although investigator bias and errors (i.e., in the interpretation of results) are present to some degree in most empirical research, they are kept to a minimum partly through rigorous methodology (e.g., randomization of participants within samples), as well as through allowing one's data to be open for scrutiny by other scientists who have no personal or ideological stake in the outcome of the investigations. As studies are repeated over time by different researchers, in different locations, and with different samples—and the same pattern of findings begins to reliably emerge (and studies designed to test rival hypotheses consistently fail to support them)—then such findings gradually move from speculation into the arena of scientifically established facts.

Methods for Assessing Cultural Bias in Psychological Tests

There are a variety of statistical methods that have been used to investigate test bias. Rigorous empirical investigation of test bias begins first with a clear definition of what bias *is not* (which includes the identification of incorrect methods of determining bias). A test is not to be considered biased simply from (1) observation of group differences in the mean or variability of scores on tests; (2) subjective negative judgement of the content of particular test items; or (3) criticisms directed at the constitution of a test's standardization sample (Jensen, 1980; Reynolds & Ramsay, 2003).

Consistent with the principles discussed previously, "cultural bias" has been defined conceptually as the effects of *construct-irrelevant variance* on examinees' performance/responses on all or parts of tests (AERA, APA, & NCME, 1999). "Construct irrelevant variance" refers to something that is measured by a test that is irrelevant to the construct that the test was designed to measure, thereby creating a contaminating source of individual differences in scores. If select subgroups differ significantly in a construct that is irrelevant to what the test purports to measure, then there could be "systematic errors in the predictive validity or the construct validity of test scores of individuals that are associated with the individual's group membership" (Jensen, 1980, p. 375). Consistent with the principles discussed previously, the scientific investigation of test bias is a "purely objective, empirical, statistical, and quantitative matter entirely independent of subjective value judgements and ethical issues concerning fairness or unfairness of tests and the uses to which they are put" (Jensen, 1980, p. 375).

Psychometricians and researchers use empirical methods (some more sophisticated than others) to investigate bias in tests that are tailored to the particular research question under investigation. First, two or more racial, ethnic, language, social class, or gender groups are identified for comparison. The examination of *content bias* refers to investigating the possibility that certain groups may be unable to correctly answer test questions due to a "lack of access" to skills or knowledge necessary for successful completion (Reynolds & Carson, 2005). Content bias questions are investigated by identifying:

(1) significant differences between groups in the rank order of test item difficulties;

(2) significant Group X Item interactions identified by Analysis of Variance and related techniques;

(3) significant differences in Item X Group correlations when the influence of group membership on the total test score is removed (partial correlations); or

(4) differential item functioning (or DIF), identified through the examination of item-characteristic curves and model parameters in large samples (or contingency tables when sample sizes are limited; see Nandakumar, Glutting, & Oakland, 1993; Reynolds & Carson, 2005, for a more detailed discussion).

Construct bias occurs when a particular test is discovered to measure different psychological constructs for one group than for another, or to measure a trait with significantly reduced accuracy for one group compared to another (Reynolds & Carson, 2005). Construct bias questions are investigated by:

(1) conducting factor analyses (exploratory or confirmatory) separately for different groups under investigation, in order to determine if a different factor structure emerges for one group compared with another;

(2) correlating the factor loadings on the same test between pairs of groups, in order to determine the degree of agreement (see Georgas, van de Vijver, Weiss, & Saklofske, 2003);

(3) comparing internal consistency, alternate forms reliability, or test-retest reliability estimates across groups; or

(4) testing for the significance of the difference in the correlation, conducted separately by group, between age differences and raw test scores (see Reynolds & Carson, 2005, for a more detailed discussion).

Predictive/criterion bias occurs whenever there is a statistically significant difference between groups in the slopes, intercepts, or standard error of estimates of each groups' regression lines when test scores (corrected for unreliability) are used to predict a criterion. When test scores that are not corrected for unreliability are used, then predictive bias can be identified in significantly different regression slopes and standard error of estimates (see Jensen, 1980, for a more detailed discussion). Path analysis can be used to investigate bias in relation to multiple independent and dependent variables (both of which may involve test scores). Whenever group membership is systematically related to residual variance after model-based variance is accounted for, bias is present. In a typical application of path analytic techniques, when group membership exerts a significant influence on ability test scores over and above the influence expected from the latent variable (e.g., true ability), bias is suggested (see Reynolds & Carson, 2005, for a more detailed discussion).

External sources of bias have been defined as "[biases] that do not involve the test per se, but result from factors in the external testing situation that interact with individual or group differences to produce a systematic bias in the test scores of individuals or groups" (Jensen, 1980, p. 589). Such sources include, but are not limited to, examinee factors (e.g., effects of anxiety level, test sophistication, prior practice, behavior during the testing session); examiner factors (e.g., effects of examiner race, rapport-building efforts, coaching procedures); test administration and scoring (e.g., language of test administration, administration of reinforcers, waiving of time limits for speeded items); or characteristics of the testing environment (e.g., room lighting, ventilation).

Personality and Behavior Assessment

The assessment of mental ability involves examinees' being asked to recall information, recognize correct answers, or solve problems in response to test items (i.e., tasks, problems, questions) that are scored along a continuum of quality, or are scored as correct/incorrect, or scored as pass/fail, and that may or may not be timed. Here, examiners can observe directly the extent to which examinees can or cannot obtain scores (to a given criterion) on prescribed tasks (see additional criteria for categorizing ability measurement in Jensen, 1998, p. 51).

In contrast, the assessment of personality or behavioral constructs involves ratings of the presence, absence, and/or frequency of behaviors, thinking, feeling, or attitudes observed in oneself or in others in multiple settings. Personality and behavioral constructs do not have a general factor, but are typically reported as profiles of (positively or negatively) correlated subscales.

As with cognitive assessment, bias in personality/behavioral assessment cannot be defined simply on the basis of observed differences between subgroups in mean scores or subscale profile elevations, scatter, or shapes (Timbrook & Graham, 1994). Scale construction concerns related to linguistic equivalence, construct equivalence, psychological equivalence, and psychometric equivalence are applicable to personality/behavior scales as well (Butcher, Cabiya, Lucio, & Garrido, 2007; Graham, 2006; Reid, 1995).

However, it remains unclear how significant subscale profile differences between ethnic/racial/language subgroups should be interpreted. Some writers argue that subscale profiles can only be interpreted properly in the context of a standardization group that has the same demographic characteristics as the target child/youth (Butcher et al., 2007). This argument implies that the interpretation of a construct (along a continuum from "normality" to "clinical relevance") has no objective anchor, but is instead to be interpreted relative to a "cultural" group.

Additionally, the determination of bias in personality/behavioral assessment becomes more salient given the potential subjective nature of raters' judgements. "Lie" scales are integrated into many personality scales in order to objectively assess this issue. The assessment of bias becomes complicated when comparing differences in ratings across different informants (e.g., mother vs. father). Here, it is difficult to discern whether rating score differences are due to errors in informants' judgements, or due to actual differences in the target child/youth's behavior in different settings.

Perhaps the strongest methodology for determining bias in personality/behavior assessment involves correlating scores on these scales with external criteria, and evaluating the statistical significance of the magnitude of the correlation differences across subgroups of interest (Graham, 2006).

Testing Adaptations Across Widely Divergent Cultural Groups

When tests are used in two or more groups separated by examinees' spoken language and/or continent of habitation, test developers must adhere to established guidelines in test adaptation to ensure that factors that have a deleterious effect on test interpretation be kept at a minimum (e.g., see Georgas, Weiss, van de Vijver, & Saklofske, 2003). Sireci, Patsula, and Hambleton (2005) articulate a crucial distinction between the oft-confused concepts of "test translation" and "test adaptation." The former term refers more narrowly to the application of linguistic skills and knowledge to rewrite the purely verbal components of test items in order to enable one or more language groups to understand a test originally designed for a different language group. In contrast, the concept of "test adaptations" refers to a broader class of activities that Hambleton (2005) defines as:

> includ(ing) all the activities from deciding whether or not a test could measure the same construct in a different language and culture, to selecting translators, to deciding on appropriate accommodations to be made in preparing a test for use in a second language, to adapting the test and checking its equivalence in the adapted form. (p. 4)

The following four principles for adapting tests for use in widely divergent cultural groups have been established by large international testing associations and organizations with extensive experience in field settings (see Hambleton, Merenda, & Spielberger, 2005):

ENSURING CONSTRUCT EQUIVALENCE

Johnson (1998) summarizes more than 50 terms found in the social science literature for describing different types of "equivalence" that are of concern to cross-cultural researchers. In adapting and/or translating a test used in one cultural context to a different cultural context, the psychological construct measured by the test must be conceptually and functionally equivalent across groups. Although Hambleton (2005) opines that subjective judgement (usually by "expert" judges representing language/cultural groups) can play an important role in evaluating construct equivalence (e.g., see Hui & Triandis, 1985), the use of subjectivity in evaluating construct equivalence has been abused in the assessment literature (see next section on sociopolitical ideologies/crusades).

Individual test items can have a straightforward translation to a linguistically different population, but not have an equivalent *psychological* meaning in the different population. For example, a cognitive ability test used in America may include a general information question related to an American historical figure, but the same question translated for a Dutch population may, understandably, have a significantly higher difficulty (van de Vijver & Poortinga, 2005). Put another way, failure to respond correctly to such an item may have implications for the construct of intelligence in an American sample, whereas the same failure in a Dutch sample has little significance in assessing the intelligence construct.

TEST ADMINISTRATION PROCEDURES

Test administration procedures, such as those found on individually administered nonverbal scales of cognitive ability (e.g., Bracken & McCallum, 1998), must necessarily involve substantial modifications (such as the use of pantomime instructions rather than verbal instructions) in order to accommodate substantially diverse test-takers. Such procedures are consistent with the intended purposes of the test, and are appropriate provided that test administration is standardized for all examinees. However, some writers advocate that administration procedures for the same test be altered (e.g., removal of time constraints on timed tasks, additional repetition or alteration of test instructions to ensure comprehension, acceptance of unconventional responses to test items) for certain subgroups but not for others (Armour-Thomas & Gopaul-Mcnicol, 1998; Elliott, 1987; Gopaul-Mcnicol & Armour-Thomas, 2002). Unfortunately, when test administration procedures are not standardized for all examinees, an additional source of variance in test scores is potentially introduced that undermines test score reliability (Mpofu & Ortiz, 2009).

TEST CONTENT

According to Hambleton (2005), "choice of item formats, stimulus material for the test, vocabulary, sentence structure, and other aspects that might be difficult to translate well can all be taken into account in preparing the test specifications. Such preventive actions can minimize later problems" (p. 10). Examples of such situations are isolated and unique to specific cultural applications, and do not form a coherent pattern of universal principles. For example, Serpell (1979) found that, when compared to British children, African Zambian children were better able to reproduce patterns using wire models—while British children were better able to reproduce models using pencil and paper drawings. This finding is interpreted to suggest that the construct of "perceptual skills," assessed via pattern recognition, is best understood using response modes that are most familiar to a particular cultural group. For a more detailed discussion of ability test content adaptation factors that must be addressed in cross cultural work (particularly with developing countries), see Frisby (1999b).

Exploratory factor analysis, confirmatory factor analysis, and multidimensional scaling methods are typically used to examine factorial and/or structural similarity of the same test items across culturally different populations (e.g., see Byrne, Shavelson, & Muthen, 1989; Little, 1997; Sireci, Patsula, & Hambleton, 2005; van de Vijver & Leung, 1997; Watkins, 1989). When one-to-one correspondence in item loading patterns cannot be reasonably expected across test adaptations for groups that differ widely in cultural milieus, then the correlations between a target measures' total score and total scores for other similar or different measures (within the cultural milieu) must be examined (van de Vijver & Poortinga, 2005).

TEST TRANSLATION/ADAPTATION ISSUES

When tests or other assessment instruments (such as rating scales, surveys, and questionnaires) are translated and/or adapted to a widely differing cultural group, a number of potential problems have been identified from field observation and research. Hambleton and Kanjee (1995) discuss a variety of potential sources of problems that can occur during the selection and training of translators, as well as the linguistic difficulties that can occur when "forward-adaptation" and "back-adaptation" designs are used. Depending upon the cultural groups studied, the extent to which a source test/assessment instrument must be altered in the test adaptation process (which involves broader issues in addition to linguistic translation) varies along a continuum of least to most alterations (van de Vijver & Poortinga, 2005). At one end of the translation/adaptation continuum, test items can be linguistically translated with no loss of literal meaning and no alteration of psychological meaning. Test stimuli and procedures for administering the test remain intact. Toward the middle of this continuum, there are occasions where a literal linguistic translation of a test item does not yield equivalence in psychological meaning across two or more groups (see van de Vijver & Poortinga, 2005, p. 41, for specific examples). In these instances, the item may need to be discarded, or its translation may not match exactly the literal translation from the target source. In addition, some elements of the test instructions and/or use of examples may need to be modified somewhat (e.g., see Elbeheri, Everatt, Reid, & Mannai, 2006; Georgas, Weiss, van de Vijver, & Saklofske, 2003). Toward the opposite end of the continuum, the construct to be measured and the method for measuring it may be so inappropriate for translation from one group to another that the test developer finds it necessary to develop an entirely new instrument (see van de Vijver & Poortinga, 2005, p. 54, for a discussion of the "assembly option"). For example, Kathuria and Serpell (1999) discuss the development and use of an ability test for rural African Zambian children that requires constructing a representation of a human figure from wet clay.

Psychological Testing with Culturally Diverse Groups: Empirically Established Conclusions

The accumulation of evidence resulting from the application of these principles to the interpretation of the cognitive ability test performance of culturally diverse groups is substantial (e.g., see Chen, Keith, Weiss, Zhu, & Li, 2010; Edwards & Oakland, 2006; Frisby, 1999a, 1999b, 2007; Georgas, Weiss, van de Vijver, & Saklofske, 2003; Gottfredson, 1997,

2005; Graham, 2006; Herrnstein & Murray, 1994; Jensen, 1980, 1991, 1993, 1998, 2003; Jencks et al., 1979; Konold, Glutting, Oakland, & O'Donnell, 1995; Kush et al., 2001; Lynn & Vanhanen, 2002; Nandakumar, Glutting, & Oakland, 1993; Rushton & Jensen, 2005; Reynolds & Kaiser, 2003; Reynolds & Lowe, 2009; Reynolds & Ramsay, 2003). The most salient of these results are briefly summarized below:

1. An examination of the "surface" characteristics of test items, by itself, provides little insight into the nature of the fundamental source of individual differences in scores on the full test battery (see discussion of "the indifference of the indicator," Jensen, 1998).

2. Although a variety of mental abilities exists, it is the general mental ability factor, or "*g* factor," that is the most fundamental source of individual differences in human cognitive abilities. The *g* factor accounts for a third to half of the variance in scores on any broad battery of mental tests.

3. Despite relatively minor imperfections, commonly used individually administered IQ tests are very good measures of the *g* factor. The average *g* loading of IQ scores derived from a variety of standard IQ tests is in the .80s.

4. IQ test batteries given to a wide variety of ethnic, racial, age, and gender groups reveal measurement of the same general and specific ability factors. In addition, these same constructs are measured equally well in all ages under examination.

5. The same *g* factor has been empirically shown to be responsible for intellectual variation in North American, European, Asian, and African groups.

6. Although all human groups display a wide range of IQ scores, racial/ethnic subgroup differences in the mean (and to a lesser extent, the standard deviation) of their IQ score distributions is the rule, not the exception, worldwide. Subgroup differences remain (although to a slightly reduced degree) even when social class is controlled or when the tests are completely nonverbal. Differences between American subgroups in mean IQ distributions have been observed in samples as young as 2.5 years of age on well developed standardized tests. In the United States and other developed nations, the mean IQ of Blacks, Hispanics, Native Americans, Whites, and East Asians is approximately 85, 90, 90, 100, and 106, respectively (assuming an IQ score distribution with a mean of 100 and a standard deviation

of 15). Even finer subgroup distinctions among these broad groups may differ slightly in mean IQ.

7. The use of completely nonverbal tests in individual cognitive assessment (where the test stimuli are completely pictorial, directions are pantomimed by the examiner, and the examinee is not required to verbalize responses) continues to reveal smaller but reliable average racial/ethnic subgroup differences in total test scores.

8. Whenever statistical methods for detecting item bias in cognitive and ability tests are used (e.g., see Camilli, 2006; Reynolds & Carson, 2005), the amount of bias found is so slight and unsystematic across items as to be totally inadequate in accounting for large group differences in mean total test scores.

9. When examiners rate the testing behaviors of examinees using a behavior rating scale standardized on a specific IQ test, such rating scales reveal slight but non-significant group differences when the correlation between test session behavior ratings and IQ scores are removed (some of which show lower-scoring IQ groups displaying more *favorable* testing behavior). That is, behavioral ratings across racial/ethnic groups do not differ significantly with respect to qualitatively distinct categories of more positive or negative testing behaviors.

10. The g factor measured by cognitive tests is significantly and negatively correlated with such social problems as school dropout rates, poverty and welfare status, illegitimacy, delinquency, and crime. Thus, racial/ethnic group differences in these importance life outcomes are significantly correlated with racial/ethnic group differences in the *g* factor measured by cognitive tests. Performance on appropriately developed cognitive tests predict learning ability in school, academic and intellectual achievements during childhood and adolescence, and other important adult life outcomes equally well for all racial/ethnic groups.

Knowledge Claims from Sociopolitical Ideologies/Crusades

A second source for what many believe about test usage and interpretation with culturally diverse groups originates from the influence of sociopolitical ideologies that have come into vogue during various periods in history (Heywood, 2010; Phelps, 2009). These sociopolitical movements lay the groundwork for negative attitudes toward test use in education and psychology. At the time of this writing, "multiculturalism" is arguably the most pervasive sociopolitical ideology in education (Webster, 1997) and psychology (Pedersen, 1999), which in turn influences perceptions of psychological testing.

Multiculturalism is a sociopolitical ideology that is ubiquitous in contemporary education and applied psychology. There exists little consensus among explicit definitions for multiculturalism, as these vary considerably as a function of each writer's philosophical perspective. Nevertheless, it is easier to distill multiculturalism ideology down to a smaller number of component doctrines, each of which contributes substantially to explaining beliefs and practices associated with cultural minority groups and testing. The component doctrines of multiculturalism ideology (for an expanded treatment, see Frisby, 2005a, 2005b), followed by their application to testing, are given in the next section.

Multiculturalism Doctrines and Testing

According to the *Group Identity Doctrine*, individuals are characterized as little more than representatives of "identity" groups defined by race, ethnicity, national origin, language, social class, or religious status. This doctrine assumes that knowledge of an individual's group membership is important for understanding the psychology of the individual, and conversely, that the psychology of individuals is inextricably tied to relevant information about their identity group. Thus, when testing texts encourage professionals to be "culturally competent" test users, directives are couched in the context of test usage with particular "groups" (as opposed to individuals). The following quote typifies this doctrine (Butcher et al., 2007):

> As for criterion validity, test users must be aware of the potential for differential prediction. This may occur when the relationship between the predictor (test score) and the criterion is significantly different between groups. This may indicate that a test is invalid for a given group and that a different instrument altogether may be needed for that group. (p. 15)

As typified in this and numerous other statements from the testing literature, the individual examinee's group membership is viewed as the only necessary and sufficient condition for invalidating (or validating) test usage for that particular examinee. Following this logic, test critics can therefore explain any behavior during testing as being attributable to a person's group membership. Thus, if an examinee from a racial/ethnic minority group fails to answer correctly a question on an IQ test, the test critic can claim (on the basis of the Group Identity Doctrine) that cultural processes associated with his/her group membership are probably responsible (see Helms, 1992, 1997).

Testing ethics and standards documents (e.g., AERA, APA, & NCME, 1999) promote the Group Identity Doctrine through the implicit assumption that the design of national standardization sampling and stratification schemes or results from test-bias studies have direct implications for the appropriateness of test use with individuals belonging to identity groups on which such research is based (e.g., see item #5 under Interpretation and Application of Assessment Results, Association for Assessment in Counseling, 2003). For a related discussion of these issues and "test fairness," see discussion of the "social address model" in Camilli (2006).

Once identity groups have been defined, the *Difference Doctrine* assumes that such groups display unique, "culturally specific" thinking patterns, attitudes, and behaviors that are more or less homogeneous within groups and mutually exclusive between groups. Test critics use this doctrine to promote three distinct messages: (1) the latent psychological constructs measured by commercially popular intelligence or personality tests are presumed not to have the same meaning for different cultural groups (Armour-Thomas & GoPaul-McNicol, 1998; GoPaul-McNicol & Armour-Thomas, 2003; Greenfield, 1997; Helms, 1997; Sternberg & Grigorenko, 2008); (2) culturally distinctive characteristics are presumed to be reliably displayed by examinees in the context of cognitive testing sessions (Helms, 1997; Kwate, 2001); and (3) as a result of the first two assumptions, the behavior of members of cultural minority groups is likely to be misunderstood, misinterpreted, and therefore "misreported" by non-minority group examiners and/or raters on psychological scales (Helms, 1992, 1997). Such claims are based solely on either speculative or anecdotal evidence (for a detailed critique, see Frisby, 1999a).

The *Equity Doctrine* is rooted in the moral imperative that cultural minority groups (1) be treated similarly to non-minority groups when served by professionals in educational and psychological settings, and (2) be represented in the same proportion as their general population numbers in desirable or undesirable social, educational, occupational, or economic outcomes in society. The first assumption is not controversial, and is a value that has nearly universal consensus among professionals who serve cultural minority clients. The second assumption is controversial, as there exist wide differences of opinion as to whether proportional representation in outcomes is desirable or attainable.

As applied to testing, then, the *Equity Doctrine* has both "politicized" and "non-politicized" applications. In the non-politicized sense, psychometricians work hard to ensure that linguistic and psychometric "equivalence" is maintained whenever tests are used with widely differing cultural and or language groups (Hambleton, Merenda, & Speilberger, 2005). In the politicized sense, this doctrine holds that test selection and use can only be considered "fair" if identity groups display "equal" score distributions, which in turn would presumably lead to proportionally equal selection outcomes resulting from decisions that are based on test results (see Reynolds, 2000). If groups do not achieve equal score distributions, then something is assumed to be deficient in the design, interpretation, and use of tests for lower-scoring groups (see discussion of the "cultural test bias hypothesis" in Reynolds, 2000; see also Helms, 1992, 1997, 2006). As such, belief in the *Equity Doctrine* is the root cause responsible for driving most, if not all, criticisms of test use with cultural minority groups. Put another way, if it were possible for groups to obtain equal score distributions on standardized tests, then most test criticisms would literally vanish overnight.

The *Inclusion Doctrine* is best known by its most popular synonym, which is "diversity" (Wood, 2003). According to the Inclusion Doctrine, desirable outcomes that reflect an inclusion of persons representing a variety of arbitrarily defined groups are assumed to be morally, philosophically, or socially preferable than outcomes that do not.

As applied to testing, adherence to the Inclusion Doctrine is manifested in a test publisher's rigorous stratification of a test's standardization sample in order to most accurately represent diversity in demographic characteristics of the target population for whom the test was designed. This standard practice may (inappropriately) lead test critics to assert that tests are "biased" against certain examinees if their ethnic/racial group is not adequately represented (according to critics' subjective standards for sufficient "diversity") in a test's standardization sample (Dent, 1996). For an empirical refutation of this claim, see Fan, Willson and Kapes (1996).

In addition, tests can be criticized as a selection measure if decision-making based on test scores does not lead to selection rates that are consistent with a predetermined vision of what are "acceptable" rates of inclusion for various racial/ethnic groups (Elliott, 1987; Gottfredson, 2000; 2004a; 2004b; Jensen, 1980).

The *Sensitivity Doctrine* is the belief that researchers, educators, and applied psychological practitioners are morally obligated to avoid any research, behavior, or speech that would inadvertently "offend" members of particular ethnic/racial groups, or important individuals who style themselves as vocal "spokespersons" for a particular group. Those who violate these norms (either intentionally or unintentionally) can thus be accused of harboring nefarious motives (i.e., prejudice, racism), or are said to suffer from "cultural insensitivity" or "cultural incompetence."

A step in the development of a potentially profitable test is for test companies to send early drafts of the test to select representatives of cultural/language minority groups for the purpose of evaluating potential "item bias" (sometimes called "sensitivity reviews"; see Bond, Moss, & Carr, 1996). Typically, reviewers are instructed to examine the surface characteristics of test items (e.g., wording of item instructions, words used in item content, item pictures depicting objects, situations, or human actors doing something) and judge the extent to which particular items may be "offensive" or "insensitive" to given groups. Although there is no empirical evidence that the judgements of ethnic-minority item review experts are more valid than those of non-minority experts (e.g., see Jensen & McGurk, 1987; Sandoval & Miille, 1980), or that potentially faulty items contribute substantially to subgroup mean differences in total test scores, test companies continue to condone such practices primarily for public relations purposes.

Writings on multicultural topics are suffused with the unspoken but palpable assumption that ethnic, cultural, or language minority status is a necessary condition for credibility and expertise on issues related to minority populations, and that those with non-minority status have a structurally imposed limitation (or inability) for understanding the culture and behavior of culturally different individuals. Thus, it is assumed implicitly that cultural minority groups have *sovereignty* in defining how psychological concepts such as "intelligence" and "psychopathology" are conceptualized, measured, and interpreted for the group of which they are designated representatives. Thus, the *Sovereignty Doctrine* assumes that ethnic, cultural, or language minority academicians have special knowledge, unavailable to non-minority academicians, on the interaction of minority status and attitudinal or behavioral responses to test item content (e.g., see Helms, 1992, 1997).

As stated previously, the fundamental issue that fuels criticism of testing is the observation of reliable differences in cognitive test score means between representative samples of racial, ethnic, language, and socioeconomic status groups. Therefore, anti-test advocates must advance knowledge claims that generate doubt and suspicion about the manner in which tests are used and interpreted with diverse cultural groups. The essential difference between knowledge claims advanced through empirical research, versus those advanced through anti-test sociopolitical advocacy, is succinctly articulated by Gottfredson (2009), who writes:

> Advocacy is different from science.... For the zealous advocate, cause and effect are predetermined to serve one's interests. An advocate need not even believe a cause or effect that she claims; her goal is to persuade others to believe it. An advocate searches not for probable causes and effects but, rather, for merely plausible ones—ones that others are willing to believe... the desired outcome is neither truth nor understanding, but conversion—getting others to view a situation in a manner that serves one's own interests. (p. 250)

Evidence for Gottfredson's observation can be clearly seen in Helms' (1997) attempts to advance a plethora of "plausible" shortcomings of intelligence tests, in order to undermine confidence in their use and interpretation with African Americans. Helms lists a number of "hypothesized" biases in tests (e.g., "language and stylistic differences *may be* misinterpreted," "Examiners of a different race *may be* suspect") absent any hard data that actually document their existence empirically (see Helms, 1997, p. 521).

Sociopolitical advocacy manifests itself as a morality play pitting the forces of "good" (those who oppose "traditional" test use and interpretation with cultural minority groups) against the forces of "evil" (those who defend traditional test use and interpretation with cultural minority groups). According to Phelps (2005), "anti-testing" advocacy:

> ... view(s) testing generally as an impediment to reform, an antiquated technology that reflects an antiquated view of teaching, learning, and social organization, perpetuates inequality, and serves the ends of cultural, political and educational oppression. (p. xi)

The goal of sociopolitical advocacy is to sow seeds of doubt about traditional test usage and interpretation with examinees from cultural minority groups, and to advocate one or more of the following practices:

1. The complete prohibition of "traditional" test use with certain racial/ethnic groups (e.g., Williams, Dotson, Dow, & Williams, 1980), which may or may not involve the substitution of assessments that are better aligned with an ideological viewpoint, but are characterized by inferior construct measurement and/or psychometric quality (Gottfredson, 2004b).

2. Altering the manner in which "traditional" tests are administered to certain racial/ethnic groups—typified by the incorporation of unstandardized procedures such as task coaching and/or relaxed time standards (e.g., Feuerstein, Feuerstein, & Gross, 1997; Hilliard, 1987; Lidz, 1997).

3. Including subtests in multi-test IQ batteries that are constructed (either intentionally or unintentionally) to have significantly reduced g loadings, which has the effect of artificially reducing the size of subgroup differences in mean total scores (Jensen, 1984b).

4. Allowing "traditional" test administration for certain racial/ethnic groups, but requiring adoption of an additional set of elaborate assessments and/or problem-solving rubrics that supplement test interpretation (e.g., Armour-Thomas & GoPaul-McNicol, 1998; Rhodes, Ochoa, & Ortiz, 2005).

5. Altering the manner in which "traditional" test scores are interpreted, most often by using group-specific norms to reinterpret the same scores differently for certain racial/ethnic groups than for other groups (see Figueroa, 1979, for an example involving children; see Gottfredson, 1994a, for application to adults).

An Analysis of Sociopolitical Advocacy Anti-Test Arguments

As sociopolitical advocates gain power and influence in academia, the media, and the legal system, this ignites an "anti-testing" sentiment (e.g., see Phelps, 2003, 2005), in which "unfairness" to cultural minority groups is trumpeted as one of many negative consequences of test use. The political interests of the anti-test movement are to reduce or eliminate test use in society, and to undermine the credibility and traditional interpretation of test scores (particularly for cultural minority groups in the context of high-stakes decision making). In attempting to accomplish these goals, the knowledge claims advanced by anti-test sociopolitical ideologies have the following characteristics:

1. *Using implicit definitions of "culture" (and its related derivatives) that are built on narrow, simplistic assumptions.* Cultural variation among human populations worldwide is extremely vast in scope and complex in its nuances (e.g., see Kitayama & Cohen, 2007). The "cultural backgrounds" of individuals are shaped by differences in parental childrearing practices, the nature of religious upbringing, political beliefs, parochial differences in the region of the country in which one is raised, a family's economic status, as well as life experiences shaped indirectly by a person's racial, ethnic, and language group membership. Unfortunately, the word "culture" has become synonymous with racial and ethnic status *alone*, such that persons who belong to different racial and ethnic groups are assumed implicitly to belong to homogeneous, mutually exclusive "cultural" groups. The reality is that many different "ethno-cultural groups" exist within any given racial group, and conversely, many different racial groups exist within any given cultural group. This results in a tremendous degree of overlapping in "cultural" characteristics across groups, so that any group of individuals can be thought of as being *both* culturally different *and* culturally similar *simultaneously*. On the basis of this misunderstanding, test critics continue to promote the belief that average group differences in mean scores across broad ethnic/racial groups imply that tests are deficient in their sensitivity to "cultural differences" (which implies that if they were "sensitive," then such group differences would not exist; see Helms, 1992).

2. *Asserting that a history of test criticism is in itself sufficient for doubting the efficacy of testing.* Critics merely state that "traditional" test use and interpretation with culturally different groups have been vigorously criticized in the past (either because tests do not measure up to some standard of perfection, or that test use with such groups has been "controversial"), and that this fact alone justifies either discontinuance of test use with such groups, or the preferred use of some alternative assessment/test interpretation method (e.g., see Armour-Thomas, 1992; Valencia & Suzuki, 2001). The unspoken implication here is that the absence

of criticism (and/or controversy) is a sufficient standard for approving the use of a particular assessment method with cultural groups. Test critics who use this method fail to inform their audiences of the next logical step, which is to *evaluate* the quality of test criticisms in order to determine whether such criticisms are indeed valid.

3. *Portraying established empirical findings as inconclusive or "open" to debate or alternative interpretations.* Many test critics reluctantly acknowledge that well standardized tests are not technically "biased" as gleaned from the accumulation of test bias research, yet will evoke the subjective criterion of "cultural equivalence" as grounds for criticizing commonly used tests (Helms, 1992, 1997; Valencia & Suzuki, 2001). Given the complexity of the culture concept (see previous point), such hypotheses are literally impossible to test or evaluate in a conceptually coherent or empirically rigorous manner. Not only do "cultural equivalence" explanations fail to explain differential gaps in test performance that very as a function of test characteristics (parsimoniously explained by Spearman's hypothesis; see Jensen, 1998), but no adequate "cultural equivalence" explanation has been advanced to explain the bewildering pattern of slight and unsystematic DIF (differential item functioning) findings in individual items on cognitive and achievement tests (Bond, 1994; Reynolds & Lowe, 2009).

4. *Advancing anti-test arguments riddled with cognitive or logical fallacies.* As previously mentioned in the Gottfredson (2009) quote, the goal of anti-test advocacy is to generate distrust and hostility toward tests through verbal persuasion. When coupled with an ignorance of the empirical literature, naïve audiences are susceptible to this persuasion when they are either unwilling or unable to identify the cognitive or logical fallacies inherent in common arguments against testing. A sampling of anti-test arguments, and their associated logical/cognitive fallacies, are shown in Table 7.1.

5. *Selective reporting of research results.* Sometimes preliminary empirical findings superficially appear to support a desired interpretation, but upon closer inspection such findings are either unpersuasive, misinterpreted, or have not been replicated by a systematic program of empirical research (e.g., see discussions of "stereotype threat" research in Jensen, 1998; Sackett, Hardison, & Cullen, 2004). Sociopolitical

Table 7.1 Common Cognitive/Logical Fallacies Associated with Psychological Test Development, Administration, and Interpretation/Usage with Culturally Diverse Groups

Cognitive/ Logical Fallacy	Definition	Citations Illustrating Advocacy for the Fallacy	Citations Identifying and/or Refuting the Fallacy
Psychological Test Development			
"Vehicle Equals Construct" Test Design Fallacy	Superficial characteristics of test items reflect the inner essence of the construct they measure	Helms (1992); Kwate (2001); Sternberg, Wagner, Williams, & Horvath, 1995	Gottfredson (2009); Jensen (1984a; 1998)
Guilt by Association	Some test researchers and developers in the past have held or voiced offensive ideas about the capabilities of minority groups, therefore modern test interpretation and usage is motivated by the same ill-will toward minority groups	Gould (1996) Valencia & Suzuki (2001)	Jensen (1982)
Standardization Fallacy	If the standardization sample for a test is not composed of a sufficient percentage of a given subpopulation, it is, by this fact, "biased" or "unfair" when used with that subpopulation	Dent (1996)	Fan, Willson, & Kapes (1996); Jensen (1980)
Psychological Test Administration			
Behavior Generality Fallacy	"Cultural" behaviors presumed to occur outside of the test administration context are reliably manifested within the test administration context	Helms (1997)	Glutting, Oakland, & McDermott (1988)
Outgroup Homogeneity Bias	Groups that are not English-speaking, white, and/or middle class are believed to manifest homogeneous behavioral/cognitive tendencies, particularly during test administration	Helms (1997); Kwate (2001)	Camilli (2006); Frisby (1999a); Frisby & Osterlind (2007); Mullen & Hu (1989)
Psychological Test Interpretation/Usage			
Dangerous Consequences Fallacy	Scientific conclusions judged to be socially divisive (e.g., group differences in intelligence) are so dangerous that they should not be entertained until proved beyond all possible doubt	(See discussion of unnamed sources in Gottfredson, 1994b)	Gottfredson (2007, 2009)
Appeal to Non-equivalent Exemplars	Wide differences between two culturally distinct groups (in test validity) justifies the *a priori* assumption of wide differences between any different pair of culturally distinct groups	Greenfield (1997)	Frisby (1999a)
Standard of Evidence Fallacy	Valid, unbiased cognitive ability and academic achievement tests should not be used for making decisions about individuals until the tests are made "error-free"	FairTest (2007)	Gottfredson (2009)
Egalitarian Fallacy	If population subgroups do not show equal distributions of test scores, then the test is "biased" in favor of the higher-scoring groups and against lower-scoring groups	Alley & Foster (1978); Williams (1971)	Jensen (1980); Rushton & Jensen (2005)

(continued)

Table 7.1 (Continued)

Cognitive/ Logical Fallacy	Definition	Citations Illustrating Advocacy for the Fallacy	Citations Identifying and/or Refuting the Fallacy
Confirmation Bias	If minority groups achieve lower scores on cognitive tests after being given anxiety-producing directions, then this presumably illustrates "stereotype threat," and is assumed to not reflect real differences in the trait measured	Steele & Aronson (1995, 1997)	Jensen (1998; pp. 513–516); Nickerson (1998); Sackett, Hardison, & Cullen (2004)
Culture-Bound Fallacy	Test "bias" or test "unfairness" can be determined subjectively by a visual inspection of specific test items	Helms (1992, 1997)	Jensen (1980); Jensen & McGurk (1987); Sandoval & Miille (1980);
Specificity Doctrine	Intelligence tests measure isolated bits of knowledge gained from prior learning and experience; therefore group differences in intelligence test scores merely reflect different opportunities to acquire such knowledge	Eells, Davis, Havighurst, Herrick, & Tyler (1951); Dent (1996)	Jensen (1984a, 1992a,1992b)

ideologies highlight research findings that appear to support the ideology, which in turn presents a dilemma for how to handle research results that do not support the ideology. Typically, contrary research results are summarily dismissed or ignored. When research that is favorable to testing is overwhelming, however, the problem for sociopolitical ideologies is doubled (Gottfredson, 2000).

6. *Advancing hypotheses or knowledge claims that are impossible to test or evaluate empirically.* Some have suggested that the scientific community should remain agnostic about the very existence of the construct of intelligence until everyone agrees on its definition (see Armour-Thomas & GoPaul-McNicol, 1998; Sternberg & Grigorenko, 2008), a condition was has never existed (Thorndike, 1921; Sternberg, 1985; Sternberg, Conway, Ketron, & Bernstein, 1981; Sternberg & Detterman, 1986) and will most likely never exist. Similarly, Helms (1992) makes the argument that test developers have not conducted adequate research to investigate the extent to which test items have a different "cultural meaning" for different racial and ethnic groups—which, in her view, will presumably enable tests to have "cultural equivalence." Ignoring the fact that cognitive tests continue to show the same degree of predictive validity for English-speaking American-born groups (Gottfredson, 2005; Jensen, 1998)—such a proposal assumes (1) a (heretofore elusive) consensus among researchers on the meaning and measurement of

"culture," and (2) that it is somehow possible to assign cultural "meaning" to individual test items.

7. *Quick promotion of "alternative" assessment techniques before they have been thoroughly vetted.* "Alternative" test procedures burst on the scene with much fanfare and hope for equalizing score distribution outcomes for subgroups. As examples, the System of Multicultural Pluralistic Assessment (SOMPA) was touted in the late 1970s as a fairer method of taking into account "sociocultural" variables in assessing cognitive functioning of different American subgroups (see Figueroa, 1979). Similarly, the Learning Potential Assessment Device (Feuerstein, Rand, & Hoffman, 1979) was marketed in the 1980s as an innovative "paradigm shift" in assessment that incorporated "innovative" theories of structural cognitive modifiability and mediated learning (Feuerstein, Feuerstein, & Gross, 1997). At the time of this writing, both of these assessment methods have largely disappeared from the psychometric scene, having been exposed to withering conceptual and empirical criticisms by researchers and disappointing outcomes from field research (Frisby, 1992; Glutting & McDermott, 1990; Goodman, 1979; Oakland, 1979; van de Vijver & Phalet, 2004; Wurtz, Sewell, & Manni, 1985). Whenever this happens, however, there is no corresponding well-publicized explanation from authors as to why the "innovative" method failed, or any attempt to revise the underlying theory. As time passes, another highly publicized "fad"

quickly captures the public's interest as a promising challenge to traditional testing.

8. *Generating fear of real or imagined negative social consequences of high stakes testing for culturally diverse minority groups.* Whether intentionally or unintentionally, test critics communicate the message that the general public has something to fear when tests are used with cultural minority groups, particularly those who tend to score lower relative to other groups (e.g., Samuda, 1998). Hale-Benson (1986) claims that, unless the "black community" of educational and psychological scholars discover their own "culturally specific" methodologies for defining and using intelligence tests for black children, the dire consequences will be that "the majority of black children... [will] continue to struggle through special classes, educable mentally retarded labels, SAT and GRE scores to make it in this society" (p. 4). Skiba, Knesting, and Bush (2002) acknowledge that the empirical research demonstrating significant test bias for African Americans is weak. Thus, they seek sources of racial bias in various aspects of public schooling (e.g., curricula, teacher expectations, school discipline practices), for fear that disproportionate results from IQ testing may lead to "a conclusion of unequal ethnic aptitude" or "genetic inferiority" (p. 66).

Ethical/Legal Professional Standards

Psychologists, educators, test developers, and researchers are represented by one or more professional organizations who advocate that tests be used responsibly, ethically, and within legal guidelines with examinees from culturally diverse groups. *Ethics* generally refers to "a system of principles of [appropriate] conduct that guide the behavior of an individual" (Jacob & Hartshorne, 2007, p. 2), and the application of ethical principles to problems that arise in professional practice is called *applied professional ethics* (Beauchamp & Childress, 2001). Applied professional ethics principles for test construction, interpretation, and use are generally embedded in professional ethics codes and professional standards documents—or are found in separate "stand-alone" documents that specifically govern testing. Such documents serve the dual purpose of protecting the public and promoting the self-interests of the profession (Jacob & Hartshorne, 2007).

Professional ethics codes involving testing and cultural minority groups are not bound by law. However, many ethics codes require professionals to know and respect the law, generally, as well as specific

law that is applicable to their professional areas. At times, professional ethics codes may advocate adherence to decisions that are more stringent than those required by law (Jacob & Hartshorne, 2007).

At the time of this writing, perhaps the most well-known document that outlines criteria for evaluating test development, the psychometric properties of tests, and test use is *Standards for Educational and Psychological Testing*, published by the American Educational Research Association, the American Psychological Association, and the National Council on Measurement in Education (AERA, APA, & NCME, 1999). In addition, there are a variety of professional standards and guidelines for test use that are associated with professional organizations for psychologists, counselors, and test publishers (see p. 105 in Phelps, 2007; Exhibit 2, p. 7, in Phelps, 2009). The most well-known ethics and "best practices" guideline documents governing test use for educators, psychologists, and counselors—as these interface with cultural/ethnic minority groups—are given in Table 7.2.

General Themes in Professional Ethics Codes Governing Test Use with Ethnically and Linguistically Diverse Populations

As derived from documents listed in Table 7.2, guidelines for selecting, using, and interpreting tests for diverse groups generally fall into three categories: (1) practices that are encouraged, (2) practices that are to be avoided, (3) and areas in which "caution" is required. Although recommendations in testing ethics documents are often suggested for test developers (e.g., see Standards 7.1, 7.3, 7.4, 9.2, 9.4, 9.6, 9.7, and 9.9 in AERA, APA, & NCME, 1999) and test researchers (e.g., see Standard 7.6 in AERA, APA, & NCME, 1999), only recommendations for test users are discussed here.

PRACTICES THAT ARE ENCOURAGED

According to Standard 9.3 in the *Standards for Educational and Psychological Testing* (hereafter referred to as SEPT; AERA, APA, & NCME, 1999),

> when testing an examinee proficient in two or more languages for which the test is available, the examinee's relative language proficiencies should be determined. The test generally should be administered in the test taker's most proficient language, unless proficiency in the less proficient language is part of the assessment. (p. 98)

Furthermore, Standard 9.10 states that "inferences about test takers' general language proficiency should be based on tests that measure a range of

Table 7.2 Standards Documents in Education, Counseling, and Psychology Relevant to the Interface of Testing and Cultural Minorities

Generic Ethics Documents for Professional Organizations That Include References to Testing/Assessment and Cultural Minority Subgroups

- American School Counselor Association (2010). Ethical standards for school counselors. Alexandria, VA: ASCA. Accessed January 2013 from HYPERLINK "http://www.schoolcounselor.org/files/EthicalStandards2010.pdf" www.schoolcounselor.org/files/EthicalStandards2010.pdf (see Standard A.9.f)

Documents Designed Specifically for Testing/Assessment Issues That Include References to Cultural Minority Subgroups

- American Counseling Association. (2003). Standards for qualifications of test users. Alexandria, VA: Author (see Standard 6)
- American Educational Research Association, American Psychological Association, & National Council of Measurement in Education (1999). *Standards for educational and psychological testing*. Washington, DC: AERA, APA, & NCME (see Chapters 7, 9)
- American School Counselor Association & Association for Assessment in Counseling (1998). *Competencies in assessment and evaluation for school counselors*. Alexandria, VA: Author (see Competency 4d.)
- Association for Assessment in Counseling (4th Edition, 2012). *Standards for multicultural assessment*. Alexandria, VA: American Counseling Association (see entire document)
- Eyde, I. D., Robertson, G. J., Moreland, K. L., Robertson, A. G., Shewan, C. M., Harrison, P.L., et al. (1993). *Responsible test use: Case studies for assessing human behavior*. Washington, DC: American Psychological Association. (See Section 3, Case #37; Section 4, Case #69, #73)
- International Test Commission (2000). *International guidelines for test use*. Accessed February 2013 from http://www.intestcom.org/guidelines/index.php (see especially sections 2.3, 2.7)
- Accessed June 2010 from http://www.intestcom.org/upload/sitefiles/41.pdf (see especially sections 2.3, 2.7)
- International Test Commission (2005). *International guidelines on computer-based and internet delivered testing*. Accessed February 2013 from http://www.intestcom.org/guidelines/index.php (see Section 2.f)
- http://www.intestcom.org/Downloads/ITC%20Guidelines%20on%20Computer%20-%20version%202005%20approved.pdf (see Section 2.f)
- International Test Commission (2010). *International Test Commission guidelines for translating and adapting tests*. Accessed February 2013 from http://www.intestcom.org/guidelines/index.php (see entire document)
- Joint Committee on Testing Practices (2000). *Rights and responsibilities of test takers: Guidelines and expectations*. Accessed February 2013 from http://www.apa.org/science/programs/testing/rights.aspx# (see "Guidelines for Testing Professionals," Points #2, #3)
- Joint Committee on Testing Practices (2004). *Code of fair testing practices in education*. Accessed February 2013 from http://www.apa.org/science/programs/testing/committee.aspx (See Points #7, #14, #15)
- National Association of School Psychologists (NASP) (2003). *Position statement on using large-scale assessment for high stakes decisions*. Bethesda, MD: NASP (see paragraph "Who Is Assessed" under section "Interpreting Results from Large Scale Assessments: Cautions and Considerations")

Document Designed Specifically for Cultural Minority Issues That Include References to Testing/Assessment

- American Psychological Association (2010). *Guidelines for providers of psychological services to ethnic, linguistic, and culturally diverse populations*. Accessed February 2013 from http://www.apa.org/pi/oema/resources/policy/provider-guidelines.aspx (under "Guidelines", see Point 2d.)

language features, and not on a single linguistic skill" (p. 99). Standard 11.23 states,

> If a test is mandated for persons of a given age or all students in a particular grade, users should identify individuals whose disabilities or linguistic background indicates the need for special accommodations in test administration and ensure that these accommodations are employed. (AERA, APA, & NCME, 1999, p. 118)

A common application of this standard involves the use of interpreters for instances in which an English-language test is individually administered to an examinee who is not fluent in the English language. These same standards stipulate that when an interpreter is used, the interpreter should be fluent in both the language of the test and also the language of the examinee, as well as having a basic understanding of the assessment process (Standard 9.11, AERA, APA, & NCME, 1999). According to Standard 11.22, "When circumstances require that a test be administered in the same language to all examinees in a linguistically diverse population, the test user should investigate the validity of the score interpretations for test takers believed to have limited proficiency in the language of the test." (p. 118).

Some directives from testing-standards documents are worded in vague generalities that leave much "wiggle room" for a variety of interpretations. For example, the American School Counselor Association and Association for Assessment in Counseling (ASCA & AAC, 1998) encourage professionals to "evaluate their own strengths and limitations in the use of assessment instruments and in assessing students with disabilities or linguistic or cultural differences. [Counselors] know how to identify professionals with appropriate training and experience for consultation" (ASCA & AAC, 1998). The American Counseling Association (2003) encourages counselors to interpret test scores " in light of the cultural, ethnic, disability, or linguistic factors that may impact an individual's score" (American Counseling Association, 2003). Similarly, under "Interpretation and Application of Assessment Results," Guideline Number 5 states, in part, "the test user should evaluate how the test taker's gender, age, ethnicity, race, socioeconomic status, marital status, and so forth, impact on the individual's results" (Association for Assessment in Counseling, 2003, p. 7).

Another example illustrating the use of vague terminology is the frequent use of the term "test fairness." Although Jensen (1980) cautioned audiences to avoid misinterpretations and misapplications of this term, some testing-standards documents encourage test users to be "committed to fairness in every aspect of testing" (American Counseling Association, 2003) and "select tests that are fair to all test takers" (Association for Assessment in Counseling, 2003, p. 3).

The Standards for Educational and Psychological Testing (AERA, APA, & NCME, 1999, p. 74) articulate four interpretations of the concept of "test fairness." Two interpretations (i.e., absence of psychometric bias in tests and equitable treatment in the testing process) have broad consensus among psychometricians and test users. However, characterizations that define "test fairness" as "equal test score outcomes across groups" are rejected. Characterizations that define test fairness as "equal opportunity to learn the material covered in tests" are judged as "clearly relevant to some uses…(but) clearly irrelevant to others" (p. 74)—with the proviso that "disagreement might arise as to the relevance of opportunity to learn to test fairness in some specific situations" (p. 74).

PRACTICES TO AVOID

SEPT states that a test should not be used for subgroups for which credible research reports differences in the effects of construct-irrelevant variance on at least some part of the test (AERA, APA, & NCME, 1999).

Under "Interpretation and Application of Assessment Results" from the "Standards for Multicultural Assessment," Point #4 states, "When test results are influenced by irrelevant test-taker characteristics (e.g., gender, age, ethnic background, cheating, availability of test preparation programs) the use of the resulting information is invalid and potentially harmful" (Association for Assessment in Counseling, 2003, p. 7).

AREAS REQUIRING CAUTION

Under "Selection of Assessment Instruments" from the "Standards for Multicultural Assessment," Point #13 urges counselors to be cautious when selecting tests for culturally diverse populations to avoid inappropriateness of testing that may be outside of socialized behavioral or cognitive patterns (Association for Assessment in Counseling, 2003, p. 3).

Test users are encouraged in the SEPT to include "cautionary statements" in their public reports whenever test scores are disaggregated by ethnic groups and credible research suggests that such scores may not have comparable meaning across groups (Standard 7.8, AERA, APA, & NCME, 1999).

When there are reports of group differences in average scores for a test, and relevant "contextual information" that would enable "meaningful interpretation" of these differences is not available, test users "should be cautioned against misinterpretation" (Standard 15.12, AERA, APA, & NCME, 1999, p. 169).

Another frequent admonition in testing ethics codes is for professionals to "use caution" when using tests with, and/or interpreting scores from, individuals representing groups that were not represented in the tests' standardization sample (American Counseling Association, 2003; American School Counselor Association, 2004).

Influence, Compatibility, and Conflict Between Knowledge Claim Sources: Blurred Boundaries

For pedagogical purposes, the three sources of knowledge claims (empirical, sociopolitical, and professional/ethical guidelines) are discussed as mutually exclusive and separate categories. In reality, the lines of demarcation between these sources are somewhat blurred, particularly as these relate to the appropriateness of test use and interpretation with culturally diverse groups. For example, sociopolitical ideologies are, by their very nature, resistant to acknowledging that their central tenets are contradicted by rigorous empirical data. Gottfredson (2009) summarizes this point as follows:

> That the testing controversy is today mostly a proxy battle over fundamental political goals explains why no amount of scientific evidence for the validity of intelligence tests will ever satisfy the tests' critics.... Tests may be legitimately criticized, but they deserve criticism for their defects, not for doing their job. (p. 14)

Further complicating matters, Marxist-inspired sociopolitical ideologies have often argued that the notion of an objective empirical science is itself an illusion. Jensen (1982) summarizes this view as follows:

> In [the Marxist] view, science is motivated to promote that form of socioeconomic class structure that most favors the privileged elite, reinforcing its position of political and economic power. By the same token, any unwitting biases of scientists are deemed most prone to line up against the socially underprivileged and economically disadvantaged classes. Presumably, such ideological science only pretends to test its hypotheses in the idealized, objective manner we learned about in our introductory high school and college science courses. In this view, scientists actually begin with prejudices, then frame them as theories, and create only the illusion of demonstrating the validity of their hypotheses. The conclusions are... "advocacy masquerading as objectivity." This end is accomplished through "biased selection"—of data, of methods of analysis, and of various possible interpretations of evidence—such that the final outcome will confirm whatever dogma originally motivated the supposedly objective search for the truth. (Jensen, p. 122)

Marxist criticisms have been particularly aggressive when directed toward the notion of intelligence, the IQ, and tests' claim to be fairly objective measures of intelligence (Gould, 1996; Sanders, 1985).

Unfortunately, both arguments supporting and arguments criticizing tests and their use with cultural minorities are published in scholarly journals. As a result, it becomes especially difficult for naïve readers (particularly those who are prone to believe anything they read in print) to discern which (among a litany of contradictory viewpoints)

is the more credible position (absent more in-depth study of psychometrics and cognitive psychology). To help in this regard, readers would also need to familiarize themselves with the academic philosophy, reputation, and rejection rates of different journal outlets, as some manuscripts prominently featured in some journals would not see the light of day in other journals.

Professional standards and ethics documents must often walk a fine line between acknowledging results from rigorous test research and at the same time acknowledging and guarding against abuses in test use frequently voiced by sociopolitical ideologies. Often such standards attempt to "please both masters." As one among many examples, *Standards for Educational and Psychological Testing* (AERA, APA, & NCME, 1999) acknowledges the conflict between those who argue that standards for test fairness have been met through technical criteria, versus those who argue that "fairness requires more than satisfying certain technical requirements" (p. 80). They then add the vague admonition that "matters of values and public policy are crucial to responsible test use" (p. 80), with no specification as to how these issues interact in making testing decisions. The authors of the *Standards* leave the issue unresolved with the statement: "It is unlikely that consensus in society at large or within the measurement community is imminent on all matters of fairness in the use of tests" (p. 80).

The tension between the need to avoid criticism from anti-test ideologies (which claim that test use with cultural minority groups is "unfair") and the need to follow research-based testing principles arises in a variety of contexts. For example, some test developers claim that the deliberate omission of cognitive test items involving "speed" should logically reduce a test's potential for cultural bias (Bracken & McCallum, 1998). Yet at the same time, Hambleton (2005) states:

> [S]ometimes speed of performance is an integral part of the construct being measured such as it is with the ability to solve analytic reasoning problems. Then, speed is an important part of the construct, so examinees need to understand the need to work quickly. (p. 9)

Thus, if a test is not measuring speed of solving problems (in order to avoid criticisms of cultural bias), then to what extent can it be said that the full range of intelligence is truly being measured?

A similar dilemma is posed in the context of understanding the relationship between the makeup of a test's standardization sample and proper test use and score interpretation with individual test takers. Sociopolitical ideologies capitalize on the idea that administering a test to an individual belonging to a racial/ethnic group that is not adequately represented in the standardization sample, to varying degrees, compromises best practice due to the possibility of test score misinterpretation (Dent, 1996; Harrington, 1975). Driven by the need to protect the public against poor practice, *Standards for Educational and Psychological Testing* includes guidelines that address this issue. These Standards state: "Tests selected for use in individual testing should be suitable for the characteristics and background of the test taker" (Standard 12.3, p. 131). The Standards then elaborate that test selection should be based, in addition to test characteristics, on validity evidence from the population that is representative of the test taker. According to Standard 4.5, clearly described populations on which test norms are based "should include individuals or groups to whom test users will ordinarily wish to compare their own examinees."

Yet even such straightforward language raises the question, What "background" characteristics should be considered as "representative" of a particular test taker? Such standards sound good as long as these are framed as abstractions. Application is not as straightforward when applied to complex individuals. For example, suppose that a test user wanted to administer a cognitive test to a middle-class Filipino-American girl living in Hoboken, New Jersey. Although the standardization sample includes individuals from Hoboken, no Filipino-Americans of this girl's social-class strata were included in the standardization sample. Should the test user feel comfortable using this test with this particular girl on the grounds that Hoboken residents were sampled, or is this test user violating best testing practices by administering a test with no comparable Filipino-Americans in the standardization sample? Furthermore, on what basis is the test user to decide which of these two variables (ethnicity or place of residence) is most important for making these decisions?

This is where empirical research can be helpful. When compared against United States norms (which included virtually no Japanese children), Japanese children at every age group between five and 15 obtained higher average scores on the Wechsler Intelligence Scale for Children (WISC) Performance scale, compared to the mostly white American WISC standardization group (Lynn, 1977).

Fan, Willson, and Kapes (1996) conducted one of the most thorough and original empirical tests of the standardization fallacy found in the testing literature. She examined data from 190,000 eleventh-grade students who had already taken the Texas Assessment of Academic Skills (TAAS) reading and math tests. This subject pool consisted of large sub-samples of Caucasian, Black, Hispanic, and Asian students. She began by dividing this large pool into two halves, and conducted her original study on one half, followed by a replication of her methods conducted on the second half. Using the first half of the subject pool (approximately 95,000 students), Fan constructed four equal sub-samples (n = 300 in each), each of which included different proportions of ethnic representation (i.e., each sample had 60%, 30%, 10%, and 0% representation of the different ethnic groups). From subjects' scores on the TAAS, she computed item/total correlations for each item, within each of the four ethnically heterogeneous sub-samples. A high item/total correlation would indicate that the higher probability of passing an item is associated with higher test scores on the entire test. Thus, the higher the item/total correlation, the better the item.

Fan et al. (1996) selected the 24 reading test items and 30 math items that had the best item/total correlations within each sub-sample. This created four (one for each ethnically heterogeneous sample of n = 300 each) "mini-tests" of the best items from each of the four sub-samples.

Fan et al. then constructed four additional sub-samples of 200 subjects, each of which was ethnically homogeneous (i.e., 200 White, 200 Black, 200 Hispanic, 200 Asian). Within each ethnically homogeneous sample, Fan et al. calculated their scores from each of the four "minitests" (comprising items with the best item/total correlations calculated from each of the four heterogeneous samples). Her hypotheses were straightforward. If bias was present (i.e., if the standardization fallacy were true), then the ethnically homogeneous sample should manifest the highest scores on mini-tests created from the heterogeneous sample in which their group was most represented. Thus, the White homogeneous sample should "achieve" their highest score on the "minitest" made from the heterogeneous sample made up of 60% whites, the next-highest score on the "minitest" made from the heterogeneous sample of 30% whites, and so on, culminating in the lowest score "achieved" on the minitest made from the heterogeneous sample in which no whites were represented. The same predictions were then applied to the homogeneous Black, Hispanic, and Asian samples.

Fan et al. found no relationship between the ethnic composition of the "minitest" subsamples and any homogeneous groups' ability to achieve higher scores from minitests constructed on a majority of their ethnic group. Fan et al. repeated the same procedures, only instead of constructing four "minitests" from a heterogeneous mixture of ethnic groups, "minitests" were constructed from 100% ethnically homogeneous samples. Even with this modification in procedures, the standardization fallacy was not supported. Fan et al. then repeated the same procedures on the second half of the subject pool (n = 95,000), and obtained the same (lack of) results.

Implications

These examples illustrate some difficulties in providing unambiguous direction for practitioners in using tests with culturally diverse groups. Using the previous example, it can be concluded that, for some tests, ethnic representation in a test's standardization sample has no effect in "biasing" test results for examinees. However, in the light of ethical and professional test standards, using a test for subjects not represented (in terms of racial/ethnic group membership) in the standardization or item-tryout sample is not viewed as best practice. If the particular group in question is traditionally a lower-scoring group on average, sociopolitical ideologies will use this as ammunition to criticize test usage with examinees from particular groups. However, no matter how vociferous these attacks, the previous examples have shown that empirical data do not support such criticisms.

It remains unknown how many other situations represent points of conflict between empirical research, sociopolitical ideology, and test standards. Part of the problem originates from scholars' attempts to impose subjective definitions on concepts of "culture," "fairness," "equivalency," and "opportunity to learn." Progress has been achieved in our attempts to provide objective, testable definitions for "test bias"—as well as empirically based evidence that would support the existence of unbiased tests. However, even research evidence demonstrating the lack of statistical bias in tests has not stopped claims that tests are "unfair" to particular groups (e.g., see Helms, 1992, 1997, 2006).

As subjective definitions for concepts increasingly appear in the psychometric literature, the potential for perceived "unfairness" multiplies exponentially. In making the argument supporting equity in assessment and school instruction, for example, Camilli (2006) argues that "students should have an opportunity to learn all of the material on a test" and that teachers may need to "compensate for such differential access to knowledge" (pp. 247–248). Although one can easily interpret these statements in the context of achievement testing, there is no easy application of these arguments to intelligence tests (which, in theory, are composed of items that the student cannot "learn" from practice). Yet, when psychometricians openly discuss these concepts, no matter how innocently, sociopolitical ideologues will use them as an "open door" for criticizing tests and their use with select cultural minority groups. Test standards and professional ethics documents are then left to grapple (sometimes unsuccessfully) with how to interpret these terms in the context of ethical practice. Clarity in, and an achieved consensus regarding, various loaded concepts in the testing literature is not likely to resolve contentious sociopolitical value conflicts surrounding test use and interpretation with cultural minority groups. Nevertheless, there is value in first untangling the components that contribute to these debates.

References

AERA, APA, & NCME (1999). *Standards for educational and psychological testing.* Washington, DC: AERA, APA, & NCME.

Alley, G., & Foster, C. (1978). Nondiscriminatory testing of minority and exceptional children. *Focus on Exceptional Children, 9,* 1–14.

American Psychological Association (2001). Appropriate use of high stakes testing in our nation's schools. Accessed July 17, 2009, from http://www.apa.org/pubinfo/testing.html.

American Psychological Association (2002). Guidelines on multicultural education, training, research, practice, and organizational change for psychologists. Accessed July 17, 2009, from http://www.apa.org/practice/Multicultural.pdf.

Armour-Thomas, E. (1992). Intellectual assessment of children from culturally diverse backgrounds. *School Psychology Review, 21*(4), 552–565.

Armour-Thomas, E., & GoPaul-McNicol, S. (1998). *Assessing intelligence: Applying a biocultural model.* Thousand Oaks, CA: Sage.

Association for Assessment in Counseling (2003). *Standards for multicultural assessment.* Alexandria, VA: Author.

Beauchamp, T., & Childress, J. (2001). *Principles of biomedical ethics* (5th ed.). New York: Oxford University Press.

Bond, L. (1994). Comments on the O'Neill and McPeek paper. In P. W. Holland & H. Wainer (Eds.), *Differential item functioning* (pp. 277–279). Hillsdale, NJ: Lawrence Erlbaum.

Bond, L., Moss, P., & Carr, P. (1996). Fairness in large-scale performance assessment. In G. W. Phillips & A. Goldstein (Eds.), *Technical issues in large-scale performance assessment* (pp. 117–140). Washington, DC: National Center for Education Statistics.

Bracken, B. A. & McCallum, R. S. (1998). *Examiner's manual: Universal Nonverbal Intelligence Test (UNIT).* Itasca, IL: Riverside Publishing.

Byrne, B. M., Shavelson, R. J., & Muthen, B. (1989). Testing for the equivalence of factor covariance and mean structures: The issue of partial measurement invariance. *Psychological Bulletin, 105*, 456–466.

Butcher, J. N., Cabiya, J., Lucio, E., & Garrido, M. (2007). *Assessing Hispanic clients using the MMPI-2 and MMPI-A.* Washington, DC: American Psychological Association.

Camilli, G. (2006). Test fairness. In R. L. Brennan (Ed.), *Educational measurement* (4th ed.; pp. 221–256). Westport, CT: Praeger.

Chen, H., Keith, T., Weiss, L., Zhu, J., & Li, Y. (2010). Testing for multigroup invariance of second-order WISC-IV structure across China, Hong Kong, Macau, and Taiwan. *Personality and Individual Differences, 49*(7), 677–682.

Dent, H. E. (1996). Non-biased assessment or realistic assessment? In R. L. Jones (Ed.), *Handbook of tests and measurement for Black populations,* Vol. 1 (pp. 103–122). Hampton, VA: Cobb & Henry.

Edwards, O., & Oakland, T. (2006) Factorial invariance of Woodcock-Johnson III scores for African Americans and Caucasian Americans. *Journal of Psychoeducational Assessment, 24* (4), 358–366.

Eells, K., Davis, A., Havighurst, R., Herrick, V., & Tyler, R. (1951). *Intelligence and cultural differences.* Chicago, IL: University of Chicago Press.

Elbeheri, G., Everatt, J., Reid, G., & Mannai, H. (2006). Dyslexia assessment in Arabic. *Journal of Research in Special Educational Needs, 6*(3), 143–152.

Elliott, R. (1987). *Litigating intelligence: IQ tests, special education, and social science in the courtroom.* Dover, MA.: Auburn House.

FairTest (2007, Aug. 20). The ACT: Biased, inaccurate, and misused [FairTest university testing fact sheet]. Retrieved May 22, 2010, from http://www.fairtest.org/act-biased-inaccurate-and-misused.

Fan, X., Willson, V. L., & Kapes, J. T. (1996). Ethnic group representation in test construction samples and test bias: The standardization fallacy revisited. *Educational and Psychological Measurement, 56*(3), 365–382.

Feuerstein, R., Feuerstein, R., & Gross, S. (1997). The Learning Potential Assessment Device. In D. P. Flanagan, J. L. Genshaft, & P. L. Harrison (Eds.), *Contemporary intellectual assessment: Theories, tests, and issues* (pp. 297–313). New York: Guilford Press.

Feuerstein, R., Rand, Y., & Hoffman, M. (1979). *The dynamic assessment of retarded performers: Learning potential assessment device, theory, instruments, and techniques.* Baltimore, MD: University Park Press.

Figueroa, R. A. (1979). The system of multicultural pluralistic assessment. *School Psychology Digest, 8*(1), 28–36.

Frisby, C. L. (1999a). Culture and test session behavior: Part I. *School Psychology Quarterly, 14*(3), 263–280.

Frisby, C. L. (1999b). Culture and test session behavior: Part II. *School Psychology Quarterly, 14*(3), 281–303.

Frisby, C. L. (2005a). The politics of multiculturalism in school psychology: Part I. In C. L. Frisby & C. R. Reynolds (Eds.), *Comprehensive handbook of multicultural school psychology* (pp. 45–80). New York: John Wiley.

Frisby, C. L. (2005b). The politics of multiculturalism in school psychology: Part II. In C. L. Frisby & C. R. Reynolds (Eds.), *Comprehensive handbook of multicultural school psychology* (pp. 81–136). New York: John Wiley.

Frisby, C. L. (1992). Feuerstein's dynamic assessment approach: A semantic, logical, and empirical critique. *Journal of Special Education, 26*(3), 281–301.

Frisby, C., & Osterlind, S. (2007). Hispanic test session behavior on the Woodcock-Johnson Psychoeducational Battery—Third edition. *Journal of Psychoeducational Assessment, 25*(3), 257–270.

Feuerstein, R., Feuerstein, R., & Gross, S. (1997). The learning potential assessment device. In D. P. Flanagan, J. L. Genshaft, & P. L. Harrison (Eds.), *Contemporary intellectual assessment: Theories, tests, and issues* (pp. 297–311). New York: Guilford.

Georgas, J., van de Vijver, F., Weiss, L., & Saklofske, D. (2003). A cross-cultural analysis of the WISC-III. In J. Georgas, L. Weiss, F. van de Vijver, & D. Saklofske (Eds.), *Culture and children's intelligence* (pp. 277–313). New York: Academic Press.

Georgas, J., Weiss, L., van de Vijver, F., & Saklofske, D. (Eds.). (2003). *Culture and children's intelligence: Cross-cultural analysis of the WISC-III.* New York: Academic Press.

Glutting, J. J., Oakland, T., & McDermott, P. A. (1988). Observing child behavior during testing: Constructs, validity, and situational generality. *Journal of School Psychology, 27*(2), 155–164.

Glutting, J. J., & McDermott, P. A. (1990). Principles and problems in learning potential. In C. R. Reynolds & R. W. Kamphaus (Eds.), *Handbook of psychological and educational assessment of children: Intelligence and achievement* (Vol. 1, pp. 296–347). New York: Guilford Press.

Goodman, J. F. (1979). Is tissue the issue? A critique of SOMPA's models and tests. *School Psychology Digest, 8*(1). 47–62.

GoPaul-McNicol, S., & Armour-Thomas, E. (2002). *Assessment and culture: Psychological tests with minority populations.* San Diego, CA: Academic Press.

Gottfredson, L. S. (1994a). The science and politics of race-norming. *American Psychologist, 49*(11), 955–963.

Gottfredson, L. S. (1994b). Egalitarian fiction and collective fraud. *Society, 31*(3), 53–59.

Gottfredson, L. S. (1997). Editorial: Mainstream science on intelligence: An editorial with 52 signatories, history, and bibliography. *Intelligence, 24*(1), 13–24.

Gottfredson, L. S. (2000). Skills gaps, not tests, make racial proportionality impossible. *Psychology, Public Policy, and Law, 6*(1), 129–143.

Gottfredson, L. S. (2004a). Schools and the g factor. *The Wilson Quarterly,* Summer, 35–45.

Gottfredson, L. S. (2004b). Realities in desegregating gifted education. In D. Booth & J. C. Stanley (Eds.), *In the eyes of the beholder: Critical issues for diversity in gifted education* (pp. 139–155). Waco, TX: Prufrock Press.

Gottfredson, L. S. (2005). Implications of cognitive differences for schooling within diverse societies. In C. L. Frisby & C. R. Reynolds (Eds.), *Comprehensive handbook of multicultural school psychology* (pp. 517–554). New York: Wiley.

Gottfredson, L. S. (2007). Applying double standards to "divisive" ideas: Commentary on Hunt and Carlson (2007). *Perspectives on Psychological Science, 2*(2), 216–220.

Gottfredson, L. S. (2009). Logical fallacies used to dismiss the evidence on intelligence testing. In R. P. Phelps (Ed.), *Correcting fallacies about educational and psychological testing* (pp. 11–65). Washington, DC: American Psychological Association.

Gould, S. J. (1996). *The mismeasure of man.* New York: W. W. Norton & Co.

Gopaul-McNicol, S. & Armour-Thomas, E. (2002). Assessment and culture: Psychological tests with minority populations. San Diego, CA: Academic Press.

Graham, J. R. (2006). *MMPI-2: Assessing personality and psychopathology* (4th ed.). New York: Oxford University Press.

Greenfield, P. M. (1997). You can't take it with you: Why ability assessments don't cross cultures. *American Psychologist, 52,* 1115–1124.

Grigorenko, E. L. (Ed.). (2009). *Multicultural psychoeducational assessment.* New York: Springer.

Hale-Benson, J. (1986). *Black children: Their roots, culture, and learning styles.* Baltimore, MD: Johns Hopkins University Press.

Hambleton, R. K. (2005). Issues, designs, and technical guidelines for adapting tests into multiple languages and cultures. In R. K. Hambleton, P. F. Merenda, & C. D. Spielberger (Eds.), *Adapting educational and psychological tests for cross-cultural assessment* (pp. 3–38). Mahwah, NJ: Lawrence Erlbaum.

Hambleton, R. K., & Kanjee, A. (1995). Increasing the validity of cross-cultural assessments: Use of improved methods for test adaptations. *European Journal of Psychological Assessment, 11*(3), 147–157.

Hambleton, R. K., & Li, S. (2005). Translation and adaptation issues and methods for educational and psychological tests. In C. L. Frisby & C. R. Reynolds (Eds.), *Comprehensive handbook of multicultural school psychology* (pp. 881–903). New York: John Wiley.

Hambleton, R. K., Merenda, P. F., & Speilberger, C. D. (Eds.). (2005). *Adapting educational and psychological tests for cross-cultural assessment.* Mahwah, NJ: Lawrence Erlbaum.

Harrington, G. M. (1975). Intelligence tests may favour the majority groups in a population. *Nature, 258,* 708–709.

Helms, J. (1992). Why is there no study of cultural equivalence in standardized cognitive ability testing? *American Psychologist, 47,* 1083–1101.

Helms, J. (1997). The triple quandary of race, culture, and social class in standardized cognitive ability testing. In D. P. Flanagan, J. L. Genshaft, & P. Harrison (Eds.), *Contemporary intellectual assessment: Theories, tests, and issues* (pp. 517–532). New York: Guilford Press.

Helms, J. (2006). Fairness is not validity or cultural bias in racial-group assessment: A quantitative perspective. *American Psychologist, 61*(8), 845–859.

Herrnstein, R. J., & Murray, C. (1994). *The bell curve: Intelligence and class structure in American life.* New York: Free Press.

Heywood, A. (2010). *Political ideologies* (4th Ed.). Houndsmill, England: Macmillan.

Hilliard, A. G. (1987). The Learning Potential Assessment Device and Instrumental Enrichment as a paradigm shift. *Negro Educational Review, 38*(2), 200–208.

Hui, C. H., & Triandis, H. C. (1985). Measurement in cross-cultural psychology. *Journal of Cross-Cultural Psychology, 16,* 131–152.

Jacob, S., & Hartshorne, T. S. (2007). *Ethics and law for school psychologists.* Hoboken, NJ: John Wiley.

Jencks, C., Bartlett, S., Corcoran, M., Crouse, J., Eaglesfield, D., Jackson, G., et al. (1979). *Who gets ahead? The determinants of economic success in America.* New York: Basic Books.

Jensen, A. R. (1980). *Bias in mental testing.* New York: Free Press.

Jensen, A. R. (1982). The debunking of scientific fossils and straw persons. [Review of "The mismeasure of man."] *Contemporary Education Review, 1,* 121–135.

Jensen, A. R. (1984a). Test validity: g versus the specificity doctrine. *Journal of Social and Biological Structures, 7,* 93–118.

Jensen, A. R. (1984b). The Black-White difference on the K-ABC: Implications for future tests. *Journal of Special Education, 18*(3), 377–408.

Jensen, A. R. (1986). Intelligence: "Definition," measurement, and future research. In R. J. Sternberg & D. K. Detterman (Eds.), *What is intelligence? Contemporary viewpoints on its nature and definition* (pp. 109–112). Norwood, NJ.: Ablex.

Jensen, A. R. (1991). Spearman's g and the problem of educational equality. *Oxford Review of Education, 17,* 169–187.

Jensen, A. R. (1992a). Spearman's hypothesis: Methodology and evidence. *Multivariate Behavioral Research, 27,* 225–234.

Jensen, A. R. (1992b). More on psychometric g and "Spearman's hypothesis." *Multivariate Behavioral Research, 27,* 257–260.

Jensen, A. R. (1993). Psychometric g and achievement. In B. R. Gifford (Ed.), *Policy perspectives on educational testing* (pp. 117–227). Boston, MA.: Kluwer Academic Publishers.

Jensen, A. R. (1998). *The g factor: The science of mental ability.* Westport, CT: Praeger.

Jensen, A. R. (2003). Do age-group differences on mental tests imitate racial differences? *Intelligence, 31,* 107–121.

Jensen, A. R., & McGurk, F. (1987). Black-White bias in "cultural" and "noncultural" test items. *Personality and Individual Differences, 8*(3), 295–301.

Johnson, T. P. (1998). Approaches to equivalence in cross-cultural and cross-national survey research. In J. A. Harkness (Ed.), *Cross-cultural survey equivalence* (pp. 1–40). Mannheim, Germany: Zentrum für Umfragen, Methoden und Analysen (ZUMA).

Kathuria, R., & Serpell, R. (1999). Standardization of the Panga Munthu test: A nonverbal cognitive test developed in Zambia. *Journal of Negro Education, 67,* 228–241.

Kaufman, J. C. (2005). Nonbiased assessment: A supplemental approach. In C. L. Frisby & C. R. Reynolds (Eds.), *Comprehensive handbook of multicultural school psychology* (pp. 824–840). New York: John Wiley.

Kitayama, S. & Cohen, D. (Eds.). (2007). *Handbook of cultural psychology.* New York: Guilford Press.

Konold, T. R., Glutting, J. J., Oakland, T., & O'Donnell, L. (1995). Congruence of test-behavior dimensions among child groups that vary in gender, race-ethnicity, and SES. *Journal of Psychoeducational Assessment, 13*(2), 111–119.

Kush, J. C., Watkins, M. W., Ward, T. J., Ward, S. B., Canivez, G. L., & Worrell, F. C. (2001). Construct validity of the WISC-III for White and Black students from the WISC-III standardization sample and for Black students referred for psychological evaluation. *School Psychology Review, 30*(1), 70–88.

Kwate, N. (2001). Intelligence or misorientation? Eurocentrism in the WISC-III. *Journal of Black Psychology, 27*(2), 221–238.

Lidz, C. S. (1997). Dynamic assessment approaches. In D. P. Flanagan, J. L. Genshaft, & P. L. Harrison (Eds.), *Contemporary intellectual assessment: Theories, tests, and issues* (pp. 281–296). New York: Guilford.

Little, T. D. (1997). Mean and covariance structures (MACS) analyses of cross-cultural data: Practical and theoretical issues. *Multivariate Behavioral Research, 32,* 53–76.

Lynn, R. (1977). The intelligence of the Japanese. *Bulletin of the British Psychological Society, 30,* 69–72.

Lynn, R., & Vanhanen, T. (2002). *IQ and the wealth of nations.* Westport, CT: Praeger.

Maxim, P. S. (1999). *Quantitative research methods in the social sciences.* New York: Oxford University Press.

Mpofu, E., & Ortiz, S. O. (2009). Equitable assessment practices in diverse contexts. In E. L. Grigorenko (Ed.), *Multicultural psychoeducational assessment* (pp. 41–76). New York: Springer.

Mullen, B. & Hu, L. (1989). Perceptions of ingroup and out-group variability: A meta-analytic integration. *Basic and Applied Social Psychology, 10,* 233–252.

Nandakumar, R., Glutting, J. J., & Oakland, T. (1993). Mantel-Haenszel methodology for detecting item bias: An introduction and example using the Guide to the Assessment of Test Session Behavior. *Journal of Psychoeducational Assessment, 11,* 108–119.

Nickerson, R. S. (1998). Confirmation bias: A ubiquitous phenomenon in many guises. *Review of General Psychology, 2,* 175–220.

Oakland, T. (1979). Research on the Adaptive Behavior Inventory for Children and the Estimated Learning Potential. *School Psychology Digest, 8*(1), 63–70.

Pedersen, P. (1999) (Ed.). *Multiculturalism as a fourth force.* Philadelphia, PA: Brunner/Mazel.

Phelps, R. P. (2003). *Kill the messenger.* New Brunswick, NJ.: Transaction.

Phelps, R. P. (2005) (Ed.). *Defending standardized testing.* Mahwah, NJ.: Lawrence Erlbaum Association.

Phelps, R. P. (2007). *Standardized testing.* New York: Peter Lang Publishing.

Phelps, R. P. (2009) (Ed.). *Correcting fallacies about educational and psychological testing.* Washington, DC: American Psychological Association.

Reid, R. (1995). Assessment of ADHD with culturally different groups: The use of behavioral rating scales. *School Psychology Review, 24*(4), 537–560.

Reynolds, C. (2000). Why is psychometric research on bias in mental testing so often ignored? *Psychology, Public Policy, and Law, 6*(1), 144–150.

Reynolds, C., & Carson, A. (2005). Methods for assessing cultural bias in tests. In C. L. Frisby & C. R. Reynolds (Eds.), *Comprehensive handbook of multicultural school psychology* (pp. 795–823). New York: Wiley.

Reynolds, C., & Kaiser, S. M. (2003). Bias in assessment of aptitude. In C. R. Reynolds & R. W. Kamphaus (Eds.), *Handbook of psychological and educational assessment of children: Intelligence, aptitude, and achievement* (2nd ed.; pp. 519–562). New York: Guilford Press.

Reynolds, C., & Lowe, P. A. (2009). The problem of bias in psychological assessment. In T. B. Gutkin & C. R. Reynolds (Eds.), *The handbook of school psychology* (4th ed.). New York: John Wiley.

Reynolds, C., & Ramsay, M. C. (2003). Bias in psychological assessment: An empirical review and recommendations. In J. R. Graham & J. A. Naglieri (Eds.), *Handbook of psychology: Assessment psychology* (Vol. 10; pp. 67–94). Hoboken, NJ.: John Wiley.

Rhodes, R. L., Ochoa, S. H., & Ortiz, S. O. (2005). *Assessing culturally and linguistically diverse students: A practical guide.* Guilford Press, NY: Guilford Press.

Ruggiero, V. R. (2001). *Beyond feelings: A guide to critical thinking* (6th Ed.). Mountain View, CA.: Mayfield.

Rushton, J. P., & Jensen, A. R. (2005). Thirty years of research on Black-White differences in cognitive ability. *Psychology, Public Policy, & Law* (pp. 235–294).

Sackett, P. R., Hardison, C. M., & Cullen, M. J. (2004). On interpreting stereotype threat as accounting for African American–White differences on cognitive tests. *American Psychologist, 59*(1), 7–13.

Samuda, R. (1998). *Psychological testing of American minorities.* Thousand Oaks, CA.: Sage.

Sanders, J. T. (1985). Marxist criticisms of IQ: In defence of Jensen. *Canadian Journal of Education, 10*(4), 402–414.

Sandoval, J., & Miille, M. (1980). Accuracy of judgements of WISC-R item difficulty for minority groups. *Journal of Consulting and Clinical Psychology, 48*(2), 249–253.

Serpell, R. (1979). How specific are perceptual skills? *British Journal of Psychology, 70,* 365–380.

Sireci, S. G., Patsula, L., & Hambleton, R. K. (2005). Statistical methods for identifying flaws in the test adaptation process. In R. K. Hambleton, P. F. Merenda, & C. D. Spielberger (Eds.), *Adapting educational and psychological tests for cross-cultural assessment* (pp. 93–115). Mahway, NJ.: Lawrence Erlbaum.

Skiba, R. J., Knesting, K., & Bush, L. D. (2002). Culturally competent assessment: More than nonbiased tests. *Journal of Child and Family Studies, 11*(1), 61–78.

Steele, C. M., & Aronson, J. (1997).A threat in the air: How stereotypes shape intellectual identity and performance. *American Psychologist, 52*(6), 613–629.

Steele, C. M., & Aronson, J. (1995). Stereotype threat and the intellectual test performance of African Americans. *Journal of Personality and Social Psychology, 69*(5), 797–811.

Sternberg, R. J. (1985). Implicit theories of intelligence, creativity, and wisdom. *Journal of Personality and Social Psychology, 49,* 607–627.

Sternberg, R. J., Conway, B. E., Ketron, J. L., & Bernstein, M. (1981). People's conceptions of intelligence. *Journal of Personality and Social Psychology, 41,* 37–55.

Sternberg, R. J., & Detterman, D. K. (Eds.) (1986). *What is intelligence? Contemporary viewpoints on its nature and definition.* Norwood, NJ: Ablex.

Sternberg, R. J., & Grigorenko, E. L. (2008). Ability testing across cultures. In L. A. Suzuki & J. G. Ponterotto (Eds.), *Handbook of multicultural assessment: Clinical, psychological, and educational applications* (3rd ed.; pp. 449–470). San Francisco: Jossey-Bass.

Sternberg, R. J., Wagner, R. K., Williams, W. M., & Horvath, J. A. (1995). Testing common sense. *American Psychologist, 50,* 912–927.

Suzuki, L. A. & Ponterotto, J. G. (Eds.) (2008). *Handbook of multicultural assessment: Clinical, psychological, and educational applications.* New York: John Wiley.

Throrndike, E. L. (1921). Intelligence and its measurement: A symposium. *Journal of Educational Psychology, 12,* 123–147, 195–216, 271–275.

Timbrook, R. E., & Graham, J. R. (1994). Ethnic differences on the MMPI-2? *Psychological Assessment, 6,* 212–217.

Valencia, R. R., & Suzuki, L. A. (2001). *Intelligence testing and minority students: Foundations, performance factors, and assessment issues.* Thousand Oaks, CA.: Sage.

van de Vijver, F. & Leung, K. (1997). *Methods and data analysis for cross-cultural research.* Newbury Park, CA: Sage.

Van de Vijver, R. & Phalet, K. (2004). Assessment in multicultural groups: The role of acculturation. *Applied Psychology: An international review, 53,* 215–236.

van de Vijver, F., & Poortinga, Y. (2005). Conceptual and methodological issues in adapting tests. In R. K. Hambleton, P. F. Merenda, & C. D. Spielberger (Eds.), *Adapting educational and psychological tests for cross-cultural assessment* (pp. 39–64). Mahwah, NJ: Lawrence Erlbaum.

Watkins, D. (1989). The role of confirmatory factor analysis in cross-cultural research. *International Journal of Psychology, 24*, 685–701.

Webster, Y. O. (1997). *Against the multicultural agenda: A critical thinking alternative.* Westport, CT: Praeger.

Williams, R. L. (1971). Abuses and misuses in testing black children. *Counseling Psychologist, 2*, 62–77.

Williams, R. L., Dotson, W., Dow, P., & Williams, W. S. (1980). The war against testing: A current status report. *Journal of Negro Education, 49*, 263–273.

Wood, P. (2003). *Diversity: The invention of a concept.* San Francisco, CA.: Encounter Books.

Wurtz, R., Sewell, T., & Manni, J. (1985). The relationship of estimated learning potential to performance on a learning task and achievement. *Psychology in the Schools, 22*(3), 293–302.

Methods for Translating and Adapting Tests to Increase Cross-Language Validity

Ronald K. Hambleton *and* Minji Kang Lee

Abstract

Translating and adapting tests for use in multiple language and cultural groups has become immensely important to psychologists and cross-cultural researchers. Psychologists want to use popular tests from one language and culture in others; cross-cultural researchers need tests they are interested in to be available in multiple languages and cultures; and credentialing agencies often need to make their tests available in multiple languages. Unfortunately, the methodology for conducting translation and adaptation studies is more comprehensive than is often assumed, and many myths about the process itself exist, and so all too often, the process is handled poorly. In this chapter, three goals will be addressed: (1) several of the popular myths will be described, (2) steps for translating and adapting tests will be presented, and (3) the International Test Commission Guidelines for Test Adaptation will be introduced.

Key Words: backward translation design; forward translation design; International Test Commission (ITC) guidelines for test adaptation; judgmental review; measurement invariance; multiple indicator and multiple cause model; partial invariance; structural equating modeling

With the substantially increasing number of tests being translated and adapted into many languages, for example, tests used in international assessments such as TIMSS and PISA are normally translated and adapted into more than 30 languages, and many popular intelligence tests and personality tests are now available in over 75 languages, it is important to use the best methods to maximize the validity of adapted tests. In two recent issues of the *European Journal of Psychological Assessment* (Issues 3 and 4, 2011), nearly 40 percent of the articles involved test translation or adaptation. With other journals reporting research studies that are in an international context, the percentages are often higher—see for example, the *Journal of Cross-Cultural Psychology* and the *International Journal of Testing*.

Prominent examples of test adaptation projects in the United States include adaptation efforts to prepare Spanish versions of College Board's Scholastic

Assessment Test (SAT), ACE's General Educational Development (GED) Test, and the United States Department of Education's National Assessment of Educational Progress (NAEP). Also, in many states, school achievement tests in mathematics and science are available to students in both English and Spanish. Substantially more test adaptations can be expected in the future as (1) international exchanges of tests become more common, (2) more credentialing exams are adapted into multiple languages (Hambleton & Patsula, 1999), and (3) interest in cross-cultural research grows (Matsumoto & van de Vijver, 2011). On this last point, van de Vijver (2009) reported that the number of test adaptation studies had increased by a factor of four in just five years between 2000 and 2005!

Test adaptations, if they are properly carried out, can increase fairness in testing—in Israel, for example, high school students can take their graduation tests in their choice of any of five languages; test adaptations permit important constructs such as intelligence, personality, and school achievement to be studied in new populations (Matsumoto & van de Vijver, 2011); and test adaptations create possibilities for more cross-cultural research (Hambleton, Merenda, & Spielberger, 2005).

Translating and adapting tests into multiple languages and cultures has a long history in education and psychology—beginning with the French psychologist Alfred Binet's famous intelligence test in the early 1900s. Unfortunately, these translation and adaptation initiatives (e.g., "back translations") have not always been successful, thus reducing the validity of the intended uses of these tests in additional languages. The reasons for the many failures of test translations/adaptations include (1) lack of appreciation by researchers for the technical challenges that arise in the test translation/adaptation process (for example, a belief that someone who knows the languages can do the translations); (2) limited time and resources committed to doing the test adaptation properly (an all too common problem among test publishers and researchers); and (3) lack of awareness among researchers of the necessary steps and methodologies that can be used. For example, it is a common belief that a good translator and judgmental reviews of the translation/adaptation itself are sufficient to validate a translated/adapted test. But there are many examples in the testing literature showing that a good translation is not sufficient technical justification for insuring validity of the target language version of a test. *The International Test Commission Guidelines for Test Adaptation* (see Hambleton, 2005) certainly are much more demanding of researchers, and emphasize that both judgmental and empirical evidence are needed to support a test being valid in a second language and culture (see www.intestcom.org).

Often, too, what researchers think is correct about the test adaptation process is not, and this misinformation further exacerbates the problem. Misunderstandings and myths are rampant in the field. Interestingly, many of the current methodological advances such as structural equation modeling, item response theory, and differential item functioning (DIF) studies are highly relevant, but these technical methods are not well known in the field.

The goals of this chapter are:

1. to describe several of the myths associated with translating and adapting tests (e.g., that almost anyone with knowledge of another language can prepare a good translation; or that judgmental reviews of a translated test are sufficient to establish the validity of scores from a test in a second language);

2. to offer steps for translating and adapting tests, along with a discussion of the methodology associated with several of the more technically challenging steps (e.g., translation designs, comparison of test structures in multiple languages, and the identification of potential item-level bias across language versions of a test); and

3. to provide the guidelines for translating and adapting tests that were prepared by the International Test Commission (and these guidelines require testing agencies and researchers to compile both judgmental evidence and statistical evidence).

Numerous examples will be provided throughout the chapter to highlight good and not so good test adaptation practices.

Before going further, we would like to mount a case for using the term *test adaptation* rather than the more popular and frequently used term *test translation*. The former term is broader and actually reflects what should happen in practice when preparing a test constructed in one language and culture for use in a second language and culture. Test adaptation includes everything from deciding whether an adapted test could measure the same construct in a different language and culture, to selecting qualified translators, to deciding on appropriate accommodations to be made in preparing a test for use in a second language, to adapting the test and then checking its equivalence in the adapted form. Test translation, on the other hand, is only one of several steps in the process of test adaptation, and even at this step, *adaptation* may be a more suitable term than *translation* to describe the process that actually takes place—for example, item formats may need to be revised, new words and concepts may need to be substituted, directions can be revised, and even the time limit may need to be changed (see for example, Hambleton, Merenda, & Spielberger, 2005). In the remainder of this chapter, we will use the term "test adaptation" rather than "test translation" to describe the process of making a test valid for use in a second language and culture. Also, we will use the term "test" to represent a wide array of terms that are used to describe data collection methods in education and psychology, including "instrument," "assessment," "scale," "survey," and "questionnaire."

Popular Myths About the Test Adaptation Process

Five popular myths about test adaptation will be addressed next.

The Preferable Strategy Is Always to Adapt an Existing Test

Translating and adapting a test is typically faster and cheaper than the alternative, which is to build a new test and validate that new test in the target language of interest. It could take several years to define the construct in an acceptable way, and then develop, field-test, and ultimately finalize a test with norms and a technical manual. This alternative is not even a possibility if the goal is to make comparisons across cultural and language groups. A new test in the second language group would raise major questions about the meaningfulness of the comparability of scores—is the new target language test measuring exactly or nearly the same construct? Are the score scales for the two tests comparable, or can the scores from the two tests be placed on a common scale so that comparisons can be made?

Many researchers, too, feel a sense of security that comes with adapting an established test that is being used in one culture and language group. The security comes from knowing that the source language test has usually been validated for many possible uses (as is the case with many popular American tests of intelligence and personality). The standard view is that a good adaptation will lead to that test's being useful again, this time in the new language. Of course, that adapted test still needs to go through the validation process, but the expectation is that the results are more likely to be successful than validating a newly constructed test.

The Minnesota Multiphasic Personality Inventory (MMPI) is an example of a personality inventory that has been widely adapted for use in multiple cultures and languages. When using an existing test, there are often a number of studies which can be compared with newly acquired data. This is an important advantage to consider. Comparing the results from one study to results from others can increase both the generalizability and even the credibility of the findings. "Such comparisons allow a literature to be built up around a commonly shared set of concepts and operational definitions, an advantage admittedly more difficult to achieve if different researchers use different instruments" (Brislin, 1986, p. 138).

At the same time, if the goal is to have a test to measure a construct in a second language for the purpose of doing research in that language group only, a case could be made for developing and validating a new test (see Tanzer, 2005). One major advantage would be that then it would be possible to revise the definition of the construct to fit local needs and conditions. One example would be the construct of "quality of life." In some cultures of the world, the construct may have to do with meeting basic health needs and having sufficient food. In others, quality of life may have to do with having sufficient money for travel and ready access to stores and doctors. Test adaptation of a quality of life measure from one language and culture to another would be possible, but unless that test is chosen carefully, the construct itself may not be relevant in the target language culture, and so the adapted test will be of limited or possibly no value at all. Developing a new test from an acceptable definition of the construct, and with a format familiar to respondents, may be the preferred choice.

On the other hand, for cross-national, cross-language, and/or cross-ethnic comparative studies, adapted tests are required. Such studies have become popular in recent years, as many countries strive to set world-class educational standards and want to compare their progress to that of other countries. The TIMSS project is a good example. Tests prepared in each country, even using the same test specifications, would be sufficiently different that valid comparisons across countries could not be made. Test adaptation is essential.

In summary, there are typically good reasons for and against adapting an existing test compared to developing a new test in that second language and cultural group. It should not be a certainty that a test that is needed can be adapted from another language and culture. Often the intended use of the information dictates the final decision.

Know Two Languages and You Can Be a Translator

Ype Poortinga, a world-class cross-cultural psychologist and a past editor of the *Journal of Cross-Cultural Psychology*, once reported that he felt a high percentage of the papers published before 1990 were fundamentally flawed because of a failure of researchers to take the test adaptation process seriously. The myth in practice is that if you know a second language you can do at least an adequate job of translating a test from one language and culture to another. But the International Test Commission Guidelines for Test Adaptation (2005) are very clear on this point: A good translator must know not only the languages, but the cultures, too, and often it is very helpful if the translator has subject-matter knowledge and knowledge of how tests are developed. (These latter two skills are not common among test translators, so some modest training can be provided to close the gap in knowledge and skills needed to do an effective translation.) For example, one common mistake of translators of multiple-choice questions is to translate the correct answer very precisely, often making the correct answer choice longer. The goal of the translator clearly is be sure that the correct answer remains correct in the translation, but the extra precision can make the answer choice longer, giving a clue to the correct answer to test-wise candidates. Good translators are essential to the test adaptation process but they need to know much more than languages, and the process of test adaptation is much more than translation.

A Good Translation Guarantees Validity

We have observed test publishers working hard to find translators and then giving them time to do their work. But often tests may not have content validity in the second language group, perhaps because of different curricula (see Hambleton, Yu, & Slater, 1999) and/or culture. We have also found that if that second language group performs very well on a test, test scores may be so homogeneous that score reliability is low, and its predictive validity is limited. There is more to ensuring validity of test scores in a second language than simply a good translation. We have even found that a translation of items in the multiple-choice format may not be meaningful (i.e., valid) if the item format is unknown to translators, or only minimally familiar to examinees in the second language group.

A good example of the misinterpretations that can follow from poor adaptations is the following (the example was passed on from Richard Wolf when he was at Columbia Teachers College and actively involved with one of the international assessment studies). In an international comparative study of reading, American students were asked to consider pairs of words and identify them as similar or different in meaning: *sanguine—pessimistic* was one of the pairs of words where American student performance was only slightly above chance (i.e., 50% in the case of this binary scored item). In the country ranked first in performance, about 98 percent of the students answered the question correctly. In the process of attempting to better understand the reason for the huge difference in performance,

it was discovered that "sanguine" had no equivalent word in the language of this top-performing country, so the equivalent of the English word "optimistic" was used. This substitution made the question considerably easier, and it would have been answered correctly by a high percentage of the American students as well, had they been presented with the pair *optimistic—pessimistic*. The point of this example is to highlight the danger in drawing conclusions from international studies without strong evidence that the test adaptation process resulted in two equivalent tests. A careful empirical analysis would have spotted the problem, and we suspect that the item would have been deleted from the assessment or revised, preferably following a field test administration.

Psychological Constructs Are Universal

The fields of psychology and education are full of examples of studies where it was found that constructs can have different definitions in different cultures—*intelligence, quality of life,* and *depression* are three examples. For example, the construct of *intelligence* in the United States includes a big component of *speed of performance.* In many cultures, speed of performance does not play nearly as important a role in the definition of the construct. *Quality of life* researchers have found that the construct can have very different meanings across the world. *Depression* is another construct that may take on a different meaning in some cultures (see some of Spielberger's research, for example).

A Judgmental Review of the Adaptation Is Sufficient Evidence to Justify the Use of the Test

Certainly, using qualified translators can be a very important step in the test adaptation process. At the same time, it is a mistake to think that this first step in the process is sufficient for insuring a valid test in a second language. Problems arise that can only be spotted through field-testing the adapted test items. In one study recently, it was discovered that, in translation, the test items were longer and required more time to read. It was learned only after the test became operational that the target-language version of the test was speeded up for examinees, an unintended consequence of the translations process and the language itself. The fact was that the words themselves were simply longer in German than they were in English. Field test work can be used to spot problematic test items or statements, inappropriate item formats, test timing issues, unintended multi-dimensionality, and so on. Rarely would these analyses, from our experience, not reveal shortcomings in the adapted test that could be fixed before the test is used operationally or in a research study. PISA and TIMSS, for example, routinely carry out field test studies prior to finalizing tests for use in these international studies of achievement.

Summary

Each of the five myths can have a negative impact on the utility of tests in a second language and culture. Sometimes it may be best not to embark on an adaptation process—perhaps because of the intended use of the test in the second language group (an adapted test may not be needed), or because the construct itself may have a different meaning in that second language and cultural group. Good translators of the language are valuable, but the translators need more than simply the language skills to be effective, and a good language translation of a test may not be what is needed. Most importantly, empirical evidence (e.g., reliability and validity evidence) is needed to support a test adaptation. A good judgmental review is rarely sufficient and should be criticized when it is the sole piece of evidence (important as it is) to support the validity of scores from an adapted test.

Steps for Conducting a Test Adaptation Study

Over the years, steps have been advanced for testing agencies and researchers to follow in enhancing the validity of a test adaptation. In this chapter, steps from a paper by Hambleton and Patsula (1999) have been edited and updated.

Step 1. *Ensure content equivalence exists in the two language and cultural groups*. Before embarking on a major test adaptation initiative, the researcher should do some checking to be sure that the construct definition in one language and culture is applicable in the other. This step can be accomplished by compiling judgmental evidence from psychologists and educators who know both cultures and understand the definition of the construct in the source language.

Step 2. *Decide whether to adapt an existing test or to develop a new test*. This step was discussed in some detail earlier in the chapter. The more similar the construct is in the two language groups, the more likely it is that an adaptation would be successful. The final decision regarding this step surely requires (1) some reasonable level of assessment expertise, (2) knowledge of just what might be involved in conducting an adaptation, (3) knowledge of the relevant literature and the validity of the source language version of the test, and (4) some knowledge of the language and culture of the target language version of the test.

Step 3. *Select well-qualified translators*. A broader definition of "well-qualified" must be adopted to suffice. Knowing the two languages is only the first criterion to be met. Knowledge of the culture is second. Also, knowledge of the construct being measured and testing practices is helpful, too. As few translators can meet these criteria, often some training may be helpful. Without it, awkward translations can result, and good testing practices can be violated. Using multiple translators is also a good idea so that they can share their knowledge and insights.

Step 4. *Adapt the test*. Often this step is what is called the "translation process," but often it is more than that. Test directions may need to be revised, answer sheets may need to be redesigned to accommodate the background of the respondents, etc. The presence of multiple translators can also greatly aid the process of obtaining an acceptable adaptation.

Step 5. *Conduct a judgmental review of the adapted test and revise the test adaptation as necessary*. Of course this is one of the critical steps in the process, and for some agencies, this may be the last step. At least two judgmental designs are popular: backward translation designs and forward translation designs.

With the backward translation design, one group of translators signs off on the adaptation, and then a second group back-translates the test. Finally, a new group compares the original source language test and the back-translated version. Any problems that are identified can be fixed in the target language version of the test. The design has merit, and many problems in the adaptation can usually be identified. The downside is that the target-language version of the test is not investigated. Researchers like the design because they do not need to be bilingual to judge the similarity of the two source-language versions of the test.

The forward-translation design involves a comparison by translators of the source and target-language versions of the test. This design has more merit than the first because the target-language version of a test is reviewed. In many comprehensive studies of test adaptation, a back-translation design is used to spot and fix problems in the target language version, and then the second design is used to further the evaluation. But the consensus among experts is that the second design is preferable to the first, if only one is to be used, because of the review of the target-language version of the test. In many studies today, both designs are used.

Step 6. *Conduct a small tryout of the target language version of the test.* This step can be used to detect problems in the target language version of the test, prior to investing considerable time and expense in carrying out more ambitious reliability and validity studies. Clarity of directions, the suitability of the test format, and the time limit (if one exists) can be studied and fixed. A small-scale item analysis and reliability study can also be insightful.

With respect to the item-review process itself, Hambleton and Zenisky (2011) published a chapter in which they described an item translation and adaptation review form they designed. The review form contains 25 questions organized into five categories that address the test items in the target language version of the test: General (4 questions), Item Format (5 questions), Grammar and Phrasing (6 questions), Passages (if present; 4 questions), and Culture (5 questions). The 25 questions were all associated with problems that have arisen in practice, and documentation for the importance of each question is contained in their chapter. A sample of the questions follows:

• Does the item have the same or highly similar meaning in the two languages?
• Is the item format, including physical layout, the same in the two versions of the test?
• Are there any grammatical clues that might make this item easier or harder in the target language version?
• Are there any words in the item that, when translated, change from having one meaning to having more than one common meaning?

The item review form should help to standardize the item review process for translators and other reviewers but it can also be used to alert test translators to problems that may arise in their adaptation initiatives. Knowledge of these problems in advance can help to improve the adaptation process as well.

Step 7. *Design and carry out a more substantial study to investigate test reliability and validity.* At this step, the testing agency or researcher has many options. The goal is to compile additional evidence for validity of the scores with the target language version of the test. Here is a partial list of analyses that could be carried out:

1. Conduct a reliability study (e.g., internal consistency, test-retest). It is basic information, but it is useful to establish.

2. Conduct an item analysis with a suitably sized sample.

3. Conduct an analysis, item by item, comparing performance on the source- and target-language versions of the test (e.g., Holland & Wainer, 1993; Sireci, 2011)—these are often called "differential item functioning (DIF)" studies, and the two language groups are often called "reference" and "focal" groups (corresponding to the source language and target language groups).

4. Check the factorial structure of the target language version of the test and compare to the source language version. Often it is here that "structural equation modeling" is used, and this topic will be considered in more detail in the next section.

5. Carry out a "linking" study if the goal is to report scores from the source- and target-language versions of the test on a common reporting scale (see Angoff & Cook, 1988; Cook & Schmitt-Cascallar, 2005).

For more details on possible methodologies, see the next section and Hambleton, Merenda, and Spielberger (2005), van de Vijver and Tanzer (1997) and special issues of *Language Testing* (Issue 2, Volume 20, in 2003) and the *International Journal of Testing* (Issue 2, Volume 9, in 2009).

Step 8. *Prepare technical and user documentation, and continue monitoring the target language version of the test adaptation.* A paper trail documenting the process of adapting the test, how certain problems may have been handled, and the design and validity results can be invaluable to those interested in checking the validity of the target-language version of the test. Of course, details for the test user administration are needed, too, so that this portion of the process can be standardized across language groups. Finally, if the test adaptation continues to be used, periodically compiling validity evidence would be valuable as well.

Checking the Equivalence of the Source- and Target-Language Versions of a Test

Structural equation modeling (SEM) is one of the most widely applied statistical methods for testing the comparability of how different language or cultural groups perform on the source- and target-language versions of an educational or psychological test (see for example, Byrne & van de Vijver, 2010). One strength of SEM is that it allows one to assess a global hypothesis regarding *measurement invariance* across the different groups. For example, the loadings of a factor model (i.e., the relationship between an item and a factor) can be constrained to be equal across groups, and the relationships between items (or sets of items or parcels) and the latent variables across groups can be examined in the same analysis. Because this type of analysis has become common in addressing the equivalence of a test across two (or even more) language versions, SEM will be described in detail next. Other popular statistical methods such as DIF can be found in the writings of many researchers. See for example, the recent publication of Sireci (2011).

Testing Measurement Invariance with SEM

Both exploratory and confirmatory factor analysis can be conducted in the SEM framework. In exploratory factor analysis, one does not have an *a priori* theory about the test structures. Whenever one does exploratory factor analysis in SEM, it is advised that cross-validation with different samples be conducted to guard against chance findings (Boomsma, 2000). In the test adaptation context, however, one would often be interested in testing whether the structure underlying the original tests carries over to their adapted versions. That is, one already has a theory of the test structure that one wants to validate in other language or culture groups; the appropriate approach for carrying out this validation is multi-group confirmatory factor analysis (MG-CFA; Byrne & van de Vijver, 2010; Gierl, 2000; Konishi et al., 2009; Loner & Peri, 2009). In particular, MG-CFA based on mean and covariance structures (MACS) instead of the more commonly used covariance structure (CS) analysis is advocated to check for increasingly stringent levels of measurement invariance (Wu, Li, & Zumbo, 2007; Gregorich, 2006).

A regression equation that represents the factor analysis model incorporating MACS can be written as follows:

$$y_{ij} = \tau_j + \lambda_{j1}\eta_{1i} + \lambda_{j1}\eta_{1i} + \cdots + \lambda_{jp}\eta_{pi} + \varepsilon_{ij},$$

where y_{ij} denotes the ith person's score ($i = 1, \ldots, N$) on the jth indicator ($j = 1, \ldots, J$). Each person's indicator score is a linear combination of the intercept (τ_j), one or more factors (η_{pi}, $p = 1, \ldots, P$), and a normally distributed random residual (ε_{ij}). Each λ_{jp} is the loading of indicator j on factor p, and τ_j is the indicator score when the factor scores are zero.

A prerequisite to testing measurement invariance is *configural invariance*, in which one investigates whether the same number of factors and the same pattern of free and fixed factor loadings hold across groups. Lack of configural invariance demonstrates that different constructs were measured across groups. Once configural invariance is satisfied, one can proceed to check the more demanding criterion of *weak invariance* by placing equality constraints on factor loadings (λ_{jp}) across groups. If these constraints do not significantly worsen model–data fit, then weak invariance is supported. This allows one to set the unit of measurement equal across groups. That is, one unit change in the factor results in the same change in the indicator, regardless of group membership. In addition to the equality of factor loadings, *strong invariance* requires equality of the intercepts (τ_j), which is tested by the application of MACS. A finding of strong invariance allows one to make comparisons of the group means of latent variables. Finally, *strict invariance* requires the equality of residual variances ($\text{Var}(\varepsilon_{ij})$) in addition to that of factor loadings and intercepts. One might argue that strict invariance is not necessary for test scores to be comparable across groups. The residual ε_{ij} is composed of two parts: A stable unique part that indicator j measures in addition to the common factor, and a random error. An indicator might fail a check for strict invariance because the two groups have different variances in either part of the residual. For example, one group might have a larger residual variance because its members are more diverse in their exposures to specific bits of knowledge required to do well on a particular test; that is, one group has greater variance in the stable unique part measured by that test. If this is the case, then it does not seem that the failure of strict invariance is a shortcoming of the test. However, it is also possible that one group has a larger residual variance because the random errors tend to be larger for members of that group, and this *does* seem to be a shortcoming of the test. For this reason it is desirable to test the hypothesis of strict invariance. In this way, all four levels of the nested hierarchy of measurement invariance can be tested to investigate the comparability of test performance across different language or cultural groups.

Partial Invariance

It is quite possible that one often finds a lack of invariance, given the stringent nature of the hypotheses of invariance. In this case, it can be more meaningful to check the degree of partial measurement invariance. If a better fit can be obtained by freeing some estimates, then one should document the proportion of freed parameters when reporting the degree of invariance. Although there is no strict rule of an acceptable degree of partial invariance, less than 20% freed parameters are recommended for many practical applications (Dimitrov, 2010).

Multiple Indicator and Multiple Cause (MIMIC) Model

MIMIC is a special case of MG-CFA. A MIMIC model examines whether different groups have the same intercepts in the regression of indicator scores on the common factor. Note that there can only be two levels in the grouping variable. The MIMIC model can be written as

$$X_j = \alpha_j + \delta_j G + \lambda_j \theta + \varepsilon_j,$$

in which X_j denotes the jth parcel score, α_j denotes the intercept, δ_j denotes the difference in intercepts between the groups, G denotes the group dummy variable, λ_j denotes the factor loading, θ denotes factor score, and ε_j denotes the error. The MIMIC model uses a path from the grouping variable to the common factor to account for the average difference of the common factor in the two groups. The significant path from the group variable to the common factor means that the two groups differ on average in the value of the common factor. This is permissible as far as the measurement is concerned, because the fact that the two groups differ in abilities does not necessarily mean that there is something wrong with the test. However, if there is a significant path from the group variable to an indicator, that means that there is something wrong with that indicator. Someone from one group with the same value of the common factor as someone from the other group is still expected to obtain a different score on the indicator. We can say that the indicator is *biased*. This is analogous to the lack of intercept equality, or differential item functioning with group differences in item difficulty.

Methodological Challenges

Some methodological challenges for the construct validation of a test across different language groups are small sample size and distributions differing greatly in shape or central tendency. Small sample size will lead to larger estimation errors and overestimation of goodness-of-fit indices, especially

when the sample size is less than 200 (Dimitrov, 2010). If the ranges or shapes of the two score distributions are different, then any differences in obtained parameter estimates may reflect either true group differences or simply one group's being located at a part of the score scale where any kind of statistical estimation is problematic.

A study by Sireci and Wells (2009) shows how they dealt with this problem. They randomly matched the examinees in the bigger sample to those in the smaller sample based on proficiency so that their distributions perfectly overlapped.

International Test Commission Guidelines for Test Adaptation

In 2005, the International Test Commission (ITC) published a set of guidelines for translating and adapting educational and psychological tests (see Hambleton, 2005). Several organizations assisted the ITC in preparing the guidelines: the European Association of Psychological Assessment, the European Test Publishers Group, the International Association for Cross-Cultural Psychology, the International Association of Applied Psychology, the International Association for the Evaluation of Educational Achievement, the International Language Testing Association, and the International Union of Psychological Science, and their assistance helped enhance both the importance of the guidelines as well as the quality of the guidelines themselves. The guidelines were organized into four categories, and the guidelines are reported below, organized by category:

Context

C.1 Effects of cultural differences that are not relevant or important to the main purposes of the study should be minimized to the extent possible.

C.2 The amount of overlap in the construct measured by the test or instrument in the populations of interest should be assessed.

Test Development and Adaptation

D.1 Test developers/publishers should insure that the adaptation process takes full account of linguistic and cultural differences among the populations for whom adapted versions of the test or instrument are intended.

D.2 Test developers/publishers should provide evidence that the language use in the directions, rubrics, and items themselves as well as in the handbook are appropriate for all cultural and language populations for whom the test or instrument is intended.

D.3 Test developers/publishers should provide evidence that the choice of testing techniques, item formats, test conventions, and procedures are familiar to all intended populations.

D.4 Test developers/publishers should provide evidence that item content and stimulus materials are familiar to all intended populations.

D.5 Test developers/publishers should implement systematic judgmental evidence, both linguistic and psychological, to improve the accuracy of the adaptation process and compile evidence on the equivalence of all language versions.

D.6 Test developers/publishers should ensure that the data collection design permits the use of appropriate statistical techniques to establish item equivalence between the different language versions of the test or instrument.

D.7 Test developers/publishers should apply appropriate statistical techniques to (1) establish the equivalence of the different versions of the test or instrument, and (2) identify problematic components or aspects of the test or instrument that may be inadequate to one or more of the intended populations.

D.8 Test developers/publishers should provide information on the evaluation of validity in all target populations for whom the adapted versions are intended.

D.9 Test developers/publishers should provide statistical evidence of the equivalence of questions for all intended populations.

D.10 Non-equivalent questions between versions intended for different populations should not be used in preparing a common scale or in comparing these populations. However, they may be useful in enhancing content validity of scores reported for each population separately.

Administration

A.1 Test developers and administrators should try to anticipate the types of problems that can be expected, and take appropriate actions to remedy these problems through the preparation of appropriate materials and instructions.

A.2 Test administrators should be sensitive to a number of factors related to the stimulus materials, administration procedures, and response modes that can moderate the validity of the inferences drawn from the scores.

A.3 Those aspects of the environment that influence the administration of a test or instrument should be made as similar as possible across populations of interest.

A.4 Test administration instructions should be in the source and target languages to minimize the influence of unwanted sources of variation across populations.

A.5 The test manual should specify all aspects of the administration that require scrutiny in a new cultural context.

A.6 The administrator should be unobtrusive and the administrator-examinee interaction should be minimized. Explicit rules that are described in the manual for administration should be followed.

Documentation/Score Interpretations

I.1 When a test or instrument is adapted for use in another population, documentation of the changes should be provided, along with evidence of the equivalence.

I.2 Score differences among samples of populations administered the test or instrument should not be taken at face value. The researcher has the responsibility to substantiate the differences with other empirical evidence.

I.3 Comparisons across populations can only be made at the level of invariance that has been established for the scale on which scores are reported.

I.4 The test developer should provide specific information on the ways in which the socio-cultural and ecological contexts of the populations might affect performance, and should suggest procedures to account for these effects in the interpretation of results.

The guidelines themselves have been adopted for use in many countries and by many testing agencies. A second edition is now being developed and is likely to be released for use in 2013. For more details on the guidelines, readers can refer to Hambleton (2005) or check www.intestcom.org.

References

Angoff, W. H., & Cook, L. L. (1988). *Equating the scores of the Prueba de Aptitud Academica and the Scholastic Aptitude Test* (Report No. 88-2). New York: College Entrance Examination Board.

Boomsma, A. (2000). Reporting analyses of covariance structures. *Structural Equation Modeling, 7*(3), 461–483.

Brislin, R. W. (1986). The wording and translation of research instruments. In W. J. Lonner & J. W. Berry (Eds.), *Field methods in cross-cultural psychology* (pp. 137–164). Newbury Park, CA: Sage Publications.

Byrne, B. M., & van de Vijver, F. J. R. (2010). Testing for measurement and structural equivalence in large-scale cross-cultural studies: Addressing the issues of nonequivalence. *International Journal of Testing, 10*(2), 107–132.

Cook, L. L., & Schmitt-Cascallar, A. P. (2005). Establishing score comparability for tests given in different languages. In R. K. Hambleton, P. Merenda, & C. Spielberger (Eds.), *Adapting educational and psychological tests for cross-cultural assessment* (pp. 139–170). Mahwah, NJ: Lawrence Erlbaum Associates, Publishers.

Dimitrov, D. M. (2010). Testing for factorial invariance in the context of construct validation. *Measurement and Evaluation in Counseling and Development, 43*(2), 121–149.

Gierl, M. J. (2000). Construct equivalence on translated achievement tests. *Canadian Journal of Education, 25*(4), 280–296.

Gregorich, S. E. (2006). Do self-report instruments allow meaningful comparisons across diverse population groups? *Medical Care, 44*(11), S78–S90.

Hambleton, R. K. (2005). Issues, designs, and technical guidelines for adapting tests into multiple languages and cultures. In R. K. Hambleton, P. Merenda, & C. Spielberger (Eds.), *Adapting educational and psychological tests for cross-cultural assessment* (pp. 3–38). Mahwah, NJ: Lawrence Erlbaum Associates, Publishers.

Hambleton, R. K., Merenda, P., & Spielberger, C. D. (Eds.). (2005). *Adapting educational and psychological tests for cross-cultural assessment.* Mahwah, NJ: Lawrence Erlbaum Associates, Publishers.

Hambleton, R. K., & Patsula, L. (1999). Increasing the validity of adapted tests: Myths to be avoided and guidelines for improving test adaptation practices. *Applied Testing Technology, 1*(1), 1–16.

Hambleton, R. K., Yu, J., & Slater, S. (1999). Field test of the ITC guidelines for adapting educational and psychological tests. *European Journal of Psychological Assessment, 15*(3), 270–276.

Hambleton, R. K., & Zenisky, A. L. (2011). Translating and adapting tests for cross-cultural assessments. In D. Matsumoto & F. J. R. van de Vijver. (Eds.), *Cross-cultural research methods in psychology* (pp. 46–70). New York: Cambridge University Press.

Holland, P. W., & Wainer, H. (Eds.). (1993). *Differential item functioning.* Hillsdale, NJ: Lawrence Erlbaum Publishers.

Konishi, C., Hymel, S., Zumbo, B. D., Li, Z., Taki, M., Slee, P., et al. (2009). Investigating the comparability of a self-report measure of childhood bullying across countries. *Canadian Journal of School Psychology, 24*(1), 82–93.

Loner, E., & Peri, P. (2009). Ethnic identification in the former Soviet Union: Hypotheses and analyses. *Europe-Asia Studies, 61*(8), 1341–1370.

Matsumoto, D., & van de Vijver, F. J. R. (Eds.). (2011). *Cross-cultural research methods in psychology.* New York: Cambridge University Press.

Sireci, S. G. (2011). Evaluating test and survey items for bias across languages and cultures. In D. Matsumoto & F. J. R. van de Vijver. (Eds.), *Cross-cultural research methods in psychology* (pp. 216–243). New York: Cambridge university Press.

Sireci, S. G., & Wells, C. S. (2009). *Evaluating the comparability of English and Spanish video accommodations for English language learners* (Final Report). Harrisburg, PA: Pennsylvania Department of Education.

Tanzer, N. (2005). Developing tests for use in multiple languages and cultures: A plea for simultaneous development. In R. K. Hambleton, P. Merenda, & C. Spielberger (Eds.), *Adapting educational and psychological tests for cross-cultural assessment* (pp. 235–264). Mahwah, NJ: Lawrence Erlbaum Associates, Publishers.

van de Vijver, F. J. R. (2009). *Translating and adapting psychological tests for large-scale projects.* An invited presentation at the 11th European Congress of Psychology, Oslo, Norway.

van de Vijver, F. J. R., & Tanzer, N. (1997). Bias and equivalence in cross-cultural assessment. *European Review of Applied Psychology, 47*, 263–279.

Wu, A. D., Li, Z., & Zumbo, B. D. (2007). Decoding the meaning of factorial invariance and updating the practice of multi-group confirmatory factor analysis: A demonstration with TIMSS data. *Practical Assessment, Research, & Evaluation, 12*(3), 1–26.

Diagnosis, Classification, and Screening Systems

R. W. Kamphaus, Erin Dowdy, Sangwon Kim, *and* Jenna Chin

Abstract

This chapter serves as a primer devoted to the main issues involved in the diagnostic and classification process of children, including an overview of widely used nosological systems and the empirical support associated with them. New directions and systems of classification and diagnosis are also presented in some detail. An overview of concepts and issues in behavioral and emotional problem screening assessment associated with prevention and early intervention concludes the chapter. Two primary conclusions are drawn. First, the amount of unsupportive evidence associated with currently used systems requires that radical changes be made to these systems going forward. Second, the newfound emphasis on early identification and screening associated with prevention practice and science requires the incorporation of classification of risk and subsyndromal problems into new and revised classification systems.

Key Words: classification, diagnosis, screening, assessment

Classification and Diagnosis

Classification of phenomena is necessary to advance any discipline, whether applied or theoretical (Kamphaus & Campbell, 2006). A "diagnostic system" is a specific type of classification system, one designed to describe clinical phenomena for research, treatment, administrative, or other purposes. "Diagnosis," the type of classification that is the focus of this text, refers to a process of classifying an individual as having a particular disease state or set of diseases. Although the diagnostic process dates from antiquity (DuBois, 1965), the modern process of psychiatric diagnosis traces its roots to the work of Emil Kraepelin, who proposed that a system be created for classifying mental illnesses according to their symptoms, causes (i.e., etiologies), and course (i.e., progression of symptomatology) (Kraepelin, 1896). In the medical sciences, conditions such as heart disease and high blood pressure are classified as separate diseases. Analogously, borderline

personality disorder is classified separately from schizophrenia in psychiatric classification. Therefore, diagnosis may be considered a specialized type of classification, one concerned with the categorization of diseases.

In spite of various objections to mental health diagnosis per se and its imperfect nature (Frick, Burns, & Kamphaus, 2009), the majority of mental health professionals concur that the basic purposes and inherent advantages of classification support its use and further development (Cantwell, 1996). Related to this assumption, Blashfield (1998) has described five primary purposes for classification in psychopathology that also serve to illustrate its utilitarian properties: (1) creation of a common professional nomenclature; (2) organization of information; (3) clinical description; (4) prediction of outcomes and treatment utility; and (5) the development of concepts upon which theories may be based. These goals, although sound and pragmatic, have yet to be obtained by any one classification system. The predominant diagnostic classification schemes do attempt to provide a common nomenclature, organize information, and clinically describe syndromes or patterns of behavior. Nevertheless, the reliability and validity of prevailing models have not been adequately demonstrated, supportive evidence varies greatly from one diagnosis to another, nor has a clear line of research established expediency with regard to treatment and theory development (Frick et al., 2009; Edelbrock & Achenbach, 1980).

Worldwide, the diagnosis of child and adolescent psychopathology has traditionally been based on the *Diagnostic and Statistical Manual of Mental Disorders* (DSM) system, now in its fifth edition. Given its status as the premier worldwide standard and its influence on the conduct of research, it is important to know and understand the basic assumptions of this system in particular, along with its limitations. This initial section will discuss widely used classification systems focusing on the DSM, as well as alternative classification approaches, including a dimensional and a person-oriented approach. This section will also address recent research trends and promising future directions that are important for further developing classification systems for child and adolescent behavioral and emotional adjustment, developmental status, competency, and mental health. Specifically, promising research based on cognitive neuroscience and genetics will be presented. In addition, a strength-based approach to mental health will be discussed, which provides a broader perspective on assessing and treating problems in children and adolescents. Lastly, the issue of culture in diagnosis, which has not been as well studied, despite its potential impact on diagnosis, will be given some attention. The field of screening will also be discussed in the latter half of the chapter, as screening can play an integral role in the early steps of classification and diagnosis, and subsequent early intervention.

Classification Systems and Approaches
SYSTEMS IN WIDESPREAD USE: THE DSM AND ICD

The two major sanctioned classification systems of child and adolescent disorders in use at this time are the American Psychiatric Association's *Diagnostic and Statistical Manual of Mental Disorders* (DSM) and the World Health Organization's International Classification of Diseases (ICD). While these classification systems are used in clinical settings, typically outside of public school settings, different classification systems are often used in school settings (e.g., Individuals with Disabilities Educational Improvement Act, or IDEIA, in the United States). However, psychologists working in schools sometimes still utilize the DSM classification system for case conceptualization and treatment planning. Additionally, practitioners often have opportunities to engage in communication and collaboration across settings as part of their work with child and adolescent populations. Therefore, although this section will primarily focus on a discussion of the DSM system, work with children and adolescents requires knowledge of both the ICD and IDEIA systems.

The DSM has undergone several revisions, with the anticipated publication of its fifth edition this year. When the DSM was first published in 1952, no specific section for child and adolescent disorders existed; instead, childhood and adolescence were considered only as a specific condition for some categories (e.g., "schizophrenic reaction, childhood type"; special symptom reactions such as learning disturbance, enuresis, and somnambulism). DSM-II (American Psychiatric Association, 1968), however, made major progress by adding a new section titled "Behavior Disorders of Childhood and Adolescence." This section including seven disorders, such as hyperkinetic reaction of childhood (or adolescence) and overanxious reaction of childhood (or adolescence), was expanded into "Disorders Usually First Evident in Infancy, Childhood, or Adolescence" in DSM-III (American Psychiatric Association, 1980). Under this title, DSM-III listed nine childhood disorders, including mental retardation, attention-deficit disorder, and conduct disorder; additionally, the DSM-III provided specific developmental disorders, such as reading disorder. The basic structure of the DSM-III was maintained in the subsequent revision of the third edition (DSM-III-R: American Psychiatric Association, 1987). Furthermore, the more recent revisions (DSM-IV and DSM-IV-TR; American Psychiatric Association, 1994, 2000) represented a section named "Disorders Usually First Diagnosed in Infancy, Childhood, or Adolescence," under which there are 10 categories of disorders such as learning disorders, communication disorders, and attention-deficit and disruptive behavior disorders. Although the DSM revisions show the continuing development and refinement of child and adolescent disorders, it is important to note that a separate section for childhood and adolescence is provided for convenience of use only, without conceptualizing child disorders as distinct from adult disorders (American Psychiatric Association, 1994).

The DSM is based on a medical model that posits that disorders reside within an individual child (Frick, Burns, & Kamphaus, 2009). In the DSM diagnostic system, disorders are conceptualized in a dichotomous way: as either present or absent within a child. This categorical premise, however, has not been empirically supported by evidence of cutoff points that can accurately distinguish individuals with a disorder from those without it (Kendell, 2002). The questionable existence of discontinuities in child and adolescent disorders has led to attempts to conceptualize mental disorders as dimensions rather than categories, which will be discussed later in this section. The all-or-nothing conceptualization of disorders also makes it difficult to identify children who present sub-threshold symptoms and may need interventions. From a preventative perspective, the failure to provide mental health services in a timely manner increases the risk for developing disorders. Hence, it is important to have a classification system that helps to assess risk status of individual children and, when necessary, intervene early before problems become severe.

As an alternative to a medical model, a biopsychosocial model has been proposed that encompasses biological, psychological, social, and cultural aspects of child and adolescent disorders. This comprehensive approach has provided a framework on which some of the recent classification systems have been based. For example, the World Health Organization developed The International Classification of Functioning, Disability and Health (World Health Organization, 2001), in which a disability is defined in terms of impairment of structure and function, restriction of activities, and environmental factors that include both facilitators of and barriers to an individual's functioning.

Another important issue pertaining to the concept of mental disorders is that the DSM defines mental disorders with symptoms, not etiology. In fact, for the most part, the causes of mental disorders remain unknown. Moreover, the DSM relies on experts' consensus in developing the concept of specific disorders, though it has moved toward an emphasis on empirical foundations. Due to the provisional nature of DSM disorders, the diagnostic process is affected by a clinician's subjectivity (Jablensky, 1999). Therefore, having balance between clinical judgment and empirical assessment data can be helpful in making a more precise diagnosis (Achenbach, 2001; Doucette, 2002). On another level, it is noted

that, in a sense, DSM disorders are social constructs, as decisions on whether and to what extent a certain behavior or symptom is inappropriate involves making social judgments (Wakefield, 1999).

There are other challenges that remain unresolved by the latest version of the DSM system. The premise that the high levels of comorbidity observed in diagnostic practice reflect true comorbidity is doubtful. The fact that no significant body of evidence supports the DSM disorders as distinct categories (e.g., Meehl, 1995) suggests the possibility that the apparent comorbidity is spurious. For this reason, it has been suggested to replace the term *comorbidity* with *co-occurrence* (Lilienfeld, Waldman, & Israel, 1994). Additionally, the DSM system does not adequately recognize the heterogeneity of children with the same diagnosis (e.g., Hinshaw & Lee, 2003), with some exceptions (e.g., ADHD subtypes and pervasive developmental disorders). A failure to recognize subgroups of a disorder hinders the search for differentiated causes, consequences, and treatments (Quay, 1987).

Lastly, reliability of the DSM diagnoses has improved, while validity evidence is lacking. Although less than the desired diagnostic reliability threshold of .90 (Nunnally, 1978), the reliability of some DSM diagnoses has been improved, in part due to the provision of operational definitions of disorders and the development of structured diagnostic interviews (Kendell, 2002; Schmidt, Kotov, & Joiner, 2004). Hence, the challenge the DSM system faces mostly is the lack of sufficient validity evidence in support of the accuracy of the child and adolescent diagnoses. In studying validity, researchers should give attention to clinical validity in addition to other types of validity. Clinical validity is related to practical issues, one important aspect of which is how much a diagnosis provides guidance on appropriate treatment (Kendell, 2002). As the ultimate purpose of classification of mental disorders lies in treating the identified disorder, the link of diagnosis to intervention is critical for establishing a clinical validity argument (Messick, 1989).

The aforementioned disadvantages of the DSM system have led to proposals for alternative classification approaches in child and adolescent psychopathology. The following section will focus on two of these: dimensional and person-oriented classification systems.

Dimensional Approach

The relative value of categorical (e.g., the DSM-IV-TR) and dimensional (e.g., Edelbrock & Achenbach, 1980) classification methods has been frequently debated (Fletcher, 1985). However, an increasing body of literature has described the advantages of dimensional models (LaCombe, Kline, Lachar, Butkus, & Hillman, 1991). For example, Achenbach and McConaughy (1992) noted that the yes/no nature of categorical methods does not necessarily account for children whose problems vary in degree or severity. As a result, the shift between "normalcy" and psychopathology cannot be well understood with categorical methods, since most high-prevalence problem behaviors in children, such as inattention and hyperactivity, are not classifiable when below diagnostic threshold levels. Substantial evidence is emerging to suggest that child behavior problems such as inattention, hyperactivity, depression, and conduct problems, in fact, fall along continua in the population. Therefore, the continuous nature of these child behaviors is more appropriately measured with dimensional scales (Hudziak, Wadsworth, Heath & Achenbach, 1999) rather than with categorical systems (Scahill, et al., 1999).

In this classification approach, child and adolescent disorders are conceptualized as dimensions, rather than categories, based on the assumption that normality and abnormality range along a continuum. In other words, the difference between persons with a disorder and persons without a disorder is quantitative rather than qualitative. Empirical findings have supported the dimensional nature of childhood disorders for various symptoms, including hyperactivity/impulsivity, inattention, conduct problems, depression, and anxiety (Deater-Deckard, Reiss, Hetherington, & Plomin, 1997; Fergusson & Horwood, 1995; Hudziak et al., 1999; Nease, Volk, & Cass, 1999).

Statistical techniques such as exploratory factor analysis are used to group a number of descriptive variables (e.g., symptoms) into a small number of dimensions (Blashfield, 1998). Put differently, a *dimension* means "a set of correlated descriptive variables" (Blashfield, p. 70). Rating scales, which are frequently used in psychological assessment of children and adolescents, exemplify the dimensional approach. For example, parent ratings of child behavior from the Behavior Assessment System for Children, 2nd edition (BASC-2; Reynolds & Kamphaus, 2004) consist of 15 scales (or dimensions), which are grouped into three composites of internalizing problems (e.g., depression), externalizing problems (e.g., aggression), and adaptive skills (e.g., social skills).

The dimensional classification approach can solve some of the problems inherent within the DSM system. By allowing simultaneous elevations on several dimensions, this approach addresses the comorbidity or co-occurrence issue in that "diagnoses" are not mutually exclusive. In addition, dimensions may have better predictive power than categories. In a study of adolescents' disruptive behaviors, Fergusson and Horwood (1995) found that dimensions were more predictive of substance abuse, juvenile offending, and school dropout than DSM diagnoses. This is not surprising, however, because categories inevitably cause a loss of information or variability, which, in turn, results in a corresponding loss of predictive power (Kim, Kamphaus, & Baker, 2006).

Despite the possibility of adopting a dimensional approach in future revisions of the DSM for some disorders, especially personality disorders (Widiger & Trull, 2007), the DSM will probably remain categorical, as categories are more effective than dimensions for communication and day-to-day decisions about treatments (Blashfield, 1998; Kendell, 2002). Also, there is an inherent problem associated with dimensions: being variable-oriented, they do not recognize the dynamic nature of human behavior. In addressing those limitations, some have proposed a person-oriented approach that creates categories of persons based on the specific patterns of dimensionally scaled variables (Bergman & Magnusson, 1997). Although the dimensional approach has problems, it is still a useful research tool and can be complementary to the DSM system in clinical practice as well.

Person-Oriented Approach

According to Blashfield (1998), a person-oriented approach that forms groups of persons is simply a specialized type of a categorical classification system. Though the DSM classification is often called a "categorical" approach, this is inaccurate because the categorical approach refers to categories of persons, not disorders (Blashfield). One way to apply this approach to classifying child and adolescent psychopathology is through cluster analysis and related techniques, which create population subgroups based on a configuration of dimensional variables (Bergman, 2000). Cluster or latent class analysis of dimensional scales is a promising classification approach that may best address the issues of comorbidity and sub-threshold symptoms (Cantwell, 1996).

Several attempts have been made to create typologies of childhood psychopathology using clustering procedures (Curry & Thompson, 1985; Edelbrock & Achenbach, 1980; Lessing, Williams, & Gil, 1982). Among these studies, some produced a comprehensive classification of child behavior using representative national samples. For example, McDermott and Weiss (1995), using the national standardization sample of the Adjustment Scales for Children and Adolescents (ASCA; McDermott, Marston, & Stott, 1993), identified 22 clusters that ranged from the absence of behavior problems to clinically diagnosable problems. In McDermott and Weiss' study, 77% of the sample were classified as well or marginally adjusted, and approximately 21% were at risk or maladjusted. In another study, Kamphaus, Huberty, DiStefano and Petoskey (1997) obtained seven clusters based on teacher ratings of the Behavioral Assessment System for Children (BASC; Reynolds & Kamphaus, 1992): 53% of the national sample were classified as adjusted with no subclinical or clinical problems (i.e., Well-Adapted, Average), 43% in the subclinical range (i.e., Mildly Disruptive, Disruptive Behavior Disorder, Learning Disorder, Physical Complaints, and Worry), and 4% at the clinical level (i.e., Severe Problems). This seven-cluster work has been supported by evidence of internal validity (Huberty, DiStefano, & Kamphaus, 1997) and external validity (DiStefano, Kamphaus, Horne, & Winsor, 2003). It has been also replicated across cultural groups (Kamphaus & DiStefano, 2001) and with at-risk samples of children and adolescents (Distefano et al.; Kim et al., 2006; Kim, Orpinas, Martin, Horne, Sullivan, et al., 2010).

The utility of a cluster analytic classification of child psychopathology should be evaluated with regard to its predictive value. To date, only a few studies have examined and compared the predictive validity of cluster analytic and dimensional classifications of child behavior in schools. Haapasalo, Tremblay, Boulerice, and Vitaro (2000) conducted a cluster analysis of five teacher-rated scales and identified eight clusters. It was found that clusters and dimensions were equally predictive of later outcomes, including delinquency, social withdrawal, and school placement. Furthermore, Kim et al. (2006) created seven clusters based on teacher ratings of 14 dimensions in first grade. They reported that, while both clusters and dimensions significantly predicted a variety of school outcomes in second grade (academic achievement, absenteeism, discipline reports, and pre-referral intervention), the former were more powerful than the latter. These findings provide support for the viability of a cluster analytic classification of child behavior in school settings. Yet continuing research is warranted to accumulate evidence that verifies the predictive validity of clusters, especially in clinical settings.

Future research also needs to examine the stability of clusters over time, using longitudinal data. Given developmental predictability and malleability, it is reasonable to predict both stability and change in cluster membership. Developmental processes are complex as a result of dynamic interactions between persons and environments, and we should always be mindful of unexpected changes. Yet, it is predicted that most individuals, if there is change, would likely move to a cluster similar or adjacent to their previous cluster membership in terms of the phenomenology of their adjustment. Using the clusters identified in the national study of Kamphaus et al. (1997) as examples, children who were initially classified as adjusted would most likely remain members of a relatively healthy cluster, rather than become behaviorally problematic: moving from Well-Adapted to Average, or vice versa. Along with stability and change, it will also be important to understand child and environmental factors that could influence changes in cluster membership over time. This kind of knowledge can be used in planning interventions designed for enhancing adjustment and/or preventing behavioral problems (Kim et al., 2010).

With regard to treatments, clusters may have important utility as a means of designing and evaluating interventions. Although the concept of clusters has been present in the literature for some time, the development of interventions for specific clusters and the evaluation of program effectiveness by cluster have been virtually nonexistent. Traditionally, program developers and researchers select children who are in need of social, academic or behavioral interventions based on a single characteristic. The majority of current intervention efforts evaluate whether the intervention reduces symptoms in relation to a control group. However, clustering may provide a more specific tool by evaluating whether effects differ by child cluster membership (Kim et al., 2010).

Although the person-oriented classification approach appears promising, its direct application to diagnostic practice seems to be limited at the present time, requiring further research. One of the problems that a cluster analytic method has is that clustering is more likely to identify disorders relatively common in children and adolescents, leaving rare disorders unclassifiable by such a framework (Cantwell, 1996).

Recent Trends and Future Directions
HYBRID MODELS
A rapprochement between DSM, dimensional, and person-oriented methods has been emerging

in the form of "composite" or "hybrid" models of classification, as espoused by Skinner (1981, 1986). According to Skinner, for example, a composite classification system that adopts the strengths from each source system offers considerable potential for the integration of seemingly disparate theories of abnormal behavior; those that emphasize quantitative versus qualitative differences between individuals classified. Composite classification systems, such as the class-quantitative structure, may provide a framework for integrating the distinctive merits of each approach. In Skinner's words, "Perhaps a real breakthrough in our understanding of psychiatric disorders awaits the skillful use of composite models" (p. 72).

COGNITIVE NEUROSCIENCE AND GENETICS

The classification approaches discussed previously, though imperfect, have made substantial progress in defining and measuring symptoms. However, this symptom-oriented approach offers limited knowledge of mental disorders by itself. Thus it is essential to integrate classification with advances in cognitive neuroscience and genetics that have enhanced our understanding of the structures and functions of the human brain associated with disorders. As noted previously, the etiology of most child and adolescent disorders is unknown, and it is hoped that those new areas of research will shed light on etiology in the next decades (Merikangas, 2002).

Neurobiological studies employing functional neuroimaging techniques have shown that specific symptoms are mediated by specific brain regions or circuits (Epstein, Isenberg, Stern, & Silbersweig, 2002). In addition, there is substantial evidence that suggests significance of genetic factors in mental disorders. For example, family studies have demonstrated that family history is the most powerful risk factor for developing most mental disorders (Merikangas & Swendsen, 1997). Although those recent studies offer promising explanations regarding mental disorders, the expression of genes is a complex process, and it is necessary to consider gene–environment interactions (Merikangas, 2002).

Based on the concept of gene–environment interactions, child and adolescent psychopathology should be understood as a result of an intertwined relationship between genes and environments, rather than nature versus nurture (Hudziak, 2008). Longitudinal twin studies conducted in the Netherlands revealed the interplay between genetic factors and the environment, which can vary as a function of problems. Specifically, for internalizing problems, a decrease in the genetic influence and an increase in the influence of the shared family environment were found from ages three to 12 years. In contrast, the influence of genetic factors increased across childhood for externalizing problems. Lastly, the genetic influence for attention problems remained rather high over time (Boomsma, van Beijsterveldt, Bartels, & Hudziak, 2008).

STRENGTH-BASED APPROACHES

A traditional approach to the classification of child and adolescent disorders overemphasizes psychopathology, neglecting the significant role that resilience plays in understanding and treating disorders. Although it is now common practice to evaluate both maladaptive and adaptive behavior of children and adolescents, especially through behavior rating scales (e.g., the ASEBA), the DSM and other official classification systems have not incorporated the assessment of the strengths of an individual child, save for the International Classification of Functioning of the ICD.

Recently, the concept of "mental health" has been broadened to include psychological well-being as well as psychopathology. In other words, mental health is defined as, not only the absence of psychopathology, but also the presence of psychological well-being. This dual-factor model of mental health has been supported by empirical evidence. In a study of middle-school students, Suldo and Shaffer (2008) identified two clinical groups of adolescents who presented high levels of clinical symptoms and yet differed in their level of subjective well-being: The *Troubled* group showed low levels of happiness, whereas the *Symptomatic but Content* group showed high levels of happiness. They also differed from each other in that the symptomatic but content adolescents perceived themselves as having more positive relationships with peers and more social support from adults than did their troubled counterparts. These findings suggest that the two clinical groups, despite the similar level of pathological symptoms, might require different approaches to treatment (Suldo & Shaffer).

As illustrated above, when both the psychopathology and strengths of an individual child are considered together, they provide more comprehensive assessment of the child's problems, which can purportedly lead to more effective treatment planning. Although the DSM multi-axial diagnostic system allows for assessing psychosocial and environmental aspects of an individual child, especially through Axis IV, it focuses only on symptoms. It may be that Axis IV will be expanded to identify not only problems but also strengths in psychosocial and environmental aspects of an individual child (Doucette, 2002). Additionally, strength-based approaches appear useful for prevention and enhancement of mental health in children and adolescents (Kim & Esquivel, 2011).

CULTURE AND DIAGNOSIS

For the most part, the DSM system assumes the universality of mental disorders. In contrast, the relativistic view posits that the culture of an individual defines normality and abnormality of behavior and shapes the expression of symptoms (Mezzich, Kleinman, Fabrega, & Parron, 1996). Unfortunately, there is a lack of empirical evidence to address whether and how culture influences the manifestation and presentation of symptoms for particular child and adolescent disorders (Cuéllar & Paniagua, 2000). However, data so far suggest that neurologically based disorders (e.g., autism, schizophrenia) are more likely to be universal, whereas other disorders (e.g., conduct disorder, oppositional defiant disorder) are more likely to vary across cultures (Canino & Alegría, 2008). Hence, these findings seem to support the combined relativistic and universalistic view (Rutter & Nikapota, 2002).

Compared to the DSM-III-R, the DSM-IV made progress in acknowledging the significance of culture in the diagnosis of mental disorders. Specifically, the DSM-IV provides an outline for cultural formulation and culture-bound syndromes in the Appendix. However, cultural considerations are treated as supplemental to the multi-axial DSM diagnostic system, rather than systematically incorporated (Alarcon, 1995). Despite the lack of formal recognition of culture's role, it is crucial to understand how the dominant cultural norms, a child's culture, and a clinician's culture interact with one another, affecting the diagnostic process. In adult psychopathology, research has demonstrated diagnostic bias associated with ethnicity of patients. For example, despite the similar presentation of symptoms, African Americans and Hispanics are more likely to be diagnosed with schizophrenia, whereas Caucasians are diagnosed with psychotic mood disorder (Garb, 1997). Similarly, the assessment of ethnic and linguistic minority children and adolescents requires cultural sensitivity to avoid misdiagnosis, over-diagnosis, or under-diagnosis. For example, in a prevalence study conducted with a community sample of Puerto Rican children, about half of the sample were found to have significant psychiatric problems when the DSM-III criteria were used without cultural considerations (Bird et al., 1988). In the assessment of child and adolescent psychopathology, adults such as parents and teachers take an active role in seeking mental health services and reporting problems. Therefore, it is important to understand the cultural meaning and interpretation of symptoms, not only from the child's perspective, but also from the adult's perspective, taking into account the influences of larger social contexts (e.g., school, community; Parron, 1997).

The issue of culture and diagnosis is becoming more important with the increasing diversity of North American and other populations with high immigration rates. At present, there is insufficient evidence that examines the cross-cultural validity of mental disorders, especially for children and adolescents. In advancing our knowledge and understanding of cultural influences on diagnosis, future research needs to address the following questions: Does a particular disorder indeed exist across cultures? Are the diagnostic criteria biased against a certain cultural group? To what extent are gene–environment interactions related to a specific disorder? Do differences in cultural backgrounds and social status between the child and the clinician cause bias? Are assessment tools culturally fair and sensitive? (Canino & Alegría, 2008; Nathan & Langenbucher, 2006).

Conclusion

This section discussed issues, advances, and future directions related to the classification and diagnosis of child and adolescent psychopathology. Although the field has not reached consensus on how to best classify disorders in children and adolescents, practitioners seem to support the idea that the DSM system should continue to be further refined as it serves several purposes, including facilitating ease of communication and providing a common nomenclature. Specifically, future revisions of the current classification system will need to address several problems such as comorbidity, validity of disorders, and links to treatment. We envision that the study of classification systems is an endeavor in "bootstrapping." This process is iterative in that a new approach is compared to a known imperfect method (the DSM) until the accumulation of evidence for a new approach becomes so compelling that it becomes the new "gold standard." Similarly, a single breakthrough investigation that resolves many issues about the utility of screening, the next topic, is not likely to occur (Schmidt et al., 2004).

Screening

While psychologists have long viewed classification and diagnosis to be essential components of service delivery, screening has not received the same widespread attention and adoption (VanDeventer & Kamphaus, in press). However, due to the renewed attention being given to proactive early identification and intervention for academic, behavioral, and emotional problems, screening, as a component of a multi-tier model of service delivery, has risen to the forefront of considerations for many psychologists and educators. Screening within the educational realm has burgeoned following the 2004 reauthorization of the Individuals with Disabilities Education Act, which emphasized a response-to-intervention (RtI) approach (Ikeda, Neesen, & Witt, 2008). Similarly, screening for mental health problems has received increased attention following reports that the current state of child and adolescent mental health services is a "public health crisis" in part due to the high percentage of children who are both unidentified and untreated for mental, emotional, and behavioral disorders (Campaign for Mental Health Reform, 2005). Both the RtI approach and the public health model consider screening to be an integral step in the process of reducing or eliminating academic and psychological problems. As psychologists and other professionals are examining ways to improve upon the current educational and health care system, screening is now more commonly being advocated as an essential component to identify those in need of services and to provide them with targeted prevention and early intervention services (Glover & Albers, 2007).

The increasing attention paid to the need for universal screening, prevention, and early intervention services across a variety of governmental, research, and educational agencies obviates the need for guidance regarding optimal screening procedures. Thus far, the complexities of diagnosis have been explained, in which the process of giving a diagnosis has been introduced in several ways; including as a continuum of quantitative dimensions of a disorder, or as an interplay of genes, environment, and culture. Since the act of diagnosing is complex, screening, which can act as a preceding or preventative step to diagnosing, is consequently also complex. Although, screening approaches may be complex, and are certainly still being developed and debated, there are several foundational elements to be aware of. Therefore, the following section has two goals: First, it is aimed at providing practitioners with a solid foundation on the central tenets of screening

so that they can better understand and utilize screening as a critical component in a multi-tiered service delivery model; second, it is intended to synthesize research findings and suggest areas of future research that are needed to move the field of screening forward. The primary focus will be on school-based screening, because children and adolescents spend the majority of their time in schools, and schools are often where problems are both identified and addressed (Skalski & Smith, 2006). However, the tenets and issues presented are applicable to screening in a wide range of settings, including primary care clinics and mental health clinics. Toward those ends, definitions of screening will be offered, followed by a discussion of current practices and practical issues to be considered when implementing or evaluating a screening program. Additional research that is needed to further refine the screening process is discussed as well.

Definitions and Background
SCREENING FOR RISK VS. SCREENING FOR DIAGNOSIS

"Screening" is generally defined as testing or examining for the presence of a problem. The "problem" can be defined as a specific diagnostic disorder, such as depression or post-traumatic stress disorder, or it could be defined as the risk for developing a disorder. For example, a screening can test for cardiovascular disease (i.e., the presence or absence of a heart condition); alternatively, the screening could test for the presence of risk for developing a heart condition. The distinction between screening for risk versus screening for a diagnosis is an important consideration to be made prior to embarking on a screening process.

Screening for risk is a preventative technique that has the intention of establishing early interventions. To screen for the risk of cardiovascular disease, a screener would ask questions about the person's current body condition and involvement in any activities that are linked to the later development of cardiovascular disease, such as age, body weight, exercise, and diet (Natarajan & Nietert, 2003). Alternatively, a doctor might take a patient's blood pressure at every appointment. These methods are not informative enough to establish a diagnosis; rather, they are assessing for "red flags" that may lead to later diagnosis. If a patient is found at risk for cardiovascular disease, the doctor will recommend some changes in behavior and lifestyle, which can serve as an early interventions to prevent a later, more serious problem. Screening for risk usually corresponds with brief and efficient screening methods, which can range from a five-minute pencil and paper rating scale, an informal question from a doctor, or a quick procedure like a reflex test or taking one's temperature. It is not intended to be diagnostic. Identifying and preventing problems before they have already fully developed is a more cost-effective and efficient method of service delivery than focusing solely on diagnosis and treatment (Levitt, Saka, Romanelli, & Hoagwood, 2007).

While screening for risk has numerous benefits, it is not an intention that is agreed upon in the screening literature. Many screeners are designed to assess for diagnosis rather than risk. As discussed earlier in this chapter, *diagnosis* refers to identifying a person as meeting sufficient criteria to be given a specific medical or clinical label, such as attention deficit/hyperactivity disorder or a specific learning disability. In contrast, *risk* is described as the likelihood or vulnerability one has to develop such a diagnosis. Two-hour clinical diagnostic interviews at a mental health clinic, an expensive scan or blood test, or a rating scale with multiple questions ascertaining functioning on each symptom criteria of the DSM-IV are aimed at diagnosis. They are comprehensive procedures that provide enough information to give or inform a diagnosis. This poses the question, when developing a screening process, should the process be designed with the intention of finding and treating incidents of diagnoses? Or should the process be designed to assess for risk, to help inform the clinician what early interventions could prevent the diagnoses from later occurring?

The confusion and controversy over the intention of screening is just one of the many ambiguities and debates related to the purpose and process of screening. Similar to the discussion of different approaches to diagnosis, there is a variety of competing definitions for "screening," and this word is used with reference to various intentions, processes, and contexts. The term "screening" conveys a variety of different meanings (Mills et al., 2006) making consensus difficult and, as a result, some have suggested alternative definitions. Crowell (2005), for example, suggested that, in lieu of the term "screening," the terms "early identification" and "early intervention" should be used. However, this appears to be based on the assumption that one is screening for risk, as opposed to diagnosis, since early identification and intervention are more aligned with the goal of reducing risk. In recognition that the term "screening" is still likely to be widely utilized, it is important for practitioners to recognize that, although the use of the term varies, the core purpose for screening should be carefully considered and *a priori* decisions about the purpose of screening should be made.

UNIVERSAL, SELECTIVE, OR INDICATED SCREENING

In addition to the lack of correspondence regarding the definitions and purpose of screening, an area that brings forth further confusion is which population will be involved in the screening process. Namely, a decision to conduct screening at the universal, selective, or indicated level must be determined. Based on the public health model of service delivery, a multi-tiered approach provides varying levels of services and support based on the level of documented need. Briefly, *universal* services are provided to all youth; *selected* services are provided to youth who are deemed at-risk; and *indicated* interventions are targeted for youth demonstrating the greatest level of need or impairment (Durlak, 1997). Under a public health approach, a systematic screening would be conducted at a universal level so that all youth have the opportunity to be identified and thus receive follow-up services as needed. However, screenings are often conducted on a population that is decidedly less than universal.

The definitions of universal screening are operationalized in various ways in the literature, making this topic even more blurred and unclear. Universal screening attempts to administer the screener to every person in the relevant population: "the relevant population" meaning every person who has a possible risk of having the problem. For example, men would not be included in the relevant population for screening for breast cancer. However, for mental health screening, the entire population could be considered relevant since there are no groups that are excluded from possible risk of poor mental health; similarly, academic screenings would include all students.

As opposed to a universal screening, a selected screening method would not attempt to screen all individuals in the relevant population but would instead focus on a population that is already deemed to be at risk. For instance, in intimate-partner violence screening, selective screening methods are often used, in which only females who appear injured and/or are perceived at being at high risk for intimate-partner violence are asked about intimate-partner violence (Phelan, 2007). Males or other females are still in the "relevant population," since anyone who has a partner could potentially be a victim of intimate-partner violence, but this is clearly not a universal approach to screening. The same could be true in mental health clinics, where individuals are not screened for depression until they seek out services, whether it be for depression or for a related problem. Or with knowledge of the link between mental health and educational outcomes, a student may only be screened for emotional or behavioral risk following a referral for reading problems (United States Public Health Service, 2000).

Indicated screening would be conducted with individuals who have already been diagnosed or identified as having a mental health problem, and would probably be a part of a comprehensive clinical assessment (Levitt et al., 2007). The goal would not be early identification of and early intervention with a problem, but rather to identify the particular needs of an individual for treatment planning or the presence of a co-occurring condition, or to prevent the occurrence of more deleterious outcomes associated with the disorder. This level of service is reserved for only the individuals at the highest level of risk and has been suggested to be viewed as a form of treatment (Durlak, 1997).

There is debate in the literature as to which approach—universal, selective or indicated screening—is superior (Levitt et al., 2007). The ultimate decision about which approach to utilize is also likely to depend on the resources available.

Current Practices and Considerations for Implementation

Following a decision regarding the purpose of screening (risk level or diagnosis) and a decision of who will be screened (universal, selected, or indicated), there are numerous additional decisions to be made and many practical issues to consider. Considerations such as the timing, setting, and administration of implementation, as well as the plan for follow-up with individuals who are screened as being at risk, should be well thought out prior to embarking on a screening program. Overall, psychologists making decisions about screening and the implementation of a screening system should recognize that screening should be a part of a comprehensive service delivery plan and work to develop a team that can be involved throughout the process (Dowdy, Furlong, Eklund, Saeki, & Ritchey, 2010). Without the vision of how screening can ultimately lead to targeted prevention or early intervention services, the result could simply be a list of individuals in need of follow-up. However, if screening is well integrated within a service delivery system, with thoughtful decisions determined prior to implementation, screening can allow for the early treatment of problems prior to the problems' becoming exacerbated and potentially being more difficult to treat. This section provides readers with information about the current state of screening practices and guides readers through a set of issues to consider when designing or implementing a screening program.

A MULTIPLE-GATING APPROACH

Currently, screening is often implemented through a *multiple-gating approach*. This approach is consistent with the multi-tiered approach to service delivery advocated by prevention scientists (Weisz, Sandler, Durlak, & Anton, 2005) in that it narrows down the population and only provides more intensive assessment to those identified as being in need of it. In a multiple-gating approach, the first "gate" generally entails all children's being screened, which provides for a universal screening (universal assessment). Then the children who are identified as "at risk" by the first gate screener pass into a second gate, in which an additional assessment is provided (*selected assessment*). The selected assessment strategy often utilizes a more comprehensive, thorough tool such as a full omnibus behavior rating scale, or an additional screener utilizing a different rater or informant. Finally, the children who continue to be identified as having significant risk through the selected assessment strategy are then evaluated with a more comprehensive, individualized assessment as a third gate assessment (*indicated assessment*). This indicated, comprehensive assessment would be more aligned with a full diagnostic assessment and could result in a diagnosis or determine eligibility for services being offered. This multiple-gating approach allows for progressively more precise, specific, and intensive assessments to be provided to students with increased levels of risk. This type of procedure has been shown to increase identification and diagnostic accuracy as well as reduce costs due to inefficient identification (Hill, Lochman, Coie, Greenberg, & The Conduct Problems Prevention Research Group, 2004; Walker & Severson, 1992; Lochman & The Conduct Problems Prevention Research Group, 1995).

One example of a multiple-gating screening procedure is the Systematic Screening for Behavior Disorders (SSBD; Walker & Severson, 1992). The SSBD utilizes a three-stage process including teacher training and rankings (i.e., nomination), teacher ratings of child behavior, and classroom observations. The first stage consists of teachers' rank-ordering all the students in their classroom on both externalizing and internalizing behavior dimensions. While all students are supposed to be considered, only the top ten students in each dimension (externalizing and internalizing) are nominated and ranked in terms of the severity of their symptoms. Out of the ten students nominated, the top three students in each category proceed through the first gate into the second gate assessment. The second gate assessment requires teachers to complete two rating scales: the Critical Events Index, to discern if the student has engaged in various significantly disruptive activities, such as being physically cruel to animals; and the Combined Frequency Index, to gather information about adaptive and maladaptive behaviors. Students who exceed normative cut points on these two instruments proceed to stage three. The third gate assessment involves systematically observing the students in naturalistic school environments, including assessing for academic engaged time in the classroom and positive social interactions while on the playground. The results from this stage three assessment are used to determine the next level of assessment or intervention that is appropriate, such as a referral for special education testing.

An additional example of a multi-stage screening process involves the use of a multi-disorder screening instrument as a first gate assessment: the Behavioral and Emotional Screening System (BESS; Kamphaus & Reynolds, 2007). The BESS was developed under the awareness that, for a screener to be truly time-efficient and effective, it should assess multiple areas of problems and strengths, including internalizing problems, externalizing problems, school problems, and adaptive skills. The BESS consists of brief screening measures, designed to be completed in five minutes or less with no training required, that can be completed by teachers, parents, and students to identify behavioral and emotional strengths and weaknesses in youth ranging from preschool through high school (Kamphaus & Reynolds). Following the administration of the BESS, children and youth who are identified as "at risk" then proceed to the second gate in which the Behavior Assessment System for Children–Second Edition (BASC-2; Reynolds & Kamphaus, 2004) is given. The BASC-2 is a comprehensive, omnibus rating scale that provides additional information regarding the specific areas that might be problematic for the individual who was screened to be at risk by the BESS. For example, through this second gate assessment, it might become apparent that the student is experiencing significant problems with anxiety as opposed to hyperactivity. A third gate assessment could entail a more comprehensive, individualized assessment incorporating multiple sources of information to aid in diagnosis and treatment planning.

The number of stages a screening process requires and the amount of personnel time required at each stage highlight the practical limitations of multiple-gating approaches. Practitioners should consider the time and resources that are available prior to implementing a screening system. It is still unknown whether multiple screening gates are, in fact, superior to single stage screenings, and the optimal number of gates to be utilized is still undecided. Multiple factors, only one of which is diagnostic accuracy, should be considered, including the feasibility and cost-effectiveness of multiple gating procedures. In fact, Lane et al. (2009) found the seven-item Student Risk Rating Scale (SRSS; Drummond, 1994) to perform comparably to the three-stage SSBD for the identification of externalizing problems. Therefore, brevity may not denote inferiority. However, a study investigating a two-stage screening process using the BESS and the BASC-2 demonstrated that adding a comprehensive behavior rating scale as the second gate significantly improved their identification accuracy over a single-gate procedure (VanDeventer & Kamphaus, in press). Furthermore, these questions require further research because many screening studies have estimated the effect of using multiple gates rather than implementing a real-world multiple gate screening procedure (VanDeventer & Kamphaus, in press).

INSTRUMENTATION

The screening instrument to be utilized is a decision that will have an impact on subsequent decisions. When evaluating a screening instrument for potential adoption and use, the instrument should be evaluated for its technical adequacy, including investigation into an instrument's norm adequacy, reliability, and validity. Screening instruments will not be absolutely accurate (i.e., correctly classify every student), and although some error is unavoidable, it is generally recommended that decisions be made in a way that is the least likely to be harmful (Ikeda et al., 2008).

There are four possible outcomes that can result from using a predictor (e.g., screener) to classify individuals according to a criterion (e.g., at risk or not at risk; diagnosed or not diagnosed): true positives, false positives, true negatives, and false negatives. The goal of a screener is to maximize the number of true positives and negatives and minimize the number of false positives and negatives. However, it is important to realize that when the number of false negatives is reduced, it conversely increases the number of false positives, necessitating a prioritization of which result is more tolerable. In screening, a higher number of false positives is often tolerated in favor of more false negatives. This is because a child classified as a false negative would be "missed" and therefore not have the opportunity to receive further assessment or services. However, under a multi-gating screening approach, children identified as false positives would simply undergo additional assessment to determine which children are identified but do not, in fact, have a disorder or risk of the disorder.

Screening instruments often report their technical adequacy in terms of their sensitivity and specificity. *Sensitivity* refers to the proportion of individuals with the disorder who are correctly identified by the instrument as having the disorder; in other words, true positives. *Specificity* refers to the proportion of individuals without the disorder who are correctly identified as not having the disorder, or true negatives. Additionally, the positive predictive value (PPV) of a screener is often reported, and this is calculated as the proportion of students correctly identified as at risk (true positives) out of all students identified as at risk on the screener. When the PPV is low, a large number of false positives is present, which is tolerated and expected in most screening scenarios (Levitt et al., 2007), given that, when the PPV is optimized, false positives are minimized at the risk of missing true cases. The negative predictive value (NPV) of the instrument is the proportion of students correctly identified as not at risk (true negatives) out of all of the students identified as not at risk on the screener. When the NPV is low, a large number of false negatives results.

It is also recommended to interpret the PPV and NPV in light of information on the base rate of the outcome of interest, as the base rate will significantly affect the PPV and NPV of a screener (Meehl & Rosen, 1955). As Hill and colleagues (2004) explained, "Sensitivity and specificity of tests may sound impressive when reported without reference to PPV, NPV, and base rates. For example, a test with sensitivity of .80 and specificity of .95 has a PPV of about 74% if the base rate is 15%, but the PPV is reduced to 46% if the base rate is 5%" (p. 810). When considering emotional and behavioral problems, for example, prior research suggests that an annual base rate would be around 20% (Campaign for Mental Health Reform, 2005; Friedman,

Katz-Leavy, Manderscheid, & Sondheimer, 1996; Hill et al., 2004), and this base rate will be lower when considering a single disorder.

In addition to technical adequacy, further considerations for evaluating screening instruments have been outlined by Glover and Albers (2007) and include ensuring that the screening instrument is appropriate for the intended use and is practical for use. In regard to practicality, Glover and Albers recommend that the screening instrument be evaluated in terms of the following: (1) cost, (2) feasibility of administration, (3) acceptability to multiple stakeholders, (4) infrastructure for collecting and interpreting screening data, (5) appropriateness of use for entire targeted population, and (6) utility of the information obtained to provide improved treatment decisions.

SETTINGS

Practitioners will also need to determine where screenings will occur. In this chapter, school-based screening is the primary focus. Schools have been advocated as an ideal setting for the delivery of academic, behavioral, and emotional screening services, not only because children and adolescents spend the majority of their time in schools, but also because schools are often where problems are both identified and addressed (Skalski & Smith, 2006). Although academic screenings seem to be more aligned with the primary mission of schools to educate all children, schools should also be considered as an ideal setting for large-scale, broad-based mental health screening of children and adolescents (Wu et al., 1999) due to the relationship between mental health problems and academic achievement. Recent studies indicate that mental health problems can be significant barriers to learning, and, conversely, positive behavioral and emotional health is associated with academic success (Atkins, Frazier, Adil, & Talbott, 2003; Bradley, Doolittle, & Bartolotta, 2008; Catalano, Haggerty, Oesterle, Fleming, & Hawkins, 2004; United States Public Health Service, 2000; Wagner, Kutash, Duchnowski, & Epstein, 2005).

Additionally, the fact that school-based mental health services are the most commonly accessed services for youth with mental health problems (Burns et al., 1995; Farmer, Burns, Phillips, Angold, & Costello, 2003) suggests that schools might be more ecologically valid, as early intervention should follow early identification. Considering that many children are not seen in primary healthcare settings, in particular children from impoverished backgrounds who are at high risk for poor behavioral outcomes, schools often become the de facto mental health care system (Kelleher, Moore, Childs, Angelilli, & Comer, 1999). In fact, 20% of all students receive some type of school-supported mental health or social services (Kutash, Duchnowski, & Lynn, 2006). Unfortunately, however, very few schools currently engage in a systematic screening process for emotional or behavioral problems (Romer & McIntosh, 2005). This trend might change with the availability of practical screening instruments and large-scale studies that are currently underway investigating screening within schools (Kamphaus, DiStefano, & Dowdy, 2009).

While schools do appear to be practical and effective settings for screening, the suggestion to conduct screening in schools is not implying that behavior and information drawn from other settings and resources is not valuable. For instance, it is also important to consider home and cultural influences, just as these influences are important aspects of diagnosis. However, conducting screening in schools is an effective starting point, since students are easily accessible and resources are available in the schools for assessment and evaluation.

INFORMANTS

Even after determining the setting for implementation, practitioners have decisions regarding who within that setting will provide the information to be included in the screening. There are varying opinions and research evidence regarding the number and type of informants who will provide the optimal amount and types of information in a mental health screening system. Although it is often recommended to collect ratings from multiple informants (Frick, Burns, & Kamphaus, 2009), and the "more is always better" stance dominates contemporary thinking (Jensen et al., 1999; Power et al., 1998, Verhulst, Dekker, & van der Ende, 1997), research findings are conflicting. There are several studies that suggest that gathering information from an additional informant adds little variance to the identification process above and beyond what was provided by the first informant (Biederman, Keenan, & Faraone, 1990; Jones, Dodge, Foster, Nix, & Conduct Problems Prevention Research Group, 2002; Lochman and the Conduct Problems Prevention Research Group, 1995). Jones and colleagues found that the effect of combining parent and teacher ratings was equal to or minimally better than that of the teacher-only rating. Mattison, Carlson, Cantwell, and Asarnow (2007) found that teachers rate externalizing and internalizing problems as well as or better than parents. In direct contrast, Goodman, Ford, Corbin, and Meltzer (2004) found that prediction was best when both caregiver and teacher ratings were combined. As explained above, environment and setting can play an important role in both diagnosis and classification. Similarly, it is also important to consider the relationship between settings and sources when selecting the number and type of informants.

There is often a lack of consistency among raters (Achenbach, McConaughy, & Howell, 1987), suggesting that perhaps different raters provide different, yet still valuable, information. In addition to parents' and teachers' being valuable sources of information, there is some evidence that supports the use of child and adolescent self-report measures of externalizing and internalizing symptomatology (Grills & Ollendick, 2003). More research is needed, however, since there is some evidence to suggest that adolescents fail to identify their own risk, at least in one sample of incarcerated males (Vreugdenhil, van den Brink, Ferdinand, Wouters, & Doreleijers, 2006). Self-report screeners, however, have been recommended as instruments of choice for middle, junior, and high school–aged students (Levitt et al., 2007). One must also consider the time and expense incurred to include additional informants. There is no current consensus on the number of informants and the type of informants that should be included in the screening process, and additional research is needed to investigate "the value of different informants at various stages of the assessment process" (Johnston & Murray, 2003).

Academic screenings typically involve students completing brief curriculum-based measures (CBMs; Shinn, 1989). CBMs have been used in universal screenings and, if they are aligned with academic benchmarks, they can be ideal for screenings due to their ease of administration, scoring, and interpretation (Ikeda et al., 2008). For example, the Dynamic Indicators of Basic Early Literacy Skills (DIBELS; Good & Kaminski, 2002) is routinely used to screen for early literacy problems and monitor the development of early literacy skills (Brunsman, 2003). Unlike in behavioral and emotional screenings, students are usually the sole informants. However, teachers can, and frequently do, refer students with academic problems for more intensive assessment and additional academic intervention.

TIMING

A practitioner interested in screening should also consider when the screener should be administered. For instance, in the context of screening in schools, a common time-point may be as a student enters a new school, such as before entrance to kindergarten, or as the student transitions to middle school or high school. Stoep and colleagues (2005), for example, targeted students during their transition from elementary to middle school in the Developmental Pathways Screening Program (DPSP), suggesting that this was a critical transitional stage. Preschool screeners are also available, highlighting the need to identify problems early in their developmental trajectories (DiStefano & Kamphaus, 2007; Kamphaus & Reynolds, 2007). Time points involving transitions are also chosen for practical reasons, since often other paperwork or screeners are commonly administered at these times. Additionally, schools can get a sense of the potential problems that the new student body may have at an early stage, so early interventions can be planned accordingly. Research also shows that children may be particularly vulnerable to emotional or behavioral problems when they move to a new school (Csorba et al., 2001; Stoep et al., 2005), which gives sufficient reason to screen for problems at this time.

It is also essential to consider what the screener is designed to look for, to aid the decision of when the screener should be implemented. It is more common to have depression in adolescence when there is an 8% to 12% prevalence rate, versus in childhood when there is a 2% to 3% prevalence rate (California Adolescent Health Collaborative, 2000). Therefore, it might be more sensible to screen for depression in junior high versus elementary school to avoid missing the majority of students who develop depression after elementary school. However, if the screening is designed to assess for the precursors to depression, as opposed to a diagnosis of depression, it might be more sensible to screen earlier so that preventative techniques can be implemented prior to exacerbating symptomatology. Therefore, a variety of factors should be considered when deciding when the screener should be implemented.

ADMINISTRATION

A logistical choice that needs to be made is in what context the screener should be administered. If the screener requires parental involvement, it can either be administered in person to parents, such as at Back-to-School nights or parent-teacher conferences, or it can be sent home, either by mail or with the student to give to the parents. The response rate tends to be lower when forms are sent home (Esbensen, Melde, Taylor, & Peterson, 2008), and parents may be less likely to consent to it or take the initiative to

ask questions they may have if a screener administrator is not available in person. However, parents may feel more comfortable completing a screener at home, and time will not be taken away from the event the parent is attending at school. For a screener completed by students, the screener can be implemented either by pulling students out of class, be administered within the classroom during a regular school day, or take place alongside state testing. There are advantages and limitations to each approach, and determinations will probably depend on administrative decisions and the amount of buy-in by the community in which the screening will occur.

INTERPRETATION AND FOLLOW-UP

Prior to implementing a screening program, considerable thought should be given to the process that will occur following an initial screening. As stated previously, screening is not an activity that should be undertaken by one individual or a small group of individuals; rather, it should be a part of an organized effort, with structures in place so that individuals identified as in need of additional services can be promptly attended to. Within a school screening context, school psychologists could oversee a universal screening administration for a variety of problems, including academic, mental health, and harmful behavior problems. For a screener for reading problems, the school psychologist may decide that the results of the screening suggest programmatic, instructional deficiencies due to a wide range of students' performing below benchmarks. Or the school psychologist may determine that there are only a few students who are primarily at risk for developing reading failure. However, the decision-making process has only begun at this point, with further decisions needed regarding the best course of action and the person to be in charge. Who, for example, is the most appropriate person to design an intervention for each of the students: the school psychologist, the teacher, or a reading specialist? Who decides whether all of the at-risk students should be given the same intervention, or whether individualized interventions will ensue? Surely, the number of at-risk students, the number of staff available, and the amount of resources available for intervention affects the answers to these questions. And how will the answers to these questions differ if the problem is mental health–related or drug-use–related? It is important to consider the context of the problem, the knowledge of the staff available, and the practicality of how much time, money, and staff are available.

LEGAL AND SOCIAL CONSIDERATIONS

In addition to practical implementation considerations, there are some social and legal considerations that deserve mention, including the consent process and the supposed link to medication. First, the process of obtaining parental consent and student assent for screening remains controversial and conflicted, particularly with regard to mental health screening. Informed consent may be either active or passive (Eaton, Lowry, Brener, Grunbaum, & Kann, 2004), and whether to screen is commonly decided by the respective school districts and how they interpret the Protection of Pupil Rights Amendment (PPRA; Chartier et al., 2008). The PPRA "seeks to ensure that schools and contractors obtain written parental consent before minor students are required to participate in any U.S. Department of Education funded survey, analysis, or evaluation that reveals information concerning…" a variety of sensitive behaviors, such as political affiliation and sexual behavior and attitudes. One area included is "mental and psychological problems potentially embarrassing to the student and his/her family" (U.S. Department of Education, 2005). These guidelines can be interpreted in various ways; therefore, it is important to evaluate the differences between active and passive consent for mental health screening. Active consent requires that the written consent form be returned with a signature from the student's parent. Passive consent requires that the parent return the consent form only if they do *not* want their child to participate in the study; if the consent form is not returned, it is assumed that the parent has given consent. There are benefits and drawbacks for each of these methods.

The explicit parent consent received through active consent provides solid assurance of parent approval. However, while this method appears legally sound, the sometimes lengthy and complicated process of distributing and collecting signed consent forms can introduce an element of bias in the sample, which may undermine the effectiveness of a universal screening approach wherein all individuals have equal opportunity for follow-up and resulting interventions. Active consent processes yield varying return rates from 34% to 67% (Eaton et al.; Esbensen et al., 1996). The decreased sample can be disadvantageous, as students who would benefit from the screener and/or services associated with it may miss out due to the active consent process. While it is important that parents be informed of and have control over what their children are subjected to, consent forms are frequently not returned

for a variety of reasons, and the children might be adversely affected. Chartier et al. (2008) found that, after switching the school-based depression screening process from passive consent to active consent, the participant rate decreased from 85% to 66%. The decrease in participation was not equivalent across subgroups of students, and the percentage of students positively screened for depression was significantly reduced. This illustrates how more stringent consent procedures can potentially reduce the effectiveness of the screener, in which at-risk populations can be less likely to be identified and served. Therefore, this brings up the question that, if the goal of screening is to identify students at risk, in an attempt to provide them help; if active consent is hurting this process, is the "less legally sound" approach of passive consent better?

Mental health screening also frequently comes under scrutiny due to the supposedly direct link to medication. The term "mental health" commonly has a negative connotation, and one of the most frequent ideas associated with "mental health problems" is medication. From the widespread knowledge of the growing practice of prescribing psychostimulants for students with ADHD, or antidepressants to teenagers who have depressive symptoms, the general population is quick to associate "mental health" with "medication." It is common for the general population to believe that children are being over-medicated and that the medications have negative long-term effects on development (Pescosolido, Perry, Martin, McLeod, & Jensen, 2007). This controversial issue becomes relevant when people associate mental health screening with a system to aid medicating or over-medicating children.

Some organizations express their concerns about the potential over-medication of children as a result of mental health screening funded by psychiatric drug industries (e.g., MindFreedom International, 2005). Therefore, while the practice of mental health screening carries with it some controversial viewpoints, it is important to stress that the sole focus of mental health screening is *not* to medicate individuals. Instead, as stated before, mental health screening is a process for identifying students at risk of developing emotional and behavioral problems so interventions can be set in place to prevent such problems from developing or getting worse. However, it is prudent for those interested in implementing a screening process to be aware of some of the controversies associated with screening so they can work to inform their constituencies.

Conclusions and Future Directions

Although the field of screening is far from mature, active early screening for emotional, behavioral, and academic problems has intuitive appeal and is generally regarded as a potentially fruitful approach to early identification and prevention (Severson, Walker, Hope-Doolittle, Kratochwill, & Gresham, 2007). The issues highlighted herein provide a critical look at many of the current practice and research considerations regarding screening. However, there are many areas in which additional research is needed regarding both the efficacy and the effectiveness of screening and screening instrumentation (Levitt et al., 2007). Due to the relationship between screening and diagnosis, it is also necessary to consider the potential upcoming changes in approaches to diagnosis to further understand the best approaches to screening. Studies investigating the long-term predictive validity and utility of screening instruments are needed, as previous studies have produced discrepant results regarding the accuracy and validity of screening procedures (Dowdy et al., 2010). Additional studies investigating the cost-effectiveness of screening (Chatterji, Caffray, Crowe, Freeman, & Jensen, 2004) and the practicality of its implementation (Shirk & Jungbluth, 2008) could help bridge the gap between the science of screening and its practical administration. Similar to concerns regarding the "unappreciated paucity of empirical support for RTI and an overly optimistic view of its practical, problematic issues" (Reynolds & Shaywitz, 2009, p. 130), the support for screening is still in its nascent stage. Psychologists interested in screening are encouraged to critically evaluate the emerging screening research and to make determinations regarding implementation based on solid evidence. However, there is enough known now about the value of early identification and intervention that action, as opposed to waiting for further refinement of the screening process, is recommended (Dowdy et al., 2010). In much the same way that the diagnostic systems of DSM and IDEA will continue to benefit from further revision, screening systems will certainly profit and improve due to continued research and refinement.

Chapter Conclusions and Future Directions

This chapter differs considerably from many other previously published chapters on classification and diagnosis for two reasons. First, up until the last two decades, the chorus of DSM detractors was relatively small, and their concerns were primarily conceptual and theoretical. Now there is sound empirical evidence, cited throughout this chapter, to suggest that future versions of the DSM will have to respond with a classification system that addresses well-documented problems. Thus, this chapter includes substantial sections on alternative approaches to diagnosis that have some evidence of empirical support.

Second, the timing of this chapter makes mandatory a thorough discussion of classification associated with prevention practice and science via screening. The long-awaited emphasis on prevention and early intervention in child services and schooling requires new classification technologies specifically related to these practices. Consequently, screening dictates the need to change classification and diagnostic systems further, to include classification of various types of "normality" or "typicality," and classification of risk status.

These two areas of classification science are likely to be the focus of intensive research efforts and conceptual breakthroughs for the foreseeable future. We look forward to the outcomes, for they portend better service to children.

Author Note

Please address correspondence to R. W. Kamphaus, Ph.D., Distinguished Research Professor, Georgia State University, 30 Pryor Street, Atlanta, Georgia, 30302–3980. Electronic mail: rkamphaus@gsu.edu.

Further Reading

Dowdy, E., Furlong, M., Eklund, K., Saeki, E., & Ritchey, K. (2010). Screening for mental health and wellness: Current school based practice and emerging possibilities. In B. Doll (Ed.), *Handbook of youth prevention science* (pp. 70–95). New York: Routledge.

Frick, P. J., Burns, C., & Kamphaus, R. W. (2009). *Clinical assessment of child and adolescent personality and behavior* (2nd ed.). New York: Springer.

Kamphaus, R. W., & Campbell, J. C. (2006). *Psychodiagnostic assessment of children: dimensional and categorical methods.* New York: Wiley.

VanDeventer, M. C., & Kamphaus, R. W. (in press). *Mental health screening at school: Instrumentation, implementation, and critical issues.* New York: Springer.

References

Achenbach, T. (2001). Challenges and benefits of assessment, diagnosis, and taxonomy for clinical practice and research. *Australian & New Zealand Journal of Psychiatry, 35* (3), 263–271.

Achenbach, T. M., McConaughy, S. H., & Howell, C. T. (1987). Child/adolescent behavioral and emotional problems: implications of cross-informant correlations for situational specificity. *Psychological Bulletin, 101*(2), 213–232.

Achenbach, T. M., & McConaughy, S. H. (1992). Internalizing disorders in children and adolescents. In W. M. Reynolds (Ed.), *Wiley series on personality processes* (pp. 19–60). Oxford, England: John Wiley & Sons.

Alarcon, R. D. (1995). Culture and psychiatric diagnosis: Impact on DSM-IV and ICD-10. *Psychiatric Clinics of North America, 18*, 449–465.

American Psychiatric Association (1968). *Diagnostic and statistical manual of mental disorders, second edition* (DSM-II). Washington, DC: American Psychiatric Association.

American Psychiatric Association (1980). *Diagnostic and statistical manual of mental disorders, third edition* (DSM-III). Washington, DC: American Psychiatric Association.

American Psychiatric Association (1987). *Diagnostic and statistical manual of mental disorders, third revised edition* (DSM-III-R). Washington, DC: American Psychiatric Association.

American Psychiatric Association (1994). *Diagnostic and statistical manual of mental disorders, fourth edition* (DSM-IV). Washington, DC: American Psychiatric Association.

American Psychiatric Association (2000). *Diagnostic and statistical manual of mental disorders, fourth text revision* (DSM-IV-TR). Washington, DC: American Psychiatric Association.

Atkins, M. S., Frazier, S. L., Adil, J. A., & Talbott, E. (2003). Handbook of school mental health: Advancing practice and research. In M. D. Weist, S. W. Evans, & N. A. Lever (Eds.), *Issues in clinical child psychology*. New York: Kluwer Academic/Plenum Publishers, 165–178.

Bergman, L. R. (2000). The application of a person-oriented approach: Types and clusters. In L. R. Bergman, R. B. Cairns, L. Nilsson, & L. Nystedt (Eds.), *Developmental science and the holistic approach* (pp. 137–154). Mahwah, NJ: Erlbaum.

Bergman, L. R., & Magnusson, D. (1997). A person-oriented approach in research on developmental psychopathology. *Development & Psychopathology, 9*, 291–319.

Biederman, J., Keenan, K., Faraone, S. V. (1990). Parent-based diagnosis of attention deficit disorder predicts a diagnosis based on teacher report. *Journal of the American Academy of Child & Adolescent Psychiatry, 29*(5), 698–701.

Bird, H. R., Canino, G., Rubio-Stipec, M., Gould, M. S., Ribera, J., Sesman, M., et al. (1988). Estimates of the prevalence of childhood maladjustment in a community survey in Puerto Rico. The use of combined measures. *Archives of General Psychiatry, 45*, 1120–1126.

Blashfield, R. K. (1998). Diagnostic models and systems. In A. A. Bellack, M. Hersen, & C. R. Reynolds (Eds.), *Comprehensive clinical psychology: Vol. 4, Assessment* (pp. 57–80). New York: Elsevier Science.

Boomsma, D. I., van Beijsterveldt, C. E. M., Bartels, M., & Hudziak, J. J. (2008). Genetic and environmental influences on anxious/depression: A longitudinal study in 3- to 12-year-old children. In J. J. Hudziak (Ed.), *Developmental psychopathology and wellness: Genetic and environmental influences* (pp. 161–190). Arlington, VA: American Psychiatric Publishing.

Bradley, R., Doolittle, J. & Bartolotta, R. (2008). Building on the data and adding to the discussion: the experiences and outcomes of students with emotional disturbance. *Journal of Behavioral Education, Special Issue: Emotional & Behavioral Disorders, 17*, 4–23.

Brunsman, B. A. (2003). Review of the DIBELS: Dynamic Indicators of Basic Early Literacy Skills, Sixth Edition. In B. S. Plake, J. C. Impara & R. A. Spies (Eds.), *The fifteenth mental measurements yearbook* (pp. 307–310). Lincoln, NE: Buros Institute of Mental Measurements.

Burns, B. J., Costello, E. J., Angold, A., Tweed, D., Stangl, D., Farmer, E. M. Z., et al. (1995). Children's mental health service use across service sectors. *Health Affairs, 14*, 149–159.

California Adolescent Health Collaborative. (2000). *Investing in adolescent health: a social imperative for California's future.* San Francisco, CA: Clayton, Brindis, Hamor, Raiden-Wright, & Fong.

Campaign for Mental Health Reform. (2005). A public health crisis: Children and adolescents with mental disorders. [Congressional briefing].

Canino, G., & Alegría, M. (2008). Psychiatric diagnosis—is it universal or relative to culture? *Journal of Child Psychology & Psychiatry, 49*, 237–250.

Cantwell, D. P. (1996). Classification of child and adolescent psychopathology. *Journal of Child Psychology & Psychiatry, 37*, 3–12.

Catalano, R. F., Haggerty, K. P., Oesterle, S., Fleming, C. B., & Hawkins, J. D. (2004). The importance of bonding to school for healthy development: Findings from the Social Development Research Group. *Journal of School Health, 74*, 252–261.

Chartier, M., Stoep, A. V., McCauley, E., Herting, J. R., Tracy, M. & Lymp, J. (2008). Passive versus active parental permission: implications for the ability of school-based depression screening to reach youth at risk. *Journal of School Health, 78* (3), 157–164.

Chatterji, P., Caffray, C. M., Crowe, M., Freeman, L., & Jensen, P. (2004). Cost assessment of a school-based mental health screening and treatment program in New York City. *Mental Health Services Research, 6*(3), 155–166.

Crowell, R. (2005). *Promoting and preserving early intervention services for children.* Paper presented at the National Mental Health Association Fall Policy Conference, Washington, D.C.

Csorba, J., Rozsa, S., Vetro, A., Gadoros, J., Makra, J., Somogyi, E., et al. (2001). Family and school related stresses in depressed Hungarian children. *European Psychiatry, 16*(1), 18–26.

Cuéllar, I., & Paniagua, F. A. (Eds.). (2000). *Handbook of multicultural mental health: Assessment and treatment of diverse populations.* San Diego: Academic Press.

Curry, J. F., & Thompson, R. J. (1985). Patterns of behavioral disturbance in developmentally disabled and categorically referred children: A cluster analytic approach. *Journal of Pediatric Psychology, 10*, 151–167.

Deater-Deckard, K., Reiss, D., Hetherington, E. M., & Plomin, R. (1997). Dimensions and disorders of adolescent adjustment: A quantitative genetic analysis of unselected samples and selected extremes. *Journal of Child Psychology & Psychiatry, 38*, 515–535.

DiStefano, C., Kamphaus, R. W., Horne, A. M., & Winsor, A. P. (2003). Behavioral adjustment in the U.S. elementary school: Cross-validation of a person-oriented typology of risk. *Journal of Psychoeducational Assessment, 21*, 338–357.

DiStefano, C. A., & Kamphaus, R. W. (2007). Development and validation of a behavioral screener for preschool-age children. *Journal of Emotional & Behavioral Disorders, 15*(2), 93–102.

Doucette, A. (2002). Child and adolescent diagnosis: The need for a model-based approach. In L. E. Beutler, & M. L. Malik (Eds.), *Rethinking the DSM: A psychological perspective* (pp. 201–220). Washington, DC: American Psychological Association.

Dowdy, E., Furlong, M., Eklund, K., Saeki, E., & Ritchey, K. (2010). Screening for mental health and wellness: Current school-based practices and emerging possibilities. In B. Doll (Ed.), *Handbook of youth prevention science* (pp. 70–95). New York: Routledge.

Drummond, T. (1994). *The Student Risk Screening Scale (SSRS)*. Grants Pass, OR: Josephine County Mental Health Program.

DuBois, P. H. (1965). With few whips. In E. G. Boring (Ed.), *Contemporary Psychology: APA Review of Books* (p. 489). St Louis, MO: American Psychological Association.

Durlak, J. A. (1997). *Successful prevention programs for children and adolescents.* New York: Plenum Press.

Eaton, D. K., Lowry, R., Brener, N. D., Grunbaum, J. A., & Kann, L. (2004). Passive versus active parental permission in school-based survey research: does the type of permission affect prevalence estimates of risk behaviors? *Evaluation Review, 28*, 564–577.

Edelbrock, C., Achenbach, T. M. (1980). A typology of child behavior profile patterns: Distribution and correlates for disturbed children aged 6–16. *Journal of Abnormal Child Psychology, 8*, 441–470.

Epstein, J., Isenberg, N., Stern, E., & Silbersweig, D. (2002). Toward a neuroanatomical understanding of psychiatric illness. In J. E. Helzer & J. J. Hudziak (Eds.), *Defining psychopathology in the 21st century: DSM-V and beyond* (pp. 57–70). Arlington, VA: American Psychiatric Publishing.

Esbensen, F. A., Deschenes, E. P., Vogel, R. E., West, J. Arboit, K., & Harris, L. (1996). Active parental consent in school-based research: an examination of ethical and methodological issues. *Evaluation Review, 20*, 737–753.

Esbensen, F., Melde, C., Taylor, T. J., & Peterson, D. (2008). Active parental consent in school-based research: how much is enough and how do we get it? *Evaluation Review, 32*(4), 335–362.

Farmer, E. M. Z., Burns, B. J., Phillips, S. D., Angold, A., & Costello, E. J. (2003). Pathways into and through mental health services for children and adolescents. *Psychiatric Services, 54*(1), 60–66.

Fergusson, D. M., & Horwood, J. (1995). Predictive validity of categorically and dimensionally scored measures of disruptive childhood behaviors. *Journal of Clinical Child & Adolescent Psychology, 32*, 396–407.

Fletcher, J. M. (1985). External validation of learning disability typologies. In B. P. Rourke (Ed.), *Neuropsychology of learning disabilities: Essentials of subtype analysis* (pp. 187–211). New York: Guilford Press.

Frick, P. J., Burns, C., & Kamphaus, R. W. (2009). *Clinical assessment of child and adolescent personality and behavior* (2nd ed.). New York: Springer.

Friedman, R., Katz-Levy, J., Manderscheid, R., & Sondheimer, D. (1996). Prevalence of serious emotional disturbance in children and adolescents. In R. Manderscheid & M. Sonnenschein (Eds.), *Mental health in the United States, 1996* (pp. 71–89). Washington, DC: U.S. Government Printing Office.

Garb, H. N. (1997). Race bias, social class bias, and gender bias in clinical judgment. *Clinical Psychology: Science & Practice, 4*, 99–120.

Grills, A. E., & Ollendick, T. H. (2003). Multiple informant agreement and the Anxiety Disorders Interview Schedule for Parents and Children. *Journal of the American Academy of Child & Adolescent Psychiatry, 42*(1), 30–40.

Glover, T., & Albers, C. (2007). Considerations for evaluating universal screening assessments. *Journal of School Psychology, 45*(2), 117–135.

Good, R. H., & Kaminski, R. A. (Eds.). (2002). *Dynamic indicators of basic early literacy skills* (6th ed.). Eugene, OR: Institute for the Development of Education Achievement. Available at http://dibels.uoregon.edu.

Goodman, R., Ford, T., Corbin, T., & Meltzer, H. (2004). Using the Strengths and Difficulties Questionnaire (SDQ) multi-informant algorithm to screen looked-after children for psychiatric disorders. *European Child & Adolescent Psychiatry, 13*(2), 25–31.

Haapasalo, J., Tremblay, R. E., Boulerice, B., & Vitaro, F. (2000). Relative advantages of person- and variable-based approaches for predicting problem behaviors from kindergarten assessments. *Journal of Quantitative Criminology, 16*, 145–168.

Hill, L. G., Lochman, J. E., Coie, J. D., Greenberg, M. T., & The Conduct Problems Prevention Research Group (2004). Effectiveness of early screening for externalizing problems: Issues of screening accuracy and utility. *Journal of Consulting & Clinical Psychology, 72*, 809–820.

Hinshaw, S. P., & Lee, S. S. (2003). Conduct and oppositional defiant disorders. In E. J. Mash, & R. A. Barkley (Eds.), *Child psychopathology* (pp. 144–198). New York: Guildford.

Huberty, C. J., DiStefano, C., & Kamphaus, R. W. (1997). Behavioral clustering of school children. *Multivariate Behavioral Research, 32*(2), 105–134.

Hudziak, J. J. (Ed.). (2008). *Developmental psychopathology and wellness: Genetic and environmental influences.* Arlington, VA: American Psychiatric Publishing, Inc.

Hudziak, J. J., Wadsworth, M. E., Heath, A. C., & Achenbach, T. M. (1999). Latent class analysis of child behavior checklist attention problems. *Journal of American Academy of Child & Adolescent Psychiatry, 38*, 985–991.

Ikeda, M. J., Neesen, E., & Witt, J. C. (2008). Best practices in universal screening. In A. Thomas & J. Grimes (Eds.), *Best practices in school psychology V* (pp. 103–114). Bethesda, MD: National Association of School Psychologists.

Jablensky, A. (1999). The nature of psychiatric classification: Issues beyond ICD-10 and DSM-IV. *Australian & New Zealand Journal of Psychiatry, 33*, 137–144.

Jensen, P. S., Rubio-Stipec, M., Canino, G., Bird, H. R., Dulcan, M. K., Schwab-Stone, M. E., et al. (1999). Parent and child contributions to diagnosis of mental disorder: Are both informants always necessary? *Journal of the American Academy of Child & Adolescent Psychiatry, 38*, 1569–1579.

Johnston, C., & Murray, C. (2003). Incremental validity in the psychological assessment of children and adolescents. *Psychological Assessment, 15*(4), 496–507.

Jones, D., Dodge, K. A., Foster, E. M., Nix, R., & Conduct Problems Prevention Research Group. (2002). Early identification of children at risk for costly mental health service use. *Prevention Science, 3*, 247–256.

Kamphaus, R. W., & Campbell, J. C. (2006). *Psychodiagnostic assessment of children: dimensional and categorical methods.* New York: Wiley.

Kamphaus, R. W., & DiStefano, C. (2001). Evaluación multidimensional de la psicopatología infantil. *Revista de Neuropsicología, Neuropsyqiatría y Neurociencias, 3*, 85–98.

Kamphaus, R. W., DiStefano, C., & Dowdy, E. (2009, June). *Universal screening of student behavior: Preliminary results of a wide-scale screening program.* Poster presented at the annual meeting of the Institute of Education Sciences, Washington, D.C.

Kamphaus, R. W., & Reynolds, C. R. (2007). *Behavior Assessment System for Children—Second Edition (BASC-2): Behavioral and Emotional Screening System (BESS)*. Bloomington, MN: Pearson.

Kamphaus, R. W., Huberty, C. J., DiStefano, C., & Petoskey, M. D. (1997). A typology of teacher-rated child behavior for a national U.S. sample. *Journal of Abnormal Child Psychology, 25*, 453–463.

Kelleher, K. J., Moore, C. D., Childs, G. E., Angelilli, M. L., & Comer, D. M. (1999). Patient race and ethnicity in primary care management of child behavior problems: a report from PROS and ASPN. *Medical Care, 37*(11), 1092–1104.

Kendell, R. E. (2002). Five criteria for an improved taxonomy of mental disorders. In J. E. Helzer & J. J. Hudziak (Eds.), *Defining psychopathology in the 21st century: DSM-V and beyond* (pp. 3–17). Arlington, VA: American Psychiatric Publishing.

Kim, S., & Esquivel, G. (2011). Adolescent spirituality and resilience: Theory, research, and educational practices. *Psychology in the Schools, 48*, 755–765.

Kim, S., Kamphaus, R. W., & Baker, J. A. (2006). Short-term predictive validity of cluster analytic and dimensional classification of child behavioral adjustment in school. *Journal of School Psychology, 44*, 287–305.

Kim, S., Orpinas, P., Martin, R. P., Horne, A. M., Sullivan, T. N., & Hall, D. B. (2010). A typology of behavioral adjustment in ethnically diverse middle school students. *Journal of Psychoeducational Assessment, 28*(6), 524–535.

Kraepelin, E. (1902/1896). *Clinical psychiatry: A text-book for students and physicians* (6th ed., translated by A. R. Diefendorf). London: Macmillan.

Kutash, K., Duchnowski, A. J., & Lynn, N. (2006). *School-based mental health: An empirical guide for decision-makers.* Tampa: University of South Florida, Louis de la Parte Florida Mental Health Institute, Dept. of Child and Family Studies, Research and Training Center for Children's Mental Health.

LaCombe, J. A., Kline, R. B., Lachar, D., Butkus, M., & Hillman, S. B. (1991). Case history correlates of a Personality Inventory for Children (PIC) profile typology. *Psychological Assessment: A Journal of Consulting & Clinical Psychology, 3*(4), 678–687.

Lane, K. L., Little, M. A., Casey, A. M., Lambert, W., Wehby, J., & Weisenbach, J. L. (2009). A comparison of systematic screening tools for emotional and behavior disorders. *Journal of Emotional & Behavioral Disorders, 17*(2), 93–105.

Lessing, E. E., Williams, V., & Gil, E. (1982). A cluster-analytically derived typology: Feasible alternative to clinical diagnostic classification of children. *Journal of Abnormal Child Psychology, 10*, 451–482.

Levitt, J. M., Saka, N., Romanelli, L. H., & Hoagwood, K. (2007). Early identification of mental health problems in schools: the status of instrumentation. *Journal of School Psychology, 45*, 163–191.

Lilienfeld, S. O., Waldman, I. D., & Israel, A. C. (1994). A critical examination of the use of the term "comorbidity" in psychopathology research. *Clinical Psychology: Science & Practice, 1*, 71–83.

Lochman, J. E., & The Conduct Problems Prevention Research Group. (1995). Screening of child behavior problems for prevention programs at school entry. *Journal of Consulting & Clinical Psychology, 63*, 549–559.

Mattison, R. E., Carlson, G. A., Cantwell, D. P., & Asarnow, J. R. (2007). Teacher and parent ratings of children with depressive disorders. *Journal of Emotional & Behavioral Disorders, 15*(3), 184–192.

McDermott, P. A., & Weiss, R. V. (1995). A normative typology of healthy, subclinical, and clinical behavior styles among American children and adolescents. *Psychological Assessment, 7*, 162–170.

McDermott, P. A., Marston, N. C., & Stott, D. H. (1993). *Adjustment scales for children and adolescents.* Philadelphia, PA: Edumetric and Clinical Science.

Meehl, P. E. (1995). Bootstraps taxometrics: Solving the classification problems in psychopathology. *American Psychologist, 50*, 266–275.

Meehl, P. E., & Rosen, A. (1955) Antecedent probability and the efficiency of psychometric signs, patterns, or cutting scores. *Psychological Bulletin, 52,* 194–216.

Merikangas, K. R. (2002). Implications of genetic epidemiology for classification. In J. E. Helzer & J. J. Hudziak (Eds.), *Defining psychopathology in the 21st century: DSM-V and beyond* (pp. 195–209). Arlington, VA: American Psychiatric Publishing, Inc.

Merikangas, K. R., & Swendsen, J. (1997). The genetic epidemiology of psychiatric disorders. *Epidemiologic Review, 19,* 1–12.

Messick, S. (1989). Educational measurement (3rd ed.). In R. L. Linn (Ed.), *The American Council on Education/Macmillan series on higher education* (pp. 13–103). New York; England: Macmillan Publishing Co.

Mezzich, J. E., Kleinman, A., Fabrega, H., & Parron, D. L. (Eds.). (1996). *Culture and psychiatric diagnosis: A DSM-IV perspective.* Washington, DC: American Psychiatric Press.

Mills, C., Stephan, S. H., Moore, E., Weist, M. D., Daly, B. P., & Edwards, M. (2006). The President's New Freedom Commission: Capitalizing on opportunities to advance school-based mental health services. *Clinical Child & Family Psychology Review, 9*(3), 149–161.

MindFreedom International. (2005). *Introductory FAQs about MFI.* Retrieved June 25, 2009, from the MindFreedom International Web site: http://www.mindfreedom.org/.

Natarajan, S., & Nietert, P. J. (2003). National trends in screening, prevalence, and treatment of cardiovascular risk factors. *Preventive Medicine, 36*, 389–397.

Nathan, P. E., & Langenbucher, J. (2006). Diagnosis and classification. In F. Andrasik (Ed.), *Comprehensive handbook of personality and psychopathology: Vol. 2: Adult psychopathology* (pp. 3–26). Hoboken, NJ: John Wiley & Sons.

National Adolescent Health Information Center. (2006). *Fact sheet on suicide: adolescents and young adults.* Retrieved May 30, 2009, from the University of San Francisco National Adolescent Health Information Center web site: http://nahic.ucsf.edu/downloads/Suicide.pdf.

Nease, D. E., Volk, R. J., & Cass, A. R. (1999). Investigation of a severity-based classification of mood and anxiety symptoms in primary care patients. *Journal of the American Board of Family Practice, 12*(1), 21–31.

Nunnally, J. C. (1978). *Psychometric theory.* New York: McGraw-Hill.

Parron, D. L. (1997). The fusion of cultural horizons: Cultural influences on the assessment of psychopathology on children. *Applied Development Science, 1*, 156–159.

Pescosolido, B. A., Perry, B. L., Martin, J. K., McLeod, J. D., & Jensen, P. S. (2007). Stigmatizing attitudes and beliefs about treatment and psychiatric medications for children with mental illness. *Psychiatric Services, 58*(5), 613–618.

Phelan, M. B. (2007). Screening for intimate partner violence in medical settings. *Trauma, Violence, & Abuse, 8*(2), 199–213.

Power, T. J., Andrews, T. J., Eiraldi, R. B., Doherty, B. J., Ikeda, M. J., DuPaul, G. J., et al. (1998). Evaluating attention deficit hyperactivity disorder using multiple informants: the incremental utility of combining teacher with parent reports. *Psychological Assessment, 10,* 250–260.

Quay, H. C. (1987). Patterns of delinquent behavior. In H. C. Quay (Ed.), *Handbook of juvenile delinquency* (pp. 118–138). New York: Wiley.

Reynolds, C. R., & Kamphaus, R. W. (1992). *Behavior Assessment System for Children.* Circle Pines, MN: American Guidance Service.

Reynolds, C. R., & Kamphaus, R. W. (2004). *Behavior Assessment System for Children–Second Edition (BASC-2).* Circle Pines, MN: AGS.

Reynolds, C. R., & Shaywitz, S. E. (2009). Response to intervention: Ready or not? Or, from wait-to-fail to watch-them-fail. *School Psychology Quarterly, 24,* 130–145.

Romer, D., & McIntosh, M. (2005). The roles and perspectives of school mental health professionals in promoting adolescent mental health. In D. L. Evans, E. B. Foa, R. E. Gur, H. Hendin, C. P. O'Brien, M. E. P. Seligman et al. (Eds.), *Treating and preventing adolescent mental health disorders: What we know and what we don't know* (pp. 598–615). New York: Oxford University Press.

Rutter, M., & Nikapota, A. (2002). Culture, ethnicity, society and psychopathology. In M. Rutter & E. Taylor (Eds.), *Child and adolescent psychiatry* (4th ed.; pp. 277–286). Oxford, England: Blackwell Publications.

Scahill, L., King, R. A., Schultz, R. T., & Leckman, J. F. (1999). Selection and use of diagnostic and clinical rating instruments. In J. F. Leckman & D. J. Cohen (Eds.), *Tourette's syndrome—tics, obsessions, compulsions: developmental psychopathology and clinical care* (pp. 310–324). Hoboken, NJ: John Wiley & Sons.

Schmidt, N. B., Kotov, R., & Joiner, T. E. (2004). *Taxometrics: toward a new diagnostic scheme for psychopathology.* Washington, DC: American Psychological Association.

Severson, H. H., Walker, H. M., Hope-Doolittle, J., Kratochwill, T. R., & Gresham, F. M. (2007). Proactive, early screening to detect behaviorally at-risk students: issues, approaches, emerging innovations, and professional practices. *Journal of School Psychology, 45*(2), 193–223.

Shaffer, D., Gould, M., Hicks, R., Fisher, P., Greenberg, T., Kraft, A., et al. (2007, March 14). *Teen suicide fact sheet.* Retrieved May 30, 2009, from the TeenScreen National Center for Mental Health Checkups at Columbia University web site: http://www.teenscreen.org/images/_getinformed/pdfs/GI4D_PDF_TeenSuicideFactSheet.pdf.

Shinn, M. R. (Ed.). (1989). *Curriculum-based measurement: Assessing special children.* New York: Guilford Press.

Shirk, S. R., & Jungbluth, N. J. (2008). School-based mental health checkups: ready for practical action? *Clinical Psychology: Science & Practice, 15*(3), 217–223.

Skalski, A., & Smith, M. (2006, Sept.). Responding to the mental health needs of students. Principal leadership. Retrieved from www.nasponline.org/resources/principals/School-Based%20Mental%20Health%20Services%20NASSP%20Sept%202006.pdf.

Skinner, H. A. (1981). Toward the integration of classification theory and methods. *Journal of Abnormal Psychology, 90,* 68–87.

Skinner, H. A. (1986). Construct validation approach to psychiatric classification. In T. Millon & G. L. Klerman (Eds.), *Contemporary directions in psychopathology: Toward the DSM-IV* (pp. 307–331). New York: Guilford Press.

Stoep, A. V., McCauley, E., Thompson, K. A., Herting, J. R., Kuo, E. S., Stewart, D. G., et al. (2005). Universal emotional health screening at the middle school transition. *Journal of Emotional & Behavioral Disorders, 13*(4), 213–223.

Suldo, S. M., & Shaffer, E. J. (2008). Looking beyond psychopathology: The dual-factor model of mental health in youth. *School Psychology Review, 37,* 52–68.

U.S. Department of Health and Human Services. (2005). *Title 45 Code of Federal Regulations Part 46, Protection of Human Subjects. Subpart A: Basic HHS Policy for Protection of Human Research Subjects 70 FR 36328.* Washington, DC: DHHS, June 23.

U.S. Department of Education. (2005). *Protection of Pupil Rights Amendment (PPRA). 20 U.S.C., & 1232h; 34 CFR Part 98.* Washington, DC: Family Policy Compliance Office, February 17.

United States Public Health Service. (2000). *Report of the Surgeon General's conference on children's mental health: A national action agenda.* Washington, DC: Department of Health and Human Services.

VanDeventer, M. C., & Kamphaus, R. W. (in press). *Mental health screening at school: instrumentation, implementation, and critical issues.* New York: Springer.

Verhulst, F. C., Dekker, M. C., & van der Ende, J. (1997). Parent, teacher, and self-reports as predictors of signs of disturbance in adolescents: whose information carries the most weight? *Acta Psychiatrica Scandinavica, 96*(1), 75–81.

Vreugdenhil, C., van den Brink, W., Ferdinand, R., Wouters, L., & Doreleijers, T. (2006). The ability of YSR scales to predict DSM/DISC-C psychiatric disorders among incarcerated male adolescents. *European Child & Adolescent Psychiatry, 15*(2), 88–96.

Wakefield, J. C. (1999). Evolutionary versus prototype analyses of the concept of disorder. *Journal of Abnormal Psychology, 108,* 374–399.

Wagner, M., Kutash, K., Duchnowski, A. J., & Epstein, M. H. (2005). The special education elementary longitudinal study and the national longitudinal transition study: Study designs and implications for children and youth with emotional disturbance. *Journal of Emotional & Behavioral Disorders, 13*(1), 25–41.

Walker, H. M., & Severson, H. H. (1992). *Systematic screening for behavior disorders* (2nd ed.). Longmont, CO: Sopris West.

Weisz, J. R., Sandler, I. N., Durlak, J. A., & Anton, B. S. (2005). Promoting and protecting youth mental health through evidence-based prevention and treatment. *American Psychologist, 60,* 628–648.

Widiger, T. A., & Trull, T. J. (2007). Plate tectonics in the classification of personality disorder. *American Psychologist, 62,* 71–83.

World Health Organization. (2001). *International classification of functioning, disability and health (ICF).* Geneva: WHO.

World Health Organization. (2005). *International classification of diseases and health related problems: ICD-10* (2nd ed.). Geneva: WHO.

Wu, P., Hoven, C., Bird, H., Moore, R., Cohen, P., Alegria, M., et al. (1999). Depressive and disruptive disorders and mental health service utilization in children and adolescents. *Journal of the American Academy of Child & Adolescent Psychiatry, 38,* 1081–1090.

The ICF-CY: A Universal Taxonomy for Psychological Assessment

Rune J. Simeonsson *and* Andrea Lee

Abstract

Assessment is central to psychological practice but has lacked an inclusive framework of health, functioning, and behavior. This chapter advances the International Classification of Functioning, Disability, and Health for Children and Youth—ICF-CY (WHO, 2007) as a new framework for guiding psychological assessment, from conceptualization of needs through documentation of intervention outcomes. In the ICF-CY taxonomy, the components of Body Functions, Body Structures, and Activities/Participation encompass different manifestations of child health and functioning defined in terms of physical, personal, and social dimensions. A unique contribution of the ICF-CY to psychological assessment is inclusion of the component of Environmental Factors for documenting the aspects of the environment that facilitate a child's functioning and participation and those that may serve as barriers. The universal and comprehensive scope of the ICF-CY provides a standard for classifying dimensions of functioning in children with disorders and disabilities complementing diagnostic and etiological information. Assignment of the universal qualifier to codes in the different components of the ICF-CY can indicate the nature and extent of disability or disorder defined in terms of impairments of functioning, activity limitations, or participation restrictions. The use of the ICF-CY is compatible with current psychological assessment methods, tools, and data sources, yielding an efficient profile for summarizing a child's functional status within a child-environment interaction perspective. As a universal tool, the ICF-CY is consistent with perspectives on children's rights and offers a common language for documentation of childhood disability and disorders not only within psychological practice, but also across disciplines and related service systems.

Key Words: children's rights, child functioning, assessment, activity, participation, impairment, disability, environmental factors, ICF-CY

Introduction

Assessment of human functioning is a central activity of the profession of psychology. It is a professional activity that is distinguished from that of other disciplines in that the focus is on assessment of subjective phenomena and their expression. From early methods of observation and interviews to the broad spectrum of standardized tests and inventories of current practice, the purpose of psychological assessment has been to identify the nature and dimensions of an individual's mental, affective,

and behavioral functioning. Such assessment is not carried out for its own sake, but as in medical assessment, serves an end of deriving diagnoses, identifying treatment options, and/or monitoring the progression of a condition or to document treatment outcome.

The aim of this chapter is to advance the practice of comprehensive psychological assessment by presenting a new tool for use. The chapter begins with consideration of the place of psychological assessment, including goals and pitfalls for psychologists who work with children and youth. The International Classification of Functioning, Disability, and Health for Children and Youth (ICF-CY; WHO, 2007) is presented as a new tool for guiding psychological assessment, from conceptualization of goals through documentation of intervention outcomes. After presenting the ICF-CY and its applicability for assessment, the chapter provides a detailed overview of an assessment approach using the ICF-CY framework, including applied examples of the approach based on vignettes. In its entirety, this chapter provides a systematic overview of how to use the ICF-CY in the practice of comprehensive assessment to document children's abilities and needs in order to enhance their functioning while minimizing the impact or presence of barriers to meaningful participation in the environment.

Challenges in Psychological Assessment

> **David** is a six-year-old boy referred to an outpatient mental health clinic for concerns regarding his delayed language development and "odd behaviors."
>
> **Jane** is a 12-year-old pre-adolescent girl referred to the psychologist at her school for "acting out." Her teachers would like insight into "what's wrong with her" so they can respond to her needs. They tell the psychologist they suspect an emotional or behavioral disorder.

On initial consideration of the vignettes above, the referral questions reflect the need for assessment in the search for a diagnosis for David and the determination of appropriate school services and supports for Jane. In each case we ask, What should be the focus of assessment; what are the measures, approaches, and strategies that should be included in the assessment? A typical approach with David might be to focus on assessment to confirm or rule out a diagnosis of autism spectrum disorder (ASD). For Jane, the approach might be to follow the sequence of steps required to determine her eligibility for special education under a designated diagnostic category. Such assessment, however, would not be sufficient to address the complexity of their presenting problems. These challenges are multiplied given the dramatic increase in the number of children identified with health conditions and disorders (Woliver, 2008). Carrying out assessment with these children in a comprehensive

and developmentally appropriate manner is associated with many significant challenges involving the process of assessment, the scope of assessment measures, and the object of assessment.

In contrast to assessment in medicine, a significant challenge in psychological assessment is that the process of assessing psychological and behavioral characteristics generally requires that the person is alert and responsive. Assessment of mental, affective, and behavioral functioning in most cases requires that the individual not only be alert, but actively cooperate in the assessment. That is, without the willingness of the individual to respond to questions, perform tasks, and engage in observable behaviors, it is difficult to document the normality or deviation of functioning. With children, this challenge is increased in that not only are their verbal and skill repertoires more limited, but so is their motivation to participate in the give-and-take of the typical assessment tasks. This challenge is exacerbated for children whose limitations are more pronounced and more pervasive, but who have the greatest need for valid assessment; that is, children with developmental disabilities or mental disorders. A critical element of this challenge is the need for an approach to assessment that both expands the view of human functioning and fosters an active process of assessment.

A second challenge is diversity in the scope of measures, tools, and procedures available for psychological assessment, described in *Tests in Print* (Murphy, Spies, & Plake, 2006) and *Burros Mental Measurements Yearbook* (Spies, Carlson, & Geisinger, 2010). The most substantial inventory of measures relates to the assessment of cognitive ability, particularly intelligence. This is a domain with well-standardized, robust measures, tracing its developmental history to the early 1900s and work of Binet and Simon. Closely related to the domain of cognitive measures are tools to assess processes such as perception, memory, and language, and the products of cognition in the form of academic achievement and performance tests. Adequate measures are available to assess interpersonal behavior as well as adaptive behavior, although the latter measures have focused more on activities of daily living than on adaptation to physical and social demands and "coping" in a broader sense. Although the domain of affective and intrapersonal functioning is perhaps the one with the greatest need for effective assessment measures, it is the one with a less well-developed inventory of measures. This variability in measures, tools, and procedures reflects a diverse, rather than integrated assessment domain.

A third and related challenge in psychological assessment is the need to expand the object of assessment beyond the child. An underlying premise of psychological theory of human functioning and development is that behavior and personal functioning are the products of ongoing person–environment interaction. However, a systematic analysis and assessment of environmental dimensions is not characteristic of much assessment practice. This is reflected by the fact that there are relatively few measures of the person's physical, social, or psychological environment.

There has been an absence of an inclusive framework for assessment of human functioning in psychology, defining typical and variant functioning and behavior. Practices and measurement in psychological assessment have thus evolved outside a unified and integrated perspective of dimensions of functioning and behavior of children and adults. Instruments and procedures have often emerged in response to meeting a specific need, such as defining the characteristics of a diagnosis or establishing eligibility criteria for intervention and services. Furthermore, when frameworks have been used, these have been based on conceptions of medical pathology in the International Statistical Classification of Diseases and Related Health Problems-ICD-10 (WHO, 1992), or psychiatric disorders in the Diagnostic and Statistical Manual of Mental Disorders, 4th Edition Text Revision-DSM-IV-TR (APA, 2000) and DSM-V (Andrews, Pine, Hobbs, Anderson, & Sunderland, 2012). The limitations of these classifications for comprehensiveness and for developmental sensitivity have resulted in the continued development of yet other classifications of childhood disability and disorders, such as Diagnostic and Statistical Manual–Primary Care (Wolraich, Felice, & Drotar,1996; Drotar, 2004) for children and youth, and Zero to Three (Wieder, 1994) for very young children. This approach has contributed to use of diagnosed conditions as a way to describe or document child status, a common practice in psychology's past, albeit a practice that has faced criticism over time.

Hobbs (1975) was a prominent voice in describing the stigma of labels, which "often depicted the child in negative terms" (p. 102), conveyed little information, and "suggested only vaguely the kind of help a child may need," (p. 102). As discussed in Florian et al. (2006), there are many problems in approaches utilizing disability status as a primary mechanism for describing a child. Disability labels mask individual differences in functioning, cannot capture the complexity of an individual's varied skills and needs, and may stigmatize an individual in a way that impairs others' abilities to see a child for who he or she is, and his or her uniqueness (Florian et al., 2006). Leonardi, Bickenbach, Ustun, Kostanjsek, and Chatterji (2006) challenged researchers and practitioners to consider the role of definitions of disability as they advocated for a definition allowing conceptualization of disability as a dynamic interplay between individuals and their environment. In their paper, Leonardi et al. (2006) proposed that *disability* could be conceptualized as "a difficulty in functioning at the body, person, or societal levels, in one or more life domains, as experienced by an individual with a health condition in interactions with contextual factors" (p. 1220). This view is in contrast to the traditional approach to assessment framed within a perspective of intra-individual pathology without adequate recognition of the influence of the environment on ongoing behavior (Simeonsson, 2006).

An inclusive framework of human functioning that integrates the role of the environment could address the challenges noted above and contribute to more comprehensive psychological assessment of children and adults. As a broad framework of human functioning, it would also lend itself to the interdisciplinary nature of efforts to assess children's functional characteristics of relevance for planning intervention and documenting outcomes. The WHO International Classification of Functioning, Disability and Health—ICF (WHO, 2001) and the derived version for children and youth, ICF-CY (WHO, 2007), offer a framework to enhance the practice and instruments of psychological assessment of children (Simeonsson, 2009).

ICF-CY: a New Tool for Psychology

The need for a common conceptualization and language of "disease" was first recognized in the nineteenth century with the introduction of a classification of causes of death (WHO, 1992). More than a century and a half passed before a comparable universal classification of health and functioning was recognized. The World Health Organization first published a taxonomy for documenting individual functioning in 1980, with the publication of a trial version of the International Classification of Impairments, Disabilities, and Handicaps (ICIDH; WHO, 1980). This classification was revised over time, and in 2001, WHO introduced the International Classification of Functioning, Disability, and Health (ICF) as its newest addition to the Family of International Classifications (FIC). The 2001 publication of the

ICF formalized a comprehensive conceptual model and taxonomy to classify health, functioning, and disability as universal human characteristics. The ICF reflected a change in paradigms from a medical model in which disability was viewed as a problem within the person to one in which disability is multidimensional in nature and affected by interactions with the environment. This view is consistent with a biopsychosocial model of health and illness (Engel, 1983, 1992), emphasizing a dynamic, interactive view of health and functioning.

As a taxonomy, the ICF provides comprehensive language to describe individual functioning based on a holistic, integrated framework of health and disability. The ICF allows the documentation of an individual's functioning in interaction with the environment, a marked departure from the use of diagnoses or labels to describe characteristics of a person. The taxonomy utilizes a common language and is sufficiently broad and inclusive to describe functioning across multiple skill domains and domains of living, with multidisciplinary applicability. In addition, the information found within the ICF is applicable across countries, societies, and cultures. The ICF is thus a universal tool for documenting the nature and scope of an individual's functioning.

The ICF provides a framework for documenting the interaction of health dimensions with environmental factors depicted schematically in Figure 10.1. The language of the ICF is important, as it reflects a framework for documenting the person's "functioning," with "disability" defined as an "impairment" or a limitation in the performance of an activity or restriction of participation. In this framework, disability can be seen as a lack of "fit" between the person's functional characteristics and the resources found within the environment to carry out activities or to participate.

There are two parts to the ICF classification. The first conveys functioning and disability; the second, contextual factors. The dimensions of the person are defined by the components of Body Structures, Body Functions, and Activities/ Participation, and the contextual dimensions by the physical, social, and psychological environment. This is reflected in the ICF, in which the term *disability* is an umbrella term that refers to impairments of body functions or structures, activity limitations, and participation restrictions. As illustrated in the conceptual model (Figure 10.1) and reflected in the taxonomical structure, the ICF thus also presents a multidimensional framework and classification of disability.

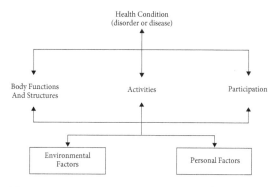

Figure 10.1 Interaction Between Components of the ICF-CY. (Adapted from WHO, 2007.)

Following its publication in 2001, the value of the ICF has been recognized as a common language for disciplinary and interdisciplinary applications by the health and health-related professions. Recognition of the potential of ICF for psychology and allied health disciplines such as occupational, physical, and speech therapy is evidenced by the development of a practice manual by the American Psychological Association (Reed et al., 2005). Of particular promise has been documentation using ICF codes in assessment measures (Ogonowski, Kronk, Rice, & Feldman, 2004), health records, and patient care in health and health-related settings. At broader policy levels, three of 18 major recommendations have been advanced for the ICF to guide initiatives of U.S. government agencies (National Academy of Sciences, 2007).

Although the content of the four domains of the ICF was extensive and suitable for covering documentation of adult functioning, it was not sufficiently inclusive of functional characteristics of children and their environments. Given that many mental disorders and disabilities have their origin in and are manifested in childhood (DSM-IV TR, 2000), the need for content to classify developmental dimensions of disability was recognized at the time that the revision of the earlier International Classification of Impairments, Disabilities, and Handicaps was underway (Simeonsson et al, 2000). That recognition continued with the publication of the ICF, emphasizing the need for a version that would encompass characteristic of children's functioning in the first two decades of life (Simeonsson et al., 2003). In response to the need for content with sufficient breadth and depth to capture the unique aspects of the developing child, WHO implemented a task force to address these needs, and the group expanded the ICF in scope and content, resulting in the ICF for Children and Youth

ICF-CY. The content of the ICF-CY provided a comprehensive classification of functional characteristics of children from infancy through age 17, as well as content-inclusive codes for precursors of more mature functioning already listed in the ICF.

The ICF-CY was published in 2007 with expanded content and increased specificity of detail reflecting characteristics of the developing child as a "moving target." Additions to the ICF were made in strong consideration of Bronfenbrenner and Ceci's (1994) ecological model conceptualizing *adaptation* as an interactive process between a child and the environment over time. The nature and organization of domains and the hierarchical structure of codes within chapters of the ICF-CY was identical to that of the ICF, with expansions taking the form of adding items to unused codes, modifying inclusion and exclusion criteria, and broadening the qualifier to include the concept of developmental delay. In addition to expanding the content to cover developmental aspects of body functions and structures, activities, and participation displayed by infants, toddlers, children, and adolescents, the added content was also suitable to capture levels of functioning of individuals beyond the childhood and adolescent periods. The Activities/Participation domain was most affected by changes made by the task force, with more new codes added in this domain than any other.

ICF-CY Organization and Structure

As shown earlier in Figure 10.1, the ICF-CY components of Body Functions, Body Structures, and Activities/Participation represent different manifestations of child health and functioning defined in terms of physical, personal, and social dimensions. The component of Environmental Factors defines elements of the physical and social environment and broader services and systems surrounding the child. Contextual factors also include a Personal Factors component, which is referenced in the text and schematic framework, but there is no associated classification of codes. An alphanumeric coding system is used for documentation and coding. Letters represent each of the four components. Body Functions are represented by "b"; Body Structures represented by "s"; Activities/Participation by "d"; and "e" represents Environmental Factors. Throughout the classification, codes within b, Body Functions, describe the physiological functions of body systems, and codes within s, Body Structures, identify parts of the body or anatomical structures. The ICF-CY defines *activity* as the "execution of a task by an individual"

(WHO, 2007, p. 9), and participation as "involvement in a life situation" (WHO, 2007, pp. xvi, 9). Thus, the Activities/Participation domain, d, contains codes describing functioning within society and at an individual level. Environmental Factors are defined as "the physical, social and attitudinal environment in which people live and conduct their lives" (WHO, 2007, pp. xvi, 9).

Each component contains multiple chapters, represented by one-digit numbers and representing relevant information to the domain. The one-level classification of the four domains is presented in Table 10.1. Content encompassing each chapter is defined in taxonomic codes presented in neutral terms. Codes contain three- to five-digit numbers, beginning with the number associated with the chapter and expanded in subcodes reflecting subsections of content. The codes are presented in a hierarchical structure, with major codes defining the central characteristic of function, structure, activities, or participation, followed by subcodes providing additional detail. For example, within component d, Activities/Participation, codes d130 to d159 describe Basic Learning. The construct represented in d131 is Learning Through Actions with Objects, which is further expanded upon with more specific subcodes describing ways in which the child would use objects to learn. Attempts were made to arrange the subcodes in the ICF-CY according to increasing levels of sophistication or toward more mature forms. In the case of use of objects in play, for example, d1310 describes Learning Through Simple Actions with a Single Object (i.e., banging, dropping); while d1314 captures Learning Through Pretend Play (i.e., substituting a novel object; pretending an object is another object). In this example, all of the codes are found within the Activities/Participation component (d), in the first chapter (represented by the initial 1 in the alphanumeric sequence), within the block of codes captured by Learning Through Actions with Objects (d131).

In the listing of codes under the components of Body Function and Activities/Participation, the ICF-CY is a classification of human health and associated environmental factors. When a universal qualifier is applied to codes, the ICF-CY provides a classification of disability documenting the extent of structural or functional problems at the body level, or functional limitations at the person level. It is also a classification of environmental barriers and facilitators when the universal qualifier is applied to document the negative or positive effects,

Table 10.1 One-Level Classification of Chapters Within ICF-CY Components

Body Functions	Body Structures
1. Mental functions	1. Structures of the nervous system
2. Sensory functions and pain	2. The eye, ear and related structures
3. Voice and speech functions	3. Structures involved in voice and speech
4. Functions of the cardiovascular, hematological, immunological, and respiratory systems	4. Structures of the cardiovascular, hematological, immunological, and respiratory systems
5. Functions of the digestive, metabolic, and endocrine systems.	5. Structures related to the digestive, metabolic, and endocrine systems.
6. Genitourinary and reproductive functions	6. Structures related to the genitourinary and reproductive systems
7. Neuromusculoskeletal and movement-related functions	7. Structures related to movement
8. Functions of the skin and related structures	8. Skin and related structures

Activities and Participation	Environmental Factors
1. Learning and applying knowledge	1. Products and technology
2. General tasks and demands	2. Natural environment and human-made changes to environment
3. Communication	3. Support and relationships
4. Mobility	4. Attitudes
5. Self-care	5. Services, systems and policies
6. Domestic life	
7. Interpersonal interactions and relationships	
8. Major life areas	
9. Community, social, and civic life	

respectively, of the environment experienced by the individual. The universal qualifier is central to the use of the ICF-CY in that the "codes are only complete with the presence of a *qualifier*, which denotes a magnitude of the level of health (e.g., severity of the problem; WHO, 2007, p. 20). The universal qualifier is defined by ordinal scale of values; *mild* = 1, *moderate* = 2, *severe* = 3 or *complete* = 4. The qualifier value 0 is typically not documented, as it indicates a typical level of functioning that is the expected default value. The ordinal value is entered following the decimal point in the code to indicate the extent or severity of restriction or limitation of functioning. Application of the universal qualifier requires evidence to support the assignment of a particular scale value. Although clinical judgment can serve as evidence for assigning a qualifier value to a code, standardized scores from tests and measures used in psychological assessment can facilitate matching of derived score from tests with the ordinal scale of the universal qualifier. In another context, we have proposed the matching of clinical and normative data with the ordinal values of the universal qualifier scale (Simeonsson Sauer-Lee, Granlund Björck-Åkesson, 2010).

To illustrate the application of the universal qualifier, if it was established that David had difficulties with energy and drive functions (b130), significant problems with impulse control (b1304) that could be coded as b1304.2, with the value of "2" reflecting moderate difficulties. Similarly, if evidence was available from records or assessment, Jane's presenting problems of emotion functions (b152) could be noted as severe, with the value of "3" for the specific code of b1521.3 (Regulation of Emotion). When the universal qualifier is applied to problems of body functions or structures, they are identified as impairments. Coding problems with impulse control and regulation of emotion for David and Jane, respectively, provides a standard language for documenting impairments of their mental functions. As impairments of these mental functions disorders are likely to be associated with difficulties with performing activities or participation, David, for example, may have problems in managing his behavior (d250) documented as moderate "2" with regard to "adapting activity level" (d2504.2). For Jane, impairments of emotional functioning may be likely to affect her complex interactions with others (d720), specifically noted as severe "3" for "regulating behaviors with others" (d7202.3). Problems experienced in these areas are defined as activity limitations and participation restrictions respectively. A major contribution of the ICF-CY is thus that it offers codes to document how different dimensions of disorders or disabilities are manifested at the level of mental functions as well as in everyday life activities and relationships with others. Of particular significance for children and youth is the conceptualization and classification of participation (Forsyth & Jarvis, 2002).

Given the ICF-CY framework of disability as a product of interactions of the child with a health condition with the environment, the domain of Environmental Factors provides codes to classify the nature and extent of the impact of the environment experienced by a child. In that the nature and severity of mental disorders or disabilities may be impacted or exacerbated by the environment, the ICF-CY provides means to classify the aspects of the environment that may impede or facilitate functioning. For environmental barriers, values of the universal qualifier can be applied following the decimal number of the environmental factor code, to quantify the extent to which environmental factors may affect Body Functions as well as Activities/Participation. For David, with severe impairment of impulse control, for example, existing educational policies (e5852.4) may serve as a barrier to his participation in a regular classroom. To document the facilitating role of the environment, a plus sign would be placed following the decimal point followed by the value of the universal qualifier. Thus, the availability of a special education classroom with appropriate placement for David could be documented as full facilitation (e5853.+4). A significant environmental barrier to participation in school experienced by Jane might be attitudes of rejection by acquaintances and peers (e425.3). For this child, a facilitating environmental factor might be the availability of supportive health services (e5800.+4) to provide therapeutic support.

The universal and comprehensive scope of the ICF-CY provides a standard for classifying dimensions of functioning in children with disorders and disabilities independent of diagnoses or underlying etiology. The ICF-CY can be applied to classify impairments of body structures and body functions, and limitations of the activity and participation of children with various health conditions, as well as defining environmental factors influencing their condition or indicated in their treatment and care. In that the ICF-CY includes developmental indicators, it is well suited to document the onset of disorders in infancy and early childhood as well as their manifestation with maturity (Lollar & Simeonsson,

2005), a feature of value in documenting conditions whose onset is during the developmental period. In addition, the ICF-CY may be particularly useful in meeting the challenge of defining characteristics of functioning in children who are dually diagnosed or identified with comorbid conditions (Jensen, Knapp, & Mrazek, 2006).

Contributions of the ICF-CY to Psychological Practice

The implications of the ICF have been advanced for psychological practice in clinical settings (Peterson, 2010) and for rehabilitation psychology (Mpofu & Oakland, 2010). An important contribution of the ICF-CY for children with disabilities and chronic conditions is to address current challenges in approaching intervention, treatment, and habilitation. The heterogeneity of developmental disorders and limitations of the existing taxonomies of ICD and DSM to define such disorders have been identified as barriers to effective interdisciplinary practice and research (Reiss, 2009). The comprehensive framework of human function defined by the ICF-CY (WHO 2007) offers a model for specifying the characteristics of the child, the environment and child–environment interaction and a common language for interdisciplinary work. As such, it provides an integrated perspective for assessment of the child's cognitive, communicative, social, and behavioral functioning. The publication of the ICF-CY formalized a comprehensive conceptual model and a common, universal language shared across disciplines and service settings to define children with developmental disabilities and disorders (Colver, 2005). The ICF-CY reflected a change from viewing and classifying disability and disorder as simply a medical problem within the child, to the recognition of disability and disorders as manifestations of child–environment interactions reflected in problems of body functions, activity limitations, and participation restrictions. The applicability and interdisciplinary utility of the ICF and ICF-CY framework and taxonomy of codes have been described in habilitation, early childhood (Bjorck-Akesson et al., 2010), clinical services (McDougall et al., 2008), and educational settings (DePolo et al., 2009).

In its current form, the ICF-CY is not intended to be the only or exclusive tool for documenting or describing human functioning and disability across all disciplines and all settings. Although the ICF-CY may be used as a primary classification, it may also be used in concert with other WHO-FIC tools, such as the ICD-10 (WHO, 1992). Diagnoses of disorders or diseases can be appropriately documented using the ICD-10, with the individual's functional characteristics across settings and environments documented using the ICF-CY. The ICF-CY could also be used to complement other classifications like the DSM-IV-TR (American Psychiatric Association, 2000), or related classifications such as the DSM-PC (Wolraich et al., 1996), or Zero to Three (Wieder, 1994). It could also be used with specialty classifications such as that produced by the American Association on Intellectual and Developmental Disabilities to document disorders of development. Although the categorical approach for defining disability in schools in the United States under the Individuals with Disabilities Education Act (IDEA; 2004) is not tied to a specific taxonomy, the ICF-CY holds promise as a tool to document educational disability within school-related eligibility requirement for special education (Simeonssson, Simeonsson, & Hollenweger, 2008).

The introductory section of the ICF-CY describes a number of potential uses, including applications to clinical, administrative, surveillance, policy, research, statistical, and educational sections (WHO, 2007, pp. xviii, 5). The goal of this section is to focus on a framework for utilizing the ICF-CY in psychological assessment of characteristics of children and youth. Such assessment takes into account that the developing child is a "moving target" and that, while a diagnosis remains static, the nature and level of functioning is dynamic, influenced by the child's experiences over time.

This section will focus on the application of the ICF-CY in assessment, from referral through measurement, documentation, and data collection surrounding intervention. The following sections describe using the ICF-CY framework (detailed above) to describe and document human functioning in clinical psychological practice. The dimensional approach of the ICF-CY provides a model for comprehensive assessment of development and psychological functioning and related environmental contexts associated with adaptation of the child. Building on the integrated approach of the ICF-CY, psychological and developmental assessment can help define the focus on the dimensions of functioning unique to children with specific disabilities and disorders. The ICF-CY can serve to provide the common language required to structure an assessment system that has utility in the development of individualized treatment plans and in the design of intervention programs. This integrated approach to

functional assessment provides a common language across disciplines and yields documentation of classification codes relevant for planning and evaluating clinical interventions. It can also yield summary data for administrative records.

In psychological assessment, the ICF-CY can provide a functional base for defining the nature and extent of a disorder and disability, and link this identification with the needed intervention. An added value is that assessment based on the common language of the ICF facilitates interdisciplinary communication and collaboration. The lack of a common language in interdisciplinary child services related to assessment and intervention is evidenced by the unique measures associated with different disciplines (i.e., psychology, education, and allied health and social services), resulting in disparate descriptors of children. A shared framework and language would constitute a clear metric permitting disciplines engaged in services for children and adolescents a shared perspective of functional aspects of behavior and development.

Applying the ICF-CY in Psychological Assessment

The ICF-CY offers contributions to assessment practice specific to the orientation for assessment, establishment of assessment goals, and uses of assessment data. These contributions are summarized in Table 10.2 and expanded upon in the following sections. A major focus of assessment practice in psychology has been to specify the nature of psychological deficits or psychopathology, rather than forming a holistic view of functioning of the individual. Each of the contributions of the ICF-CY to assessment in psychology noted below emphasizes the value of an integrated view of the individual child in which health and functioning, as well as the nature of impairments and functional impact of problems, are of interest.

To demonstrate the application of the ICF-CY to psychological assessment, the two brief vignettes discussed in the opening to this chapter are used as a platform to illustrate the way the comprehensive framework of human functioning of the ICF-CY can guide psychological services from the time of referral through documentation of outcomes as a result of intervention. The reader will recall that *David* is a six-year-old boy referred to an outpatient mental health clinic for concerns regarding his delayed language development and "odd behaviors." The second vignette involved *Jane*, a 12-year-old pre-adolescent girl referred to the psychologist at

Table 10.2 Applying the ICF-CY in Psychological Assessment

Aspect of Psychological Assessment	Contributions of the ICF-CY
Orientation to assessment	1. Use of conceptual framework to guide assessment
	2. Identifying levels of evidence needed to document codes within ICF-CY domains
	3. Identifying measures corresponding to form and level evidence
Purpose of assessment	4. Identifying environmental factors influencing child functioning
	5. Generating profiles of functioning
	6. Confirming functional criteria for eligibility
Application of assessment	7. Providing basis for intervention/ treatment planning
	8. Monitoring intervention implementation and outcomes

her school for "acting out." Her teachers would like insight into "what's wrong with her" so they can respond to her needs. They have told the psychologist they suspect that Jane has an emotional or behavioral disorder.

1. Use of Conceptual Framework to Guide Assessment

Within the ICF-CY framework, the skills, abilities, and needs of individuals reflect their ongoing interactions with the environment over time. This universal perspective facilitates the assessment and documentation of human functioning without resorting to labels, providing the groundwork for altering practices in making or receiving referrals for psychological assessment. A referral requesting information of a child's profile of functioning across multiple domains is quite different from a focused referral for an "autism diagnostic" or identification of a diagnosis inclusive of "acting out" behavior. While both referrals may involve common instruments, methods of assessment, and similar areas of development, their difference lies in an integrated

perspective of an individual's overall functioning, including strengths and challenges, as opposed to confirmation of a diagnostic label that describes only aspects of the individual's impaired functioning.

How does one transition to such a referral process? In many ways, the transition involves the expansion and reframing of existing practices, as opposed to completely altered processes. In the instance when a clinician questions whether a child meets the diagnostic criteria of an autism spectrum disorder (ASD), the clinician is already considering the multifaceted, multiple-domain nature of an ASD diagnosis (Simeonsson, 2003) and would be considering functioning in communication, social relationships, and behaviors. The conceptual framework illustrated earlier in Figure 10.1 could be applied to identify the nature, focus, and means of psychological and developmental assessment. With reference to the components of the model shown in Figure 10.1, assessment of sensory, mental, or psychosomatic characteristics would relate to the domains of Body Functions and Body Structure. Characteristics related to the child's physical, social, and psychological adaptation to home, school, and community would be defined by codes in the domain of Activities/Participation. Characteristics of the child's environment and the extent to which it impedes or facilitates functioning would be covered by Environmental Factors.

As an example, we can return to David and consider the continuation of the referral process and its potential expansion for generating a plan for assessment.

David: The psychologists at the outpatient clinic interview David's parents to understand their perceptions of David, his interests, and how he functions in a typical day. His parents describe David as six years old and full of energy. David's pediatrician and his parents jointly referred him to the outpatient mental health clinic based on concerns about David's "language development." They have "moderate" concerns, as David will speak in only two to three meaning-unit phrases. Further questioning reveals David was a late talker and has always had a tendency to speak louder and in more of a monotone compared to other children. On reflection, his mother confides that David seems to struggle when talking about specific types of human experiences, such as feelings and friendship.

David's parents also note several other behaviors and skills for their son. David can jump, run, and climb as well as his peers, and his ability to use his hands seems age-appropriate. He has full functional use of his body, though his parents remember having great difficulty toilet-training David. He loves trains and building long tracks for the cars. When he is happy to be playing with his trains, David will move his arms and hands very excitedly. If David's play is stopped without warning, he becomes very agitated and will have difficulty transitioning to the next activity. His parents describe him as "shy" and note that he prefers to play alone. He is able to sort colors and shapes but does not name them. He can rote count to 30 and loves numbers. Except for ear infections as a toddler, David has been a healthy child.

Using the ICF-CY as a conceptual framework, the brief interview with David's parents allows the practitioner to expand the focus from a referral for language development and behavioral concerns to an assessment plan based on questions regarding David's overall functioning. As is common practice, caregivers working with David want to know if he perceives the world accurately, and will thus request information regarding his hearing, vision, and sensory processing. It is unclear from the parent interview whether David's cognitive ability is of concern, so additional information will need to be gathered regarding his global mental functions. Several important issues for further exploration are immediately apparent from the referral and David's parents' comments; these include David's limited general communication skills and ability to interact with others. He seems to have emerging pre-academic skills, but the pattern of his skills warrants further exploration as well. David's parents report that he struggled to master toileting skills and responds somewhat atypically to changes in routine. Each of these areas needs to be explored fully by assessing his skills and challenges in self-care and meeting demands in his daily environment. Table 10.3 provides an overview of the process of expanding a referral to questions for assessment of David anchored in the ICF-CY taxonomy.

Thus, translating the ASD diagnostic referral question into an approach consistent with the ICF-CY would involve expansion of the word "autism" to conceptualizing which ICF-CY domains, chapters, and codes capture salient aspects of the individual's functioning and interaction with the environment. For example, assessment might reveal that relevant codes for capturing the functioning unique to a child such as David, suspected of experiencing difficulties related to autism, would be likely to include codes across Body Functions such as b122 (Global Psychosocial Functions), b1252 (Activity Level) and b163 (Basic Cognitive Functions). In the domain of Activities/Participation, relevant codes are likely to include d175 (Solving Problems), d240 (Handling Stress and Other Psychological Demands), and d335 (Producing Nonverbal Messages). Codes in the Environmental Factors component would probably include facilitators such as e310 (Immediate Family Supports), e410, (Individual Attitudes of Immediate Family Members) and barriers in the form of limited servicese535 (Communication Services, Systems, and Policies).

The advantage of utilizing ICF-CY codes to help capture the information needed is that the psychologist already knows which pieces of information speak to specific areas of functioning, and which are the same areas to be targeted for intervention, providing a direct link from referral through intervention development. In this way, the ICF-CY framework provides both the framework and the structure for clear, systematic, purposeful documentation throughout the assessment process and into intervention. In many ways, an assessment approach oriented to the ICF-CY as both framework and taxonomy involves the process of expanding the focus beyond conceptualization of disorder to allow for needed documentation of both skills and areas of challenge for later planning of intervention. Using the ICF-CY as a framework, the psychologist explicitly broadens the conceptualization of the child and his or her needs, considering an expansive set of codes important for documenting the child's level of functioning. The link between the nature of assessment and the framework can also be illustrated with a consideration of the referral concerns for Jane.

The psychologist at Jane's school reviewed the referral and realized she knew very little about Jane or her skills. After interviewing Jane's teacher and mother, the psychologist learned that Jane is considered quite bright. Her teachers believe she is capable of higher achievement, but she receives poor grades in school. Jane has difficulty attending in class and often does not complete assignments on time. She has few friends and has difficulties relating to peers or teachers. Jane's teachers indicate that she gets

Table 10.3 Matching Assessment Questions Within ICF-CY Domains

Expanding Focus	Step 1: Identify Applicable Domains and Codes	Step 2: Level of Evidence	Step 3: Assessment Approach and Measures
What are the characteristics of David's vision, hearing, and other sensory functioning?	Body Functions, Chapter 2: Sensory functions and pain	Percent problem and clinical judgment Standard scores	Vision and hearing screening Short sensory profile (Dunn, 1999)
How does David understand information compared to other children his age?	Body Functions, Chapter 1: Mental functions	Clinical judgment Standard scores	Observation and interview Wechsler Intelligence Scale for Children–Fourth Edition (WISC-IV; Wechsler, 2003)
How does David communicate? What is his communication style? What is the developmental quality of his speech and language?	Activities/Participation, Chapter 3: Communication	Description Clinical judgment Standard scores	Parent interview Observation in natural setting Clinical Evaluation of Language Fundamentals–4 (CELF-4; Semel, Wiig, & Secord, 2003) Aspects of the Vineland Adaptive Behavior Scales–2nd ed. (VABS-II; Sparrow, Cicchetti, & Balla, 2005)
How does David interact with others? What are his relationships like?	Activities/Participation, Chapter 7: Interpersonal interactions and relationships	Clinical judgment Description Standard scores	Autism Diagnostic Observation Schedule (ADOS; Lord, Rutter, DiLavore, & Risi, 1999) Observations and interview Aspects of the Vineland Adaptive Behavior Scales–2nd ed.
How does David respond and behave in his environment? How does he respond to demands and transition?	Activities/Participation, Chapter 2: General tasks and demands	Description and clinical judgment Standard scores	Observations and interview Aspects of the Vineland Adaptive Behavior Scales-2nd Edition
How does David learn? What are the characteristics of his learning style?	Activities/Participation, Chapter 1: Learning and applying knowledge	Descriptive terms Standard scores	Classroom artifacts and teacher interview Woodcock Johnson Tests of Achievement–3rd ed. (WJ-III; Woodcock, McGrew, & Mather, 2001)
What level of support does David need in regards to adaptive functioning?	Activities/Participation, Chapter 5: Self-care	Clinical judgment Standard scores	Observation and interview Vineland Adaptive Behavior Scales–2nd ed.

upset easily and acts out, with the result that she often finds herself in trouble at school.

Interviewing Jane, the psychologist finds out that she complains of not having an appetite and experiences difficulty sleeping. She has missed school many days in the last several years for a variety of physical complaints. At home, her mother reports that Jane acts out when asked to help with routine household tasks.

The psychologist using the ICF-CY as a framework would be able to capture the complex set of difficulties reported by this youngster in direct assessment (Young, Yoshida, Wlliams, Bobardier, & Wright, 1995) documenting areas of her functioning, and in consideration of the environmental context. Based on the interviews conducted, the psychologist may plan an evaluation protocol based on functioning related to the domain of Body Functions, such as codes for b1251 (Responsivity), b1261 (Agreeableness), b1521 (Regulating Emotion), b1302 (Appetite), b134 (Sleep Functions) and b1644 (Insight). In the domain of Activities/Participation, relevant codes defining Jane's difficulties are likely to include d2501 (Responding to Demands), d2502 (Approaching Persons or Situations), d7104 (Social Cues in Relationships), and d 7202 (Regulating Behaviors within Relationships). Negative attitudes of people in positions of authority (e430) and peers and others (e425) in school and community toward Jane may be barriers to her social functioning, whereas professional support (e355) and social support from friends (e320) could serve facilitating roles. In the development of an assessment plan, the practitioner may choose to frame concerns in a question format. Aligning the questions to ICF-CY chapters or codes will help organize the process and allow for systematic documentation of skills and needs throughout the assessment process.

2. Identifying Evidence Needed to Document Codes Within ICF-CY Domains

Beginning the assessment approach with a careful review of all information needed, and how to collect this information for the purpose of documentation of functioning, is an important step facilitated by use of the ICF-CY framework. After identifying a set of codes that are likely to describe an individual and his or her needs, the psychologist must identify sources of evidence to document their functioning and consider how this functioning will be quantified or captured for the purposes of interpretation. This process is particularly important for the later process of utilizing assessment data to design specific, individualized interventions that enhance the individual's functioning.

As a central purpose of assessment is to document an individual's functioning in terms of both their strengths and needs, it is important to select measures that allow for documentation of the severity (including possible absence) of any disorder or disability, utilizing the ICF-CY universal qualifier. As previously described, the universal qualifier can be assigned to document impairment, limitation, or restriction of functioning with values ranging from 0, "no impairment/limitation," to 4, "complete impairment/limitation." Values of 2 and 3 represent "moderate" and "severe impairment/limitation of functioning" respectively. If standardized tools are used in assessment of a

child's functioning, assigning values for the qualifier to document severity of limitation or impairment can be done with standard scores, scaled scores, T-scores, standard deviations, and percentile ranks (Simeonsson, et al., 2010). It is possible to document clinical judgment utilizing the universal qualifier as well, with the same advantages and limitations to the reliability and validity of the documentation as are inherent whenever clinical judgment is used as a primary mechanism for evaluating functioning. The important point is to systematically decide how the data resulting from the assessment approach will be applied to the activity of documenting the child's functioning and characteristics, and to do so during the process of selecting measures to ensure that the highest-quality data possible are collected during the assessment process. Here, it will be important to consider whether eligibility determination is a goal of the assessment process. If so, the psychologist must recognize the importance of matching the level of evidence required for eligibility to the level of evidence selected for the assessment. For example, eligibility criteria may require a child to demonstrate a discrepancy of a certain number of standard deviations or standard score points between areas of functioning measured, so it would be necessary to incorporate that knowledge into planning for assessment.

Returning to David's vignette, the psychologist designing an assessment approach and battery will need to consider the ultimate goal of the assessment process. David is of school age and attends a school system that provides free school-based services for children with disabilities, as long as the child meets specific eligibility criteria. The criteria are defined, in large part, by differences in a child's scores on standardized measures from those of other same-age children, or large intra-individual discrepancies on areas of functioning. Large discrepancies are typically characterized by a specific number of standard deviations or standard score points, and as such, there is a heavy reliance on standardized measures in assessment. As all assessments incorporate clinical judgment, and some skill sets are not easily measured by formal tests, the psychologist will need to identify which areas of functioning can be captured by standard scores and which will be based on clinical judgment of the child's functioning supplementing evidence for tests. The psychologist's choice of level of evidence for each area of functioning can be seen in Table 10.3 for David.

3. Identifying Measures Corresponding to Desired Level of Evidence for Use with ICF-CY

With the referral question expanded and described using a set of ICF-CY codes capturing children's functioning across domains and in interaction with the environment, along with the identification of level of evidence required of the assessment data, the next step is to select the actual measures that will be used to capture estimates of a child's skills and needs. This third step presents a central challenge in the field of psychology, in that tools themselves have served as the standard for describing phenomena difficult to observe directly. That is, the goal of many tools is to elicit responses from a child assumed to measure constructs such as intelligence, but the items that compose such measures may lack a conceptual framework integrating domains of functioning. A related concern is that measurement is often focused on performance of specific tasks rather than aspects of functioning such as attending, learning, and problem-solving that underlie such achievement and are prerequisites for developmental and academic readiness. Another issue pertains to the fact that although child–environment interaction is a central tenet of developmental theory and research, systematic attention to the child in context is limited in screening and assessment measures. This is a limitation in that understanding the child–environment interaction forms the foundation for the provision of required support and intervention (Sameroff & Fiese, 2000). These and other limitations are consistent with recommendations advanced to address the need for improved measurement of young children's functioning and development. It is important for psychologists to be cognizant of the limitations of their own tools, particularly when these tools are used to "measure" a child's skills to determine their eligibility for services and design interventions to meet their "measured" needs. Also note that there are many resources available to help guide psychologists' tasks of reviewing the reliability, validity, and general adequacy of a particular instrument to capture information regarding a specific individual, given factors such as his or her age, gender, education, sociocultural background, and the presence and/or relative severity of particular impairments. These resources include the *Mental Measurements Yearbooks* (Buros, by year) and the *Standards for Educational and Psychological Testing* (AERA, APA, & NCME, 1999).

In practice, then, the third step involves the careful and thoughtful selection of existing tools and informal measures that can best and most accurately capture a child's functioning for the later purpose of noting the level of limitation/impairment for designing individualized interventions matched to the child's unique pattern of skills and needs (Lollar, Simeonsson, & Nanda, 2000). These measures must not only capture the area of functioning in question, but they must also result in the level of evidence selected during Step 2. As most assessment tools were not developed with reference to the ICF-CY component framework, sources identifying tests or measures covering specific component content are available (see, for example, selected measures capturing emotional functioning by Lee, 2012) and will probably continue to emerge.

For assessment of cognitive, social, and affective functioning, a psychologist would need to carefully consider which available tools would be appropriate for a child of a particular age and background, which are designed to estimate levels of functioning in a particular area, and which will meet the pre-identified level of evidence. The psychologist would also need to consider if any measure could capture functioning in multiple areas, so as to limit the number of measures to administer in consideration of cost, time, and fatigue. In reference to David's case described in this chapter, the psychologist selected the Vineland Adaptive Behavior Scales–Second Edition (VABS-II; Sparrow, Cicchetti, & Balla, 2005) because of its utility in capturing estimates of functioning from parent and teacher reports in multiple areas of functioning, including communication skills, interpersonal or social skills, adaptability to changes in the environment or routine, and general self-care skills. The Strengths and Difficulties Questionnaire, a recently normed measure in the United States (Bourdon et al., 2005) and a number of other countries (Obel et al., 2004) may offer an efficient way for parents and teachers to report aspects of child functioning that correspond with some content under Mental Functions and Activities and Participation domains in the ICF-CY.

4. Identifying Environmental Factors Influencing Child Functioning

A unique contribution of the ICF-CY to assessment is inclusion of the Environmental Factors classification allowing documentation of the aspects of the environment that facilitate a child's functioning and participation and those that may serve as barriers. Until the introduction of the ICF, there was no standard way to document the role of environmental factors in a systematic, clear manner that would be understandable to caregivers and professionals involved with the child.

Two central aspects of the environment that are important to document during assessment are *barriers* and *facilitators*. In the process of planning interventions, psychologists readily recognize that it is as important to know what resources, services, and aspects of the environment are available for enhancing a child's functioning and participation as it is to know which aspects of environment serve as barriers to the child's ability to live and function as meaningfully as possible. Indeed, a central theme in designing interventions involves consideration of what can be altered in the environment, what can be added in, and what can be removed. However, recognition of the role of environmental influences on child functioning has probably been based more on informal observations by the psychologist than on assessment using specific tools.

The importance of documenting both the child's skills as well as characteristics of the environment is exemplified by considering a child in a resource-impoverished environment. A child may have the foundational abilities necessary to read but is not developing reading skills, given limited access to formal schooling (ICF-CY, Chapter 5 of Environmental Factors) and the lack of books and reading materials (ICF-CY, Chapter 1 of Environmental Factors) in the home environment. In this context, it is important not only to assess the child's limited reading skills, but also to assess factors in the child's environment that restrict or provide opportunities for learning, while documenting the skills the child does have that create the groundwork for later skill development.

Just how does one measure environmental factors? Person–environment interaction (Bronfenbrenner & Ceci, 1994) has been central to psychological assessment as a concept, but a standard approach to measurement of the environment and associated tools to capture physical and social qualities of the environment has been limited. This is in contrast to the measures that have been developed to assess specific aspects of interaction with the environment, such as child–teacher interaction, classroom environment, or parent–child interaction within the home. When considering how to best measure and describe facilitators, psychologists should consider not only if an aspect of the environment is available, but also if it is accessible, reasonable in terms of cost and time, and if it would be acceptable to the child and family. The quality is also important—including issues such as structural integrity, dependability, and a general sense of whether the quality is poor or good. Barriers, on the other hand, may affect a child because of either their presence or their absence. Other important issues to consider in relation to barriers include how frequently they hinder the individual, when they occur, if they can be avoided, and the relative strength of the barrier in terms of its impact on the child. Drawing on chapters of the Environmental Factors domain of the ICF-CY, a psychologist may identify barriers and/or facilitators involving products and technology (Chapter 1), natural environment and human-made changes to the environment (Chapter 2), support and relationships (Chapter 3), attitudes (Chapter 4), and services, systems, and policies (Chapter 5). These environmental factors can be summarized as relating to physical aspects (Chapters 1–2), social supports and attitudes (Chapters 3–4), or infrastructures and systems (Chapter 5) in the environment.

Compared to the wide array of psychometric tools for measuring cognitive, social, psycho-educational, and neuropsychological functioning, a significant problem is that there are relatively few measures for systematically assessing the environments of children. In a recent review of 43 measures commonly used to assess children with acquired brain injury, Ehrenfors, Borell, and Hemmingson (2009) found that 30 measures addressed the ICF domain of Body Functions, 13 addressed the domain of Activities and Participation, but none related to Environmental Factors domain. Measures that do exist are typically focused on documenting physical dimensions of children's environments, such as home, day care, and kindergarten settings (Bradley et al.,2001), or measurement of the school environment (Trickett, Leone, Fink & Braaten 1993). Interest in assessment of environments is increasing with the development of tools measuring children's activity environments (Hume, Ball, & Salmon, 2006) with content that may be mapped to some items in the Environmental Factors domain of the ICF-CY. It may also be important to assess needs related to specific assistive or augmentative devices of children with physical or motor impairments. As the latter may be unfamiliar to psychologists, they may want to team with an occupational or physical therapist or another professional trained in the use of such devices to determine how to identify which environmental factors are important for planning interventions.

While more tools to measure the environment corresponding to the ICF-CY classifications are a priority, psychologists do have skills in informal assessment that can be helpful in documenting environmental factors. These skills include objective observation and interviewing. Careful and thorough observation of a child in his or her environments, across many settings and contexts, cannot be overvalued in terms of its contribution to identify and describe environmental factors that can serve as barriers or facilitators. Interviewing the child, caregivers, and peers is also very important, particularly given the significance of attitudes of those working and living with the child and how they may facilitate or inhibit the child's participation and functioning. Returning to David and his story, Table 10.4 illustrates how a psychologist could (on his or her own) identify and document salient facilitators and barriers pertinent to David's life and functioning.

5. Generating Profiles of Functioning

The classification of codes and qualifiers is the essential contribution of the ICF-CY, offering for the first time a universal language for communication, not only within psychological practice, but also across disciplines, service systems, and countries. Implementation of this universal language of functioning, disability, and health in practice takes the form of assigning ICF-CY codes to assessment results for a child. The assessment of the child to address questions and concerns defined in Table 10.3

will yield results documenting characteristics of the child's functioning and environment. Those results then serve as evidence for assigning ICF-CY codes and qualifiers corresponding to the nature and extent of impairments of body functions, activity limitations, and restrictions of participation characterizing the child. The array of resulting ICF-CY codes constitutes a profile of functioning unique to that child at that point of time. The profile should also include codes documenting environmental factors influencing such functioning. In each case, the profiles should reflect the nature and severity of functional problems unique to David and Jane in their respective environments and at specific developmental stages.

The profile of codes does not take the place of test results and clinical data, but provides a common language to profile the functional status of the child and corresponding needs for intervention or support. Furthermore, in that it is based on description rather than diagnosis, it is in keeping with a holistic and non-stigmatizing approach to defining disorder and disability. The utility of functional profiles based on the ICF has been demonstrated in the documentation of school inclusion of students with disabilities in a regional study in Italy (Fusaro, Maspoli, & Vellar, 2009). Beyond an efficient description of the individual child, the code profiles can be aggregated across children to summarize the characteristics of children served by a clinic, school system, agency, or larger entity. In addition, the systematic use of codes

Table 10.4 Identifying Environmental Barriers and Facilitators

ICF-CY Environmental Factors Code	Data Source	Facilitator (+) or Barrier (–) and Level Using Qualifier
Chapter 1: Products and Technology	Observations and interviews	e11521+2: access to specialized/adapted play materials e1251+2: access to assistive communication devices, such as communication boards e1301.1: few assistive educational products available to child e310+3: very supportive immediate family prepared to adapt environment
Chapter 3: Support and Relationships	Observations and interviews	e355: health professionals are available to the child through the school system if he qualifies for services
Chapter 4: Attitudes	Observations and interviews	e410+3: immediate family members are supportive and understanding of child's needs e460.1: family impacted by negative societal stereotypes of mental health
Chapter 5: Services, Systems, and Policies	Observations and interviews	E5854: special education and training services available to child if he qualifies for services

can also be useful in studies of disability prevalence (Mudrick, 2002) and in national surveys (McDougall & Miller, 2003). For these kinds of applications, it would be important to establish a uniform list or set of codes that would portray the distribution of problems in the population. An example of a minimal list of codes has been proposed in Annex 9 of the ICF-CY for surveys and information systems. As the ICF-CY is implemented, code sets will be designed for documentation of developmental characteristics (Ellingsen & Simeonsson, 2010) or applications for specific settings such as clinics or schools.

6. Confirming Functional Criteria for Eligibility

Codes in the ICF-CY document disability when the universal qualifier is assigned to indicate the extent of disability or disorder, defined in terms of impairments of functioning, activity limitations, or participation restrictions. In contexts specifying criteria for a child's eligibility for intervention, receipt of specialized services, or referral for care, documentation has typically been based on a medical model encompassing etiological or diagnostic indicators derived from ICD-10 or DSM-IV-TR. In early-childhood intervention in the United States for example, a young child's eligibility under Part C of IDEA for early intervention is based on evaluation results that meet the criteria for assigning the child to one of three categories: "manifested developmental delay," "established medical condition," and the status of "at risk for delay" (U.S.C. §1432, as amended by IDEA, 2004). As it is problems of functioning that identify children in need of intervention and support, the ICF-CY may be particularly useful in shifting the focus of eligibility criteria from a medical to a biopsychosocial framework. Thus, whether eligibility is to be determined for receipt of assistive technology, special education, or therapy, the basis for defining criteria would be reframed in terms of activity limitations and participation restrictions. In the case of young children with development delays, applicable codes could be found in the Activities/ Participation domain of learning (Chapter 1) communication (Chapter 3), mobility (Chapter 4), personal care (Chapter 5), interpersonal relationships (Chapter 7), and major life areas (Chapter 8).

7. Providing a Base for Intervention/ Treatment Planning

An assessment approach organized with ICF-CY facilitates the process of using assessment to specify interventions. The assessment itself allows identification of the nature and extent of problems and delays in functional performance. In contrast to documentation of underlying impairments, assessment on the basis of functional limitations provides a correspondence with the nature of the needed interventions. Within the framework of the ICF-CY, the identification of functional limitations can serve as the basis for the development of individualized interventions. Such interventions recognize the child's interaction with the environment as the unit for assessment, and the design of programs of supports and treatments based on the child's profile of functioning defined by Activities/ Participation (Simeonsson, Leonardi et al., 2003; Simeonsson, Pereira et al., 2003). In other words, intervention planning subsequent to assessment organized by the ICF-CY can focus on increasing skills in completing activities and participating in important life situations and experiences.

The focus on functioning, as opposed to diagnosis, is a distinct advantage of using the ICF-CY to frame assessment. Too often, interventions are selected from a list because they are thought to address the diagnosis describing the child's impairments. While common, this approach often is not followed with efforts to individualize the intervention to meet the child's specific needs while capitalizing on the child's specific strengths. For example, selecting "an intervention for children with autism" utilizing a schedule of verbal activities would be inappropriate for a nonverbal child or a child who does not read. Concern regarding the lack of individualized assessment and individualized intervention has been expressed for decades, including remarks made by Donald Campbell in 1969 as he addressed fellow psychologists of the American Psychological Association, and in the special-education literature in the United States, which has encouraged use of a problem-solving assessment model to facilitate the implementation of individualized interventions based on data gathered on each individual child (see, for example, Deno, 1989, 2002). The ICF-CY-based approach to assessment provides the practitioner with functional information as well as identification of factors in the environment that play a role in the interventions or that must be intervened upon.

In David's example, his parents are important environmental resources and supports and may provide more individualized support than the school system, should he not qualify for services at school. Therefore, interventions focused on enhancing parental knowledge of David's unique patterns of skills and needs and providing them with training on intervention techniques helpful to David would be a prudent approach to providing intervention. The focus of intervention will depend on the results from his assessment. Areas of primary focus may include the areas of David's profile reflecting significant limitations, with the goal of decreasing the relative severity of his impairment and/or improving his actual level of functioning.

8. Monitoring Intervention Implementation and Outcomes

Interventions should be monitored frequently and over time in order to ensure that the intervention is implemented correctly and adjusting the nature or process of the intervention if necessary to ensure optimal outcomes for the child. Monitoring interventions by documenting outcomes with the ICF-CY qualifier or codes should be an ongoing process (Loe & Feldman, 2007). Changes attributed to intervention can be documented with the ICF-CY by noting either a change in qualifier or a change in functioning as denoted by a change in actual code. A change in the qualifer would denote a reduction in the severity level of impairment of limitation within an area of functioning as captured by the code. For example, if the universal qualifier decreases from 3 (i.e., b1342.3), describing *severe impairment*, to 1 (i.e., b1342.1), describing *mild impairment*, then there is documentation of the severity of impairment decreasing over time. There may also be a change in functioning that could be documented based on noting a shift in the hierarchy of the codes, from a lower- to higher-level code. For example, a child may improve from walking short distances with moderate impairment (d4500.2) to walking long distances with moderate impairment (d4501.2), representing an increase in functioning but no notable decrease in the severity of impairment.

In this way, data monitoring becomes part of the child's record, and documentation with the ICF-CY allows ongoing evidence of progress to be included in the child's educational, health, social services, medical, or other files. If continued systematically, documentation within the child's files would provide measurement of outcomes, including clear documentation of the child's needs for services (as identified at the beginning of the intervention process) through documentation of the impact of interventions that were identified to meet the child's individual's needs based on clear identification of impairments or limitations in functioning clearly documented in the child's profile of functioning.

In David's case, let us consider the scenario where he had moderate impairments in comprehending simple spoken messages (d3101.2). Interventions were designed to help David increase his ability to communicate with others. More specifically, David's parents minimized the number of meaning units ("David, sit" instead of "David, you need to sit down") in their own communication with him to provide David greater opportunity to understand their meaning. After three months, David was responding to their requests, and assessment results indicated that he understood simple spoken messages with only mild impairment (d3101.1). After one year, he could understand simple spoken messages with no impairment (d3101.0), and his parents were guided to increase the number of meaning units in their communication with him. Over the course of his elementary school years, David still had moderate impairments with understanding complex spoken language (d3102.2), but he had advanced in his receptive communication abilities. David's teachers maintained a log of codes with qualifiers describing his progress in comprehending spoken messages. This provided documentation of his progress, which could be traced back to the original assessment that estimated his level of communication functioning. Table 10.5 below provides an example of ongoing documentation of interventions for David and functional outcomes defined by changes in qualifier level and shifting of codes.

Conclusions

Although the health, functioning, and well-being of the individual are central to the practice of psychology, a corresponding classification of these domains has not been available to the profession prior to the publication of the ICF in 2001. As the two primary members of the WHO family of classifications, the ICD-10 and the ICF contribute complementary classification of disease and health, respectively. With the publication of the ICF-CY, it contributes a universal language defining elements of health, functioning, and well-being essential for all children and youth. In this context, the ICF-CY can be seen as a reference for defining these elements as children's rights, complementing the United Nations Convention on the Rights of the Child (United Nations General Assembly, 1989). Drawing on the principles of equality of opportunity, participation, and independence, the Convention articulates rights of children, such as the right to be heard; to have access to care, education, and support; and to be secure from harm, neglect, and exploitation (Corker & Davis, 2000; Dalton, 2002; Lansdown, 2000). It can also serve

Table 10.5 Documenting Intervention Implementation and Outcomes

Date	Description of Intervention	David's Level of Functioning	Description of Progress
March 2012	Use two meaning-unit phrases when speaking to David	D3101.2	Initial assessment
June 2012	Use two to three meaning-units phrases when speaking to David	D3101.1	Decrease in severity of impairment
March 2013	Use two simple sentences (three to five meaning units) to communicate with David	(D3101.0) D3102.3	Decrease in severity of impairment Shift in hierarchy of codes/increase in spoken message complexity
June 2013	Use two or more simple sentences (three to five meaning units) to communicate with David	D3102.2	Decrease in severity of impairment

as a reference for related documentation of rights and standards for equality of opportunity (United Nations General Assembly, 1993).

To the extent that psychology and related disciplines are committed to insuring that these rights are met for children (Simeonsson, Björck-Åkesson, & Bairrao, 2006), the ICF-CY extends beyond existing diagnostic classifications by providing a structure for practice, interdisciplinary collaboration, and communication (Lollar & Simeonsson, 2005). This chapter has advanced the framework and the taxonomy of the ICF-CY as an approach to enhance the assessment of physical, social, and personal functioning of children and youth. The use of the ICF-CY is compatible with current assessment methods, tools, and data sources, yielding an efficient profile summarizing a child's functional status within a child–environment interaction perspective. In this way, the ICF-CY can facilitate synergistic efforts to match children's needs with environmental supports through a common interdisciplinary language.

Future Directions

Since their respective publications, the growth of interest in the implementation of the ICF (2001) and the ICF-CY (2007) has been substantial, reflected in a wide range of clinical, policy, and research applications. As that interest continues to grow, several priorities can be identified for research and development with particular reference to implementation of the ICF-CY in psychological services for children and youth.

1. As the development of most existing assessment tools was often purpose-specific and not referenced to a comprehensive framework of human

functioning, implementation of the ICF-CY has required "back-coding" of instruments, that is, examining the extent to which their content can be matched to ICF-CY codes. Instruments are being developed based on the ICF-CY framework (Saigal et al., 2005; Wells & Hogan, 2003), but there is a need for more measures that yield evidence corresponding directly to ICF-CY codes.

2. The Environmental Factors domain of the ICF-CY represents an essential focus for assessment, but it is a domain that is largely lacking coherent conceptualization as an area for assessment as well as valid measurement tools. To this end, there is a priority for the development of tools to assess the physical, social, and infrastructure environments that are compatible with the ICF-CY taxonomy.

3. Current diagnostic practice with children is problematic in that there are issues of instability and fluidity of diagnoses and comorbidity and practices are discipline-specific, for example the use of DSM-IV TR in mental health and IDEA categories in special education in the United States. A particular limitation of diagnostic approaches with children is that signs and symptoms are collapsed into a single diagnosis, masking intra- and inter-individual differences. An area for further work is the application of the ICF-CY separately or in combination with other classification systems to complement diagnostic data with profiles of the child's functioning and the environmental factors that may influence such functioning.

References

AERA, APA, & NCME. (1999). *Standards for educational and psychological testing*. Washington, DC: American Educational Research Association.

American Psychiatric Association (2000). Diagnostic and statistical manual of mental disorders: DSM-IV-TR. Washington, DC: Author.

Anderson, G., Pine, D. S., Hobbs, J., Anderson, T. M., & Sunderland, M. (2012). Neurodevelopmental disorders: cluster 2 of the proposed meta-structure for DSM-V and ICD-11. *Psychological Medicine, 39*, 2013–2023.

Bjorck-Akesson, E., Wilder, J., Granlund, M., Pless, M., Simeonsson, R., Adolfsson, M., , & et al. (2010). The International Classification of Functioning, Disability and Health and the version for children and youth as a tool in child habilitation/early childhood intervention—feasibility and usefulness as a common language and frame of reference for practice. *Disability & Rehabilitation, 32*(S1), S125–S138.

Bourdon, K. H., Goodman, R., Rae, D., Simpson, G., & Koretz, D. S. (2005). The strengths and difficulties questionnaire: U.S. normative data and psychometric properties. *Journal of the American Academy of Child & Adolescent Psychiatry, 44*(6), 557–564.

Bradley, R. H., Corwynm, R. F., McAdoo, H. P., Coll. C. G. (2001). The home environments of children in the United States part 1: variations by age, ethnicity and poverty status. *Child Development 72(6)* 1844–67.

Bronfenbrenner, U., & Ceci, S. J. (1994). Nature-nurture reconceptualized in developmental perspective: a bioecological model. *Psychology Review, 101*(4), 568–586.

Campbell, D. T. (1969). Reforms as experiments. *American Psychologist, 24*, 409–429.

Colver, A. (2005). A shared framework and language for childhood disability. *Developmental Medicine & Child Neurology, 47*, 780–784.

Corker, M., & Davis, J. M. (2000). Disabled children: (Still) Invisible under the law. In J. Cooper (Ed.), *Law, rights, and disability* (pp. 217–238). London: Jessica Kingsley Publishers, Ltd.

Dalton, M. A. (2002). Education rights and the special needs child. *Child & Adolescent Psychiatric Clinics of North America, 11*, 859–868.

Deno, S. L. (1989). Curriculum-based measurement and special education services: A fundamental and direct relationship. In M. R. Shinn (Ed.), *Curriculum-based measurement: Assessing special children* (pp. 1–17). New York: Guilford Press.

Deno, S. L. (2002). Problem solving as "best practice." In A. Thomas & J. Grimes (Eds.), *Best practices in school psychology IV* (pp. 37–56). Bethesda, MD: National Association of School Psychologists.

DePolo, G., Pradal, M., Bortlot, S., Buffoni, M., & Martinuzzi, A. (2009). Children with disability at school: the application of the ICF-CY in the Veneto region. *Disability & Rehabilitation, 31*(S1), S67–S73.

Drotar, D. (2004). Detecting and managing developmental and behavioral problems in infants and young children: The potential role of the DSM-PC. *Infants & Young Children, 17*, 114–124.

Dunn, W. (1999). *Short sensory profile.* San Antonio, TX: Harcourt Assessment.

Ehrenfors, R., Borell, L., & Hemmingson, H. (2009). Assessments used in school-aged children with acquired brain injury: Linking to the international classification of functioning, disability and health. *Disability & Rehabilitation, 31*(17), 1392–1401.

Ellingsen, K. M., & Simeonsson, R. J. (2011). *WHO ICF-CY Developmental Code Sets.* Retrieved December 21, 2012, from http://www.icf-cydevelopmentalcodesets.com/

Engel, G. L. (1983). The biopsychosocial model and family medicine. *Journal of Family Practice, 16*, 409–413.

Engel, G. L. (1992). How much longer must medicine's science be bound by a seventeenth century world view? *Psychotherapy & Psychosomatics, 57*, 3–16.

Florian, L., Hollenweger, J., Simeonsson, R. J., Wedell, K., Riddell, S., Terzi, L., et al. (2006). Cross-cultural perspectives on the classification of children with disabilities: Part I. Issues in the classification of children with disabilities. *Journal of Special Education, 40*, 3–45.

Forsyth, R., & Jarvis, S. (2002). Participation in childhood. *Child: Care, Health & Development, 28*, 277–279.

Fusaro, G., Maspoli, M., & Vellar, G. (2009). The ICF-based functioning profiles of school children in care with the neuropsychiatric community services in the Piedmont region: Evidence for better caring and programming. *Disability & Rehabilitation, 31* (S1), S61–S66.

Hobbs, N. (1975). *The future of children.* San Francisco, CA: Jossey-Bass.

Hume, C., Ball, K., & Salmon, J. (2006). Development and reliability of a self-report questionnaire to examine children's perceptions of the physical activity environment at home and in the neighborhood. *International Journal of Behavioral Nutrition and Physical Activity. 3*, 16. doi: 10.1186/1479-5868-3-16

Individuals with Disabilities Education Act. (2004). P. L. No. 108–446, 118 Stat. 2647.

Jensen, P. S., Knapp, P., & Mrazek, D. A. (2006). *Toward a new diagnostic system for child psychopathology.* New York: The Guilford Press.

Lansdown, G. (2000). Implementing children's rights and health. *Archives of Disease in Childhood, 83*, 286–288.

Lee, A. L. (2012). *Specific mental functions: Emotional functions, experience of self/time. Measures for children with developmental disabilities: Framed by the ICF-CY.* London: Mac Keith Press.

Leonardi, M., Bickenbach, J., Ustun, T. B., Kostanjsek, N., & Chatterji, S. (2006). The definition of disability: What is in a name? *The Lancet 368*, 1219–1221. Retrieved May 10, 2008, from www.thelancet.com.

Loe, I. M., & Feldman, H. M. (2007). Academic and educational outcomes of children with ADHD. *Journal of Pediatric Psychology, 32*, 643–654.

Lollar, D. J., & Simeonsson, R. J. (2005). Diagnosis to function: classification of children and youth. *Journal of Developmental & Behavioral Pediatrics, 26* (4), 323–330.

Lollar, D. J., Simeonsson, R. J., & Nanda, U. (2000). Measures of outcomes for children and youth. *Archives of Physical Medicine & Rehabilitation, 81*(2 Suppl 2), S46–S52.

Lord, C., Rutter, M., DiLavore, P. C., & Risi, S. (1999). *Autism diagnostic observation schedule.* Los Angeles, CA: Western Psychological Services.

McDougall, J., & Miller, L. T. (2003). Measuring chronic health conditions and disability as distinct concepts in national surveys of school aged children in Canada: A comprehensive review with recommendations based on the ICD-10 and ICF. *Disability & Rehabilitation, 25*, 922–939.

McDougall, J., Horgan, K., Baldwin, P., Tucker, M. A., & Frid, P. (2008). Employing the International Classification of Functioning, Disability and Health to enhance services for children and youth with chronic physical health conditions and disabilities. *Paediatric Child Health, 13*(3), 173–178.

Mpofu, E., & Oakland, T. (Eds.). *Rehabilitation and health assessment: applying ICF guidelines.* New York: Springer.

Mudrick, N. R. (2002). The prevalence of disability among children: paradigms and estimates. *Physical Medicine & Rehabilitation Clinics of North America, 13*, 775–792.

Murphy, L. L., Spies, R. A., & Plake, B. S. (Eds.). (2006). *Tests in print VII: An index to tests, test reviews, and the literature on specific tests.* Lincoln, NE: University of Nebraska Press.

Ogonowski, J., Kronk, R., Rice, C., & Feldman, H. (2004). Inter-rater reliability in assigning ICF codes to children with disabilities. *Disability & Rehabilitation, 26*, 353–361.

Peterson. D. (2010). *Psychological aspects of functioning, disability and health.* New York: Springer Publishing Company.

Reed, G. M., Lux, J. B., Bufka, L. F., Trask, C., Peterson, D. B., Stark, S., et al. (2005). Operationalizing the International Classification of Functioning Disability and Health (ICF) in clinical settings. *Rehabilitation Psychology, 50*, 122–131.

Reiss, A. L. (2009). Childhood developmental disorders: an academic and clinical convergence point for psychiatry, neurology, psychology and pediatrics. *Journal of Child Psychology & Psychiatry, 50*(1–2), 87–98.

Saigal, S., Rosenbaum, P., Stoskopf, B., Hoult, L, Furlong, W., Feeny, D., et al. (2005). Development, reliability and validity of a new measure of overall health for preschool children. *Quality of Life Research, 14*, 243–257.

Sameroff, A. J., & Fiese, B. (2000). Transactional regulation: The developmental ecology of early intervention. In J. P. Shonkoff & S. J. Meisels (Eds.), *Handbook of early childhood intervention* (pp. 135–159). New York: Cambridge University Press.

Semel, E., Wiig, E. H., & Secord, W. A. (2003). *Clinical evaluation of language fundamentals—Fourth edition.* San Antonio, TX: Pearson Education.

Simeonsson, R. J. (2003). Communication disabilities in children and youth; issues in classification and measurement. *International Journal of Audiology, 42*(Suppl.1), S2–S8.

Simeonsson, R. J. (2006). Defining and classifying childhood disability. In Institute of Medicine (Ed.), *Workshop on disability in America* (pp. 67–87). Washington, DC: National Academy Press.

Simeonsson, R. J. (2009). ICF-CY: a universal for documentation of disability. *Journal of Policy & Practice in Intellectual Disabilities, 6*, 70–72.

Simeonsson, R. J., Björck-Åkesson, E., & Bairrao, J. (2006). Children's rights. In G. L. Albrecht (Ed.), *Encyclopedia of disability* (pp. 257–259). Thousand Oaks, CA: Sage Publications.

Simeonsson, R. J., Lollar, D., Hollowell, J., & Adams, M. (2000). Revision of the International Classification of Impairments, Disabilities and Handicaps: developmental issues. *Journal of Clinical Epidemiology, 53*, 113–124.

Simeonsson, R. J., Leonardi, M., Lollar, D., Björck-Åkesson, E., Hollenweger, J., & Martinuzzi, A. (2003). Applying the International Classification of Functioning, Disability and Health (ICF) to measure childhood disability. *Disability & Rehabilitation, 25*, 602–610.

Simeonsson, R. J., Pereira, S., & Scarborough, A. S. (2003). Documenting delay and disability in early development with the WHO-ICF. *Psicologia, 17*, 31–41.

Simeonsson, R. J., Sauer-Lee, A., Granlund, M., & Bjorck-Akesson, E. (2010). Developmental and health assessments in habilitation with the ICF-CY. In E. Mpofu & T. Oakland (Eds.), *Rehabilitation and health assessment: Applying ICF guidelines* (pp. 27–46). New York: Springer.

Simeonsson, R. J., Simeonsson, N. E., & Hollenweger, J. (2008). International classification of functioning, disability and health: a common language for special education. In L. Florian & M. McLaughlin (Eds.), *Disability classification in education.* New York: Corwin Publishers.

Sparrow, S. S., Cicchetti, D. V., & Balla, D. A. (2005). *Vineland adaptive behavior scales, second edition.* San Antonio, TX: Pearson Education, Inc.

Spies, R. A., Carlson, J. F., & Geisinger, K. F. Eds. (2010). *The eighteenth mental measurements yearbook.* Lincoln, NE: University of Nebraska Press.

Trickett, E. J., Leove, P. E., Fink C. M., & Braaten S. L. (1993). The perceived environment of special education classrooms for adolescents: a revision of the classroom environmental scale. *Exceptional children, 59*(5), 411–420.

United Nations General Assembly. (1989). *Convention on the rights of the child (A/Res/44/25).* New York: UN.

United Nations General Assembly. (1993). *The standard rules on equalization of opportunities for persons with disabilities (A/48/96).* New York: UN.

Wechsler, D. (2003). *Wechsler Intelligence Scale for Children* (4th ed). San Antonio, TX: Psychological Corporation.

Wells, T., & Hogan, D. (2003). Developing concise measures of childhood activity limitations. *Maternal & Child Health Journal, 7*, 115–126.

Wieder, S. (Ed.). (1994). *Diagnostic classification of mental health and developmental disorders of infancy and early childhood.* Washington, DC: Zero to Three: National Center for Infants, Toddlers, and Families.

Woliver, R. (2008). *Alphabet kids—from ADD to Zellweger syndrome.* London: Jessica Kingsley, Publishers.

Wolraich, M. L., Felice, M. E., & Drotar, D. (1996). *The classification of child and adolescent mental diagnoses in primary care: Diagnostic and statistical manual for primary care (DSM-PC) child and adolescent version.* Elk Grove Village, IL: American Academy of Pediatrics.

Woodcock, R. W., McGrew, K. S., & Mather, N. (2001). *Woodcock-Johnson III tests of achievement.* Itasca, IL: Riverside Publishing.

World Health Organization. (1980). *International classification of impairments, disabilities and handicaps.* Geneva, Switzerland: WHO.

World Health Organization. (1992). *International statistical classification of diseases and related health problems* (10th rev.). Geneva, Switzerland: WHO.

World Health Organization. (2001). *International classification of functioning, disability and health.* Geneva, Switzerland: WHO.

World Health Organization. (2007). *International classification of functioning, disability and health—children and youth version.* Geneva, Switzerland: WHO.

Young, N. L., Yoshida, K. K., Williams, I., Bombardier, C., & Wright, J. G. (1995). The role of children in reporting their physical disability. *Archives of Physical Medicine & Rehabilitation, 76*, 913–918.

Responsible Use of Psychological Tests: Ethical and Professional Practice Concerns

Jonathan W. Gould, David A. Martindale, *and* James R. Flens

Abstract

Psychologists bring to the task of assessing children and adolescents their knowledge of psychometrics and their skills in psychological testing. Ethical standards and professional practice guidelines admonish psychologists to select psychological assessment techniques that are reliable and valid as well as suitable for use with the population being assessed. In this chapter, we argue that when selecting psychological tests to be administered in an evaluation, psychologists must employ, not set aside, their knowledge of psychometrics: unreliable projective techniques should be eliminated from consideration.

Key Words: projective tests, projective techniques, psychological testing, ethical standards, *Daubert*, rules of evidence

Among the most important distinctions between clinical psychology practice and other forms of mental health practice is the use of formal assessment using psychometrically sound assessment techniques. Historically, clinical psychologists have employed projective techniques as part of a comprehensive approach to diagnostic assessments, and these techniques have been considered particularly useful in the comprehensive assessment of children (Chandler, 2003). McClure, Kubiszyn, and Kaslow (2002) suggest that "less well-validated assessment techniques, including projectives ... can provide rich data about the older child's internal life and inform the clinician more fully about developmental, relational, cultural, and contextual variables" (p. 131).

On the other hand, the use of projective techniques in the assessment of children has come under fire. In response to McClure et al., Lee and Hunsley (2003) comment that the recommendation to use projective techniques as part of an evidence-based assessment model for the evaluation of children is "particularly troubling" (p. 112) because many of the projective techniques recommended for use in child assessments "have consistently failed to meet scientific standards for psychological tests" (p. 112).

Over the past several decades, there has been a decline in the use of "time-intensive, clinician administered instruments that have historically defined personality practice" (Meyer, Finn, Eyde, Kay, Moreland, Dies, et al., 2001, p. 128). Despite this decline, the use of projective techniques, which are of questionable reliability and validity, continues to be widespread (Chandler, 2003). For example, the second edition of this volume contained an entire section, comprising six chapters, describing various projective techniques, including projective story telling, projective drawings, sentence completion, and the Holtzman Inkblot Technique.

The theoretical foundation upon which the use of projective techniques rests is the projective hypothesis (Chandler, 2003; Martindale, 2008). Important elements of the projective hypothesis have never been supported by empirical examination, however.

As Chandler (2003), a supporter of the use of projective techniques in children's assessment, reminds us: "Until there is some agreement as to what constitutes an appropriate outcome when projective techniques are used in clinical assessment, validity problems will remain, and projective techniques will continue to be poorly understood" (p. 56).

Why *Daubert v. Merrell* Is Important to Clinicians As Well As to Forensic Practitioners

Our approach to the selection of psychological tests is influenced by our work in the forensic arena. When conducting an evaluation for the courts, psychologists need to select psychological tests that are grounded in the methods and procedures of science, with appropriate validation. As discussed in the next section, on ethical standards, we argue that the selection of psychological tests must be grounded in the methods and procedures of science, such as the emphasis on reliable and valid techniques discussed in Ethical Standard 9.01 (a) addressing assessment (APA, 2002).

Although we have identified no research examining the selection, administration, scoring, and interpretation of psychological tests used in child assessment, we have observed that psychologists often base their test selections on the frequency with which various tests are used, on the basis of what tests were used during their graduate education and training, and on the frequency with which various tests are alluded to in journals articles or books (Bow, Gould, Flens, & Greenhut, 2006). That is, psychologists seem to select tests for use in a psychological assessment based on their familiarity or popularity rather than on their reliability and validity.

The criteria articulated in the Supreme Court's decision in *Daubert* (*Daubert v. Merrell Dow Pharmaceuticals Inc.* 509 US 579 [1993]) to assist judges in determining the admissibility of scientific evidence are, in our judgment, useful criteria to consider when choosing psychological tests to be used in clinical psychological assessments as well as in forensic psychological assessments.

The first criterion to be considered is whether the underlying theory upon which the test has been developed has been subjected to testing examining its falsifiability [*Daubert* at 580]. As applied to the selection of psychological tests in child assessment, the first issue to consider is whether the underlying theory upon which the test rests has been subjected to empirical examination through rigorous challenge.

The second criterion articulated in *Daubert* is whether the underlying theory has been subjected to critical peer review and publication [*Daubert* at 580]. When examining the degree to which a test has received support, one might consult independent peer review publications such as the Buros Mental Measurement Yearbook's "Test Reviews Online."

Not all peer review procedures are equal (see for example, Dickersin, 1990; Dickersin, Chan, Chalmers, Sacks, & Smith, 1987; Kerr, 1998; Rosenthal, 1979). It is our position that, in the process of establishing expertise, professionals whose publications have appeared in peer-reviewed journals or in texts that have included a peer review element in the editorial procedure are quick to point this out. In doing so, they indirectly suggest that peer review is a procedure that yields scholarly contributions and eliminates foolishness. It turns out that this is true only if one's peers are scholars and not fools. The right of fools to publish their foolishness is protected by our Constitution. We delude ourselves when we think of peer-reviewed journals as scholarly periodicals requiring that each article submitted for publication be judged by an independent panel of scholarly or scientifically minded peers, who will reject submitted articles that are lacking in scholarship. Though the process of peer review (sometimes referred to as "refereeing") subjects authors' work to examination by others, when fools examine the work of their colleagues, we cannot expect foolish work to be eliminated in the screening process. The purpose of peer review is to require that authors meet the standards of their respective disciplines; but what if those who run a particular journal and those who submit articles are all members of a generally unrecognized discipline? Won't contributors to the *Journal of Unsupported Theories*, the *Journal of Sophistry & Silliness*, and the *Journal of the Wildly Whimsical* all assert that their published works have been peer-reviewed? Members of the editorial boards of journals are ordinarily well-respected members of their respective fields of study; however, not all fields of study are worthy of respect.

The third criterion articulated in the *Daubert* decision is whether the theory has a known or potential error rate [*Daubert* at 580]. To date, there has been little case law regarding addressing error rate. In two federal appellate cases it was suggested that the error rate involved the error in classification based on the scientific methodology, such as a false positive or false negative classification (*United States v. Smith,* 869 F.2d 348 [U.S. App. Dist. 7, 1989]; *United*

States v. Williams, 583 F.2d 1194 [U.S. App. Dist. CA2 1978]). Both of these federal cases predated the *Daubert* opinion, but they offer some understanding of how error rate might be applied to psychological testing; specifically, whether a test score can accurately classify an individual, and what the rate of error might be in that classification attempt. In the reporting of intelligence and achievement test performance, it is common to see scores combined with confidence intervals. The psychometrically savvy reader will recall that the calculation of psychological test scores involves the assumption of error in the score, whether it is in the form of standard deviation, standard error of measurement, or confidence intervals. All of these methods involve the use of a score's anticipated error. A reported test score is actually an estimate of an individual's true score on a particular scale. By reporting confidence intervals along with scores, evaluators provide to the readers of their reports information concerning the likely range of accuracy for any given reported score.

The fourth criterion is whether there are standards controlling the technique's operation [*Daubert* at 580]. Does the test have a manual with standard instructions for administration and scoring? Some practitioners who use the Thematic Apperception Test (TAT), for example, tend to administer the technique using a personally developed set of ideas about which cards are most likely to elicit useful responses, sometimes administering different sets of cards to different people, depending upon the issues being assessed (Ackerman & Kane, 2002; Dana, 1996). It has been our experience in the forensic setting that, often, practitioners do not own the most current edition of the manuals for tests that they are using, or they have not read test manuals prior to administering tests. Some practitioners develop their own set of administration procedures, deliberately ignoring the procedures prescribed in manuals (Ackerman & Kane, 2002; Gould, Martindale, & Flens, 2009).

The fifth criterion is whether the theory is generally accepted in the field in which it is being offered for use [*Daubert* at 580]. General acceptance is often reflected in favorable reviews in respected, peer-reviewed journals. Elsewhere, we (Martindale & Gould, 2008) and others (Zeedyk & Raitt, 1998) have suggested that, generally, acceptance is not as useful a criterion as it might appear to be.

Although these criteria were developed for use by judges so that they might more effectively rule on the admissibility of proffered scientific evidence, the quality of assessments conducted by psychologists would increase if psychologists were to consider these criteria when selecting and administering psychological tests.

Ethical Standards

Important companions to the criteria identified above are the ethical standards guiding the work of psychologists drawn from the American Psychological Association's Ethical Code of Conduct. Competence is the first stepping-stone in developing an ethical framework for the psychological assessment of children.

Competence

Those familiar with Federal and State Rules of Evidence will note that the psychological ethical standard defining *competence* is similar to the definition used in Federal Rule 702 regarding qualifying expert witnesses. In both psychology and law, a list of the defining characteristics of expertise begins with education, training, supervised experience, consultation, and study.

Though the foregoing characteristics are necessary, they are not sufficient when the expertise at issue involves psychological testing. Psychologists are responsible for demonstrating the reliability and validity of methodology used to generate data upon which psychologists base their opinions. "[S]ocial scientists will be called upon to demonstrate the validity of the premises that lie behind their testimony" (Faigman, Kaye, Saks, & Sanders, 2002, p. 52).

Again, we stress a dominant theme of this chapter: The law requires scientists to be good scientists first and good expert witnesses second (Faigman et al., 2002). Just as the task of an expert witness is to regulate the supply of facts to a jury or judge in a manner that "states a preference for science as the preeminent method for discovering facts" (Faigman et al., 2002, p. 47), it is our contention that psychologists engaged in psychological assessment have a parallel responsibility to their clients. Treating practitioners must regulate the supply of facts to clients in a manner that gives evidence of a preference for scientific rigor and integrity as the preeminent method for discovering useful psychological information.

In a 2006 study, Bow, Flens, Gould, and Greenhut (2006) found that child custody evaluators who administered psychological tests were often unfamiliar with important elements of the tests. For example, almost half of the Bow et al. sample of forensic practitioners underestimated the required reading level for the Minnesota Multiphasic Personality Inventory 2 (MMPI-2) and Millon Clinical Multiphasic Inventory 3rd Edition (MCMI III); 25 percent of respondents allowed examinees to take the tests in the lobby of their offices; only a slight majority of respondents were aware of the MCMI III cutoff for the presence and prominence of a trait/syndrome; and 42 percent of respondents interpreted subscale scores whether or not the parent scales were elevated.

To the best of our knowledge, no similar study has been undertaken investigating psychologists' use of psychological tests in child assessment. We presume, however, that forensic practitioners are more likely than clinical practitioners to be aware that their work product may be critically reviewed by others and, as a result, may be more likely to be familiar with the tests they use in forensic assessment.

We foresee as an increased need for those practicing in the forensic arena to be well versed in psychological testing. Bow et al. (2006) wrote:

> [W]e believe there will be increased legal scrutiny about the use of psychological testing in child custody evaluations. Consequently, psychologists will need to be well versed in the properties of psychological testing in such evaluations, along with the legal issues that may arise from a *Daubert* challenge. (p. 26)

ETHICAL STANDARD 2.01 (C)

Psychologists planning to provide services, teach, or conduct research involving populations, areas, techniques, or technologies new to them undertake relevant education, training, supervised experience, consultation, or study.

We have observed, on clinical and forensic online listservs in which we participate, that mental health colleagues often accept assignments to conduct evaluations and then post queries about test selection and test administration relating to assessment devices they are unfamiliar with and that they have never used. It is clear from their inquiries that their endeavor to interpret the data from these tools will be their first.

Psychologists asked to conduct evaluations that will involve the use of psychological tests or techniques they are unfamiliar with should consider the APA Ethical Standard 2.01 (c), which admonishes psychologists to undertake relevant education, training, supervised experience, consultation, or study. With specific reference to consultation, we recommend developing a formal consultative relationship with a colleague who is more knowledgeable and experienced and who can offer assistance in the selection of appropriate instruments and the interpretation of assessment data.

2.03: MAINTAINING COMPETENCE

Psychologists should undertake ongoing efforts to develop and maintain their competence.

Maintaining competence in psychological assessment and keeping up with current empirical research and professional practice in the use of psychological tests enables psychologists to base their work on established scientific principles and the professional knowledge of the discipline.

Ethical Standard 2.04 admonishes psychologists to base their work on established scientific principles and on the professional knowledge of the discipline. There is a parallel between the criteria established in the *Daubert* decision and Ethical Standard 2.04, in which both the legal rule and the psychological standard focus attention on the need for psychological opinions to be based upon established scientific principles and on the professional knowledge of the discipline.

Psychologists have an ethical obligation to know about the laws governing their work, including state and federal laws about the creation of records, retention of records, release of records, confidentiality, and other relevant areas that affect clinical practice. Psychologists working in the forensic arena are admonished to be reasonably familiar with the judicial or administrative rules governing their roles.

Once competence has been developed, Ethical Standard 2.03 directs psychologists to maintain competence. Often, we have been witness to depositions or trials in which aggressive cross examination of clinicians who conducted psycho-educational or psychological evaluations of children revealed that the evaluators under scrutiny had not kept up with research and practice in the use of the psychological tests administered as part of their evaluations, had not attended continuing education courses aimed at maintaining competence in the tests administered, and had not sought peer supervision or peer consultation relating to tests they utilized. These evaluators appear to have taken the position that once psychological tests have been learned in graduate school, there is no reason to engage in ongoing efforts to maintain their competence in relevant areas of psychological assessment.

Multiple Relationships

Whether one works in the clinical or forensic arena, it is important that psychologists be transparent in all aspects of their professional evaluative work. The 1992 APA ethics code contained an ethical standard emphasizing the importance of transparency in record keeping. Standard 1.23 (b) read as follows:

> When psychologists have reason to believe that records of their professional services will be used in legal proceedings involving recipients of or participants in their work, they have a responsibility to create and maintain documentation in the kind of detail and quality that would be consistent with reasonable scrutiny in an adjudicative forum.

Although no similar admonition appears in the 2002 ethics code, it is our position that records of all aspects of psychological evaluations should be created in reasonable detail, should be legible, should be stored in a manner that makes expeditious production possible, and should be made available in a timely manner to those with the legal authority to inspect them or possess copies of them. (The foregoing wording has been adapted from Model Standard 3.2 (b) of the Association of Family and Conciliation Courts' *Model Standards for Child Custody Evaluation* [AFCC, 2007]).

Ethical Standard 6.01: Documentation of Professional and Scientific Work and Maintenance of Records Psychologists create, and to the extent the records are under their control, maintain, disseminate, store, retain, and dispose of records and data relating to their professional and scientific work in order to:

- facilitate provision of services later by them or by other professionals;
- allow for replication of research design and analyses;
- meet institutional requirements;
- ensure accuracy of billing and payments;
- ensure compliance with law.

Whether an evaluation of a child is conducted at the request of a parent, is the result of government-mandated programs, or is conducted as the result of a court order, the integrity of the evaluative process is dependent upon transparency and the degree to which actions by the evaluator is subject to scrutiny. Unless otherwise informed by the court or mandated by the government, evaluators should presume that everything in their files is subject to disclosure. Withholding or destroying components of our files undermines our work.

Transparency is an essential element of our system of justice. Courts, not psychologists, decide what is and what is not discoverable. The willingness of the public to view us and our work products as trustworthy is dependent upon the transparency that characterizes our work.

The term *transparency*, as used in this chapter, is intended to describe a philosophy from which a pattern of professional behavior logically follows. The philosophy guides us in our roles as evaluators and, subsequently, in our roles as consulting psychologists to families and as testifying experts to courts.

(1) *As evaluators*, in order to gather information helpful to triers of fact and to the families being assessed, psychologists must be unencumbered by personal or philosophical agendas; must be committed to a balanced approach in their work; and, must be alert to phenomena that adversely affect decision making.

(2) *As consultants to families or as testifying experts to the court*, in order to be effective, psychologists must be credible; must recognize that credibility is earned and that complete openness is one means by which an expert establishes credibility; and, must respect the rights of those wishing to question a consultant's or expert's opinions and the manner in which they were formulated. The pattern of behavior that flows from the stated philosophy includes: (a) prior to commencing an evaluation, actively disclosing any prior or current relationships with the participants; (b) being diligent in the creation and maintenance of one's records; and (c) producing, in response to a legally permissible request, the complete contents of one's file in the matter being litigated to those who are the legal authority to review the file.

The Initial Contact

In any type of psychological evaluation, a file should be created at the time of the initial contact. Ideally, messages left by those seeking an evaluator's services should be noted and responded to quickly. If one is engaged in a psychological evaluation for the courts, it may be wise to have a member of the office staff respond to messages. When this is not possible, only the most basic information should be taken during an initial phone contact, but all information should be recorded with care. If an evaluation is litigation-related, it is important to maintain precise records of all contacts. It is not uncommon (nor is it unreasonable) for a cross-examining attorney to inquire concerning all contacts that litigants, collateral sources, and others have had with an evaluator.

An evaluator's records should indicate when and by whom the initial contact was made and what information was provided. Before agreeing to accept an assignment, an evaluator should determine who the participants will be and disclose prior involvements with any of them and with individuals with significant ties to them. From our perspective, disclosure is a no-lose endeavor. Keeping track of contacts is relatively easy (but not a topic for this chapter); making such contacts known sets the stage for an open process; and, pre-evaluation disclosure eliminates one of the more unpleasant avenues of cross-examination. We also encourage those engaged in clinical (as contrasted to forensic) work to maintain a similar set of records.

Information Gathering

A discussion of the types of information likely to be useful to an evaluator and the means by which to gather such information is beyond the scope of this chapter. It must be emphasized, however, that under no circumstances whatsoever should an evaluator take possession of information offered without first having made it clear to the provider(s) of the information that it will be shared with others. All information accepted by an evaluator must be open for discussion with the person for whom or organization for which the evaluation is being conducted, whether that is a parent, a school district, or a court. Exceptions are rare, and evaluators must be familiar with any state laws that prohibit or place specific limitations on disclosure. Particularly when parents or school administrators have had previous involvements with mental health professionals, they should be reminded that the principles of confidentiality that may have applied in earlier interactions with mental health professionals are not applicable in contexts such as those in which forensic evaluations are conducted.

Preservation of Records

With the exceptions of dishonesty and displays of ignorance, there is no greater threat to a psychologist's credibility than the appearance that s/he has endeavored to shield from scrutiny any aspect of the manner in which s/he has conducted her/his professional activities.

The American Psychological Association's Record Keeping Guidelines (Committee on Professional Practice and Standards, American Psychological Association, 2007, p. 995) remind psychologists that they have "a professional and ethical responsibility to develop and maintain their records."

It is our view that the most useful guidance concerning the creation, maintenance, and release of records is to be found in the previously referenced AFCC *Model Standards*. Though the document was developed for custody evaluators, there is no element of the AFCC's guidance relating to records that is not equally helpful to mental health professionals performing other types of evaluations, including evaluations performed in a health service context.

Model Standard 3.2 admonishes evaluators to create all records expeditiously and to presume that their records are created, maintained, and preserved in anticipation of their review by others who are legally entitled to possess them and/or to review them. Model Standard 3.2 (b) declares that records should be created in reasonable detail, should be legible, should be stored in a manner that makes expeditious production possible, and should be made available in a timely manner to those with the legal authority to inspect them or possess copies of them.

It is important to recognize that distinctions often made in clinical contexts between progress notes and process notes or between a client's file and a treating practitioner's personal file are distinctions that are not recognized in forensic mental health evaluations. Mental health professionals whose previous evaluative tasks have been conducted within a treatment context should recognize that, in a litigation context, several ground rules are different. For example, regardless of the form in which information is presented, once evaluators take possession of an item, it must be retained, and reasonable care must be taken to prevent its loss or destruction. More often than not, evaluators who offer testimony are required to produce items that were considered by them in the course of their evaluations, even if, after having considered certain items, decisions were made not to rely upon them. For those conducting clinical evaluations, maintaining information in the file that was influential in forming their opinions is also important.

The responsibilities alluded to above are all tied to the concept of transparency. Evaluators cannot be effectively cross-examined if appropriate records have not been created; if handwritten documents are illegible; or if records that might form the basis of cross-examination have been concealed, destroyed, or returned to the litigants or others. Federal Rule of Evidence #705 reminds expert witnesses of the obligation to disclose the facts or data that form the basis for their opinions.

Though psychologists who have conducted their evaluations in forensic contexts are called upon to explain and defend their findings and the opinions formulated on the basis of those findings, treatment providers should not presume that they will never have to shoulder the burden of justifying their methods. All providers of liability coverage for health professionals stress the importance of creating reasonably detailed records and preserving those records. It is foolhardy for clinicians to embrace the flawed notion that whatever records they create are created and maintained only for their own use and, for that reason, do not have to be created with the possibility of their inspection by others in mind.

"The Full Monty"

Without access to evaluators' complete files, those wishing to challenge our data or question our interpretations of those data are put at a significant disadvantage in their endeavors to shed light on deficiencies in our work. When evaluators' alteration, concealment, or destruction of portions of the file inhibits or interferes with a thorough exploration of their methods and procedures, there is an increased risk that errors will go undetected.

Those who conduct psychological evaluations in forensic contexts implicitly accept several responsibilities. Among them is the responsibility to familiarize ourselves with the ways in which ineradicable biases and the lacunae in psychology's knowledge base limit the precision of our assessments. Education and training make us aware of the sources of bias, and various professional guidelines urge us to reduce the effects of these biases by seeking corroboration of information relied upon and to generate and explore alternative hypotheses. We must, however, be mindful of the fact that our best efforts may bring our biases to an irreducible level, but education, training, and significant effort do not eliminate them.

Protecting Privacy

We have reviewed clinical evaluations and forensic evaluations that contain information that has no relevance to matters under investigation. Standard 4.04 of our Ethics Code (American Psychological Association, 2002) instructs us to minimize intrusions on privacy. "Psychologists include in written and oral reports and consultations, only information germane to the purpose of which the communication is made." Psychologists may elect to exclude from their reports information reasonably viewed as not germane to the matter at hand. Though evaluators have the authority to omit information not deemed pertinent from their reports, all information must be preserved, and, when the evaluator is asked for it, its existence must be made known.

There are times when mental health professionals are reasonably expected to protect their records (or portions of their records) from disclosure in order to prevent unwarranted intrusions into the privacy of others who are owed a duty of care. When psychologists are in possession of material that they reasonably believe should be protected from disclosure, their concerns should be raised with the proper authorities. In a forensic context, this may mean making application to the court and respecting the court's decision-making authority. For forensic practitioners, though it is likely that the procedures to be followed vary somewhat from state to state, the process is outlined in the Federal Rules of Civil Procedure [specifically, Fed. R. Civ. P. 26(b)(5)(C), 2001, p. 33], the language of which has been adopted by many of the states. For clinical psychologists.

There may be times when you are faced with the need to protect your records to prevent unwarranted intrusions into the privacy of others to whom you owe a duty of care. When a psychologist is in possession of material that she reasonably believes should be protected from disclosure, she may raise such a concern with the proper authorities. In a clinical context, the proper authorities whom one may need to consult include attorneys representing organizations in which evaluations have been conducted.

Staying Within What We Know

Among the most common errors we have observed among the reports we have reviewed is the offering of opinions based on insufficient information or based on psychological assessment techniques with little or no evidence of reliability and/or validity. Psychology is a social science, and, as such, is presumed to have developed a foundation of knowledge derived from empirical research. The methods and procedures developed for use in empirical research are presumed to have psychometric integrity; that is, the assessment techniques used in empirical research are expected to have demonstrated reasonable reliability and validity.

Shuman and Sales (1998) identified four types of expert testimony, and we believe that these four types of expert testimony are useful categories to use when examining the presentation of psychological testing results both inside and outside of a court context. The first type of expert opinion is based on clinical judgment because there is no scientific research available. We propose that offering such an opinion is inconsistent with psychologists' code of ethical conduct. Psychologists have an ethical responsibility to offer professional opinions for which there is sufficient support from reliable and valid scientific research. This is discussed more fully below.

The second type of expert opinion is based on clinical judgments where there is research evidence available on the issue that is contrary to the clinical judgment. Similar to the concern voiced above, we believe that offering of such an opinion is inconsistent with psychologists' code of ethical conduct.

The third type of expert opinion is based on presentation of results of scientific research and includes opinions based on clinical judgments that go beyond the results of current research. Psychologists have an ethical responsibility not to over-interpret—or under-interpret—psychological findings.

The fourth type of expert opinion is based on the results of scientific research (Shuman & Sales, 1998, p. 1230). Opinions based on results of scientific research reflect the spirit and intention of psychologists' code of ethical conduct.

Bases for Assessment

Ethical Standard 9.01 (a) addresses the need for psychologists to "base the opinions contained in their recommendations, reports, and diagnostic or evaluative statements, including forensic testimony, on information and techniques sufficient to substantiate their findings." A foundation of contemporary psychology is the development of reliable and valid procedures to assess human behavior. When psychologists are engaged to conduct psychological evaluations of children, it is presumed is that they will employ psychological assessment procedures that are scientifically based; that the data generated from those assessment procedures are reliable and valid; and that the interpretations of these reliable and valid data are sufficient to support the opinions that will subsequently be expressed by the evaluators.

In reviewing the work of psychologists who have been appointed or retained to conduct psychological assessments of children, we often encounter evidence of inattentiveness to Ethical Standard 9.01

(b) and offer opinions about people who they have neither met nor evaluated. Specifically, reports are prepared in which psychologists offer opinions on the matter of a child's psychological best interests when they have failed to evaluate both parents. In such reports, it is not uncommon to find very specific statements about the psychological characteristics of individuals who have not been evaluated.

Psychologists have traditionally been trained in service models derived from clinical treatment. Psychotherapy has been conceived as a process initiated by the client, on the basis of the client's own perception of a need to make changes in his or her life. The psychotherapist-patient privilege is presumed to facilitate open communication by decreasing the risk that a client's thoughts, feelings, or behavior will be revealed to others without the client's permission. Implicit in the psychotherapy process is the assumption that the client will be motivated to provide as much *accurate* information to the therapist as possible, so that the therapist's ability to assist the client will be maximized (Greenberg, Martindale, Gould, & Gould-Saltman, 2004).

Greenberg et al. (2004) argued that many psychotherapists adopt a mindset that leads to the uncritical acceptance of information provided by their clients—adults and children alike. Therapists are often trained to accept, support, and advocate for the needs of their clients. This orientation may lead to a reluctance to challenge a client's assumptions, interpretations, or dysfunctional behavior. Therapists who adopt this perspective may also underestimate the level of bias in information they receive from their clients.

When a psychologist is appointed or retained to conduct a psychological evaluation of a child whose parents are involved in conflict over custodial placement, the assumptions underlying clinical assessment and treatment become inapplicable. Particularly in high-conflict cases, parents may become consumed with their desire to prevail in the custody conflict to such a degree that it impairs their ability to perceive situations accurately and support their children's independent needs. Constructive motives ordinarily encountered in the psychotherapy process, such as the desire to be candid in the reporting of information, may be subordinated to the parent's desire to prevail in the litigation. This issue is complicated by the fact that in high-conflict disputes, the litigating parents often believe that the parenting arrangement that they seek is the arrangement that best serves the child's interests. Quite often the arrangement is one in which the role of the other parent is dramatically minimized. Thus, even where a particular parent has been the one to seek an evaluation, the parent is motivated by a desire to prevail in the legal matter. The desire to identify and alter problematic attitudes and behaviors—the desire ordinarily present in a psychotherapy context—is not present. In such situations, even when parents engage in efforts to improve their parenting skills or address emotional issues identified by evaluators or the court, it appears that they are often motivated by a wish to be perceived more favorably.

Adults who are intent on achieving a particular outcome may (intentionally or otherwise) alter, or may teach their children to alter, their interaction with mental health professionals in order to achieve their overall goals. While even young children are capable of reporting events accurately if they are not exposed to suggestive questioning (Ceci, Kulkofsky, Klemfuss, Sweeney, & Bruck, 2007), children at the center of a custody conflict are often exposed to significant adults (including parents) whose perceptions and interpretations of events have been distorted by bias. Children often respond to biased questioning, or to an interviewer with a strong opinion or emotional agenda, by producing the information the adult is seeking (Martindale, 2005a).

Where litigation is involved, all of these factors must be considered as decisions are made concerning what weight should be attached to children's reported perceptions, behaviors, and statements either to evaluators or to therapists. Opinions expressed by evaluators that are based on children's stated perceptions of parents who have never been evaluated are likely to have been formulated based on unreliable information or upon information whose reliability has not been ascertained.

Ethical Standard 9.01 (c): When psychologists conduct a record review or provide consultation or supervision, and an individual examination is not warranted or necessary for the opinion, psychologists explain this and the sources of information on which they base their conclusions and recommendations.

Most psychological assessment techniques that have been developed for psycho-educational assessment tend to have manuals that contain useful information about the reliability and validity of the instrument. As discussed above, our survey data suggest that a minority of psychologists do not administer tests in a manner consistent with the instructions in the manual. In general, however, we have observed that assessments examining psycho-educational functioning appear to have fewer problems than assessments examining psychological and emotional functioning.

Among the commonly used assessment procedures of many child and clinical psychologists are projective techniques. Many of those who utilize these techniques attach to them a misleading aura of precision by identifying them as psychological "tests." *Standards for Educational and Psychological Testing* (American Psychological Association, American Educational Research Association, & National Council on Measurement in Education, 1999), in the introductory section, offers a definition of "test": "A test is an evaluative device or procedure in which a sample of an examinee's behavior in a specified domain is obtained and subsequently evaluated and scored using a standardized process" (p. 3).

Chapters in previous editions of this text have supported the use of projective techniques in the psychological assessment of children (e.g., Chandler, 2003; Knoff, 2003). It is our position that consumers of our professional services are being misled when projective techniques are identified as psychological tests. As discussed extensively below, there is no support in current research for the notion that projective techniques constitute a scientifically informed psychological assessment procedure.

Chandler and Knoff are not the only colleagues who encourage the use of projective techniques in the psychological assessment of children. McClure, Kubiszyn, and Kaslow (2002) have argued that there is an urgent need for empirical validation of techniques used in the psychological assessment of children and point to a number of articles that they believe support such a use of projective techniques. Most of the articles they refer to, however, focus on the Rorschach test (see Hilsenroth, Fowler, & Padawer, 1998; Meyer et al., 2001), rather than more commonly used projective techniques.

It should be noted that, in commenting on the use of the Rorschach with children, Exner (1980, p. 569) has stated: "It would be very erroneous to assume that test findings developed from a record of a younger child can be used as indicators of 'things to come.'" Exner, Thomas, and Mason (1985, pp. 17 & 18) stated: "The magnitude of the many changes [that take place in children] argues against the decision to make long-term *predictive descriptions* [emphasis in original] concerning a child from a Rorschach taken prior to age 14." In addition, there are concerns about the Comprehensive System's normative data for children. The Comprehensive System's existing normative data, for example, may overpathologize psychologically healthy children (see for example, Shaffer, Erdberg, & Meyer, 2007).

Chapters in the previous edition of this volume describe the projective hypothesis as the theoretical foundation for projective techniques (e.g., Chandler, 2003); various projective techniques such as storytelling (Dupree & Prevatt, 2003); drawings (Knoff, 2003); sentence completion (Haak, 2003); the Rorschach, and, in particular, the Exner Comprehensive System, with children (Allen & Hollifield, 2003); and the Holtzman Inkblot Technique with children (Holtzman & Swartz, 2003). Writing about the use of the TAT, Dupree and Prevatt (2003) declare, "Despite the fact that there appears to be no consistently used, psychometrically sound scoring system for it, the TAT continues to enjoy widespread usage in academic training programs, internships, and clinical practice" (p. 71).

Reviews of research on the psychometric integrity of projective drawings reveal concerns that are similar to those that have been alluded to by Dupree and Prevatt with respect to the TAT. Knoff (2003) reported that any analysis of the usefulness of projective drawings is virtually impossible because of the multitude of methodologies used in such studies. He concludes that "these studies provide such widely differing methodological details that one cannot assume that results are clinically accurate and socially valid without additional validation and replication" (p. 101). Knoff concludes that interpretations of projective drawings are characterized by poor test-retest reliability and poor internal consistency. Citing a review of the psychometric literature on the Kinetic Family Drawing Technique (Handler & Habenicht, 1994), Knoff concludes that "few, if any, recent studies have specifically evaluated the reliability of projective drawings" (p. 101). In light of the fact that psychologists with favorable views of projective techniques acknowledge their psychometric deficiencies, we are perplexed by their continued use and by the frequent labeling of these techniques as psychological tests. Knoff (2003) suggests that projective drawing techniques (a) be used only for the generation of social, emotional, or behavioral hypotheses; (b) never be used as a sole basis of clinical diagnoses; and (c) never be used as the sole basis for conclusions.

The distinction between a "psychological test" and an "interview aid" is significant, and it is one that psychologists should take great care to make.

When the writer of a report identifies an assessment procedure or device as a "psychological test," readers of the report are likely assume that the procedure or device rests on a scientific foundation. Projective techniques are based on the projective hypothesis, which has never been validated. With the possible exception of the Rorschach, scored using the Exner system and the recently developed Rorschach Performance Assessment System[1] (Meyer, Viglione, Mihura, Erard, & Erdberg, 2011), not one of the projective techniques currently in use has been shown to have psychometric integrity. Therefore, we believe it is inappropriate to include such techniques on the lists of psychological tests that customarily appear in the opening sections of reports outlining the findings of comprehensive psychological assessments. It is our contention that, with the possible exception of the Exner-scored Rorschach and the newer Rorschach Performance Assessment System, no projective techniques have demonstrated reliability and validity sufficient to justify their use as anything other than interview aids (see, e.g., Mihura, Meyer, Dumitrascu, & Bombel, 2012). When we reflect on the reports we have reviewed over the years, it is our impression that only a small percentage of the evaluators who employ projective techniques describe the strengths and limitations of the interpretations they have generated.

More often than not, the readers of reports that have been prepared in a clinical context are not informed of the limitations of interpretations based on psychometrically unsound assessment techniques. In our judgment, the failure to include a discussion of the limitations of projective techniques violates both the letter and the spirit of the ethical code.

> Ethical Standard 9.02 (b): Psychologists use assessment instruments whose validity and reliability have been established for use with members of the population tested. When such validity or reliability has not been established, psychologists describe the strengths and limitations of test results and interpretation.

When parents are in the process of choosing pediatricians, the parents are entitled to know whether the pediatricians practice conventional, mainstream medicine that includes administering scientifically developed medical tests, or use holistic or Far Eastern approaches to maintaining health. When pediatricians use unconventional treatment methods that do not enjoy scientific support in the medical literature yet find support in holistic, alternative treatment literature, parents are entitled to the information that will enable them to make informed decisions in selecting health care practitioners for their children.

In 2006, Trubitt, recognizing the unreliability of assessments of children that rely on interpretations of the children's drawings or play, nevertheless advised play therapists to "continue to use play therapy methods" (Trubitt, 2006, p. 5). She opined: "We do not have to mention [our] use [of these methods]" (p. 5). Our perspective contrasts sharply with Trubitt's. In our view, when psychologists use projective techniques and utilize interpretations of responses to projective stimuli in diagnosing children, the psychologists have an ethical responsibility to inform parents of the known psychometric deficiencies in projective assessment techniques. Standard 9.03 (a) of the Psychologists' Ethics Code admonishes psychologists to "obtain informed consent for assessments, evaluations, or diagnostic services...." One cannot give informed consent to any procedure (including an assessment procedure) without first having been provided with all pertinent information. In particular, psychologists should disclose the risks known to be associated with their favored assessment procedures and should discuss alternative assessment methods.

We have found evaluators who believe children's drawings can be helpful even though they lack psychometric integrity. For example, the following was taken from a report reviewed by one of the authors:

> The House-Tree-Person test is based on the premise that unconscious aspects of the personality are exposed through the person's drawings of familiar items. Children who are in stressful situations are often hesitant to respond to direct questioning about this experience. Researchers have studied the H-T-P to determine if these children produce discrete indicators of their situation, however the test's validity and reliability have not been proven. Despite this lack of psychometric support, the test can be very valuable in providing general information about a child's personality.

Such an approach is consistent with the "broken clock" approach to psychometric integrity: Even a broken clock is accurate twice a day.

Many of our psychodynamically oriented colleagues believe strongly in the usefulness of psychodynamic concepts and believe that projective techniques shed light on unconscious processes, filling a void that is created by the use of self-report inventories. Our position, quite simply, is that when using assessment procedures that lack an empirically supportable theoretical foundation and lack demonstrable reliability and validity, psychologists have a responsibility under Ethical Standard 9.03 (a) to provide full information concerning the techniques, so that those with decision-making authority (parents, school administrators, courts) are able to make informed decisions.

It is our position that if one fully understands the concept of projection, one is more likely than not to conclude that drawings cannot possibly be viewed as a reliable source of information concerning children's perceptions of themselves, their families, the dynamics within their families, or anything else. Even if it could be demonstrated that the dynamic of projection consistently operates as children produce these drawings, there would still be no basis for conceptualizing interpretations of drawings as a reliable data source. The early proponents of projective techniques made it clear that we cannot be certain what perceptions, attitudes, fears, or wishes are being projected.

Practitioners who request that children "draw a person" are generally in agreement that the same-sex figure should be conceptualized as a "self" figure. Even if we presume that drawings "tell" us something about the psychology of children who have produced drawings, it must be recognized that the "self" figure may represent a child's perception of himself or herself (with emphasis either on physical or psychological attributes); may represent what s/he wishes himself or herself to be (again, with emphasis either on physical or psychological attributes); or, to complicate things further, the drawing may symbolically portray physical or psychological impairment, compensation for a real or perceived shortcoming, or a combination of these factors.

If these cautionary statements are applied to family drawings, it follows that if a child produces a drawing in which she places herself close to her father, this may represent a projection of her perception of her relationship with her father, but it may also represent a wish rather than a perception. The child with a father who is either physically absent or emotionally distant might draw the father close to the child. An older child whose drawing skills are somewhat better might draw himself being cared for by a parent who, in reality, provides deficient care.

Other complicating factors must also be considered. Even if children's family drawings reflected the children's perceptions of family relationships as accurately as thermometers measure temperature, there is no basis whatsoever for presuming that such perceptions are stable over time. How a particular child views his parents and his relationship with each of them today may be dramatically different from how he will view his parents and his relationship with them six months from today. Finally, even if we could presume that it is always a perception (as opposed to a wish) that is being projected, and even if we could presume that such perceptions are reasonably stable over time, there is no basis for presuming that children's perceptions of family dynamics are accurate. Neither is there a basis for presuming that if children's perceptions are inaccurate, it does not matter, because it is only their perceptions that are of concern to us. Reality matters.

There are no data demonstrating that children's drawings display temporal stability (test/retest reliability) and there is no evidence that different experts viewing the same drawing will formulate the same opinions concerning the information provided by the drawing. Though some of those who wish to employ drawings in their assessments have endeavored to create standardized processes, there is no evidence to suggest that any of the systems designed to date demonstrate acceptable inter-judge reliability.

The standardized processes alluded to above involve utilization of what is known as the "sign approach" to figure-drawing interpretation, in which certain features in the drawings are viewed as signs (indicators) of various life experiences or personality characteristics. In commenting on the sign approach, several well-respected writers have concluded that the advocates of the sign method often disagree among themselves concerning what a particular feature indicates (Lally, 2001).

Richard Dana (1996), a psychologist who has written extensively on projective techniques, has called attention to the fact that interpretations of responses to projective stimuli are vulnerable to *eisegesis*—distortion stemming from projection by the examiner (as opposed to the examinee) deriving from the examiner's theoretical biases, emotional investment in certain hypotheses, etc. The late Anne Anastasi (Anastasi & Urbina, 1997), one of psychology's leaders in the field of assessment, opined that the interpretation of responses to projective stimuli "may reveal more about the theoretical orientation, favorite hypotheses, and personality idiosyncrasies of the examiner than it does about the examinee's personality dynamics."

Though no published data are available for reference, it is our impression that more often than not, practitioners who rely upon drawings as an assessment technique offer no statements in their reports that might alert readers to the deficiencies in the technique. In the 1999 edition of *Standards for Educational and Psychological Testing* (APA et al., 1999), the following admonition appears: "Professionals are expected to make every effort to be aware of evidence of validity and reliability that supports or does not support their inferences and to place appropriate limits on the opinions rendered." In reviews of drawing techniques prepared for The Buros Institute and published in the *Mental Measurements Yearbook*, reviewers have consistently concluded that there are no empirical data to support the use of drawings.

Some clinicians and forensic evaluators have utilized drawings produced by a child for the purpose of identifying the child as a member of a specific group (for example, sexually abused children). There are no data to support the notion that interpretations of drawings can be effectively used for the purpose of discriminating between two classes of examinees. Research has repeatedly shown drawings to be lacking in discriminant validity. Even if there were research findings supporting the contention that a certain feature is often observed in drawings produced by abused children, detection of this feature would be useful only if research also demonstrated that the specified feature is observed exclusively in the drawings of abused children and is not observed in the drawings of non-abused children.

The methods employed both by treatment providers and by evaluators in gathering information from children differ dramatically from the methods employed in gathering information from adults. Statements made by individuals of any age are viewed as a data source, and mental health professionals interviewing children often find that play, building tasks, drawing tasks, and similar activities facilitate constructive oral interaction. When drawings are utilized as a stimulus for conversation and where it is the statements made that are conceptualized as the data source, it is unlikely that any harm is created by the use of drawings. We contend, however, that significant risk of harm is created when no inquiry is conducted and when the drawings themselves and the mental health professional's interpretations of those drawings are viewed as a data source.

The psychologists' Ethical Standard 9.02 (a) reads: "Psychologists administer, adapt, score, interpret, or use assessment techniques, interviews, tests, or instruments in a manner and for purposes that are appropriate *in light of the research on or evidence of the usefulness and proper application of the techniques* [emphasis added]." Section (b) reads, in pertinent part: "Psychologists use assessment instruments *whose validity and reliability have been established* [emphasis added] for use with members of the population tested." It is our position that projective assessment techniques do not meet the criteria alluded to in the ethics code.

Notes

1. The Rorschach Research Council began in 1997 with the goal to improve the research of the Comprehensive System. Following Exner's death in 2006, several members of the original Rorschach Research Council developed the Rorschach Performance Assessment System, also known as the R-PAS. The goal of this group was to expand on the evidence-based scoring and interpretation of the Comprehensive System. The R-PAS group developed a more structured administration procedure, a detailed scoring system and kept only those scores and indices with solid research foundations. Their work relied heavily on a meta-analytic review of the Comprehensive System's variables (Mihura, Meyer, Dumitrascu, & Bombel, 2012). At this point, the R-PAS has an extensive manual, a computer-assisted scoring system that utilizes an extensive international reference group, and uses research-based interpretive strategies.

References

Ackerman, M. J., & Kane, A. W. (2002). *Psychological experts in divorce actions* (4th ed.). New York: Aspen Law & Business.

Allen, J. C., & Hollifield, J. (2003). Using the Rorschach with children and adolescents: The Exner comprehensive system. In C. R. Reynolds & R. W. Kamphaus (Eds.), *Handbook of psychological and educational assessment of children: Personality, behavior, and context* (2nd ed.; pp. 182–197). New York: Guilford Press.

American Educational Research Association, American Psychological Association & National Council on Measurement in Education. (1999). *Standards for educational and psychological testing*. Washington, DC: American Psychological Association.

American Psychological Association. (2002). Ethical principles of psychologists and code of conduct. *American Psychologist, 57*, 1060–1073.

Anastasi, A., & Urbina, S. (1997). *Psychological testing* (7th ed.). Upper Saddle River, NJ: Prentice-Hall.

Association of Family and Conciliation Courts. (2007). *Model standards of practice for child custody evaluations*. Madison, WI: AFCC.

Bow, J., Gould, J., Flens, J., & Greenhut, D. (2006). Testing in child custody evaluations—Selection, usage, and *Daubert* admissibility: A survey of psychologists. *Journal of Forensic Psychology Practice, 6*(2), 17–38.

Bow, J., Flens, J., Gould, J. W., & Greenhut, D. (2006). An analysis of administration, scoring, and interpretation of the MMPI-2 and MCMI-III in child custody evaluations. *Journal of Child Custody, 2*(4), 1–22.

Ceci, S. J., Kulkofsky, S., Klemfuss, J. Z., Sweeney, C. D., & Bruck, M. (2007). Unwarranted assumptions about children's

testimonial accuracy. *Annual Review of Clinical Psychology, 3*, 311–328.

Chandler, L. A. (2003). The projective hypothesis and the development of projective techniques for children. In C. R. Reynolds & R. W. Kamphaus (Eds.), *Handbook of psychological and educational assessment of children: Personality, behavior, and context (2nd ed.*; pp. 51–65). New York: Guilford Press.

Committee on Professional Practice and Standards, American Psychological Association. (2007). *Record keeping guidelines*. Washington, DC: Author.

Dana, R. H. (1996). The thematic apperception test (TAT). In C. S. Newmark (Ed.), *Major psychological assessment instruments* (2nd ed.). Boston: Allyn & Bacon.

Daubert v. Merrell Dow Pharmaceuticals Inc. 125 L.Ed.2d. 469 [1993].

Dickersin, K. (1990). The existence of publication bias and risk factors for its occurrence. *Journal of the American Medical Association, 263*(10), 1385–1359.

Dickersin, K., Chan, S., Chalmers, T. C., Sacks, H. S., & Smith, H. (1987). Publication bias and clinical trials. *Controlled Clinical Trials, 8*(4), 343–353.

Dupree, J. L. & Prevatt, F. (2003). Projective storytelling techniques. In C. R. Reynolds & R. W. Kamphaus (Eds.), *Handbook of psychological and educational assessment of children: Personality, behavior, and context* (2nd ed.; pp. 66–90). New York: Guilford Press.

Exner, J. E., Jr. (1980). But it's only an inkblot. *Journal of Personality Assessment, 44*, 563–577.

Exner, J. E., Jr., Thomas, E. A., & Mason, B. (1985). Children's Rorschachs: Description and prediction. *Journal of Personality Assessment, 49*, 13–20.

Faigman, D. L., Kaye, D. H., Saks, M. J., & Sanders, J. (2002). *Science in the law: Standards, statistics, and research issues*. St. Paul, MN: West Group.

Federal Rules of Civil Procedure. United States Code.

Federal Rules of Evidence. United States Code. Title 28.

Gould, J. W. (2006). *Conducting scientifically crafted child custody evaluations* (2nd ed.). Sarasota, FL: Professional Resource Press.

Gould, J. W., Martindale, D. A., & Flens, J. R. (2009). Use of psychological tests in child custody evaluations. In R. M. Galatzer-Levy, L. Kraus, & J. Galatzer-Levy. *Scientific basis of child custody decisions* (2nd ed., pp. 85–124). New York: Wiley.

Greenberg, L. R., Martindale, D. A., Gould, J. W., & Gould-Saltman, D. J. (2004). Ethical issues in child custody and dependency cases: Enduring principles and emerging challenges. *Journal of Child Custody, 1*(1), 9–32.

Haak, R. A. (2003). The sentence completion as a tool for assessing emotional disturbance. In C. R. Reynolds & R. W. Kamphaus (Eds.), *Handbook of psychological and educational assessment of children: Personality, behavior, and context* (2nd ed.; pp. 159–181). New York: Guilford Press.

Handler, L., & Habenicht, D. (1994). The kinetic family drawing technique: A review of the literature. *Journal of Personality Assessment, 62*(3), 440–464.

Hilsenroth, M. J., Fowler, J. C., & Padawer, J. R. (1998, June). The Rorschach Schizophrenia Index (SCZI): An examination of reliability, validity, and diagnostic efficiency. *Journal of Personality Assessment, 70*(3), 514–534.

Holtzman, W., & Swartz, J. D. (2003). Use of the Holtzman inkblot technique with children. In C. R. Reynolds & R. W. Kamphaus (Eds.), *Handbook of psychological and educational assessment of children: Personality, behavior, and context* (2nd ed.; pp. 198–215). New York: Guilford Press.

Kerr, N. L. (1998). HARKing: Hypothesizing after the results are known. *Personality and Social Psychology Review, 2*(3), 196–217. doi: 10.1207/s15327957pspr0203_4

Knoff, H. M. (2003). Evaluation of projective drawings. In C. R. Reynolds & R. W. Kamphaus (Eds.), *Handbook of psychological and educational assessment of children: Personality, behavior, and context* (2nd ed.; pp. 91–158). New York: Guilford Press.

Lally, S. J. (2001). Should human figure drawings be admitted into court? *Journal of Personality Assessment, 76*(1), 135–149.

Lee, C. M., & Hunsley, J. (2003). Evidence-based assessment of childhood mood disorders: Comment on McClure, Kubiszyn, and Kaslow (2002). *Professional Psychology: Research & Practice, 34*(1), 112–113.

Martindale, D. A. (2005a). Confirmatory bias and confirmatory distortion. *Journal of Child Custody, 2*(2), 31–48.

Martindale, D. A. (2008). One picture may not be worth 1,000 words. *The Matrimonial Strategist,* Available at http://www.lawjournalnewsletters.com retrieved on October 10, 2010.

Martindale, D. A., & Gould, J. W. (2008). Failure of peer review. *The Matrimonial Strategist*, February. Available at www.lawjournalnewsletters.com retrieved on November 26, 2012.

McClure, E. B., Kubiszyn, T., & Kaslow, N. J. (2003). Evidence-based assessment of childhood mood disorders: Reply to Lee and Hunsley (2003). *Professional Psychology: Research & Practice, 34*(1), 113–114.

McClure, E. B., Kubiszyn, T., & Kaslow, N. J. (2002). Advances in the diagnosis and treatment of childhood disorders. *Professional Psychology: Research & Practice, 33*(2), 125–134.

Meyer, G. J., Finn, S. E., Eyde, L. D., Kay, G. G., Moreland, K. L., Dies, R. R., et al. (2001). Psychological testing and psychological assessment: A review of evidence and issues. *American Psychologist, 56*(2), 128–165.

Meyer, G. J., Viglione, D. J., Mihura, J. L., Erard, R. E. & Erdberg, P. (2011). *Rorschach Performance Assessment System: Administration, coding, interpretation, and technical manual.* Toledo: Rorschach Performance Assessment System.

Shuman, D. W., & Sales, B. D. (1998). The admissibility of expert testimony based upon clinical judgment and scientific research. *Psychology, Public Policy & Law, 4*(4), 1226–1252.

Mihura, J. L., Meyer, G. J., Dumutrascu, N., & Bombel, G. (2012). The validity of the individual Rorschach variables: Systematic reviews and meta-analyses of the Comprehensive System. *Psychological Bulletin.* August 27, 2012. doi: 10.1037/a0029406.

Rosenthal, R. (1979). The file drawer problem and tolerance for null results. *Psychological Bulletin, 86*(3), 638–641.

Shaffer, T. W., Erdberg, P., & Meyer, G. J. (Eds.) (2007). International reference samples for the Rorschach Comprehensive System [Special issue]. *Journal of Personality Assessment, 89*(Suppl. 1), S2–S6.

Trubitt, A. (2006). Workshop outline for To play or not to play in child custody evaluations: Recent challenges in current practice. Workshop presented Oct. 13, 2006, at the Association for Play Therapy Conference in Toronto, Canada.

United States v. Smith, 869 F.2d 348 [U. S. App. Dist. 7, 1989].

United States v. Williams, 583 F.2d 1194 [U. S. App. Dist. CA2 1978]).

Zeedyk, M. S., & Raitt, F. E. (1998). Psychological evidence in the courtroom: Critical reflections on the General Acceptance Standard. *Journal of Community & Applied Social Psychology, 8*, 23–39.

PART 2

Models of Assessment

Cognitive Assessment: Progress in Psychometric Theories of Intelligence, the Structure of Cognitive Ability Tests, and Interpretive Approaches to Cognitive Test Performance

Dawn P. Flanagan, Vincent C. Alfonso, Samuel O. Ortiz, *and* Agnieszka M. Dynda

Abstract

This chapter highlights the progress that has been made in theories of intelligence (particularly psychometric theories), the structure of cognitive ability batteries, and methods of cognitive ability test interpretation over the past century. Early theories of intelligence revolved around notions of a single general factor, or *g*, but steadily advanced into two-factor models (e.g., original *Gf–Gc*), early multiple-factor models (e.g., Thurstone's Primary Mental Abilities), and eventually to current, multiple-factor models (e.g., Cattell-Horn-Carroll [CHC] theory). Also discussed is the fact that cognitive batteries seldom kept pace with developments in theory, but they nevertheless have shown significant growth and development overall, particular within the last decade. The latter half of the chapter provides a discussion of refinements to CHC theory at both the broad and narrow ability levels, application of CHC theory to academic outcomes research, integration of CHC and neuropsychological theories, and greater emphasis on flexible battery approaches. We conclude that contemporary cognitive assessment allows for sufficient illustration of the links between abilities (e.g., cognitive and academic) and neuropsychological processes such that avenues for instruction, intervention, and treatment of individuals who struggle to learn will not only be clear, but also empirically supported.

Key Words: psychometric theories, CHC theory, cognitive assessment, cross-battery, flexible battery, intelligence, neuropsychological assessment

Introduction

As the measurement of cognitive abilities with standardized, norm-referenced tests passes its first century of practice, it seems appropriate to write about the progress that has been made in psychometric theories of intelligence, the structure of cognitive ability tests, and interpretive approaches to cognitive test performance. Indeed much has changed since the days of Spearman's general intelligence or *g* factor and the Stanford-Binet Intelligence Scale (Terman, 1916). Although progress in psychometric theories of intelligence was steady and proceeded gradually over a period of decades, measurement and interpretation of cognitive abilities did not keep pace. Despite 100 years of psychological assessment, the most significant changes in the practice of the measurement and interpretation of cognitive abilities occurred recently and over an astonishingly short period of time.

In a review of the state of the art in cognitive assessment prior to 2000, Flanagan and colleagues (Flanagan, Ortiz, Alfonso, & Dynda, 2008) pointed out a number of major concerns with cognitive assessment that existed at the time. For example, they noted that nearly all intelligence (or cognitive) batteries available prior to 2000 were mainly "based on either outdated (psychometric) theory or no theory at all" (p. 633). Historically, psychological testing was more concerned with practical issues than theoretical ones, apart from vague notions of Spearman's g (see Wasserman, 2012). Thus, even up to the brink of the twenty-first century, practitioners were routinely using intelligence tests that were not, in fact, based on the most current and credible scientific evidence (Carroll, 1993a; Flanagan & Ortiz, 2001; Horn, 1991; Kamphaus, 1993; McGrew & Flanagan, 1998; Shaw, Swerdlik, & Laurent, 1993).

Flanagan and colleagues (2008) also pointed out that the major contribution of intelligence tests was the intelligence quotient itself (or Full Scale IQ [FSIQ] as defined by the popular Wechsler scales) (e.g., Flanagan, McGrew, & Ortiz, 2000). The term *IQ* worked its way into the common vernacular quickly and, since the publication of the Wechsler-Bellevue in 1939, became central and critical to virtually all clinical, educational, and neuropsychological conclusions, diagnoses, and decisions (Kamphaus, Winsor, Rowe, & Kim, 2005, 2012). Despite the prominence and ubiquity of IQ, many researchers questioned whether such a reputation was deserved and whether IQ had significant relevance for differential diagnosis and treatment (e.g., Carroll, 1993a; Flanagan et al., 2000; Lezak, 1995; Reschly & Grimes, 1995; Sternberg, 1993). By the 1990s, there was considerable debate regarding the utility of IQ in psychological evaluations, with one camp arguing its superiority over analysis of lower-order composites and subtests (e.g., McDermott, Fantuzzo, & Glutting, 1990) and the other camp arguing that IQ should be de-emphasized or replaced with an evaluation of multiple, theory-based ability composites (e.g., Horn & Blankson, 2005; Keith, Kranzler, & Flanagan, 2001; McGrew, Flanagan, Keith, & Vanderwood, 1997). While both camps have continued this debate (see Canivez, this volume; and Reynolds, Keith, Flanagan, & Alfonso, in press), current intelligence tests (now more popularly known as "cognitive" tests) are, nevertheless, on the whole more firmly grounded in contemporary psychometric theory and research than their predecessors.

The purpose of this chapter is to describe the progress that has been made in: (a) psychometric theories of intelligence or the structure of cognitive abilities; (b) the structure of cognitive ability tests; and (c) interpretive approaches to cognitive test performance. Figure 12.1 highlights the progress that has been made in each of these areas via three continua. It is important to recognize that the three continua presented in Figure 12.1 do not represent linear timelines; rather, they portray developments in the three broad categories of theories, tests, and interpretive approaches. Also noteworthy is the fact that the specific theories, tests, and interpretive approaches listed in Figure 12.1 are examples and, therefore, the figure does not contain a complete list in any of the three continua. This chapter discusses each continuum and concludes with a description of the current state-of-the-art of cognitive assessment.

Progress in Psychometric Theories of Intelligence

There is perhaps only one irrefutable law or truth in psychology—the law of individual differences (cf. McGrew & Flanagan, 1998). Accordingly, "individuals differ from one another in their ability to understand complex ideas, to adapt effectively to the environment, to learn from experience, to engage in various forms of reasoning, to overcome obstacles by taking thought" (Neisser et al., 1996, p. 77). The construct of *intelligence* has been offered to explain and clarify this particular constellation of abilities, and tests were developed to account for individual differences among them.

Attempts to define the construct of intelligence and to explain individual differences in intellectual functioning have been characterized by much variability over the period of several decades (e.g., Carroll, 1993b; Gustafsson & Undheim, 1996; Horn, 1991; McGrew, 1997, 2005; Schneider & McGrew, 2012; Taylor, 1994; Thorndike, 1997). The significant differences between theories of intelligence are exemplified by the various multiple intelligences models that have been offered and revised recently to explain the structure of intelligence; namely, the Cattell-Horn Fluid-Crystallized (*Gf-Gc*) theory (Horn & Blankson, 2005), Carroll's three-stratum theory of cognitive abilities (Carroll, 1993b, 1997), Gardner's Theory of Multiple Intelligences (Chen & Gardner, 2012), the Luria-Das model of information processing (Naglieri, Das, & Goldstein, 2012), Sternberg's Triarchic Theory of Intelligence (Sternberg, 2012), and the Cattell-Horn-Carroll (CHC) theory of cognitive abilities (McGrew, 2005; Schneider & McGrew, 2012). Each of these theories provides a framework for understanding the

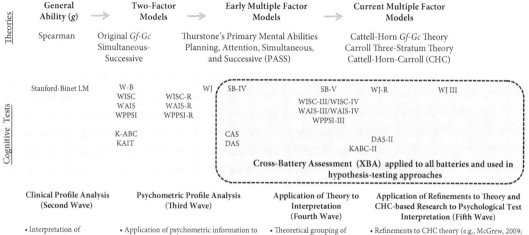

Figure 12.1 Progress in psychometric theories of intelligence, the structure of cognitive ability tests, and interpretive approaches to cognitive test performance.

Note: This figure is an adaptation and extension of Woodcock's (1994) "Continuum of Progress in Theories of Multiple Intelligences" and Flanagan, McGrew, and Ortiz's (2000) "Progress in Psychometric Theories and Applied Measures of Intelligence." The second, third, and fourth waves of interpretation included in this figure were described by Kamphaus, Petoskey, and Morgan (1997). The first wave of interpretation (quantification of general level) is omitted from this figure due to space limitations.

multi-differentiated structure of cognitive abilities and the interrelationships among them. For a comprehensive description of these theories, the reader is referred to Flanagan and Harrison (2005, 2012). This chapter will focus specifically on the *psychometric* or structural approach to understanding individual differences.

The psychometric approach "attempts to measure performance along dimensions which are purported to constitute the fundamental structure of the psychological domain" (Taylor, 1994, p. 185). The psychometric approach relies on psychological tests that yield scores on qualitative scales that may be analyzed by correlative and factor-analytic methods to identify ability dimensions that form the structure of individual differences in cognitive ability (Gustafsson & Undheim, 1996; Keith, 2005; Keith & Reynolds, 2010, 2012; McGrew, 1997, 2005). As compared to other theoretical and research traditions (e.g., information processing, cognitive modifiability; see Taylor, 1994, for an overview), the psychometric approach is the oldest, most research-based and best established (Daniel, 1997; Gustafsson & Undheim). Additionally, the psychometric approach led to the most economically efficient and practical tests for measuring intelligence in applied settings (Neisser et al., 1996). Space limitations preclude the presentation of a detailed summary of the history and evolution of the dominant psychometric theories of intelligence (see Wasserman, 2012, for more information). Instead, we provide here a general description of the progress in psychometric approaches, as depicted in the top portion of Figure 12.1.

Spearman's *g*-Factor Theory

The genesis of the psychometric research tradition, by and large, is considered to have begun with Spearman's (1904, 1927) development of factor analytic techniques with which he offered a *general* or *g*-factor that became synonymous with the concept of general intelligence. Although Spearman's model refers rightly to a two-factor theory (i.e., *g*, the general factor to which all tests contribute, and *s*, the specific information provided by each test), the general factor was always considered to be preeminent and *s* factors were always subordinate, so that the theory was seen largely as a single-factor model of intelligence. His application of factor analytic methods to general mental ability measures provided the basis for defining both the substance of general intelligence and the tests that were developed to measure it (Jensen, 1998). Spearman's *g* is thus a theory of general intelligence, a single factor that accounts for the performance of individuals on nearly all types of cognitive tasks.

Despite the view that Spearman's *g* represents a single-factor theory, Spearman himself did not entirely let go of the possible significance of the *s* factors, which he believed could represent independent and unique factors apart from the group factor known as *g*. In fact, together with Karl Holziner, he developed a "bi-factor" model that may have been the beginning of a recognition of *s* factors as being more than merely subordinate to general ability but perhaps important in their own right. According to Carroll (1993b), if Spearman had lived beyond 1945, he most likely would have converged on a multiple-abilities model similar to the ones proposed by other researchers (e.g., Thurstone's [1938] "primary mental abilities"), although unlike Thurstone and others, he would have probably retained the notion of *g* as a measure of general intelligence.

Two-Factor Theories and Models

The demise of Spearman's general factor and bi-factor models might have begun as early as 1909, primarily as a result of the evidence presented by Sir Cyril Burt in favor of *group factors*. According to Jensen (1998), by 1911, Burt's data had convinced most psychologists that it was more reasonable to accept the existence and importance of independent group factors, *s*, in addition to *g*. The evidence for factors beyond *g* resulted in a variety of attempts to develop theories and measures of independent vs. general group factor abilities. The recognition that a complete understanding of intelligence required the measurement and interpretation of abilities beyond *g* set the stage for the eventual development and interpretation of new intelligence tests. It is important to note, however, that Burt did not deny the existence of a general ability factor nor its cardinal position among factors, because it was necessary for support of the prevailing hereditarian views on intelligence. Burt suggested only that there did appear to be some significance to the lesser, but

independent factors, of which there appeared to be at least two promising candidates—verbal and quantitative abilities.

One of the early factor models of intelligence that did not involve a pyramidal hierarchy was developed by Raymond Cattell (1941, 1957) and included a framework that identified two independent but equally important abilities, which he named *fluid* (*Gf*) and *crystallized* (*Gc*). Cattell, who earned his doctoral degree under Spearman, believed his data suggested that *g* was not a unitary or general trait at all, but rather a composite of two different types of specific factors or abilities representing novel problem-solving (*Gf*) and consolidated knowledge (*Gc*) (Jensen, 1998). His model became known simply as *Gf-Gc* theory, and it formed the foundation for advancements in intelligence theory that still underlie research in the present day, despite not providing support for a single, supreme general ability factor (i.e., *g*).

Another framework that relied on a similar two-factor view of intelligence was later offered by Russian neuropsychologist A. R. Luria (1966, 1970, 1973, 1980), who utilized the prevailing information processing theory in the development of a "simultaneous-successive" processing model. According to Luria, *simultaneous* processing is involved in the integration or synthesis of stimuli into groups when the individual components of the stimuli are interrelated, and is primarily associated with the right hemisphere (Kaufman, 1994; Naglieri, 1997). In contrast, *successive* processing is involved when the individual stimuli are processed in a serial order and there is no point in time at which the stimuli are interrelated. This type of processing is typically associated with left-hemisphere functioning. Luria's model became and remains heavily influential as the guiding paradigm in the neuropsychological assessment arena, and like Cattell's model, it does not rely on any notion of general intelligence or *g*.

Early Multiple Intelligences Theories

Early investigations of the concept of intelligence were not limited to only two independent factors. As stated above, Thurstone, for example, proposed a factor analytic–based theory composed of seven *primary mental abilities* (PMAs; Thurstone, 1938; Thurstone & Thurstone, 1941). Thurstone's PMA theory suggested that, rather than being a function of *g*, performance on psychometric tests of cognitive ability was due to a number of primary mental abilities or faculties, such as spatial visualization (S), perceptual speed (P), number (N, computational), verbal comprehension (V), word fluency (W), associative memory (M), and inductive reasoning (R) (Gould, 1996; Kamphaus, 1993). Because of its complexity and range at the time, Thurstone's PMA model was not directly operationalized by any particular battery of tests. Nevertheless, whether by intention or not, many modern-day tests are constructed in a manner that is similar to that which Thurstone proposed (Taylor, 1994). Other examples of factor-analytically based models are seen in the works of Burt (1949), although, unlike Thurstone, who saw abilities as independent in an egalitarian manner, Burt continued to insist that secondary abilities beyond *g* were subordinate to it. Other models were later proposed by French, Eckstrom, and Price (1963), and Vernon (1961), but did not receive much attention. Given the benefit of hindsight, the generation of "multiple" intelligences theories described thus far are seen as relatively "limited" (Flanagan et al., 2008; McGrew & Flanagan, 1998).

As depicted in Figure 12.1, even the simultaneous/successive processing model ultimately evolved into four constructs and became known as the Planning, Attention, Simultaneous, and Successive model (PASS; Das & Naglieri, 1997; Naglieri, Das, & Goldstein, 2012). Planning is one of a number of activity-related executive functions used to identify and organize steps required to achieve a goal or carry out an intention. It is characterized by "forward thinking," the generation of alternatives, the weighing and making of choices, and the development of a framework or structure that provides direction in the completion of a plan (Lezak, 1995). Planning is associated with the prefrontal lobe region of the brain. Attention involves the processes that allow individuals to focus and respond to a particular stimulus while concurrently ignoring "competing" stimuli (Naglieri, 1997) and is associated with the brainstem region.

Current Multiple Intelligences Theories

Psychometric intelligence theories converged in recent years on a more complete multiple intelligences taxonomy, reflecting syntheses of factor-analytic research conducted over the past 60 to 70 years. The most recent representation of this taxonomy is reflected by the Cattell-Horn-Carroll theory of the structure of cognitive abilities. CHC theory is an integration of Horn's *Gf-Gc* and Carroll's three-stratum theories of intelligence.

Original Gf-Gc Theory and the Cattell-Horn Expanded Gf-Gc Theory: First Precursors to CHC Theory

The original concept of intelligence developed by Cattell in the early 1940s, *Gf-Gc* theory, was essentially a dichotomous view of human cognitive ability. Cattell based his theory on his own factor-analytic work as well as that of Thurstone, conducted in the 1930s. Cattell believed that fluid intelligence (*Gf*) included inductive and deductive reasoning abilities that were influenced by biological and neurological factors, as well as incidental learning through interaction with the environment. He postulated further that crystallized intelligence (*Gc*) consisted primarily of acquired knowledge abilities that reflected, to a large extent, the influences of acculturation (Cattell, 1957, 1971).

In 1965, Cattell's student John Horn reanalyzed Cattell's data and expanded the dichotomous *Gf-Gc* model to include four additional abilities; namely, visual perception or processing (*Gv*), short-term memory (short-term acquisition and retrieval— SAR or *Gsm*), long-term storage and retrieval (tertiary storage and retrieval—TSR or *Glr*), and speed of processing (*Gs*). Later Horn also added auditory processing ability (*Ga*) to the theoretical model and refined the definitions of *Gv, Gs,* and *Glr* (Horn, 1968; Horn & Stankov, 1982). By the early 1990s, Horn had added a factor representing an individual's quickness in reacting (reaction time) and making decisions (decision speed). The decision speed factor was labeled *Gt* (Horn, 1991). Finally, factors for quantitative ability (*Gq*) and broad reading/writing ability (*Grw*) were added to the model, based on the research of Horn (1991) and Woodcock (1994), respectively. As a result of the work of Horn and his colleagues, *Gf-Gc* theory expanded into an 10-factor model that became known as the Cattell–Horn *Gf-Gc* theory, or sometimes as *modern Gf-Gc theory* (Horn, 1991; Horn & Blankson, 2005; Horn & Noll, 1997).

Carroll's Three-Stratum Theory: Second Precursor to CHC Theory

In his seminal review of the world's literature on human cognitive abilities, Carroll (1993b) proposed that the structure of cognitive abilities could be understood best via three strata that differ in breadth and generality. The broadest and most general level of ability is represented by stratum III. According to Carroll, stratum III represents a general factor consistent with Spearman's (1927) concept of *g* and subsumes both broad (stratum II) and narrow (stratum I) abilities. The various broad (stratum II) abilities are denoted with an uppercase *g* followed by a lowercase letter(s), much as they had been written by Cattell and Horn (e.g., *Gf* and *Gc*). The eight broad abilities included in Carroll's theory subsume a large number of narrow (stratum I) abilities (Carroll, 1993b; see also Carroll, 1997).

The Cattell–Horn and Carroll Theories: Similarities and Differences

Figure 12.2 provides a comparison of the Cattell–Horn *Gf-Gc* theory and Carroll's three-stratum theory (with only broad abilities shown). These theories are presented together in order to highlight the most salient similarities and differences between them. It is readily evident that the theories have much in common, as each posits multiple broad (stratum II) abilities that, for the most part, have names and abbreviations that are either similar or identical. But there are at least four major structural differences between the two models that bear noting. First, Carroll's theory includes a general ability factor (stratum III) whereas the Cattell–Horn theory does not (see Schneider & McGrew, 2012, for a more detailed discussion regarding *g* in this context). Second, the Cattell–Horn theory includes quantitative reasoning as a distinct broad ability (i.e., *Gq*), whereas Carroll's theory includes

quantitative reasoning as a narrow ability subsumed by *Gf*. Third, the Cattell–Horn theory includes a distinct, broad reading/writing (*Grw*) factor. Carroll's theory includes reading and writing as narrow abilities subsumed by *Gc*. And fourth, Carroll's theory includes short-term memory with other memory abilities, such as associative memory, meaningful memory, and free-recall memory, under *Gy*, whereas the Cattell–Horn theory separates short-term memory (*Gsm*) from associative memory, meaningful memory, and free-recall memory, because the latter abilities are purported to measure long-term retrieval (*Glr* in Figure 12.2). Notwithstanding these differences, Carroll (1993b) concluded that the Cattell–Horn *Gf-Gc* theory represents the most comprehensive and reasonable approach to understanding the structure of cognitive abilities currently available.

A Decade of CHC Theory (2001–2011)

In the late 1990s, McGrew (1997) attempted to resolve some of the differences between the Cattell–Horn and Carroll models. On the basis of his research, McGrew proposed an "integrated" *Gf-Gc* theory, and he and his colleagues used this model as a framework for interpreting the Wechsler scales (Flanagan et al., 2000). This integrated theory became known as the "CHC theory of cognitive

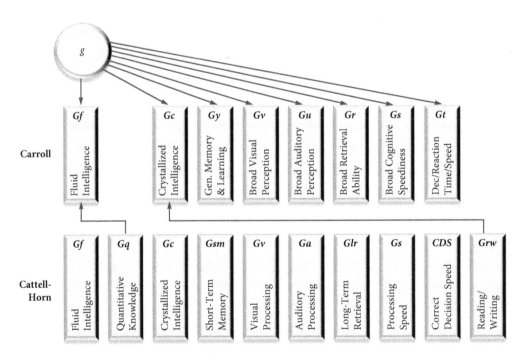

Figure 12.2 Comparison of the Cattell-Horn and Carroll theoretical models.

Note: This figure was reproduced with permission from the authors, Flanagan, McGrew, and Ortiz (2000). All rights reserved.

abilities" shortly thereafter (see McGrew, 2005), and the Woodcock-Johnson III Tests of Cognitive Abilities (WJ III COG; Woodcock, McGrew, & Mather, 2001) was the first cognitive battery to be based on this theory. The components of CHC theory are depicted in Figure 12.3. This figure shows that CHC theory consists of 10 broad cognitive abilities and more than 70 narrow abilities.

The CHC theory presented in Figure 12.3 omits a *g* or general ability factor, primarily because the utility of the theory (as it is employed in assessment-related disciplines) is in clarifying individual cognitive and academic strengths and weaknesses, which are understood best through the operationalization of broad (stratum II) and narrow (stratum I) abilities (Flanagan, Ortiz, & Alfonso, 2007, 2013). Others, however, believe that *g* is the most important ability to assess because it predicts the lion's share of the variance in multiple outcomes, both academic and occupational (e.g., Canivez & Watkins, 2010; Glutting, Watkins, & Youngstrom, 2003). Notwithstanding one's position on the importance of *g* in understanding various outcomes (particularly academic), there is considerable evidence that both broad and narrow CHC cognitive abilities explain a significant portion of variance in specific academic abilities, over and above the variance accounted for by *g* (e.g., Floyd, McGrew, & Evans, 2008; McGrew et al., 1997; Vanderwood, McGrew, Flanagan, & Keith, 2002).

The various revisions of and refinements to the original theory of fluid and crystallized intelligence over the past several decades, along with its mounting network of validity evidence, only began to influence intelligence test development relatively recently—that is, in the middle to late 1980s (see Schneider & McGrew, 2012). In the past decade, however, nearly every intelligence test developer and author acknowledged the importance of CHC theory in defining and interpreting cognitive ability constructs, and most have used this theory to guide directly the development of their cognitive tests. The increased importance given to CHC theory in intelligence test development is summarized next.

Progress in the Structure of Cognitive Ability Batteries

The middle portion of Figure 12.1 highlights progress in the structure of intelligence and cognitive ability batteries. Although there was substantial evidence supporting at least eight or nine broad cognitive CHC abilities by the late 1980s, intelligence tests of that era did not reflect this diversity in measurement. As such, there was a notable theory–practice gap in assessment practice (Flanagan & McGrew, 1997). For example, Table 12.1 shows that, from a CHC theoretical perspective, the popular ability tests such as the Wechsler Preschool and Primary Scale of Intelligence – Revised (WPPSI-R), Kaufman Assessment Battery for Children (KABC), Kaufman Adolescent and Adult Intelligence Test (KAIT), Wechsler Adult Intelligence Scale – Revised (WAIS-R), and Cognitive Assessment System (CAS) only measured two or three broad abilities adequately (Alfonso, Flanagan, & Radwan, 2005). The WPPSI-R primarily measured *Gv* and *Gc*. The K-ABC primarily measured *Gv* and *Gsm*, and to a much lesser extent, *Gf*, while the KAIT primarily measured *Gc* and *Glr*, and to a much lesser extent, *Gf* and *Gv*. The CAS measured *Gs*, *Gsm*, and *Gv*. Finally, while later tests, such as the Differential Ability Scales (DAS), Stanford-Binet Intelligence Scales – Fourth Edition (SB:FE), and Wechsler Intelligence Scale for Children –Third Edition (WISC-III) also failed to provide sufficient coverage of abilities to narrow the gap between contemporary theory and practice, their comprehensive measurement of approximately four CHC abilities was nonetheless an improvement over the aforementioned batteries. Table 12.1 shows that even as the new millennium dawned, only the Woodcock-Johnson Psycho-educational Battery – Revised (WJ-R) included tests that measured nearly all of the broad cognitive abilities depicted in Figure 12.3 (i.e., 9 out of 10) as compared to the other batteries available at that time, which measured far fewer broad abilities adequately (i.e., between 2 and 4; Alfonso et al., 2005; McGrew & Flanagan, 1998).

In general, Table 12.1 highlights the fact that many CHC abilities, namely *Gf*, *Gsm*, *Glr*, *Ga*, and *Gs*, were not measured well by the majority of intelligence and cognitive ability tests published prior to 2000. Therefore, it is clear that test authors did not make routine use of contemporary psychometric theories of the structure of cognitive abilities to guide the development of their tests. As such, the theory-practice gap continued; that is, theories of the structure of cognitive abilities were far in advance of the instruments used to operationalize them. In fact, prior to the mid 1980s, theory seldom played a fundamental role in intelligence test development. The numerous dashes in Table 12.1 exemplify the "theory-practice gap" that existed in the field of psychological assessment at that time (i.e., prior to

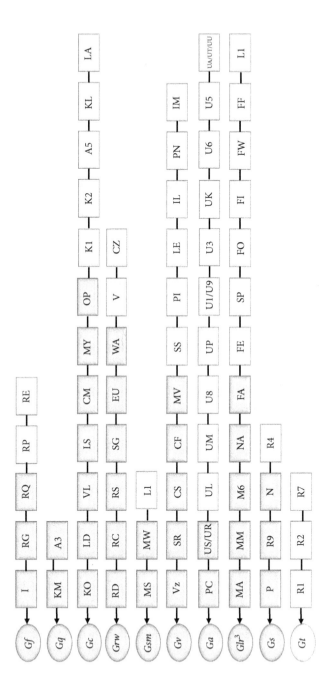

Figure 12.3 The Cattell-Horn-Carroll (CHC) model of cognitive abilities that guided intelligence test construction in the first decade of the millennium.

Note: Broad abilities appear as ovals and narrow abilities appear as rectangles in this figure. The shaded broad and narrow abilities are those that are measured most consistently on current and widely used cognitive and achievement tests. *Gf* = Fluid Intelligence; *Gq* = Quantitative Knowledge; *Gc* = Crystallized Intelligence; *Grw* = Reading/Writing Ability; *Gsm* = Short-Term Memory; *Gv* = Visual Processing; *Ga* = Auditory Processing; *Glr* = Long-Term Storage and Retrieval; *Gs* = Processing Speed; *Gt* = Decision Speed/Reaction Time. I = Induction; RG = General Sequential Reasoning; RQ = Quantitative Reasoning; RP = Piagetian Reasoning; RE = Speed of Reasoning; KM = Math Knowledge; A3 = Math Achievement; K0 = General (verbal) Knowledge; LD = Language Development; VL = Lexical Knowledge; LS = Listening Ability; CM = Communication Ability; MY = Grammatical Sensitivity; OP = Oral Production and Fluency; K1 = General Science Information; K2 = Information about Culture; A5 = Geography Achievement; KL = Foreign Language Proficiency; LA = Foreign Language Aptitude; RD = Reading Decoding; RC = Reading Comprehension; RS = Reading Speed; SG = Spelling Ability; EU = English Usage Knowledge; WA = Writing Ability; V = Verbal (printed) Language Comprehension; CZ = Cloze Ability; MS = Memory Span; MW = Working Memory; L1 = Learning Abilities; Vz = Visualization; SR = Spatial Relations; CS = Closure Speed; CF = Flexibility of Closure; MV = Visual Memory; SS = Spatial Scanning; PI = Serial Perceptual Integration; LE = Length Estimation; IL = Perceptual Illusions; PN = Perceptual Alternations; IM = Imagery; PC = Phonetic Coding; US/UR = Speech Sound Discrimination/ Resistance to Auditory Stimulus Distortion; UL = Sound Localization; UM = Memory for Sound Patterns; U8 = Maintaining and Judging Rhythm; U1/U9 = Musical Discrimination and Judgment; U3 = General Sound Discrimination; UK = Temporal Tracking; U6 = Sound-Intensity/Duration Discrimination; U5 = Sound-Frequency Discrimination; UA/UT/UU = Hearing and Speech Threshold Factors; MA = Associative Memory; MM = Meaningful Memory; M6 = Free Recall Memory; NA = Naming Facility; FA = Associational Fluency; FE = Expressional Fluency; SP = Sensitivity Problems; FO = Originality/ Creativity; FI = Ideational Fluency; FW = Word Fluency; FF = Figural Fluency; P = Perceptual Speed; N = Number Facility; R4 = Semantic Processing Speed; R1 = Simple Reaction Time; R2 = Choice Reaction Time; R7 = Mental Comparison Speed.

Table 12.1 Cognitive Subtests Representing Broad CHC Abilities on Nine Intelligence Batteries Published Prior to 2000

	Gf	Gc	Gv	Gsm	Glr	Ga	Gs
WISC-III	–	Vocabulary Information Similarities Comprehension	Block Design Object Assembly Picture Arrangement Picture Completion Mazes	Digit Span	–	–	Symbol Search Coding
WAIS-R	–	Vocabulary Information Similarities Comprehension	Block Design Object Assembly Picture Completion Picture Arrangement	Digit Span	–	–	Digit-Symbol
WPPSI-R	–	Vocabulary Information Similarities Comprehension	Block Design Object Assembly Picture Completion Mazes Geometric Design	Sentences	–	–	Animal Pegs
KAIT	Mystery Codes Logical Steps	Definitions Famous Faces Auditory Comprehension Double Meanings	Memory for Block Designs	–	Rebus Learning Rebus Delayed Recall Auditory Delayed Recall	–	–
K-ABC	Matrix Analogies	–	Triangles Face Recognition Gestalt Closure Magic Window Hand Movements Spatial Memory Photo Series	Number Recall Word Order	–	–	–

2000; Alfonso et al., 2005; Flanagan & McGrew, 1997).

Despite the persistent gap between theory and practice, much has changed in the past decade to narrow the gap. Particularly, CHC theory had a significant impact on the revision of nearly all cognitive tests that were revised in the 2000's. There are likely various reasons for this "collective psychometric epiphany" (Flanagan et al., 2008) in the field of psychological assessment, such as the wealth of research supporting CHC theory and the well-established relationships among its component parts and various outcomes (e.g., academic). In addition, advances in training standards, better operationalization and definitions of learning disabilities, and the rise in popularity of systematic, theoretically, and psychometrically defensible interpretive approaches (e.g., the cross-battery approach [XBA]; Flanagan et al., 2001, 2007, 2013; McGrew & Flanagan, 1998; this method of assessment is discussed in the last section of this chapter) facilitated the field's convergence on CHC theory to guide practice. As a result, a wider range of broad and narrow abilities is now represented on current intelligence batteries than that which was represented on any and all previous editions of these tests. Table 12.2 provides several salient examples of the impact that CHC theory and the XBA CHC classifications have had on intelligence test development in recent years. In addition, Table 12.2 lists the major intelligence tests in the order in which they were revised, beginning with those tests with the greatest number of years between revisions (i.e., K-ABC) and ending with newly revised tests (i.e., WPPSI-IV). As is obvious from a review of Table 12.2, CHC theory and the CHC XBA classifications have had a significant impact on recent test development (Alfonso et al., 2005).

Of the seven intelligence batteries that were published since 2000, the test authors of four explicitly used CHC theory and the CHC XBA classifications as the foundation upon which to guide test construction and development (i.e., WJ III, SB5, KABC-II, and DAS-II). Only in the case of the Wechsler Scales (i.e., WPPSI-III, WPPSI-IV, WISC-IV, WAIS-IV) is there no direct reference as to whether CHC theory was used as a guide for revision. Nevertheless, the authors of the Wechsler Scales do acknowledge the research of Cattell, Horn, and Carroll in their most recent manuals (Wechsler, 2002, 2003, 2008, 2012) and it would appear that CHC theory played an important role in shaping the final versions of each test whether so stated or not. The information contained in Table 12.2 demonstrates that all intelligence and cognitive tests in current use with some regularity subscribe either explicitly or implicitly to CHC theory (Alfonso et al., 2005; Flanagan et al., 2007, 2012).

Additional information and data regarding the convergence of recent intelligence and cognitive ability tests toward the incorporation of CHC theory is presented in Table 12.3. This table is similar to Table 12.1, except that it includes all the major intelligence and cognitive ability tests published after 2000, including the revisions of many of the tests from Table 12.1. This table also includes the *narrow* CHC abilities that are measured by the subtests within each of the batteries. A comparison of Tables 12.1 and 12.3 shows that many of the gaps in measurement of *broad* cognitive abilities have now been filled. Specifically, the majority of tests published after 2000 now measure four to five broad cognitive abilities and do so adequately (see Table 12.3), as compared to measuring only two to four (see Table 12.1) and not always in adequate fashion. Specifically, Table 12.3 shows that the WISC-IV, WAIS-IV, WPPSI-III, KABC-II, and SB5 measure four to five broad CHC abilities. The WISC-IV and WAIS-IV measure *Gf, Gc, Gv, Gsm,* and *Gs,* while the KABC-II measures *Gf, Gc,* and *Gv* adequately, and to a lesser extent *Gsm* and *Glr.* The WPPSI-III measures *Gc, Gv,* and *Gs* adequately, and to a lesser extent *Gf.* The DAS-II measures *Gf, Gc, Gv, Gsm,* and *Glr* adequately, and to a lesser extent *Gs* and *Ga.* Finally, the SB5 measures four CHC broad abilities adequately (i.e., *Gf, Gc, Gv, Gsm*; Alfonso et al., 2005). Table 12.3 also shows that the WJ III measures seven broad cognitive abilities adequately.

In addition, comparison of Tables 12.1 and 12.3 indicates that two broad abilities not measured by many intelligence and cognitive ability tests prior to 2000 are now measured by the majority of these tests available today; that is, *Gf* and *Gsm.* It seems likely that these broad abilities may be better represented on current intelligence and cognitive ability batteries because of the accumulating research evidence regarding their importance in overall academic success (see Flanagan, Alfonso, & Mascolo, 2011; Flanagan, Ortiz, Alfonso, & Mascolo, 2006; McGrew & Wendling, 2010). Finally, despite the significant improvements in the number of abilities measured and the increased adequacy of construct representation, Table 12.3 reveals that intelligence and cognitive ability batteries continue to fall short in their measurement of three CHC broad abilities;

Table 12.2 Impact of CHC Theory and XBA CHC Classifications on Intelligence Test Development

Test (Year of Publication) CHC and XBA Impact	Revision (Year of Publication) CHC and XBA Impact
K-ABC (1983) No obvious impact.	**KABC-II (2004)** Provided a second global score that includes fluid and crystallized abilities; Included several new subtests measuring reasoning; Interpretation of test performance may be based on CHC theory or Luria's theory; Provided assessment of five CHC broad abilities.
SB:FE (1986) Used a three-level hierarchical model of the structure of cognitive abilities to guide construction of the test: the top level included general reasoning factor or "*g*"; the middle level included three broad factors called crystallized abilities, fluid-analytic abilities, and short-term memory; the third level included more specific factors including verbal reasoning, quantitative reasoning, and abstract/visual reasoning.	**SB5 (2003)** Used CHC theory to guide test development; Increased the number of broad factors from 4 to 5; Included a Working Memory Factor based on research indicating its importance for academic success.
WPPSI-R (1989) No obvious impact.	**WPPSI-III (2002)** Incorporated measures of Processing Speed that yielded a Processing Speed Quotient based on recent research indicating the importance of processing speed for early academic success; Enhanced the measurement of fluid reasoning by adding the Matrix Reasoning and Picture Concepts subtests.
WJ-R (1989) Used modern *Gf-Gc* theory as the cognitive model for test development; Included two measures of each of eight broad abilities.	**WJ III (2001; Normative Update, 2007)** Used CHC theory as a "blueprint" for test development; Included two or three qualitatively different narrow abilities for each broad ability; The combined cognitive and achievement batteries of the WJ III include 9 of the 10 broad abilities subsumed in CHC theory.
WISC-III (1991) No obvious impact.	**WISC-IV (2003)** Eliminated Verbal and Performance IQs; Replaced the Freedom from Distractibility Index with the Working Memory Index; Replaced the Perceptual Organization Index with the Perceptual Reasoning Index; Enhanced the measurement of fluid reasoning by adding Matrix Reasoning and Picture Concepts; Enhanced measurement of Processing Speed with the Cancellation subtest.
DAS (1990) No obvious impact.	**DAS-II (2007)** CHC broad abilities are represented in the DAS-II subtests and composites
WAIS-III (1997) No obvious impact.	**WAIS-IV (2008)** Eliminated Verbal and Performance IQs; Replaced the Perceptual Organization Index with the Perceptual Reasoning Index; Enhanced the measurement of fluid reasoning by adding the Figure Weights and Visual Puzzles subtests; Enhanced measurement of Processing Speed with the Cancellation subtest. Enhanced measurement of memory with the Working Memory Index.
WPPSI-III (2002) Incorporated measures of Processing Speed that yielded a Processing Speed Quotient based on recent research indicating the importance of processing speed for early academic success; Enhanced the measurement of fluid reasoning by adding the Matrix Reasoning and Picture Concepts subtests.	**WPPSI-IV (2012)** Eliminated Verbal and Performance IQs; Enhanced measures of visual memory, processing speed and inhibitory control.

Table 12.3 Broad and Narrow CHC Ability Representation on Seven Current Intelligence Batteries

	Gf	*Gc*	*Gv*	*Gsm*	*Glr*	*Ga*	*Gs*
WISC-IV	Matrix Reasoning (I) Picture Concepts (I) Arithmetic (RQ, *Gsm*-MW, *Gq*-A3)	Vocabulary (VL) Information (K0) Similarities (VL, *Gf*-I) Comprehension (K0) Word Reasoning (VL, *Gf*-I)	Block Design (Vz) Picture Completion (CF, *Gc*-K0)	Digit Span (MS, MW) Letter-Number Sequencing (MW)	**Not Measured**	**Not Measured**	Symbol Search (P) Coding (R9) Cancellation (P)
WAIS-IV	Matrix Reasoning (I) Arithmetic (RQ, *Gsm*-MW, *Gq*-A3) Figure Weights (RQ)	Vocabulary (VL) Information (K0) Similarities (VL, *Gf*-I) Comprehension (K0)	Block Design (Vz) Picture Completion (CF, *Gc*-K0) Visual Puzzles (Vz)	Digit Span (MS, MW) Letter-Number Sequencing (MW)	**Not Measured**	**Not Measured**	Symbol Search (P) Coding (R9) Cancellation (P)
WPPSI-III	Matrix Reasoning (I)	Picture Concepts (*Gc*-K0, *Gf*-I) Vocabulary (VL) Information (K0) Similarities (VL, *Gf*-I) Comprehension (K0) Receptive Vocabulary (VL) Picture Naming (VL) Word Reasoning (VL, *Gf*-I)	Block Design (VZ) Object Assembly (CS) Picture Completion (CF, *Gc*-K0)	**Not Measured**	**Not Measured**	**Not Measured**	Coding (R9) Symbol Search (P)
KABC-II	Pattern Reasoning (I)[1] Story Completion (RG, *Gc*-K0)[2]	Expressive Vocabulary (VL) Verbal Knowledge (VL, K0) Riddles (VL, *Gf*-RG)	Face Recognition (MV) Triangles (Vz) Gestalt Closure (CS) Rover (SS, *Gf*-RG) Block Counting (Vz) Conceptual Thinking (Vz, *Gc*-K0, *Gf*-I)	Number Recall (MS) Word Order (MS, MW) Hand Movements (MS, *Gv*-MV)	Atlantis (MA) Rebus (MA) Atlantis Delayed (MA) Rebus Delayed (MA)	**Not Measured**	**Not Measured**
WJ III	Concept Formation (I) Analysis-Synthesis (RG)	Verbal Comprehension (VL, *Gf*-I) General Information (K0)	Spatial Relations (Vz) Picture Recognition (MV) Planning (SS, *Gf*-RG)	Memory for Words (MS) Numbers Reversed (MW) Auditory Working Memory (MW)	Visual-Auditory Learning (MA) Retrieval Fluency (FI) Visual-Auditory Learning Delayed (MA) Rapid Picture Naming (NA)	Sound Blending (PC) Auditory Attention (UR) Incomplete Words (PC)	Visual Matching (P) Decision Speed (P) Pair Cancellation (P)

SB5	Nonverbal Fluid Reasoning (I) Verbal Fluid Reasoning (I, RG, Gc-CM) Nonverbal Quantitative Reasoning (RQ, Gq-A3) Verbal Quantitative Reasoning (RQ, Gq-A3)	Nonverbal Knowledge (K0, LS, Gf-RG) Verbal Knowledge (VL,K0)	Nonverbal Visual-Spatial Processing (Vz) Verbal Visual-Spatial Processing (Vz, Gc-VL, K0)	Nonverbal Working Memory (MS, MW) Verbal Working Memory (MS, MW)	**Not Measured**	**Not Measured**	**Not Measured**
DAS-II	Matrices (I) Picture Similarities (I) Sequential & Quantitative Reasoning (RQ)	Early Number Concepts (VL, Gq-KM) Naming Vocabulary (VL) Word Definitions (VL) Verbal Comprehension (LS) Verbal Similarities (VL, GfI)	Pattern Construction (Vz) Recall of Designs (MV) Recognition of Pictures (MV) Copying (Vz) Matching Letter-Like Forms (Vz)	Recall of Digits-Forward (MS) Recall of Digits-Backward (MW) Recall of Sequential Order (MW)	Rapid Naming (NA)[3] Recall of Objects-Immediate (M6) Recall of Objects-Delayed (M6)	Phonological Processing (PC)	Speed of Information Processing (P)

Note. CHC classifications are based on the literature and primary sources such as Carroll (1993); Flanagan & Ortiz (2001); Flanagan, Ortiz, & Alfonso (2007, 2012); Flanagan, Ortiz, Alfonso, & Mascolo (2006); Horn (1991); Keith, Fine, Taub, Reynolds, & Kranzler (2006); McGrew (1997); and McGrew & Flanagan (1998). WISC-IV = Wechsler Intelligence Scale for Children–Fourth Edition (Wechsler, 2003); WAIS-IV = Wechsler Adult Intelligence Scale–Fourth Edition (Wechsler, 2008); WPPSI-III = Wechsler Preschool and Primary Scale of Intelligence–Third Edition (Wechsler, 2002); KABC-II = Kaufman Assessment Battery for Children–Second Edition (Kaufman & Kaufman, 2004); WJ III = Woodcock-Johnson III Normative Update Tests of Cognitive Abilities (Woodcock, McGrew, & Mather, 2001, 2007); SB5 = Stanford-Binet Intelligence Scales–Fifth Edition (Roid, 2003); DAS-II = Differential Ability Scales–Second Edition (Elliot, 2007). Gf= Fluid Intelligence; Gc = Crystallized Intelligence; Gv = Visual Processing; Gsm = Short-Term Memory; Glr = Long-Term Storage and Retrieval; Gs = Processing Speed; Gq = Quantitative Knowledge; RQ = Quantitative Reasoning; I = Induction; RG = General Sequential Reasoning; VL = Lexical Knowledge; K0 = General (verbal) Knowledge; LS = Listening Ability; MV = Visual Memory; Vz = Visualization; SS = Spatial Scanning; CF = Flexibility of Closure; CS = Closure Speed; MW = Working Memory; MS = Memory Span; MA = Associative Memory; F1 = Ideational Fluency; NA = Naming Facility; M6 = Free Recall Memory; PC = Phonetic Coding; UR = Resistance to Auditory Stimulus Distortion; P = Perceptual Speed; R9 = Rate-of-Test-Taking; KM = Math Knowledge; A3 = Math Achievement.

[1]Pattern Reasoning appears to be a measure of Gv-Vz only at ages 5–6 years.

[2]Gc-K0 appears to be the primary ability measured by Story Completion at ages 5–6 years. At older ages (i.e., ages 7+), the primary ability measured by Story Completion appears to be Gf-RG.

[3]Elliot (2007) places Rapid Naming under the construct Gs based on the results of factor analysis. The current authors place this test under the construct Glr based on theory.

specifically, *Glr*, *Ga*, and *Gs*. Moreover, current intelligence and cognitive ability tests do not provide adequate measurement of most specific or narrow CHC abilities—many of which are important in predicting academic achievement (Flanagan et al, 2007, 2012; McGrew & Wendling). Thus, although there is greater coverage and better adequacy in measurement of CHC broad abilities now than there was just a few years ago, practitioners interested in measuring the full range of cognitive abilities will probably need to supplement testing in some manner (e.g., use of the XBA approach), since a significant number of narrow abilities remains inadequately measured by current intelligence tests (Alfonso et al., 2005; Flanagan et al., 2012, 2013).

Progress in Approaches to Interpreting Cognitive Test Performance

Kamphaus and colleagues (1997, 2005, 2012) provided a detailed historical account of the major approaches that have been used to interpret an individual's performance on intelligence and cognitive ability tests since their inception. These authors describe the history of intelligence test interpretation in terms of four "waves": (1) quantification of general level; (2) clinical profile analysis; (3) psychometric profile analysis; and (4) application of theory to intelligence test interpretation. Kamphaus and colleagues' organizational framework is used here to illustrate the evolution of test interpretation (see bottom portion of Figure 12.1), which was based largely on the Wechsler scales and efforts to derive meaning without the aid of theory. In addition, we offer a discussion on what we believe to be the current, fifth wave of interpretation—application of refinements to theory and CHC-based research to psychological test interpretation.

The First Wave: Quantification of General Level

Intelligence tests, particularly the "gold standard" Stanford-Binet, as proclaimed by Lewis Terman, garnered widespread use in psychology and a variety of other applied fields, largely because they appeared to offer an objective method of differentiating and rank ordering individuals on the basis of their general intelligence. According to Kamphaus and colleagues (2012), this was the first wave of intelligence test interpretation and was driven by practical considerations regarding the need to classify individuals into distinct groups that shared the same level of this attribute (e.g., mentally retarded, now called intellectual disability).

During the first wave, the omnibus IQ (so named after the original mental age score was replaced by a ratio quotient) was the focus of intelligence test interpretation. The prevalent influence of Spearman's *g* theory of intelligence and the age-based Stanford-Binet scale, coupled with the fact that budding factor-analytic and other psychometric methods were not yet widely available for investigating multiple cognitive abilities, contributed to the almost exclusive use of global IQ for classification purposes. Hence, a number of classification systems were proposed for organizing individuals according to their global IQs.

Early classification systems included labels that had already entered into the medical and legal lexicon, including "idiot," "imbecile," and "moron" (Levine & Marks, 1928). Although the Wechsler scales did not contribute to the early classification efforts during most of the first wave of test interpretation, David Wechsler eventually made his contribution by proposing a classification system that relied less on evaluative labels (although it still contained the terms "defective" and "borderline," presumably "borderline moron") and more on meaningful deviations from the mean as specified by the deviation IQ, which he believed more accurately reflected the "prevalence of certain intelligence levels in the country at that time" (Kamphaus et al., 1997, p. 35). With some refinements over the years, interpretation of intelligence tests continue to be based largely on the deviation IQ metric and similar descriptive classification systems that rely on characterizations of performance relative to others in general. That is, distinctions are still made between individuals who are intellectually disabled versus average, or those who are intellectually gifted versus average, for example. But the difference in intelligence between individuals in one of these groups versus those in another is more precisely described by a score (IQ) that is based on the individual's relative standing in the general population as determined by the normal probability distribution. As such, current classification categories are quite different from earlier ones, as may be seen in Table 12.4.

His pioneering of the deviation IQ aside, it appears that Wechsler accepted the prevailing ideas regarding *g* and the conceptualization of intelligence as a global entity, consistent with those already put forth by Terman, Binet, Spearman, and others (Reynolds & Kaufman, 1990). This is evident in the definition of intelligence he offered as underlying his own scales. According to Wechsler (1939), *intelligence* is "the aggregate or global capacity of the

Table 12.4 Comparison of Selected Historical and Current Test Score Classification Systems

Levine & Marks (1928) Classifications			Wechsler Scales (1944) IQ Classifications			Flanagan, Ortiz, & Alfonso (2007) XBA Classifications		
Normative Classification	Standard Score Range	Percentile Range	Normative Classification	Standard Score Range	Percentile Range	Normative Classification	Standard Score Range	Percentile Range
Idiot	0–24	<.02						
Imbecile	25–49	.02nd to .04th						
Moron	50–74	.05th to 4th	Defective	≤ 65	≤ 1st	Lower Extreme	< 70	<2nd
Borderline	75–84	5th to 14th	Borderline	66–79	1st to 8th	Below Average – Normative Weakness	70–84	2nd to 14th
Dull	85–94	16th to 35th	Dull Normal	80–90	9th to 25th	Low Average	85–89	16th to 23rd
Average	95–104	38th to 62nd	Average	91–110	27th to 75th	Average	90–110	25th to 75th
Bright	105–114	65th to 83rd	Bright Normal	111–119	77th to 89th	High Average	111–115	77th to 84th
Very Bright	115–124	84th to 95th	Superior	120–127	91st to 97th	Above Average – Normative Strength	116–129	86th to 97th
Superior	125–149	95th to 99.94th	Very Superior	≥ 128	≥ 97th	Upper Extreme	>130	≥98th
Very Superior	150–174	99.95th to 99.99th						
Precocious	>175	>99.99						

individual to act purposefully, to think rationally and to deal effectively with his environment" (p. 3). He concluded that this definition "avoids singling out any ability, however esteemed (e.g., abstract reasoning), as crucial or overwhelmingly important" (p. 3) and implied that any one intelligence subtest is readily interchangeable with another. In this way, Wechsler was also minimizing the importance of the manner in which he had constructed his tests; that is, subtests that were categorized as either "verbal" or "performance." Given his experiences during World War I with the Army Mental Tests (Alpha and Beta) as well as his interactions with Yerkes, Terman, Brigham, and others, Wechsler recognized the importance of attempts to measure intelligence in various modalities, but it seems clear that, at least initially, he did not see the Verbal IQ (VIQ) or Performance IQ (PIQ) as constructs unto themselves or as scores that merited individual interpretation. Nevertheless, the clinical need for assigning meaning to test results eventually led to subsequent interpretive methods that included use of both the VIQ and PIQ, particularly the difference between them.

The Second Wave: Clinical Profile Analysis

Kamphaus and colleagues (1997, 2005, 2012) identified the second wave of interpretation as *clinical profile analysis* and stated that the publication of the Wechsler-Bellevue (W-B; Wechsler, 1939) was pivotal in spawning this approach to interpretation. Clinical profile analysis was a method designed to go beyond global IQ and interpret more specific aspects of an individual's cognitive capabilities through the analysis of patterns of subtest scaled scores.

The Wechsler-Bellevue Intelligence Scale, Form I (W-B I), published in 1939 (an alternate form, the W-B II, was published in 1946), represented an approach to intellectual assessment in adults that was clearly differentiated from other instruments available at that time (e.g., the Binet scales). The W-B was composed of 11 separate subtests, namely Information, Comprehension, Arithmetic, Digit Span, Similarities, Vocabulary, Picture Completion, Picture Arrangement, Block Design, Digit Symbol, and Coding. (The Vocabulary subtest was an alternate for W-B I.)

As stated previously, perhaps the most notable feature introduced with the W-B, which advanced interpretation beyond classification of global IQ, was the grouping of subtests into Verbal and Performance composites. The Verbal-Performance dichotomy represented an organizational structure that was based on the notion that intelligence could be expressed and measured through both verbal and nonverbal communication modalities. To clarify the Verbal-Performance distinction, Wechsler asserted that this dichotomy "does not imply that these are the only abilities involved in the tests. Nor does it presume that there are different kinds of intelligence (e.g., verbal, manipulative). It merely implies that these are different ways in which intelligence may manifest itself," again, a lesson probably learned from his experiences with the Army Alpha and Army Beta tests (Wechsler, 1958, p. 64, cf. Flanagan & Kaufman, 2009).

Another important feature pioneered in the W-B revolved around the construction and organization of subtests. At that time, the Stanford-Binet scale was ordered and administered sequentially according to developmental age, irrespective of the task. In contrast, Wechsler utilized only 11 subtests, each scored by points rather than age, and each with sufficient range of item difficulties to encompass the entire age range of the scale.

In his later writings, Wechsler often shifted between conceptualizing intelligence as either a singular entity (the first wave) or possibly as a collection of specific mental abilities (the second wave). At times he appeared to encourage the practice of subtest-level interpretation, suggesting that each subtest measured a relatively distinct cognitive ability (McDermott et al., 1990). To many, this position appeared to contradict his prior attempts not to equate general intelligence with the sum of separate cognitive or intellectual abilities. This shift in viewpoint may have been responsible, in part, for the development of interpretive methods that characterize the second and third waves, notably profile analysis (Flanagan, 2000).

Without a doubt, the innovations found in the W-B were impressive, practical, and in many ways, superior, to other intelligence tests available in 1939. More importantly, the structure and organization of the W-B scale provided the impetus for Rapaport, Gill, and Schafer's (1945–1946) approaches to test interpretation, which included an attempt to understand the meaning behind the shape of a person's profile of scores. This notion may have been prompted in part by the manner in which the 11 tests on the W-B were organized on the scoring protocol (6 verbal vs. 5 performance). By grouping the verbal and performance tests relatively independently, it tended to suggest that the VIQ and PIQ were distinct constructs in their own right. Likewise, the scoring protocol provided a graph wherein the arrangement explicitly encouraged practitioners to connect the obtained subtest scaled scores via lines that effectively produced a visual "profile." Whatever its original intent, the ubiquitous visual profile available on every scored W-B protocol easily supported and facilitated the search for enduring and similar "patterns" of test score performance that would be associated with specific pathologies or diagnoses. According to Kamphaus and colleagues (1997, 2005, 2012), a new method of test interpretation had been developed under the assumption that "patterns of high and low subtest scores could presumably reveal diagnostic and psychotherapeutic considerations" (Kamphaus et al., 1997, p. 36). Thus, during the second wave of intelligence test interpretation, the W-B (1939) was the focal point from which a variety of clinical interpretations were developed for deriving diagnostic and prescriptive meaning from the shape of subtest profiles and the difference between Verbal and Performance IQs.

In addition to the scope of Rapaport and colleagues' (1945–1946) diagnostic suggestions, their approach to understanding profile shape led to a flurry of investigations that sought to identify the psychological functions underlying an essentially infinite number of profile patterns and their relationships to each other. Perhaps as a consequence of the clinical appeal of Rapaport and colleagues' approach, the availability of the W-B (and its later incarnation, WAIS, and siblings WISC and WPPSI) helped relegate general-level assessment to the back burner while increasing the heat on clinical profile analysis (Flanagan & Kaufman, 2009).

Although the search for diagnostic meaning in subtest profiles and IQ differences was a more sophisticated approach to intelligence test interpretation as compared to the interpretive method of the first wave, it also created methodological problems. For example, with enough practice, just about any astute clinician could provide a seemingly rational interpretation of an obtained profile to fit the known functional and dysfunctional patterns of the examinee. Not surprisingly, analysis of profile shape and IQ differences never actually resulted in any increased diagnostic validity for the WISC (e.g., Glutting, McDermott, & Konold, 1997; Watkins, Glutting & Youngstrom, 2005). Despite its failings, the next wave in intelligence test interpretation sought to address the methodological flaws in the clinical-profile analysis method in hopes of still advancing it as a viable and valid interpretive method (Kamphaus et al., 2012).

The Third Wave: Psychometric Profile Analysis

In 1955, the original W-B was revised and updated, and its new name, Wechsler Adult Intelligence Scale (WAIS; Wechsler, 1955), was aligned with the existing child version (i.e., WISC) which had been created by Wechsler in 1949. Major changes and revisions included (1) incorporating Forms I and II of the W-B into a single scale with a broader range of item difficulties; (2) realigning the target age range to include ages 16 years and older (which eliminated overlap with the WISC, creating a larger and more representative norm sample); and (3) refining the subtests to improve reliability (Flanagan & Kaufman, 2004, 2009).

Within this general time period, eventual technological developments in the form of computers and statistical software to assist with intelligence test interpretation provided the impetus for what Kamphaus and colleagues (1997, 2005, 2012) called the "third wave" of interpretation—*psychometric profile analysis*. The work of Cohen (1959), which was based primarily on the WISC and the WAIS, sharply criticized the clinical-profile analysis tradition that had defined the second wave. For example, Cohen's factor-analytic procedures revealed a viable three-factor solution for the WAIS that challenged the prevailing dichotomous verbal-performance model and remained the *de facto* standard for the Wechsler scales for decades. The labels used by Cohen for the three Wechsler factors that emerged in his factor analysis of the WISC subtests (i.e., Verbal Comprehension, Perceptual Organization, and Freedom from Distractibility) were the names of the Indexes on two subsequent editions of this test (WISC-R and WISC-III), spanning more than two decades (Flanagan & Kaufman, 2009).

By examining and removing the variance shared between subtests, Cohen demonstrated that the majority of Wechsler subtests had very poor *specificity* (i.e., reliable, specific variance). Thus, the frequent clinical practice of interpreting individual subtests as reliable measures of a *presumed* construct was not supported. Kamphaus and colleagues (1997, 2005, 2012) summarize Cohen's significant contributions, which largely defined the third wave of test interpretation, as threefold: (1) empirical support for the FSIQ based on analysis of shared variance between subtests; (2) development of the three-factor solution for interpretation of the Wechsler scales; and (3) revelation of limited subtest specificity, questioning individual subtest interpretation.

The most vigorous and elegant application of psychometric profile analysis to intelligence test interpretation occurred with the revision of the venerable WISC as the Wechsler Intelligence Scale for Children–Revised (WISC-R; Wechsler, 1974). Briefly, the WISC-R utilized a larger, more representative norm sample than its predecessor; included more contemporary-looking graphics and updated items; eliminated some content that was differentially familiar to specific groups; and included improved scoring and administration procedures. "Armed with the WISC-R, Kaufman (1979) articulated the essence of the psychometric profile approach to intelligence test interpretation in his seminal book, *Intelligent Testing with the WISC-R* (which was superseded by *Intelligent Testing with the WISC-III*; Kaufman, 1994)" (Flanagan et al., 2000, p. 6). Kaufman had been Wechsler's primary collaborator on the revision of the WISC and as such had a great deal of insight into the test as well as into potential methods for appropriate interpretation.

Kaufman emphasized flexibility in interpretation and provided a logical and systematic approach that utilized principles from measurement theory. He applied these principles to clinical profile analysis and thereby provided the very name for this third wave of interpretation—psychometric profile analysis. His approach was more complex than previous ones and required the examiner to have a greater level of psychometric expertise than might ordinarily be possessed by the average psychologist (Flanagan et al., 2000). Anastasi (1988) lauded this and recognized that "the basic approach described by Kaufman undoubtedly represents a major contribution to the clinical use of intelligence tests. Nevertheless, it should be recognized that its implementation requires a sophisticated clinician who is well informed in several fields of psychology" (p. 484).

In some respects, publication of Kaufman's work can be viewed as an indictment against the poorly reasoned and unsubstantiated interpretation of the Wechsler scales that had sprung up in the second wave (clinical profile analysis; Flanagan et al., 2000). Kaufman's ultimate message centered on the notion that interpretation of Wechsler intelligence test performance must be conducted with a higher than usual degree of psychometric precision and based on credible and dependable evidence, rather than merely the clinical lore that surrounded earlier interpretive methods (Anastasi, 1988; Flanagan & Kaufman, 2009; Flanagan et al., 2000).

Despite the enormous body of clinical, case study, and anecdotal literature that has mounted

steadily over the years arguing in support of the use of profile analysis with the Wechsler scales, this form of interpretation, even when upgraded with the rigor of psychometrics, has been regarded as a perilous endeavor primarily because it lacks empirical support and is not grounded in a well-validated theory of intelligence. With over 75 different profile types discussed in a variety of areas, including neuropsychology, personality, learning disabilities, and juvenile delinquency (McDermott et al., 1990), there is considerable temptation to believe that the findings of this type of analysis alone are reliable. Nevertheless, many studies (e.g., Hale, 1979; Hale & Landino, 1981; Hale & Saxe, 1983) demonstrated consistently that "profile and scatter analysis is not defensible" (Kavale & Forness, 1984, p. 136; also see Glutting, McDermott, Watkins, Kush, & Konold, 1997).

In a meta-analysis of 119 studies of the WISC-R subtest data, Mueller, Dennis, and Short (1986) concluded that using profile analysis with the WISC-R in an attempt to differentiate various diagnostic groups is clearly not warranted. Subsequent evaluations regarding the merits of psychometric profile analysis produced similar results (e.g., Glutting, McDermott, Watkins, et al., 1997; Kamphaus, 1993; McDermott, Fantuzzo, Glutting, Watkins, & Baggaley, 1992; Watkins et al., 2005; Watkins & Kush, 1994).

The Fourth Wave: Application of Theory to Interpretation

Although the third wave of intelligence test interpretation did not meet with any real degree of success in terms of establishing validity evidence for profile analysis, the psychometric approach provided the foundation necessary to catapult the field into the fourth wave of intelligence test interpretation. This wave is described generally by Kamphaus and colleagues (1997, 2005, 2012) as "application of theory." Although the need to integrate theory and research into the intelligence test interpretation process appeared obvious to those involved in theory development, it was not until Kaufman's book *Intelligent Testing with the WISC-R* was published in 1979 that practitioners began to understand the need for this connection. Specifically, Kaufman observed that problems with intelligence test interpretation went beyond psychometric deficiencies and could be attributed largely to the lack of a specific theoretical base to guide interpretive practices. He suggested that it was possible to enhance interpretation significantly by reorganizing subtests into clusters specified by a particular theory. In fact, Kaufman's test, the K-ABC (Kaufman & Kaufman, 1983), was the first cognitive battery to be based on theory (i.e., Luria's Simultaneous-Successive theory of information processing; Luria, 1973). The WJ-R (Woodcock & Johnson, 1989) is also a good example of a test that was explicitly designed to yield clusters that represented theoretical constructs—in this case, constructs specified by the Cattell-Horn *Gf-Gc* theory. In essence, the end of the third wave of intelligence test interpretation and the beginning of the fourth wave was marked by Kaufman's pleas for practitioners to ground their interpretations in theory, as well as by his efforts to demonstrate the importance of linking intellectual measurement tools to empirically supported and well-established conceptualizations of human cognitive abilities (Flanagan & Kaufman, 2004, 2009; Flanagan et al., 2000; Woodcock, Werder & McGrew, 1991).

In response to Kaufman's calls to narrow the theory–practice gap in intelligence test development and interpretation by applying theory, Flanagan and colleagues (Flanagan & Ortiz, 2001; Flanagan et al., 2000; McGrew & Flanagan, 1998) developed a method for measurement and interpretation called the "cross-battery approach" (XBA) and applied it to the Wechsler scales and other major intelligence and cognitive ability tests available at that time (i.e., the late 1990s). This method was intentionally grounded in *Gf-Gc* (and later CHC) theory and provided a series of systematic steps and rigorous guidelines that were designed to ensure that science and practice are closely linked in the measurement and interpretation of cognitive abilities. According to McGrew (2005), the cross-battery approach "infused CHC theory into the minds of assessment practitioners and university training programs, regardless of their choice of favorite intelligence battery...." (p. 149). Kaufman's (2000) description of the cross-battery approach as an interpretive method that (1) has "research as its foundation," (2) "adds theory to psychometrics," and (3) "improves the quality of the psychometric assessment of intelligence" (p. xiii) is consistent with Kamphaus and colleagues' fourth wave of intelligence test interpretation.

In comparison to prior waves, where the strong need and desire for assigning meaning to scores meant relatively quick and easy acceptance of "new" interpretive schemes, theory-driven interpretive approaches (e.g., XBA) did not fare especially well early on. Despite their availability and applicability for interpreting the most popular intelligence and cognitive ability tests available (including the WISC-III), the inertia of tradition remained strong, and practitioners largely continued using interpretive methods based on the second and third waves (Flanagan & Kaufman, 2004). This is not to say that there was no recognition of problems with or concern about the theoretical structure, or lack thereof, of many tests. For example, evaluations of the WISC-III upon its publication were anything but positive, and the conclusions offered by a wide range of reviewers were remarkably similar—the newly published WISC-III was *outdated*. According to Kamphaus (1993), "The WISC-III's history is also its greatest liability. Much has been learned about children's cognitive development since the conceptualization of the Wechsler scales, and yet few of these findings have been incorporated into revisions" (p. 99). Similarly, Shaw, Swerdlik, and Laurent (1993) concluded, "Despite more than 50 years of advancement of theories of intelligence, the Wechsler philosophy of intelligence...written in 1939, remains the guiding principle of the WISC-III.... [T]he latest incarnation of David Wechsler's test may be nothing more than a new and improved dinosaur" (p. 163).

Eventually the message seemed to get through—practitioners slowly began to recognize the theoretical and psychometric limitations of measurement tools and interpretive approaches, which probably made them more receptive to alternatives (e.g., XBA; Flanagan & Ortiz, 2001; Flanagan et al., 2007). Whatever the reasons, and there were no doubt many, the advent of the twenty-first century was accompanied by a dramatic rise in the popularity of CHC theory (and the tests and interpretive methods based on it). Apart perhaps from Spearman's *g*, never before in the history of intelligence testing had any theory played so prominent a role in test development and interpretation. Amidst the publication of CHC-based instruments was the latest revision of the Wechsler scales—the WISC-IV—which, although not explicitly based on CHC theory, nevertheless represented the most sweeping structural revision of any Wechsler scale in the history of the Wechsler lineage, due primarily to its closer alliance with theory.

As noted previously, CHC theory became the foundation for the revision of most major cognitive ability tests, the majority of which were published after 2000. At the same time, measurement and interpretive methods, such as XBA, have also gained considerable popularity among practitioners, particularly school psychologists. Whether the former promoted the latter or vice versa, it is clear that there has been a significant change in the manner in which measurement and interpretation of cognitive abilities are conducted (see Flanagan & Harrison, 2012; Sotelo-Dynega & Cuskley, 2011).

The Fifth Wave: Application of Refinements in Theory and CHC-based Research to Psychological Test Interpretation

As the fourth wave continues to unfold, it is our belief that the beginnings of the next wave have already begun to emerge. Indeed, specific programs of research in cognitive psychology, neuropsychology, neuroscience, and learning disabilities, for example, will converge in the next decade, resulting in more defensible and clinically meaningful interpretations of cognitive test performance. It is beyond the scope of this chapter to discuss the range of research programs that will lead to better test interpretation in the future. The interested reader is referred to the work of Keith and Reynolds (2010, 2012) for information on their rigorous program of research on factorial invariance within the CHC taxonomy, as their work will continue to shed light on the construct validity of cognitive batteries and lead to refinements of theories on the structure of cognitive abilities. Also, the ongoing work of Berninger and colleagues (see Berninger, 2011) and Fletcher and colleagues (e.g., Fletcher, Lyon, Fuchs, & Barnes, 2007) will continue to demonstrate how converging research programs (including their own) enhance test interpretation and, therefore, should be followed closely. For the purpose of this chapter, we limit our discussion of the fifth wave of intelligence and cognitive ability test interpretation to the following areas: (a) refinements and extensions to CHC theory; (b) CHC theory applied to academic outcomes research; (c) integrating CHC and neuropsychological theories to enhance test interpretation; and (d) greater emphasis on flexible battery approaches to assessment and interpretation.

Refinements and Extensions to CHC theory

Recently, Schneider and McGrew (2012) reviewed CHC-related research and provided a summary of the CHC abilities (broad and narrow) that have the most evidence to support them. In their attempt to provide a CHC overarching framework that incorporates the best-supported cognitive abilities, they articulated a 16-factor model containing over 80 narrow abilities (see Figure 12.4). Because of the greater number of abilities represented by CHC theory now, compared to past CHC models (e.g., Figure 12.3), the broad abilities in Figure 12.4

have been grouped conceptually into six broad categories, in a manner similar to those suggested by Schneider and McGrew, to enhance comprehensibility (i.e., Reasoning, Acquired Knowledge, Memory and Efficiency, Sensory, Motor, and Speed and Efficiency). Space limitations preclude a discussion of all the ways in which CHC theory has evolved and the reasons why certain refinements and changes have been made (see Schneider & McGrew for a discussion). However, to assist the reader in transitioning from the 10-factor CHC model (Figure 12.3) to the 16-factor CHC model (Figure 12.4), the following brief explanations are offered.

Of the 10 CHC factors depicted in Figure 12.3, all were refined by Schneider and McGrew (2012), except *Gq*. First, with regard to *Gf*, Piagetian Reasoning (RP) and Reasoning Speed (RE) were de-emphasized (and, therefore, are not included in Figure 12.4), primarily because there is little evidence that they are distinct factors. Second, four narrow abilities (Foreign Language Proficiency [KL], Geography Achievement [A5], General Science Information [K1], and Information about Culture [K2]) were moved to a different CHC broad ability, called Domain-Specific Knowledge (*Gkn*; defined below). Also, within the area of *Gc*, Foreign Language Aptitude (LA) was dropped, as it is a combination of abilities designed for the purpose of predicting one's success in learning foreign languages, and, as such, is not considered a distinct ability. The final refinement to *Gc* involved dropping the narrow ability of Oral Production and Fluency (OP) because it is difficult to distinguish it from the narrow ability of Communication Ability (CM). Nevertheless, OP continues to be represented in Figure 12.4 because several tests and subtests have been classified as OP in existing resources (e.g., Flanagan et al., 2007; Flanagan, Ortiz, Alfonso, & Mascolo, 2006).

Third, in the area of *Grw*, Verbal (Printed) Language Comprehension (V) was dropped because it appears to represent a number of different abilities (e.g., reading decoding, reading comprehension, reading speed) and, therefore, is not a distinct ability. Likewise, Cloze Ability (CZ) was dropped from *Grw* because it is not meaningfully distinct from reading comprehension. Rather, CZ appears to be an specific method of measuring reading comprehension. As such, tests like those formally classified as CZ (e.g., WJ III Passage Comprehension) should be classified (or reclassified) as "RC" or Reading Comprehension. The final refinement to *Grw*

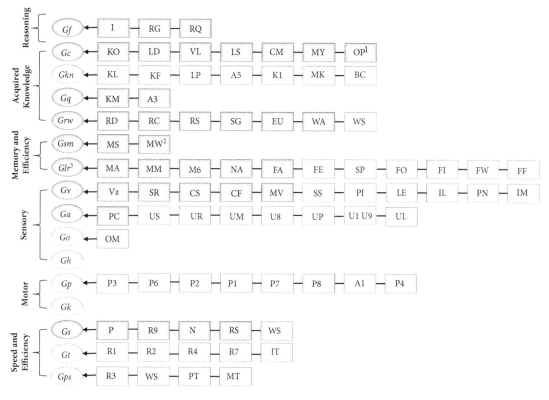

Figure 12.4 Current Cattell-Horn-Carroll (CHC) model of cognitive abilities.

Note: The current CHC model depicted in this figure contains 16 broad abilities and over 80 narrow abilities as specified by Schneider and McGrew (2012). Abilities encompassing the domains of "Reasoning," "Acquired Knowledge," "Memory and Efficiency," "Speed and Efficiency," and "Motor" are grouped according to function and "Sensory" abilities are grouped conceptually, following the logic of Schneider and McGrew. Broad and narrow abilities represented by gray shaded ovals and rectangles, respectively are those most commonly measured by contemporary cognitive and achievement batteries.

[1]The narrow ability of Oral Production and Fluency (OP) is difficult to distinguish from the narrow ability of Communication Ability (CM). Therefore, Schneider and McGrew recommended that OP be dropped from the CHC model. However, OP continues to be represented in this model because several tests and subtests have been classified as OP in existing resources (e.g., Flanagan, Ortiz, & Alfonso, 2007; Flanagan, Ortiz, Alfonso, & McGrew, 2006).

[2]Working Memory is now called Working Memory Capacity.

[3]The narrow abilities comprised by *Glr* may be divided into two categories—Learning Efficiency (MA, MM, M6) and Retrieval Fluency (which includes the remaining narrow *Glr* abilities listed in this figure). Note that Figural Flexibility (FX) was not listed in this figure due to space limitations.

Gf = Fluid Intelligence; *Gc* = Crystallized Intelligence; *Gkn* = General (Domain-Specific) Knowledge Ability; *Gq* = Quantitative Knowledge *Grw* = Reading/Writing Ability; *Gsm* = Short-Term Memory; *Glr* = Long-Term Storage and Retrieval; *Gv* = Visual Processing; *Ga* = Auditory Processing; *Go* = Olfactory Abilities; *Gh* = Tactile Abilities; *Gp* = Psychomotor Abilities; *Gk* = Kinesthetic Abilities; *Gs* = Processing Speed; *Gt* = Decision Speed/Reaction Time; *Gps* = Psychomotor Speed; I = Induction; RG = General Sequential Reasoning; RQ = Quantitative Reasoning; K0 = General (verbal) Knowledge; LD = Language Development; VL = Lexical Knowledge; LS = Listening Ability; CM = Communication Ability; MY = Grammatical Sensitivity; OP = Oral Production and Fluency; KL = Foreign Language Proficiency; KF = Knowledge of Signing; LP = Skill in Lip-reading; A5 = Geography Achievement; K1 = General Science Information; MK = Mechanical Knowledge; BC = Knowledge of Behavioral Content; KM = Math Knowledge; A3 = Math Achievement; RD = Reading Decoding; RC = Reading Comprehension; RS = Reading Speed; SG = Spelling Ability; EU = English Usage Knowledge; WA = Writing Ability; WS = Writing Speed; MS = Memory Span; MW = Working Memory Capacity; MA = Associative Memory; MM = Meaningful Memory; M6 = Free Recall Memory; NA = Naming Facility; FA = Associational Fluency; FE = Expressional Fluency; SP = Sensitivity Problems; FO = Originality/Creativity; FI = Ideational Fluency; FW = Word Fluency; FF = Figural Fluency; FX = Figural Flexibility; Vz = Visualization; SR = Speeded Rotation; CS = Closure Speed; CF = Flexibility of Closure; MV = Visual Memory; SS = Spatial Scanning; PI = Serial Perceptual Integration; LE = Length Estimation; IL = Perceptual Illusions; PN = Perceptual Alternations; IM = Imagery; PC = Phonetic Coding; US = Speech Sound Discrimination; UR = Resistance to Auditory Stimulus Distortion; UM = Memory for Sound Patterns; U8 = Maintaining and Judging Rhythm; UP = Absolute Pitch; U1U9 = Musical Discrimination and Judgment; UL = Sound Localization; OM = Olfactory Memory; P3 = Static Strength; P6 = Multilimb Coordination; P2 = Finger Dexterity; P1 = Manual Dexterity; P7 = Arm-hand Steadiness; P8 = Control Precision; A1 = Aiming; P4 = Gross Body Equilibrium; P = Perceptual Speed; R9 = Rate-of-Test-Taking; N = Number Facility; RS = Reading Speed; WS = Writing Speed; R1 = Simple Reaction Time; R2 = Choice Reaction Time; R4 = Semantic Processing Speed; R7 = Mental Comparison Speed; IT = Inspection Time; R3 = Speed of Limb Movement; WS = Writing Speed; PT = Speed of Articulation; MT = Movement Time.

involved adding the narrow ability of Writing Speed (WS), as this ability appears to cut across more than one broad ability (see Schneider & McGrew, 2012).

Fourth, several refinements were made to the broad memory abilities of *Glr* and *Gsm*. Learning Abilities (L1) was dropped from both *Glr* and *Gsm*. It appears that Carroll conceived of L1 as a superordinate category consisting of different kinds of long-term learning abilities. Schneider and McGrew (2012) referred to this category (i.e., L1) as "*Glr*-Learning Efficiency," which includes the narrow abilities of Free Recall Memory, Associative Memory, and Meaningful Memory. The remaining *Glr* narrow abilities are referred to as "Retrieval Fluency" abilities (see Figure 12.4). In the area of *Gsm*, the name of the Working Memory (MW) narrow ability was changed to *Working Memory Capacity*, as Schneider and McGrew believe the latter term is more descriptive of the types of tasks that are used most frequently to measure MW (e.g., Wechsler Letter-Number Sequencing).

Fifth, in the area of *Gv*, one refinement was made. That is, the narrow ability name Spatial Relations (SR) was changed to "Speeded Rotation" (also "SR") to more accurately describe this ability. Speeded Rotation is the *ability to solve problems quickly using mental rotation of simple images* (Schneider & McGrew, 2012, p. 129). This ability is similar to visualization because it involves rotating mental images, but it is distinct because it has more to do with the speed at which mental rotation tasks can be completed (Lohman, 1996; Schneider & McGrew; Lohman, 1996). Also, Speeded Rotation tasks typically involve fairly simple images. It is likely that the majority of tests that were classified as Spatial Relations in the past should have been classified as measures of Vz *only* (rather than SR, Vz) (see Flanagan et al., 2013).

Sixth, in the area of *Ga*, Temporal Tracking (UK) tasks are thought to measure Attentional Control within working memory. As such, UK was dropped as a narrow ability comprising *Ga*. In addition, six *Ga* narrow abilities (General Sound Discrimination [U3], Sound-Intensity/Duration Discrimination [U6], Sound-Frequency Discrimination [U5], and Hearing and Speech Threshold [UA, UT, UU]) were considered to represent sensory acuity factors, which fall outside the scope of CHC theory and, therefore, were dropped (Schneider & McGrew, 2012).

Seventh, in the area of *Gs*, Reading Speed (RS) and Writing Speed (WS) were added. Although tasks that measure these abilities clearly fall under the broad ability of *Grw*, they demand quick, accurate performance and are, therefore, also measures of *Gs*. The narrow *Gs* ability of Semantic Processing Speed (R4) was moved to *Gt*. Also, the narrow ability of Inspection Time (IT) was added to the broad ability of *Gt* (see Schneider & McGrew, 2012, for details).

In addition to the within-factor refinements just mentioned, the CHC model has been expanded to include six additional broad abilities, namely General (Domain-Specific) Knowledge (*Gkn*), Olfactory Abilities (*Go*), Tactile Abilities (*Gh*), Psychomotor Abilities (*Gp*), Kinesthetic Abilities (*Gk*) and Psychomotor Speed (*Gps*). A brief description of these broad abilities is found in a subsequent section of this chapter. Noteworthy is the fact that the major intelligence tests do not measure most (or any) of these additional factors directly. The reason for this is probably related to the fact that these abilities (with the possible exception of *Gkn*) do not contribute much to the prediction of achievement, which is a major purpose of intelligence and cognitive ability tests. However, many of these factors appear to be assessed by neuropsychological instruments because these tests are intended, in part, to understand the sensory and motor manifestations of typical and atypical fine and gross motor development, traumatic brain injury, and other neurological disorders. For example, several tasks of the Dean-Woodcock Neuropsychological Battery (Dean & Woodcock, 2003) appear to measure *Gh* (e.g., tactile examination: finger identification; tactile examination: object identification; tactile examination: palm writing; tactile identification: simultaneous localization; see Flanagan et al., 2013, for additional examples). Also noteworthy is the fact that, with rare exceptions, there do not appear to be any commercially published and commonly used intelligence or neuropsychological batteries that measure *Go*, *Gt*, or *Gps*.

In sum, despite the number of refinements and extensions that have been made to CHC theory recently, approximately nine broad cognitive abilities and 35–40 narrow abilities are measured consistently by popular cognitive and achievement tests. These commonly measured abilities are shaded gray in Figures 12.3 and 12.4. Researchers have already begun classifying tests according to the CHC extensions discussed by McGrew (2005; e.g., Flanagan et al., 2010). Without question, our next generation of psychological tests and CHC test classifications will correspond more closely to current CHC theory as it is depicted in Figure 12.4 (e.g., Flanagan et al., 2013).

CHC Theory Applied to Academic Outcomes Research

Because practitioners often use intelligence and cognitive ability tests to gain insight into the underlying causes of learning difficulty and academic failure, it is important to understand the cognitive correlates to specific academic skills. Research on the relations between cognitive abilities, cognitive processes, and academic outcomes has mounted over the years (see Flanagan, et al., 2006; Fletcher et al., 2007; and McGrew & Wendling, 2010 for summaries). Much of the recent research on cognitive-academic relationships has been interpreted within the context of CHC theory (e.g., Flanagan, Alfonso, & Mascolo, 2011). In addition, statistical analyses, such as structural equation modeling, has been used to understand the extent to which specific cognitive abilities explain variance in academic skills above and beyond the variance accounted for by *g* (e.g., Floyd et al., 2008; McGrew et al., 1997; Vanderwood, McGrew, Keith, & Flanagan, 2002). Finally, many valuable resources summarize the research on cognitive and neurobiological processes associated with specific academic skill deficits (e.g., Fletcher et al., 2007; Miller, 2010; Fletcher-Janzen & Reynold, 2008).

The research summarized in this section is limited to the relations among the various CHC cognitive abilities and processes and the major areas of achievement—namely, reading, math, and writing. Tables 12.5 and 12.6 provide two sets of findings from two different literature reviews (i.e., Flanagan et al., 2006; and McGrew & Wendling, 2010). Because the literature reviews yielded some differences with regard to which abilities and processes are most relevant to academic achievement, these tables include a "Comments" section that offers some possible explanations for the differences. Likewise, Table 12.7 provides a summary of the literature on the relations between CHC cognitive abilities and processes and writing achievement (Flanagan et al., 2006). The information in Tables 12.5—12.7 is discussed below.

Cognitive Abilities and Reading Achievement

A review of the literature suggests a number of conclusions regarding the relations between CHC abilities and reading achievement (see Table 12.5). First, narrow abilities subsumed by *Ga*, *Gc*, *Glr*, *Gsm*, and *Gs* displayed the most consistent significant relations with reading achievement. Measures

of phonological processing or awareness (e.g., Phonetic Coding [PC], which is subsumed by *Ga*) showed strong and consistent relations with reading achievement across many studies, especially during the early elementary school years. *Gc* abilities, which were typically represented by measures of Lexical Knowledge (VL), Listening Ability (LS), Language Development (LD), and General Information (KO), were also significantly related to reading achievement. As reported in some studies (e.g., Evans, Floyd, McGrew, & Leforgee, 2001; Garcia & Stafford, 2000; McGrew, 1993; McGrew et al., 1997), the significant effects of *Ga* and *Gc* on reading were present even after the powerful effect of *g* was accounted for in the analyses. That is, specific CHC abilities contributed significantly to the explanation of reading above and beyond the significant and large effect of *g*.

Many studies that included *Gsm* indicated that *Gsm* most likely contributes to reading achievement through working memory processes. Nevertheless, significant relationships between Memory Span and reading achievement have also been documented (see McGrew & Wendling, 2010). Taken as a whole, independent, comprehensive reviews of the reading achievement literature suggest that *Gsm*, including working memory and memory span, contributes significantly to the prediction of reading achievement (e.g., Flanagan et al., 2006; Feifer, 2011; McGrew & Wendling).

The relationship between *Glr* and reading achievement is consistent across most of the school age range (e.g., 6–13 years). Associative Memory and Naming Facility are important during the elementary years; Meaningful Memory is important at ages 9–13 years, particularly for reading comprehension (McGrew & Wendling, 2010). In addition, several studies found a strong relation between Perceptual Speed (P), a narrow *Gs* ability, and reading achievement across the school age range (6–19 years) (e.g., McGrew, 1993; McGrew et al., 1997). The effect of *Gs* was present even after the effect of *g* on reading achievement was accounted for in the McGrew and colleagues' (1997) study. This finding was replicated by Evans et al. (2001) who found *Gs* to be significantly related to both basic reading skills and reading comprehension in the early years. Thus, as with *Ga* and *Gc* abilities, *Gs* abilities (viz., perceptual speed) explain significant variance in reading achievement above and beyond the variance explained by *g*.

It appears that *Gf* and *Gv* abilities are less related to reading achievement as compared to *Gc*, *Ga*,

Table 12.5 Important Findings on Relations Between CHC Abilities and Reading Achievement

CHC Ability	Flanagan, Mascolo, Alfonso, & Ortiz (2006) General Reading Review (116 independent studies)	McGrew & Wendling (2010) Basic Reading Skills and Reading Comprehension Findings[1] (19 CHC/WJ studies)	Comments
Gf	Inductive (I) and General Sequential Reasoning (RG) abilities play a moderate role in reading comprehension.	Quantitative Reasoning (RQ) is tentative/speculative at ages 6–8 and 14–19 years for Basic Reading Skills (BRS).[2] Broad *Gf* is tentative/speculative at ages 14–19 years for Reading Comprehension (RC).	The lack of a relationship between *Gf* abilities and reading in the McGrew and Wendling summary may be related to the nature of the dependent measures. For example, RC was represented by the WJ Passage Comprehension and Reading Vocabulary tests, both of which draw minimally on reasoning (e.g., they do not require an individual to draw inferences or make predictions).
Gc	**Language Development (LD), Lexical Knowledge (VL), and Listening Abilities (LS) are important. These abilities become increasingly important with age.**	LS is moderately consistent at ages 6–8 years for BRS. LS is highly consistent at ages 6–19 years for RC. General Fund of Information (KO) is consistent at ages 6–8 and moderately consistent at ages 9–19 years for BRS. KO is highly consistent at ages 6–19 years for RC. Broad *Gc* is moderately consistent at ages 6–13 and highly consistent at ages 14–19 years for BRS. Broad *Gc* is highly consistent at ages 6–19 years for RC.	The findings across the Flanagan et al., and McGrew and Wendling summaries are quite similar given that Broad *Gc* in the McGrew and Wendling summary is defined primarily by the narrow abilities of LD and VL. However, Flanagan et al. did not find a consistent relationship between the narrow ability of KO and reading, as KO was not well represented in the studies they reviewed.
Gsm	Memory Span (MS) is important especially when evaluated **within the context of working memory.**	Working Memory (MW) is moderately consistent at ages 6–19 years for BRS and highly consistent for RC at ages 6–19 years. MS is tentative/speculative at ages 6–8 and moderately consistent at ages 9–19 years for BRS. MS is consistent at ages 6–13 and moderately consistent at ages 14–19 years for RC. Broad *Gsm* is consistent at ages 6–8 and highly consistent at ages 9–19 years for BRS. Broad *Gsm* is consistent at ages 6–8 and 14–19 years for RC.	Both the Flanagan et al. and McGrew and Wendling summaries highlight the importance of *Gsm* for reading.

Gv	Orthographic processing	Visual Memory (MV) is moderately consistent at ages 14–19 years for RC. Broad Gv is not consistently related to BRS or RC.	One possible explanation for the lack of a Gv relationship with BRS in the McGrew and Wendling summary is that the types of tasks used to measure visual processing in the studies they reviewed (e.g., spatial relations) do not measure the visual aspects of reading (e.g., orthographic processing). Orthographic processing or awareness (the ability to rapidly map graphemes to phonemes) may be more related to the perceptual speed tasks found on cognitive tests (e.g., Symbol Search on the Wechsler scales).
Ga	**Phonetic Coding (PC) or phonological awareness/processing is very important during the elementary school years.**	PC is moderately consistent at ages 6–13 and consistent at ages 14–19 years for BRS. PC is consistent at ages 6–8 and 14–19 years; tentative/speculative at ages 9–13 years for RC. Speech Sound Discrimination and Resistance to Auditory Stimulus Distortion (US/UR) are consistent at ages 9–19 years for BRS. Broad Ga is not consistently related to BRS. Broad Ga is moderately related at ages 6–8 years for RC.	Interestingly, and in contrast to Flanagan et al.'s summary, McGrew and Wendling's summary does not show a strong relationship between PC/phonological processing and reading at any age level. Given the wealth of research on the relations between PC/phonological processing and reading coupled with the neuroimaging research showing normalization of brain function in response to effective interventions for PC/phonological processing deficits, a reasonable assumption is that PC/phonological processing plays an important role in reading development during the early elementary school years. The relationship between PC/phonological processing and reading may be more prominent in students with reading difficulties, a population not included in the McGrew and Wendling samples.

(continued)

Table 12.5 (Continued)

CHC Ability	Flanagan, Mascolo, Alfonso, & Ortiz (2006) General Reading Review (116 independent studies)	McGrew & Wendling (2010) Basic Reading Skills and Reading Comprehension Findings[1] (19 CHC/WJ studies)	Comments
Glr	**Naming Facility (NA) or *rapid automatic naming* is very important during the elementary school years.** Associative Memory (MA) was also found to be related to reading at young ages (e.g., age 6 years).	MA is consistent at ages 6–8 years for BRS. Meaningful Memory (MM) is highly consistent at ages 9–19 years for RC. NA is consistent at ages 14–19 and moderately consistent at ages 9–13 years for RC. Broad *Glr* is consistent at ages 6–8 years for BRS. Broad *Glr* is consistent at ages 9–13 years for RC.	The lack of a significant relation between NA and BRS in the early elementary school years (ages 6–8 years) in the McGrew and Wendling summary is surprising, as rapid automatized naming or rate has always been implicated in young children who struggle with reading achievement, particularly reading fluency. However, the outcome measures in the studies reviewed by McGrew and Wendling may not have measured reading fluency well or at all.
Gs	**Perceptual speed (P) is important during all school years, particularly the elementary school years.**	P is consistent at ages 6–8 and 14–19 years and moderately consistent at ages 9–13 years for BRS. P is consistent at ages 14–19 and moderately consistent at ages 6–13 years for RC.	Flanagan et al.'s summary shows a stronger relationship between *Gs* and reading than McGrew and Wendling's summary. Nevertheless, the findings of both investigations show that *Gs* and P, in particular, are important for reading.

Note: For a discussion of the limitations of the findings reported in this table, see McGrew and Wendling (2010).
[1] Qualitative descriptors of *consistency* for McGrew and Wendling (2010) analyses were coded as follows: The label "highly consistent" means that a significant finding was noted in 80% or more of the studies reviewed; "moderately consistent" means that a significant finding was noted in 50% to 79% of the studies reviewed; and "consistent" means that a significant finding was noted in 30% to 49% of the studies reviewed.
[2] *Tentative speculative* results were those that were: (a) between 20%–29% in consistency, (b) based on a very small number of analyses (e.g., n = 2), and/or (c) based only on McGrew's (2007) exploratory multiple regression analysis of manifest WJ III variables at the individual IV test level (McGrew & Wendling, 2010).

Table 12.6 Important Findings on Relations Between CHC Abilities and Mathematics Achievement

CHC Ability	Flanagan, Mascolo, Alfonso, & Ortiz (2006) General Math Review1 (32 independent studies)	McGrew & Wendling (2010) Basic Math Skills and Math Reasoning Findings[2] (10 CHC/WJ studies)	Comments
Gf	**Inductive (I) and general sequential (RG) reasoning abilities are consistently related to math achievement at all ages.**	Quantitative Reasoning (RQ) highly consistent at ages 6–19 years. RG highly consistent at ages 14–19 years for Math Reasoning (MR) and consistent at ages 6–19 years for Basic Math Skills (BMS).	Broad *Gf* is highly consistent at ages 6–13 and moderately consistent at ages 14–19 years for MR and moderately consistent at ages 6–19 years for BMS. In McGrew & Wendling's analyses, Induction was part of the RQ tasks and also was subsumed by *Gf*.
Gc	**Language development (LD), lexical knowledge (VL), and listening abilities (LS) are important. These abilities become increasingly more important with age.**	LD and VL are consistent at ages 9–13 and highly consistent at ages 14–19 years for BMS. LD and VL are consistent at ages 6–8, moderately consistent at ages 9–13 and highly consistent at ages 14–19 years for MR. LS is consistent at ages 6–8 and highly consistent at ages 9–19 years for MR. LS is highly consistent for BMS at ages 6–19 years. K0 is moderately consistent up to age 13 and highly consistent at ages 14–19 years for MR only.	The lack of a relationship between LD/VL and BMS at ages 6–8 years in McGrew and Wendling is surprising, as elementary math contains several language concepts (e.g., less than, greater than, sum, in all, together). This finding is likely related to the nature of the math tasks used in the studies reviewed. General Fund of Information (K0) was either not represented or did not demonstrate a consistent relationship with math achievement in the Flanagan et al. review. Broad *Gc* is moderately consistent at ages 9–19 years for BMS. Broad *Gc* is consistent at ages 6–8 years, moderately consistent at ages 9–13 and highly consistent at ages 14–19 years for MR.
Gsm	Memory span (MS) is important especially when evaluated **within the context of working memory.**	Working Memory (MW) is highly consistent at ages 6–19 years. MS is consistent at ages 6–8 years for MR only.	Broad *Gsm* is consistent at ages 14–19 years for MR only.
Gv	May be important primarily for higher level or advanced mathematics (e.g., geometry, calculus).	Spatial Scanning (SS) is consistent at ages 6–8 years for BMS only.	*Gv* abilities related to math achievement are either not measured or not measured adequately by current intelligence batteries. Alternatively, the importance of an adequately measured *Gv* ability may be masked by the presence of other important variables (e.g., *Gc*, *Gsm*) included in the analyses (McGrew & Wendling).

(continued)

Table 12.6 (Continued)

CHC Ability	Flanagan, Mascolo, Alfonso, & Ortiz (2006) General Math Review[1] (32 independent studies)	McGrew & Wendling (2010) Basic Math Skills and Math Reasoning Findings[2] (10 CHC/WJ studies)	Comments
Ga		Phonetic Coding (PC) is consistent at ages 6–13 years for BMS. PC is moderately consistent at ages 9–19 years and consistent at ages 6–8 and consistent at ages 9–19 years for MR. Speech Sound Discrimination and Resistance to Auditory Stimulus Distortion (US/UR) are moderately consistent at ages 9–13 years for MR only.	The relationship in the McGrew and Wendling study between PC and BMS reflects the use of Sound Blending as the PC indicator. Memory span is necessary for optimal performance on Sound Blending, which may account for the presence of the relationship.
Glr		Meaningful Memory (MM) is moderately consistent at ages 14–19 years for MR. MM is moderately consistent at ages 9–13 years for BMS. Associative Memory (MA) is consistent at ages 6–8 years for BMS. NA is consistent at ages 6–19 years for BMS only.	MM and MA was either not represented or did not demonstrate a consistent relationship with math achievement in the Flanagan et al. review. The relationship between Naming Facility (NA) and BMS would likely be more robust if the cognitive task stimuli involved the rapid naming of numbers rather than pictures.
Gs	Speed of Processing (*Gs*) and, more specifically, Perceptual Speed (P) is important during all school years, particularly during elementary school.	Broad *Gs* is moderately consistent at ages 6–13 and consistent at ages 14–19 years for BMS. Broad *Gs* is consistent at ages 6–8 and moderately consistent at ages 9–13 years for MR. AC/EF is consistent at ages 6–8 years for BMS. AC/EF is highly consistent for ages 9–13 and consistent for ages 14–19 years for BMS. P is highly consistent at ages 6–19 years for BMS and moderately consistent at ages 6–19 years for MR.	In McGrew and Wendling's summary of the relations between *Gs* and math, P is also described as Attention–Concentration/Executive Functioning (AC/EF).

Note: For a discussion of the limitations of the findings reported in this table, see McGrew and Wendling (2010).

[1] The absence of comments for a particular CHC ability and achievement area (e.g., *Ga* and mathematics) in the Flanagan et al. review indicates that the research reviewed either did not report any significant relationships between the respective CHC ability and the achievement area, or if significant findings were reported, they were only for a limited number of studies. Comments in bold represent the CHC abilities that demonstrated the strongest and most consistent relationship to mathematics achievement.

[2] Qualitative descriptors of *consistency* for McGrew & Wendling (2010) analyses were coded as follows: The label "highly consistent" denotes that a significant finding was noted in 80% or more of the studies reviewed; "moderately consistent" denotes that a significant finding was noted in 50% to 79% of the studies reviewed; and "consistent" denotes that a significant finding was noted in 30% to 49% of the studies reviewed.

Table 12.7 Important Findings on Relations Between CHC Abilities and Writing Achievement

CHC Ability	Writing Achievement
Gf	Inductive (I) and general sequential reasoning abilities are related to basic writing skills primarily during the elementary school years (e.g., 6–13) and consistently related to written expression at all ages.
Gc	**Language development (LD), lexical knowledge (VL), and general information (KO)[1] are important primarily after age 7. These abilities become increasingly more important with age.**
Gsm	**Memory span (MS) is important to writing, especially spelling skills whereas working memory has shown relations with advanced writing skills (e.g., written expression).**
Gv	Orthographic Processing
Ga	**Phonetic coding (PC) or "phonological awareness/processing" is very important during the elementary school years for both basic writing skills and written expression (primarily before age 11).**
Glr	Naming facility (NA) or "rapid automatic naming" has demonstrated relations with written expression, primarily the fluency aspect of writing. Associative Memory.
Gs	**Perceptual Speed (P) is important during all school years for basic writing and related to all ages for written expression.**

Note: Comments in bold represent the CHC abilities that showed the strongest and most consistent relation to writing achievement. Information in this table was reproduced from Flanagan, Ortiz, Alfonso, & Mascolo (2006) with permission from John Wiley and Sons. All rights reserved.
[1]Includes orthographic knowledge and knowledge of morphology, which contribute to spelling and written expression.

Glr, *Gsm*, and *Gs* abilities. The significant and most consistent *Gf* findings were between inductive and deductive reasoning and reading comprehension (e.g., see Flanagan et al., 2006, for a discussion). This suggests that the comprehension of text may draw on an individual's reasoning abilities, depending on the demands of the comprehension task (e.g., tasks that require drawing inferences and making predictions).

Very few studies reported a significant relation between *Gv* and reading achievement, although McGrew and Wendling (2010) reported a consistent relationship between Visual Memory and reading comprehension at ages 14–19 years. Overall it appears that *Gv* abilities do not play a significant role in reading achievement. This does not mean that visual processing abilities are not involved during reading. The lack of significant *Gv*/reading research findings indicates that the contribution of *Gv* abilities (as measured by the major intelligence batteries) to the explanation and prediction of reading achievement is so small that, when compared to other abilities (e.g., *Ga*), it is of little practical significance. However, it is important not to over generalize this conclusion to all visual abilities. As pointed out by Berninger (1990), visual perceptual abilities should not be confused with abilities that are related to the coding of visual

information in printed words (i.e., orthographic code processing)—visual processes thought to be important during reading. Indeed, Flanagan and her colleagues (2006) found in their review of the literature a consistent relationship between orthographic processing and reading achievement (i.e., basic reading skills).

In summary, narrow abilities in seven broad CHC domains appear to be related significantly to reading achievement. The findings of two independent, comprehensive literature reviews (i.e., Flanagan et al., 2006; McGrew & Wendling, 2010) suggest that abilities subsumed by *Gc* (Language Development, Lexical Knowledge, Listening Ability, General Information), *Gsm* (Memory Span, Working Memory), *Ga* (Phonetic Coding), *Glr* (Associative Memory, Naming Facility, Meaningful Memory), and *Gs* (Perceptual Speed) are related significantly to reading achievement. Furthermore, developmental results suggest that the *Ga*, *Gs*, and *Glr* relations with reading are strongest during the early elementary school years, after which they systematically decrease in strength (e.g., Flanagan et al.; McGrew, 1993). In contrast, the strength of the relations between *Gc* abilities and reading achievement increases with age. The *Gv* abilities of orthographic processing and visual memory are related to reading achievement. Finally, *Gf* abilities appear related primarily to reading comprehension from childhood to young adulthood.

Cognitive Abilities and Math Achievement

Similar to reading, both literature reviews (i.e., Flanagan et al., 2006; McGrew & Wendling, 2010) found that *Gc*, *Gsm* (particularly working memory), and *Gs* are related significantly to math achievement. In contrast to reading, stronger evidence of the relations between *Gf* and *Gv* abilities and math achievement was found.

In some of the more comprehensive studies of the relations between CHC abilities and math achievement (e.g., McGrew & Hessler; 1995), *Gf*, *Gc*, and *Gs* abilities correlated consistently and significantly with basic math skills and math problem-solving. However, there were developmental differences. The *Gc* relation with mathematics achievement increased monotonically with age, whereas the *Gs* relation was strongest during the elementary school years, after which it decreased (although the relationship remained significant well into adulthood). *Gf* was related consistently to mathematics achievement at levels higher than all other CHC abilities (except *Gc*) across all ages. As in the reading achievement research just mentioned, certain specific abilities (*Gf*, *Gs*, *Gc*) were found to be related significantly to mathematics achievement above and beyond the contribution of *g* (e.g., McGrew et al., 1997).

With one exception (i.e., a consistent relation between Spatial Scanning and basic math skills), no significant relations between *Gv* and mathematics achievement were found. Likewise, very few studies reported a significant relationship between *Glr* and mathematics achievement (Floyd et al., 2003; Geary, 1993; Geary, Hoard, & Bailey, 2011). According to McGrew and Wendling (2010), the *Glr* narrow ability of Meaningful Memory is related to basic math skills at ages 9–13 years and math reasoning at ages 14–19 years; Associative Memory and Naming Facility are related to basic math skills at ages 6–8 years and 6–19 years, respectively. Moreover, Swanson and Beebe-Frankenberger (2004) found that long-term memory is important in predicting mathematical problem-solving solution accuracy beyond that predicted by other abilities (e.g., *Gsm*, *Gs*).

Cognitive Abilities and Writing Achievement

A review of Table 12.7 demonstrates that several CHC domains are related to writing achievement. Specifically, researchers have documented relations between cognitive abilities and writing achievement across the seven CHC domains listed in Table 12.7 (*Gf*, *Gc*, *Gsm*, *Gv*, *Ga*, *Glr*, and *Gs*). However, the limited number of studies in certain CHC domains clearly suggests that the consistency of relations differs markedly across areas. For instance, only one study demonstrated a relation between *Gf* abilities and writing achievement. Specifically, McGrew and Knopik (1993) found that fluid reasoning abilities (i.e., induction and general sequential reasoning) were related significantly to basic writing skills primarily during the elementary school years (i.e., ages 6 to 13) and significantly related to written expression across all ages.

Similarly, the study by McGrew and Knopik (1993) provided evidence for the role of *Gs* abilities in writing. More specifically, this study demonstrated that the *Gs* cluster (comprised of measures of perceptual speed) "was significantly related to Basic Writing Skills during the school years . . . after which it decreased in strength of association" (p. 690) with age. The relations between *Gs* and written expression were more consistent in strength across ages. As explained by McGrew and Knopik, "Given the timed nature of the [WJ-R] Writing Fluency tests that comprises one-half of the [WJ-R] Written Expression cluster, the finding of consistently significant associations between Processing Speed and this writing achievement criterion was not surprising" (p. 692). This finding is also not surprising in light of the recent refinements to CHC theory, particularly the addition of Writing Speed (WS) as a narrow *Gs* ability (see Figure 12.4).

Similar to McGrew and Knopik's (1993) findings, Floyd and colleagues (2008) and Williams and colleagues (1993) also reported significant relations between *Gs* and writing abilities. For example, the latter study demonstrated relations between the WISC-III Coding subtest (a measure of Rate of Test Taking) and the WJ-R Writing Fluency test. Likewise, Hargrave (2005) found that, in addition to other CHC broad abilities, *Gs* significantly predicted performance on the WJ III ACH Broad Written Language Cluster. Given these findings, it seems likely that processing speed is important in terms of writing automaticity as well as more general writing ability. Although only a few studies found a relation between *Gs* and writing achievement, the strength of the *Gs* effects demonstrated in the aforementioned studies is significant and warrants continued attention and investigation (Floyd et al., 2008).

Research on the relations between *Gv* and writing achievement is sparse, suggesting the need for continued study (see Berninger, 1999). Because only one study in Flanagan and colleagues' (2006) review reported a significant relation between *Gv* and writing achievement (Aaron, 1995), it may be that *Gv* abilities as assessed by the major intelligence batteries do not play a significant role in writing achievement. This is not to say that *Gv* abilities are unimportant for writing. In fact, orthographic processing, is particularly influential in basic writing tasks (e.g., spelling; see Berninger, 2009). As defined by Aaron (1995), orthography refers to the visual patterns of the written language. However, "orthographic processing ability is not the same as visual memory even though visual memory may play a role in it" (Aaron, p. 347). Specifically, some researchers have indicated that a certain type of memory for orthographic units may play a role in spelling words that cannot be accurately spelled using the rules of pronunciation alone (see Kreiner & Gough, 1990, for a more in-depth discussion). Despite the role that orthographic knowledge plays in basic writing tasks, this relationship is not evident in Table 12.7, primarily because CHC theory does not currently have a narrow ability category corresponding to this type of processing. Many of the existing *Gv* abilities that comprise CHC theory (e.g., visualization, spatial relations; closure speed) appear to be minimally related to writing achievement. It is likely that *Gv*-type abilities, such as orthographic processing, that are related to writing (and reading) achievement will be incorporated within the CHC theoretical framework in the near future, particularly as this research base mounts (Flanagan et al., 2006).

The research on the relations between *Glr* and *Gc* and writing achievement is also sparse. The fact that only a handful of studies have documented a significant relation between *Glr* and writing to date suggests that either *Glr* abilities are of limited importance to the writing process or the importance of *Glr* in writing ability has not been investigated thoroughly. Nevertheless, the narrow ability of Associative Memory (MA) appears to be involved in mapping sounds to their corresponding letters (e.g., Mather & Wendling, 2011). In terms of *Gc*, McGrew and Knopik (1993) and Floyd et al. (2008) found significant relations among language development (LD), lexical knowledge (VL), general information (K0), and writing abilities (i.e., basic writing skills and written expression). Although the *Gc* research is also limited, there are certainly stores of knowledge (*Gc*) that are necessary for successful writing. For example, knowledge of orthography and morphology as well as lexical knowledge contribute to spelling and written expression (Mather & Wendling).

Despite the limited research on the relations between CHC abilities and writing achievement, Table 12.7 shows that *Gc* and *Gsm* displayed the most consistent significant relations with overall writing achievement. Additionally, Phonetic Coding, a narrow *Ga* ability, and Perceptual Speed, a narrow *Gs* ability, were found to have strong and consistent relations with writing achievement across many studies, especially during the early elementary school years (e.g., Berninger et al., 1994; Johnson, 1993; Joshi, 1995; McGrew & Knopik, 1993). Finally, the majority of studies that found a relationship between *Gsm* and writing achievement suggested that memory span is an important predictor of early writing achievement.

Overall, several CHC abilities are related significantly to writing achievement. Among these, the most consistent relations appear to be with *Ga* (phonetic coding), *Gsm* (memory span), *Gs* (perceptual speed), and *Gc* (lexical knowledge, language development, and general information, the latter of which includes orthographic knowledge and knowledge of morphology). The relatively limited research on the relations between cognitive abilities and writing achievement may be related, in part, to the fact that writing research has taken a tertiary position to reading and math research. That is, although the early pioneering literature on learning disabilities emphasized both writing and reading disabilities, the subsequent learning disabilities literature has given more attention to reading than writing (Berninger, 1997, 2011). Given the importance of writing throughout one's educational (and often, professional) careers, the field would benefit from additional research within this domain.

In summary, Tables 12.5, 12.6, and 12.7 presented the available literature on the relations between cognitive abilities (and processes) and reading, math, and writing achievement, respectively, based largely on two independent, comprehensive reviews of the literature (Flanagan et al., 2006; McGrew & Wendling, 2010). Narrow abilities subsumed by *Gc* (lexical knowledge, language development, listening ability, general information), *Gsm* (memory span, working memory), *Ga* (phonetic coding), *Glr* (associative memory, meaningful memory, naming facility), and *Gs* (perceptual speed) were found to be significantly and most consistently related to reading achievement. Similarly, narrow abilities within these same broad abilities were found to be related to writing achievement. Narrow abilities within the areas of *Gf*, *Gc*, *Gsm*, *Glr*, and *Gs* were found to relate significantly to math achievement, with *Gf* (induction and general sequential reasoning) showing a stronger relation to this academic area than either reading or writing.

Integrating CHC and Neuropsychological Theories to Enhance Test Interpretation[1]

With the emergence of the field of school neuropsychology (e.g., Fletcher-Janzen & Reynolds, 2008; Hale & Fiorello, 2004; Miller, 2007, 2010) came the desire to link CHC theory and neuropsychological theories. Understanding how CHC theory and neuropsychological theories relate to one another will expand the options available for interpreting cognitive test performance in particular and will improve the quality and clarity of test interpretation in general, as a much wider research base will be available to inform practice.

Although scientific understanding of the manner in which the brain functions and how mental activity is expressed on psychometric tasks has increased dramatically in recent years, there is still much to be learned. All efforts to create a framework that guides test interpretation benefit from diverse points of view. For example, according to Fiorello et al. (2008), "the compatibility of the neuropsychological and psychometric approaches to cognitive functioning suggests converging lines of evidence from separate lines of inquiry, a validity dimension essential to the study of individual differences in how children think and learn" (p. 232). Their analysis of the links between the neuropsychological and psychometric approaches not only provides validity for both, but also suggests that each approach may benefit from knowledge of the other. As such, a framework that incorporates the neuropsychological and psychometric approaches to cognitive functioning holds the promise of increasing knowledge about the etiology and nature of a variety of disorders (e.g., specific learning disability) and the manner in which such disorders are treated. This type of framework should not only connect the elements and components of both assessment approaches, but it should also allow interpretation of data within the context of either model. In other words, the framework should serve as a "translation" of the concepts, nomenclature, and principles of one approach into their similar counterparts in the other. A brief discussion of one such framework, developed by Flanagan, Alfonso, Ortiz, and Dynda

(2010), is presented in the following section. This framework is illustrated in Figure 12.5 and represents an integration based on psychometric, neuropsychological, and Lurian perspectives.

The interpretive framework shown in Figure 12.5 draws upon prior research and sources, most notably Dehn (2006); Fiorello et al. (2007); Fletcher-Janzen and Reynolds (2008); Miller (2007); and Strauss, Sherman, and Spreen (2006). In understanding the manner in which Luria's blocks, the neuropsychological domains, and CHC broad abilities may be linked to inform test interpretation and mutual understanding among assessment professionals, Flanagan and colleagues pointed out four important observations that deserve mention. First, there is a hierarchical structure among the three theoretical conceptualizations. Second, the hierarchical structure parallels a continuum of interpretive complexity, spanning the broadest levels of cognitive functioning, where mental activities are "integrated," to the narrowest level of cognitive functioning where mental activity is reduced to more "discrete" abilities and processes (see far left side of Figure 12.5). Third, all mental activity takes place within a given ecological and societal context and is heavily influenced by language as well as other factors external to the individual. As such, the dotted line surrounding Figure 12.5 represents "language and ecological influences on learning," which includes factors such as exposure to language, language status (English learner vs. English speaker), opportunity to learn, and socioeconomic status (SES). Fourth, because the administration of cognitive and neuropsychological tests should not typically be conducted in the schools (for students suspected of having a learning disability) unless a student fails to respond as expected to evidence-based instruction and intervention, a rectangle is included at the top of Figure 12.5 that is labeled, "Difficulty with Classroom Learning and Failure to RTI." Thus, the framework in Figure 12.5 is a representation of the cognitive constructs that may be measured and the manner in which they relate to one another.

According to Flanagan and colleagues (2010), arrows leading from the "Difficulty with Classroom Learning and Failure to RTI" rectangle to Luria's three functional units of the brain (represented as large circles in Figure 12.5) demonstrate the beginning of a school-based hypothesis-generation, testing, and interpretation process. Luria's functional units are depicted in Figure 12.5 as overarching cognitive concepts. The interaction between, and the interconnectedness among, the functional units

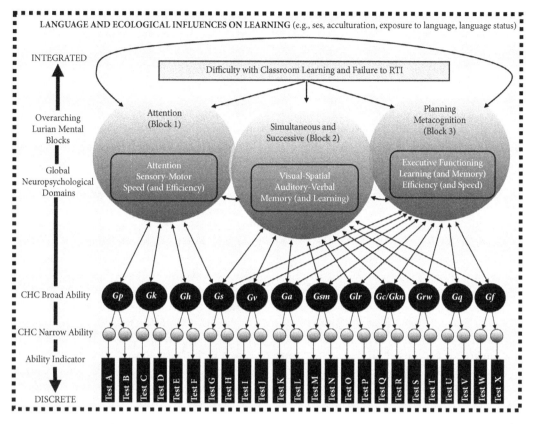

Figure 12.5 An integrative framework based on psychometric, neuropsychological, and Lurian perspectives.

Note: Reproduced with permission from Wiley. Copyright 2010. All rights reserved.

are represented by double-headed arrows. Because Luria's functional units are primarily descriptive concepts designed to guide applied clinical evaluation practices, neuropsychologists have had considerable independence in the manner in which they align their assessments with these concepts (Flanagan et al., 2010).

Although a few psychoeducational batteries have been developed to operationalize one or more of Luria's functional units, for the most part, neuropsychologists have couched Luria's blocks within clinical and neuropsychological domains. In doing so, the Lurian blocks have been transformed somewhat from overarching concepts to domains with more specificity (Flanagan et al., 2010). These domains are listed in rectangles within each of the three functional units (large circles) in Figure 12.5. For example, the neuropsychological domains include: *attention, sensory-motor, and speed (and efficiency)*, corresponding to Block 1; *visual-spatial, auditory-verbal, memory (and learning)*, corresponding to Block 2; and *executive functioning, learning (and memory)*, and *efficiency (and speed)*

corresponding to Block 3. Noteworthy is the fact that the memory and learning domain spans Blocks 2 and 3, and its placement and use of parentheses is intended to convey that memory may be associated primarily with Block 2 (simultaneous/successive) whereas the learning component of this domain is probably more closely associated with Block 3 (planning/metacognition). Likewise, speed and efficiency spans Blocks 1 and 3, and its placement and use of parentheses denote that speed may be associated more with Block 1 (i.e., attention) whereas efficiency seems to be associated more with Block 3 (Flanagan et al., 2010).

Perhaps the most critical juncture of Flanagan and colleagues' (2010) integrative framework is the distinction between functioning at the neuropsychological domain level and functioning at the broad CHC level. As compared to the neuropsychological domains, CHC theory allows for greater specificity of cognitive constructs. Because of structural differences in the conceptualization of neuropsychological domains and CHC broad abilities vis-à-vis factorial complexity, it is not possible to provide a precise, one-to-one correspondence between these conceptual levels. This is neither a problem nor an obstacle, but simply the reality of differences in perspective among these two lines of inquiry.

As compared to the neuropsychological domains, CHC constructs within the psychometric tradition tend to be relatively distinct because the intent is to measure a single broad ability as purely and independently as possible. This is not to say, however, that the psychometric tradition has completely ignored shared task characteristics in favor of a focus on precision in measuring relatively distinct cognitive constructs. For example, Kaufman provided a "shared characteristic" approach to individual test performance for several intelligence tests including the KABC-II (Kaufman & Kaufman, 2004) and the various Wechsler scales (Kaufman, 1979; see also McCloskey, 2009, McGrew & Flanagan, 1998 and Sattler, 1998). This practice has often provided insight into the underlying cause(s) of learning difficulties, and astute practitioners continue to make use of it. Despite the fact that standardized, norm-referenced tests of CHC abilities were designed primarily to provide information about relatively discrete constructs, performance on these tests can still be viewed within the context of the broader neuropsychological domains. That is, when evaluated within the context of an entire battery, characteristics that are shared among groups of tests on which a student performed either high or low, for example, often provide the type of information necessary to assist in further understanding the nature of an individual's underlying cognitive function or dysfunction, conceptualized as neuropsychological domains (Flanagan et al., 2010).

The double-headed arrows between neuropsychological domains and CHC abilities in Figure 12.5 demonstrate that the relationship between these constructs is bidirectional. That is, one can conceive of the neuropsychological domains as global entities that are composed of various CHC abilities, just as one can conceive of a particular CHC ability as involving aspects of more than one neuropsychological domain. Flanagan and colleagues' (2010) conceptualization of the relations between the neuropsychological domains and the CHC broad abilities follows. For the purpose of parsimony the neuropsychological domains are grouped according to their relationship with the Lurian blocks and thus, these domains are discussed as clusters, rather than discussed separately.

Correspondence Between the Neuropsychological Domains and CHC Broad Abilities

According to Flanagan and colleagues (2010), at least six CHC broad abilities compose the *Attention/Sensory-Motor/Speed (and Efficiency)* neuropsychological cluster, including Psychomotor Abilities (*Gp*), Tactile Abilities (*Gh*), Kinesthetic Abilities (*Gk*), Decision/Reaction Time or Speed (*Gt*)[2], Processing Speed (*Gs*), and Olfactory Abilities (*Go*)[3]. *Gp* involves the ability to perform body movements with precision, coordination, or strength. *Gh* involves the sensory receptors of the tactile (touch) system, such as the ability to detect and make fine discriminations of pressure on the surface of the skin. *Gk* includes abilities that depend on sensory receptors that detect bodily position, weight, or movement of the muscles, tendons, and joints. Because *Gk* includes sensitivity in the detection, awareness, or movement of the body or body parts and the ability to recognize a path the body previously explored without the aid of visual input (e.g., blindfolded), it may involve some visual-spatial processes, but the input remains sensory-based and thus better aligned with the sensory-motor domain. *Gt* involves the ability to react and/or make decisions quickly in response to simple stimuli, typically measured by chronometric measures of reaction time or inspection time. *Gs* is the ability to automatically and fluently perform relatively easy or overlearned cognitive tasks, especially when high mental efficiency is required. As measured by current intelligence tests (e.g., WISC-IV Coding, Symbol Search, and Cancellation), *Gs* seems to capture the essence of both speed and efficiency, which is why there are double headed arrows from *Gs* to Block 1 (where *Speed* is emphasized) and Block 3 (where *Efficiency* is emphasized) in Figure 12.5. *Go* involves abilities that depend on sensory receptors of the main olfactory system (nasal chambers). Many of the CHC abilities comprising the Attention/Sensory-Motor/Speed (and efficiency) cluster are measured by neuropsychological tests (e.g., Dean-Woodcock; Flanagan et al., 2010).

Prior research suggests that virtually all broad CHC abilities may be subsumed by the *Visual-Spatial/Auditory-Verbal/Memory (and Learning)* neuropsychological cluster. That is, the vast majority of tasks on neuropsychological, intelligence, and cognitive ability tests require either visual-spatial or auditory-verbal input. Apart from tests that relate more to discrete sensory-motor functioning and that utilize sensory input along the kinesthetic, tactile, or olfactory systems, all other tests will necessarily rely either on visual-spatial or auditory-verbal stimuli. Certainly, visual (*Gv*) and auditory (*Ga*) processing are measured well on neuropsychological and cognitive instruments. Furthermore, tests of Short-Term Memory (*Gsm*) and Long-Term Storage and Retrieval (*Glr*) typically rely on visual (e.g., pictures) or verbal (digits or words) information for input. Tasks that involve reasoning (*Gf*), stores of acquired knowledge (viz., *Gc*), and even speed (*Gs*) also use either visual-spatial and/or auditory-verbal channels for input. Furthermore, it is likely that such input will be processed in one of two possible ways—simultaneously or successively (Flanagan et al., 2010).

And last, Flanagan and colleagues (2010) believe that prior research suggests that the *Executive Functioning/Learning (and Memory)/Efficiency (and Speed)* neuropsychological cluster is thought to correspond well with perhaps eight broad CHC abilities, including Fluid Intelligence (*Gf*), Crystallized Intelligence (*Gc*), General (Domain-Specific) Knowledge Ability (*Gkn*), Quantitative Knowledge (*Gq*), Broad Reading and Writing Ability (*Grw*), Processing Speed (*Gs*), Short-Term Memory (*Gsm*), and Long-Term Storage and Retrieval (*Glr*). *Gf* generally involves the ability to solve novel problems using inductive, deductive, and/or quantitative reasoning and, therefore, is most closely associated with executive functioning. *Gc* represents one's stores of acquired knowledge (e.g., vocabulary, general information) or "learned" information and is entirely dependent on language, the ability that Luria believed was necessary to mediate all aspects of learning. In addition, Domain-Specific Knowledge (*Gkn*), together with knowledge of Reading/Writing (*Grw*) and Math (*Gq*), reflect the *learning* component of "memory and learning." Therefore, *Gc, Gkn, Grw,* and *Gq* are included as part of this cluster. *Gsm,* especially working memory, and *Glr* appear to require executive functions, such as planning and organizing.

As may be seen in Figure 12.5, Flanagan and colleagues (2010) have placed the CHC *narrow* abilities at the *discrete* end of the integrated–discrete continuum. Noteworthy is the fact that narrow ability deficits tend to be more amenable to remediation, accommodation, or compensatory strategy interventions as compared to broad and more overarching abilities. For example, poor memory span, a narrow ability subsumed by the broad ability, *Gsm,* can often be compensated for effectively via the use of strategies such as writing things down or recording them in some manner for later reference. In contrast, when test performance suggests more pervasive dysfunction, as may be indicated by deficits in one or more global neuropsychological domains, for example, the greater the likelihood that intervention will need to be broader, perhaps focusing on the type of instruction being provided to the student and how the curriculum ought to be modified and delivered to improve the student's learning (Flanagan et al., 2011; Fiorello et al., 2008). An example of the applicability of this framework may be seen in Table 12.8, which includes an example of how the WISC-IV was classified via the framework depicted in Figure 12.5 (Flanagan, Alfonso, Mascolo, & Hale, 2011; for classifications of other intelligence and neuropsychological batteries, see Flanagan et al., 2010).

Greater Emphasis on Flexible Battery Approaches

As our understanding of cognitive abilities continues to unfold and as we begin to gain a greater understanding of how school neuropsychology will influence the practice of intelligence and cognitive ability test interpretation, it seems clear that the breadth and depth of information we can garner from our tests is ever increasing. In light of the recent expansion of CHC theory and the integration of this theory with neuropsychological theories, it will remain unlikely that an individual intelligence, cognitive ability, or neuropsychological battery will provide adequate coverage of the full range of abilities and processes that may be relevant to any given evaluation purpose or referral concern. The development of a battery that fully operationalizes CHC theory, for example, is likely to be extremely labor-intensive and prohibitively expensive for the average practitioner, school district, clinic, or university training program. Therefore, flexible battery approaches are likely to remain essential within the repertoire of practice for most professionals. By definition, flexible battery approaches offer an efficient and practical method by which practitioners may evaluate a broad range of human cognitive abilities and processes. In this section, we summarize one such flexible battery approach, XBA, because it is grounded in CHC theory and is based on sound psychometric principles and procedures.

The XBA was introduced by Flanagan and her colleagues about 15 years ago (Flanagan & McGrew, 1997; Flanagan, McGrew, & Ortiz, 2000;

Table 12.8 Lurian, Neuropsychological, and Cattell-Horn-Carroll (CHC) Classifications of Wechsler Intelligence Scale for Children–Fourth Edition (WISC-IV) Subtests

Subtest	Lurian Block			Neuropsychological Domains								CHC Broad and Narrow Abilities				
	Attention	Simultaneous or Successive	Planning and Metacognition	Sensory-Motor	Speed and Efficiency	Attention	Visual-Spatial (RH) and Detail (LH)	Auditory-Verbal	Memory and/or Learning	Executive	Language	Gf	Gc	Gsm	Gv	Gs
Arithmetic	✓	✓	✓			✓		✓	✓	✓	✓R	✓ (RQ)		✓ (MW)		
Block Design		✓	✓	✓			✓			✓					✓ (Vz)	
Cancellation	✓	✓	✓	✓	✓	✓	✓			✓						✓ (P)
Coding	✓	✓	✓	✓	✓	✓	✓		✓	✓						✓ (R9)
Comprehension		✓	✓					✓	✓		✓E/R		✓ (K0)			
Digit Span	✓	✓	✓			✓		✓	✓					✓ (MS,MW)		
Information		✓	✓					✓	✓		✓E/R		✓ (K0)			
Letter-Number Sequencing	✓	✓	✓			✓		✓	✓	✓				✓ (MW)		
Matrix Reasoning		✓	✓				✓			✓		✓ (I,RG)				

Picture Completion	✓	✓				✓						✓ (K0)	✓ (CF)
Picture Concepts		✓	✓			✓					✓ (I)		
Similarities		✓		✓		✓	✓ E				✓ (I)	✓ (VL)	
Symbol Search	✓		✓	✓	✓	✓							✓ (P)
Vocabulary		✓				✓	✓ E					✓ (VL)	
Word Reasoning		✓	✓			✓	✓ E/R				✓ (I)	✓ (VL)	

Note. Gf = Fluid Intelligence; Gc = Crystallized Intelligence; Gsm = Short-Term Memory; Gv = Visual Processing; Gs = Processing Speed. RQ = Quantitative Reasoning; MW = Working Memory; SR = Spatial Relations; Vz = Visualization; P = Perceptual Speed; R9 = Rate-of-Test-Taking; K0 = General (verbal) Knowledge; MS = Memory Span; I = Induction; RG = General Sequential Reasoning; CF = Flexibility of Closure; VL = Lexical Knowledge. The following Cattell-Horn-Carroll (CHC) broad abilities are omitted from this table because none is a primary ability measured by the WISC-IV: Gh (Tactile Abilities); Gk (Kinesthetic Abilities); Gp (Psychomotor Abilities); Gkn (General [domain-specific] Knowledge); Gq (Quantitative Knowledge); Gt = (Decision/Reaction Time or Speed); Grw (Reading and Writing Ability); Go (Olfactory Abilities); and Gps (Psychomotor Speed). Most CHC test classifications are from *Essentials of Cross-Battery Assessment, 2nd edition* (Flanagan, Ortiz, & Alfonso, 2007). Classifications according to neuropsychological domains were based on the authors' readings of neuropsychological texts (e.g., Fletcher-Janzen & Reynolds, 2008; Hale & Fiorello, 2004; Lezak, 1995; Miller, 2007).

Flanagan & Ortiz, 2001; McGrew & Flanagan, 1998). It provides practitioners with the means to make systematic, reliable, and theory-based interpretations of cognitive batteries and to augment them with other cognitive ability subtests, including subtests from academic and neuropsychological instruments, to gain a more complete understanding of an individual's strengths and weaknesses (Flanagan et al., 2007, 2013). Moving beyond the boundaries of a single cognitive, achievement, or neuropsychological battery by adopting the theoretically and psychometrically defensible XBA principles and procedures allows practitioners the flexibility necessary to measure the cognitive constructs and neurodevelopmental functions that are most germane to referral concerns (e.g., Carroll, 1998; Decker, 2008; Kaufman, 2000; Wilson, 1992).

According to Carroll (1997), the CHC taxonomy of human cognitive abilities "appears to prescribe that individuals should be assessed with respect to the total range of abilities the theory specifies" (p. 129). However, because Carroll recognized that "any such prescription would of course create enormous problems," he indicated that "[r]esearch is needed to spell out how the assessor can select what abilities need to be tested in particular cases" (p. 129). Flanagan and colleagues' XBA approach was developed specifically to "spell out" how practitioners can conduct assessments that approximate the total range of cognitive and academic abilities and neuropsychological processes more adequately than what is possible with any collection of co-normed tests.

In a review of the XBA approach, Carroll (1998) stated that it "can be used to develop the most appropriate information about an individual in a given testing situation" (p. xi). More recently, Decker (2008) stated that the XBA approach "may improve school psychology assessment practice and facilitate the integration of neuropsychological methodology in school-based assessments...[because it] shift[s] assessment practice from IQ composites to neurodevelopmental functions" (p. 804).

Noteworthy is the fact that assessment professionals "crossed" batteries well before Woodcock (1990) recognized the need to do so and before Flanagan and her colleagues introduced the XBA approach in the late 1990s, following his suggestion. Neuropsychological assessment has long adopted the practice of crossing various standardized tests in an attempt to measure a broader range of brain functions than that offered by any single instrument (Lezak, 1976, 1995; Lezak, Howieson, & Loring, 2004; also see Wilson, 1992 for a review). Nevertheless, several problems with crossing batteries plagued assessment-related fields for years. Many of these problems have been circumvented by Flanagan and colleagues' XBA approach (see Table 12.9 for examples). But unlike the XBA model, the various so-called cross-battery techniques applied within the field of neuropsychological assessment, for example, are not typically grounded in a systematic approach that is theoretically and psychometrically sound. Thus, as Wilson (1992) cogently pointed out, the field of neuropsychological assessment was in need of an approach that would guide practitioners through the selection of measures that would result in more specific and delineated patterns of function and dysfunction—an approach that provided more clinically useful information than one that was "wedded to the utilization of subscale scores and IQs" (p. 382). Indeed, all fields involved in the assessment of cognitive and neuropsychological functioning have some need for an approach that would aid practitioners in their attempt to "touch all of the major cognitive areas, with emphasis on those most suspect on the basis of history, observation, and on-going test findings" (Wilson, 1992, p. 382). The XBA approach has met this need. A brief definition of and rationale for XBA is presented next.

Definition of the XBA Approach

The XBA approach is a method of assessing cognitive and academic abilities and neuropsychological processes that is grounded mainly in CHC theory and research. It allows practitioners to measure reliably a wider range (or a more in depth but selective range) of ability constructs than that represented by any given stand-alone assessment battery. The XBA approach is based on three foundational sources of information (Flanagan et al., 2007, 2013) that together provide the knowledge base necessary to organize theory-driven, comprehensive assessments of cognitive, achievement, and neuropsychological constructs.

The Foundation of the XBA Approach

The foundation of the XBA approach rests on contemporary CHC theory and the broad and narrow CHC ability classifications of all subtests that comprise current cognitive, achievement, and selected neuropsychological batteries. Because CHC theory was described previously, we will focus here on the classifications of tests.

Table 12.9 Parallel Needs in Cognitive Assessment–Related Fields Addressed by the XBA Approach

Need Within Assessment-Related Fields[1]	Need Addressed by the XBA Approach
School psychology, clinical psychology, and neuropsychology have lagged in the development of conceptual models of the assessment of individuals. There is a need for the development of contemporary models.	The XBA approach provides a contemporary model for measurement and interpretation of cognitive and academic abilities and neuropsychological processes.
It is likely that there is a need for events external to a field of endeavor to give impetus to new developments and real advances in that field.	Carroll and Horn's *Fluid-Crystallized* theoretical models (and more recently, Schneider and McGrew's CHC model) and research in cognitive psychology and neuropsychology provided the impetus for and continued refinements to the XBA approach and led to the development of better assessment instruments and interpretive procedures.
There is a need to utilize a conceptual framework to direct any approach to assessment. This would aid in both the selection of instruments and methods, and in the interpretation of test findings.	The XBA approach to assessment is based mainly on CHC theory, but also neuropsychological theory. Since the XBA approach links all the major intelligence and achievement batteries as well as selected neuropsychological instruments to CHC theory, in particular, both selection of tests and interpretation of test findings are made easier.
It is necessary that the conceptual framework or model underlying assessment incorporates various aspects of neuropsychological and cognitive ability function that can be described in terms of constructs which are recognized in the neuropsychological and cognitive psychology literature.	The XBA approach incorporates various aspects of neuropsychological and cognitive ability functions that are described in terms of constructs that are recognized in the literature. In fact, a consistent set of terms and definitions within the CHC literature (e.g., Schneider & McGrew, 2012) and the neuropsychology literature (e.g., Miller, in press) underlie the XBA approach.
There is a need to adopt a conceptual framework that allows for the measurement of the full range of behavioral functions subserved by the brain. Unfortunately, in neuropsychological assessment there is no inclusive set of measures that is standardized on a single normative population.	XBA assessment allows for the measurement of a wide range of broad and narrow cognitive abilities specified in CHC theory and neuropsychological processes specified by neuropsychology theory and research. Although an XBA norm group does not exist, the crossing of batteries and the interpretation of assessment results are based on sound psychometric principles and procedures.
Because there are no truly unidimensional measures in psychological assessment, there is a need to select subtests from standardized instruments that appear to reflect the neurocognitive function of interest. In neuropsychological assessment, the aim, therefore, is to select those measures that, on the basis of careful task analysis, appear mainly to tap a given construct.	The XBA approach is defined, in part, by a CHC classification system. The majority of subtests from the major intelligence and achievement batteries as well as selected neuropsychological instruments were classified empirically as measures of broad and narrow CHC constructs (either via CHC within- or cross-battery factor analysis or expert consensus, or both). In addition, the subtests of intelligence and neuropsychological batteries were classified according to several neuropsychological domains (e.g., attention, visual-spatial, auditory-verbal, speed and efficiency, executive). Use of evidence-based classifications allows practitioners to be reasonably confident that a given test taps a given construct.
It is clear that an eclectic approach is needed in the selection of measures, preferably subtests rather than the omnibus IQs, in order to gain more specificity in the delineation of patterns of function and dysfunction.	The XBA approach ensures that two or more relatively pure, but qualitatively different, indicators of each *broad* cognitive ability are represented in a complete assessment. Two or more qualitatively similar indicators are necessary to make inferences about specific or *narrow* CHC abilities. This process is eclectic in its selection of measures.
There is a need to solve the potential problems that can arise from crossing normative groups as well as sets of measures that vary in reliability.	In the XBA approach, one can typically achieve baseline data in cognitive functioning across seven to nine CHC broad abilities through the use of only two well-standardized batteries, which minimizes the effects of error due to norming differences. Also, since interpretation of both broad and narrow CHC abilities is made at the cluster (rather than subtest) level, issues related to low reliability are less problematic in this approach. Finally, because cross-battery clusters are generated using estimated median reliabilities and intercorrelations, the data yielded by this approach are psychometrically sound.

1. Information obtained, in part, from Wilson, B.C. (1992). The neuropsychological assessment of the preschool child: A branching model. In I. Rapin & S. I. Segalowitz (Eds.), *Handbook of neuropsychology: Child neuropsychology* (Vol. 6) (pp. 377–394).

CHC BROAD (STRATUM II) CLASSIFICATIONS OF COGNITIVE, ACHIEVEMENT, AND NEUROPSYCHOLOGICAL TESTS

Based on the results of a series of cross-battery confirmatory factor analysis studies of the major intelligence batteries (see Keith & Reynolds, 2010, for a review) and the task analyses of many cognitive test experts, Flanagan and colleagues classified all the subtests of the major cognitive and achievement batteries, as well as selected neuropsychological batteries according to the particular CHC broad abilities they measured (e.g., Flanagan et al., 2006, 2007, 2013; McGrew, 1997; McGrew & Flanagan, 1998; Reynolds, Keith, Flanagan, & Alfonso, in press). To date, more than 100 batteries and 700 subtests have been classified according to the CHC broad and narrow abilities they measure, based in part on the results of these studies (see Flanagan et al., 2013). The CHC classifications of cognitive, achievement, and neuropsychological batteries assist practitioners in identifying measures that assess the various broad and narrow abilities represented in CHC theory.

Classification of tests at the broad ability level is necessary to improve the validity of cognitive assessment and interpretation. Specifically, broad ability classifications ensure that the CHC constructs that underlie assessments are minimally affected by *construct-irrelevant variance* (Messick, 1989, 1995). In other words, knowing which tests measure what abilities enables clinicians to organize tests into *construct-relevant* clusters—clusters that contain only measures that are *relevant to* the construct or ability of interest (McGrew & Flanagan, 1998).

To clarify, *construct-irrelevant variance* is present when an "assessment is too broad, containing excess reliable variance associated with other distinct constructs...that affects responses in a manner irrelevant to the interpreted constructs" (Messick, 1995, p. 742). For example, the WISC-IV Perceptual Reasoning Index (PRI) contains construct-irrelevant variance because, in addition to its two indicators of *Gf* (i.e., Picture Concepts, Matrix Reasoning), it has an indicator of *Gv* (i.e., Block Design). Therefore, the PRI is a *mixed* measure of two relatively distinct, broad CHC abilities (*Gf* and *Gv*); it contains reliable variance (associated with *Gv*) that is irrelevant to the interpreted construct of *Gf*. Through CHC-driven confirmatory factor analysis (CFA), Keith et al. (2006) showed that a five-factor model that included *Gf* and *Gv* (in lieu of PRI) fit the WISC-IV standardization data well. As a result of their analysis, *Gf* and *Gv* composites for the WISC-IV were provided in Flanagan and Kaufman (2004, 2009) and are recommended in the XBA approach because they contain only construct-*relevant* variance (Flanagan et al., 2013). The ongoing cross-battery CFAs conducted by Keith and colleagues will continue to lead to improvements in how cognitive subtests are classified in general, and organized within the context of XBA in particular (e.g., Reynolds et al., in press).

CHC NARROW (STRATUM I) CLASSIFICATIONS OF COGNITIVE, ACADEMIC AND NEUROPSYCHOLOGICAL TESTS

Narrow ability classifications were originally reported in McGrew (1997), then later reported in McGrew and Flanagan (1998) and Flanagan, McGrew, and Ortiz (2000) following minor modifications. Flanagan and her colleagues continued to gather content validity data on cognitive ability tests and expanded their analyses to include tests of academic achievement (Flanagan et al., 2002; 2006) and more recently tests of neuropsychological processes (Flanagan et al., 2010, 2013). Classifications of cognitive ability tests according to content, format, and task demand at the narrow (stratum I) ability level were necessary to improve further upon the validity of intellectual assessment and interpretation (see Messick, 1989). Specifically, these narrow ability classifications were necessary to ensure that the CHC constructs that underlie assessments are well represented (McGrew & Flanagan). According to Messick (1995), *construct underrepresentation* is present when an "assessment is too narrow and fails to include important dimensions or facets of the construct" (p. 742).

Interpreting the WJ III Concept Formation (CF) test as a measure of Fluid Intelligence (i.e., the broad *Gf* ability) is an example of construct underrepresentation. This is because CF measures *one* narrow aspect of *Gf* (viz., Inductive Reasoning). At least one other *Gf* measure (i.e., subtest) that is qualitatively different from Inductive Reasoning is necessary to include in an assessment to ensure adequate representation of the *Gf* construct (e.g., a measure of General Sequential [or Deductive] Reasoning). Two or more qualitatively different indicators (i.e., measures of two or more narrow abilities subsumed by the broad ability) are needed for adequate construct representation (Comrey, 1988; Keith & Reynolds, 2012; Messick, 1989, 1995). The aggregate of CF (a measure of Inductive Reasoning at the narrow ability level) and the WJ III Analysis-Synthesis test (a measure of Deductive Reasoning at the narrow ability level), for example, would provide an adequate estimate of the broad *Gf* ability because these tests are strong measures of *Gf* and represent qualitatively different aspects of this broad ability (see Flanagan et al., 2013 for additional examples).

In short, the classifications of tests at the broad and narrow ability levels of CHC theory guard against two ubiquitous sources of invalidity in assessment: construct-irrelevant variance and construct underrepresentation. In addition, these classifications augment the validity of test performance interpretation. Taken together, the CHC classifications of tests that underlie the XBA approach provide the necessary foundation upon which to organize assessments and interpret assessment results in a manner that is comprehensive and supported by theory and research.

Application of the XBA Approach
GUIDING PRINCIPLES

In order to ensure that XBA procedures are theoretically and psychometrically sound, it is recommended that practitioners adhere to several guiding principles (McGrew & Flanagan, 1998). First, select a comprehensive ability battery as your core battery in assessment. It is expected that the battery of choice will be one that is deemed most responsive to referral concerns. These batteries may include, but are certainly not limited to, the major intelligence, cognitive, academic, and neuropsychological batteries. It is important to note that the use of co-normed tests, such as the WJ III tests of cognitive ability and tests of achievement and the KABC-II and KTEA-II, may allow for the widest coverage of broad and narrow CHC abilities and processes.

Second, use subtests and *clusters/composites* from a single battery whenever possible, to represent broad CHC abilities. In other words, best practices involve using actual norms whenever they are available, in lieu of various other methods of aggregating scores (e.g., averaging, use of formulae). Because the development of current intelligence and cognitive ability batteries benefited greatly from CHC theory and research, the practice of averaging scores or using formulae to create cross-battery composites is seldom necessary at *the broad ability level*. However, aggregating scores across batteries continues to be necessary at the narrow ability level and when testing hypotheses about aberrant performance within broad ability domains. In these circumstances, Flanagan and colleagues provide a psychometrically defensible method for aggregating scores from different batteries that is based on formulae that incorporate test reliability and test intercorrelations (see Flanagan et al., 2013, for details).

Third, when constructing CHC broad and narrow ability clusters, select tests that have been classified through an acceptable method, such as through CHC theory-driven within-battery or preferably cross-battery factor analyses and/or expert consensus content validity studies. All test classifications included in the works of Flanagan and colleagues have been classified through these methods (Flanagan et al., 2007, 2013). Furthermore, to ensure appropriate construct representation when constructing broad (stratum II) ability composites, *two or more qualitatively different,* narrow (stratum I) ability indicators should be included to represent each domain. Of course, it seems likely that the more broadly an ability is represented (i.e., through the derivation of composites based on *multiple* qualitatively different, narrow ability indicators), the more confidence one would have in drawing inferences about the broad ability underlying a composite. A minimum of two qualitatively different indicators per CHC broad ability is recommended in the XBA approach mainly for practical reasons (i.e., time-efficient assessment). Noteworthy is the fact that most commonly used intelligence tests include at least two qualitatively different indicators (subtests) to represent broad abilities, which is why constructing broad ability clusters in the XBA approach is seldom necessary.

Fourth, when at least two qualitatively different indicators of a broad ability of interest are not available on the core battery, then supplement the core battery with at least two qualitatively different indicators of that broad ability from another battery. In other words, if an evaluator is interested in measuring Auditory Processing (*Ga*), and the core battery includes only one or no *Ga* subtests, then select a *Ga cluster* from another battery to supplement the core battery. This practice ensures that actual norms are used when interpreting broad ability performance.

Fifth, when crossing batteries (e.g., augmenting a core battery with relevant CHC clusters from another battery) or when constructing CHC broad or narrow ability clusters using tests from different batteries, select tests that were developed and normed within a few years of one another to minimize the effect of spurious differences between test scores that may be attributable to the "Flynn effect" (Flynn, 1984; Kaufman & Weiss, 2010). The tests that have been recommended by Flanagan and her colleagues in their most recent XBA books include only those that were normed within 10 years of one another (Flanagan et al., 2006, 2007, 2012).

Sixth, select tests from the smallest number of batteries to minimize the effect of spurious differences between test scores that may be attributable to differences in the characteristics of independent norm samples (McGrew, 1994). In many cases, using selected tests from one battery to augment the constructs measured by any other comprehensive ability battery is sufficient to represent a significant breadth of broad cognitive abilities adequately (i.e., about seven broad abilities), as well as to allow for at least three qualitatively different narrow ability indicators of the broad abilities (Flanagan et al., 2007).

Seventh, establish ecological validity for any and all test performances that are suggestive of normative weaknesses or deficits. The finding of a cognitive weakness or deficit is largely meaningless without evidence of how the weakness is manifested in activities of daily living, including academic achievement (Flanagan et al., 2011, 2013). The validity of test findings is bolstered when clear connections are made between the cognitive dysfunction (as measured by standardized tests) and the educational impact of that dysfunction; for example, as observed in classroom performance and as may be gleaned from a student's work samples.

When the XBA guiding principles are implemented systematically and the recommendations for development, use, and interpretation of clusters are adhered to, the potential error introduced through the crossing of norm groups is negligible (Flanagan et al., 2007). Additionally, the authors of *Essentials of Cross-Battery Assessment* (2nd and 3rd editions) included software with their books to facilitate the implementation of the XBA method and aid in the interpretation of cross-battery data (see Flanagan et al., 2007, 2013).

The XBA Approach in Perspective

The XBA approach is a method that allows practitioners to augment or supplement any ability battery to ensure measurement of a wider range of cognitive and academic abilities, and neuropsychological processes, in a manner consistent with contemporary theory and research. The foundational sources of information upon which the XBA approach was built (e.g., the classifications of ability batteries according to CHC theory) along with its guiding principles and steps provide a way to systematically construct a theoretically driven, comprehensive, and valid assessment of abilities and processes. For example, when the XBA approach is applied to the Wechsler Intelligence Scales, it is possible to measure important abilities and processes

that would otherwise go unassessed (e.g., *Ga, Glr, orthographic processing, executive functions*)—abilities and processes that are important in understanding acquisition of certain basic academic skills and school learning (e.g., Flanagan et al., 2013).

The XBA approach allows the measurement of the major cognitive areas specified in CHC theory with emphasis on those considered most critical on the basis of history, observation, and available data sources. The CHC classifications of a multitude of ability tests bring stronger content and construct validity evidence to the evaluation and interpretation process. As test development continues to evolve and becomes increasingly more sophisticated (psychometrically and theoretically), batteries of the future will undoubtedly possess stronger content and construct validity. Notwithstanding, it is unrealistic from an economic and practical standpoint to develop a battery that operationalizes contemporary CHC theory fully (Carroll, 1998; Flanagan et al., 2007, 2013). Therefore, it is likely that the XBA approach will become increasingly useful as the empirical support for CHC theory mounts (Reynolds et al., in press).

Summary

The purpose of this chapter was to highlight the progress that has been made in theories of intelligence (particularly psychometric theories), the structure of cognitive ability batteries, and methods of cognitive ability test-interpretation over the past century. The initial part of this chapter traced such influences in each of these areas back to Galton, Burt, Spearman, and others. Early theories of intelligence revolved around notions of a single general factor, or g, but steadily advanced into two-factor models (e.g., original Gf-Gc), early multiple-factor models (e.g., Thurstone's PMAs), and eventually to current multiple-factor models (e.g., CHC theory).

Cognitive batteries have seldom kept pace with developments in theory, but they nevertheless have shown significant growth and development overall, particularly within the last decade. Whereas the original Stanford-Binet was the first test designed to measure general intelligence or g, other tests such as the Wechsler-Bellevue and subsequent Wechsler scales, K-ABC and KACB-II, CAS, DAS and DAS-II, and WJ-R and WJ III continued to expand the range of options available to practitioners in their quest to measure abilities and processes beyond general intelligence.

Not surprisingly, as cognitive batteries expanded and incorporated contemporary theory, methods of interpretation advanced accordingly. It was discussed that test interpretation began with evaluation of a single factor (*g*) because that was all that was offered by the Stanford-Binet. But as new batteries were developed and later expanded, methods of interpretation followed suit and shifted toward clinical profile analysis, followed by psychometric profile analysis, and on to the present wave, where current theory and its related research base are applied to the understanding of test results.

The latter half of the chapter provided a discussion of what we believe to be an emerging interpretive wave—the fifth wave—which includes refinements to CHC theory at both the broad and narrow ability levels, application of CHC theory to academic outcomes research, integration of CHC and neuropsychological theories, and greater emphasis on flexible battery approaches. The fifth wave is likely to lead to a clearer "road map" for assessment that will allow practitioners to either expand or selectively focus their evaluations as may be necessary and appropriate in the search for underlying causal explanations for learning problems and neurodevelopmental disorders, difficulties in academic skill development, and application of academic skills to acquire content knowledge. But the major result of the fifth wave is likely to be a growing body of research related to outcomes that are predictable and explainable via empirically related abilities and processes. That is, contemporary cognitive assessment within this wave should allow for sufficient illustration of the links between abilities (e.g., cognitive and academic) and neuropsychological processes such that avenues for instruction, intervention, and treatment of individuals who struggle to learn will not only be clear, but also empirically supported.

Notes

1. This section of the chapter was adapted from Flanagan, Alfonso, Ortiz, and Dynda (2010) with permission from Wiley. 2010. All rights reserved.

2. G*t* is omitted from Figure 12.5 because commonly used intelligence and neuropsychological batteries do not measure this ability.

3. G*o* is omitted from Figure 12.5 because commonly used intelligence and neuropsychological batteries do not measure this ability and the cognitive and perceptual aspects of this ability have not been studied extensively (McGrew, 2005).

References

Aaron, P. G. (1995). Differential diagnosis of reading disabilities. *School Psychology Review, 24*, 345–360.

Alfonso, V. C., Flanagan, D. P., & Radwan, S. (2005). The impact of the Cattell-Horn theory on test development and interpretation of cognitive and academic abilities. In D. P. Flanagan & P. L. Harrison (Eds.), *Contemporary intellectual assessment: Theories, tests, and issues* (pp. 185–202). New York: Guilford Press.

Anastasi, A. (1988). *Psychological testing* (6th ed.). New York: Macmillan.

Berninger, V. W. (1990). Multiple orthographic codes: Key to alternative instructional methodologies for developing the orthographic-phonological connections underlying word identification. *School Psychology Review, 19*, 518–533.

Berninger, V. W. (1997). Introduction to interventions for students with learning problems: Myths and realities. *School Psychology Review, 26*, 326–332.

Berninger, V. W. (1999). Coordinating transcription and text generation in working memory during composing: Automatic and constructive processes. *Learning Disability Quarterly, 22*, 99–112.

Berninger, V. W. (2009). Highlights of programmatic, interdisciplinary research on writing. *Learning Disabilities Research & Practice, 24*, 69–80.

Berninger, V. W. (2011). Evidence-based differential diagnosis and treatment of reading disabilities with and without comorbidities in oral language, writing, and math: Prevention, problem-solving consultation, and specialized instruction. In D. P. Flanagan & V. C. Alfonso (Eds.), *Essentials of specific learning disability identification* (pp. 203–232). Hoboken, NJ: John Wiley & Sons.

Berninger, V. W., Cartwright, A. C., Yates, C. M., Swanson, H. L., & Abbott, R. D. (1994). Developmental skills related to writing and reading acquisition in the intermediate grades: Shared and unique functional systems. *Reading & Writing, 6*, 161–196.

Burt, C. (1949). Alternative methods of factor analysis and their relations to Pearson's method of principal axes. *British Journal of Psychology, Statistical Section, 2*, 98–121.

Canivez, G. L., & Watkins, M. W. (2010). Exploratory and higher-order factor analyses of the Wechsler Adult Intelligence Scale-Fourth Edition (WAIS–IV) adolescent subsample. *School Psychology Quarterly, 25*, 223–235.

Carroll, J. B. (1993a). What abilities are measured by the WISC-III? *Journal of Psychoeducational Assessment, 11*, 134–143.

Carroll, J. B. (1993b). *Human cognitive abilities: A survey of factor-analytic studies.* New York: Cambridge University Press.

Carroll, J. B. (1997). The three-stratum theory of cognitive abilities. In D. P. Flanagan, J. L. Genshaft, & P. L. Harrison (Eds.), *Contemporary intellectual assessment: Theories, tests, and issues* (pp. 122–130). New York: Guilford Press.

Carroll, J. B. (1998). Foreword. In K. S. McGrew & D. P. Flanagan, *The intelligence test desk reference: Gf-Gc cross-battery assessment* (pp. xi–xii). Boston, MA: Allyn & Bacon.

Cattell, R. B. (1941). Some theoretical issues in adult intelligence testing. *Psychological Bulletin, 38*, 592.

Cattell, R. (1957). *Personality and motivation structure and measurement.* New York: World Book.

Cattell, R. (1971). *Abilities, their structure, growth and action.* Boston, MA: Houghton Mifflin.

Chen, J. Q., & Gardner, H. (2012). Assessment of intellectual profile: A perspective from multiple intelligences theory. In D. P. Flanagan & P. L. Harrison (Eds.), *Contemporary intellectual assessment: Theories, tests, and issues* (3rd ed., pp. 145–155). New York: Guilford.

Cohen, J. (1959). The factorial structure of the WISC at ages 7–7, 10–6, and 13–6. *Journal of Consulting Psychology, 23*, 285–299.

Comrey, A. L. (1988). Factor-analytic methods of scale development in personality and clinical psychology. *Journal of Consulting and Clinical Psychology, 56*, 754–761.

Daniel, M. H. (1997). Intelligence testing: Status and trends. *American Psychologist, 52*, 1038–1045.

Das, J. P., & Naglieri, J. A. (1997). *Cognitive Assessment System.* Itasca, IL: Riverside.

Dean, R. S., & Woodcock, R. W. (2003). *Dean-Woodcock Neuropsychological Battery.* Itasca, IL: Riverside Publishing.

Decker, S. L. (2008). School neuropsychology consultation in neurodevelopmental disorders. *Psychology in the Schools, 45*, 799–811.

Dehn, M. J. (2006). *Essentials of processing assessment.* New York: John Wiley.

Elliott, C. D. (1990). *Differential Ability Scales.* San Antonio, TX: The Psychological Corporation.

Elliott, C. D. (2007). *Differential Ability Scales* (2nd ed.). San Antonio, TX: Harcourt Assessment.

Evans, J. J., Floyd, R. G., McGrew, K. S., & Leforgee, M. H. (2001). The relations between measures of Cattell-Horn-Carroll (CHC) cognitive abilities and reading achievement during childhood and adolescence. *School Psychology Review, 31*, 246–262.

Feifer, S. (2011). How SLD manifests in reading. In D. P. Flanagan & V. C. Alfonso (Eds.), *Essentials of specific learning disability identification* (pp. 21–42). Hoboken, NJ: John Wiley & Sons.

Fiorello, C. A., Hale, J. B., Holdnack, J. A., Kavanagh, J. A., Terrell, J., & Long, L. (2007). Interpreting intelligence test results for children with disabilities. Is global intelligence relevant? *Applied Neuropsychology, 14*, 2–12.

Fiorello, C. A., Hale, J. B., Snyder, L. E., Forrest, E., & Teodori, A. (2008). Validating individual differences through examination of converging psychometric and neuropsychological models of cognitive functioning. In S. K. Thurman & C. A. Fiorello (Eds.), *Applied cognitive research in K–3 classrooms* (pp. 232–254). New York: Routledge.

Flanagan, D. P. (2000). Wechlser-based CHC cross-battery assessment and reading achievement: Strengthening the validity of interpretations drawn from Wechsler test scores. *School Psychology Quarterly, 15*, 295–229.

Flanagan, D. P., & Alfonso, V. C., & Mascolo, J. T. (2011). A CHC-based operational definition of SLD: Integrating multiple data sources and multiple data-gathering methods. In D. P. Flanagan & V. C. Alfonso (Eds.), *Essentials of specific learning disability identification* (pp. 233–298). Hoboken, NJ: John Wiley & Sons.

Flanagan, D. P., Alfonso, V. C., Mascolo, J. T., & Hale, J. B. (2011). The Wechsler Intelligence Scale for Children–Fourth Edition in Neuropsychological Practice. In A. S. Davis (Ed.), *Handbook of pediatric neuropsychology* (pp. 397–414). New York: Springer Publishing Company.

Flanagan, D. P., Alfonso, V. C., Ortiz, S. O., & Dynda, A. M. (2010). Best practices in cognitive assessment for school neuropsychological evaluations. In D. C. Miller (Ed.), *Best practices in school neuropsychology: Guidelines for effective practice, assessment, and evidence-based intervention* (pp. 101–140). New York: John Wiley and Sons.

Flanagan, D. P., Ortiz, S. O., & Alfonso, V. C. (2012). The cross-battery assessment approach: Past, present, and future. In D. P. Flanagan & P. L. Harrison, *Contemporary intellectual assessment: Theories, tests, and issues* (3rd ed., pp. 643–669). New York: Guilford.

Flanagan, D. P., Ortiz, S. O., Alfonso, V. C., & Dynda, A. M. (2006). Integration of response to intervention and norm-referenced tests in learning disability identification: Learning from the Tower of Babel. *Psychology in the Schools, 43*, 1–19.

Flanagan, D. P., & Harrison, P. L. (Eds.). (2005). *Contemporary intellectual assessment: Theories, tests, and issues* (2nd ed.). New York: Guilford.

Flanagan, D. P., & Harrison, P. L. (Eds.). (2012). *Contemporary intellectual assessment: Theories, tests, and issues* (3rd ed.). New York: Guilford.

Flanagan, D. P., & Kaufman, A. S. (2004). *Essentials of WISC-IV assessment.* New York: John Wiley & Sons.

Flanagan, D. P., & Kaufman, A. S. (2009). *Essentials of WISC-IV assessment* (2nd ed.). New York: John Wiley & Sons.

Flanagan. D. P., & McGrew. K. S. (1997). A cross-battery approach lo assessing and interpreting cognitive abilities: Narrowing the gap between practice and cognitive science. In D. P. Flanagan, J. L. Genshaft, & P. L. Harrison (Eds.), *Contemporary intellectual assessment: Theories, tests, and issues* (pp. 314–325). New York: Guilford.

Flanagan, D. P., McGrew, K. S., & Ortiz, S. O. (2000). *The Wechsler Intelligence Scales and Gf-Gc theory: A contemporary approach to interpretation.* Boston: Allyn & Bacon.

Flanagan, D. P., & Ortiz, S. O. (2001). *Essentials of cross-battery assessment.* New York: John Wiley.

Flanagan, D. P., Ortiz, S. O., & Alfonso, V. C. (2013). *Essentials of cross-battery assessment* (3rd ed.). New York: John Wiley.

Flanagan, D. P., Ortiz, S. O., & Alfonso, V. C. (2007). *Essentials of cross-battery assessment* (2nd ed.). New York: John Wiley.

Flanagan, D. P., Ortiz, S. O., Alfonso, V. C., & Dynda, A. M. (2008). Best practices in cognitive assessment. In A. Thomas & J. Grimes (Eds.), *Best practices in school psychology V* (pp. 633–660). Washington, DC: National Association of School Psychologists.

Flanagan, D. P., Ortiz, S. O., Alfonso, V. C., & Mascolo, J. T. (2006). *Achievement test desk reference: A guide to learning disability identification* (2nd ed.). New York: John Wiley.

Fletcher, J. M., Lyon, G. R., Fuchs, L. S., & Barnes, M. A. (2007). *Learning disabilities: From identification to intervention.* New York, NY: Guilford.

Fletcher-Janzen, E., & Reynolds, C. R. (Eds.). (2008). *Neuropsychological perspectives on learning disabilities in the era of RTI: Recommendations for diagnosis and intervention.* New York: John Wiley & Sons.

Floyd, R. G., Evans, J. J., & McGrew, K. S. (2003). Relations between measures of Cattell-Horn-Carroll (CHC) cognitive abilities and mathematics achievement across the school-age years. *Psychology in the Schools, 40*, 155–171.

Floyd, R. G., McGrew, K. S., & Evans, J. J. (2008). The relative contributions of the Cattell-Horn-Carroll cognitive abilities in explaining writing achievement during childhood and adolescence. *Psychology in the Schools, 45*, 132–144.

French, J. W., Eckstrom, R. B., & Price, L. A. (1963). *Manual and kit of reference tests for cognitive factors.* Princeton, NJ: Educational Testing Service.

Garcia, G. M., & Stafford, M. E. (2000). Prediction of reading by *Ga* and *Gc* specific cognitive abilities for low-SES White and Hispanic English-speaking children. *Psychology in the Schools, 37*, 227–235.

Geary, D. C. (1993). Mathematical disabilities: Cognitive, neuropsychological, and genetic components. *Psychological Bulletin, 114*, 345–362.

Geary, D. C., Hoard, M. K., & Bailey, D. H. (2011). How SLD manifests in mathematics. In D. P. Flanagan & V. C. Alfonso (Eds.), *Essentials of specific learning disability identification* (pp. 43–64). Hoboken, NJ: John Wiley & Sons.

Glutting, J. J., McDermott, P. A., & Konold, T. R. (1997). Ontology, structure, and diagnostic benefits of a normative subtest taxonomy from the WISC-III standardization sample. In D. P. Flanagan, J. L. Genshaft, & P. L. Harrison (Eds.), *Contemporary intellectual assessment: Theories, tests, and issues* (pp. 349–372). New York: Guilford.

Glutting, J. J., McDermott, P. A., Watkins, M. M., Kush, J. C., & Konold, T. R. (1997). The base rate problem and its consequences for interpreting children's ability profiles. *School Psychology Review, 26*, 176–188.

Glutting, J. J., Watkins, M. W., & Youngstrom, E. A. (2003). Multifactored and cross-battery ability assessments: Are they worth the effort? In R. Reynolds & R. W. Kamphaus (Eds.), *Handbook of psychological and educational assessment: Vol. 1. Intelligence and achievement* (2nd ed.; pp. 343–373). New York: Guilford Press.

Gould, S. J. (1996). *The mismeasure of man* (revised and expanded). New York: W. W. Norton & Company.

Gustafsson, J. E., & Undheim, J. O. (1996). Individual differences in cognitive functions. In D. C. Berliner & R. C. Cabfee (Eds.), *Handbook of educational psychology* (pp. 186–242). New York: Macmillan.

Hale, J. B., & Fiorello, C. A. (2004). *School neuropsychology: A practitioner's handbook*. New York: Guilford Press.

Hale, R. L. (1979). The utility of the WISC-R subtest scores in discriminating among adequate and underachieving children. *Multivariate Behavioral Research, 14*, 245–253.

Hale, R. L., & Landino, S. A. (1981). Utility of the WISC-R subtest analysis in discriminating among groups of conduct problem, withdrawn, mixed, and non-problem boys. *Journal of Consulting & Clinical Psychology, 41*, 91–95.

Hale, R. L., & Saxe, J. E. (1983). Profile analysis of the Wechsler Intelligence Scale for Children–Revised. *Journal of Psychoeducational Assessment, 1*, 155–162.

Hargrave, J. L. (2005). The relationship between executive functions and broad written language skills in students ages 12 to 14 years old. *Dissertation Abstracts International, 65*(8- B). University Microfilms International.

Horn, J. L. (1968). Organization of abilities and the development of intelligence. *Psychological Review, 75*, 242–259.

Horn, J. L. (1991). Measurement of intellectual capabilities: A review of theory. In K. S. McGrew, J. K. Werder, & R. W. Woodcock (Eds.), *Woodcock-Johnson technical manual* (pp. 197–232). Chicago: Riverside.

Horn, J. L., & Blankson, N. (2005). Foundations for better understanding of cognitive abilities. In D. P. Flanagan & P. L. Harrison (Eds.), *Contemporary intellectual assessment: Theories, tests, and issues* (2nd ed., pp. 41–68). New York: Guilford Press.

Horn, J. L., & Noll, J. (1997). Human cognitive capabilities: Gf-Gc theory. In D. P. Flanagan, J. L. Genshaft, & P. L. Harrison (Eds.), *Contemporary intellectual assessment: Theories, tests, and issues* (pp. 53–91). New York: Guilford Press.

Horn, J. L., & Stankov, L. (1982). Auditory and visual factors of intelligence. *Intelligence, 62*, 165–185.

Jensen, A. R. (1998). *The g factor: The science of mental ability*. Westport, CT: Praeger Publishers.

Johnson, D. J. (1993). Relationship between oral and written language. *School Psychology Review, 22*, 595–609.

Joshi, R. M. (1995). Assessing reading and spelling skills. *School Psychology Review, 24*, 361–375.

Kamphaus, R. W. (1993). Review of the WISC-III [WISC-III Monograph]. *Journal of Psychoeducational Assessment, 94*–104.

Kamphaus, R. W., Petoskey, M. D., & Morgan, A. W. (1997). A history of intelligence test interpretation. In D. P. Flanagan, J. L. Genshaft, & P. L. Harrison (Eds.), *Contemporary intellectual assessment: Theories, tests, and issues* (pp. 32–51). New York: Guilford.

Kamphaus, R. W., Winsor, A. P., Rowe, E. W., & Kim, S. (2005). A history of intelligence test interpretation. In D. P. Flanagan & P. L. Harrison (Eds.), *Contemporary intellectual assessment: Theories, tests, and issues* (2nd ed.; pp. 23–38). New York: Guilford.

Kamphaus, R. W., Winsor, A. P., Rowe, E. W., & Kim, S. (2012). A history of intelligence test interpretation. In D. P. Flanagan & P. L. Harrison (Eds.), *Contemporary intellectual assessment: Theories, tests, and issues* (3rd ed., pp. 56–72). New York: Guilford.

Kaufman, A. S. (1979). *Intelligent testing with the WISC-R*. New York: Wiley & Sons.

Kaufman, A. S. (1994). *Intelligent testing with the WISC-III*. New York: Wiley & Sons.

Kaufman, A. S. (2000). Foreword. In D. P. Flanagan, K. S. McGrew, & S. O. Ortiz, *The Wechsler intelligence scales and Gf-Gc theory: A contemporary approach to interpretation* (pp. xiii–xv). Boston, MA: Allyn & Bacon.

Kaufman, A. S., & Kaufman, N. L. (1983). *Kaufman assessment battery for children*. Circle Pines, MN: American Guidance Service.

Kaufman, A. S., & Kaufman, N. L. (1993). *The Kaufman adolescent and adult intelligence test*. Circle Pines, MN: American Guidance Service.

Kaufman, A. S., & Kaufman, N. L. (2004). *Kaufman assessment battery for children* (2nd ed.). Circle Pines, MN: American Guidance Service.

Kaufman, A. S., & Weiss, L. G. (Eds.) (2010). The Flynn effect [Special Issue]. *Journal of Psychoeducational Assessment, 28*, 379–381.

Kavale, K. A., & Forness, S. R. (1984). A meta-analysis of the validity of Wechsler scale profiles and recategorizations: Patterns and parodies. *Learning Disabilities Quarterly, 7*, 136–156.

Keith, T. Z. (2005). Using confirmatory factor analysis to aid in understanding the constructs measured by intelligence tests. In D. P. Flanagan & P. L. Harrison (Eds.), *Contemporary intellectual assessment: Theories, tests, and issues* (2nd ed.; pp. 581–614). New York: Guilford.

Keith, T. Z., Fine, J. G., Reynolds, M. R., Taub, G. E., & Kranzler, J. H. (2006). Hierarchical, multi-sample, confirmatory factor analysis of the Wechsler Intelligence Scale for Children–Fourth edition: What does it measure? *School Psychology Review, 35*, 108–127.

Keith, T. Z., Kranzler, J. H., & Flanagan, D. P. (2001). What does the cognitive assessment system (CAS) measure? Joint confirmatory factor analysis of the CAS and the Woodcock-Johnson tests of cognitive ability–third edition. *School Psychology Review, 30*, 89–119.

Keith, T. Z., & Reynolds, M. R. (2010). CHC and cognitive abilities: What we've learned from 20 years of research. *Psychology in the Schools, 47*, 635–650.

Keith, T. Z., & Reynolds, M. R. (2012). Using confirmatory factor analysis to aid in understanding the constructs measured by intelligence tests. In D. P. Flanagan & P. L. Harrison (Eds.), *Contemporary intellectual assessment: Theories, tests, and issues* (3rd ed., pp. 758–799). New York: Guilford.

Kreiner, D. S., & Gough, P. B. (1990). Two ideas about spelling: Rules and word-specific memory. *Journal of Memory & Language, 29*, 103–118.

Lezak, M. D. (1976). *Neuropsychological assessment.* New York: Oxford University Press.

Lezak, M. D. (1995). *Neuropsychological assessment* (3rd ed.). New York: Oxford University Press.

Lezak, M. D., Howieson, D. B., & Loring, D. W. (2004). *Neuropsychological assessment* (4th ed.). New York: Oxford University Press.

Levine, A. J., & Marks, L. (1928). *Testing intelligence and achievement.* New York: Macmillan.

Lohman, D. F. (1996). Spatial ability and *G*. In I. Dennis & P. Tapsfield (Eds.), *Human abilities: Their nature and assessment* (pp. 97–116). Hillsdale, NJ: Erlbaum.

Luria, A. R. (1966). *Human brain and psychological processes.* New York: Harper & Row.

Luria, A. R. (1970). The functional organization of the brain. *Scientific American, 222*, 66–78.

Luria, A. R. (1973). *The working brain: An introduction to neuropsychology.* New York: Basic Books.

Luria, A. R. (1980). *Higher cortical functions in man* (2nd ed., rev. and expanded). New York: Basic Books.

Mather, N., & Wendling, B. J. (2011). How SLD manifests in writing. In D. P. Flanagan & V. C. Alfonso (Eds.), *Essentials of specific learning disability identification* (pp. 65–88). Hoboken, NJ: John Wiley & Sons.

McCloskey, G. (2009). The WISC-IV integrated. In D. P. Flanagan & A. S. Kaufman, *Essentials of WISC-IV assessment* (2nd ed.; pp. 310–467). Hoboken, NJ: John Wiley & Sons.

McDermott, P. A., Fantuzzo, J. W., & Glutting, J. J. (1990). Just say no to subtest analysis: A critique on Wechsler theory and practice. *Journal of Psychoeducational Assessment, 8*, 290–302.

McDermott, P. A., Fantuzzo, J. W., Glutting, J. J., Watkins, M. W., & Baggaley, R. A. (1992). Illusions of meaning in the ipsative assessment of children's ability. *Journal of Special Education, 25*, 504–526.

McGrew, K. S. (1993). The relationship between the WJ-R *Gf-Gc* cognitive clusters and reading achievement across the lifespan. *Journal of Psychoeducational Assessment, Monograph Series: WJ-R Monograph*, 39–53.

McGrew, K. S. (1994). *Clinical interpretation of the Woodcock-Johnson Tests of Cognitive Ability-Revised.* Boston, MA: Allyn & Bacon.

McGrew, K. S. (1997). Analysis of the major intelligence batteries according to a proposed comprehensive *Gf-Gc* framework. In D. P. Flanagan, J. L. Genshaft, & P. L. Harrison (Eds.), *Contemporary intellectual assessment: Theories, tests, and issues* (pp. 151–180). New York: Guilford Press.

McGrew, K. S. (2005). The Cattell-Horn-Carroll theory of cognitive abilities: Past, present, and future. In D. P. Flanagan & P. L. Harrison (Eds.), *Contemporary intellectual assessment: Theories, tests, and issues* (2nd ed.; pp. 136–182). New York: Guilford Press.

McGrew, K. S., & Flanagan, D. P. (1998). *The intelligence test desk reference (ITDR): Gf-Gc cross-battery assessment.* Boston, MA: Allyn & Bacon.

McGrew, K. S., Flanagan, D. P., Keith, T. Z., & Vanderwood, M. (1997). Beyond *g*: The impact of *Gf-Gc* specific cognitive abilities research on the future use and interpretation of intelligence tests in the schools. *School Psychology Review, 26*, 189–210.

McGrew, K. S., & Hessler, G. L. (1995). The relationship between the WJ-R *Gf-Gc* cognitive clusters and mathematics achievement across the life-span. *Journal of Psychoeducational Assessment, 13*, 21–38.

McGrew, K. S., & Knopik, S. N. (1993). The relationship between the WJ-R *Gf-Gc* cognitive clusters and writing achievement across the life-span. *School Psychology Review, 22*, 687–695.

McGrew, K. S., & Wendling, B. J. (2010). Cattell-Horn-Carroll cognitive-achievement relations: What we have learned from the past 20 years of research. *Psychology in the Schools, 47*, 651–675.

McGrew, K. S., Werder, J. K., & Woodcock, R. W. (1991). *WJ-R technical manual.* Chicago: Riverside Publishing Company.

Messick, S. (1989). Validity. In R. Linn (Ed.), *Educational measurement* (3rd ed., pp. 104–131). Washington, DC: American Council on Education.

Messick, S. (1995). Validity of psychological assessment: Validation of inferences from persons' responses and performances as scientific inquiry into score meaning. *American Psychologist, 50*, 741–749.

Miller, D. C. (2007). *Essentials of school neuropsychological assessment.* Hoboken, NJ: John Wiley & Sons.

Mueller, H. H., Dennis, S. S., & Short, R. H. (1986). A meta-exploration of WISC-R factor score profiles as a function of diagnosis and intellectual level. *Canadian Journal of School Psychology, 2*, 21–43.

Naglieri, J. A. (1997). Planning, attention, simultaneous, and successive theory and the cognitive assessment system: A new theory-based measure of intelligence. In D. P. Flanagan, J. L. Genshaft, & P. L. Harrison (Eds.), *Contemporary intellectual assessment: Theories, tests, and issues* (pp. 247–267). New York: Guilford.

Naglieri, J. A., & Das, J. P. (1997). *Cognitive Assessment System.* Itasca, IL: Riverside Publishing.

Naglieri, J. A., Das, J. P., & Goldstein, S. (2012). PASS: A cognitive processing based theory of intelligence. In D. P. Flanagan & P. L. Harrison (Eds.), *Contemporary intellectual assessment: Theories, tests, and issues* (3rd ed.). New York: Guilford.

Neisser, U., Boodoo, G., Bouchard, T. J., Boykin, A. W., Brody, N., Ceci, S. J., et al. (1996). Intelligence: Knowns and unknowns. *American Psychologist, 51*, 77–101.

Rapaport, D., Gill, M. M., & Schafer, R. (1945–46). *Diagnostic psychological testing* (2 vols.). Chicago: Yearbook Publishers.

Reschly, D. J., & Grimes, J. P. (1995). Best practices in intellectual assessment. In A. Thomas & J. Grimes (Eds.), *Best practices in school psychology–III* (pp. 763–774). Washington, DC: The National Association of School Psychologists.

Reynolds, C. R., & Kaufman, A. S. (1990). Assessment of children's intelligence with the Wechsler Intelligence Scale for Children—Revised (WISC-R). In C. R. Reynolds & R. W. Kamphaus (Eds.), *Handbook of psychological and educational assessment of children: Intelligence and achievement* (pp. 127–165). New York: Guilford.

Reynolds, M., Keith, T. Z., Flanagan, D. P., & Alfonso, V. C. (in press). A cross-battery, reference variable, confirmatory factor analytic investigation of the CHC taxonomy. *Journal of School Psychology.*

Roid, G. (2003). *Stanford Binet Intelligence Scales, Fifth Edition.* Itasca, IL: Riverside.

Sattler, J. M. (1988). *Assessment of children* (3rd ed.). San Diego, CA: Author.

Schneider, J. W., & McGrew, K. S. (2012). The Cattell-Horn-Carroll model of intelligence. In D. P. Flanagan & P. L. Harrison (Eds.), *Contemporary intellectual assessment: Theories, tests, and issues* (3rd ed., pp. 99–144). New York: Guilford.

Shaw, S. R., Swerdlik, S. E., & Laurent, J. (1993). Review of the WISC-III [WISC-III Monograph]. *Journal of Psychoeducational Assessment*, 161–164.

Sotelo-Dynega, M., & Cuskley, T. (2011). *Cognitive assessment: A survey of current school psychologists' practices*. Poster session presented at the annual meeting of the National Association of School Psychologists, San Francisco, CA.

Spearman, C. E. (1904). "General Intelligence," objectively determined and measured. *American Journal of Psychiatry*, *15*, 201–293.

Spearman, C. E. (1927). *The abilities of man, their nature and measurement*. New York: Macmillan.

Sternberg, R. J. (1993). Rocky's back again: A review of the WISC-III [WISC-III Monograph]. *Journal of Psychoeducational Assessment*. 161–164.

Sternberg, R. J. (2012). The triarchic theory of successful intelligence. In D. P. Flanagan & P. L. Harrison (Eds.), *Contemporary intellectual assessment: Theories, tests, and issues* (3rd ed., 156–177). New York: Guilford.

Strauss, E., Sherman, E. M. S., & Spreen, O. (2006). *A compendium of neuropsychological tests: Administration, norms, and commentary* (3rd ed.). New York: Oxford University Press.

Swanson, H. L., & Beebe-Frankenberger, M. (2004). The relationship between working memory and mathematical problem solving in children at risk and not at risk for math disabilities. *Journal of Education Psychology*, *96*, 471–491.

Taylor, T. R. (1994). A review of three approaches to cognitive assessment, and a proposed integrated approach based on a unifying theoretical framework. *South African Journal of Psychology*, *24*, 183–193.

Terman, L. S. (1916). *The measurement of intelligence: An explanation of and a complete guide for the use of the Stanford revision and extension of the Binet-Siman Scale*. Boston: Houghton Mifflin.

Thorndike, R. M. (1997). The early history of intelligence testing. In D. P. Flanagan, J. L. Genshaft, & P. L. Harrison (Eds.), *Contemporary intellectual assessment: Theories, tests and issues* (pp. 3–16). New York: Guilford.

Thorndike, R. L., Hagen, E. P., & Sattler, J. M. (1986). *The Stanford-Binet Intelligence Scale: Fourth Edition*. Itasca, IL: Riverside Publishing.

Thurstone, L. L. (1938). *Primary mental abilities*. Chicago: University of Chicago Press.

Thurstone, L. L., & Thurstone, T. G. (1941). *Factorial studies of intelligence*. Chicago: University of Chicago Press.

Vanderwood, M. L., McGrew, K. S., Flanagan, D. P., & Keith, T. Z. (2002). The contribution of general and specific cognitive abilities to reading achievement. *Learning & Individual Differences*, *13*, 159–188.

Vernon, P. E. (1961). *The structure of human abilities* (2nd ed.). London: Methuen.

Wasserman, J. D. (2012). A history of intelligence assessment: The unfinished tapestry. In D. P. Flanagan & P. L. Harrison (Eds.), *Contemporary intellectual assessment: Theories, tests, and issues* (3rd ed., pp. 3–55). New York: Guilford.

Watkins, M. W., Glutting, J. J., & Youngstrom, E. C. (2005). Issues in subtest profile analysis. In D. P. Flanagan & P. L. Harrison (Eds.), *Contemporary intellectual assessment: Theories, tests, and issues* (2nd ed.; pp. 251–268). New York: Guilford Press.

Watkins, M. W., & Kush, J. C. (1994). Wechsler subtest analysis: The right way, the wrong way, or no way? *School Psychology Review*, *23*, 640–651.

Wechsler, D. (1939). *The measurement of adult intelligence*. Baltimore, MD: Williams & Wilkins.

Wechsler, D. (1958). *The measurement and appraisal of adult intelligence* (4th ed.). Baltimore, MD: Williams & Wilkins.

Wechsler, D. (1955). *Wechsler Adult Intelligence Scale-Revised*. San Antonio, TX: The Psychological Corporation.

Wechsler, D. (1974). *Wechsler Intelligence Scale for Intelligence--Revised*. San Antonio, TX: The Psychological Association.

Wechsler, D. (1989). *Wechsler Preschool and Primary Scale of Intelligence–Revised*. San Antonio, TX: The Psychological Association.

Wechsler, D. (1991). *Wechsler Intelligence Scale for Children–Third Edition*. San Antonio, TX: The Psychological Corporation.

Wechsler, D. (1997). *Wechsler Adult Intelligence Scale–Third Edition*. San Antonio, TX: The Psychological Corporation.

Wechsler, D. (2002). *Wechsler Preschool and Primary Scale of Intelligence–Third Edition*. San Antonio, TX: The Psychological Association.

Wechsler, D. (2003). *Wechsler Intelligence Scale for Children–Fourth Edition*. San Antonio, TX: The Psychological Association.

Wechsler, D. (2008). *Wechsler Adult Intelligence Scale–Fourth Edition*. San Antonio, TX: The Psychological Corporation.

Williams, J., Zolten, A. J., Rickert, V. I., Spence, G. T., & Ashcraft, E. W. (1993). Use of nonverbal tests to screen for writing dysfluency in school-age children. *Perceptual & Motor Skills*, *76* (3, Pt. 1), 803–809.

Wilson, B. C. (1992). The neuropsychological assessment of the preschool child: A branching model. In I. Rapin & S. I. Segalowitz (Eds.), *Handbook of neuropsychology: Child neuropsychology* (Vol. 6, pp. 377–394). Amsterdam: Elsevier.

Woodcock, R. W. (1990). Theoretical foundations of the WJ-R measures of cognitive ability. *Journal of Psychoeducational Assessment*, *8*, 231–258.

Woodcock, R. W. (1994). Measures of fluid and crystallized theory of intelligence. In R. J. Sternberg (Ed.), *Encyclopedia of human intelligence* (pp. 452–456). New York: Macmillan.

Woodcock, R. W., & Johnson, M. B. (1989). *Woodcock-Johnson Psycho-Educational Battery–Revised*. Rolling Meadows, IL: Riverside Publishing.

Woodcock, R. W., McGrew, K. S., & Mather, N. (2001, 2007). *Woodcock-Johnson III Tests of Achievement*. Rolling Meadows, IL: Riverside Publishing.

Woodcock, R. W., McGrew, K. S., & Mather, N. (2001, 2007). *Woodcock-Johnson III Tests of Cognitive Abilities*. Rolling Meadows, IL: Riverside Publishing.

Principles of Assessment of Aptitude and Achievement

W. Joel Schneider

Abstract

An idiosyncratic account of the assessment of achievement and aptitudes is presented. Major theories of cognitive abilities are reviewed briefly, with emphasis on the Cattell-Horn-Carroll theory of cognitive abilities. Procedures for combining scores in a statistically and theoretically sound manner are shown. The use of multiple regression applied to individuals is explained. Recommendations about psychological report writing are offered.

Key Words: aptitude, achievement, cognitive abilities, psychological assessment, psychological reports

The principles of assessment are like a set of unruly and loosely affiliated wandering tribes. There is no established hierarchy of rules, no "Prince of Principles," and no royal family. There is no Senate, no Supreme Court, no United Nations. Yet, some members are esteemed by all. Others play partisan politics. Some are pompous windbags, others meek speakers of truth. Some are brilliant but impractical, others practical but limited. Some go unnoticed because they are subtle, others because they are so obvious. Some are widely misunderstood and some have outlived their usefulness. Some appear to be senselessly confining but actually protect us from our own excesses and foibles.

This review will not be a comprehensive account of the principles of assessment of aptitudes and achievement. Were it even feasible, such an account would be too large and detailed to be useful to anyone. Instead, I have focused on essential, practical, or curious aspects of assessment that may have been underemphasized, oversimplified, or simply omitted by the instructor of an introductory cognitive assessment course (or under-appreciated, misunderstood, or dimly remembered if not forgotten by

the students!). I will make a good faith effort in this idiosyncratic account to be candid when I am aware that my opinions may not be widely held.

Aptitudes and Achievement: Definitions, Distinctions, and Difficulties

"Achievement" typically refers to knowledge and skills that are formally taught in academic settings. However, this definition of achievement can be broadened to include any ability that is valued and taught in a particular cultural setting (e.g., hunting, dancing, or computer programming). "Aptitude" refers to an individual's characteristics that indicate the potential to develop a culturally valued ability, given the right circumstances. The difference between aptitudes and achievement at the definitional level is reasonably clear. However, at the measurement level, the distinction becomes rather murky.

Potential, which is latent within a person, is impossible to observe directly. It must be inferred by measuring characteristics that either are typically associated with an ability or are predictive of the future development of the ability. Most of the time, aptitude is assessed by measuring abilities that are considered to be necessary precursors of achievement. For example, children who understand speech have greater aptitude for reading comprehension than do children who do not understand speech. Such precursors may themselves be a form of achievement. For example, it is possible for researchers to consider students' knowledge of history as an outcome variable that is intrinsically valuable. However, some researchers may measure knowledge of history as a predictor of being able to construct a well-reasoned essay on politics. Thus, aptitude and achievement tests are not distinguished by their content, but by how they are used. If we use a test to measure current mastery of a culturally valued ability, it is an achievement test. If we use a test to explain or forecast mastery of a culturally valued ability, it is an aptitude test.

IQ tests are primarily used as aptitude tests. However, an inspection of the contents of most IQ tests reveals that many test items could be repurposed as items in an achievement test (e.g., vocabulary, general knowledge, and mental arithmetic items). Sometimes the normal roles of reading tests and IQ tests are reversed, such as when neuropsychologists estimate loss of function following a brain injury by comparing current IQ to performance on a word-reading test.

A simple method to distinguish between aptitude and achievement is to ask, "Do I care about whether a child has the ability measured by this test because it is inherently valuable or because it is associated with some other ability (the one that I actually care about)?" Most people want children to be able to comprehend what they read. Thus, reading tests are typically achievement tests. Most people are not particularly concerned about how well children can reorder numbers and letters in their heads. Thus, the WISC-IV Number-Letter Sequencing subtest is typically used as an aptitude test, presumably because the ability it measures is a necessary component of being able to master algebra, program computers, follow the chain of logic presented by debating candidates, and other skills that people in our culture care about.

Mean-spirited Mono-*g*-ists vs. Muddleheaded Poly-G-ists

I hate the impudence of a claim that in fifty minutes you can judge and classify a human being's predestined fitness in life. I hate the pretentiousness of the claim. I hate the abuse of scientific method which it involves.

I hate the sense of superiority which it creates, and the sense of inferiority which it imposes.

—Walter Lippmann, in a 1923 essay on Lewis Terman and the IQ testers

Most of us have uncritically taken it for granted that children who attend school eight or ten years without passing the fourth grade or surmounting long division are probably stupider than children who lead their classes into high school at twelve years and into college at sixteen. Mr. Lippmann contends that we can't tell anything about how intelligent either one of these children is until he has lived out his life. Therefore, for a lifetime at least, Mr. Lippmann considers his position impregnable!

—Lewis Terman, in response to Walter Lippmann

Spearman's (1904, 1927) little *g* caused a big stir when it was first proposed, and it has, for over a century now, been disrupting the natural state of harmony that would otherwise prevail amongst academics. Many a collegial tie has been severed, many a friendship has soured, perhaps even engagements broken off and marriages turned into dismal, loveless unions because of the rancor this topic provokes. I have seen otherwise mild-mannered professors in tweed jackets come to blows in bars over disagreements about *g*.[1]

It all began when Spearman observed that mental abilities that he measured were all positively correlated. This observation has been replicated by thousands of studies. No one who is familiar with this gigantic body of evidence doubts that essentially all cognitive abilities are positively correlated. This statistical regularity is typically referred to as the *positive manifold*.[2] You could become an academic superstar (i.e., admired by six or seven other academics) if you were to find a pair of cognitive abilities that are negatively correlated with each other. So far, no one has.[3] Thus, everyone in the know agrees with Spearman on this point. What some people hate is his explanation for it.

Spearman believed (and invented some very fancy statistical procedures to support his argument)[4] that abilities are correlated because all abilities are influenced by a common cause, *g* (general intelligence). Spearman was careful to note that he did not know for certain what *g* was but was not shy about speculating about its nature. He thought that it might be a kind of mental energy, and that some people had a lot of it and some had very little.

The essential points of contention in the Byzantine quarrels between Spearmanian mono-*g*-ists and anti-Spearmanian poly-G-ists[5]

have not changed much over the decades. There is some diversity within both groups, but the lines between them are fairly clear. Not only do the mono-g-ists insist that g be acknowledged as an ability, but they believe that it should be esteemed above all others. Some appear to believe that no ability other than g even matters. Some poly-G-ists will grant that g exists but deem it inconsequential compared to the myriad other abilities that influence the course of a human life. Other poly-G-ists deny that g exists and are disgusted by the very idea of it.

It turns out that these two groups are not merely on opposite sides of an intellectual debate—they are members of different tribes. They speak different dialects, vote for different candidates, and pray to different gods. Their heroic tales emphasize different virtues, and their foundation myths offer radically different but still internally consistent explanations of how the world works. If you think that the matter will be settled by accumulating more data, you have not been paying attention for the last hundred years.

Poly-G-ists do not merely believe that mono-g-ists are mistaken but that they are mean-spirited, perhaps evil, or at the very least, Republicans. In their view, the course of human history can be summed up in this manner:

> Since the dawn of time up to the beginning of the twentieth century, humans lived in a paradise of loving harmony and high self-esteem. Then Spearman invented g and ruined everything. Previously, Live White Males (for back then they were not yet dead) had been content to be equal to everyone else and were really rather decent fellows. However, many of them were corrupted by Spearman's flattery and convinced themselves they had more g than other people. The deceived began to call themselves Fascists and went around disempowering people with nasty labels. Though eventually defeated by George Lincoln King, Jr., in the Civil Liberties War, Fascists still wield influence via college aptitude tests. If we rid the world of all standardized tests, people will no longer label one another, low self-esteem will be eradicated, and a new Utopia will be established.

On the other side, mono-g-ists know that poly-G-ists have seen the same data and read the same studies as they have. They believe that the poly-G-ists are simply too muddle-headed to understand the data, too blinded by their ideological wishes to see the world as it is, or too fearful of social consequences to proclaim publicly that the emperor has no clothes. In the short epic tragedy *The Spearmaniad*, mono-g-ists find this account of how things came to be:

> In the dark mists of prehistory, life was nasty, brutish, and short. Worse, it was almost impossible to tell the common folk from their betters, and some very mediocre presidents were elected. When the goddess of mathematics looked upon the chaos of the world, she cried crystal tears of pure correlation coefficients. Now Spearman was a mighty statistician, and he gathered the correlations up and arranged them in matrices. From these matrices, he invented factor analysis, from which flowed new knowledge: first IQ tests, then writing, then the wheel. All that was done with factor analysis was beautiful, virtuous, and true. But the brief flowering of civilization that followed was ended when a cabal of ignorant do-gooders objected to the use of IQ tests, presumably because they (or their ugly, talentless children) performed poorly on them. We now stand on the brink of disaster. Giving up IQ tests will be followed immediately by a rapid descent into barbarism. College aptitude tests may postpone or soften the impact of this catastrophe for a little while but cannot avert it entirely.

The theoretical status of g will not cease to be controversial until something extraordinary happens to the field. I do not pretend to know what this might be. Maybe a breakthrough from biology will resolve the matter. Maybe divine intervention. Until then, I feel no need to join either tribe. I will remain agnostic and I will not get too excited the next time really smart people eagerly announce that finally, once and for all, they have proof that the other side is wrong. This has happened too many times before.

How to Assess Aptitudes If You Are a Mono-g-ist

For the mono-g-ist, the assessment of aptitudes is rather simple: measure g and be done with it. Other abilities may have a little predictive validity beyond g, but not enough to make it worth all the additional effort needed (Glutting, Watkins, Konold, & McDermott, 2006). This advice is simple enough, but how does one measure g well?

The first step is to select a set of highly g-loaded tests. The term *highly g-loaded* simply means "to correlate strongly with statistical g." This raises an important question. If the existence of g is in doubt, how can we know if a test correlates with it? To the poly-G-ist, this might sound like studying the environmental impact of unicorn overpopulation. The problem is resolved by distinguishing between two different meanings of g. First, there is theoretical g, a hypothetical entity thought to have causal relationships with many aspects of daily functioning. This is the *g* that many doubt exists. Second, there is statistical *g*, which is not in question. It is typically defined by a statistical procedure called *factor analysis* (or a closely related procedure called *principal components analysis*). All scholars agree that statistical *g* can be extracted from a correlation matrix and that virtually all cognitive tests correlate positively with it to some degree. Thus, a *g*-hating poly-G-ist can talk about a *g*-loaded test without fear of self-contradiction. A highly *g*-loaded test simply has a strong correlation with statistical *g*. A highly *g*-loaded test, then, is by definition highly correlated with many other tests. This means that it is probably a good predictor of academic achievement tests, which are, for the most part, also highly *g*-loaded. A cognitive test with a low *g*-loading (e.g., WJ III Planning or WISC-IV Cancellation) does not correlate with much of anything except itself. Mono-*g*-ists avoid such tests whenever possible (but Poly-g-ists love them—if they can be found to be uniquely predictive of an important outcome).

The second step to estimate *g* is to make sure that the highly *g*-loaded tests you have selected are as different from each other as possible in terms of item content and response format. To select highly similar tests (e.g., more than one vocabulary test) will contaminate the estimate of *g* with the influence of narrow abilities, which, to the mono-*g*-ist, are unimportant.

Fortunately, cognitive ability test publishers have saved us much trouble and have assembled such collections of subtests to create composite scales that can be used to estimate *g*. Such composite scores go by many different names,[6] but I will refer to them as IQ scores. These operational measures of *g* tend to correlate strongly with one another, mostly in the range of 0.70 to 0.80 but sometimes as low as 0.60 or as high as 0.90 (Kamphaus, 2005). Even so, they are not perfectly interchangeable. If both tests have the traditional mean of 100 and standard deviation of 15, the probability that the two scores will be within a certain range of each other can be found in Table 13.1.[7] For example, for a person who takes two IQ tests that are correlated at 0.80, there is a 29% chance that the IQ scores will differ by 10 points or more.

If a person has two or more IQ scores that differ by a wide margin, it does not necessarily mean that something is wrong. To insist on perfect correlations between IQ tests is not realistic and not fair.[8] However, when a child has taken two IQ tests

Table 13.1 What Is The Probability That a Person's Scores on Two IQ Tests Will Differ by the Specified Amount or More?

Difference	Probability if the IQ tests correlate at r =			
	0.60	0.70	0.80	0.90
> 5	0.71	0.67	0.60	0.46
> 10	0.46	0.39	0.29	0.14
> 15	0.26	0.20	0.11	0.03
> 20	0.14	0.09	0.03	0.003
> 25	0.06	0.03	0.01	0.0002

recently and the scores are different, it raises the question of which IQ is more accurate.

Can't Decide Which IQ Is Best? Make a Composite Score[9]

A man with a watch knows what time it is. A man with two watches is never sure.
—Segal's Law

Suppose you have been asked to settle a matter with important implications for an evaluee. A young girl was diagnosed with mental retardation three years ago. Along with low adaptive functioning, her Full Scale IQ was a 68, two points under the traditional line used to diagnose mental retardation. Upon re-evaluation two months ago, her IQ, derived from a different test, was now 78. Worried that their daughter would no longer qualify for services, the family paid out of pocket to have their daughter evaluated by another psychologist, and the IQ came out as 66. Because of your reputation for being fair-minded and knowledgeable, you have been asked to decide which, if any, is the real IQ. Of course, there is no such thing as a "real IQ," but you understand what the referral question is.

You give a different battery of tests, and the girl scores a 76. Now what should be done? It would be tempting to assume that "other psychologists are sloppy, whereas my results are free of error." However, you are fair-minded. You know that all scores have measurement error, and you plot the scores and their 95% confidence intervals as seen in Figure 13.1.

It is clear that Test C's confidence interval does not overlap with those of Tests B and D. Is this kind of variability in scores unusual?[10] There are two tests that indicate an IQ in the high 60s

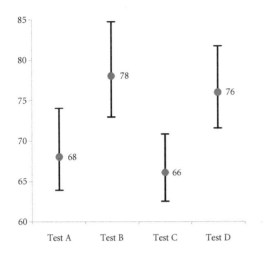

Figure 13.1 Recent IQ Scores and Their 95% Confidence Intervals from the Same Individual.

and two tests that indicate an IQ in the high 70s. Which pair of tests is correct? Should the poor girl be subjected to yet another test that might act as a tie breaker?

Perhaps the fairest solution is to treat each IQ test as a subtest of a much larger "Mega-IQ Test." That is, perhaps the best that can be done is to combine the four IQ scores into a single score and then construct a confidence interval around it.

Where should the confidence interval be centered? Intuitively, it might seem reasonable to simply average all four IQ results and say that the IQ is 72. However, this is not quite right. Averaging scores gives a rough approximation of a composite score, but it is less accurate for low and high scorers than it is for scorers near the mean. An individual's composite score is further away from the population mean than the average of the individual's subtest scores. About 3.1% of people score a 72 or lower on a single IQ test (assuming perfect normality). However, if we were to imagine a population of people who took all four IQ tests in question, only 1.9% of them would have an average score of 72 or lower. That is, it is more unusual to have a mean IQ of 72 than it is to score a 72 IQ on any particular IQ test. It is unusual to score 72 on one IQ test, but it is even more unusual to score that low on more than one test on average. Another way to think about this issue is to recognize that the mean score cannot be interpreted as an IQ score, because it has a smaller standard deviation than IQ scores have. To make it comparable to IQ, it needs to be rescaled so that it has a "standard" standard deviation of 15.

Here is a good method for computing a composite score and its accompanying 95% confidence interval. It is not nearly so complicated as it might seem at first glance. This method assumes that you know the reliability coefficients of all the scores and you know all the correlations between the scores. All scores must be index scores ($\mu = 100$, $\sigma = 15$). If they are not, they can be converted using this formula:

$$\text{Index Score} = 15\left(\frac{X - \mu}{\sigma}\right) + 100$$

Computing a Composite Score

Step 1: Add up all of the scores.
In this case,

$$68 + 78 + 66 + 76 = 288$$

Step 2: Subtract the number of tests times 100.
In this case there are 4 tests. Thus,

$$288 - 4 * 100 = 288 - 400 = -112$$

Step 3: Divide by the square root of the sum of all the elements in the correlation matrix.
In this case, suppose that the four tests are correlated as follows:

	Test A	Test B	Test C	Test D
Test A	1	0.80	0.75	0.85
Test B	0.80	1	0.70	0.71
Test C	0.75	0.70	1	0.78
Test D	0.85	0.71	0.78	1

The sum of all 16 elements, including the ones in the diagonal, is 13.18. The square root of 13.18 is about 3.63. Thus,

$$-112 / 3.63 = -30.85$$

Step 4: Complete the computation of the composite score by adding 100.
In this case,

$$-30.82 + 100 = 69.18$$

Given the four IQ scores available, assuming that there is no reason to favor one above the others, the best estimate is that her IQ is 69. Most of the time, there is no need for further calculation. However, we might like to know how precise this estimate is by constructing a 95% confidence interval around this score.

Confidence Intervals of Composite Scores

Calculating a 95% confidence interval is more complicated than the calculations above, but not overly so.

Step 1: Calculate the composite reliability.

Step 1a: Subtract the number of tests from the sum of the correlation matrix.

In this case, there are 4 tests. Therefore,

$$13.18 - 4 = 9.18$$

Step 1b: Add in all the test reliability coefficients.

In this case, suppose that the four reliability coefficients are 0.97, 0.96, 0.98, and 0.97. Therefore,

$$9.18 + 0.97 + 0.96 + 0.98 + 0.97 = 13.06.$$

Step 1c: Divide by the original sum of the correlation matrix.

In this case,

$$13.06 / 13.18 \approx 0.9909$$

Therefore, in this case, the reliability coefficient of the composite score is higher than that of any single IQ score. This makes sense: given that we have four scores, we should know what her IQ is with greater precision than we would if we only had one score.

Step 2: Calculate the standard error of the estimate by subtracting the reliability coefficient squared from the reliability coefficient and taking the square root. Then, multiply by the standard deviation, 15.

In this case,

$$15\sqrt{.9909 - 0.9909^2} \approx 1.4247$$

Step 3: Calculate the 95% margin of error by multiplying the standard error of the estimate by 1.96.

In this case,

$$1.96 * 1.44247 \approx 2.79$$

The value 1.96 is the approximate z-score associated with the 95% confidence interval. If you want the z-score associated with a different margin of

error, then use the following Excel formula. Shown here is the calculation of the z-score for a 99% confidence interval:

$$=NORMSINV(1-(1-0.99)/2)$$

Step 4: Calculate the estimated true score by subtracting 100 from the composite score, multiplying the reliability coefficient, and adding 100. That is,

Estimated True Score = Reliability Coefficient * (Composite − 100) + 100

In this case,

$$0.9909 * (69.18 - 100) + 100 = 69.46$$

Step 5: Calculate the upper and lower bounds of the 95% confidence interval by starting with the estimated true score and then adding and subtracting the margin of error.

In this case,

$$69.46 \pm 2.79 = 66.67 \text{ to } 72.25$$

This means that we are 95% sure that her IQ is between about 67 and 72. Assuming that other criteria for mental retardation are met, this is in the range to qualify for services in most states. It should be noted that this procedure can be used for any kind of composite score, not just for IQ tests.

Potential Misconceptions about Potential

If you are a mono-*g*-ist, you can use the estimate of *g* (IQ) to get an idea of what is the typical range of achievement scores for a child with that IQ. Not every child with the same IQ will have the same achievement scores.[11] Not even mono-*g*-ists believe that. Also, it is simply not true that achievement cannot be higher than IQ. Equally false is the assumption that if achievement is higher than IQ, then the IQ is wrong. These misconceptions are based on two premises: one true, the other false. If potential is the range of all possible outcomes, it is logically true that people cannot exceed their potentials. The false premise is that IQ and achievement tests are measured on the "potential scale." By analogy, if I say, "This thermometer reads −10 degrees. I know from my understanding of physics that Brownian motion never stops and thus no temperature dips below zero. Therefore, this thermometer is incorrect." My premise is true, if the thermometer is on the Kelvin scale. However, it is on the Celsius scale, so there is no reason to believe that something is amiss. IQ and achievement simply are not measured on the "potential scale." They are measured with standard scores, which are transformed deviations from a population mean. Because of this, about half of all people have academic achievement scores that are higher than their own IQ. There is nothing wrong with this.

Predicted Achievement Using Simple Linear Regression

There are two ways to make an estimate of a person's abilities. A *point estimate* (a single number) is precise but usually wrong, whereas an *interval estimate* (a range of numbers) is usually right but can be so wide that it is nearly useless. Confidence intervals combine both types of estimates in order to balance the weaknesses of one type of estimate with the strengths of the other. If I say that Suzie's expected reading comprehension is 85 ± 11, the 85 is the point estimate (also known as the "expected score," or the "predicted score," or just "Ŷ"). The ± 11 is called the *margin of error*. If the confidence level is left unspecified, by convention we mean the 95% margin of error. If I add 11 and subtract 11 to get a range from 74 to 96, I have the respective lower and upper bounds of the 95% confidence interval.

Calculating the Predicted Achievement Score

I will assume that both the IQ and achievement scores are index scores ($\mu = 100$, $\sigma = 15$) to make things simple. The predicted achievement score is a point estimate. It represents the best guess we can make in the absence of other information. The equation below is called a *regression equation*.

$$\hat{Y} = \sigma_Y r_{XY} \frac{X - \mu_X}{\sigma_X} + \mu_Y$$

If X is IQ, $\hat{Y}$ is the predicted Achievement score, and both scores are index scores ($\mu = 100$, $\sigma = 15$), the regression equation simplifies to:

Predicted achievement = (Correlation between IQ and Achievement) (IQ − 100) + 100

Calculating the Confidence Interval for the Predicted Achievement Score

Whenever you make a prediction using regression, your estimate is not exactly right very often. It is expected to differ from the actual achievement score by a certain amount (on average). This amount is called the *standard error of the estimate*. It

is the standard deviation of all the prediction errors. Thus, it is the *standard* to which all the *errors* in your *estimates* are compared. When both scores are index scores, the formula is:

Standard error of the estimate
$$= 15\sqrt{1 - \text{Correlation}^2}$$

To calculate the margin of error, multiply the standard error of the estimate by the z-score that corresponds to the degree of confidence desired. In Microsoft Excel, the formula for the z-score corresponding to the 95% confidence interval is:

$$= \text{NORMSINV}(1 - (1 - 0.95)/2)$$
$$\approx 1.96$$

For the 95% confidence interval, multiply the standard error of the estimate by 1.96. The 95% confidence interval's formula is:

95% Confidence Interval = Predicted Achievement ± 1.96 * Standard Error of the Estimate

This interval estimates the achievement score for 95% of people with the same IQ as the child. About 2.5% will score lower than this estimate, and 2.5% will score higher.

You can use Excel to estimate how unusual it is for an observed achievement score to differ from a predicted achievement score in a particular direction by using this formula,

$$= \text{NORMSDIST}(-1*\text{ABS}(\text{Observed-Predicted})/$$
$$(\text{Standard error of the estimate}))$$

If a child's observed achievement score is unusually low, it does not automatically mean that the child has a learning disorder. Many other things need to be checked before that diagnosis can be considered valid. However, it does mean that an explanation for the unusually low achievement score should be sought.

Aptitude Assessment Using CHC Theory

There is much more to talk about once you have decided that you are interested in more than just *g*. First, you have to decide which abilities are relevant to the assessment question. In order to do that, you have to decide, at least tentatively, which abilities even exist. There are many models of the structure of cognitive abilities, but most are historical relics with no living supporters. For example, in the end, even Spearman rejected his Two-Factor Theory (Horn & Blankson, 2005). There are a few theories that are still alive in the sense that they are taken seriously by active researchers. Chief among them is the Cattell-Horn-Carroll theory of cognitive abilities (CHC theory; McGrew, 2005; Schneider & McGrew, 2012).

CHC theory is the child of two titans, Carroll's (1993) lumbering leviathan, the Three-Stratum Theory of Cognitive Abilities, and Cattell and Horn's two-headed giant, G*f*-G*c* Theory (Horn & Cattell, 1966). Given that Horn was as staunchly anti-*g* as they come (Horn & Blankson, 2005) and that Carroll was a dedicated *g*-man (though not of the *g*-and-only-*g* variety; Carroll, 2003), it surprising that these theories even had a courtship, much less a marriage. From 1986 to the late 1990s, in a series of encounters initiated and chaperoned by test developer Richard Woodcock, Horn and Carroll discussed the intersections of their theories and eventually consented to have their names yoked under a single framework (McGrew, 2005). Although the interfaith ceremony was officiated by Woodcock, the product of their union was midwifed primarily by McGrew (1997). Woodcock, McGrew, and colleagues' ecumenical approach has created a space in which mono-*g*-ists and poly-G-ists can engage in civil dialogue, or at least ignore one another politely. CHC theory puts *g* atop a three-stratum hierarchy of cognitive abilities, but *g*'s role in the theory is such that poly-G-ists can ignore it to the degree that they see fit. By 2005, it was clear that revisions to almost all of the major cognitive tests batteries were being influenced, partially

if not primarily, by the development of CHC theory (Alfonso, Flanagan, & Radwan, 2005). In the intervening years, this trend has not changed.

Broad Overview of CHC Theory

Performance on cognitive ability tests is influenced by many cognitive functions operating simultaneously. If performance on two tests is influenced by more or less the same subset of cognitive functions, the scores on the two tests will be highly correlated. If test performance on the two tests is influenced by only a few cognitive functions in common, the correlation between the tests is likely to be low.

CHC theory distinguishes among abilities at three levels: Stratum I (narrow abilities), Stratum II (broad abilities), and Stratum III (*g*). The words *broad* and *narrow* are so versatile that it is easy to forget that they are being used as metaphors in this case. What is meant by the distinction between broad and narrow is not typically made explicit, but there are at least two interpretations that can be considered. Of course, these interpretations are not mutually exclusive.

Broad vs. Narrow: Different Levels of Generality

The distinction between broad and narrow that is implied by Figure 13.2 is that broad abilities are cognitive functions that influence performance in a wide variety of tasks. Narrow abilities are functions that influence performance in a smaller subset

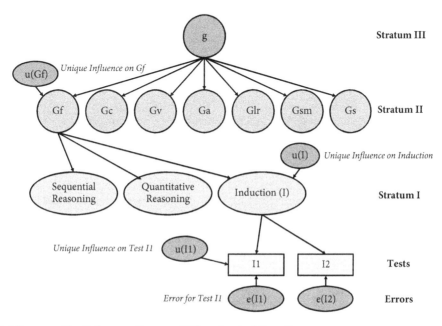

Figure 13.2 Influences on Test Performance Operate at Different Levels of Generality.

of tasks. Thus, from this perspective, broad abilities (including the broadest of abilities, *g*) are not fundamentally different from narrow abilities. They are all abilities in the same sense. They simply differ in their generality.

Consider the difference between two physical abilities, the ability to walk and the ability to hurl a shot in shot put. They are both learned, they require practice, and some people are better at them than are others. However, walking is an ability that can be used to achieve a much larger set of goals than can throwing the shot. In this sense, walking is a broad ability and throwing the shot is a narrow one. If you cannot walk, many other activities are difficult. If you cannot throw the shot very far but are otherwise healthy, the consequences for you are slight.

In Figure 13.2, it is clear that there are multiple ways in which people might obtain the same level of performance on the hypothetical measure of inductive reasoning, Test *I*1. Performance on Test *I*1 could be described as

$$I1 = g + u(Gf) + u(I) + u(I1) + e(I1)$$

Where

*I*1 = Score on Test *I*1

g = The sum of all factors that influence all test scores

u(*Gf*) = The sum of all factors that influence all *Gf* tests, controlling for *g*

u(*I*) = The sum of all factors that influence all Induction tests, controlling for *g* and *u*(*Gf*)

u(*I*1) = The sum of all stable influences on Test *I*1, controlling for *g*, *u*(*Gf*), and u(*I*)

e(*I*1) = The sum of all unstable influences on Test *I*1

A person might score well on *I*1 because of luck (a form of error), previous exposure to very similar tasks (a kind of unique influence on *I*1), specific training in inductive reasoning (a unique influence on the narrow ability of inductive reasoning), cultural emphasis on abstract reasoning (a unique influence on the broad ability of fluid intelligence), or a lifetime of having been fed well and protected from large brain injuries and exposure to neurotoxins (different kinds of influences that would affect the functioning of the whole brain and thus would affect *g*).

Broad vs. Narrow: Different Levels of Abstraction[12]

A second meaning of the distinction between broad abilities and narrow abilities is that we can conceive of abilities as existing at different levels of abstraction. Certain tasks are inherently complex in that they require the coordinated actions of multiple cognitive functions simultaneously or in sequence. To use another example involving track and field events, performing well on the 100-meter hurdles requires, among other things, sprinting and jumping in a well-timed alternating sequence. We could measure sprinting speed by having people sprint for 100 meters. We could measure jumping by having people stand still and then jump over the hurdle. However, it is hard to argue that this is the same kind of jumping (and an argument could be made that it is not same kind of sprinting if one is not expected to hurdle). Thus, running the 100-meter hurdles requires an ability that is not merely the sum of sprinting and jumping abilities, but a non-additive combination of the skills.

That hurdling requires sprinting and jumping is obvious, because we are able to observe athletes as they run and jump. When people perform cognitive tasks, it is not always so obvious which cognitive functions contribute to performance. Thus, the components of performance must be inferred statistically.

In Figure 13.3, a hypothetical set of tests that are intended to measure different facets of ability are shown. Although it was the intention of the hypothetical researchers to measure the five narrow abilities in the figure with two tests each, it is impossible to measure one and only one ability at a time, and there is considerable overlap. For example, a General Information test inherently requires language development. Furthermore, fluid reasoning plays a role in acquiring knowledge because most of what we know is not explicitly taught. For example, if I notice that a word is used only by snobby people, I might use inductive reasoning to infer that using the word makes one sound snobby. Because I know that there are no settlements on the moon, I can deduce that there are no fast food restaurants there…yet!

What is being illustrated in Figure 13.3 is that *g*, *Gf*, and inductive reasoning are not distinct abilities that differ in terms of their generality. Rather, they exist at different levels of abstraction. *Gf* is a legitimate category because a certain subset of narrow abilities is bundled together in ways that are difficult, if not impossible, to separate. In a sense, *Gf* is not really an ability at all. One can see this clearly by an analogy to vision. It is perfectly acceptable to talk about "the ability to see." However, a moment's reflection will reveal that *seeing* is not a single ability but many abilities (to list but a few: the ability to distinguish light and dark, color vision, the ability

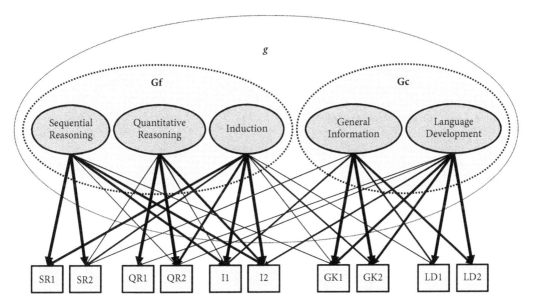

Figure 13.3 Abilities Conceptualized at Different Levels of Abstraction.

to focus, the ability to move one's eyes to follow an object, the ability to see distinct stimuli as forming a gestalt, and so forth[13]). What makes it legitimate to talk about vision as an ability is that the various sub-abilities work together as a functional unit. In the same sense, fluid intelligence (G*f*) is an ability (and so too, possibly, is the dreaded *g*).

Fluid Intelligence (G*f*)

Mentioning fluid intelligence at cocktail parties as if it were a perfectly ordinary topic of conversation carries with it a certain kind of cachet that is hard to describe unless you have experienced it for yourself. Part of G*f*'s mystique can be attributed to Cattell's (1987) assertions that G*f* is linked to rather grand concepts such as innate ability, genetic potential, biological intelligence, mass action, and the overall integrity of the whole brain.[14] Heady stuff indeed!

At the measurement level, G*f* tests require reasoning with abstract symbols such as figures and numbers.[15] Good measures of G*f* are novel problems that require mental effort and controlled attention to solve. If a child can solve the problem without much thought, the child is probably making use of prior experience. Thus, even though a test is considered a measure of fluid intelligence, it does not measure fluid intelligence to the same degree for all children. Some children have been exposed to matrix tasks and number series in school or in games. Fluid intelligence is about novel problem–solving and, as Kaufman (1994, p. 31) noted, wryly pointing out the obvious, a test is only novel once.

The second time a child takes the same fluid intelligence test, performance typically improves (by about 5 points or 1/3 standard deviation, Kaufman & Lichtenberger, 2006). This is why reports that fluid intelligence can be improved with training (Jaeggi, Buschkuehl, Jonides, & Perrig, 2008) cannot be taken at face value.[16] Just because performance has improved on "G*f* tests" because of training does not mean that G*f* is the ability that has improved.

At the core of G*f* is the narrow ability of *induction*. Inductive reasoning is the ability to figure out an abstract rule from a limited set of data. In a sense, inductive reasoning represents a person's capacity to acquire new knowledge without explicit instruction. Inductive reasoning allows a person to profit from experience. That is, information and experiences are abstracted so that they can be generalized to similar situations. *Deductive* reasoning is the ability to apply a rule in a logically valid manner to generate a novel solution. In CHC theory, deductive reasoning is called "general sequential reasoning." Although logicians have exquisitely nuanced vocabularies for talking about the various sub-categories of inductive and deductive reasoning, it will suffice to say that everyday problem-solving typically requires a complex mix of the two.

Inductive and deductive reasoning can be found in multiple places in CHC theory. Whenever inductive and deductive reasoning are applied to quantitative content, they are called "quantitative reasoning." For mysterious reasons, inductive and deductive reasoning with quantitative stimuli tend to cluster together in factor analyses. Inductive and deductive reasoning also make an appearance in Gc. Whenever inductive and deductive reasoning tasks rely primarily on past experience and previous knowledge, they are classified as measures of crystallized intelligence. Many researchers have supposed that the Similarities subtest in the Wechsler tests contains an element of fluid reasoning because inductive reasoning is used to figure out how two things or concepts are alike. If the question is something like, "How are a dog and a cat alike?" then it is very unlikely that a child arrives at the correct answer by reasoning things out for the first time. Instead, the child makes an association immediately based on prior knowledge.

Researchers are not satisfied with accepting Gf as a given. They wish to know the origins of Gf and to understand why some people are so much more adept at abstract reasoning than other people are (Conway, Cowan, Bunting, Therriault, & Minkoff, 2002). One hypothesis that is still being explored is that fluid reasoning has a special relationship with working memory. *Working memory* is the ability to hold information in mind while using controlled attention to transform it in some way (e.g., rearranging the order of things or applying a computational algorithm). Many researchers have noted that tests of fluid reasoning, particularly matrix tasks (e.g., WISC-IV Matrix Reasoning), can be made more difficult by increasing the working memory load required to solve the problem. Kyllonen and Christal (1990) published the provocative finding that individual differences in Gf could be explained entirely by individual differences in working memory. Many studies have attempted to replicate these finding but have failed. Most studies find that Gf and working memory are strongly correlated (about 0.6) but are far from identical (Kane, Hambrick, Tuholski, Wilhelm, Payne, & Engle, 2004).

Just as we have distinguished between statistical *g* and theoretical *g*, it is important to note that there is a difference between the Gf that is measured by Gf tests and the Gf that is written about by theorists. Some of Cattell's hypotheses about Gf have stood the test of time, whereas others have not held up very well. For example, the heritability of Gf is not higher than that of Gc, as Cattell's theory predicts. I mention this because it is probably not justified to claim that because a child scores well on Gf tests, the child has high innate talent or that the child's biological intelligence is high.

Table 13.2 Measures in the Gf Domain

Narrow Abilities	Measures
Inductive Reasoning	CAS Nonverbal Matrices
	DAS-II Matrices
	KABC-II Pattern Reasoning
	KAIT Mystery Codes
	RIAS Odd-Item Out
	SB5 Nonverbal Fluid Reasoning
	WISC-IV Matrix Reasoning
	WJ III Concept Formation
General Sequential Reasoning	KAIT Logical Steps
	WJ III Analysis-Synthesis
Quantitative Reasoning	DAS-II Sequential & Quantitative Reasoning
	SB5 Nonverbal Quantitative Reasoning
	SB5 Verbal Quantitative Reasoning
	WAIS-IV Figure Weights
	WJ III Number Matrices
	WJ III Number Series

Most of the effects of Gf on academic achievement are mediated by Gc (i.e., better reasoning leads to more knowledge, which leads to higher achievement). However, Gf seems to have a special relationship with complex problem–solving in mathematics. Because Gf tests measure abstract reasoning, it is unsurprising that they would predict performance in an abstract domain such as mathematics (Floyd, Evans, & McGrew, 2003).

Examples of tests that measure narrow abilities in the Gf domain can be found in Table 13.2.

Crystallized Intelligence (Gc)

Sir, the man who has vigour, may walk to the east, just as well as to the west, if he happens to turn his head that way.

—Samuel Johnson, arguing that Edmund Burke would have achieved greatness in any field

Broadly speaking, *crystallized intelligence* refers to the ability to use culturally sanctioned knowledge and problem-solving methods to achieve culturally sanctioned goals (Hunt, 2000). In Cattell's (1941) original theory, there were two general factors of intelligence, g_f and g_c.[17] General fluid intelligence (g_f) represented potential, whereas crystallized intelligence (g_c) represented the realization of potential. In what came to be known as *investment theory*, Cattell observed that children with more potential to learn tend to acquire more knowledge. Thus, Cattell called statistical g "historical g_f" because it represents the aggregate effects of g_f on g_c over a person's lifetime ("...this year's crystallized ability level is a function of last year's fluid ability level..."; Cattell, 1987, pp. 139). This may be the reason that g_f is indistinguishable from g in some samples (Gustafsson & Undheim, 1996).

Fortunately for people with low g_f, it is possible for differences in learning to occur that have nothing to do with g_f. Cattell called any intentional effort to enhance g_c "investment." That is, g_f is "invested" in activities that enhance g_c. Investment takes many forms, including parental investment of time and energy to teach children, societal investment to educate the next generation with public schooling and special programs to help children with intellectual gifts or deficits, and personal investment to educate oneself via the personality traits of conscientiousness (some children learn more because they are more obedient in school), ambition (some children learn more because they hope to accomplish more), and intellectual curiosity (some children learn more because they enjoy learning more). This theory predicts that, to the degree a society provides equal opportunity to all its citizens, g_f and g_c will be more correlated and harder to distinguish.

Cattell (1987) invoked the metaphor of the fluid/crystallized distinction to suggest that talent was inchoate, whereas knowledge had definite form resulting from specific experiences.[18] In later years, Horn de-emphasized the conceptualization of fluid intelligence as potential and saw it more as a person's current capacity for abstract thought. Thus, he believed that not only did fluid intelligence affect the growth of crystallized intelligence but also that education and other forms of experience might affect one's capacity for abstraction (Horn & Blankson, 2005).

In my experience, a kind of sincere but misguided egalitarianism leads many graduate students to esteem Gf and to disdain Gc. In their minds, Gf is *real* intelligence, whereas Gc is merely the result of opportunity. Thus, contemplating a person whose opportunities to learn have been limited, students wish to ignore the person's lack of knowledge and focus instead on things that "actually matter," like potential. Although this position is not entirely wrong, it turns out that knowledge matters quite a bit. Almost all of IQ's predictive validity in the workplace is mediated by specific job knowledge. That is, although bright people learn faster, more efficiently, and more deeply, it is the job knowledge itself that primarily determines competence (Gottfredson,

1997).[19] Students assume that if a child has high fluid ability but low crystallized intelligence, the child will be fine (eventually), either because raw talent will carry the day or because the child's high Gf will cause accelerated knowledge acquisition in the future. The question they fail to ask is, "Why hasn't this happened already?" There may be hidden factors at work, and these knowledge-inhibiting factors are not likely to change unless the right intervention is implemented.

Crystallized intelligence is the best Stratum II predictor of every kind of academic achievement (Benson, 2008; Evans, Floyd, McGrew, & Leforgee, 2002; Floyd, Evans, & McGrew, 2003). The exact nature of the relationship between the narrow facets of Gc and mathematics is not clear. For example, it is doubtful that knowing the capital of Australia (Canberra!) helps children with long division. It is unlikely that knowing about oxymorons will unlock the secrets of geometry. Nevertheless, Gc predicts mastery of mathematics even after controlling for all other abilities, probably because the link between calculation and quantitative reasoning is typically mediated via language. Verbal concepts (e.g., integers, perfect squares, right triangles) are just as much a part of mathematics as they are of any other academic domain. There is no reason to suppose that learning them is radically different from learning other verbal concepts. Thus, Gc is an essential precursor ability to mathematics achievement.

What constitutes adequate measurement of Gc in practice is not entirely settled; it seems best to discuss only the aspects that are widely accepted as belonging in this domain and are measured clearly by the major cognitive test batteries.

Lexical Knowledge

If *lexical knowledge* is simply memorizing the definitions of fancy words, then, at best, it is a trivial ability valued by academics, pedants, and fuddy-duddies. At worst, its elevation by elitists is a tool of oppression. There is some truth to these views of lexical knowledge, but they are myopic. I will argue that vocabulary tests are rightfully at the center of most assessments of language and crystallized intelligence. Some words have the power to open up new vistas of human experience. For example, when I was thirteen, learning the word "ambivalence" clarified many aspects of interpersonal relationships that were previously baffling.

A word is an abstraction. The need for labels of simple categories is perfectly clear. Knowing the word "anger" (or its equivalent in any other language) frees us from having to treat each encounter with the emotion as a unique experience. Being able to communicate with others about this abstract category of experience facilitates self-awareness and the understanding of interpersonal relations. We can build up a knowledge base of the sorts of things that typically make people angry and the kinds of reactions to expect from angry people.

It is less obvious why "anger" has so many synonyms and near-synonyms, some of which are a bit obscure (e.g., iracund, furibund, and zowerswopped!). Would it not be easier to communicate if there were just one word for every concept? It is worthwhile to consider the question of why words are invented. At some point in the history of a language, a person thought that it would be important to distinguish one category of experience from others, and that this distinction merited its own word. Although most neologisms are outlived even by their inventors, a few of them are so useful that they catch on and are used by enough people for enough time that they are considered "official words" and are then taken for granted as if they had always existed.[20] That is, people do not adopt new words with the primary goal of impressing one another. They do it because the word succinctly captures an idea or a distinction that would otherwise be difficult or tiresome to describe indirectly. Rather than saying, "Because Shelly became suddenly angry, her sympathetic nervous system directed her blood away from her extremities toward her large muscles. One highly visible consequence of this redirection of blood flow was that her face turned white for a moment and then became discolored with splotches of red." It is simply more economical to say that "Shelly was livid with rage." By convention, the use of the word "livid" signals that Shelly is probably not thinking too clearly at the moment, and that the next thing that Shelly says or does is probably going to be impulsive and possibly hurtful.

Using near-synonyms interchangeably is not merely offensive to word nerds and the grammar police. It reflects, and possibly leads to, an impoverishment of thought and a less nuanced understanding of the world. For example, *jealousy* is often used as a substitute for *envy*. They are clearly related words, but they are not at all the same. In fact, in a sense, they tend to be experienced by people on opposite sides of a conflicted relationship. Envy is the painful, angry awareness that someone else enjoys some (probably undeserved) advantage that we covet. Jealousy is the angry, often vigilant, suspicion we may lose our beloved to a rival.

Unaware of this distinction, it would be difficult to benefit from or even make sense of the wisdom of Rochefoucauld's observation that "Jealousy is born with love, but does not die with it."

Lexical knowledge is obviously important for decoding words while reading. If you are familiar with a word, it is easier to decode. It is also obviously important for reading comprehension. If you know what a word means, it is easier to comprehend the sentences in which it appears. It is probably the case that reading comprehension also influences lexical knowledge. Children who comprehend what they read are more likely to enjoy reading and thus read more. Children who read more expose themselves to words that rarely occur in casual speech but whose meaning can be inferred from how they are used in the text. Finally, lexical knowledge is important for writing. Children with a rich understanding of the distinctions between words will not only be able to express what they mean more precisely, but their knowledge of certain words will enable them to express thoughts that they might not otherwise have had. For example, it seems to me unlikely that a student unfamiliar with the word "paradox" would be able to write an essay about two ideas that appear to be contradictory at first glance but at a deeper level are consistent with each other.

Language Development

Time flies like an arrow; fruit flies like a banana.
   —Groucho Marx

While he was declaring the ardour of his passion in such terms, as but too often make vehemence pass for sincerity, Adeline, to whom this declaration, if honourable, was distressing, and if dishonourable, was shocking, interrupted him and thanked him for the offer of a distinction, which, with a modest, but determined air, she said she must refuse.

   —Ann Radcliffe, in *Romance of the Forest* (1791), describing the heroine's response to an unwelcome sexual advance

Language development refers to the complexity of one's understanding and use of language. Without a deep understanding of language, neither of the above quotes can be understood, much less admired for their genius. There is no sharp distinction between lexical knowledge and language development. Indeed, Carroll (1993) considered "lexical knowledge" to be a subcomponent of "language development." In their initial application of CHC theory to major test batteries, McGrew and Flanagan (1998) labeled many subtests from major cognitive ability batteries (e.g., WISC-III Comprehension) as primarily measures of language development. More recently, almost all of these subtests have been reclassified to other areas (primarily to General Information and to Lexical Knowledge). However, the secondary loading to language development is still noted on the most recent cross-battery worksheets (Flanagan, Ortiz, & Alfonso, 2007). Specialized measures of syntax (e.g., CELF-4 Sentence Assembly) and nonliteral language comprehension (e.g., CASL Nonliteral Language) are more direct measures of language development. McGrew and I (Schneider & McGrew, 2012) have drawn attention to Carroll's original conception of language development as an intermediate category between Gc and narrow language abilities such as lexical knowledge, grammatical sensitivity, listening ability, and oral production.

General Verbal Information

There is much pleasure to be gained from useless knowledge.
　　—Bertrand Russell

When critics look though the items in a general verbal information test, they, with some justification, sometimes sneer at the usefulness of the content. Is there any money in being able to reel off the names of the planets? Can I oppose injustice, armed with my knowledge of state capitals? Will any babies be saved because I know who Julian the Apostate was? Probably not. Many (most?) facts I have learned are unlikely to ever be of practical use. If I knew which ones they were, I might happily surrender them to forgetfulness. However, because it is impossible to know what might be useful in the future, I will hang onto my useless and pointless knowledge for a little while longer, thank you very much.

When Francis Bacon wrote parenthetically that "knowledge itself is a power…" in the context of an argument attempting to discredit the theological beliefs of certain religious sects, he probably did not mean the phrase in the sense that it is invoked today (i.e., that knowledge *confers* power). However, the phrase "knowledge is power" has survived because it resonates with our experience and pithily expresses something that is increasingly true in an age that gives increasing returns to those who can profit from information.

Good items in a General Information test should not be about random facts. Easy items should not be *merely* easy (e.g., "What is the color of the sky?").

Rather, they should test for knowledge of information considered essential for living independently in our culture. A person who does not understand why dishes should be washed is not ready to live unsupervised. More difficult items should not be *merely* difficult (e.g., "What is the largest city in Svalbard?" "How many teeth does an orca whale have?"). Rather, they should measure knowledge that is relevant to what are considered core aspects of our culture (e.g., "Why do banks loan people money?" "Why do people still learn Latin and ancient Greek?" "Who was Isaac Newton?" "What is the purpose of the United Nations?").

Just as language development consists of many narrow abilities, there are many sub-categories in general information. Typically these sub-categories consist of academic domains such as knowledge of the humanities and knowledge of the sciences. These categories have further subdivisions (e.g., physics, chemistry, biology, and so forth)—and each of these, in turn, has further subdivisions.

General information consists of knowledge that each person in a culture is expected to be familiar with (or would be admired for if he or she knew). However, much (if not most) of a person's knowledge is not of this sort. For example, although it is expected that everyone in this culture should know what airplanes are, only pilots are expected to know how to fly them. In CHC theory, knowledge that is expected to be known only to members of a particular profession or enthusiasts of a particular hobby, sport, or other activity is classified as Domain-Specific Knowledge (Gkn). Most subject-specific academic achievement tests (e.g., European history, geology, contemporary American literature) would be considered measures of Gkn, not Gc. That is, typically (but not always), achievement measures are the relevant outcomes we wish to explain, not explanatory aptitudes. In contrast, measures of general information (e.g., WISC-IV Information) are intended to be estimates of the body of knowledge from which a person can draw to solve a wide range of problems.

Like lexical knowledge, general information has a bi-directional relationship with reading comprehension. Very little of what is written is fully self-contained; authors presume that readers have considerable background knowledge and often do not bother to explain themselves. Drout (2006) describes how difficult and amusing it is to explain to non-native speakers of English what newspaper headlines such as "Under Fire from G.O.P.,

White House Hunkers Down" mean.[21] Children who know more understand more of what they read. Understanding more makes reading more enjoyable. Reading more exposes children to more knowledge, much of which is inaccessible via oral culture.

Examples of tests that measure narrow abilities in the Gc domain can be found in Table 13.3.

Visual-Spatial Processing (G*v*)

G*v* and G*a* (auditory processing) are two broad abilities linked to specific sensory modalities. There are efforts to expand CHC theory to include abilities linked to other senses (olfactory, gustatory, tactile, and kinesthetic) but it is not yet clear what the abilities are and how distinct they are from other abilities already included in CHC theory (Danthiir, Roberts, Pallier, & Stankov, 2001; Stankov, Seizova-Cajic, & Roberts, 2001). It is confusing to parents to talk about visual-spatial processing (or about auditory processing) because we are not used to thinking about visual-spatial processes divorced from the sensory experience of vision. I like to explain the difference between vision and visual-spatial processing like this:

> Vision is the ability to see something, and visual-spatial processing helps you make sense of what you see. Vision is the ability to see what is there. Visual-spatial processing is the ability to see what is not there, too, in a sense. With good vision you can see what something looks like; with good visual-spatial processing you can imagine what something would look like if you turned it around or if you were standing somewhere else, or if something else was covering part of it. With good vision, you can see objects; with good visual-spatial processing, you can see how they might fit together. With good vision, you can see a bunch of lines and splotches of colors; with good visual-spatial processing, you can see how those lines and splotches of color form meaningful patterns. This is the ability that sculptors, painters, designers, engineers, and architects need. It comes in pretty handy for the rest of us, too.

Within the domain of G*v*, there are many narrow abilities. Few of them are well understood, and they seem to be defined more by the kind of test used to measure them than by the underlying psychological processes needed to perform on the tests. Most of them are not measured directly by the major cognitive test batteries and thus they have been omitted from this discussion.

Spatial Relations and Visualization

In Carroll's (1993) theory, *spatial relations* and *visualization* were distinguished from each other in the following manner. "Spatial relations" was defined by tests in which participants had to answer as many questions as possible as quickly as possible by mentally rotating simple visual figures in order to deduce the correct answer.[22] The "visualization" factor was defined by tests in which time pressure was less of an issue and the spatial reasoning tasks were more complex. Visualization tests require children to imagine what something might look like from a different angle, to manipulate a visual image in the mind's eye, and to assemble objects to fit them together. Visualization tests tend to be more *g*-loaded and, in the minds of many theorists and test developers, good markers of G*f* (more accurately, of Cattell's original fluid intelligence factor g_f). Although the theoretical distinction between spatial relations and visualization may be important, there are no commercially available test batteries designed

Table 13.3 Measures in the G*c* Domain

Narrow Abilities	Measures
Communication Ability	KTEA-II Oral Expression
	WIAT-III Oral Expression
General Information	KAIT Famous Faces
	SB5 Nonverbal Knowledge
	WISC-IV Comprehension
	WISC-IV Information
	WJ III Academic Knowledge
	WJ III General Information
Lexical Knowledge	DAS-II Similarities
	DAS-II Word Definitions
	KABC-II Expressive Vocabulary
	KABC-II Riddles
	KABC-II Verbal Knowledge
	KAIT Definitions
	KAIT Double Meanings
	SB5 Verbal Knowledge
	WISC-IV Similarities
	WISC-IV Vocabulary
	WJ III Picture Vocabulary
	WJ III Verbal Comprehension
Listening Ability	KAIT Auditory Comprehension
	KTEA-II Listening Comprehension
	WIAT-III Listening Comprehension
	WJ III Oral Comprehension
	WJ III Understanding Directions

to help clinicians to distinguish between these factors. Specifically, no commercially available subtest resembles the highly speeded mental rotation tasks that define the Spatial Relations factor as described originally by Carroll.[23] Although McGrew and Flanagan (1998) tentatively speculated that some subtests from major test batteries might be influenced by spatial relations to some degree, they were always clear that all such tests at least had a strong secondary loading on visualization. To my knowledge, no evidence exists that would make the distinction between spatial relations and visualization clinically vital for any purpose. It is therefore my recommendation not to worry about the distinction. Instead, I recommend selecting measures of spatial relations/visualization that have differing formats to minimize the effects of format-specific factors.

After controlling for g, this factor of ability does not typically have substantial relationships with achievement tests (Floyd, Evans, & McGrew, 2003). One of the reasons for this is that most academic achievement tests de-emphasize aspects of learning that require visual-spatial reasoning. It is quite possible that achievement tests could be devised that draw on this ability, but few test developers do so. At any rate, there is ample reason to suspect that visual-spatial reasoning is an important predictor of success in certain fields. For example, visual-spatial ability (primarily visualization) measured in childhood was a strong predictor of educational and occupational outcomes for mathematically precocious students (Shea, Lubinski, & Benbow, 2001). In particular, strong visual-spatial ability predicted choosing careers in the physical sciences and mathematics. These effects were important even after controlling for verbal and quantitative ability.

Closure Speed

In *closure speed* tasks, a child is given a distorted picture of a real object and must guess what it is. It is not exactly clear to me where speediness factors into Closure Speed tasks unless bonus points are awarded for faster responses.[24] It seems that French's (1951) term *Gestalt perception* would be a better name for what is being measured.

In both commercially available tests of closure speed (KABC-II Gestalt Closure and WJ III Visual Closure), the test g-loadings are low. In addition, closure speed tests often have low correlations with other Gv tests and can have substantial loadings on Gc (Reynolds, Keith, Fine, Fisher, & Low, 2007; Woodcock, McGrew, Schrank, & Mather, N., 2007). Presumably, closure speed tasks load

on Gc because the distorted image is compared to images stored in long-term memory to see if there is a match. To my knowledge, no study has ever identified any clinically relevant outcome that is better predicted by closure speed than by some other narrow ability.

Visual Memory

It is obvious that such a thing as "visual memory" exists. However, it is unclear how distinct the visual memory factor is from other abilities. One of the problems with the measurement of visual memory is that people employ a wide variety of strategies on visual memory tasks, and these strategies alter which abilities are employed. In most visual memory tasks, children are shown a complex visual stimulus and are asked to reproduce the stimulus from memory or to recognize it from an array of similar pictures.[25] Many children verbalize what they see ("Three circles inside a square"), converting the task into a verbal memory test. Some children encode the stimulus analytically (part by part), whereas others encode it holistically. The more children can encode the stimulus as broken into larger units, the lower the load on memory, and the higher the load on visual-spatial ability. Carroll was unsure about the theoretical status of this factor. Furthermore, he was not aware of any research on the usefulness of visual memory tasks in predicting educational or occupational success (Carroll, 1993, p. 184). In the intervening years, no study I am aware of has shown the usefulness of this factor.

Examples of tests that measure narrow abilities in the Gv domain can be found in Table 13.4.

Auditory Processing (G*a*)

> ME: *Tell me about why you decided to be evaluated.*
> ADULT CLIENT: *I think I might have HDHD and dahlexia.*
> ME (unsure): *You think you might have ADHD and dyslexia?*
> ADULT CLIENT (embarrassed): *Right, ADHD… but I think I have dahlexia, too.*

Auditory processing problems are among the hardest problems to explain. If you were to give parents a simple, technically correct definition of *auditory processing* (e.g., the ability to perceive patterns in sound), you are likely to be misunderstood. Parents know that "auditory" has something to do with hearing and are likely to think that their child has a hearing problem or has difficulty understanding

Table 13.4 Measures in the G*v* Domain

Narrow Abilities	Measures
Spatial Relations/ Visualization	CAS Verbal-Spatial Relations
	DAS-II Pattern Construction
	KABC-II Block Counting
	KABC-II Triangles
	SB5 Nonverbal Visual-Spatial Processing
	SB5 Verbal Visual-Spatial Processing
	WAIS-IV Visual Puzzles
	WISC-IV Block Design
	WJ III Block Rotation
	WJ III Spatial Relations
Closure Speed	KABC-II Gestalt Closure
	WJ III Visual Closure
Visual Memory	CAS Figure 13.Memory
	DAS-II Recall of Designs
	RIAS Nonverbal Memory
	WJ III Picture Recognition

speech. "Auditory processing" is the ability that I spend the most time explaining so that I do not cause confusion. If a child has auditory processing problems, I say something like this to the parents:

Auditory Processing is not the ability to hear. Your daughter can hear just fine. The problem that she has is difficult to explain, so I am going to start by comparing her problem to vision problems (She does not have a vision problem, either. I am just comparing the two problems.) Nearsighted people are not blind. Up close, they see well. Things that are far away, however, are blurry. Making lights brighter does not help; nearsighted people need glasses. In the same way that someone who is nearsighted is not blind, your daughter is not deaf; she is not even hard of hearing. However, for her, speech sounds are a little blurry for her. It is as if she needs glasses for her ears, to make sounds clearer. Unfortunately, no such thing exists. A hearing aid would not help because it is not the volume of the sound that is the problem.

The problem is that the sounds in words are hard for her to distinguish. I'll explain what I mean. Words are made of different sounds blended together. We usually think of the word "cat" as one big blob of sound— /cat/. However, whenever we need to, we can break "cat" into three separate sounds— /c/ /a/ /t/. With a word like *cat*, this is easy to do, and even your daughter does not have much trouble with it. However, when she hears a long word or a word

with a lot of consonants bunched together, it is hard for her to break the word into individual sounds. For example, the word "strength" has only one syllable but it has six sounds—/s/ /t/ /r/ /e/ /η/ /θ/. With "cat" there are three letters, one for each sound. With "strength" it gets complicated because the *n* and the *g* form a single sound /η/ and the *t* and the *h* make the sound /θ/. If I pronounce both the *n* and the *g* separately–/stren/ /g/ /θ/–it sounds strange. With a word like "strength," your daughter can hear the first sound and the last sound but gets lost in the middle and starts leaving sounds out or guessing wrong sounds.

Now, if you say the word "strength" out loud, she can hear it and she understands it. She is not confused. She can even pronounce the word correctly Why? I'll make another comparison to vision. When you are driving and you see a road sign from far away, you might not be able to see every letter on the sign distinctly. However, you might be able to make out the shape of the word, and because you know what different signs are likely to say, you can tell someone what the word on the sign is. This is sort of like what you daughter can do. She hears the word and can say what it is based on the overall features of the word. However, she has difficulty hearing each of the sounds as distinct from each other.

If the only thing that were wrong was that she could not split words into different sounds, there would be no cause for concern. However, it turns out that this ability to hear the sounds in words as distinct rather than as big blobs of sound is really important to learning to read. If you can hear the different sounds in words, you can hear why the words are spelled as they are (if they are words with regular spelling). If you are reading and you come across a new word, you can sound it out like they do on *Sesame Street*.

Children who have difficulty hearing speech sounds distinctly often have trouble learning to spell and to read. Most children learn their letters and the sounds they make and then can figure out how to read and spell most words (at least the ones with regular spelling). Without the ability to sound out a word, learning to read and spell depends mostly on memorizing each word one by one. New words have to be taught explicitly to the child. Some children with this problem figure out how to work around it; some have help. When children with this problem fall behind in their ability to read, we call the problem *dyslexia*.

I want to be clear what dyslexia is and what it is not. You may have heard that dyslexia is when children see words backwards. This is not true. I have been doing this for a long time, and I have seen many children with dyslexia. Not one of those children saw anything backwards. However, many of them jumble their letters and, like younger children, sometimes they write their letters backwards. This is not due to *seeing* things backwards. Instead, these mistakes are due to ordinary memory errors. If you give me a long list of groceries to buy, I might remember most of the items on the list, but I might not remember them in the right order. When children with dyslexia learn a new word, they might remember which letters were in the word but might forget their order. They will probably remember the first and last letters but might mix up the middle letters. If they could sound out the words, they would be able to see that the order was wrong, but that does not happen as often as it otherwise would.

The reason that young children often write letters backward is that letters are very unusual. Most things have the same name no matter what angle we view them from [*I demonstrate with a pen, rotating it and turning it*]. This pen is called a *pen* no matter what I do with it. Letters are not like that. The letter *b* changes its name, depending on how it is rotated or flipped. It can be a *d*, a *p*, or even a *q*. A backwards *j* does not even have a name. This is weird for children, and it takes a while for them to get the hang of it. Children with dyslexia have a bit of a problem remembering which sounds go with which letters, and thus continue making these sorts of errors longer than do most children. The problem is blurry sounds, not backwards vision.

There are many narrow abilities within the auditory processing domain. They include abilities that are important for achievement in music (e.g., judging differences in volume, pitch, and rhythm). Other abilities have to do with tracking the temporal sequencing of sound, localizing sound, and deciphering sound under distorted conditions (e.g., understanding a conversation in a noisy room, recorded with a bad microphone). The most important predictor of academic achievement in this domain is *phonetic coding* (also known as *phonological processing* and *phonemic awareness*). Sometimes (e.g., Flanagan, Ortiz, Alfonso, & Mascolo, 2006) phonetic coding is divided into *analytic phonetic coding* (the ability to hear a word and distinguish among its phonemes) and *synthetic phonetic coding* (the ability to hear disconnected phonemes and assemble them into a pronounceable word). This distinction is primarily useful in selecting tests that have differing task demands. To my knowledge, there is no clinical utility in knowing which ability is higher.

Phonetic coding is clearly relevant to the acquisition of reading decoding skills. Its predictive validity is most evident in children who are just learning to read (Evans, Floyd, McGrew, & Leforgee, 2002). It is likely that there is something of a threshold effect at work. To learn to decode words, it is advantageous to have a certain level of phonological processing ability. However, there is probably little to be gained by reading decoding and reading comprehension once a person has passed that threshold. Imagine that, at age six, only the bottom 10% of children have phonetic decoding problems that are severe enough to hamper reading decoding skills. By age 10, almost all of those children have reached the threshold at which they have surpassed the bottom 10% of six-year-olds (Woodcock, McGrew, Schrank, & Mather, 2007). If children are still poor readers by age 10, it is probably for reasons other than their current phonological processing. This may be hard for clinicians to accept because they have been trained to view phonological processing problems as the primary cause of reading problems. Try this thought experiment: If a child has a WJ III Comprehension-Knowledge (*Gc*) score of 100 and a WJ III Phonemic Awareness score of 70, what is the likeliest score on Basic Reading Skills? What is the probability that the child's Basic Reading Skills score is poor (< 85), given that, among all children, about 16% have scores this low or lower? These questions can be answered approximately using the correlations from the WJ III NU manual (Woodcock, McGrew, Schrank, & Mather, 2007), and creating a multiple regression equations for different age groups.[26] Until I worked out the calculations myself, my estimates would have been wildly off from the answers presented in Table 13.4. I would never have guessed that only 24% of children aged six to eight with those predictor scores would have Basic Reading Skills scores less than 85, and that half of them would score over 94.

I was prompted to run these estimates when I tested a teenager with extremely low *Ga* but with average *Gc* and reading skills. I remember explaining to his mother, "It is as if he has a dyslexic's brain, but without the dyslexia." I wondered how common this was and ran some estimates. I was shocked. I wondered why I had not seen more children like this before. A moment's reflection revealed the answer: I probably had. If the initial interview

Table 13.5 Predicted WJ III Basic Reading Skills for Children with Various Combinations of WJ III Comprehension-Knowledge and WJ III Phonemic Awareness.

	Age Ranges		
	6 to 8	9 to 13	14 to 19
Intercept	34.42	32.21	24.03
Slope for PA	0.45	0.53	0.56
Slope for Gc	0.21	0.15	0.20

Predictor Scores	$\hat{Y}$	% < 85	$\hat{Y}$	% < 85	$\hat{Y}$	% < 85
Gc = 100, PA = 55	91	32	93	25	91	28
Gc = 100, PA = 70	94	24	95	19	94	20
Gc = 100, PA = 85	97	16	98	14	97	13
Gc = 100, PA = 100	100	11	100	10	100	8

Note: Gc = WJ III Comprehension-Knowledge; PA = WJ III Phonemic Awareness; $\hat{Y}$ = Predicted Score for WJ III Basic Reading Skills. Regression equations derived from correlations in Appendix E in the *Woodcock-Johnson III Normative Update Technical Manual*.

does not suggest that reading is a problem, I typically skip measuring Ga and therefore do not see this pattern as often as it occurs in the population. In addition, good readers with poor Ga are less likely to be evaluated in the first place.

The main point of Table 13.5 is that the adequate Gc/low Ga pattern associated with phonological dyslexia does not doom a person to having poor reading skills. Most people with reasonable Gc but low Ga actually do learn to read. However, the risk of reading decoding problems increases substantially if Ga is low.

Examples of tests that measure narrow abilities in the Ga domain can be found in Table 13.6.

Memory

If any one faculty of our nature may be called more wonderful than the rest, I do think it is memory. There seems something more speakingly incomprehensible in the powers, the failures, the inequalities of memory, than in any other of our intelligences. The memory is sometimes so retentive, so serviceable, so obedient: at

Table 13.6 Measures in the Ga Domain

Narrow Abilities	Measures
Phonetic Coding: Analysis	WJ III Incomplete Words WJ III Sound Awareness DAS-II Phonological Processing
Phonetic Coding: Synthesis	KTEA-II Phonological Awareness WJ III Sound Blending
Speech/ General Sound Discrimination	WJ III Auditory Attention WJ III Sound Patterns—Voice WJ III Sound Patterns—Music

others, so bewildered and so weak; and at others again, so tyrannic, so beyond control! We are, to be sure, a miracle every way—but our powers of recollecting and of forgetting do seem peculiarly past finding out.
—Jane Austen, Mansfield Park

It is clear that there are individual differences in abilities related to memory. It is also clear that there are many different kinds of memory. If you have had a recent course in cognitive psychology or have kept abreast of developments in the study of memory, you might be surprised at how little overlap cognitive psychology and CHC theory have in terms of theoretical constructs. There are several reasons for this. Cognitive psychologists are typically not interested in the individual differences of memory. They wish to understand how memory works in general. They are less interested in why some individuals have better memory than others, unless such differences shed light on how memory works in general. By analogy, engineers who design automobiles and mechanics who repair them have much knowledge in common. However, mechanics have a specialized knowledge of the parts of the car that tend to break down and how to replace them, whereas engineers may have an exquisite understanding of how those parts work (but may not be competent at diagnosing your car's problem). Psychologists who diagnose memory problems use tests that are sensitive to those problems. They are not typically designed to measure all of the complex processes that cognitive psychologists study. It is possible that memory assessment will become increasingly aligned with the field of cognitive psychology, but for now, the borrowings are meager and crude. This is not a criticism of our field. It is extremely difficult to measure many aspects of memory, and in many cases it is not yet clear if it would be worth the effort even if we could.

Of all the Stratum II abilities in CHC theory, the two memory abilities are the least settled. It is not clear how separate they should be considered to be, and it is not yet clear where some narrow factors belong. In Carroll's (1993) theory, the fundamental distinction was between learning and the fluency of recall. Short-term memory and long-term memory (learning) were grouped together in a factor called General Memory and Learning. Carroll also named a factor "Broad Retrieval Ability." In G*f*-G*c* Theory, the distinction is between short-term and long-term retrieval. What is meant by *long-term* is a period of hours or more (Horn & Blankson, 2005).

In CHC theory, the two broad memory factors have varied considerably from the source theories. The distinction between short- and long-term memory is maintained, but "long-term" seems to mean any amount of time in which the information is no longer expected to be maintained in one's immediate awareness (less than 15–30 seconds). This means that *associative memory*, *free recall memory*, and *meaningful memory* had to be relocated to the long-term factor, even though tests measuring such abilities require children to answer immediately after the stimuli are presented. The reasons for the differences in theory reflect, I believe, some of the inherent difficulties in distinguishing between memory processes that typically work as a functional whole. Information must have been retained over the short term in order for it to be retained over the long term. Thus, even if the short-term/long-term distinction is valid, short- and long-term memory processes are inherently intertwined on any memory test. There does seem to be an important distinction, too, between the amount of information one can retain and the fluency with which it can be retrieved. This is one manifestation of the speed/power distinction that is pervasive in intelligence research. Both Cattell (1987) and Carroll (1993) agreed that there is a sense in which speed is an important aspect of all of the broad abilities, but they were unclear about how speed should be integrated into the theory.

Short-Term Memory (G*sm*)
Memory Span

Memory span refers to the ability to hold information in mind just long enough to use it. For example, looking up a telephone number and holding it in mind until it has been dialed is an example of the use of memory span. Memory span can be compared to a computer's random-access memory (RAM) because it is a temporary holding space for information that can be accessed rapidly. Unlike RAM, however, information in short-term memory is very fragile. Unless you engage in deliberate mental rehearsal, the information is lost quickly. Typically, information in short-term memory decays spontaneously within 15 to 30 seconds. If your concentration is disrupted, the information in short-term memory is likely to be lost much sooner.

The size of a person's memory span is the number of elements that can be held in short-term memory. This is not really a fixed number. It varies considerably depending on a person's state of mind; fatigue, worry, intoxication, and many other disruptive influences shorten memory span considerably. Aspects of the stimuli in memory matter as well. People perform on tests with real words better than pseudo-words (e.g., gub, ril, stad); monosyllabic words better than polysyllabic words (longer articulation times impede performance); phonologically dissimilar lists (e.g., bed, puck, cup, fill) better than phonologically similar lists (e.g., bid, bet, but, bit, bed, bud); and semantically related words (e.g., bed, pillow, blanket) better than semantically unrelated words (e.g., bell, willow, ticket; Baddeley, 2006).

Memory span tests can be constructed so that they have very low *g*-loadings. In fact, Spearman believed that rote-memory tasks had little to do with intelligence (Carroll, 1993, p. 249). It is not uncommon for children with mental retardation to have memory spans approaching the average range (Conners, Carr, & Willis, 1998). Likewise, children with very high IQs often have memory spans that are much lower than the rest of their abilities (Wilkinson, 1993).

However, much can be done to increase the *g*-loadings of memory span tests. This is desirable if the goal is to measure *g*, but not if the goal is to measure memory span. To make a measure that is a purer measure of memory span, it is necessary to reduce the influence of previously learned information. There are two ways of doing this: to use stimuli that are equally familiar to all (simple words, numbers, or letters) or to use stimuli that are equally unfamiliar to all (pseudo-words or simple visual stimuli). Children with high G*c* or G*f* will have an advantage on memory span tasks if it occurs to them to group stimuli in easily remembered *chunks* (yes, this is the technical term for it!). This advantage can be minimized by ensuring that the test stimuli do not have obvious relationships. For example, it is much easier to remember "table chair kitten puppy" than "kitten table pink candy." However, subtle relationships may be found by some children. Using the last example, many children may visualize a kitten on a table with pink candy. Simply reordering the words can make such visualizations harder (e.g., "table kitten candy pink"). Even with digits, subtle effects can happen. I once lived in a city in which the telephone area code matched the first three digits in a difficult item on the WISC-III. For children who recognized this, the item was much easier than it was intended to be. Some children will enhance their performance via mental rehearsal. Minimizing the effects of Gc and Gf (or g, if you are a mono-g-ist) can be accomplished by instructing all children to employ the same mental rehearsal strategy. Another way to accomplish this is to prevent rehearsal altogether by having children say "the" repeatedly or to present the stimuli so quickly that rehearsal is not possible. With these considerations in mind, I believe that the purest commercially available measure of memory span is the CTOPP Memory for Digits subtest. It is like a traditional digit span test—except that two digits per second are presented (via audio recording) instead of one digit per second.[27] The CTOPP Non-Word Repetition subtest is also an interesting measure of memory span because it uses unfamiliar stimuli. The pseudo-words vary in syllable length and are spoken as if they were a single word, minimizing chunking. Unfortunately, it is unclear to what degree this subtest depends on auditory processing in addition to memory span. It is my impression that many children fail the difficult items not so much because of short-term memory problems, but because they did not encode the word properly in the first place because of difficult phoneme combinations. It would be interesting to compare the factor loadings of a test in which the pseudo-words were easily pronounceable (e.g., kanumisa) with a test in which they were difficult to encode and pronounce (e.g., statishraflirsks).

It is not yet clear how relevant memory span is to predicting academic outcomes. The evidence is mixed. It is possible that the predictive validity of memory span tests comes from the sources of contamination discussed in the previous paragraph. It is possible that the predictive validity of these tests comes from the overlap with working memory. It seems reasonable that memory span is important for comprehending complex forms of speech in which distant parts of sentences (or even paragraphs) have to be held in mind and then linked in order for the meaning to be clear. However, most evidence suggests that working-memory measures are much more highly correlated with reading and speech comprehension (Just, & Carpenter, 1992).

Working Memory

When reading the research and applied literature about working memory, it is helpful to remember that the term *working memory* is invoked to mean two closely related but distinct things: either a complex theoretical construct or performance on complex span tasks.

When the term *working memory* is used, it is typically meant to refer to the theoretical construct proposed by Baddeley and Hitch (1974). Over the decades, it has undergone considerable elaboration but has retained most of its essential features (Baddeley, 2006). The theoretical construct of working memory is broad and is meant to explain a wide variety of memory-related phenomena. It encompasses all of what is called *short-term memory* and is integrated with Norman and Shallice's (1986) concept of the Supervisory Attentional System.

Much of the time, our actions are automatic and require little thought. If I am walking toward my house, I am not usually thinking about the subtle ways in which my balance is maintained, the care my neighbor puts in into maintaining her yard, the feel of the breeze on my face, or a thousand other things that I am capable of noticing but do not. I typically continue walking, guided by habit (schemas and scripts), until I reach my door. However, if something unusual happens, such as being confronted by a barking dog, my attention quickly focuses so that my actions can be guided by the demands of the moment instead of by habit. The Supervisory Attentional System is the hypothetical set of mental structures that monitor goal attainment (i.e., it is "aware" of which parts of a problem have been solved and which have not in order to reach a goal) and focus attention when something unusual happens or when some non-habitual response is required. Specifically, Norman and Shallice (1986) list five kinds of situations in which the Supervisory Attentional System is active:

1. When planning or decision making
2. When troubleshooting
3. When enacting novel (or not yet mastered) sequences of actions
4. When enacting dangerous or technically difficult sequences of actions
5. When overcoming a strong habitual response or resisting temptation

Baddeley (1986) inserted Norman and Shallice's Supervisory Attentional System into his model of working memory, grafting it onto his concept of the "central executive." It has all of the features described above but also allows a person to manipulate and transform information in short-term memory. It links current sensory information with schemas stored in long-term memory and then uses the available information to take action.

How can one wonderful mechanism do so many wonderful things? Indeed, Baddeley's central executive has been criticized as a being a *homunculus*.[28] Baddeley's (2002, p. 246) response is instructive:

> I have to confess however, that I am rather fond of homunculi, sharing Attneave's (1960) view that they can be very useful, if handled with care. They are, in particular, helpful in allowing one to put on one side important but currently intractable problems, while concentrating on more manageable issues. It is of course important to recognise that they do not offer a solution to a problem, merely serving a holding function.

Baddeley used the concept of the *central executive* as a holding container for all that he did not yet understand so that he could concentrate on describing other aspects of working memory. He and others are now working to "fractionate" the central executive, to divide it up into understandable pieces. However, this work has only just begun. Therefore, when you, as a clinician, say something like, "Johnny is impulsive because his central executive does not function properly." you should know that not even the central executive's inventor thinks that you are explaining anything. This statement essentially boils down to a tautology: "Johnny is impulsive because he is unable to control his impulses." "Central executive dysfunction" works perfectly well as a descriptive term but not as an explanatory one. Lamentably, this criticism is easily applied to many other terms in cognitive ability research and in psychological theory in general.

One influential preliminary step in fractionating the central executive identified three distinct but still related executive functions: *inhibit, shift*, and *update* (Miyake, Friedman, Emerson, Witzki, Howerter, & Wager, 2000). "The inhibit function" refers to the central executive's role in "deciding" when to inhibit one's habitual behavior (termed the *prepotent response*) and produce a novel behavior instead. A classic measure of this function is the Stroop test, in which an examinee is asked to look at color words ("red") that are printed in non-matching colors (e.g., the color blue) and name the color of the ink instead reading the color word. It requires controlled attention to inhibit the urge to read the word and name the color of the ink instead.

"The shift function" refers to deliberately shifting the focus of one's attention back and forth to different tasks. Not intuitively obvious is that, for the shift to occur, a person must inhibit the urge to engage in the previous activity (failure to do so is called *perseveration*) and initiate a new activity (failure to do so is called *akinesia*, a common symptom of Parkinson's disease). It is not clear to what degree there is a difference between self-initiated shifts of attention (such as the shift of mental set required to perform well on the Wisconsin Card Sorting Test) and the task-driven back-and-forth shifting of mental set required by tasks such as the Trails B component of the Trail Making Test.

"The update function" refers to updating the contents of working memory. The central executive "decides" which information to hold onto and which can be let go. This is typically what is measured in complex span tasks.

In CHC theory, "working memory" refers simply to individual differences in performance on complex span tasks. What distinguishes memory span tasks from complex span tasks is that, instead of simply retaining information, the examinee must simultaneously store and process information in short-term memory. In the classic memory span paradigm, Digits Forward, no processing is required. The Digits Backward paradigm is a complex span task because the digits must be retained in memory while they are sorted in reverse order. Laboratory measures of working memory are usually modeled on the Daneman and Carpenter (1980) Reading Span measure in which the examinee reads a series of sentences aloud and must recall the final word of each sentence. Many variations on this paradigm have been used in research, including the Operation Span test (Conway et al., 2002), in which the examinee must remember a word or number after performing simple calculations. The only commercially available working memory test to use this paradigm is the SB5 Verbal Working Memory subtest in which the examinee must answer a series of questions correctly and then remember the final word in the questions. This is an ingenious improvement over the laboratory measures that required reading or math ability. It also requires the examinee to pay attention to the question instead of simply mentally rehearsing the words.

Working memory measures have a robust relationship with many aspects of academic achievement.[29] It is believed that working memory is important in reading comprehension for a variety of reasons, not all of them obvious (Cain, Oakhill, & Bryant, 2004). If a sentence is long, the full intent of the author may not be clear until the reader has reached the end of the sentence. Thus, the first part of the sentence has to be held in working memory and then linked to the last part of the sentence. In the quote below, consider the necessity of working memory in understanding Cicero's use of the *zeugma*, a literary form in which a series of phrases are linked by a common noun or verb. Cicero is trying to shame a would-be dictator into backing down, sparing the citizenry of Rome the horrors of civil war.

> Does not the nightly watch of the Palatine, does not the guard of the city, does not the fear of the people, does not the union of all good men, does not the holding of the Senate in this most defensible place, do not the looks and faces of these people move you?
> —Marcus Tullius Cicero, *In Catilinam I–IV*

Often an author leaves it to the reader to make appropriate inferences. Children with poor working memory are presumed to have fewer attentional resources to make such inferences. It is believed that working memory facilitates vocabulary acquisition via informal inferences about the meanings of words (Gathercole & Baddeley, 1993). If reading were a simple act of decoding words, even children with low working memory could eventually become skilled enough at decoding that there would be sufficient attentional resources left over. However, reading comprehension does not consist of simply decoding words successively. Instead, it is a complex process that involves constant prediction of what is coming next. As children read, they anticipate what is about to happen, and they update their predictions based on whether their expectations have been confirmed or not. Here is an example of a pair of sentences in which the first sentence causes a predictive inference that is confirmed in the second sentence:

> As Brad pulled out the blue math worksheet he had worked on so hard last night, he noticed that everyone else was turning in a yellow worksheet. He had done the wrong homework assignment by accident!

Calvo (2005) measured where readers' eyes moved as they read sentences like these. Three distinct cognitive abilities were associated with different patterns of eye movements. Readers with poor decoding skills, not surprisingly, had long-lasting eye gazes, meaning that they took a long time to figure out what the words were. Readers with poor working memories often finished the second sentence and had to go back and read the first sentence. It appears that readers with poor working memories

could not retain the entire representation of the sentence or phrase from which the prediction was generated, and thus they had to double-check to see if their confirmation was correct. Readers with poor vocabularies often had to go back and read the first sentence again even before moving on to the second sentence. It appears that they had trouble making succinct inferences in the first place. Thus, if Calvo is correct, both vocabulary and working memory are related to making predictive inferences while reading, but they are important at different stages of the inferential process. Vocabulary facilitates the ease and speed of making initial inferences, whereas working memory facilitates the "tying together" of new information with initial inferences. This predictive inference process is not just an idle pastime. It is a form of deep processing that facilitates recall. Children with poor working memory have difficulty decoding words and making predictive inferences at the same time. Their reading experiences tend to be effortful, inefficient, and choppy instead of automatic, flowing, and pleasant. Furthermore, being less able to make predictive inferences diminishes one of the great pleasures of reading: authors delight us by playing with our expectations using foreshadowing, humor, and irony.

Working memory also plays a role in comprehension-monitoring while reading (Cain, 2006; Pressley, 2002). We have all had the experience of "reading" (sounding out words in our heads) and then discovering that we have not been paying attention to what we have been reading for about a page or two. Part of comprehension-monitoring is to ask, "Am I still understanding this? Where was the last part where I stopped paying attention?" Readers with poor comprehension-monitoring fail to notice inconsistencies in the text (and therefore miss irony and humor). Reading while juggling all these concerns requires working memory. Without sufficient attentional resources, readers with poor working memory have a less engaging experience with rich narratives.

Although it is certain that there is a relationship between working memory and competence in mathematics, much less is known about the mechanisms underlying this relationship (Bull & Espy, 2006). In the various Wechsler IQ tests, mental arithmetic is used as a measure of working memory. In order to perform mental calculations, information must be held in memory and transformed. This fits the definition of a working memory test: simultaneous storage and processing.[30] However, the role of working memory in computation is more complex than this.

In a process analogous to that of comprehension monitoring in reading, working memory plays an important part in solving complex, multi-step math problems. Consider the example of using algebra to solve simultaneous linear equations such as:

$$2x + y = 12$$
$$4x - 2y = 0$$

Arriving at the solutions (x = 3, y = 6) requires many intermediate steps. It is easy to lose one's place in the middle of the sequence and for things to go awry. Without adequate working memory, it is hard to monitor where one is in the process, what is already known, and what still needs to be accomplished.

One final note about the domain of short-term/working memory. Baddeley and Hitch (1974) conceived of working memory as consisting of the central executive, which processed stimuli from all sensory modalities, and modality-specific "slave systems" that acted as temporary storage structures. For verbal/phonological information, the phonological/articulatory loop replays information in a continuous loop of high-fidelity imagined sound. For visual-spatial information, the visuospatial sketchpad holds information for the "mind's eye" to look at. Most of the linkages between individual differences in working memory capacity and academic outcomes are based on auditory measures. The role of nonverbal working memory in academic achievement is not yet clear. Therefore, it is my recommendation to administer and interpret auditory working memory tests and to de-emphasize nonverbal working memory unless the child has hearing problems or there is a highly specific referral question that requires the administration of nonverbal working memory.

Examples of tests that measure narrow abilities in the Gsm domain can be found in Table 13.7.

Long-Term Memory Storage and Retrieval (G*lr*)

As the name of this broad ability implies, there is an important distinction between measures of long-term storage and measures of long-term retrieval (fluency). However, they are grouped together because it impossible to measure one process without measuring the other, at least to some degree.

Meaningful Memory

Humans are particularly good at remembering large amounts of information if it is presented in

Table 13.7 Measures in the *Gsm* Domain

Narrow Abilities	Measures
Memory Span (Auditory)	DAS-II Recall of Digits—Forward KABC-II Number Recall WISC-IV Digits Forward WISC-IV Letter Span Non-rhyming WISC-IV Letter Span Rhyming WJ III Memory for Sentences WJ III Memory for Words TOMAL-2 Digits Forward TOMAL-2 Letters Forward WRAML-2 Number Letter WRAML-2 Sentence Memory
Memory Span (Visual-Spatial)	KABC-II Hand Movements WISC-IV Spatial Span Forward TOMAL-2 Manual Imitation WRAML-2 Finger Windows
Working Memory (Auditory)	DAS-II Recall of Digits—Backward DAS-II Recall of Sequential Order KABC-II Word Order* SB5 Verbal Working Memory* TOMAL-2 Digits Backward TOMAL-2 Letters Backward WISC-IV Digits Backward WISC-IV Letter-Number Sequencing WJ III Auditory Working Memory WJ III Numbers Reversed WJ III Understanding Directions WRAML-2 Verbal Working Memory
Working Memory (Visual-Spatial)	SB5 Nonverbal Working Memory* WISC-IV Spatial Span Backward WRAML-2 Symbolic Working Memory

*These tests measure memory span in the easy items and then shift to working memory.

a narrative form. After hearing a story just once, most people can retell the gist of it fairly accurately. Unfortunately, few commercially available measures are designed to measure long-term memory of the gist of a story (the KAIT Auditory Comprehension Delayed is an important exception). Instead, examiners tell a story to the child and ask the child to tell the story back, word for word. The stories are often filled with details that are not relevant to the gist of the story (e.g., "On Monday, October 14th, a man named Frank Forbes walked six blocks down Market Street and then turned on Washington Avenue. There he saw an old man in a blue blazer selling balloons, books, and games. Before buying a balloon for his son Carl, Frank asked the cashier...")." Such details make these tests more like memory span tests and less like gist memory tests. It is perhaps for this reason (and the fact that the child retells the story immediately) that both Carroll and Horn and Cattell grouped meaningful memory with short-term memory. However, immediate recall and delayed recall of stories are so closely related (Tulsky, Ivnik, Price, & Wilkens, 2003) that it is hard to conceive of them as being on separate broad factors.

It is important to note that Meaningful Memory tests often have strong secondary (if not primary) loadings on Gc (listening ability). In a sense, Gc is the historical record of the child's use of meaningful memory. However, the influence is not unidirectional. Children who have more background knowledge can chunk more information together while listening to a story because they have a richer, more nuanced, more integrated, and broader framework on which to hang new information (Hirsch, 2006). Thus, knowing more leads to remembering more.

The relevance of meaningful memory for academic achievement is obvious. Remembering stories is vital for the accumulation of knowledge about most academic fields, even in disciplines such as chemistry or physics. It is much easier to remember important scientific theories when they are embedded in narratives of scientists working to explain puzzling or controversial phenomena.

Associative Memory

Some information is not embedded in a narrative. It must be memorized by brute force (e.g., math facts are typically learned in this manner). *Associative memory* is the ability to remember the links between facts or pieces of information that have been paired (e.g., Einstein–Relativity, "th" – /θ/, mammals–milk).

There are two primary methods of measuring this ability. In the paired-associates paradigm, pairs of unrelated words (e.g., Book–Door, Candle–Fence) are presented in the learning phase of the task. Then the examiner names one of the words of each pair, and the child must identify the other member of the pair. If there is just one opportunity to learn the pairs, this task is actually a short-term memory task. However, most commercially available variants of this task have multiple learning phases in which the word pairs are presented again and recall is tested each time to measure how quickly the child can remember all the word pairs correctly. After a delay of at least 20 minutes, recall is tested again in a delayed condition.

In the structured learning paradigm, the effects of individual differences in short-term memory are minimized because each new item is presented individually and then tested. The procedure begins with teaching a single association (between two words, between two symbols or pictures, or between a word or name and a symbol or picture). For example, in the WJ - III Memory for Names subtest, the child is shown a picture of a space alien and is told its name. The child then points to the picture and says the name. The child is shown a new alien and is taught the name. The examiner shows both aliens and asks the child to name them both. This process is repeated many times. Each time a new alien's name is taught, memory for the name of that alien is tested first, and then the child is asked to name each of the other aliens. Each time the child makes an error, the examiner gives the correct name. In this way, an early memory failure does not result in a total loss of points for all subsequent test phases. It is clear that the structured learning paradigm is a purer way of measuring long-term memory processes because it minimizes the role of short-term memory. However, the paired-associates paradigm allows for the observation of a child's learning strategy that would not be apparent in the structured learning paradigm.

Delayed conditions of associative memory tests do not typically reveal additional information that was not already apparent in the immediate-recall conditions (Tulsky, Ivnik, Price, & Wilkens, 2003). An important exception to this generalization is in the assessment of dementia (not a concern for most children, thankfully), in which the delayed scores are much lower than the immediate scores (Delis, Jacobson, Bondi, Hamilton, & Salmon, 2003). It is unclear if there are other special populations in which this pattern is common.

Associative memory is known to be an important predictor of both math and reading achievement, particularly in the first few years of school, when basic reading decoding skills and math facts and calculation skills are being acquired (Evans, Floyd, McGrew, & Leforgee, 2002; Floyd, Evans, & McGrew, 2003). That is, skilled readers shift from phonologically decoding each word to recognizing familiar words automatically. To be skilled in math, something similar must occur with math facts. To be good at algebra, you have to stop counting on your fingers and develop effortless recall of all the basic math facts (Fleischner, Garnett, & Shepherd, 1982). Effortless recall of math facts frees working memory resources for complex problem-solving.

Free Recall Memory

This factor, like several other narrow abilities in CHC theory, has a name that describes the kind of tests that measure the factor rather than a name that describes a psychological process. The fact that a theorist as knowledgeable as Carroll could not think of a theoretical construct to link this factor to makes me suspicious that what emerged in the factor analysis was a method factor rather than a distinct psychological ability. With apologies to E. G. Boring, free recall memory is what free recall memory tests test.[31]

Free recall memory tests typically begin with a presentation of a list of words, pictures, or other stimuli. This list's length is designed to exceed the child's memory span (hence the term *supraspan* tests). The child immediately attempts to recall as many items as possible. The number recalled is an estimate of memory span. However, the list is presented again and the child has another chance to recall the entire list. This process is repeated several times (typically four times in all). After a long delay, the child is asked to recall the list one more time.

It is probably safe to say that performance on free recall memory tests predicts performance on exams in which lists need to be memorized (What are the five pillars of Islam? Name all 50 states.). However, I am aware of no such study that has demonstrated this effect nor of any other specific effect of Free Recall Memory on academic achievement.

Retrieval Fluency

There are about nine or so different kinds of retrieval fluency in CHC theory. I will not describe them all because few of them are measured by major test batteries. Fluency measures have been used extensively by creativity researchers because the ability they measure is thought to be a precursor to the creative production of ideas.

Ideational fluency is the ability to produce many examples related to a specific topic. The classic ideational fluency test is to name as many animals (or foods, furniture, names, sports, and so forth) as possible in a specified time limit. Cattell originally placed this ability in the G*c* broad factor. He was not wrong about this. He used very generous time limits on his tests so that the speed of retrieval was unimportant and instead the breadth of the examinee's knowledge was tested. In contrast, most variations of ideational fluency tests given in commercially available tests have very short time limits and thus measure the fluency of responding. Ideational fluency tests measure what Guilford (1967) would call

divergent production ability (as opposed to *convergent production ability*) because there is not a single correct answer, but a large pool of correct answers that can be offered. Ideational fluency tests are sensitive to brain injuries and have long been used by neuropsychologists to measure word-finding problems (dysnomia). I am unaware of any specific relationships ideational fluency has with academic achievement.

Word fluency is very similar to ideational fluency, except that the examinee is told to generate as many words as possible that have a common orthographic or phonological characteristic, such as words that begin with a "t" or end with "tion." Word fluency tests are also used to assess for dysnomia, a common effect of brain injuries.

Naming facility is also known as *rapid automatic naming*. It is the ability to recall the name of an object or symbol as quickly and fluently as possible. Tests of naming facility consist of an array of objects or symbols that are well known to the examinee. The object of the test is to name the elements in the array as quickly as possible. This ability is quite different from ideational fluency and typically has low correlations with it (Woodcock, McGrew, Schrank, & Mather, N., 2007). Naming facility tests are what Guilford (1967) would call *convergent production tests* because the examinee "converges" on a single answer, which is judged to be correct or not. Naming facility is known to be an important independent predictor of reading decoding, fluency, and comprehension. In a sense, reading is the act of naming words fluently. However, there is some controversy about whether the effect of rapid automatic naming on reading only occurs in rapid digit-naming and rapid letter-naming tasks, or if it is a more general effect of the ability to name any object fluently (Bowey, McGuigan, & Ruschena, 2005).

A comprehensive investigation of memory-related abilities requires specialized knowledge that is beyond the scope of this chapter. There is not a single ability called "memory" but rather a loose affiliation of memory abilities. It requires a bit of detective work to deduce the source of memory problems. The correlations of most narrow abilities within G*lr* are so low that it is not reasonable to expect scores from different domains to converge to a single number in most examinees. If there are concerns about long-term memory processes, it is probably best to use a comprehensive memory battery such as the Children's Memory Scale, the Test of Memory and Learning,

Second Edition (TOMAL-2), or the Wide Range Assessment of Memory and Learning, Second Edition (WRAML-II) and then conduct follow-up testing with more specialized measures as needed. If there are no specific concerns about long-term memory, a story memory subtest (e.g., WJ III Story Recall), a structured learning subtest (e.g., KABC-II Rebus Learning) and a rapid naming subtest (e.g., DAS-II Rapid Naming) can act as a good screener for common memory problems.

I addressed long-term visual memory somewhat in the Gv section. This area is not well defined in CHC theory (nor really anywhere else). It is not clear what the utility of measures of visual memory is either. Tests that measure recognition of faces, however, measure a highly specialized and distinct cognitive function that may have special utility in understanding social cognition deficits common in autistic spectrum disorders (Klin, Sparrow, de Bildt, Cicchetti, Cohen, & Volkmar, 1999).

Examples of tests that measure narrow abilities in the Glr domain can be found in Table 13.8.

Table 13.8 Measures in the *Glr* Domain

Narrow Abilities	Measures
Meaningful Memory	CMS Family Pictures
	CMS Stories
	RIAS Verbal Memory
	TOMAL-2 Memory for Stories
	WJ III Story Recall
	WRAML-2 Story Memory
Associative Learning	CMS Word Pairs
	KABC-II Atlantis
	KABC-II Rebus
	KAIT Rebus Learning
	TOMAL-2 Paired Recall
	WJ III Memory for Names
	WJ III Visual-Auditory Learning
	WRAML-2 Sound-Symbol Learning
Free Recall	CMS Word Lists
	TOMAL-2 Object Recall
	TOMAL-2 Word Selective Reminding
	WRAML-2 Verbal Learning
Naming Facility	DAS-II Rapid Naming
	KTEA-II Naming Facility
	WJ III Rapid Picture Naming
Ideational Fluency	KTEA-II Associational Fluency
	WJ III Retrieval Fluency

Processing Speed (G*s*)

It is important to note that *processing speed* is probably too broad a term for what this factor entails. It is not the speed at which all mental processing occurs. Indeed, CHC Theory has three broad factors related to different kinds of mental processing speed and several narrow factors in other domains that have to do with speed as well (Schneider & McGrew, 2012). G*s* is narrower; it is the speed and fluency at which very simple repetitive tasks (typically involving visual perception) can be performed. In Mirsky's (1987) taxonomy of attention-related abilities, the *focus-execute* aspect of attention is primarily measured by tests that load on the G*s* factor. Were I to rename the G*s* factor, I might call it something like "Attentional Fluency," because tests that measure this factor require sustained concentration and fluent control of attentional focus as each stimulus is engaged and disengaged successively.

The *perceptual speed* narrow factor measures the speed at which a child can compare and distinguish between simple visual stimuli. The *rate of test taking* narrow factor is the speed at which a child can perform very simple tasks such as sorting objects. There may be other narrow abilities in this domain, such as *visual scanning, number facility, speed of reasoning,* and *pattern recognition* (McGrew, 2005). Although it is clear that G*s* is an important domain of cognitive ability, there is no research of which I am aware that demonstrates that it is important to distinguish between the various subfactors of G*s*.[32]

Processing speed is a good predictor of performance once the skill has become overlearned and automatized. It not only has considerable predictive utility in predicting academic outcomes but also performance in many job categories, particularly jobs that require repetitive work (e.g., sewing; Ackerman & Cianciolo, 2000). Unlike the effect of G*a* on reading abilities, the effect of G*s* seems to increase with age (Benson, 2008), presumably because reading decoding has become relatively automatic. G*s* also showed substantial relationships with math calculation and math reasoning (Floyd, Evans, McGrew, 2003), probably for the same reasons as with reading comprehension.

Examples of tests that measure narrow abilities in the G*s* domain can be found in Table 13.9.

Abilities Not Well Accounted For by CHC Theory

Attention and executive functions are not addressed very thoroughly in CHC Theory, possibly

Table 13.9 Measures in the G$_s$ Domain

Narrow Abilities	Measures
Perceptual Speed	WISC-IV Cancellation
	WISC-IV Symbol Search
	WJ III Cross Out
	WJ III Pair Cancellation
	WJ III Visual Matching
Rate-of-Test Taking	DAS-II Speed of Information Processing
	WISC-IV Coding
Speed of Reasoning	WJ III Decision Speed

because our measures in these domains are relatively crude and no dominant theory has emerged from which we could construct a well-founded taxonomy of attention and executive functions. There are many attention and executive function tests available (e.g., Conners's Continuous Performance Test II, Delis-Kaplan Executive Function System, NEPSY-2, and many others). These tests and test batteries contain measures that are clear markers of working memory and naming facility. However, many aspects of these tests are simply not well understood and thus have not yet been incorporated into major theories of intelligence.

There are many alternative theories to CHC theory that contain intriguing ideas. In Planning-Attention-Simultaneous-Successive Theory (PASS; Naglieri & Das, 1988), there is a distinction between tests that require simultaneous processing and tests that require successive processing. The terms *simultaneous* and *successive processing* were not first used by Luria (e.g., Bitterman, Tyler, & Elam, 1955). However, Luria's (1966) conceptualization of these terms has directly influenced at least two major cognitive assessment batteries (CAS and KABC-II). When cognitive psychologists use these terms, they typically are trying to figure out which types of perception rely on serial processing (each process completed one at a time, successively) and which rely on parallel processing (coordinated processes that operate simultaneously). It is known that the time it takes to find certain primitive features in a visual field does not increase so much as the number of distracters increases (Treisman & Gelade, 1980). For example, people can find a red X on a computer screen in about the same time whether there are 10 distracters (blue X's) or 20. This means that people do not typically have to scan each part of the screen

in successive fashion; the red X is brought to one's attention immediately because of simultaneous processes. However, when people have to find a red Y in a field of red X's and blue Y's, the search time increases with the number of distracters. This means that successive search processes had to occur.

Tests such as the CAS are intended to measure individual differences in successive and simultaneous processing. Thus the focus is not on *whether* simultaneous or successive processes are engaged to solve the task but on *how well* or *how fast* to those processes operate. That said, Das, Naglieri, and Kirby (1994, pp. 64–65) are careful to point out that there are not two abilities called "simultaneous processing" and "successive processing." Rather, these terms refer to two different categories of processing. The simultaneous processing used to complete a certain verbal task may be quite distinct from the simultaneous processing used to complete a spatial reasoning task. Thus, the theory does not predict that simultaneous and successive processing will necessarily emerge in a factor analysis. This subtlety is probably hard to keep in mind given that the CAS, which operationalizes the four basic cognitive processes in PASS theory, provides a composite score called *Successive* and another composite score called *Simultaneous*. With a single number, it is easy to think of these concepts as unitary abilities, even though the theory says that they are not.

If clinicians wish to interpret CAS subtests in terms of CHC theory, there is ample justification for doing so. Indeed, the CAS appears to have a factor structure that fits in with CHC theory better than a direct mapping of CAS subtests to PASS constructs (Keith, Kranzler, & Flanagan, 2001; Kranzler, & Keith, 1999). However, this does not mean that the CAS measures CHC constructs and CHC constructs only. The CAS subtests may measure aspects of cognitive functions that are not included in CHC theory, given that the CAS appears to out-predict some of the traditional cognitive batteries (Naglieri, 1999; Naglieri, De Lauder, Goldstein, & Schwebach, 2006). That said, it is likely that CAS subtests, ingeniously crafted as they are, probably are mixed measures of CHC abilities and PASS constructs, and it is a live hypothesis as to whether the CAS measures these extra-CHC sources of variance with sufficient reliability to be useful to the clinician. Thus far, Das, Naglieri, and colleagues have amassed an impressive and diverse body of validity data for their model, and for the CAS in particular (Das, Naglieri & Kirby, 1994; Naglieri & Das, 2005). It is likely that future validation efforts will result in a synthesis of the distinctive aspects of PASS and CHC theory. The dual PASS/CHC interpretive framework of the KABC-II (Kaufman & Kaufman, 2004) is a step in this direction, but the links are, for now, more assumed than proven.

Several theories present a very broad view of cognitive abilities, so broad that the traditional boundaries between cognitive abilities, personality, interests, and motivation are blurred. Ackerman's (1996) Intelligence as Process, Personality, Interests, Intelligence as Knowledge (PPIK) theory integrates intelligence as process (akin to Cattell's original g_f factor), Big 5 Personality factors, Holland's Interests, and intelligence as knowledge (akin to Cattell's original g_c factor with emphasis on specialized knowledge that is difficult to test). Sternberg's (2005) Triarchic Theory of Successful Intelligence is broader still. His theory is so complex that it is unlikely that there will ever be a comprehensive battery that operationalizes all of the components of the theory. However, one of the intriguing aspects of Sternberg's work is his emphasis on *implicit knowledge*, the informal skills and unstated rules for success in highly specific domains of achievement. It might be very helpful in increasing our ability to assess aptitude if measures of implicit knowledge were commercially available.

Custom Composite Scores

Closely tied to CHC Theory, the Cross-Battery Assessment approach (Flanagan & McGrew, 1997; Flanagan, Ortiz, & Alfonso, 2007) uses the taxonomy from CHC theory to classify subtests from diverse cognitive test batteries under the same interpretive framework, allowing clinicians to integrate diverse sources of information in a consistent manner. Flanagan and colleagues offer a comprehensive set of guidelines for selecting subtest across batteries. I will focus on just a few of them.

If you are designing an initial battery of tests to give to a particular individual, it is generally best to select subtests that are maximally different in terms of test format while still measuring the same broad ability. For the most part, it is best to estimate abilities at the broad ability level rather than the narrow ability level. (Glr is probably an exception to this rule. There is little point in getting an average long-term memory score when the narrow abilities are so loosely related.) It is helpful to be mindful of subtests' narrow ability classifications so that broad ability composites can be constructed with minimal overlap.

If a child's test results are unexpected (too high, too low, or too inconsistent), follow-up tests should be given to confirm that the results are real instead of random errors or fluctuations of ability. When a person's profile of scores is strange, the results are not typically replicated with follow-up testing. What is not stable in testing situations is unlikely to generalize to anything else in the child's life. It is therefore usually best not to interpret findings that are not replicated. However, if scores within a broad domain are consistently different from each other, it is acceptable to interpret the scores at the narrow ability level. Even so, given the state of our knowledge of the incremental validity of narrow abilities, it is important to be modest in interpreting narrow ability differences within Stratum II broad ability clusters.

Good Composites Are Theoretically Plausible

It is important to group subtests by theory, not by intuition. As brilliant as Kaufman's (1994) Intelligent Testing system was, there is little evidence that any of the hundreds of subtle influences on test performance he lists has ever been measured with any reliability. Fly low to the ground and stick with a well-validated interpretive framework such as CHC theory (or simply IQ if you are a mono-g-ist).

Good Composites Are Either Unidimensional or Well Balanced

If you wish to measure a single narrow ability, you can create composite scores that are reasonably unidimensional. However, it is important not to select measures that use the same format (e.g., multiple versions of the digits forward paradigm) or the scores will be overly influenced by format-specific factors that have little predictive validity.

A measure of a multidimensional construct such as g or any of the broad abilities should be measured with a well balanced selection of subtests. That is, you should not measure Gc with three vocabulary tests and a General Information test. It would be better to have two of each type, or, better still, four measures of four different Gc narrow abilities.

Good Composites Produce Reliable Scores

With Gc subtests, a very reliable composite score usually can be created with just two or three subtests. With less reliable or less correlated scores (e.g., some measures of Gv), four or five subtests are necessary to measure abilities accurately. The less reliable the composite score, the more modest the interpretation must be. There are a number of guidelines about acceptable levels of reliability. It is sometimes said that one should base high-stakes decisions only on scores with reliability coefficients of 0.98 or better, base substantive interpretations on scores with reliability coefficients of 0.90 or better, and base decisions to give more tests or not on scores with reliability coefficients of 0.80 or more. This is not bad advice, but I believe that reliability coefficients are not intuitively informative. When I say that the reliability coefficient for a particular population is 0.77, I find it hard to grasp exactly how unstable the score is. Instead, I recommend paying close attention to confidence intervals around the test scores and you will save yourself (and the children you assess) from over-interpreting test results. The more reliable the score is, the narrower the confidence interval will be. The 95% confidence interval of a score with a 0.80 reliability coefficient is about 26 index score points wide! That is, the true score for a particular individual might be, for example, anywhere between 64 and 90! The 95% confidence interval with a score with a 0.98 reliability coefficient is still about 8 index score points wide.

An additional point to remember is that reliability is not constant for all individuals. People with unusual test-taking behavior or extreme scores may require more subtests to measure their abilities accurately. For most tests, only one confidence interval width is provided for each age range. However, in truth, confidence interval widths are typically (though not necessarily) larger for children who score very high or very low on the test. The WJ III is one of the few individually administered cognitive ability tests to calculate different confidence intervals for different levels of performance.

Reliable Measurement Is Not Necessarily Construct-Relevant Measurement

It is possible for subtests with reasonably high internal consistency estimates (e.g., Cronbach's α > 0.80) to be added together to form a composite score with an even higher internal consistency coefficient. However, it is quite possible that much of the reliability of the composite comes from reliable but construct-irrelevant variance (i.e., variance not related to the ability we intend to measure).

Imagine that there are two subtests, A and B, that are influenced by the factors depicted in Figure 13.4. Both are intended to be measures of the same construct and their results are added to

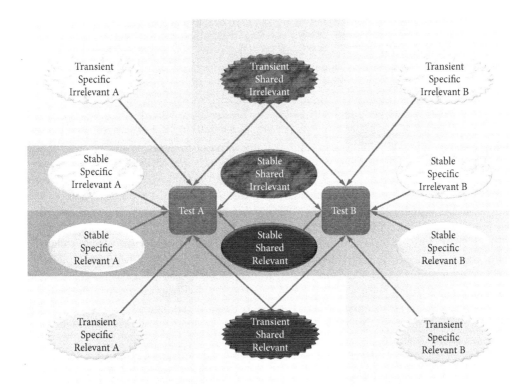

Figure 13.4 Types of Influence on Tests A and B: Relevant vs. Irrelevant, Shared vs. Specific, and Stable vs. Transient.

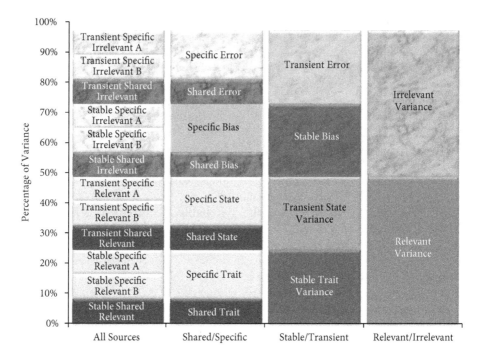

Figure 13.5 Types of Influence on the Composite Score Formed from Tests A and B.

form a composite score. As shown in Figure 13.5, the sources of variance in the composite score can be shared or specific, be relevant to the construct or irrelevant, and be stable or transient. Many discussions of validity consider only the possibility of stable, shared, construct-relevant variance, but it is possible to have specific construct-relevant sources of variance if the construct is multidimensional and different tests are designed to differentially operationalize different aspects of the construct. For example, the construct of simple arithmetic could be measured by forming a composite score consisting of four tests, one for each arithmetic operation (addition, subtraction, multiplication, and division). Undoubtedly, the four tests would be correlated because of shared construct-relevant variance. However, each test would contain reliable specific variance that is no less relevant to the construct of arithmetic than the shared variance.

In cognitive measures, we typically only consider stable sources of construct-relevant variance, but it is possible for construct-relevant variance to be transient for some constructs. For example, when I am fatigued, my working memory capacity is lessened, and a good measure of working memory capacity will reflect this if I take a test in such a state. A good clinician would, of course, be alert to my fatigue and would readminister the measure on a different day. In Figure 13.4, the distinction between stable

and transient is dichotomous. In reality, everything is in a state of flux, but some things are more stable than others.

Not all shared variance is relevant to the construct the measures are intended to measure. Shared construct-irrelevant variance can result from any influence on both scores that has nothing to do with the construct of interest, such as method variance. Method variance arises from tests that are highly similar in their testing format and item content in ways that are unrelated to the construct. For example, in two speeded tests of General Information, the effect of the speed requirement on both tests is method variance. Method variance and other stable construct-irrelevant influences bias test scores in a particular direction, depending on how the test influence affects the particular evaluee. Transient shared construct-irrelevant influences are usually called "shared measurement error." When a child takes subtests A and B from the same examiner, any effects the examiner might have (e.g., sloppy administration or unusually poor rapport) are shared by both tests.

Some stable construct-irrelevant variance is specific to one test. For example, the WAIS-IV Working Memory Index consists of the Digit Span and Arithmetic subtests. Both subtests require familiarity with numbers (a potential shared construct-irrelevant influence) but only for Arithmetic does achievement in mathematics give a substantial benefit. This specific and stable factor is not relevant to the construct of working memory.

It should be pointed out that construct-irrelevant variance (both specific and shared) can have predictive validity. For example, if children with higher Gf use better strategies on certain subtests intended to measure Gv, some of the composite's predictive validity will come from the Gf contamination. If the Gf component of the "Gv composite" is unrecognized, the added predictive validity of the composite will be misattributed to Gv. The WAIS-IV Working Memory Index may be used to explain math performance, but some of its predictive validity may be due to the specific construct-irrelevant influence from the Arithmetic subtest.[33]

The ratio of stable (reliable) variance to total variance is measured by a reliability coefficient. There are many different measures of reliability, and unfortunately, none is perfect for all situations. It is important to remember that reliability coefficients are not measures of validity. It is frequently claimed that the validity of a test is no higher than its reliability. This is only true if all valid variance is stable. The idea that reliability is an upper limit to validity is further complicated by the fact that there are many different ways of measuring reliability and that they sometimes give substantially different estimates of reliability. Which reliability coefficient is the upper limit to validity? It is not always easy to tell.

The correlation between the same test given at different times is the test-retest reliability coefficient. The test-retest reliability coefficient can be misleading high or low if there are shared construct-irrelevant sources of variances such as practice effects, memory effects, and fatigue effects or if there are transient construct-relevant sources of variance (e.g., developmental effects). The correlation between alternate forms of the same test is called the *alternate-form reliability coefficient*. The correlation can also be misleadingly high or low, depending on how successfully the test developers made the tests to be truly parallel. Internal consistency measures of reliability measure how correlated the test items are and estimate the ratio of shared variance to total variance in the total score of all the items. These types of measures are popular (especially Cronbach's α) because they require no additional data collection. Internal consistency measures are lowered when there is specific construct-relevant variance and raised by shared construct irrelevant variance.

This discussion of test reliability is further complicated by the likely possibility that tests are not equally reliable for all populations. Typically, test publishers present a variety of reliability estimates and present the case that the test scores are sufficiently reliable in most circumstances and populations.

The ratio of shared variance to total variance can be measured using a statistic called "McDonald's (1999) ω." What we would really like is a "validity coefficient," the ratio of construct-relevant variance to total variance. However, this is not easily obtained, so we must satisfy ourselves with a statistic like McDonald's ω, which can be estimated using subtest loadings from factor analysis. McDonald's ω can range between the internal consistency coefficient and the validity coefficient. Thus, it puts an upper limit to validity. That is, it gives an estimate of the construct-relevant variance to total variance ratio in the best-case scenario in which there is no construct-irrelevant shared variance.

Even Good Composites Do Not Always Function as Intended

The previously mentioned fact that a Gf test taken a second time is a suboptimal measure of Gf is a special case of a much broader principle: not every test measures what it is intended to measure for every individual. For example, I rock at the Tower of Hanoi. You could give me a stack of as many discs as you like, and I can move the whole stack from one peg to the other without any hesitation and without a single error. I don't mean to be immodest about it, but it's true. My performance is like 11.8 standard deviations above the mean, which by my calculations is so rare that if a million people were born every second ever since the Big Bang, there is still only a 2.7% chance that I would have been born by now. I feel very lucky (and honored) to be here. You would be forgiven for thinking that I had excellent planning ability but not if you voiced such an opinion out loud, within earshot of my wife, causing her to die of laughter—I would miss her very much. No, it is not by preternatural planning ability that I compete with only the gods in Tower of Hanoi tournaments-in-the-sky. In fact, the first time I tried it, my score was not particularly good. I am not going say what it was, but the manual said that I ranked somewhere between the average Darwin Award winner and the person who invented English spelling rules. After giving the test some thought, however, I realized that each movement of the discs is mechanically determined by a simple rule. I will not say what the rule is for fear of compromising the validity of the test for more people. The rule is not so simple that you would figure it out while taking the test for the first time, but it is simple enough that once you learn it, you will be surprised how easy the test becomes.

All kidding aside, it is important for the clinician to be mindful of the process by which a child performs well or poorly on a test. For me, the Tower of Hanoi does not measure planning. For others, it might. Edith Kaplan (1988) was extremely creative in her methods of investigating how people performed on cognitive tests. Kaplan-inspired tools such as the WISC-IV Integrated provide more formal methods of assessing strategy use. However, careful observations and even simply asking children how they approached a task (after the tests have been administered according to standard procedures) is often enlightening and can save time during the follow-up testing phase. For example, I once read about an otherwise low-performing boy who scored very well on the WISC-IV Block Design subtest. When asked how he did so well on it, he said that he had the test at home and that he practiced it often. The clinician doubted this very much, but his story turned out to be true! His mother was an employee at a university and saw someone from the Psychology Department throwing outdated WISC-III test kits into the garbage. She was intrigued and took one home for her children to play with.

I once gave the WAIS-III to a woman who responded to the WAIS-III Vocabulary subtest as if it were a free-association test. I tried to use standard procedures to encourage her to give definitions to words, but the standard prompts ("Tell me more") just made it worse. Finally, I broke with protocol and said, "These are fabulous answers and I like your creativity. However, I think I did not explain myself very well. If you were to look up this word in the dictionary, what might it say about what the word means?" In the report I noted the break with protocol, but I believe that the score she earned was much more reflective of her lexical knowledge than would have been the case had I followed procedures more strictly. I do not wish to be misunderstood, however; I never deviate from standard procedures except when I must. Even then, I conduct additional follow-up testing to make sure that the scores are correct.

Discrepant Subtest Scores Do Not (Necessarily) Invalidate the Composite

A widely held view among clinicians is that if two or more subtests in a composite score differ widely, the composite score is not valid (Fiorello, Hale, McGrath, Ryan, & Quinn, 2002). This seems reasonable at first, but there are many problems with this belief. First, imperfectly correlated scores can differ because of error and specific variance, sometimes

by several standard deviations. Because these deviations just as likely to be positive as they are negative, the best estimate of the true score is actually the composite score. Second, the composite's predictive validity does not change whether its component subtest scores are consistent or discrepant (Watkins, Glutting, & Lei, 2007). Third, if you follow this recommendation to its logical conclusion, you should not interpret subtest scores if there is significant variability in the item scores. This recommendation ignores the whole reason that we aggregate scores in the first place: to distill true score variance from error variance. The point is that within-composite variability does not, by itself, invalidate the composite. Random error is to be expected. Of course, if you have reason to believe that one or more scores is incorrect, then by all means conduct more tests to estimate the ability with more precision. You may be surprised, however, how often the original composite score was not that far off the mark.

Calculating Custom Composite Scores

A quick-and-dirty way to calculate a custom composite score is simply to convert all the scores to index scores and then average them. This will be reasonably accurate for most purposes, including for on-the-spot profile interpretations. However, the procedure for combining IQ scores described earlier can be applied to any composite score to ensure maximum accuracy. The true composite score will always be more extreme than the average score. That is, if the average is below 100, the true composite score will be lower than the average of the subtest scores. If the average is above 100, the true composite will always be higher than the average of the subtest scores. The difference between the average and the true composite score is usually small, within a few index score points. However, the difference grows larger at the extremes and is larger for composite scores made from subtests with low inter-correlations. A more complete discussion of these issues can be found in a freely available position paper (Schneider & McGrew, 2011).

Predicted Achievement Using Multiple Regression[34]

If you believe that there are multiple cognitive abilities that influence academic achievement, you need some way of determining how unusual a child's achievement is, given the child's cognitive abilities. You can use *multiple regression* for this purpose if you know the correlations among all the predictors and the correlations between the achievement score and each of the predictors. Multiple regression, as described here, assumes that all relationships among the predictors and the criterion are linear. Modeling non-linear relationships with multiple regression is possible, but it is unlikely that test manuals will give enough information to construct such models.

You might think that you need raw data from the standardization sample to make regression models. This is not so. Knowing the variables' means, standard deviations, and correlation matrix is all that is required. This information is typically included in test manuals.

Calculating regression coefficients is much simplified if all test scores are converted to index scores:

$$\text{Index Score} = 15 * (\text{Original Score} - \text{Original Mean}) / \text{Original SD} + 100$$

For example, a scaled score (Mean = 10, SD = 3) of 14 is converted to an index score of 120, like so:

$$120 = 15 * (14 - 10) / 3 + 100$$

The advantage of making all scores on the same metric is that the unstandardized regression coefficients equal the standardized coefficients, which are easier to calculate and to interpret. Standardized coefficients have this formula:

$$\beta = R_p^{-1} r_c$$

Where

β is the column vector of standardized regression coefficients

R_p is the correlation matrix of the predictors

r_c is the column vector of the correlations between the criterion variable and each of the predictors

With a program such as Microsoft Excel, it is easy to calculate regression coefficients with just a correlation matrix. Suppose that we believe that performance on Applied Math ("word problems") is primarily determined by Gc, Gf, and working memory (WM).[35] This is certainly too simple to be accurate, but it will do for the purposes of demonstration. If the hypothetical correlation matrix shown in Table 13.10 were in an Excel spreadsheet, the intercept and regression coefficients for Gc, Gf, and WM predicting Applied Math can be calculated as follows.

1. Select a column of three cells outside of the correlation matrix (e.g., J2:J4).

2. Type "=MMULT(MINVERSE(B2:D4),A2:A4)" (without the quotes). The correlation matrix of the predictors "B2:D4" is inverted with the MINVERSE function, then the MMULT function post-multiplies it by the column of correlations of the criterion variable with each of the predictors "A2:A4."

3. While simultaneously holding the Control and Shift keys, press Enter. The result will show the three standardized regression coefficients in the three cells selected in Step 1. The coefficient for Gc is 0.4886. The coefficient for Gf is 0.2386. The coefficient for WM is 0.1364.

4. Because all variables are index scores, the intercept is easy to calculate. Add up all of the coefficients and multiply the sum by 100. Now subtract this number from 100. In this example, the intercept is:

$$\text{Intercept} = 100 - 100 * (0.4886 + 0.2386 + 0.1364) = 13.64$$

Table 13.10 Correlation Matrix of Hypothetical Measures of Cognitive and Academic Abilities

Variable		AP	Gc	Gf	WM	BC	MFF
		A	B	C	D	E	F
Applied Math (AP)	1	1	0.7	0.6	0.5	0.6	0.5
Crystallized Intelligence (Gc)	2	0.7	1	0.6	0.5	0.5	0.4
Fluid Intelligence (Gf)	3	0.6	0.6	1	0.5	0.5	0.4
Working Memory (WM)	4	0.5	0.5	0.5	1	0.4	0.3
Basic Calculation (BC)	5	0.6	0.5	0.4	0.4	1	0.5
Math Fact Fluency (MFF)	6	0.5	0.4	0.3	0.3	0.5	1

Note: The non-standard formatting of this correlation matrix, with numbers and letters in the left and top margins, is intended to imitate how it might appear in a spreadsheet program.

5. Thus, the resulting regression equation is:

Predicted Applied Math = 13.64 + 0.4886 * Gc
+ 0.2386 * Gf + 0.1364 * WM

The difference between the predicted Applied Math score and the observed Applied Math score is the prediction error.

Prediction Error = Observed Applied
Math − Predicted Applied Math

The multiple R^2 is the percentage of variance in Applied Math that is explained by the three predictors. It is calculated by starting with 1 and then subtracting the determinant of the entire correlation matrix divided by the determinant of the predictor correlation matrix. That is,

$$\text{Multiple } R^2 = 1 - \frac{|R_{all}|}{|R_p|}$$

where R_{all} is the correlation matrix of all of the variables and R_p is the correlation matrix of just the predictor matrix.

For this example in Excel, the multiple R^2 is

= 1−MDETERM(A1:D4)/MDETERM(B2:D4)
=0.5534

The standard error of the estimate is the standard deviation of the prediction errors. Thus, it is the typical size of a prediction error. Its formula is, when all scores are index scores,

Standard error of the estimate
$$= 15\sqrt{1 - R^2}$$
$$= 15\sqrt{1 - 0.5534} \approx 10.0242$$

To estimate the prevalence of a prediction error of a particular size and direction, the Excel formula is the same as it was with simple linear regression.

= NORMSDIST(−1*ABS(Observed-Predicted)/
(Standard error of the estimate))

This formula assumes that all variables are normal and that there are no non-linear relationships between any of the variables. These assumptions are likely to be approximately but not strictly true with most cognitive and academic variables.

Suppose that a girl is performing poorly in math, and her score on the Applied Math test was 78. Her cognitive scores are Gc = 96, Gf = 91, and WM = 75. Without a method such as multiple regression,

we can simply observe that her math performance suffers, in part, because of her low working memory. This is a binary interpretation. Something either does or does not influence performance. With multiple regression, we can estimate how much her Applied Math performance depends on working memory (after controlling for the other predictors). In this case, her predicted Applied Math score is

Predicted Applied Math = 13.64 + 0.4886 * 96
+ 0.2386 * 91 + 0.1364 * 75 ≈ 92.49

Given the assumptions of normality and linear relationships only, about half all children with this girl's cognitive profile of Gc = 96, Gf = 91, and WM = 75 score above 92.49 on Applied Math. The prevalence of an Applied Math score of 78 is calculated in Excel like so:

= NORMSDIST(−1*ABS(78−92.49)/(10.0242))
≈ 0.074

It appears that the girl's poor math performance is still unexplained. Among children with her profile on Gc, Gf, and WM, her Math performance is somewhat unusual. Some combination of other variables (including, perhaps, measurement error) is responsible for her low performance. Without the multiple regression results, we might have reasoned as follows.

1. Her math performance is low.
2. Working memory affects math performance.
3. Her working memory is low.

∴ Her low working memory accounts for her low math performance.

With the multiple regression results, we are now not so sure about this reasoning. Working memory certainly does matter. Had the girl's WM been 90 (1 SD higher so that it is consistent with her Gf and Gc scores), the predicted Applied Math score would improve by only 2 points, to about 95.5. However, the prevalence of Applied Math of 78 or lower among children with this new profile is 0.049, which is a 34% reduction of risk. Even so, we might need to look for additional explanations, perhaps outside of the cognitive domain.

One needlessly underutilized procedure is to think of other, more basic academic abilities as aptitudes (i.e., predictors) or precursors of more complex academic abilities. In this example, solving math word problems depends on basic calculation skills (BC) and math fact recall fluency (MFF). We can add these predictors to the three that are already there. Following the procedures described previously, we select a 5 by 1 column somewhere outside the correlation matrix, type "=MMULT(MINVERSE(B2:F6),A2:A6)" and press "Enter" while holding the Control and Shift keys. The intercept is calculated by adding the six coefficients, multiplying by 100, and subtracting from 100. The regression equation now is:

$$= -2.9547 + 0.3605 * Gc + 0.2065 * Gf + 0.0786 * WM + 0.2275 * BC + 0.1566 * MFF$$

Supposing that her Basic Calculation score is 73 and her Math Fact Fluency score is 83, we can calculate a new predicted score, which is approximately 85.9. The prediction error has shrunk from −14.5 to −7.9. The prevalence of an error this size and direction is about 0.192, more than double what it was before the academic predictors were added. The multiple R^2 has increased from 0.55 to 0.63, meaning that the two academic predictors explain an additional 8% of the variance in Applied Math beyond what the three cognitive predictors could explain. These changes mean that we have a more plausible explanation than we did previously. Even so, about 37% of the variance in Applied Math is not explained by the model. Realistically, a good portion of that 37% is due to measurement error (typically from 5% to 20%, depending on the test's reliability coefficient) but the rest comes from outside the model.

If we are saying that part of the reason that the girl performed poorly in Applied Math is that she has poor calculation skills and math fact fluency,

the next question we should consider is why her more basic math skills are low. Part of the reason, undoubtedly, is that working memory is low. The model in Figure 13.6 is an example of the use of path analysis. In most cases, path analysis is a set of interlocking regression equations. As long as there are no circular effects or bidirectional causation, the coefficients in a path analysis are simply the standardized regression coefficients from one or more regression equations. In Figure 13.6, there are three standardized regression equations.

1. Math Fact Fluency = 0.36 * Gc + 0.06 * Gf + 0.12 * WM
2. Basic Calculation = 0.25 * Gc + 0.08 * Gf + 0.13 * WM + 0.34 * MFF
3. Applied Problems = 0.36 * Gc + 0.21 * Gf + 0.08 * WM + 0.16 * MFF + 0.23 * BC

Path analysis is typically unable to tell us if a particular causal model is true, but it can inform us about the nature and size of various effects once we specify the causal model we believe is reasonable. For example, if the model in Figure 13.6 can be assumed, working memory's correlation of 0.5 with applied math is partly due to a direct causal effect (0.08) and three separate indirect effects. The indirect effect via basic calculation (0.13 * 0.23 ≈ 0.03) means that working memory has an effect on basic calculation which then has an effect on applied math. Working memory has an indirect effect on applied math via math fact fluency (0.12 * 0.16 ≈ 0.02). The third indirect effect on applied

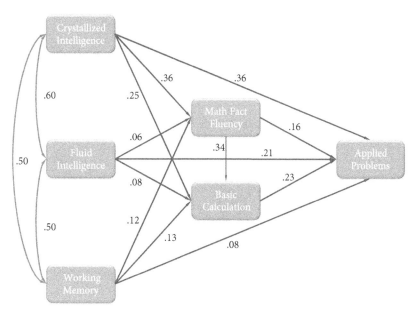

Figure 13.6 A Possible Causal Model of Math Achievement.

math comes about because working memory affects math fact fluency, which affects basic calculation, which then affects applied math ($0.12 * 0.34 * 0.23 \approx 0.01$). The indirect effects total about 0.06. The indirect and direct effects together are about 0.14, which is the same value as the direct effect of working memory in the first model without the academic predictors. The sum of indirect and direct effects means that if working memory were one standard deviation higher but Gf and Gc stayed the same, Applied Problems is expected to be 0.14 standard deviations higher (about 2 index score points). About half of this small increase is due to the higher scores expected in Basic Calculation and Math Fact Fluency when working memory is higher.

When 0.14 is subtracted from the overall correlation of working memory with applied math ($r = 0.50$), about 0.36 is not accounted for by the model. This occurs because working memory is correlated with Gf and Gc but no attempt was made to specify the causal nature of the relationships. Thus, 0.36 can be termed working memory's "unanalyzed" effect on applied math. If we were to specify a model that shows how the three cognitive variables cause one another (or are caused by one or more other variables outside of the model), the unanalyzed effect of working memory on applied math would be shown to be indirect effects via Gc and Gf or spurious effects (the parts of the correlation between working memory and applied math that are due to the fact they have one or more causes in common).

The fact that the multiple R^2 increased when the two academic predictors were added to the model suggests that Gf, Gc, and working memory are incapable of explaining all of the effects of basic calculation and math fact fluency on applied math. If we are to understand applied math in solely cognitive terms (which may not be possible), we need to look at cognitive variables beyond the three already included in the model. However, this is beyond the scope of this demonstration.

If the correlations between two particular tests are unknown, it is reasonable to estimate them from known correlations between similar tests. I hesitate to make this recommendation for fear of encouraging sloppiness, but I think it can be used responsibly. Whenever you use an estimate, your confidence in your conclusions should drop accordingly. Even so, I believe that using multiple regression in this fashion will reduce diagnostic error and overinterpretation. For users of the WJ III, these path analyses can be applied flexibly and automatically using the free software program *The Compositator* (Schneider, 2010). Using proper interpretive safeguards, this program can apply path analysis to estimate how much an academic outcome might improve if any of the precursor cognitive or academic abilities in the model were to be remediated.

Recommendations about the Assessment Process and Report Writing
Begin with the End in Mind

You would think that being mindful of the purpose of an assessment is so obvious that it need not be stated explicitly. Unfortunately, it has too often been my experience that I am asked to give a child an assessment and no one involved with the child has a well-articulated understanding of why an assessment is needed. It is easy to accept the vague responsibility to give the child an IQ test and anything else deemed interesting and then figure it all out on the fly. This approach can lead to unnecessary testing. Worse, it can lead to a failure to answer questions that are relevant to the child's difficulties.

Teachers regularly complain that psychological reports too often tell them only what they already know: This child is struggling! It is well worth the extra time it takes to talk with parents, teachers, and to the child to formulate a set of answerable questions they have. Inspired by Finn (1996), I often ask, "After the interviews are finished, after all the testing is completed, after I write up the results in a report, and after we meet to talk about what the report has to say about Suzie, what would you like to know about her that you do not know already? To which questions would it be really helpful to know the answers?"

How Allowing Yourself to Be Wrong Allows You to Be Right... Eventually

The greatest enemy of knowledge is not ignorance, it is the illusion of knowledge.
　—Stephen Hawking

It is wise to remember that you are one of those who can be fooled some of the time.
　—Laurence J. Peter

We human beings are so good at pattern recognition that sometimes we find patterns that are not even there. I have never seen a cognitive profile, no matter how unusual and outlandish, that did not inspire a vivid interpretation that explained EVERYTHING about a child. In fact, the more outlandish, the better. On a few occasions, some of the anomalous scores that inspired the vivid interpretations turned out to be anomalies due to scoring errors. In these humbling experiences, I have learned something important. I noticed that in those cases, my interpretations seemed just as plausible to me as any other. If anything, I was more engaged with them because they were so interesting. Of course, there is nothing wrong with making sense of data, and there is nothing wrong with doing so with a little creativity. Let your imagination soar! The danger is in taking yourself too seriously.

The scientific method is a system that saves us from our tendencies not to ask the hard questions after we have convinced ourselves of something. Put succinctly, the scientific method consists of not trusting any explanation until it survives your best efforts to kill it. There is much to be gained in reserving some time to imagine all the ways in which your interpretation might be wrong. The price of freedom is responsibility. The price of divergent thinking is prudence. It is better to be right in the end than to be right right now.

Time Lavished on Hypothesis Fishing Trips Is Stolen from Children We No Longer Have the Time to Help

We do what we must, and call it by the best names we can.
     —Ralph Waldo Emerson

Cheetahs are the fastest animals on land but do not always catch their prey. For about 60 seconds or so, cheetahs give it their all. After that, they give up. Why? For a cheetah to persist, the expected rewards must justify the caloric expenditure, the risk of injury, and the considerable strain on their bodies that sprinting inevitably causes. In the wild, there is no glory in Pyrrhic victories. Sometimes it is better to cut your losses, even though you could "succeed" with more effort.

There is something analogous that happens in cognitive assessment. For a time, it is worthwhile to vigorously pursue a hypothesis, to clarify an anomalous finding, or to explain a curious behavior. However, when answers are not forthcoming, there is a point at which it is wise to give up, even before all alternatives have been exhausted. The time saved can be devoted to other questions about the child that may be important. It is perfectly acceptable to write in reports that, given the available data, it is not yet possible to distinguish between alternative hypotheses about a child. It is perfectly acceptable to speculate about those hypotheses, provided that those speculations are clearly labeled as such and that it is explicitly stated

that the true explanation might not be included in the list of speculations.

It is not possible to be precise about when one should persist in seeking explanations and when one should admit defeat. Some questions are so important to answer that it is hard to imagine a good time to give up. For example, imagine that the MRI was inconclusive and the neurosurgeon needs to know where in the brain to cut in order to spare as much of the child's cognitive functioning as possible. Fortunately, psychologists are rarely faced with such awesome responsibility (not any more, at least).

Some questions are so clearly trivial that one should not bother with them at all. For example (and your mileage may vary), I never learn anything I care about from the WISC-IV Arithmetic subtest score. If the problem is poor working memory, it will show up on Letter-Number Sequencing and Digit Span. If the problem is low fluid reasoning, it will show up on Matrix Reasoning. If the problem is poor calculation skills or poor quantitative reasoning, it will show up on the achievement tests. I typically plan to assess these abilities anyway; therefore, the Arithmetic subtest provides little additional information. Furthermore, using a math test to explain math performance ("The reason you are bad at math is that you are bad at math") is just silly. Even when it is available, I barely even look at the Arithmetic subtest score.

In your decisions about whether it is a good idea to administer further testing, it is advisable to imagine all of the possible outcomes that might occur after the additional testing has been done. Ask yourself how your course of action might change in these various scenarios (e.g., the test score might be high, low, or just as expected). If you cannot state explicitly how knowing the additional information could significantly alter how a child might be helped, it is best to discontinue testing. For example, suppose a child performed poorly on the WISC-IV Cancellation subtest but well on Coding and Symbol Search. Given the current state of our knowledge, what are the realistic odds that something useful will come of confirming that this pattern is real (i.e., not due solely to measurement error) with further testing? Once confirmed, what does such a pattern mean? I can speculate just as well as anyone else, but the sad fact is that no one yet has done the hard work of empirically specifying the practical utility of this information. To proceed with further testing when I am working on the clock is simply to indulge my intellectual curiosity on someone else's dime.

Render Abstruse Jargon in the Vernacular

PRIMUS DOCTOR: Most learned bachelor whom I esteem and honor, I would like to ask you the cause and reason why opium makes one sleep.

BACHELIERUS: . . . . The reason is that in opium resides a dormitive virtue, of which it is the nature to stupefy the senses.

—from Molière's *Le Malade Imaginaire* (1673)

A man thinks that by mouthing hard words he understands hard things.

—Herman Melville

The veil of ignorance can be woven of many threads, but the one spun with the jangly jargon of a privileged profession produces a diaphanous fabric of alluring luster and bewitching beauty. Such jargon not only impresses outsiders but comforts them with what Brian Eno called "the last illusion": the belief that someone out there knows what is going on. Too often, it is a two-way illusion. Like Molière's medical student, we psychologists fail to grasp that our (invariably Latinate) technical terms typically do not actually explain anything. There is nothing wrong with technical terms *per se*; indeed, it would be hard for professionals to function without them. However, with them, it is easy to fall into logical traps and never notice. For example, saying that a child does not read well because she has dyslexia is not an explanation. It is almost a tautology, unless the time is taken to specify which precursors to reading are absent, and thus make dyslexia an informative label.

An additional and not insubstantial benefit of using ordinary language is that you are more likely to be understood. This is not to say that your communication should be dumbed down to the point that the point is lost. Rather, as allegedly advised by Albert Einstein, "Make everything as simple as possible, but not simpler."

$$\sum_{i=1}^{\infty} \left(Fact_i \right) < Useful\ Knowledge$$

I have made this [letter] longer, because I have not had the time to make it shorter.
—Blaise Pascal, "Lettres provinciales," letter 16, 1657

The secret of being a bore is to tell everything.
   —Voltaire

A little inaccuracy sometimes saves tons of explanation.
   —Saki, "The Square Egg," 1924

The observation that in every fat book there is a much better thin one trying to get out also applies to reports. By stating everything we know about a child, our reports become more accurate in a narrow sense, but such accuracy has diminishing returns and, at some point, has negative value. Student clinicians sometimes misunderstand their task. A report should not simply list the facts so that the readers can come to their own conclusions. Readers are rarely qualified to interpret raw data and cannot be expected to draw the conclusions you hint at indirectly.

Most of what is observed should not be included in a report. Many behaviors have no diagnostic value and may not even generalize to situations outside of the testing environment. A report should not describe the child in exquisite detail simply to paint a vivid picture. All descriptions should have a clear purpose. For example, it is fine to observe that the girl seemed confident on the easy math items but became a little anxious on the difficult items. But to observe without interpreting is to abandon your readers, leaving them vulnerable to wild speculations. Does the girl have performance anxiety? If she has performance anxiety, is it because she knows that she does not know how to do the hard problems and is ashamed, or is it because she knows how to do the hard problems but feels self-conscious in your presence and is thus unable to demonstrate her knowledge? Are the scores not valid estimates of her "true potential" (whatever that means)? Maybe all of the testing results are worthless! How common is it to be a little anxious? Did the anxiety *enhance* her performance, as described by the Yerkes-Dodson Law (Yerkes & Dodson, 1908)?

It is preferable to describe a child's behavior and interpret it so that the reader is better able to understand and help the child. Even if you are unsure which interpretation is correct, it is desirable to list plausible alternatives (clearly labeled as such) so that implausible and inappropriate alternatives are eliminated from consideration.

Write about People, Not Tests

At its best, the end product of a psychological assessment is that a child's life is made better because something useful and true is communicated to people who can use that information to make better decisions. How is this information best communicated? I believe that it is by the skillful retelling of the story of the child's struggle to cope with the difficulties that led to the testing referral.

Not only are humans storytelling creatures, we are also story-listening creatures. We are moved by drama, cleansed by tragedy, unified by cultural myths, and inspired by tales of heroic struggle. Most importantly, through stories we remember enormous amounts of information. Tabulated test results are inert until the evaluator weaves them together into a coherent narrative explanation that helps children and their caregivers construct a richer, more nuanced, and more organized understanding of the problem. Compare the following assessment results.

EXPLANATION 1

On a test in which Judy had to repeat words and segment them into individual phonemes, Judy earned a standard score of 78, which is in the Borderline Range. Only 7% of children performed at Judy's level or lower on this test. This test is a good predictor of the ability to read single words isolated from contextual cues. On a test that measures this ability, Judy scored an 83, which is in the 13th percentile, or in the Low Average Range. Reading single words is necessary to understand sentences and paragraphs. On a test that requires the evaluee to read a paragraph and then answer questions that test the evaluee's understanding of the text, Judy scored an 84, which is in the Low Average Range. This is in the 14th percentile. An 84 in Reading Comprehension is 24 points lower than her Full Scale IQ of 110 (75th percentile, High Average Range). This is significant at the .01 level, and only 3% of children in Judy's age range have a 24-point discrepancy or larger between Reading Comprehension and Full Scale IQ. Thus, Judy meets criteria for Reading Disorder. More specifically, Judy appears to have phonological dyslexia. *Phonological dyslexia* refers to difficulties in reading single words because of the inability to hear individual phonemes distinctly. This difficulty in decoding single words makes reading narrative text difficult because the reading process is slow and error-prone. Intensive remediation in phonics skills followed by reading fluency training is recommended.

EXPLANATION 2

For most 12-year-olds as bright as Judy is, reading is a skill that is so well developed and automatic that it becomes a pleasure. For Judy, however, reading is chore. It takes sustained mental effort for her to read each word one by one. It then requires further concentration for her to go back and figure out what these individual words mean when they are strung together in complete sentences, paragraphs, and stories. It is a slow, laborious process that is often unpleasant for Judy.

Why did Judy, a bright and delightfully creative girl, fail to learn to read fluently? It is impossible to know with certainty. However, the problem that most likely first caused Judy to fall behind her peers

is that she does not hear speech sounds as clearly as most people do. It is as if she needs glasses for her ears: The sounds are blurry. For example, although she can hear the whole word "cat" perfectly well, she might not recognize as easily as most children do that the word consists of three distinct sounds: |k|, |a|, and |t|. For this reason, she has to work harder to remember that these three sounds correspond to three separate letters: |k| = C, |a| = A, and |t| = T. With simple words like "cat," Judy's natural ability is more than sufficient to help her remember what the letters mean. However, learning to recognize and remember larger words, uncommonly used words, or words with irregular spellings is much more difficult for Judy than it is for most children.

Many children with the same difficulty in hearing speech sounds distinctly eventually learn to work around the problem and come to read reasonably well. However, Judy is a perceptive and sensitive girl. These traits are typically helpful but, unfortunately, they allowed her to be acutely aware, from very early on, that she did not read as well as her classmates. She clearly remembers that her friends and classmates giggled when she made reading errors that were, to them, inexplicable. For example, for a while she earned the nickname "Tornado Girl" when she was reading aloud in class and misread "volcano" as "tornado." She came to dread reading aloud in class and felt growing levels of shame even when she read silently to herself. She began to avoid reading at all costs. She did not read for pleasure, even when the texts were easy enough for her to read, because she felt, in her words, "dumb, dumb, and dumb." Over the next several years, she fell further behind her peers. By avoiding reading, she never developed the smooth, automatic reading skills that are necessary to make reading a pleasurable and self-sustaining activity.

Although Judy's ability to hear speech sounds distinctly is still low compared to that of her 12-year-old peers, this weakness is not what is holding her back now. Indeed, her current ability to hear speech sounds distinctly is actually better than that of most 6- and 7-year-olds, most of whom learn to read without difficulty. With extra help, Judy can learn to decode words phonetically. However, in order for her to develop her reading fluency and reading comprehension skills to the level that she is capable of, she will need to engage in sustained practice reading texts that are both interesting for her and are at the correct level of difficulty. She is likely to be willing to read only if she is helped to manage the sense of shame she feels when she attempts to read a book. This may require the collaboration of a reading specialist and a behavior specialist with expertise in the cognitive-behavioral treatment of anxiety-related problems.

Comparing Explanations

I am reasonably confident that most readers would find the second explanation to be much more useful than the first. The second explanation is not better than the first simply because it is more detailed. Explanation 1 could have been supplemented with more details if I had taken the time to fill it with even more information about test results. The second explanation is not better simply because it avoids statistical jargon that is difficult for parents and teachers to understand. Even if the jargon were removed from the first explanation and inserted into the second, the second explanation would still be better.

The second explanation is better because it is more about Judy than about her performance on tests. The narrative explanation of how her reading problem developed and how it was maintained is better because it leads to better treatment recommendations. More importantly, it leads to recommendations that will be understood and remembered by Judy's parents and teachers. One of the problems with the first explanation is, ironically, that it is not difficult to understand if it is properly explained. Most parents and teachers will nod their heads as they hear it. However, they are likely to forget the explanation as soon as they leave the room. Most of us are not accustomed to thinking about people in terms of sets of continuous variables. Without a narrative structure to hold them together, assessment details slip through the cracks of our memories quickly. It is unfortunate that a forgotten explanation, no matter how accurate, no matter how brilliant, is as helpful as no explanation at all. I hope that in listing these principles of assessment that I have made them memorable enough for them to be of use.

Those are my principles, and if you don't like them... well, I have others.
—Groucho Marx

Notes

1. Okay... not really... but I have seen some very sarcastic emails exchanged on professional listservs!

2. The term *positive manifold* at one time had a precise meaning drawn from mathematics, meaning that the correlation matrix of all tests was nearly a rank 1 matrix (i.e., a correlation matrix implied by Spearman's Two-Factor Theory). As it is currently used, the term simply means that the correlation matrix consists entirely of positive correlations.

3. Not, at least, in more than one large representative sample. From time to time, someone gets an occasional negative correlation, but other researchers have trouble replicating the finding.

4. Hence, the intense controversy is not merely a result of "lies and damned lies."

5. So named because in perhaps the most important theory to deny the existence of *g* (Horn & Cattell, 1964), the most important abilities all have names that begin with a capital letter G (G*f*, G*c*, G*v*, and so forth).

6. Full Scale IQ (WISC-IV, SB5, UNIT), Full Scale (Leiter-R, CAS), General Intellectual Ability (WJ III), General Conceptual Ability (DAS-II), Composite Intelligence Index (RIAS), Composite Intelligence Scale (KAIT), Fluid-Crystallized Index (KABC-II), and many others.

7. This table was created by calculating the standard deviation of the difference between two correlated normally distributed variables and then applying the cumulative probability density function of the normal curve.

8. "If I were to command a general to turn into a seagull, and if the general did not obey, that would not be the general's fault. It would be mine." —Antoine de Saint-Exupéry, *The Little Prince*

9. An Excel spreadsheet I wrote can calculate all of the statistics in this section and can be downloaded for free at http://my.ilstu.edu/~wjschne/tests.html.

10. This degree of profile variability is not at all unusual. In fact, it is quite typical. A statistic called the *Mahalanobis Distance* (Crawford & Allen, 1994) can be used to estimate how typical an individual profile of scores is compared to a particular population of score profiles. Using the given correlation matrix and assuming multivariate normality, this profile is at the 86th percentile in terms of profile unusualness... and almost of all of the reason that it is unusual is that its overall elevation is unusually low (*Mean* = 72). If we consider only the profiles that have an average score of 72, this profile's unusualness is at the 54th percentile (Schneider, 2012). That is, the amount of variability in this profile is typical compared to other profiles with an average score of 72.

11. And not every child with the same achievement scores will have the same IQ.

12. This section was inspired by the work of the nearly forgotten hero of the anti-*g*-ists, Godfrey Thomson. In what became known as "Bond Theory," Thomson (1939) proved mathematically that it is possible for statistical *g* to emerge without a single common entity influencing all scores. Thomson did not, however, discuss abilities in the same terms as they have been presented here.

13. Each of these abilities, of course, can be further subdivided into ever narrower categories until we begin to talk about specific neural assemblies of individual neurons. In the end, there is only one ability in the brain: the ability of a neuron to change the rate at which a few other neurons fire. Actually, that is not really the end of it. Inside each neuron there are all kinds of different organelles, each with different functions... and so this line of thinking goes until we reach the subatomic particles and on down to string theory. I am not sure it stops there, either. It might be cosmic turtles all the way down.

14. Horn (1985) tended to de-emphasize the biological/genetic interpretation of fluid intelligence.

15. Test developers have tried to create G*f* measures with verbal content (e.g., WJ-R Verbal Analogies or SB5 Verbal Fluid

Reasoning) but find that verbal G*f* tests do not always load on the same factor as traditional G*f* tests (Canivez, 2008; Woodcock, 1990). It is possible that the KAIT Logical Steps subtest may be the only commercially available verbal G*f* test that does not have substantial loadings on G*c* (Flanagan & McGrew, 1998; Immekus & Miller, 2010), possibly because it does not use the verbal analogy format.

16. See Moody (2009) for a discussion of other methodological problems that may have compromised the validity of the Jaeggi et al. (2008) study.

17. I will use g_f and g_c when discussing Cattell's original theory and G*f* and G*c*, respectively, when discussing the later developments of the theory with Horn.

18. He did not mean to imply that such knowledge, once formed, was immutable; nor did he believe that talent was a kind of fluid that flows from one part of the mind into another part of the mind where it was transformed into crystal, diminishing the available supply of fluid. Cattell (1987) played a bit with the fluid/crystallized metaphor on occasion. For example, he noted that fluid ability was everywhere in the brain yet nowhere in particular; thus damage to any part of the cortex decreased G*f* in proportion to the size of the lesion. In contrast, crystallized ability was in particular places in the brain, according to Cattell. The theory predicts that if there is a lesion in the region where a particular skill resided, the skill is lost. Otherwise the skill is spared completely.

19. IQ also has a direct effect on job performance if the job is one that requires novel problem–solving (Gottfredson, 1997).

20. Of course, dictionaries abound with antique words that were useful for a time but now languish in obscurity. For example, in our more egalitarian age, calling someone a "cur" (an inferior dog because it is of mixed breed) is not the insult that it once was. It is now used mostly for comedic effect when someone affects an aristocratic air. My favorite example of a possibly soon-to-be antique word is "decadent," which is nowadays almost exclusively associated with chocolate.

21. *Why would anyone be under a fire?* It means being shot at. *People are shooting at the White House?* No, it is just a vivid way of saying that the G.O.P. is criticizing the administration, which is symbolized by the White House, where the president lives. *Who is the G.O.P.?* It stands for "the Grand Old Party." *If they are old, why haven't I heard of them?* They are the Republicans. *Oh! Is the Democratic Party the new party?* No, they have been around longer than the Republicans. The nickname GOP was first used when the party was only a few decades old. *I don't understand.* I don't either, really. I just know that "old" is an affectionate way of describing something you have liked for a long time. *Could I say that I enjoy old ice cream?* No, that doesn't sound right. You should probably just avoid using "old" that way. *What does hunker mean?* I really have no idea. I just know that when you are under fire, you should hunker down. *If you don't know what it means, how do you know what to do?* True! I just looked it up. It means to squat, to sit on your haunches. I guess it all makes sense now. *So, when the Republicans criticize the president, he sits on his haunches?* That is an amusing image, but no. It means that you stick to your guns...er...I mean....

22. For this reason, this factor was renamed "Speeded Rotation" by McGrew and me (Schneider & McGrew, 2012), as suggested by Lohman (1996).

23. If test developers were to add such a test to a test battery, it would be a controversial decision. Speeded mental rotation tests are unusual in that there is a large gender difference

in performance (about 0.75σ to 1σ; Voyer, Voyer, & Bryden, 1995). It is not yet clear if the difference represents a cognitive ability difference, a strategy difference, a confidence difference, a socialization difference, or some mix of the these explanations (Clements-Stephens, Rimrodt, & Cutting, 2009).

24. Carroll (1993, pp. 465) wrote, "It is with some hesitation that I classify [Closure Speed] as a speed factor because some people are seemingly unable to perform very difficult items at all, even given a very generous time-limit."

25. Visual memory tests are thus different from spatial working memory tests in which the visual stimuli are simple but must recalled in a particular sequence.

26. This model assumes that all three variables are normally distributed index scores and that the relationships among them are linear.

27. The DAS-II Recall of Digits-Forward subtest also has this feature.

28. A *homunculus* is a little man. Trying to explain how we decide to do things by saying the central executive does it is no more informative than saying that there is a little man inside our brains and he makes all the decisions. Now we are begging the question, for we now have to explain how the brain of the homunculus makes decisions. Thus, calling a psychological construct a homunculus is meant as an insult: the theorist is trying to disguise what is not understood with a fancy name.

29. This review draws primarily from Cain (2006) and from Bull and Espy (2006).

30. Unfortunately, the load on working memory in such a test is much reduced with higher mathematical ability. For example, if asked to average 5, 10, and 15, it is possible arrive at the solution by adding the numbers and then dividing by 3. However, a child of high quantitative ability might recognize that the numbers are evenly spaced and thus would infer that the average is the middle number. This solution to the problem puts much less of a load on working memory. For this reason, I tend to be wary of mental arithmetic tests as measures of working memory.

31. By the way, I am really tired of writers' smugly mocking E. G. Boring for being so stupid as to say that intelligence is "what the tests test" (Boring, 1923). It is fine to disagree with the philosophical position he was espousing (operationalism), but not if you do not know what it was.

32. An important exception to this statement is when we consider the various academic fluency measures such as reading fluency, calculation fluency, and writing fluency. It is obvious that these measures should be considered separately when attempting to explain academic performance.

33. Amazingly, Arithmetic, a math test, predicts performance on other math tests.

34. Just before this chapter was finished, Professor John Crawford's excellent multiple regression computer program became available at http://www.abdn.ac.uk/~psy086/dept/psychom.htm. His program can be used to do all of the calculations explained in this section and more. The program is described fully in Crawford, Garthwaite, Denham, and Chelune (2012). For users of the WJ III, my computer program *The Compositator* (Schneider, 2010; http://www.woodcock-munoz-foundation.org/press/compositator.html) is more convenient (i.e., less data entry). It offers many additional features, including path analysis. Both programs are free.

35. These are generic labels not tied to any commercial achievement test.

References

Ackerman, P. L. (1996). A theory of adult intellectual development: Process, personality, interests, and knowledge. *Intelligence, 22*, 227–257.

Ackerman, P. L., & Cianciolo, A. T. (2000). Cognitive, perceptual speed, and psychomotor determinants of individual differences during skill acquisition. *Journal of Experimental Psychology: Applied, 6*, 259–290.

Alfonso, V. C., Flanagan, D. P., & Radwan, S. (2005). The impact of the Cattell-Horn-Carroll theory on test development and interpretation of cognitive and academic abilities. In D. Flanagan & P. L. Harrison (Eds.), *Contemporary intellectual assessment: Theories, tests, and issues* (2nd ed.; pp. 185–202). New York: Guilford.

Baddeley, A. (2002). Fractionating the central executive. In D. Stuss & R. Knight (Eds.), *Principles of frontal lobe function* (pp. 246–260). New York: Oxford University Press.

Baddeley, A. (2006). Working memory: An overview. In S. J. Pickering (Ed.), *Working memory and education* (pp. 1–31). New York: Elsevier.

Baddeley, A. D., & Hitch, G. (1974). Working memory. In G. A. Bower (Ed.), *The psychology of learning and motivation* (Vol. 8; pp. 47–89). New York: Academic Press.

Baddeley, A. D. (1986). *Working memory*. Oxford, England: Oxford University Press.

Benson, N. (2008). Cattell-Horn-Carroll cognitive abilities and reading achievement. *Journal of Psychoeducational Assessment, 26*, 27–41.

Bitterman, M. E., Tyler, D. W., & Elam, C. B. (1955). Simultaneous and successive discrimination under identical stimulating conditions. *American Journal of Psychology, 68*, 237–248.

Boring, E. G. (1923). Intelligence as the tests test it. *New Republic, 36*, 35–37.

Bowey, J. A., McGuigan, M., & Ruschena, A. (2005). On the association between serial naming speed for letters and digits and word-reading skill: Towards a developmental account. *Journal of Research in Reading, 28*, 400–422.

Bull, R., & Espy, K. A. (2006). Working memory, executive functioning, and children's mathematics. In S. J. Pickering (Eds.), *Working memory and education* (pp. 93–123). London: Academic Press.

Cain, K., Oakhill, J., & Bryant, P. E. (2004). Children's reading comprehension ability: Concurrent prediction by working memory, verbal ability, and component skills. *Journal of Educational Psychology, 96*, 31–42.

Cain, K. (2006). Children's reading comprehension: The role of working memory in normal and impaired development. In S. J. Pickering (Ed.), *Working memory and education* (pp. 62–91). San Diego: Academic Press.

Calvo M. G. (2005). Relative contribution of vocabulary knowledge and working memory span to elaborative inferences in reading. *Learning & Individual Differences, 15*, 53–65.

Canivez, G. L. (2008). Hierarchical factor structure of the Stanford-Binet Intelligence Scales–Fifth Edition. *School Psychology Quarterly, 23*, 533–541.

Carroll, J. B. (1993). *Human cognitive abilities: A survey of factor-analytical studies*. Cambridge, United Kingdom: Cambridge University Press.

Carroll, J. B. (2003). The higher-stratum structure of cognitive abilities: Current evidence supports g and about ten broad factors. In H. Nyborg (Ed.), *The scientific study of general intelligence: Tribute to Arthur R. Jensen* (pp. 5–21). New York: Pergamon Press.

Cattell, R. B. (1941). Some theoretical issues in adult intelligence testing. *Psychological Bulletin, 38*, 592.

Cattell, R. B. (1987). *Intelligence: Its structure, growth, and action*. New York: Elsevier.

Clements-Stephens, A. M., Rimrodt, S. L., & Cutting, L. E. (2009). Developmental sex differences in basic visuospatial processing: Differences in strategy use? *Neuroscience Letters, 449*, 155–160.

Conners, F. A., Carr, M. D., & Willis, S. (1998) Is the phonological loop responsible for intelligence-related differences in forward digit span? *American Journal on Mental Retardation, 103*, 1–11.

Conway, A. R. A., Cowan, N., Bunting, M. F., Therriault, D., & Minkoff, S. (2002). A latent variable analysis of working memory capacity, short term memory capacity, processing speed, and general fluid intelligence. *Intelligence, 30*, 163–183.

Crawford, J. R., & Allan, K. M. (1994). The Mahalanobis distance index of WAIS-R subtest scatter: Psychometric properties in a healthy UK sample. *British Journal of Clinical Psychology, 33*, 65–69.

Crawford, J. R., Garthwaite, P. H., Denham, K. A., & Chelune, G. J. (2012). Using regression equations built from summary data in the psychological assessment of the individual case: extension to multiple regression. *Psychological Assessment 12*, 801–14. doi:10.1037/a0027699.

Daneman, M., & Carpenter, P. A. (1980). Individual differences in working memory and reading. *Journal of Verbal Learning & Verbal Behavior, 19*, 450–466.

Danthiir, V., Roberts, R. D., Pallier, G., & Stankov, L. (2001). What the nose knows: Olfaction and cognitive abilities. *Intelligence, 29*, 337–361.

Das, J. P., Naglieri, J. A., & Kirby, J. R. (1994). *Assessment of cognitive processes: The PASS theory of intelligence*. Boston: Allyn and Bacon.

Delis, D. C., Jacobson, M., Bondi, M. W., Hamilton, J. M., & Salmon, D. P. (2003). The myth of testing construct validity using factor analysis or correlations with normal or mixed clinical populations: Lessons from memory assessment. *Journal of the International Neuropsychological Society, 9*, 936–946.

Drout, D. C. (2006). *A way with words: Rhetoric, writing and the arts of persuasion*. Prince Frederick, MD: Recorded Books, Inc.

Evans, J., Floyd, R., McGrew, K., & Leforge, M. (2002). The relations between measures of Cattell-Horn-Carroll (CHC) cognitive abilities and reading achievement during childhood and adolescence. *School Psychology Review, 31*, 246–262.

Finn, S. E. (1996). *A manual for using the MMPI-2 as a therapeutic intervention*. Minneapolis, MN: University of Minnesota Press.

Fiorello, C. A., Hale, J. B., McGrath, M., Ryan, K., & Quinn, S. (2002). IQ interpretation for children with flat and variable test profiles. *Learning & Individual Differences, 13*, 115–125.

Flanagan, D. P., & McGrew, K. S. (1997). A cross-battery approach to assessing and interpreting cognitive abilities: Narrowing the gap between practice and cognitive science. In D. P. Flanagan, J. L. Genshaft, & P. L. Harrison (Eds.), *Contemporary intellectual assessment: Theories, tests, and issues* (pp. 314–325). New York: Guilford Press.

Flanagan, D. P., & McGrew, K. S. (1998). Interpreting intelligence tests from contemporary Gf- Gc theory: Joint confirmatory factor analysis of the WJ-R and the KAIT in a non-white sample. *Journal of School Psychology*, *36*, 151–182.

Flanagan, D. P., Ortiz, S. O., & Alfonso, V. (2007). *Essentials of cross-battery assessment* (2nd ed.). New York: Wiley & Sons.

Flanagan, D. P., Ortiz, S. O., Alfonso, V. C., & Mascolo, J. T. (2006). *The achievement test desk reference* (2nd ed.) (ATDR-2). New York: Wiley.

Fleischner, J. E., Garnett, K., & Shepherd, M. J. (1982). Proficiency in basic fact computation of learning disabled and nondisabled children. *Focus on Learning Problems in Mathematics*, *4*, 47–55.

Floyd, R. G., Evans, J. J., & McGrew, K. S. (2003). Relations between measures of Cattell-Horn-Carroll (CHC) cognitive abilities and mathematics achievement across the school-age years. *Psychology in the Schools*, *40*, 155–171.

French, J. W. (1951). The description of aptitude and achievement tests in terms of rotated factors. *Psychometric Monograph 5*. Chicago: Univ. Chicago Press.

Gathercole, S. E., & Baddeley, A. D. (1993). Phonological working memory: A critical building block for reading development and vocabulary acquisition? *European Journal of Psychology of Education*, *8*, 259–272.

Glutting, J. J., Watkins, M. W., Konold, T. R., & McDermott, P. A. (2006). Distinctions without a difference: The utility of observed versus latent factors from the WISC-IV in estimating reading and math achievement on the WIAT-II. *Journal of Special Education*, *40*, 103–114.

Gottfredson, L. S. (1997). Why g matters: The complexity of everyday life. *Intelligence*, *24*, 79–132.

Guilford, J. P. (1967). *The nature of human intelligence*. New York: McGraw-Hill.

Gustafsson, J. E., & Undheim, J. O. (1996). Individual differences in cognitive functions. In D. C. Berliner & R. C. Calfee (Eds.). *Handbook of educational psychology* (pp. 186–242. New York: Simon & Schuster, Macmillan.

Hirsch, E. D. (2006). *The knowledge deficit: Closing the shocking education gap for American children*. New York: Houghton Mifflin.

Horn, J. L., & Blankson, N. (2005). Foundations for better understanding of cognitive abilities. In D. Flanagan & P. Harrison (Eds.), *Contemporary intellectual assessment: Theories, tests, and issues* (2nd ed.; pp. 41–68). New York: Guilford Press.

Horn, J. L., & Cattell, R. B. (1966). Refinement and test of the theory of fluid and crystallized general intelligences. *Journal of Educational Psychology*, *57*, 253–270.

Hunt, E. (2000). Let's hear it for crystallized intelligence. *Learning & Individual Differences*, *12*, 123–129.

Immekus, J. C., & Miller, S. J. (2010). Factor structure invariance of the Kaufman Adolescent and Adult Intelligence Test across male and female samples. *Educational & Psychological Measurement*, *70*, 91–104.

Jaeggi, S. M., Buschkuehl, M., Jonides, J., & Perrig, W. J. (2008). Improving fluid intelligence with training on working memory. *Proceedings of the National Academy of Sciences of the United States of America*, *105*, 6829–6833.

Just, M. A., & Carpenter, P. A. (1992). A capacity hypothesis of comprehension: Individual differences in working memory. *Psychological Review*, *99*, 122–149.

Kamphaus, R. (2005). *Clinical assessment of child and adolescent intelligence* (2nd Ed.). New York: Springer-Verlag.

Kane, M. J., Hambrick, D. Z., Tuholski, S. W., Wilhelm, O., Payne, T. W., & Engle, R. W. (2004). The generality of working memory capacity: A latent variable approach to verbal and visuo-spatial memory span and reasoning. *Journal of Experimental Psychology: General*, *133*, 189–217.

Kaplan, E. (1988). A process approach to neuropsychological assessment. In T. Boll & B. K. Bryant (Eds.), *Clinical neuropsychology and brain function: Research, measurement, and practice* (pp. 129–231). Washington, DC: American Psychological Association.

Kaufman, A. S. (1994). *Intelligent testing with the WISC-III*. New York: Wiley.

Kaufman, A. S., & Kaufman N. L. (2004). *Manual for the Kaufman Assessment Battery for Children–Second Edition (KABC-II) Comprehensive Form*. Circle Pines, MN: American Guidance Service.

Kaufman, A. S., & Lichtenberger, E. O. (2006). *Assessing adolescent and adult intelligence* (3rd ed.). New York: Wiley.

Keith, T. Z., Kranzler, J. H., & Flanagan, D. P. (2001). What does the Cognitive Assessment System (CAS) measure? Joint confirmatory factor analysis of the CAS and the Woodcock-Johnson tests of cognitive ability (3rd ed.). *School Psychology Review*, *30*, 89–119.)

Klin, A., Sparrow, S. S., de Bildt, A., Cicchetti, D. V., Cohen, D. J., & Volkmar, F. R. (1999). A normed study of face recognition in autism and related disorders. *Journal of Autism & Developmental Disorders*, *29*, 499–508.

Kranzler, J. H., & Keith, T. Z. (1999). Independent confirmatory factor analysis of the Cognitive Assessment System (CAS): What does the CAS measure? *School Psychology Review*, *28*, 117–144.

Kyllonen, P. C., & Christal, R. E. (1990). Reasoning ability is (little more than) working memory capacity?! *Intelligence*, *14*, 389–433.

Lohman, D. F. (1996). Spatial ability and G. In I. Dennis & P. Tapsfield (Eds.), *Human abilities: Their nature and assessment* (pp. 97–116). Hillsdale, NJ: Erlbaum.

Luria, A. R. (1966). *Human brain and psychological processes*. New York: Harper and Row.

McDonald, R. P. (1999). *Test theory: A unified treatment*. Mahwah, NJ: L. Erlbaum Associates.

McGrew, K. S. (2005). The Cattell-Horn-Carroll (CHC) theory of cognitive abilities. Past, present and future. In D. P. Flanagan & P. L. Harrison (Eds.), *Contemporary intellectual assessment. Theories, tests, and issues* (2nd ed.; pp.136–181). New York: Guilford.

McGrew, K. S. (1997). Analysis of the major intelligence batteries according to a proposed comprehensive Gf-Gc framework. In D. P. Flanagan, J. L. Genshaft, & P. L. Harrison (Eds.), *Contemporary intellectual assessment: Theories, tests, and issues* (pp. 151–179). New York: Guilford.

McGrew, K. S., & Flanagan, D. P. (1998). *The intelligence test desk reference (ITDR): Gf-Gc cross-battery assessment*. Boston, MA: Allyn & Bacon.

Mirsky, A. F. (1987). Behavioral and psychophysiological markers of disordered attention. *Environmental Health Perspective*, *74*, 191–199.

Miyake, A., Friedman, N. P., Emerson, M. J., Witzki, A. H., Howerter, A., & Wager, T. (2000). The unity and diversity of executive functions and their contributions to complex "frontal lobe" tasks: A latent variable analysis. *Cognitive Psychology*, *41*, 49–100.

Moody, D. E. (2009). Can intelligence be increased by training on a task of working memory? *Intelligence, 37*, 327–328.

Naglieri, J. A. (1999). How valid is the PASS theory and the CAS? *School Psychology Review, 28*, 145–161.

Naglieri, J. A., & Das, J. P. (1988). Planning-arousal-simultaneous-successive (PASS): A model for assessment. *Journal of School Psychology, 26*, 35–48.

Naglieri, J. A., & Das, J. P. (2005). Planning, attention, simultaneous, successive (PASS) theory: A revision of the concept of intelligence. In D. P. Flanagan & P. L. Harrison (Eds.), *Contemporary intellectual assessment: Theories, tests, and issues* (2nd ed.; pp. 120–135). New York: Guilford.

Naglieri, J., De Lauder, B., Goldstein, S., & Schwebech, A. (2006). WISC-III and CAS: Which correlates higher with achievement for a clinical sample? *School Psychology Quarterly, 21*, 62–76.

Norman, D. A., & Shallice, T. (1986). Attention to action: Willed and automatic control of behaviour. In R. Davidson, G. Schwartz, & D. Shapiro, (Eds.), *Consciousness and self regulation: Advances in research and theory* (Vol. 4; pp. 1–18). New York: Plenum.

Pressley, M. (2002). Metacognition and self-regulated comprehension. In A. E. Farstrup & S. J. Samuels (Eds.), *What research has to say about reading instruction* (3rd ed.; pp. 291–309). Newark, DE: International Reading Association.

Reynolds, M. R., Keith, T. Z., Fine, J. G., Fisher, M. E., & Low, J. A. (2007). Confirmatory factor structure of the Kaufman assessment battery for children–second edition: Consistency with Cattell-Horn-Carroll theory. *School Psychology Quarterly, 22*, 511–539.

Schneider, W. J. (2010). *The Compositator 1.0*. Olympia, WA: WMF Press.

Schneider, W. J. (2012). A geometric representation of composite scores and profile variability. Unpublished manuscript.

Schneider, W. J., & McGrew, K. S. (2011). "Just say no" to averaging IQ subtest scores. *Applied Psychometrics 101 #10*. Institute of Applied Psychometrics. Retrieved from http://www.iapsych.com/iapap101/iap10110.pdf

Schneider, W. J., & McGrew, K. S. (2012). The Cattell-Horn-Carroll model of intelligence. In D. Flanagan & P. Harrison (Eds.), *Contemporary intellectual assessment: Theories, tests, and issues* (3rd ed.; pp. 99–144). New York: Guilford.

Shea, D. L., Lubinski, D., & Benbow, C. P. (2001). Importance of assessing spatial ability in intellectually talented young adolescents: A 20-year longitudinal study. *Journal of Educational Psychology, 93*, 604–614.

Spearman, C. (1904). General intelligence, objectively determined and measured. *American Journal of Psychology, 15*, 201–293.

Spearman, C. (1927). *The abilities of man*. London: Macmillan.

Sternberg, R. J. (2005). The triarchic theory of successful intelligence. In D. P. Flanagan & P. L. Harrison (Eds.), *Contemporary intellectual assessment: Theories, tests, and issues* (2nd ed., 103–119). New York: The Guilford Press.

Stankov, L., Seizova-Cajic, T., & Roberts, R. D. (2001). Tactile and kinesthetic perceptual processes within the taxonomy of human cognitive abilities. *Intelligence, 28*, 1–29.

Thomson, G. H. (1939). *The factorial analysis of human ability*. London: University of London Press.

Treisman, A. M., & Gelade, G. (1980). A feature-integration theory of attention. *Cognitive Psychology, 12*, 97–136.

Tulsky, D. S., Ivnik, R. J., Price, L. R., & Wilkens, C. (2003). Assessment of Cognitive Functioning with the WAIS-III and WMS-III: Development of a Six-Factor Model. In D. S. Tulsky et al. (Eds.), *Clinical interpretation of the WAIS-III and WMS-III* (pp. 147–179). San Diego, CA: Academic Press.

Voyer, D., Voyer, S., & Bryden, M. P. (1995). Magnitude of sex differences in spatial abilities: A meta-analysis and consideration of critical variables. *Psychological Bulletin, 117*, 250–270.

Watkins, M. W., Glutting, J. J., & Lei, P. W. (2007). Validity of the full-scale IQ when there is significant variability among WISC-III and WISC-IV factor scores. *Applied Neuropsychology, 14*, 13–20.

Wilkinson, S. C. (1993). WISC-R profiles of children with superior intellectual ability. *Gifted Child Quarterly, 37*, 84–91.

Woodcock, R. W. (1990). Theoretical foundations of the WJ-R measures of cognitive ability. *Journal of Psychoeducational Assessment, 8*, 231–258.

Woodcock, R. W., McGrew, K. S., Schrank, F. A., & Mather, N. (2007). *Woodcock-Johnson III normative update*. Rolling Meadows, IL: Riverside Publishing.

Yerkes, R. M., & Dodson, J. D. (1908). The relation of strength of stimulus to rapidity of habit-formation. *Journal of Comparative Neurology & Psychology, 18*, 459–482.

Principles of Neuropsychological Assessment in Children and Adolescents

Cynthia A. Riccio *and* Cecil R. Reynolds

Abstract

Neuropsychological assessment is often recommended for a variety of neurodevelopmental disorders. Neurological involvement may be presumed (e.g., learning disability) or identifiable (e.g., seizure disorder). In either case, possible consequences can include impaired cognitive, sensory, motor, educational, behavioral, and psychological functioning. Neuropsychological assessment provides additional information across a range of domains to aid in case conceptualization and formulation of treatment planning. There are multiple approaches that may be applied in neuropsychological assessment, as well as various measures that may be used. This chapter identifies key principles to guide neuropsychological assessment of children and adolescents consistent with ethical and professional standards. Included is a discussion of how neuropsychological assessment complements the response to intervention (RTI) movement. Some of the continuing issues with regard to measurement and additional research needed are also highlighted.

Key Words: neuropsychological assessment, benchmarking, Luria, fixed battery, idiographic approach; process orientation

Introduction

Neuropsychological assessment is often recommended for a variety of disorders with an identified neurological basis (e.g., seizure disorder), as well as for disorders such as learning disabilities, where a neurological basis is presumed. In effect, historically, when an individual was referred for a neuropsychological assessment, oftentimes the primary purpose was to identify (or rule out) pathology. More recently, however, the emphasis has shifted to identification of strengths and weaknesses (Brickman, Cabo, & Manly, 2006; Hale et al., 2010; Riccio & Reynolds, 1998; Wong, 2006). This is in part due to the research that suggests that children with neurodevelopmental disorders are those who have, or who are at risk for, limitations in some or all life activities as a result of impairments in the central nervous system (Mudrick, 2002; Spreen, Risser, & Edgell, 1995). The possible consequences and limitations range from mild to severe cognitive, sensory, motor, educational, and behavioral/psychological impairments (Mendola, Selevan, Gutter, & Rice, 2002).

The neuropsychological approach to case conceptualization incorporates information related to various behavioral domains believed to be reflect functional neurological systems (Luria, 1980; Riccio & Reynolds, 1998). A major premise of neuropsychological assessment is that different behaviors involve differing neurological structures or functional systems (Luria, 1980; Stuss & Levine, 2002); neuropsychological assessment is intended to be comprehensive enough to address all functional systems. As such, a neuropsychological evaluation provides for consideration of a wider array of functions than is addressed in a typical psychological or psychoeducational evaluation (Dean, 1986;

Reynolds & Mayfield, 1999) and includes assessment of perceptual, motor, and sensory areas; attention; executive function (planning, organization, problem-solving); and learning and memory (Dean & Gray, 1990; Reynolds & Mayfield, 1999; Riccio, 2008; Riccio & Reynolds, 1998). Although there is no agreed-upon model or approach (Wong, 2006), a number of models have been proposed to explain the interface between brain function and behaviors associated with childhood psychopathology, including Luria's model (Korkman, 1999; Luria, 1980).

It has been suggested that neuropsychological assessment of children provides a better understanding of the ways in which neurological conditions have an impact on behavior and the translation of this knowledge into educationally relevant information (Goldstein & Naglieri, 2008). Advances in the understanding of neuroanatomical correlates, as well as neuropsychological perspectives, have improved the understanding of autism (Carter et al., 2008; Iacoboni & Mazziotta, 2007; Kleinhans, Müller, Cohen, & Courchesne, 2008; Oberman, Ramachandran, & Pineda, 2008; Verte, Geurts, Roeyers, Oosterlaan, & Sergeant, 2005), attention deficit hyperactivity disorder (ADHD; Goldstein & Naglieri, 2008; Krain & Castellanos, 2006; Martel, Nikolas, & Nigg, 2007; Seidman, 2006), language impairment (Ballantyne, Spilkin, & Trauner, 2007; Chiarello, Kacinik, Manowitz, Otto, & Leonard, 2004; Cohen, Hall, & Riccio, 1997; Cohen, Riccio, & Hynd, 1999; Im-Bolter, Johnson, & Pascual-Leone, 2006), and other disorders. These advances facilitate the development of interventions and lead to better understanding. Improved understanding of the child's strengths and weaknesses potentially can be used to identify areas that may provide difficulty for the child in the future, as well as to suggest compensatory strategies or methods to circumvent these difficulties. Furthermore, many components of neuropsychological assessment can be helpful in providing documentation of changes in behavior and development over time with regard to genetic and neurodevelopmental disorders (Reynolds & Mayfield, 1999). Thus, neuropsychological assessment may be considered appropriate whenever a child is suspected of having a neurological disorder or when it is believed that the integrity of the central nervous system (CNS) has been compromised in some way. As previously stated, the intention of such an assessment is no longer the localization of damage or dysfunction; it also is not solely for diagnostic purposes, but for identification of individual strengths and weaknesses in order to inform rehabilitation efforts. Neuropsychological assessment is "hypothesis-driven"; it involves integration of all the information obtained in the context of neurodevelopmental systems (Berkelhammer, 2008: Hale Fiorello, Bertin, & Sherman, 2003). The goal of this integration is the generation of recommendations for habilitation, accommodations, or modifications. The ultimate goal of the assessment should be to derive a case conceptualization that informs intervention or rehabilitation planning. This case conceptualization is based on the individual's performance across a variety of domains, with attention to developmental contexts, inferences about brain integrity, and application of the understanding of brain–behavior relations (Stuss & Levine, 2002). There is no single approach or combination of measures, but rather a set of principles and standards (some of which apply across all forms of assessment) that guides neuropsychological assessment. The purpose of this chapter is to present and discuss some of these principles in the context of neuropsychological assessment and theory. These principles are summarized in Table 14.1.

Ethical and Legal Considerations

As with other types of assessment and service delivery in psychology, the most basic ethical considerations and standards are taken from the American Psychological Association ethical guidelines and code of conduct (American Psychological Association, 2002). In addition to APA ethics, the first set of guidelines formally reviewed and endorsed by the American Academy of Clinical Neuropsychology (AACN) was published in 2007 (AACN Board of Directors, 2007). The Board guidelines were developed as a next step in defining the training and practice of clinical neuropsychology; they incorporate the common features of previous endeavors to establish core training requirements (Hannay et al., 1998), as well as general approaches to valid and appropriate neuropsychological assessment (Lezak, Howieson, & Loring, 2004). Although specific to the provision of neuropsychological services, the guidelines were developed to be compatible with other existing ethical and practice guidelines, including those of the APA. As with all guidelines, those developed by the AACN Board are described as a means of facilitating development of the profession, and are aspirational. At the same time, they represent a "high level of professional practice" (AACN Board, 2007, p. 281). Some, but not all, of these ethical principles will be discussed specifically as they apply to neuropsychological assessment.

Table 14.1 Principles in Neuropsychological Assessment

Principle (Source)
General ethical principles:
Obtain informed consent; ensure understanding of the purpose and scope of the evaluation; determine competency to provide consent if age 18 or older (American Psychological Association, 2002; AACN Board, 2007; Bush, 2005; Heilbrun et al., 2003; Moberg & Kniele, 2006; Wong, 2006).
Discuss issues of confidentiality, billing, release of information (American Psychological Association, 2002; Bush, 2005; Bush & Martin, 2008).
Maintain records and ensure confidentiality consistent with ethical and legal requirements (American Psychological Association, 2002; Bush, 2005; Bush & Martin, 2008).
Clarify role and relationship, for example, as expert witness or clinician (American Psychological Association, 2002; AACN Board, 2007; Heilbrun et al., 2003).
Appropriately portray competency and limits of training (American Psychological Association, 2002; AACN Board, 2007; Bush, 2005; Hartlage & Long, 2009).
Planning and organizing the assessment:
Identify the most appropriate theoretical model to guide information gathering and interpretation (Heilbrun et al., 2003).
Obtain a comprehensive developmental, educational, and medical history from which to generate *a priori* hypotheses (Reynolds & Mayfield, 1999; Riccio & Reynolds, 1998).
Use multiple methods and multiple sources for all aspects of the assessment (Heilbrun, et al., 2003; Reynolds & Mayfield, 1999).
Plan, conduct and integrate assessment so that it is informative to prevention/intervention planning (Reynolds & Mayfield, 1999; Riccio & Reynolds, 1998).
In choosing the specific measures and methods to be included:
Consider the neurodevelopmental context, as well as any medical or physical limitations of the child (Reynolds & Mayfield, 1999; Riccio & Reynolds, 1998; Simeonsson & Rosenthal, 2001).
Consider the family context and availability of family supports (Rosenthal et al., 2001).
Consideration of cultural context and primary language, both in the assessment and the design of interventions.
Consider school context through collaboration with school personnel in the assessment process (Reynolds & Mayfield, 1999; Riccio & Reynolds, 1998).
Ensure coverage of all cognitive and higher-order processes that may impact on educational performance (Reynolds & Mayfield, 1999; Riccio & Reynolds, 1998).
Ensure coverage of all four quadrants of the cortex (left, right, anterior, posterior; Reynolds & Mayfield, 1999; Riccio & Reynolds, 1998).
Consider psychometric properties of the measures to be included (reliability, validity, sensitivity, specificity; Reynolds & Mason, 2009).
Consider the extent to which the measures provide information about real world functioning (ecological validity; Rabin, Barr, & Burton, 2005; Sbordone, 2008).
Include measures to assess social, emotional, behavioral, and personality aspects (Teeter et al., 2009).

(continued)

Table 14.1 (Continued)

Principle (Source)

Inference and interpretation:

Make inferences that are based on all available evidence (Fennell & Bauer, 2009).

Identify any intact complex functional systems (Reynolds & Mayfield, 1999; Riccio & Reynolds, 1998).

Identify the child's specific deficits (Reynolds & Mayfield, 1999; Riccio & Reynolds, 1998).

Communication of results:

Provide a written report that is both comprehensive and understandable to the stakeholders who receive it (Heilbrun et al., 2003; Reynolds & Mayfield, 1999; Riccio & Reynolds, 1998).

Identify and communicate how these strengths and weaknesses relate to educational and social functioning (Reynolds & Mayfield, 1999; Riccio & Reynolds, 1998).

Make appropriate recommendations that follow from the conclusions and are consistent with the contexts in which the child functions (Reynolds & Mayfield, 1999; Riccio & Reynolds, 1998; Teeter, 2009).

Consent and Related Issues

Taken together, both APA's ethical code and the AACN Board's guidelines include similar components with respect to the need for *consideration of informed consent*. With children and adolescents, there are special considerations involved with consent to psychological assessment and services, as their parent(s) or guardian(s) usually provide(s) the consent (Jacob & Hartshorne, 2007); these considerations are also in place with neuropsychological assessment, With older adolescents, and the transfer of rights from parents to the adult child at age 18, given that neuropsychological assessment is often considered in light of known or suspected brain damage, additional concerns may be present. As yet, there are no agreed-upon criteria for determining competency of the individual to give consent; most of the discussion related to competency is related to treatment issues or forensic situations (Moberg & Kniele, 2006).

Regardless of the consenting party, it is necessary for the neuropsychologist to *establish the aim and scope of assessment* in language that is readily understood and includes agreement on any financial aspects. As with any assessment, this should include the types of procedures to be used as part of the process; any change will necessitate renegotiation of the scope, and financial agreement as appropriate, with the consenting party (AACN Board, 2007; Jacob & Hartshorne, 2007). *Roles and responsibilities need to be defined and limits of confidentiality specified*. In forensic cases, it will be necessary for the neuropsychologist to carefully define whether they are conducting the assessment as an "expert witness" or as a "clinician," as this may affect

whether they advocate for the system or for the client (AACN Board, 2007; Heilbrun et al., 2003). With children, this includes defining one's role if the assessment is conducted as part of an independent educational evaluation (IEE) (Wills, 2008).

Clinician Competency

Of the ethical considerations, probably one of the more controversial is the issue of clinician competency. Historically, there have been few formal training programs in neuropsychology, with the first documented guidelines for establishing competency in neuropsychology established by the International Neuropsychological Society (INS) in 1973 (Hartlage & Long, 2009). Since then, more formal training programs have emerged, with approximately 40 programs offering a degree in neuropsychology (Bieliauskas, 2008; Hartlage & Long, 2009), and various delineations of what should compose training for neuropsychology have been offered (Bieliauskas, 2008; Hannay et al., 1998). Definitions offered by both Division 40 of the American Psychological Association (Clinical Neuropsychology) and the National Academy of Neuropsychology (NAN) suggest at least two years of specialized training, including formal (university) training in neuropsychology and neuroscience (Division 40), or the study and practice of clinical neuropsychology and neuroscience (NAN). More detailed explanations are available from each of these organizations and in the Board document, as well as reviewed in Hartlage and Long (2009). Notably, consistent with the doctrine of the APA, the term *neuropsychologist* is presumed to be reserved to those holding a doctoral degree in psychology, with the neuropsychology and neuroscience training additional to the base competencies for the practice of psychology (AACN Board, 2007). At the same time, the Board does not state that individuals must have this training to use specific measures that may be considered "neuropsychological"; rather, both the APA ethical code and the Board guidelines reflect the need for truthful representation of whether the training of the individual is consistent with the appropriate use of the title. *More advanced clinical training is prerequisite to the inferential and interpretation process* involved in neuropsychological assessment than for the actual test administration (Hartlage & Long, 2009).

Other Ethical Considerations

All of the other issues related to confidentiality, record-keeping, billing, test security, and so on, apply similarly to typical psychological evaluations and neuropsychological assessment (APA, 2002). Application of the theoretical bases for understanding brain–behavior relations (e.g., the Lurian model) across cultures is also being considered, with more and more individuals being seen coming from a variety of cultures and linguistic backgrounds (Kotik-Friedgut, 2006); with the increasing Hispanic population, much of the discussion has focused on this population (Judd et al., 2009). Regardless of the person's language or culture, however, it is increasingly being recognized that *it is important for cultural and first-language issues to be considered in the planning process* (Byrd, Arentoft, Scheiner, Westerveld, & Baron, 2008; Harris, Wagner, & Cullum, 2007; Judd et al., 2009; Llorente, 2008; Smith, Lane, & Llorente, 2008). Of particular concern is, not only the appropriateness of some of the tasks with culturally and linguistically diverse individuals, but also the use of interpreters (APA, 1993, 2002). Additional issues relate to the model of assessment being used, the approach to test selection, and psychometrics and test standards. These are discussed in the context of the assessment process.

Planning and Organizing the Assessment

In planning and organizing the assessment, it is important that the clinician have some *theoretical model* in mind; oftentimes this is an application of Luria's model (Korkman, 1999; Luria, 1980), but it may also reflect Cattell-Horn-Carroll or other models of cognitive ability (Naglieri, Conway, & Goldstein, 2009), which may or may not be in some way related to Luria's model. Using Luria's model, for example, neuropsychological assessment

generally consists of a number of functional domains that are, based on clinical evidence, associated with functional systems of the brain. Applying Lurian principles requires that the assessment itself be organized in such a manner that the majority of the areas of functioning, as well as the various contexts in which the child is expected to function, are considered. Measures and observations need to include the various contexts in which the child functions, and the associated expectations of the child, particularly within the educational context. For this reason, regardless of the theoretical model, the neuropsychological assessment should be organized to ensure *evaluation of the majority of cognitive and higher-order processes that relate to educational functioning.* Some key features from this perspective have been identified elsewhere and will be discussed further here (Reynolds & Mayfield, 1999; Riccio & Reynolds, 1998); methods and measures are discussed in other chapters. Regardless of the approach, however, *multiple sources of information should be used for each area or domain being assessed; multiple methods also should be utilized to maximize the information garnered from the assessment process* (Heilbrun et al., 2003; Reynolds & Mayfield, 1999).

Neuropsychological assessment of a child or adolescent needs to incorporate information from a variety of sources (e.g., parents, teachers, physicians, medical records, school records, and so on). In many cases, school records may include test results from a prior psychoeducational or psychological evaluation: *whenever possible, it is recommended that the neuropsychological assessment be coordinated with the child's school district* (Reynolds & Mayfield, 1999; Riccio & Reynolds, 1998; Wills, 2008). If prior testing is not already available, it may be appropriate for school personnel (e.g., school psychologist, speech/language pathologist) to participate in the evaluation process, thus reducing the financial strain on the school system and family. Equally due consideration is the fact that schools are the second major environment in which children must function. In many ways, schools and school personnel have the greatest long-term impact on outcome, as the resources and support available from the school district will continue to follow the child through to graduation. This type of collaborative effort also can facilitate program planning for the child in the school setting in that school personnel will be intimately involved in any arrangements for school-based direct or indirect service delivery for the child (Riccio & Reynolds, 1998). Assessment of resources available in the schools, with in-service training for educators and administrators as needed, may be appropriate (Goldstein & Naglieri, 2008).

Background Information

The history and review of prior medical and educational records provide some standard information about a child and the basis for an initial hypothesis-formation. *Obtaining a comprehensive history is an important component of neuropsychological assessment,* as the complete history provides useful information to help differentiate chronic deficits or neurodevelopmental disorders from new, acute problems (Riccio & Reynolds, 1998). Information on the child's developmental and social history provides input related to the onset, duration, and intensity of the problems of concern; it provides the information needed to differentiate chronic deficits or neurodevelopmental disorders from new, acute problems (Reynolds & Mayfield, 1999). Family history and the identification of family stressors also provides information on the supports available within the family system; *as it is the primary setting in which a child functions, consideration of the family context is critical* (Rosenthal, Cohen, & Simeonsson, 2001). A number of developmental and social history forms exist for this purpose. Most of these forms can be either completed in interview format or completed independently by the parents. The Structured Developmental History form (SDH) of the Behavior Assessment System for Children–Second Edition (BASC-2; Reynolds & Kamphaus, 2004) is one example of a developmental history questionnaire. The SDH solicits information specific to the prenatal, perinatal, and postnatal early childhood development, medical problems and concerns, exposure to formal education, progress in school, and so on. It also asks for information specific to the family situation, housing, leisure activities of the child, preferred activities, and so on, that may be helpful in case conceptualization and intervention planning (Riccio & Reynolds, 1998). Family history for various disorders, disciplinary techniques used in the past, medications used in the past, and other prior treatment information can be solicited with this single form (Reynolds & Kamphaus, 2004).

Other considerations may be of importance in planning and organizing the assessment process, including *accounting for medical conditions or limitations in communication that may require special attention* (Simeonsson & Rosenthal, 2001). In particular, for individuals with chronic illness, the length of time required for neuropsychological assessment demands that fatigue be considered and assessment be broken into smaller, manageable segments. Planning and organizing the assessment includes identification of the domains to be assessed to ensure comprehensive coverage. Specific areas that are included in the neuropsychological assessment that are not usually included in depth as part of a standard psychoeducational battery include the sensory, motor, auditory/linguistic, and visual perceptual areas; as well as learning and memory; attention; and the executive functions of planning, organization, and problem-solving (Dean & Gray, 1990; Riccio & Reynolds, 1998). These domains and the range of methods available for assessment have been identified elsewhere in this volume, as well as in other texts (see Hartlage & Long, 2009; Riccio, 2008, for examples). It is also important to ensure that measures are included that will directly address any *a priori* hypotheses (i.e., hypothesis-driven assessment). The assessment process is hypothesis-driven (Berkelhammer, 2008) to the extent that the methods and measures are selected based on hypotheses regarding the underlying pathology derived from the reason for the referral, the medical history, and any developmental information obtained in advance. With all these considerations, a theoretical model, and hypotheses, the next step is the actual selection of tests to be included, and a discussion of psychometric standards, sensitivity, and specificity.

Test Selection

Cognitive and achievement measures are usually components of a psychoeducational evaluation; they are also components of a neuropsychological assessment. Many cognitive tasks (e.g., those requiring concept formation or reasoning) provide a general sense of CNS integrity. To make a determination of overall functioning, however, it is important to ensure that the results obtained allow for the *evaluation of the four major quadrants of the neocortex* (left, right, anterior, posterior; Reynolds & Mayfield, 1999). Therefore, it is important that the assessment sample the relative efficiency of the right and left hemispheres; this is important in that, to some extent, differing brain systems are involved in each hemisphere. Similarly, the anterior of the brain is generally viewed as subserving differing functions (e.g., regulatory) as opposed to the posterior region of the brain (receptivity). For this reason, anterior–posterior comparisons can provide important information for treatment planning. One reason to be sure to cover all four quadrants is that, regardless of the nature or extent of the injury or disorder, there may be a greater impact on one area of the brain as opposed to others; most cognitive measures do not necessarily tap all four quadrants of the cortex (Reynolds & Mayfield, 1999; Riccio & Reynolds, 1998). Therefore, to accomplish this goal, additional measures are included in the assessment process.

FIXED BATTERY OR FLEXIBLE BATTERY APPROACH

Many clinicians use a predetermined battery of tests for the neuropsychological assessment of children (Koziol & Budding, 2011; Riccio, 2008); this is often referred to as the "fixed battery" or nomothetic approach. Specific fixed batteries such as the Halstead-Reitan Neuropsychological Battery (HRNB; Reitan & Davison, 1974; Reitan & Wolfson, 1985), the Kaplan Baycrest Neurocognitive Assessment (Leach, Kaplan, Rewilak, Richards, & Proulx, 2000), or the Neuropsychological Investigation for the Children, Second Edition (NEPSY-2; Korkman, Kirk, & Kemp, 2007) may be used in neuropsychological assessment in conjunction with cognitive and achievement measures, as well as measures of behavior and personality. These neuropsychological batteries are designed to provide a sampling of sensory and motor functions so that information relating to left/right hemisphere differences and anterior/posterior differences are provided. Furthermore, they are intended to be compatible with the Luria model (Korkman, 1999; Luria, 1980). Of these, the HRNB continues to be one of the most widely used neuropsychological test batteries, but there are concerns with its normative data and the cultural loading of some tasks; if it is going to continue to be useful in clinical practice, it may need to be revised and updated normative data obtained across samples (Sinco, D'Amato, & Davis, 2008).

Alternatively, neuropsychologists may use a flexible battery approach (Koziol & Budding, 2010). With this approach, the neuropsychologist combines a number of tasks (some of which may come from one of the fixed batteries) based on their own training philosophy or a variation in a model; they may use a fixed battery for major components, but supplement it with additional measures. For example, other, but similar measures (e.g., a different trail-making task) may be used instead of the Trails A and B tasks of the HRNB; or specific tasks from the fixed batteries may be combined to provide additional coverage of domains of interest for a given population or related to a particular theoretical model. The selection of tests is then intended to fit that model, but it should also ensure comprehensive coverage of brain function. The theoretical model should lead to accurate predictions about the individual's ability to function in multiple contexts and inform intervention planning (Reynolds, Kamphaus, Rosenthal, & Hiemenz, 1997; Riccio & Reynolds, 1998). This is one of the core assumptions of the Comprehensive Hypothesis Testing model (Hale & Fiorello, 2004; Hale et al., 2003).

With one model, the deficit model, clinicians take a much more idiographic approach and tailor the selection of measures based on the presenting problems of the child, with other measures added based on the child's performance on initial measures (Berkelhammer, 2008; Christensen, 1975; Luria, 1973). This type of approach is intended to isolate the mechanisms that are contributing to a specific, identified problem as part of hypothesis testing. Furthermore, the more idiographic approach may fail to assess domains that are important and will subsequently have an impact on rehabilitation efforts (Riccio & Reynolds, 1998). Alternatively, good organization and planning can identify in advance appropriate measures to accomplish the comprehensive coverage. Ultimately, a clinician could begin with a fixed battery, and then adopt a more idiographic approach to ensure more in-depth coverage of the specific areas of concern or the areas that might not be covered in an existing fixed battery. A concern with regard to the idiographic and flexible battery approaches is the potentially high number of differing normative samples used in generating the scores and the added error variance that can result (Wong, 2006). In some cases, test publishers are choosing to link normative samples of various measures to help address the potential problems in using a flexible or idiographic battery, or even when supplementing the fixed battery with cognitive and achievement testing. The profession, as represented by the various professional organizations, has yet to take a strong position on the issue of whether a fixed battery, flexible battery, or idiographic approach is better; as a result, this tends to vary as a function of clinician training and choice (Wong, 2006).

As noted earlier, even with a fixed battery, there is a need to supplement the battery in order to get a complete picture, including a summary of the child's past history and family system, as well as any other factors that may explain the child's current pattern of functioning. Furthermore, regardless of the type of battery or model one uses, the assessment may or may not include naturalistic observation and informal assessment (Reynolds, 1997); the approach may be standardized or incorporate a process orientation (Kaplan, 1988, 1990; Milberg & Hebben, 2006); the orientation may be more quantitative or more qualitative. In fact, many clinicians prefer a combination of quantitative and qualitative measures to balance the strengths and weaknesses of both approaches; however, reliance on a qualitative approach is not easily replicated and inter-diagnostician agreement may be compromised (Poreh, 2006).

PSYCHOMETRIC CONSIDERATIONS

Although there is much variation in neuropsychological assessment, *it is important to attend to the psychometric properties and limitations of available measures* (Reynolds & Mason, 2009). Neuropsychology, historically, has been criticized for its failure to incorporate psychometric advances in test use and construction (Cicchetti, 1994; Ris & Noll, 1994). One major concern relates to the extent and nature of normative data for many measures used in the neuropsychological assessment of children (Reynolds, 1986a). Sound normative data provide a necessary backdrop with which to validate clinical insight and hypotheses, yet it is often lacking (Reynolds, 1997). Because of the need for adequate normative data, some clinicians advocate the interpretation of traditional measures of cognitive ability (e.g., the Wechsler scales) from a neuropsychological perspective. Concerns and criticisms arise with the re-categorization of subtests from standardized measures that (a) were not developed based on neuropsychological theory, and (b) have not been validated for this purpose (Kamphaus, Petoskey, & Rowe, 2000; Lezak, 1995; Lezak et al., 2004). Others have developed cognitive measures in alignment with neuropsychological models (Das, 2001, 2002; Reynolds et al., 1997).

Not only are normative data oftentimes a concern, but neuropsychologists may overlook the psychometric concepts of reliability and validity, making interpretations based on the "clinical" nature of the tasks. The need for the *establishment of the reliability and validity of scores with differing populations and purposes,* as well as their interpretation related to neuropsychological test performance, has been an important issue in the literature (Reynolds, 1982; Reynolds & Mason, 2009; Riccio & Reynolds, 1998). Reliability is a key component not only in that it is directly related to inter- and intra-individual differences, but also because it is

the foundation for the validity of the test results and conclusions (Reynolds, 1986b). In this regard, the reliability of cross-cultural use of measures continues to be a concern (Smith et al., 2008).

A related concern is the *developmental appropriateness of measures with children.* Unfortunately, many of the measures used with adults are not appropriate to developmental issues, and, as a result, the usefulness of the same procedures used with adults for the neuropsychological assessment of children has multiple pitfalls (Reynolds & Mayfield, 1999; Riccio & Reynolds, 1998). Neuropsychological assessment of children and adolescents requires not only measures that have sufficient empirical support for the inferences being made, but, moreover, it is important to document that the measures are consistent with neurobehavioral and neurodevelopmental functioning in children (Cohen, Branch, Willis, Weyandt, & Hynd, 1992; Reynolds & Mayfield, 1999). Thus, in addition to selecting tests based on psychometric properties, it has been suggested that measures used in the neuropsychological assessment process need to vary along a continuum of difficulty, include both rote and novel tasks, and include variations with regard to processing and response requirements within modalities (Rourke, 1994, 2005).

The sensitivity of a measure is most often in the context of detecting a disorder; in this context, "sensitivity" refers to whether the measure is sensitive to brain damage or dysfunction in a global sense. For measures that purport to reflect more specific brain function, the question is whether the measure is in fact doing just that. Several studies have investigated the "science" behind the use of specific measures (Riccio & Hynd, 2000; Riccio, Reynolds, Lowe, & Moore, 2002). For example, there is evidence that continuous performance tests (CPTs) are *sensitive* to brain dysfunction, with various components of the CPT associated with the neural substrates of attention and inhibition (Riccio et al., 2002). A related aspect is that of specificity. It is not sufficient for measures to be sensitive to brain dysfunction and neurodevelopmental changes. They also need to have *specificity* in order to facilitate differential diagnosis and the identification of specific strengths and weaknesses. For example, the Luria Nebraska Neuropsychological Battery – Children's Revision (LNNB-CR) has been found to be sensitive to deficits in language and rhythm as well as in reading and writing (Geary & Gilger, 1984), and in understanding learning problems (Tramontana, Hooper, Curley, & Nardolillo, 1990); however, the specificity of the LNNB-CR is questionable (Morgan &

Brown, 1988; Snow & Hynd, 1985). Similarly, continuous performance tests generally have a high level of sensitivity, but lack specificity (Riccio et al., 2002). Few studies have examined the sensitivity and specificity of measures cross-culturally. Thus, *it is important to consider the sensitivity and specificity of the measures and methods being used, particularly with regard to cultural and linguistic differences.*

PRACTICAL AND ECOLOGICAL CONSIDERATIONS

As noted earlier, a key principle is the collaboration with and consideration of the school and home contexts. In order to effectively link assessment to intervention in a meaningful manner, it is important to consider all contexts and the child's level(s) of functioning in those contexts. In effect, even if the measures reflect integrity of brain function (or atypicality in brain function), the information obtained may not reflect the child's day-to-day functioning, or what has been referred to as "ecological validity" (Rabin, Burton, & Barr, 2007; Ready, Stierman, & Paulsen, 2001; Sbordone, 2008). It may seem logical to presume, for example, that measures of executive or frontal lobe functioning will *reflect the real world behaviors of the child* (or adult), but in fact, there is little evidence that this is the case. For this reason, it is important to include information from others (parents, teachers) as to daily functioning in the various domains. The Behavior Rating Inventory of Executive Function (BRIEF; Gioia, Isquith, Guy, & Kenworthy, 2000) is one example of a rating scale that can be used to add to the information available from performance-based measures; it has been used effectively to examine day-to-day executive functions in several childhood disorders (Gioia, Isquith, Kenworthy, & Barton, 2002). The Behavior Assessment System for Children–Second Edition (BASC-2; Reynolds & Kamphaus, 2004) also covers these areas in detail, and if used, will negate the need for more specialized scales like the BRIEF.

SOCIAL-EMOTIONAL/PERSONALITY ASPECTS

It is important to *consider social-emotional/personality aspects as a component of the neuropsychological assessment process*, both as part of the case conceptualization and in identifying targets for intervention or treatment. Research consistently demonstrates that adjustment and behavioral problems are associated with children who have neurodevelopmental deficits secondary to, if not as a direct result of, the neurological impairment (Beitchman, Brownlie, &

Wilson, 1996; Breslau & Chilcoat, 2000; Faraone, Biederman, Weber, & Russell, 1998; Miniscalco, Nygren, Hagberg, Kadesjö, & Gillberg, 2006; Teeter et al., 2009). Given this potential for adjustment difficulties a transactional/reciprocal framework is appropriate (Batchelor, 1996; Teeter, 2009). A transactional model takes into consideration the reciprocal interactions of the child; home and family members; teacher and peers; and other social environments in which the child functions.

The family system may be disrupted as a result of a child in the family having a disability; this is most evident with traumatic brain injury (TBI), but is also evident in the family systems of those with neurodevelopmental and congenital disorders. The family may react with denial or may avoid dealing with necessary issues associated with the child's disability; parents' hopes may be discrepant from realistic expectations (Ryan, LaMarche, Barth, & Boll, 1996). The importance of the family system in the long-term recovery and adjustment, as well as the effects of the injury on the family system, have been recognized in the literature (Gan, Campbell, Gemeinhardt, & McFadden, 2006; León-Carrión, Perino, & Zitnay, 2006); although not studied as extensively as with TBI, the family system is an important component to be considered for evaluating any child with a disability (Teeter, 2009). Therefore, some type of assessment (quantitative or qualitative) is needed to determine the impact of the child's functioning level on the family system in order to determine the extent to which family-based intervention should be included as part of the intervention program. At the same time, the supports and services available through the family system need to be identified.

The most common approach to emotional and behavioral assessment relies on published rating scales. A multifaceted (i.e., multi-method, multi-source) approach that includes parent and teacher rating scales, self-report measures, direct observation, and clinical interviews provides the most comprehensive and broad-based view of the child's emotional and behavioral status (Kamphaus & Frick, 2002; McConaughy & Ritter, 2002; Reynolds & Kamphaus, 2004). For example, the BASC-2 includes not only teacher and parent forms, but also a structured observation system (SOS) and, for children over age nine, a self-report measure that can be used to assess emotional and behavioral status effectively. A major advantage to the BASC-2 (rating scales and SOS) is the inclusion of positive adaptive behaviors (e.g., social skills, adaptability to change in the environment) in addition to the more common maladaptive skills included on other rating scales. When adaptive behavior is an identified concern, completion of a more comprehensive adaptive behavior scale may be helpful for intervention planning. With the BASC's second edition, the additional content scales (e.g., Autism, Executive Function) are also helpful.

Inferences and Interpretation

When neuropsychological theory is applied to children and adolescents, the premise that their behavior can be used to make inferences about their brain function and integrity has to be modified to include consideration of neurodevelopmental differences (Hooper & Tramontana, 1997; Koziol & Budding, 2010; Riccio & Reynolds, 1998). "Inference" refers to the process one uses to reach a conclusion on the basis of all available evidence (Fennell & Bauer, 2009). There are multiple levels of inference (Fennell & Bauer, 2009; Hartlage & Long, 2009). The initial or low level of inference involves the dichotomous choice of whether brain dysfunction either is the likely cause or is the contributing factor to the impaired functioning. In contrast, higher levels of inference implicate specific neurological abnormalities (e.g., a tumor, epilepsy) as the causal factor. Most often the inferences made fall somewhere in between, such that based on the data obtained, there is an inferred level of brain integrity or dysfunction with some stated relationship to the child's cognitive or behavioral presentation (Hartlage & Long, 2009).

The inferential process should adhere to some organized set of rules that includes the type of information needed to make an inference, and *the level of inference that can be made based on the data or evidence available, as well as the logical connections that can be made between the data and the conclusions reached* (Fennell & Bauer, 2009). Following from these presumably basic rules, in neuropsychological assessment, the "data available" include all of the available information gathered as part of the assessment process to make inferences about brain function and brain integrity. The extent to which one can reasonably infer that poor performance on a given task is indicative of dysfunction in a specific neurocognitive domain, or inferred to reflect brain function, is highly dependent on the neurological validity (i.e., the extent to which the measure has been shown to reflect specific neurological substrates; or criterion validity), as well as psychological validity (i.e., the extent to which the measure has been

shown to reflect some aspect of functioning in a meaningful way; or ecological validity). Across measures and methods, the extent to which inferences like these can be made differs at various points in development (Fennell & Bauer, 2009). Most importantly, the inferences or hypotheses are generated as a result of information obtained and data obtained. Inference involves an initial hypothesis or hypotheses, which are then tested to determine which one(s) are accurate (i.e., supported by the data). This is the basis of inductive inference, and it underscores the need to include multiple measures that examine the same domain from differing perspectives. This allows the neuropsychologist to examine performance on individual tasks as differing variables that function separately or in combination with other tasks, and the congruence or incongruence of a child's performance across these tasks allows for the inferences to be made about more specific aspects of brain function. At a very simple level, tasks of math calculation, math word problems, and math fluency all target some of the same math skills, but they also vary in some key ways. One may emphasize speed while another emphasizes reasoning; one might be limited to basic math facts with single digits to 10, and one involves more complex calculation problems. Employing a process approach, a fourth task might be added that includes a multiple-choice (recognition) format; alternatively, a fifth task might allow the use of a calculator in order to ascertain if the individual understands the concepts despite not knowing the math facts. Having a combination of tasks allows for some disassociation of the possible factors associated with the area of concern; it further informs the focus of intervention or remediation.

Thus, the cumulative performances of the child on neuropsychological measures are seen as behavioral indicators of brain function (Fennell & Bauer, 2009). The additional areas of functioning included in the neuropsychological assessment are needed to support inferences about the integrity of various functional systems of the brain. Results are interpreted based on functional neuroanatomy and brain development in order to approximate (i.e., hypothesize about) the extent and nature of brain damage or dysfunction while considering the context (Berkelhammer, 2008). As such, inference is the first step in the process of interpretation. The inferential process involves an initial development of hypotheses, as well as the validation of those hypotheses (Fennell & Bauer, 1997, 2009); hence, the hypothesis-driven conceptualization of the assessment process (Berkelhammer, 2008). This inferential process needs to take into consideration not only the type of functional system(s) impaired and the number of systems impaired, but also the characteristics of the impairments (Reynolds & Mayfield, 1999; Riccio & Reynolds, 1998). Additional assumptions in neuropsychology dictate that the measures used as a basis for inference provide valid information (i.e., have demonstrated construct validity), and that the measures provide meaningful information on aspects of the individual's functioning (have ecological validity). Based on all of the data generated in the evaluation process and inferences, hypotheses are generated that are specific as to how and why the individual processes information; hypotheses are also offered as to what areas of functioning are likely to be affected in the future (Berkelhammer, 2008; D'Amato, Rothlisberg, & Rhodes, 1997; Dean, 1986). Information on strengths and weaknesses is then used to generate an appropriate rehabilitation or habilitation plan. The inferential interpretation process is heavily impacted by the neuropsychologist's clinical skills and acumen (Hartlage & Long, 2009).

One inference that may be made is a *general conclusion about integrity of brain function*. This conclusion may be based on the subject's overall performance level across tasks (Reitan, 1986, 1987). For example, one method is the use of criterion or cutoff scores, such that a score above (or below) a criterion is considered indicative of brain damage or impaired function. With increased emphasis on psychometric methods, use of normative data, and measures that provide valid and reliable results are emphasized in the contemporary literature, the use of a criterion score is not seen as strong evidence for the inference. This is particularly critical when working with individuals from diverse backgrounds and individuals who were not part of the sampling process (Llorente, 2008). With the actuarial or normative model, conclusions are reached based on a comparison of the child's overall level of performance to normative data. There are multiple problems with this model as well, including the variability among typically developing children, insensitivity for individuals with higher cognitive abilities, and a tendency to yield a high number of false positives due to the potential impact of fatigue and motivation on test performance (Nussbaum & Bigler, 1997; Reitan & Wolfson, 1985).

Another inferential model used in interpretation examines performance patterns across tasks (Reitan, 1986, 1987) as a means of differentiating functional from dysfunctional neural systems; this may incorporate examination of intra-individual differences or *asymmetry* (i.e., lateralization of function; Reitan, 1986, 1987). Examination of intra-individual differences allows for identification of strengths as well as weaknesses; emphasis on a strength model for intervention planning is viewed as more efficacious than focusing only on deficits (Reynolds et al., 1997). Again, this is usually addressed in terms of *anterior-posterior differences* or *left-right differences*, rather than on consideration of single scores, but it also may be done by comparison of auditory/linguistic, visual/spatial, and domains of function that parallel the four quadrants.

Another model of interpretation involves looking for, or identifying, what are called "pathognomonic signs or clear signs of brain damage of some kind (Fennell & Bauer, 2009; Kaplan, 1988; Lezak et al., 2004; Reitan, 1986, 1987; Spreen et al., 1995). While this method has been used reliably with adult populations, the reliability of this approach with children has not been demonstrated (Batchelor, 1996). Similarly, the reliability of profile analysis has not been consistently demonstrated (Iverson, Brooks, & Holdnack, 2008; Reynolds, 2007; Watkins, Glutting, & Youngstrom, 2005). In practice, clinicians use any one or some combination of these features (Reitan, 1986, 1987; Riccio & Reynolds, 1998) in the interpretation process, including clinical judgement. The extent to which a clinician relies on the features with less scientific basis or reliability will in turn affect the accuracy of the resulting interpretation (Fennell & Bauer, 2009).

A major component to the interpretation process is the *identification of the child's specific deficits* as well as the *identification of any intact complex functional systems*. Along with the identification of deficits, depending on their number and severity, it may be necessary to prioritize these in terms of their importance in the settings in which the child is expected to function (home and school). Consideration of strengths may help inform which specific evidence-based practices may be most likely to be successful for a given child. The specific goals and objectives, as well as recommendations for intervention, also need to be responsive to the information obtained regarding the home and school contexts, the clients' expectations, and the resources available (Riccio & Reynolds, 1998).

Communicating the Results and Recommendations

Whichever model one uses, whether measures or methods, it is important that the information obtained be understood not only by medical professionals, but by all stakeholders. A critical issue that continues to be a problem is the translation of knowledge from neuropsychology (the science component) to the contexts in which children function (the practice piece). There is a definite need to ensure that information garnered from neuropsychological assessment be useful to the consumers receiving the information—the parents, the schools, and the physician. One factor that may contribute to the impression that neuropsychological assessment does not transfer into rehabilitation programming may be that, all too often, neuropsychological reports are written expressly for medical personnel or acute-care facilities from a biomedical model (Fletcher-Janzen & Kade, 1997). Thus, *test results need to be presented in such a way that all stakeholders (including parents and educators) can understand both the abilities and the problems of their child.* Teachers, as well as parents, look to the report for information regarding the child's current status; they also may be concerned with the potential trajectory and prognosis. As noted by others (e.g., Reynolds & Mayfield, 1999), reports should be written in language that is easily understood, and concrete examples or explanations should be provided. The focus of the report should be on the child and the child's level of functioning, as opposed to the tests or psychometric studies. The report should clearly *link the strengths and weaknesses with the child's functioning in real-world situations.* This is consistent with the trend toward consideration of strengths and weaknesses in determination of specific learning disabilities (Hale et al., 2010).

Finally, based on the information gleaned, recommendations for appropriate interventions need to be provided. Recommendations need to include information specific to whether the child would seem most likely to benefit from remediation, compensatory training, or some combination of both; this may vary from one deficient skill area to another. Potential instructional materials or methods that may be best suited to the child should also be indicated. Neuropsychological results provide information relating to the appropriateness of using specific types of interventions, such as neurocognitive therapy, or for a specific group of interventions, such as cognitive behavioral therapy (Reynolds & Mayfield, 1999). Recommendations need to be viewed as flexible with a broad scope that is efficient, integrated, and promotes growth (Fletcher-Janzen & Kade, 1997). Based on assessment of the specific contexts for a given child,

environmental modifications that may facilitate the child's academic progress and that are reasonable need to be identified. These often take the form of extended time for test-taking, options for oral testing, preferential seating, and decreased extraneous information. These also may include the use of any of a number of educational support materials (e.g., computers, calculators, tape recorders, audiotapes). As noted earlier, involvement of school personnel and family members as part of the assessment process increases the likelihood of their involvement in the service delivery. Their early involvement increases the likelihood that they will be involved and work to ensure the child receives the necessary and broad-based services (Fletcher-Janzen & Kade, 1997. Recommendations provided in the neuropsychological report relating to intervention and instruction may not be exhaustive; however, enough information should be provided from the assessment to assist in developing the appropriate intervention to meet the needs of the individual child. With the current climate, it is important to identify the evidence-based practices that have support for children with neurodevelopmental disorders.

Conclusions

Neuropsychological assessment, and the field of clinical child neuropsychology in general, have much to offer in the way of understanding the learning and behavior problems of children and youth. It is important, however, that those conducting the assessment adhere to the basic ethical principles, as well as to basic principles that apply only to neuropsychological assessment. At the same time, while there have been significant advances in the knowledge base and a proliferation of measures and methods in neuropsychology, there are continued problems with the application of neuropsychological practices and perspectives to child assessment. Historically, neuropsychological assessment of children has taken its lead from research and practice with adults, and predominantly adults with acquired brain damage (Riccio & Reynolds, 1998). Issues relating to developmental issues, manifestation of developmental disorders over time, and the varying contexts in which children function, make this approach untenable. Furthermore, the continued methodological and measurement problems impede progress in the field of child neuropsychology, affect the accuracy of diagnosis, and pose serious problems for clinical practice (Reynolds, 1986a; Riccio & Reynolds, 1998).

Future Directions

Child neuropsychology has made significant contributions to our understanding of children; neuropsychological assessment has the potential to contribute in the context of special education decision-making and intervention-planning, as well as to the understanding of specific disorders (Augustyniak, Murphy, & Phillips, 2005; Feagans, Short, & Meltzer, 1991; Goldstein & Naglieri, 2008; Hale et al., 2010; Hendriksen et al., 2007; Peters, Fox, Weber, & Llorente, 2005; Riccio, Gonzales, & Hynd, 1994; Riccio & Hynd, 1995; Schwarte, 2008). Further research and study of the linkage between neuropsychological assessment of children and the provision of information that is educationally relevant rather than medically focused for intervention planning is needed. With recent trends toward a Response to Intervention (RTI) approach to identification of children with disabilities, there has been increased discussion of how neuropsychology and neuropsychological assessment will fit in this model (Fletcher-Janzen & Reynolds, 2008). At its core, the RTI model is not focusing on a specific disorder, syndrome, or disease, but whether the child makes expected gains as a result of an intervention. The RTI approach may be adequate for *describing* the child's performance, but it may fall short in terms of *explaining* the child's performance or deficits; in effect, it does not answer the question of why the child did not respond to the intervention.

Using a Lurian perspective, there are still many unanswered questions regarding the developmental progression of many functional systems. Furthermore, how the neurodevelopmental progression maps onto cognitive functioning is not fully understood. This is an area that is in need of additional research with attention to the sensitivity of various measures and methods to subtle impairments, as well as change over time. This will require longitudinal research that looks at the performance across domains not only of children with neurodevelopmental disorders, but also of those who appear to be developing normally. For prevention, as well as intervention, purposes, identification of critical developmental periods, with the establishment of basic screening (i.e., benchmarking) prior to or at these critical times may be warranted.

References

American Psychological Association (2002). *Ethical principles of psychologists and code of conduct*. Washington, DC: APA.

Augustyniak, K., Murphy, J., & Phillips, D. K. (2005). Psychological perspectives in assessing mathematics learning needs. *Journal of Instructional Psychology, 32,* 277–286.

Ballantyne, A. O., Spilkin, A. M., & Trauner, D. A. (2007). Language outcome after perinatal stroke: Does side matter? *Child Neuropsychology, 13,* 494–509.

Batchelor, E. S. (1996). Neuropsychological assessment of children. In J. E. S. Batchelor & R. S. Dean (Eds.), *Pediatric neuropsychology: Interfacing assessment and treatment for rehabilitation* (pp. 9–26). Boston: Allyn & Bacon.

Beitchman, J. H., Brownlie, E. B., & Wilson, B. (1996). Linguistic impairment and psychiatric disorder: Pathways to outcome. In J. H. Beitchman, N. J. Cohen, M. M. Konstantareas, & R. Tannock (Eds.), *Language, learning, and behavior disorders: Developmental, biological, and clinical perspectives* (pp. 493–514). New York: Cambridge University Press.

Berkelhammer, L. D. (2008). Pediatric neuropsychological evaluation. In M. Herson & A. M. Gross (Eds.), *Handbook of clinical psychology* (pp. 497–519). Hoboken, NJ: Wiley.

Bieliauskas, L. A. (2008). The preparation of the clinical neuropsychologist: Contemporary training models and specialization. In J. E. Morgan & J. H. Ricker (Eds.), *Textbook of clinical neuropsychology. Studies on neuropsychology, neurology, and cognition* (pp. 18–24). New York: Psychology Press.

Board of Directors AACN (2007). American Academy of Clinical Neuropsychology (AACN) practice guidelines for neuropsychological assessment and consultation. *The Clinical Neuropsychologist, 21,* 209–231.

Breslau, N., & Chilcoat, H. D. (2000). Psychiatric sequelae of low birth weight at 11 years of age. *Biological Psychiatry, 47,* 662–668.

Brickman, A. M., Cabo, R., & Manly, J. J. (2006). Ethical issues in cross-cultural neuropsychology. *Applied Neuropsychology, 13,* 91–100.

Bush, S. S. (2005). *A casebook of ethical challenges in neuropsychology.* New York: Psychology Press.

Bush, S. S., & Martin, T. A. (2008). Confidentiality in neuropsychological practice. In A. M. Horton & D. Wedding (Eds.), *The neuropsychology handbook* (3rd ed.; pp. 515–530). New York: Springer.

Byrd, D., Arentoft, A., Scheiner, D., Westerveld, M., & Baron, I. S. (2008). State of multicultural neuropsychological assessment in children: Current research issues. *Neuropsychology Review, 18,* 214–222.

Carter, J. C., Capone, G. T., Kaufmann, W. E. (2008). Neuroanatomic correlates of autism and stereotypy in children with Down syndrome. *NeuroReport, 19,* 653–656.

Chiarello, C., Kacinik, N., Manowitz, B., Otto, R., & Leonard, C. (2004). Cerebral asymmetries for language: Evidence for structural-behavioral correlations. *Neuropsychology, 18,* 219–231.

Christensen, A. L. (1975). *Luria's neuropsychological investigation.* New York: Spectrum.

Cicchetti, D. V. (1994). Multiple comparison methods: Establishing guidelines for their valid application in neuropsychological research. *Journal of Clinical and Experimental Neuropsychology, 16,* 155–161.

Cohen, M. J., Branch, W. B., Willis, W. G., Weyandt, L. L., & Hynd, G. W. (1992). Childhood. In A. E. Puente & R. J. McCaffrey (Eds.), *Handbook of neuropsychological assessment* (pp. 49–79). New York: Plenum.

Cohen, M. J., Hall, J., & Riccio, C. A. (1997). Neuropsychological profiles of children diagnosed as specific language impaired with and without hyperlexia. *Archives of Clinical Neuropsychology, 12,* 223–229.

Cohen, M. J., Riccio, C. A., & Hynd, G. W. (1999). Children with specific language impairment: Quantitative analysis of dichotic listening performance. *Developmental Neuropsychology, 16,* 243–252.

D'Amato, R. C., Rothlisberg, B. A., & Rhodes, R. L. (1997). Utilizing neuropsychological paradigms for understanding common educational and psychological tests. In C. R. Reynolds & E. Fletcher-Janzen (Eds.), *Handbook of clinical child neuropsychology* (2nd ed.; pp. 270–295). New York: Plenum.

Das, J. P. (2001). Reconceptualizing intelligence: Luria's contributions. *Psychological Studies, 46,* 1–6.

Das, J. P. (2002). A better look at intelligence. *Current Directions in Psychological Science, 11,* 28–33.

Dean, R. S. (1986). Lateralization of cerebral functions. In D. Wedding, A. M. Horton, & J. S. Webster (Eds.), *The neuropsychology handbook: Behavioral and clinical perspectives* (pp. 80–102). Berlin: Springer-Verlag.

Dean, R. S., & Gray, J. W. (1990). Traditional approaches to neuropsychological assessment. In C. R. Reynolds & R. W. Kamphaus (Eds.), *Handbook of psychological and educational assessment of children* (pp. 317–388). New York: Guilford.

Faraone, S. V., Biederman, J., Weber, W., & Russell, R. L. (1998). Psychiatric, neuropsychological, and psychosocial features of DSM-IV subtypes of Attention-Deficit/Hyperactivity Disorder: Results from a clinically referred sample. *Journal of the American Academy of Child & Adolescent Psychiatry, 37,* 185–193.

Feagans, L. V., Short, E., & Meltzer, L. J. (1991). *Subtypes of learning disabilities: Theoretical perspectives and research.* Hillsdale, NJ: Erlbaum.

Fennell, E. B., & Bauer, R. M. (1997). Models of inference in evaluating brain–behavior relationships in children. In C. R. Reynolds & E. Fletcher-Janzen (Eds.), *Handbook of clinical child neuropsychology.* New York: Plenum.

Fennell, E. B., & Bauer, R. M. (2009). Models of inference in evaluating brain–behavior relationships in children. In C. R. Reynolds & E. Fletcher-Janzen (Eds.), *Handbook of clinical child neuropsychology* (pp. 231–246). New York: Springer.

Fletcher-Janzen, E., & Kade, H. D. (1997). Pediatric brain injury rehabilitation in a neurodevelopmental milieu. In C. R. Reynolds & E. Fletcher-Janzen (Eds.), *Handbook of clinical child neuropsychology* (2nd ed.; pp. 452–481). New York: Plenum.

Fletcher-Janzen, E., & Reynolds, C. R. (2008). *Neuropsychological perspectives on learning disabilities in the era of RTI: Recommendations for diagnosis and intervention.* Hoboken, NJ: Wiley.

Gan, C., Campbell, K. A., Gemeinhardt, M., & McFadden, G. T. (2006). Predictors of family system functioning after brain injury. *Brain Injury, 20,* 587–600.

Geary, D. C., & Gilger, J. W. (1984). The Luria-Nebraska neuropsychological battery—children's revision: Comparison of learning disabled and normal children matched on full scale IQ. *Perceptual and Motor Skills, 58,* 115–118.

Gioia, G. A., Isquith, P. K., Guy, S. C., & Kenworthy, L. (2000). *Behavior Rating Inventory of Executive Function manual.* Odessa, FL: Psychological Assessment Resources.

Gioia, G. A., Isquith, P. K., Kenworthy, L., & Barton, R. M. (2002). Profiles of everyday executive function in acquired and developmental disorders. *Child Neuropsychology, 8,* 121–137.

Goldstein, S., & Naglieri, J. A. (2008). The school neuropsychology of ADHD: Theory, assessment, and intervention. *Psychology in the Schools, 45,* 859–874.

Hale, J., Alfonso, V., Berninger, V., Bracken, B., Christo, C., Clark, M., et al.(2010). Critical issues in response to intervention, comprehensive evaluation, and specific learning disabilities identification and intervention: An expert white paper consensus. *Learning Disability Quarterly, 33,* 1–14.

Hale, J. B., & Fiorello, C. A. (2004). *School neuropsychology: A practitioner's handbook.* New York: Guilford.

Hale, J. B., Fiorello, C. A., Bertin, M., & Sherman, R. (2003). Predicting math achievement through neuropsychological interpretation of WISC-III variance components. *Journal of Psychoeducational Assessment, 21*(4), 358–380.

Hannay, H. J., Bielasukas, L. A., Crosson, B., Hammeke, T. A., Hamsher, K. d., & Koffler, S. P. (1998). Proceedings: The Houston conference on specialty education and training in clinical neuropsychology. *Archives of Clinical Neuropsychology, 13,* 157–250.

Harris, J. G., Wagner, B., & Cullum, C. M. (2007). Symbol vs. digit substitution task performance in diverse cultural and linguistic groups. *The Clinical Neuropsychologist, 21,* 800–810.

Hartlage, L. C., & Long, C. J. (2009). Development of neuropsychology as a professional psychological specialty: History, training, and credentialing. In C. R. Reynolds & E. Fletcher-Janzen (Eds.), *Handbook of clinical child neuropsychology* (pp. 3–18). New York: Springer.

Heilbrun, K., Marczyk, G. R., DeMatteo, D., Zillmer, E. A., Harris, J., & Jennings, T. (2003). Principles of forensic mental health assessment: Implications for neuropsychological assessment in forensic contexts. *Assessment, 10,* 329–343.

Hendriksen, J. G. M., Keulers, E. H. H., Feron, F. J. M., Wassenberg, R., Jolles, J., & Vles, J. S. H. (2007). Subtypes of learning disabilities: Neuropsychological and behavioural functioning of 495 children referred for multidisciplinary assessment. *European Child & Adolescent Psychiatry, 16,* 517–524.

Iacoboni, M., & Mazziotta, J. C. (2007). Mirror neuron system: Basic findings and clinical applications. *Annals of Neurology, 62,* 213–218.

Im-Bolter, N., Johnson, J., & Pascual-Leone, J. (2006). Processing limitations in children with specific language impairment: The role of executive function. *Child Development, 77,* 1822–1841.

Iverson, G. L., Brooks, B. L., & Holdnack, J. A. (2008). Misdiagnosis of cognitive impairment in forensic neuropsychology. In R. L. Heilbronner (Ed.), *Neuropsychology in the courtroom: Expert analysis of reports and testimony* (pp. 243–266). New York: Guilford.

Jacob, S., & Hartshorne, T. S. (2007). *Ethics and law for school psychologists* (5th ed.). Hoboken, NJ: Wiley.

Judd, T., Capetillo, D., Carrión-Baralt, J., Mármol, L. M., San Miguel-Montes, L., Navarrete, M. G., et al. (2009). Professional considerations for improving the neuropsychological evaluations of Hispanics: A National Academy of Neuropsychology education paper. *Archives of Clinical Neuropsychology, 24,* 127–135.

Kamphaus, R. W., & Frick, P. J. (2002). *Clinical assessment of child and adolescent personality and behavior* (2nd ed.). Boston: Allyn & Bacon.

Kamphaus, R. W., Petoskey, M. D., & Rowe, E. W. (2000). Current trends in psychological testing of children. *Professional Psychology: Research and Practice, 31,* 155–164.

Kaplan, E. (1988). A process approach to neuropsychological assessment. In T. Boll & B. K. Bryant (Eds.), *Clinical* neuropsychology and brain function (pp. 125–167). Washington, DC: American Psychological Association.

Kaplan, E. (1990). The process approach to neuropsychological assessment of psychiatric patients. *Journal of Neuropsychiatry*, 2(1), 72–87.

Kleinhans, N. M., Müller, R.-A., Cohen, D. N., & Courchesne, E. (2008). Atypical functional lateralization of language in autism spectrum disorders. *Brain Research*, *1221*, 115–125.

Korkman, M. (1999). Applying Luria's diagnostic principles in the neuropsychological assessment of children. *Neuropsychology Review*, *9*, 89–105.

Korkman, M., Kirk, U., & Kemp, S. (2007). *NEPSY* (2nd ed.). San Antonio, TX: Pearson.

Kotik-Friedgut, B. (2006). Development of the Lurian approach: A cultural neurolinguistic perspective. *Neuropsychology Review*, *16*, 43–52.

Koziol, L. F., & Budding, D. E. (2011). Pediatric neuropsychological testing: Theoretical models of test selection and interpretation. In A. S. Davis (Ed.), *Handbook of pediatric neuropsychology* (pp. 443–455). New York: Springer.

Krain, A. L., & Castellanos, F. X. (2006). Brain development and ADHD. *Clinical Psychology Review*, *26*, 433–444.

Leach, L., Kaplan, E., Rewilak, D., Richards, P. M., & Proulx, G.-B. (2000). *Kaplan-Baycrest neurocognitive assessment manual*. San Antonio, TX: The Psychological Corporation.

León-Carrión, J., Perino, C., & Zitnay, G. A. (2006). The role of family in the rehabilitation of traumatic brain injury patients: Advocate or co-therapist. In J. León-Carrión, K. R. H. von Wild, & G. A. Zitnay (Eds.), *Brain injury treatment: Theories and practices. Studies on neuropsychology, neurology, and cognition* (pp. 513–526). Philadelphia, PA: Taylor & Francis.

Lezak, M. D. (1995). *Neuropsychological assessment*. New York: Oxford

Lezak, M. D., Howieson, D. B., & Loring, D. W. (2004). *Neuropsychological assessment*. New York: Oxford.

Llorente, A. M. (2008). *Principles of neuropsychological assessment with Hispanics: Theoretical foundations and clinical practice*. New York: Springer.

Luria, A. R. (1973). *The working brain*. New York: Basic.

Luria, A. R. (1980). *Higher cortical functions in man* (2nd ed.). New York: Basic Books.

Martel, M., Nikolas, M., & Nigg, J. T. (2007). Executive function in adolescents with ADHD. *Journal of the American Academy of Child and Adolescent Psychiatry*, *46*, 1437–1444.

McConaughy, S. H., & Ritter, D. R. (2002). Best practices in multidimensional assessment of emotional or behavioral disorders. In A. Thomas & J. Grimes (Eds.), *Best practices in school psychology IV* (pp. 1303–1320). Bethesda, MD: National Association of School Psychologists.

Mendola, P., Selevan, S. G., Gutter, S., & Rice, D. (2002). Environmental factors associated with a spectrum of neurodevelopmental deficits. *Mental Retardation and Developmental Disabilities Research Reviews*, *8*, 188–197.

Milberg, W., & Hebben, N. (2006). The historical antecedents of the Boston Process Approach. In A. M. Poreh (Ed.), *The quantified process approach to neuropsychological assessment. Studies on neuropsychology, neurology and cognition* (pp. 17–25). Philadelphia, PA: Taylor & Francis.

Miniscalco, C., Nygren, G., Hagberg, B., Kadesjö, B., & Gillberg, C. (2006). Neuropsychiatric and neurodevelopmental outcome of children at age 6 and 7 years who screened positive language problems at 30 months. *Developmental Medicine & Child Neurology*, *48*, 361–366.

Moberg, P. J., & Kniele, K. (2006). Evaluation of competency: Ethical considerations for neuropsychologists. *Applied Neuropsychology*, *13*, 101–114.

Morgan, S. B., & Brown, T. L. (1988). Luria-Nebraska Neuropsychological Battery—Children's Revision: Concurrent validity with three learning disability subtypes. *Journal of Consulting and Clinical Psychology*, *56*, 463–466.

Mudrick, N. R. (2002). The prevalence of disability among children: Paradigms and estimates. *Physical Medical Rehabilitation Clinics of North America*, *13*, 775–792.

Naglieri, J. A., Conway, C., & Goldstein, S. (2009). Using the planning, attention, simultaneous, successive (PASS) theory within a neuropsychological context. In C. R. Reynolds & E. Fletcher-Janzen (Eds.), *Handbook of clinical child neuropsychology* (pp. 783–800). New York: Springer.

Nussbaum, N. L., & Bigler, E. D. (1997). Halstead-Reitan neuropsychological test batteries for children. In C. R. Reynolds & E. Fletcher-Janzen (Eds.), *Handbook of clinical child neuropsychology* (2nd ed.; pp. 219–236). New York: Plenum.

Oberman, L. M., Ramachandran, V. S., & Pineda, J. A. (2008). Modulation of mu suppression in children with autism spectrum disorders in response to familiar and unfamiliar stimuli: The mirror neuron hypothesis. *Neuropsychologia*, *46*, 1558–1565.

Peters, S. A., Fox, J. L., Weber, D. A., & Llorente, A. M. (2005). Applied and theoretical contributions of neuropsychology to assessment in multicultural school psychology. In C. L. Frisby & C. R. Reynolds (Eds.), *Comprehensive handbook of multicultural school psychology* (pp. 841–860). Hoboken, NJ: Wiley.

Poreh, A. M. (2006). Methodological quandaries of the Quantified Process Approach. In A. M. Poreh (Ed.), *The quantified process approach to neuropsychological assessment. Studies on neuropsychology, neurology and cognition* (pp. 27–41). Philadelphia, PA: Taylor & Francis.

Rabin, L. A., Barr, W. B., & Burton, L. A. (2005). Assessment practices of clinical neuropsychologists in the United States and Canada: A survey of INS, NAN, and APA Division 40 members. *Archives of Clinical Neuropsychology*, *20*, 33–65.

Rabin, L. A., Burton, L. A., & Barr, W. B. (2007). Utilization rates of ecologically oriented instruments among clinical neuropsychologists. *The Clinical Neuropsychologist*, *21*, 727–743.

Ready, R. E., Stierman, L., & Paulsen, J. S. (2001). Ecological validity of neuropsychological and personality measures of executive function. *The Clinical Neuropsychologist*, *15*, 314–323.

Reitan, R. M. (1986). *Theoretical and methodological bases of the Halstead-Reitan Neuropsychological Test Battery*. Tucson, AZ: Neuropsychological Press.

Reitan, R. M. (1987). *Neuropsychological evaluation of children*. Tucson, AZ:: Neuropsychological Press.

Reitan, R. M., & Davison, L. A. (1974). *Clinical neuropsychology: Current status and applications*. Washington, DC: V. H. Winston.

Reitan, R. M., & Wolfson, D. (1985). *The Halstead Reitan neuropsychological battery: Theory and clinical interpretation*. Tucson, AZ: Neuropsychological Press.

Reynolds, C. R. (1982). The importance of norms and other traditional psychometric concepts to assessment in clinical neuropsychology. In R. N. Malathesha & L. C. Hartlage (Eds.), *Neuropsychology and cognition* (Vol. III; pp. 55–76). The Hague, The Netherlands: Nijhoff.

Reynolds, C. R. (1986a). Clinical acumen but psychometric naiveté in neuropsychological assessment of educational disorders. *Archives of Clinical Neuropsychology, 1,* 121–137.

Reynolds, C. R. (1986b). Transactional models of intellectual development, yes. Deficit models of process remediation, no. *School Psychology Review, 15,* 256–260.

Reynolds, C. R. (1997). Measurement and statistical problems in neuropsychological assessment of children. In C. R. Reynolds & E. Fletcher-Jantzen (Eds.), *Handbook of clinical child neuropsychology* (2nd ed.; pp. 180–203). New York: Plenum.

Reynolds, C. R. (2007). Subtest level profile analysis of intelligence tests: Editor's remarks and introduction. *Applied Neuropsychology, 14,* 1.

Reynolds, C. R., & Kamphaus, R. W. (2004). *Behavior assessment system for children* (2nd ed.). Circle Pines, MN: American Guidance Service.

Reynolds, C. R., Kamphaus, R. W., Rosenthal, B. L., & Hiemenz, J. R. (1997). Application of the Kaufman assessment battery for children (KABC) in neuropsychological assessment. In C. R. Reynolds & E. Fletcher-Janzen (Eds.), *Handbook of clinical child neuropsychology* (2nd ed.; pp. 252–269). New York: Plenum.

Reynolds, C. R., & Mason, B. A. (2009). Measurement and statistical problems in neuropsychological assessment of children. In C. R. Reynolds & E. Fletcher-Janzen (Eds.), *Handbook of clinical child neuropsychology* (pp. 203–230). New York: Springer.

Reynolds, C. R., & Mayfield, J. W. (1999). Neuropsychological assessment in genetically linked neurodevelopmental disorders. In S. Goldstein & C. R. Reynolds (Eds.), *Handbook of neurodevelopmental and genetic disorders in children* (pp. 9–37). New York: Guilford.

Riccio, C. A. (2008). A descriptive summary of essential neuropsychological tests. In R. C. D'Amato & L. C. Hartlage (Eds.), *Essentials of neuropsychological assessment: Treatment planning and for rehabilitation* (2nd ed.; pp. 207–242). New York: Springer.

Riccio, C. A., Gonzales, J. J., & Hynd, G. W. (1994). Attention-deficit hyperactivity disorder (ADHD) and learning disabilities. *Learning Disabilities Quarterly, 17,* 311–322.

Riccio, C. A., & Hynd, G. W. (1995). Contributions of neuropsychology to our understanding of developmental reading problems. *School Psychology Review, 24,* 415–425.

Riccio, C. A., & Hynd, G. W. (2000). Measurable biological substrates to verbal performance differences in Wechsler scales. *School Psychology Quarterly, 15,* 389–399.

Riccio, C. A., & Reynolds, C. R. (1998). Neuropsychological assessment of children. In C. R. Reynolds (Ed.), *Comprehensive clinical psychology* (Vol. 4; pp. 267–301). Oxford: Elsevier.

Riccio, C. A., Reynolds, C. R., Lowe, P. A., & Moore, J. J. (2002). The continuous performance test: A window on the neural substrates for attention? *Archives of Clinical Neuropsychology, 17,* 235–272.

Ris, M. D., & Noll, R. B. (1994). Long-term neurobehavioral outcome in pediatric brain-tumor patients: Review and methodological critique. *Journal of Clinical and Experimental Neuropsychology, 16,* 21–42.

Rosenthal, S. L., Cohen, S. S., & Simeonsson, R. J. (2001). Assessment of family context. In R. J. Simeonsson & S. L. Rosenthal (Eds.), *Psychological and developmental assessment* (pp. 141–152). New York: Guilford.

Rourke, B. P. (1994). Neuropsychological assessment of children with learning disabilities: Measurement issues. In G. R. Lyon (Ed.), *Frames of reference for the assessment of learning disabilities: New views on measurement issues* (pp. 475–514). Baltimore, MD: Brookes.

Rourke, B. P. (2005). Neuropsychology of learning disabilities: Past and future. *Learning Disability Quarterly, 28,* 111–114.

Ryan, T. V., LaMarche, J. A., Barth, J. T., & Boll, T. J. (1996). Neuropsychological consequences and treatment of pediatric head trauma. In E. S. Batchelor & R. S. Dean (Eds.), *Pediatric neuropsychology* (pp. 117–137). New York: Pergamon.

Sbordone, R. J. (2008). Ecological validity of neuropsychological testing: Critical issues. In A. M. Horton & D. Wedding (Eds.), *The neuropsychology handbook* (3rd ed.; pp. 367–394). New York: Springer.

Schwarte, A. R. (2008). Fragile X syndrome. *School Psychology Quarterly, 23,* 290–300.

Seidman, L. J. (2006). Neuropsychological functioning in people with ADHD across the lifespan. *Clinical Psychology Review, 26,* 466–485.

Simeonsson, R. J., & Rosenthal, S. L. (2001). Clinical assessment of children: An overview. In R. Simeonsson & S. L. Rosenthal (Eds.), *Psychological and developmental assessment* (pp. 1–16). New York: Guilford.

Sinco, S. R., D'Amato, R. C., & Davis, A. S. (2008). Understanding and using the Halstead-Reitan Neuropsychological Test Batteries with children and adults. In R. C. D'Amato & L. C. Hartlage (Eds.), *Essentials of neuropsychological assessment: Treatment planning for rehabilitation* (pp. 105–125). New York: Springer.

Smith, P., Lane, E., & Llorente, A. M. (2008). Hispanics and cultural bias: Test development and applications. In A. M. Llorente (Ed.), *Principles of neuropsychological assessment with Hispanics: Theoretical foundations and clinical practice. Issues of diversity in clinical neuropsychology* (pp. 136–163). New York: Springer.

Snow, J. H., & Hynd, G. W. (1985). A multivariate investigation of the Luria-Nebraska Neuropsychological Battery—Children's Revision with learning disabled children. *Journal of Psychoeducational Assessment, 2,* 23–28.

Spreen, O., Risser, A. H., & Edgell, D. (1995). *Developmental neuropsychology.* London: Oxford University Press.

Stuss, D. T., & Levine, B. (2002). Adult clinical neuropsychology: Lessons from studies of the frontal lobes. *Annual Review of Psychology, 53,* 401–433.

Teeter, P. A. (2009). Neurocognitive interventions for childhood and adolescent disorders: A transactional model. In C. R. Reynolds & E. Fletcher-Janzen (Eds.), *Handbook of clinical child neuropsychology* (pp. 427–458). New York: Springer.

Teeter, P. A., Eckert, L., Nelson, A., Platten, P., Semrud-Clikeman, M., & Kamphaus, R. W. (2009). Assessment of behavior and personality in the neuropsychological diagnosis of children. In C. R. Reynolds & E. Fletcher-Janzen (Eds.), *Handbook of clinical child neuropsychology* (pp. 349–382). New York: Springer.

Tramontana, M., Hooper, S. R., Curley, A. S., & Nardolillo, E. M. (1990). Determinants of academic achievement in children with psychiatric disorders. *Journal of the American Academy of Child & Adolescent Psychiatry, 29,* 265–268.

Verte, S., Geurts, H. M., Roeyers, H., Oosterlaan, J., & Sergeant, J. A. (2005). Executive functioning in children with autism and Tourette syndrome. *Development and Psychopathology, 17*, 415–445.

Watkins, M. W., Glutting, J. J., & Youngstrom, E. (2005). Issues in subtest profile analysis. In D. P. Flanagan & P. L. Harrison (Eds.), *Contemporary intellectual assessment* (pp. 251–268). New York: Guilford.

Wills, K. (2008). A pediatric neuropsychologist's lessons from "independent educational evaluations: Respect parents, listen to teachers, do your homework, but think for yourself. In R. L. Heilbronner (Ed.), *Neuropsychology in the courtroom: Expert analysis of reports and testimony* (pp. 170–198). New York: Guilford.

Wong, T. M. (2006). Ethical controversies in neuropsychological test selection, administration, and interpretation. *Applied Neuropsychology, 13*(2), 68–76.

Models for the Personality Assessment of Children and Adolescents

Donald H. Saklofske, Diana K. Joyce, Michael L. Sulkowski, *and* Emma A. Climie

Abstract

Personality theories hold a central position in the study of individual differences, from models outlining the underlying factors of personality to understanding "how we are both like others and yet unique." Notably, the effort invested by psychologists in the research of personality rivals that directed at intelligence. However, much of the focus has been on adult personality with the assumption that personality formation in childhood is more variable and thus less psychologically-relevant than other developmental domains. Conversely, research has demonstrated that personality, although somewhat dynamic in childhood and adolescence, is clearly present and measureable at these earlier ages, particularly traits such as extraversion and neuroticism. Furthermore, temperament has received considerable recent study and it is shown to be reliably defined even in very young infants. This chapter reviews the personality trait and temperament literature with particular attention to personality assessment.

Key Words: Personality assessment, children, adolescents, personality theory, temperament

Introduction

Psychological assessment of children and adolescents is challenging for many reasons. Gaining an accurate understanding of a child's psychological characteristics and traits requires that a trained clinician use appropriate methods including standardized tests, questionnaires, observation, and interviews. The significance of personality traits in a description of individual differences is as important as intelligence or conative measures such as motivation and self-efficacy. There is a pressing need to better understand the personality types of adolescents and the emerging personalities of preadolescent children, especially for those who may be experiencing psychological challenges. It is also important to understand that adolescents are not simply viewed as "mini-adults." Thus, merely modifying existing adult personality measures through simplifying and reducing the number of

questions or adapting and creating new norm sets will not provide an accurate understanding of the complexities of adolescent development (McCann, 2008).

Although personality assessment measures for children are gaining more widespread use in schools, mental health facilities, hospitals, and forensic settings, a strong theoretical understanding of the development of children's personality styles and what the research evidence indicates is important in any clinical assessment. The assessment of personality provides complex challenges as a variety of factors must be considered in the creation of personality measures. These measures must be grounded in a solid theoretical foundation that allows for individual differences in measurement and the research-based findings that personality and personality assessment differ across the lifespan. Theoretical models developed to explain adult personality such as the "Big Five" theory have become the catalyst for similar assessment constructs of personality factors in children (Kamphaus & Frick, 2002). However, there is a notable difference between adults and children in this regard. In part, this difference can be understood from research showing that some personality traits do not stabilize until adulthood (for review, see Caspi & Roberts, 2001). Therefore, personality assessments used with children and adolescents often coincide with aspects of overt behavior and sometimes psychopathology in addition to traditionally defined personality factors (Martin, Hooper, & Snow, 1986; Weis & Smenner, 2007).

Theoretical Underpinnings of Personality Assessment in Children

Personality factors in children have received considerably less research attention than have similar factors in adults. In fact, personality is not a core or central theme in the assessment and psychological description of children as it is for adults, at least not until adolescence. Certainly particular traits and behavioral descriptors such as aggression, anxiety, shyness, social skills, and self-concept are frequently assessed when children present with anger management problems, interpersonal conflicts, learning and attentional problems (e.g., Learning Disorders, Attention-Deficit/Hyperactivity Disorder, Autism Spectrum Disorder), or other problem areas that might require a comprehensive psychological assessment. But again, it is not until later adolescence that personality traits are more commonly used to describe psychological characteristics. While non-cognitive factors including both personality and conative factors are found in developmental theories of children, such affective qualities are usually linked to temperament.

No specific theories of personality focus exclusively on children. Even Freud's psychosexual stages (i.e., oral, anal, phallic, latency, genital) as they relate to the personality development of id, ego, and superego had more relevance to understanding the causes of adult "neurosis" than in focusing on the personality of the child (exceptions of course being Anna Freud and others). Certainly, the developmental theory of Maslow (1943, 1954) who proposed a hierarchy of needs in the process of leading to self-actualization has its beginnings in the early stages of infancy. Likewise, Erikson's (1963, 1982) eight stages of psychosocial development can be used as a framework for examining the personality development of children with the resolution at each stage (e.g., trust versus mistrust) laying the foundation for the next stage (e.g., autonomy versus shame and doubt) as one progresses through the life span.

The social-cognitive theories of personality presented, for example by Bandura (1986, 2006; see also Cervone, 2008) certainly have applications to the childhood and adolescent years. Trait theories such as Eysenck's "Super 3" (Eysenck, 1991) or the "Big 5" (e.g., Costa & McCrae, 2008) have been extended downward to include child and adolescent versions of their better-known and often used adult scales but without particular reference to a comprehensive theory of child personality. However, theories of temperament, focusing more on traits associated with affect, arousal, and attention, are a major focus of discussion of childhood behavior and for later adult personality. Strelau and Zawadzki (2008) define temperament as "a set of relatively stable personality traits present since infancy" (p. 352). For them, it is temperament as biologically determined traits that comprise the core of personality. Strelau and Zawadzki (2008) have also described the following characteristics of temperament: can be measured with high accuracy from a very early age, may be diagnosed in humans, are universal, have a genetic/heritable background and are related to biological mechanisms, demonstrate high temporal stability, manifest themselves in overt behavior, determine behavior in every day settings, and moderate both normal and abnormal behavior.

Again, depending on the author or researcher, personality and temperament are discussed either interchangeably or as separate but related constructs. For example, Asendorpf (2008) provides a general definition of personality that subsumes temperament and is developmental in its scope: "...includes at any age, any social-emotional characteristic of an individual that shows some stability over shorter time periods...that varies between individuals of the same culture...includes temperament (traits related to affect, arousal and attention) but does not restrict early personality to temperament" (p. 101). Thus, this chapter will examine models that are both labeled personality and temperament.

Personality must also be viewed across the lifespan and both qualitative and quantitative differences must be understood within a developmental framework. Asendorpf's (2008) argument that personality is not a collection of traits and qualities that only appear after childhood is reflected in several principles. Personality is plastic at all stages of life but especially in the early years. Roberts and DelVecchio (2000) reported that the Big Five personality traits are most variable in childhood and then become increasingly stable through adolescence and early to mid-adult years; however, it is not until 50 years of age or later that they become especially stable. The underlying causes of personality stability reflect genetic factors, selection of environments to fit or match one's personality, commitment to a stable personal identity, and resiliency (i.e., the capacity to address external challenges).

Trait Models

Trait theories tend to dominate the personality literature (Boyle, Matthews, & Saklofske, 2008a, b). Costa and McCrae (2008) have emphatically agreed with the view that "traits are alive and well, and tools for their assessment are flourishing." (p. 192). However, this viewpoint would appear to be truer of adult scales in contrast to personality trait measures for children and adolescents. Several well-established adult personality trait models have been extended downward to the childhood and adolescent years, including the descriptions of Cattell, Eysenck, and Costa and McCrae. In brief, all of these models have employed factor analytic procedures to determine the structure of personality although Eysenck's model also has a solid basis in Pavlovian respondent conditioning, behavior genetics, and brain-behavior relationships (e.g., extraversion; Saklofske, Eysenck, Eysenck, Stelmack, & Revelle, 2012)

Raymond B. Cattell

The contributions of Raymond Cattell in both describing and measuring personality are documented in his many books and articles and are more recently summarized by Boyle and Barton (2008) and Cattell and Mead (2008). There are 92 primary factors proposed by Cattell that have been reduced using factor analysis to 29 broad factors (30 with the curiosity construct). Probably best known of these is the Sixteen Personality Factor Questionnaire (16PF) that describes the constellation of 16 normal personality source traits, five global or second stratum factors (referred to as the "original Big Five" by Cattell & Mead, 2008) and two third stratum factors. This model included a broader set of second-stratum dimensions that has served as the foundation for other extensions of Cattell's various personality measures. Cattell was also most supportive of using a multi-method approach to personality measurement including life record data (L-data), questionnaire data (Q-data), and objectively derived data (T-data). However, it is the very complexity of Cattell's psychometric model that has likely limited the impact that his work and measures have had in the applied practice areas of psychology and especially psychological assessment.

While the majority of Cattell's research and the personality tests were developed for use with adults, several measures are intended for children and adolescents. Stemming from the basic 16 PF model, these downward extensions to younger age groups have a smaller number of factors as a function of the developmental differentiation in personality that occurs over the age range. The better-known personality measures for children and adolescents include the High School Personality Questionnaire (Cattell & Cattell, 1975) which has been updated and renamed the Adolescent Personality Questionnaire, the Children's Personality Questionnaire (Porter & Cattell, 1985), the Early School Personality Questionnaire (Coan & Cattell, 1959), and the Preschool Personality Questionnaire (Dreger, Lichtenstein, & Cattell, 1995).

Dynamic traits that are less stable than personality traits but more stable than transitory mood-state dimensions are assessed with the School Motivation Analysis Test (SMAT; Boyle, 1989) or the Children's Motivation Analysis Test (CMAT; Boyle & Start, 1988). The CMAT can be used with primary school age children and appears to be tapping four broad factors labeled superego, narcissism, play, and self-sentiment. However, the school orientation factor present on the SMAT was not found in the analyses conducted by Boyle and Start (1988). While gender differences have been noted on the CMAT, Boyle (2008a) concluded that "these instruments need extensive psychometric revision, not only to simplify their factor structure, but also to bring them up to date for contemporary use" (p. 263).

Boyle and Barton (2008) have also written a comprehensive overview of the various Cattellian personality measures. While the extensive and creative work by Cattell during his career has provided a most complex and detailed description of personality traits and their assessment, there seems to be less research on this work and the measures per se at present. However, a most compelling point made by Boyle and Barton is the need to continue Cattell's quest for "truly objective interactive personality tests."

Hans J. Eysenck

Hans Eysenck was another prolific researcher of personality and individual differences, although his many contributions extend to other areas of psychology ranging from intelligence and aesthetics to addictions and health (Furnham, Eysenck, & Saklofske, 2008). His first book, "Dimensions of Personality" (Eysenck, 1947), provided the foundation for applying factor analysis to determine the structure of personality along a set of quantifiable dimensions. O'Connor (2008) has described the three pillars that guided much of Eysenck's approach to analyzing and describing human behavior:

"First, adoption of a dimensional approach to quantifying individual characteristics; second, that a sufficient understanding requires a matching of correlational and experimental methods to be complete; and third, that accounting for person-situation variation is the key to building causal models of behaviour" (p. 215).

Eysenck's dimensional personality model has undergone several revisions, which are reflected in his questionnaires, beginning with the Maudsley Personality Inventory (Eysenck, 1959) to the most recent Eysenck Personality Questionnaire-Revised (EPQ-R; Eysenck & Eysenck, 1991). The children's version of the EPQ was developed under the guidance of Sybil Eysenck and has been extensively studied in many countries and cultures (Saklofske & Eysenck, 1998) The earlier MPI and Eysenck Personality Inventory (Eysenck & Eysenck, 1964) measured two of the three "super factors" proposed by Eysenck in his PEN (Psychoticism or tough-tender mindedness, Extraversion-Introversion, and Neuroticism or emotionality-stability) model but with the publication of the EPQ, all three factors were included.

Eysenck's dimensional personality model is one of the most parsimonious, focusing on the major factors of Psychoticism (P), Extraversion (E), and Neuroticism (N) although various primary factors are also noted in both his writings and measures (e.g., empathy, venturesomeness, impulsiveness). Extraversion and Neuroticism are the most studied and best known personality factors and are found on the Cattell measures as well as the Big Five. Based on cortical arousal theory, Extraversion has been extensively studied in relation to a wide range of human behaviors from academic performance to delinquency and crime. Neuroticism is tied to activation thresholds in the sympathetic nervous system and underlies very emotional expressions ranging from negative affect and anxiety to calmness. Described most fully by Eysenck and Eysenck (1976), Psychoticism has generated considerable controversy in contrast to the other two major personality factors. While the biological basis of P is linked for example to sex hormones, it has been most often studied in the context of delinquency, psychopathy, and diagnosed psychosis. More recently, Rawlings and Dawe (2008) have revisited this debate and have further explored the relationship between P and impulsivity.

The most often used of the Eysenck personality scales are the EPQ and EPQ-R, including the short forms, all of which measure P, E, and N. The Junior EPQ has been shown to have adequate psychometric properties for children as young as 7–8 years, although the P scale does manifest lower reliabilities (e.g., Eysenck & Saklofske, 1983; Saklofske & Eysenck, 1998). These results are similar to the findings for the revised EPQ. Another important finding is the cross-cultural robustness of both the EPQ across 34 countries and the Junior EPQ based on studies in over 20 countries (Furnham, Eysenck, & Saklofske, 2008).

Paul T. Costa and Robert R. McCrae

In contrast to the more expansive personality model proposed by Cattell and the very parsimonious PEN model of Eysenck, the so-called Big Five is the most often cited trait description of personality in recent years. While much of the foundations for this model can be traced to Norman (1963) and later Goldberg (1983), it is the familiar measures for assessing the Big Five that are attributed to Paul Costa and Robert McCrae (e.g., see Costa & McCrae, 2008; McCrae & Costa, 2008) that are familiar to psychologists. This model reflects the view that personality descriptions have, over time, been incorporated into our language such that a search of the lexicon will provide a listing of the key traits or personality descriptors. Building from Norman's original five-factor model and drawing from the theoretical models, research, and measurement efforts of Cattell and Eysenck as discussed above, but also others such as Digman and Inouye (1986), the Big Five personality factors are Extroversion (E), Neuroticism (N), Openness (O), Agreeableness (A), and Conscientiousness (C).

The earliest three-factor model considered by Costa and McCrae included the already well-established N and E factors but added O (Costa & McCrae, 1980). Shortly after that the NEO-PI (Costa & McCrae, 1985) and then the NEO-PI-R (Costa & McCrae, 1992) were published and added A and C to complete the Big Five personality description. An impressive number of validity and reliability as well as cross-cultural studies of these five personality traits have given it a primary place in the personality assessment literature, although not without its critics (Boyle, 2008b; Eysenck, 1991)

Although the NEO-PI has been further developed for use with children age 12 years and over, this scale and its counterparts such as the NEO-FFI are most often employed in the assessment of adults. However, research has shown that both children's personality as rated by self-report and teachers supports the Big Five description of personality (e.g., Mervielde, Buyst, & DeFruyt, 1995). More recently, McGhee, Ehrler, and Buckhalt (2007) have published the Five Factor Personality Inventory-Children (FFPI-C), which is a 75-item scale normed with children 9 to 18 years of age. Reliabilities appear to be satisfactory across various age and groups of children and results reported in the manual suggest that the FFPI-C is a valid measure of the five major personality factors in children.

Beyond Trait Theories

In contrast to the trait descriptions found in the 3-5-16 and other trait factor models of personality, many contemporary researchers have taken a more "eclectic and clinical perspective" to assessing personality characteristics of children and adolescents. The work of Theodore Millon has received considerable attention from practitioners and will be briefly outlined here (see also Millon [2008]).

Theodore Millon

Theodore Millon is a contemporary leader in personality and psychopathology theory, and also in the development and interpretation of adolescent- and preadolescent-specific measures of personality. Millon's publications over the past several decades have garnered worldwide recognition and use as they inform personality assessment.

The history of the Millon scales began with the development of Millon's Biosocial Learning Theory (Millon, 1969), a theory of psychopathology that merged together existing knowledge of personality categories with acknowledged mental disorders. This theory is an integrative approach to personality and psychotherapy and emphasizes the relationship between biological and environmental factors (Choca, 1999; Dorr, 2006). Millon theorized that personality and psychopathology emerge as a result of interactions between the self and environment and that this interaction is continuous across the lifespan. Although two children may have the same biological predisposition, a combination of environmental and biological factors help to shape, facilitate, or limit the personality development of each child resulting in two adolescents with differing personality patterns. According to the Biosocial Learning Theory, personality styles are learned strategies that are developed and implemented in order to enhance positive reinforcement and reduce punishment (Kamp & Tringone, 2008). For example, parents who value passiveness in their family may have children who develop submissive personalities.

In 1990, Millon reconceptualised his Biosocial Learning Theory to incorporate new knowledge from evolutionary biology and psychology (Choca, 1999). In general, he sought to explain the "structure and styles of personality with reference to deficient, imbalanced, or conflicted modes of survival, ecological adaptation and reproductive strategy" (Millon, 2008, pp. 666). Specifically, Millon emphasized that there are three important factors, each of which is necessary to support the evolutionary progress of organisms. The first of these factors is survival, in which organisms must make decisions that will enhance their chances of continued existence. Second, organisms must demonstrate environmental adaptation, whereby their behaviour must be modified as a result of environmental influences. Lastly, for continued existence, an organism must reproduce, allowing for new organisms to continue to grow and develop (Millon & Bloom, 2008).

Each of these factors is closely related to an individual's personality patterns and is expressed as "polarities," whereby unique personality styles result in individual personality patterns. For example, individuals seek to enhance favourable life circumstances (pleasure-producing) and reduce negative outcomes (pain-avoidance) to increase their chance of survival. To adapt to the surrounding environment, individuals must choose either to conform to the environmental circumstances (passive) or to actively influence the environment in an effort to maximize pleasure and minimize pain (active). Lastly, to support reproduction, individuals must critically decide whether they will look out for themselves, first in order to survive (self-oriented) or whether they will focus on nurturing and supporting those around them (other-oriented). Together, these personality polarities form the core of Millon's personality theory and are the guiding principles for the creation of his series of assessment measures. Table 15.1 provides a summary of each of the extremes of polarities and the corresponding *Diagnostic and Statistical Manual of Mental Disorders, 4th Edition (Text Revision)* (DSM-IV-TR; American Psychiatric Association, 2000) Axis II personality disorders.

Table 15.1 Millon's Theory-Derived Personality Disorders, table adapted from http://www.millon.net/content/evo_theory.htm

Imbalance, Deficiency, or Conflict		Pleasure versus Pain		Self versus Other		
		Pleasure (Low), Pain (Low or High)	Pleasure-Pain Reversal	Low Self, High Other	High Self, Low Other	Self-Other Reversal
DSM-IV-TR Axis II Personality Disorders	Passive versus Aggressive	Schizoid Melancholic	Masochistic	Dependent	Narcissistic	Compulsive
		Avoidant	Sadistic	Histrionic Hypomanic	Antisocial	Negativistic

An important distinction in the Millon scales from other personality measures (e.g., Cattell) involves the interpretative mechanism of these scales. Specifically, Millon utilizes base rates as a standard of comparison, which makes allowances for the frequency in which a behavioural personality pattern is present within society. Base rates take into consideration the fact that there are different prevalence rates of disorders within the population and that some disorders (e.g., depression) may occur more frequently than others (e.g., paranoid schizophrenia) (McCann, 2008; Strack, 2008).

Assessment of Adolescent and Preadolescent Children. Millon has been an instrumental leader in the development of personality measures for youth and adolescents. Though many psychologists who work with older adolescents and adults are familiar with the Millon Clinical Multiaxial Inventory-III (MCMI-III), use of the Millon scales for adolescent assessment began with the publication of the Millon Adolescent Inventory (MAI) in 1974. In 1982, the more well-known Millon Adolescent Personality Inventory (MAPI) was published, differing only slightly from the MAI. However, despite the fact that these measures were intended for use in school and mental health settings, clinical application and precision was restricted primarily due to the limited normative samples with which the measures were developed (Strack, 2008).

As a result, a new Millon scale was created and it is in widespread use today. The Millon Adolescent Clinical Inventory (MACI; Millon, 1993; Millon et al., 2006) was developed for a number of reasons. Of foremost importance, the MACI incorporated the revisions to Millon's personality theory, integrating the evolutionary perspective into the revised measure as well as provided a framework for the revised personality pattern scales. Additionally, although the MAI and MAPI had some clinical utility, it was still necessary to align the MACI with developments in research, specifically through the current version of the DSM (DSM-IV, American Psychiatric Association [APA], 1994; DSM-IV-TR, APA, 2000) and through conversations with clinicians who required more clinically-oriented scales (Strack, 2008). Lastly, it was important to create a clinical adolescent personality measure with a norming sample that is more representative of a clinical population. Specifically, the norming process of the MACI included two separate groups of males and females (aged 13 to 15 and 16 to 19 years) from Canada and the United States. These individuals were referred from a number of clinical settings in which the primary clinical focus was on forming diagnostic impressions (Millon, Millon, Davis, & Grossman, 2006).

The MACI examines psychological disturbances and concerns such as depression, anxiety, eating disorders, or substance abuse, as well as problematic interpersonal behaviours and personality disturbances such as severe introversion, excessive dependency, egocentricity, and manipulativeness (McCann, 2008). It consists of 12 Personality Pattern scales (Introversive, Inhibited, Doleful, Submissive, Dramatizing, Egotistic, Unruly, Forceful, Conforming, Oppositional, Self-demeaning, and Borderline Tendency), eight Expressed Concerns scales (Identity Diffusion, Self-Devaluation, Body Disapproval, Sexual Discomfort, Peer Insecurity, Social Insensitivity, Family Discord, and Childhood Abuse), and seven Clinical Syndromes scales (Eating Dysfunctions, Substance Abuse Proneness, Delinquent Predisposition, Impulsive Propensity, Anxious Feelings, Depressive Affect, and Suicidal Tendency).

The MACI is unique in that, although it does not perfectly align with the DSM-IV-TR (APA, 2000), it incorporates ratings from both Axis I and Axis II in its measurement and interpretation. Specifically, through the clinical syndromes scales, the MACI assesses syndromes associated with Axis I such as anxiety, depression, and eating disorders. Through the personality patterns scales, the MACI focuses on Axis II personality disorders including specific personality patterns such as avoidant personality or schizoid personality disorder (McCann, 2008; Millon et al., 2006). This will need to be revisited with the forthcoming publication of the DSM-V.

Millon also recognized the need for an assessment tool for preadolescents aged 9 to 12 years and created a measure to capture the *emerging* personality traits and patterns within this age group. The Millon Preadolescent Clinical Inventory (M-PACI; Millon, Tringone, Millon, & Grossman, 2005) was developed in order to expand the range of personality assessment to capture the personality patterns of younger children.

The M-PACI is based on the same theoretical foundations as the MACI. Within the M-PACI, there are seven Emerging Personality Patterns (Confident, Outgoing, Conforming, Submissive, Inhibited, Unruly, and Unstable) and seven Current Clinical Signs (Anxiety/Fears, Attention Deficits, Obsessions/Compulsions, Conduct Problems, Disruptive Behaviours, Depressive Mood, and Reality Distortions) that are based on Millon's three polarity model. The personality scales are referred to as *Emerging* Personality Patterns in recognition of the fact that, at this age, personality styles are emerging and are still malleable (Kamp & Tringone, 2008).

Together, the MACI and the M-PACI offer the opportunity for personality assessment with adolescents and preadolescents. The high correlations between assessed constructs on these measures and other psychological assessments (e.g., Behavior Assessment System for Children-2nd Edition, Children's Depression Inventory) along with their solid and theory-driven basis, collectively illustrate the clinical utility of these measures for assessing personality.

Omnibus Rating Scales: The Achenbach and BASC-2 Scales

The prior sections of this chapter discussed personality measures based upon theories that initially emerged to define broad adult personality variables (e.g., Super Three, Big Five, 16 Personality Factors) and were later adapted to measure some forms of adult pathology. As noted, many of these instruments also were adapted to measure the same constructs of personality and pathology in youth (e.g.,

CPI, FFPI-C, MACI). This section will continue the discussion of multivariate measures with a brief review of omnibus rating scales that were designed to assess a variety of psychopathological traits in children that have behavioural manifestations. Further, two widely accepted omnibus measures created specifically for children (e.g., the Achenbach Child Behavior Checklist [CBCL] and the Behavior Assessment System for Children [BASC]) are discussed in detail. The implications of single construct measures for assessment of specific personality variables also are reviewed. Finally, the last section of the chapter discusses temperament as a foundational substratum of personality assessment.

Internalizing and Externalizing Dimensions of Psychopathology. In 1961, Donald Peterson utilized data from teacher rating scales to describe two broad personality dimensions in children. These dimensions included *conduct problems* and *personality problems*. Peterson's problems dimensions related to specific types of psychopathology. Children with conduct problems had difficulties with following rules and they acted aggressively toward others. On the other hand, children with personality problems displayed shyness and a tendency to withdraw from social interactions. Peterson's original dimensions are still reflected in the design of many assessment instruments. In 1966, Thomas Achenbach analyzed data from case histories of outpatients and short-term inpatients to determine common factors that may explain patients' symptomology (Kamphaus & Frick, 2002). From this analysis, two primary factors emerged. The first resembled Peterson's personality problems dimension but also included conduct problems. This factor was described as an *internalizing-externalizing* dimension because of its inclusion of mixed internalizing and externalizing psychopathology. Achenbach's second identified factor was labeled as a *severe and diffuse psychopathology* dimension due to its inclusion of severe forms of psychopathology such as psychosis.

Following subsequent analysis, Achenbach divided the internalizing-externalizing dimension and found that children with conduct problems tended to display more externalizing problems whereas children with phobias, anxiety concerns, and somatic complaints tended to display more internalizing problems. Additionally, other researchers were starting to replicate this finding in studies that used parent and teacher reports (e.g., Conners, 1969; Quay, Morse, & Cutler, 1966); however, the terms *internalizing* and *externalizing* did not become part of common vernacular until

1978 when Achenbach published a paper entitled: *The Classification of Child Psychopathology: A Review and Analysis of Empirical Efforts* in the Psychological Bulletin. Children with internalizing problems were described as "over controlling" their behaviors, being highly anxious, and being excessively shy. In contrast, children with externalizing problems were described as "under controlling" their behaviours, having conduct problems, and often engaging in acting-out behaviours.

Achenbach and Edelbrock's (1978) dichotomization of psychopathology into internalizing and externalizing symptoms was incorporated into the Achenbach Child Behavior Checklist Parent and Teacher Rating Forms (Achenbach & Edelbrock, 1983). Research conducted with these rating scales has added additional support for the utility of separate internalizing and externalizing symptom dimensions (Cohen, Gotlieb, Kershner, & Wehrspan, 1985; Compas, Phares, Banez, & Howell, 1991; Gjone & Stevenson, 1997; Greenbaum & Dedrick, 1998; Massey & Murphy, 1991; McConaughy, Achenbach, & Gent, 1988).

Research also has indicated that a number of educational outcomes are associated with internalizing and externalizing characteristics. In general, students who are high in internalizing psychopathology tend to have higher intelligence scores, better executive functioning abilities, read better, utilize more adaptive coping skills when dealing with stressful situations, and to be less disruptive in educational environments when compared to youth who are high in externalizing psychopathology (Austin, Groth-Marnat, Matthews, Saklofske, Schwean, & Zeidner, 2011; Cohen et al., 1985; Massey & Murphy, 1991; Matson & Fischer, 1991; McConaughy et al., 1988).

Research from biological-based fields such as behavioral genetics also supports the independence of internalizing and externalizing symptoms. As an example, Gjone and Stevenson (1997) found higher concordance rates in children with only internalizing or externalizing problems in comparison to those with combined problems. Further, a more recent study that aimed to determine the heritability of internalizing and externalizing symptoms found genetic factors to account for about 50% of the variability in children's externalizing symptoms and 35% of the variance in internalizing symptoms in both males and females (van der Valk, van den Oord, Verhulst, & Boomsma, 2003). Therefore, similar to other relatively stable psychological traits (e.g., intelligence, extraversion), heritability also

plays a significant role in the development of internalizing and externalizing symptoms.

Following the work of Achenbach, many behaviour ratings scales including his own the Child Behavior Checklist (CBCL; Achenbach & Rescorla, 2001), have adopted a dichotomous internalizing-externalizing format due to the preponderance of research supporting this framework (Kamphaus & Frick, 2002). Other measures include the Adolescent Psychopathology Scale (Reynolds, 1998) and the Adolescent Psychopathology Scale—Short Form (Reynolds, 2000), the BASC-2 (Reynolds & Kamphaus, 2004), the Reynolds Adolescent Adjustment Screening Inventory (Reynolds, 2001) and the Devereux Scales of Mental Disorders (Naglieri, LeBuffe, & Pfeiffer, 1994). Other child omnibus measures include the Personality Inventory for Children (Lachar & Gruber, 2001) and the Personality Inventory for Youth (Lachar & Gruber, 1995).

The Use of Behavior Rating Scales. The BASC-2 (Reynolds & Kamphaus, 2004) and the CBCL (Achenbach & Rescorla, 2001) are two of the most commonly used omnibus behaviour rating assessments with children. These assessments both include broad internalizing and externalizing composites under which various behaviour symptom scales are subsumed. Although slight variations exist across ages and rating formats (teacher, parent, or self-report), internalizing problems on the BASC-2 generally include somatization, anxiety, depression, and externalizing problems include aggression, conduct problems, and hyperactivity. On the CBCL, internalizing symptoms include anxiety, depression, somatic complaints, social withdrawal, and externalizing symptoms include attention problems, rule-breaking behaviour, and aggressive behaviour (Achenbach & Rescorla, 2001; Reynolds & Kamphaus, 2004). Thus, considerable overlap exists in the internalizing and externalizing symptoms assessed across measures even though slight differences can be meaningful and help guide assessment decisions (Ostrander, Weinfurt, Yarnold, & August, 1998).

Each type of personality measure or behaviour rating scale will likely provide slightly different information about a child based on the constructs assessed (Sattler & Hoge, 2006). In addition, raters such as parents and teachers observe children in different environments with differing demands. Therefore, multiple measures should be used to assess multiple constructs, at varying time periods, and across different raters to provide reliable data and minimize assessment bias. When considering data from multiple measures, convergent evidence that particular attributes are more indicative of stable personality variables is suggested by consistency in data across settings and raters. However, when data differ significantly across settings and raters, this divergent evidence may prompt clinicians to consider other hypotheses such as various environmental variables that may better account for the child's behavior.

Recent advances in the development of brief universal behaviour screeners and behavior progress monitoring instruments may allow for even broader usage of behavior ratings scales, particularly for the early identification of problems. The BASC-2 Behavioral and Emotional Screening System (BASC-2 BESS; Kamphaus & Reynolds, 2007) is an example of a screening type of instrument. It allows for the quick assessment of behaviour problems in children and can provide tables of cross-reference scores for whole classrooms of students. This type of screener is consistent with a multiple gating approach to identifying problems in children early so intervention services are available before symptoms become chronic or severe. The multiple gating assessment approach (Walker & Severson, 1992) involves the systematic screening of all children with brief rating scales followed by more extensive progress monitoring (PM) assessment of children who are receiving interventions. Progress monitoring with the BASC-2 PM system (Reynolds & Kamphaus, 2009) offers forms for assessing internalizing and externalizing problems. Psychosocial difficulties also may be assessed with more extensive rating scales (e.g., BASC-2), behaviour observations, and clinical interviews if an intervention is not effective and/or if exceptional student education eligibility is considered (Salvia, Ysseldyke, & Bolt, 2007).

Assessment of Narrow Constructs. Single-construct behaviour rating scales and checklists also assess a variety of adaptive and maladaptive behaviours and are usually completed by the child or those who are familiar with him or her. The transition from using an omnibus measure to a single-construct measure often is driven by the need to more clearly assess a child's strengths and weakness for diagnostic or intervention purposes. Omnibus measures may provide a broad overview of a child's psychosocial functioning but do not allow for in depth assessment of many relevant symptoms that a clinician may wish to address. For example, a study by Storch and colleagues (2006) indicated that the CBCL assessed many broad symptoms of obsessive-compulsive disorder (OCD) that overlapped with other psychiatric disorders (e.g., anxiety, inattention), but the measure poorly discriminated between specific OCD symptoms and symptoms of other internalizing disorders. However, despite this noted problem, when the scores from the CBCL were compared with a clinically administered narrow measure of OCD symptoms (e.g., The Children's Yale-Brown Obsessive Compulsive Scale [Scahill et al., 1997]), reliable and consistent OCD diagnoses were achieved.

In contrast to omnibus measures, single-construct measures also may allow for the assessment of behaviour change over time. Instruments that provide norms by small age increments (e.g., 6 months, 1 year) are important for evaluating children as they develop rapidly in multiple domains in early childhood. Progress monitoring single-construct measures are designed for repeated measurement and generally are sensitive to change; therefore, they have a unique utility because they can be used as outcome measures to assess the degree to which children respond to interventions. For example, changes in overall shyness or social skills T-scores on a progress monitoring single-contract measure before and after implementation of a behaviour management plan can document school-based intervention efficacy. As a shift is made to a "response-to-intervention" (RtI) model (also called Multi-tiered System of Supports [MTSS]) for the provision of support services to children, highly sensitive, single-construct measures will be important for monitoring behaviour change in relation to implemented interventions (National Association of State Directors of Special Education [NASDSE], 2005). Additional examples of single-construct measures that assess narrow personality traits include the Social Skills Improvement System (Gresham & Elliott, 2008), the Piers Harris Children's Self-Concept Scale: Second Edition (Piers, Harris, & Herzberg, 2002), and the Tennessee Self-Concept Scale: Second Edition (Fitts & Warren, 1996).

On a final note, some behaviour rating scales combine features of omnibus and single-construct measures. For example, the Conners Third Edition (Conners-3; Conners, 2008) is designed to assess symptoms of Attention-Deficit/Hyperactivity Disorder (ADHD), but the measure also includes items that screen for internalizing disorders such as anxiety and depression. Therefore, in addition to differentiating between various ADHD symptoms and subtypes, the Conners-3 allows a clinician to assess for comorbid conditions or other problems that may need further evaluation. The short form of the Conners-3 also can be used for as a progress-monitoring instrument since it provides wide coverage of ADHD symptoms and related aspects of adjustment (e.g., learning problems, executive functioning).

Temperament as a Foundational Substratum of Personality Assessment

This final section of the chapter will discuss temperament as a foundational substratum of personality assessment. In beginning this discussion, it is important to note that temperament is not synonymous with personality; however, there is overlap in important constructs in both theoretical frameworks. Thus, temperament assessment can add additional insights in understanding personality.

In contrasting the definitions of personality and temperament, personality refers to a wide variety of personal qualities; demeanor characteristics such as social appeal and expressive energy; traits; cognitive attributions; emotional response patterns; behaviors; and temperament qualities that collectively form a unique constellation recognized by others as the individual's persona. Any of these qualities also can be identified as individual personality variables that are common to many persons. Thus, it is the unique combination and degree of expression of personality traits that is specific to the individual rather than the presence of particular traits in isolation (Joyce, 2010).

By contrast, temperament components are thought to have a biological basis that is evident earlier than the underlying basis is for personality traits. These predispositions are evident through physiological attributes and influence the reciprocal interactions between children and caregivers, eliciting particular types of responses and often are identifiable in infancy. For example, if a young child is outgoing or has a calm temperament, adults are likely to respond more positively than if the child is withdrawn or demonstrates an irritable temperament. Temperament characteristics also are subject to influence from environmental factors such as parenting styles, which may foster or stifle a child's emerging traits. Based on these premises, temperament is a foundational substrate on which later personality traits may evolve.

Temperament has been a topic of speculation for ages. Ancient Greek scholars such as Hippocrates, Plato, and Aristotle, whose writings date back to 400 B.C., have pondered human behaviour patterns (Hippocrates, trans. 1939; 1988; 1994). They noted clusters of characteristics that commonly occurred in individuals as well as pathology such as malaise or foul tempers. Rudimentary theories included four humors or temperaments: choleric, phlegmatic, melancholic, and sanguine (Galen, trans. 1916; trans. 1992). Several iterations of these classical theories of temperament emerged throughout the following centuries. However, it was not until the early 1900s that a distinctly psychological theory of temperament was established. Over the past one hundred years, two temperament paradigms have yielded a number of assessment measures for children and adolescents: the psychological type paradigm and the constitutional-based paradigm.

Psychological Temperament Assessment Paradigms

Modern psychological temperament type theory emerged in the early 1920's with the work of Carl Jung (Jung, 1921/1971). Through his hospital-based psychiatry practice in Zurich, Jung observed reoccurring patterns of behavior among his patients. He noted that patients who were generally depressed or out of touch with reality (e.g., schizophrenic) exhibited pathology related to interactions with others or were preoccupied with internal musings. In contrast, patients with intact reality testing abilities more often exhibited outward forms of pathology, such as aggression or overtly negative interactions with others. Jung termed the broader set of internally focused temperament qualities as introversion and the outgoing qualities as extraversion. He noted that all individuals have the ability to act in an introverted or extroverted manner and each dimension could be expressed either positively or negatively. However, there is a propensity within each person for either introversion or extroversion to be preferred and thus more strongly developed. As noted earlier, Donald Peterson and Thomas Achenbach's contributions to rating scale measures of internalizing and externalizing behaviours in the 1960's is similar to Jung's early conceptualizations.

Jung delineated three dichotomous temperament dimensions: introversion-extraversion, sensing-intuition, and thinking-feeling. Persons who are introverted are described as introspective, cautious toward new circumstances, keenly interested in internal thoughts, and they prefer to renew their personal energy from solitude or small group interactions. For an individual who is strongly introverted, social skills, collaboration strategies, and support networks may be limited or restricted. Persons who are extroverted are described as quick to make new friends, talkative, engaging, keenly interested in the external environment, and acquire energy from frequent interactions with others. Without developing the opposing introversion qualities, extroverts may lack self-reflection, share ideas before they are well thought-out, and intrude on others' need for privacy (Jung, 1921/1971; Wehr, 1971).

Sensing individuals are noted to learn best through tangible experiences. They prefer facts, seek specific details, enjoy fine points of information, and are pragmatic. Persons who prefer sensing styles may undervalue complexity, abstractions, and theory. In contrast, learning thorough intuition relies on quickly assimilating information that incorporates insights and hunches. Intuitive individuals prefer theories and broad patterns. They can easily overlook important details and practical implications when considering ideas (Jung, 1921/1971; Wehr, 1971).

The thinking-feeling dimension defines how individuals prefer to make decisions. A thinking style emphasizes logic, analysis of objective data, and a strong sense of justice based on unbiased and impartial values. In their eagerness for truth, individuals with a strong thinking orientation may seem blunt, calloused, critical, and insensitive although this generally is not their intention. With a feeling orientation for decision-making, subjective qualities such as empathy, mood, compassion, and prior experience are influential. As subjective qualities are variable and often in flux, feeling-based decisions may be perceived by others as unpredictable, acquiescent, and irrational. However, Jung perceived feeling as a rational quality because the decision was carefully pondered, albeit based on personal and different criteria from thinking decisions.

Katherine Briggs and Isabel Myers developed an assessment instrument based on Jung's theory and added a fourth dimension: judging-perceiving. This dichotomy reflected how individuals structure their daily lives (Myers & Myers, 1980; Quenk, 2000). Judging characteristics include the desire for a highly organized lifestyle with a need for structure, schedules, advanced planning, and routine in managing personal affairs. Persons with this propensity also seek closure and may be prone to prematurely eliminating options. On the opposite end of the spectrum, perceiving characteristics include spontaneity, last minute changes, as well as great tolerance and flexibility. This desire to keep all options open can interfere with predictability, meeting deadlines, and other's perceptions of dependability.

Table 15.2 Myers-Briggs Type Indicator (MBTI)

Myers-Briggs Type Indicator (MBTI) Psychological Types			
ISTJ	ISFJ	INFJ	INTJ
ISTP	ISFP	INFP	INTP
ESTP	ESFP	ENFP	ENTP
ESTJ	ESFJ	ENFJ	ENTJ

Note. I = introverted, E = extroverted, S = sensing, N = intuition, T = thinking, F = feeling, J = judging, P = perceiving

When utilizing the Briggs and Myers's assessment instrument, the *Myers-Briggs Type Indicator* (MBTI), T-scores are provided on each of the four dimensions, yielding a possible sixteen temperament profiles (see Table 15.2).

The MBTI can be utilized for temperament assessment with adolescents ages 14 through adulthood (Myers, McCaulley, Quenk, & Hammer, 1998). A parallel instrument, the Murphy-Meisgeier Type Indicator for Children (MMTIC; Murphy & Meisgeier, 2008) applies MBTI theory to the assessment of children ages 7 to 18 and grades 2 through 12. The Student Styles Questionnaire (SSQ; Oakland, Glutting, & Horton, 1996) is based on Jungian-Briggs theory and assesses youth ages 8 to 17 years. On this instrument, the judging-perceiving dimension is designated as organized-flexible to better reflect descriptors of the temperament qualities measured.

The MMTIC and the SSQ differ from adult measures of temperament in several ways. First, they consider school-related behaviour test items in assessing temperament and provide classroom learning applications. In addition, they support interpretations relevant to understanding and enhancing parent-child interactions. For example, some studies indicate a high prevalence of specific temperament preferences among children with particular diagnoses (e.g., oppositional defiant disorder, conduct disorders) and thus understanding these differences may help therapists remediate underdeveloped characteristics (Joyce & Oakland, 2005).

David Keirsey (1998) argued against the interpretation of the MBTI's sixteen types in favor of four clusters: sensing-perceiving, sensing-judging, intuition-thinking, and intuition-feeling. He developed the Temperament Sorter-II, which also has a student version. Unlike the parental rating scales method noted in the prior section of this chapter, psychological temperament scales for children are self-report measures with the assumption that children best understand their own preferences.

Constitutional-based Temperament Assessment Paradigms

Constitutional-based temperament assessments measure the earliest manifestations of personality traits from infancy through early childhood. Constitutional-based theories presume that characteristics have a strong biological basis. Costa and McCrae (2001) argue that behaviours exhibited by infants are the core tenets of personality as children have the least capacity for communication at that time, and thus are the least influenced by the perceptions of others. Instruments for measuring constitutional-based temperament qualities are primarily reliant on observational techniques and parent interviews. Through their New York Longitudinal Study (NYLS) research, Alexander Thomas and Stella Chess identified nine measurable behavioural characteristics: activity level, rhythmicity, approach-withdrawal, adaptability, threshold of responsiveness, intensity of reaction, quality of mood, distractibility, and attention span/persistence (Thomas & Chess, 1977; Thomas & Chess, 1989).

Activity level referred to children's ratio of active and inactive times, whereas rhythmicity referred to the regularity of the child's daily activities (e.g., sleeping pattern). Approach or withdrawal was assessed by noting the infant's adaptive or maladaptive initial responses to new persons or objects. How quickly a child habituated to new stimuli was noted as adaptability and threshold of responsiveness measured the level of stimulus needed to evoke a response. The energy of the baby's response was called intensity of reaction and quality of mood evaluated the frequency of pleasant versus unpleasant responses. A child's ability to attend despite diversion was noted as distractibility and attention span/persistence qualities. Thomas and Chess also identified three behavioural response patterns: easy, slow-to-warm, and difficult. Over time, the difficult temperament category experienced the most negative long-term outcomes and the slow-to-warm children also reported significant psychological stressors whereas the children with an easy temperament had positive outcomes (Chess & Thomas, 1984; Thomas & Chess, 1977; Thomas, Chess, & Birch, 1968).

Another important contribution from their work is the concept of goodness-of-fit. From their observations, Thomas and Chess noted that some temperament qualities were less problematic when parents had similar characteristics or high tolerance for differences. Therefore, educating parents about the innate differences between children's temperament and how these characteristics may align or misalign with those of the parent has the potential to improve parent-child interactions. Subsequent instruments based on their theory include the Parent Questionnaire and the Teacher Temperament Questionnaire.

In the following years, several researchers published measures based on the work of Thomas and Chess (e.g., Carey Revised Infant Temperament Questionnaire, the Toddler Temperament Scale, the Behavioral Style Questionnaire, and the Middle Childhood Temperament Questionnaire). Later adaptations found support for five rather than the original nine dimensions proposed (Lerner, Palermo, Spiro, & Nesselroade, 1982; Sanson, Prior, Garino, Oberklaid, & Sewell, 1987). Buss (1989) and Buss and Plomin (1975, 1984) identified only four qualities (i.e., activity, emotionality, sociability, and impulsivity) from their research and subsequently published the EASI Temperament Survey. Others argue for defining assessment of child temperament and personality through the concepts of reactivity and self-regulation, primary emotions, or over-controllers and undercontrollers as integral components of temperament (Block & Block, 1980; Goldsmith & Campos, 1986; Kagan, 2009; Kagan & Snidman, 1991; Rothbart & Derryberry, 1981; Strelau, 1983). A variety of assessment instruments have been developed for each perspective.

Validity Studies for Temperament Constucts

Psychological-Based Temperament. The validity of psychological temperament constructs is supported by heritability research, factor analyses of test instruments, and cross-cultural studies. Currently, the dimension of MBTI theory that overlaps the most with other major personality measures is introversion-extraversion (see Table 15.3). Some researchers refer to introversion-extraversion as a super trait (e.g., Saklofske, Eysenck, Eysenck, Stelmack, & Revelle, 2012) since this dimension has the strongest heritability support even when differing instruments are utilized to measure the trait (Buss & Plomin, 1984; Loehlin, 1982). Bouchard, McGue, Hur, and Horn (1998) found heritability to account for significant portions of phenotype variance for introversion-extraversion (h^2 = .60) in a study of monozygotic and dyzygotic twins that involved using the MBTI. To a lesser degree, heritability also explained considerable variance in sensing-intuition and judgment-perception traits

Table 15.3 Overlapping Constructs in Personality and Temperament Measures

Overlapping Constructs in Personality and Temperament Measures							
Big 5–16 PF!Personality Theories	Cattell, 16PF	Extraversion-Introversion	Anxiety	Tough-Mindedness		Independence	Self-Control
	Costa & McCrae, NEO-PI-R	Extraversion	Neuroticism	Openness		Agreeableness	Conscientiousness
Super 3	Eysenck, Eysenck EPQ	Extraversion	Neuroticism			Psychoticism	
MBTI	Myers, Briggs, MBTI	Extraversion—Introversion		Intuition—Sensing	Feeling—Thinking	Judging—Perception	

(h^2 approximately .40). Greater cortical arousal, limbic site activity, and heart disease among introverts as compared to extraverts have been noted in several studies (Kagan & Snidman, 1991, 2004; Shelton, 1996; Sternberg, 1990; Wilson & Languis, 1990). Higher cortical arousal among introverts may account for their propensity to need more solitude and to temporarily withdrawal from highly stimulating environments to renew their energy.

Within the brain lateralization literature, sequential processing of information, consistent with sensing temperament qualities, is considered a left hemisphere function. Holistic or simultaneous processing is thought to be primarily a right hemisphere function. Research does support greater left hemisphere brain activity for individuals with a sensing temperament. The opposite is true for persons self-reporting an intuitive temperament preference (Hartman, Hylton, & Sanders, 1997). Gender differences for the thinking-feeling scale are supported across multiple studies indicating more males prefer thinking and more females prefer feeling qualities (Myers et al., 1998; Oakland et al., 1996).

Cross-cultural research supports the reliability and construct validity for the MBTI scales in English-speaking and non-English speaking countries. Studies also support similar distributions of temperament preferences for the introversion-extroversion scale (Carlson & Levy, 1973; Kirby & Barger, 1996; Myers et al., 1998). However, these findings are based on a very limited number of cross-cultural studies. Research with students of African-American, Hispanic-American, and Euro-American ancestry within the United States that used the SSQ supports the four factor structure of temperament (Stafford & Oakland, 1996). In addition, studies of the SSQ across multiple countries (e.g., Australia, China, Costa Rica, Pakistan, Philippines, Samoa, U.S., and Zimbabwe) also found a strong fit for the four dichotomous temperament dimensions (Benson, Oakland, & Shermis, 2008; Callueng et al., 2011; Oakland, Callueng, Rizwan, & Aftab, 2011).

Constitutional-BasedTemperament. Heritability studies provide support for some constitutionally-based temperament constructs including activity level, emotionality, and sociability (Buss & Plomin, 1984; Florderus-Myrhed, Pedersen, & Rasmuson, 1980; Goldsmith & Gottesman, 1981). In research on the threshold of response factor, correlations are noted for increases in cortical arousal, larger evoked potentials, blood pressure, and heart rate when comparing high-versus low-reactive children (Kagan & Snidman, 2004). The Australian Temperament Project, a longitudinal study of infants through the age of 18, provided support for many of the early findings from Thomas and Chess (Prior, Sanson, Smart, & Oberklaid, 2000). Children with easy temperaments were noted to have more positive outcomes and children with difficult temperaments experienced more negative outcomes. Moreover, children with a more reticent temperament developed more anxiety-related symptoms.

Practical Implicatons

There are a number of implications for considering temperament dimensions as a foundational substratum of personality and thus an important evaluation component. Many qualities such as extraversion, intuition, and self-regulation have positive attributes and describe personal qualities in nonpathological language traits (Oakland & Joyce, 2006). Additionally, early temperament assessment captures data from formative years of infancy and toddlers that other measures do not, which may help with identifying risk factors. Clinicians can utilize early child temperament data to better assist parents in understanding their own child's traits as well as utilize the goodness-of-fit concept in addressing conflicting needs between the parent and child. The goodness-of-fit paradigm also has implications for assisting teachers in better understanding students' differences. Temperament qualities are considered somewhat malleable; and therefore, self-awareness of one's own strengths and lesser developed characteristics can foster personal development.

Conclusion

This chapter reviewed the major paradigms on which are based the assessment of personality in children and adolescents. Although there is no consensus on a definition of personality, most theorists agree that personality traits have a biological basis, are moderately stable over time, and can be somewhat influenced by environmental factors. The early manifestation of personality variables as well as their stability facilitates measurement of these attributes in children. Several scientific methods including lexical hypothesis and multi-variant factor analyses have provided empirical support for multiple constructs of personality.

As noted in the chapter, many of the current measurements for children and youth have been derived from earlier adult measures. However, it is important to acknowledge that throughout the developmental stages of childhood and adolescence, expressions of personality are evolving. Especially for young children, these early personality qualities may be expressed differently and thus require different measurement methods. In fact, infant measures often rely on observations or parent interview reports of physiological manifestations (e.g., startle effects or crying) whereas child and adolescent measures may include self-report or parent and teacher ratings scales. Omnibus rating scales are designed to briefly sample a wide variety of factors. In contrast, single construct scales measure a narrow set of qualities with more depth. The scales or facets within personality measures are defined by the underlying theory and can range from positive qualities of demeanor and response patterns to pathology. Temperament is considered by some theorists to be a foundational substratum upon which adult personality is built. There are a number of instruments designed specifically for the measurement of early childhood and adolescent temperament as related to personality. Temperament theories and instruments can be conceptualized in two categories: psychological type and constitutionally-based. In many cases,

clinicians will utilize more than one personality measure as part of an assessment battery, thus, providing a broader multi-dimensional understanding of the individual's persona.

References

Achenbach, T. M., & Edelbrock, C. S. (1978). The classification of child psychopathology: A review and analysis of empirical efforts. *Psychological Bulletin, 85*, 1275–1301.

Achenbach, T. M., & Edelbrock, C. S. (1983). *Manual for the Child Behavior Checklist and the Revised Child Behavior Profile.* Burlington, VT: University of Vermont, Department of Psychiatry.

Achenbach, T. M., & Rescorla, L. A. (2001). *Manual for the ASEBA School-Age Forms & Profiles.* Burlington, VT: University of Vermont, Research Center for Children, Youth, & Families.

American Psychiatric Association. (1994). *Diagnostic and statistical manual of mental disorders* (4th ed.). Washington, DC: Author.

American Psychiatric Association. (2000). *Diagnostic and statistical manual of mental disorders* (4th ed., text rev.). Washington, DC: Author.

Asendorpf, J. B. (2008). Developmental perspective. In G. J. Boyle, G. Matthews, & D. H. Saklofske (Eds.), *The SAGE handbook of personality theory and assessment, Vol 1: Personality theories and models.* (pp. 101–123). Thousand Oaks, CA, US: Sage Publications, Inc.

Austin, E., Boyle, G., Groth-Marnat, G., Matthews, G., Saklofske, D. H., Schwean, V. L., & Zeidner, M. (2011). Integrating intelligence and personality. In T. M Harwood, L.E. Beutler, & G. Groth-Marnat (Eds.), *Integrative assessment of adult personality* (3nd Ed.). (pp. 119–151), New York: Guilford.

Bandura, A. (1986). *Social foundations of thought and action: A social cognitive theory.* Engelwoods, NJ: Prentice-Hall

Bandura, A. (2006). Toward a psychology of human agency. *Perspective on Psychological Science, 1*(2), 164–180.

Benson, N., Oakland, T., & Shermis, M. (2008). Cross-national invariance of children's temperament. *Journal of Psychoeducational Assessment, 20*(10), 1–14.

Block, J. H., & Block, J. (1980). The role of ego-control and ego-resiliency in the organization of behavior. In W. A. Collins (Ed.), *Development of cognition, affect, and social relations. The Minnesota symposia on child psychology: Volume 1* (pp. 39–101). Hillsdale, NJ: Erlbaum.

Bouchard, T. J. Jr., McGue, M., Hur, Y., & Horn, J. M. (1998). A genetic and environmental analysis of the California Psychological Inventory using adult twins reared apart and together. *European Journal of Personality 12*(5), 307–320.

Boyle, G. J. (1989). Central dynamic traits measured in the School Motivation Analysis Test. *Multivariate Experimental Clinical Research, 9*(1), 11–26.

Boyle, G. J. (2008a). Simplifying the Cattellian psychometric model. In G. J. Boyle, G. Matthews, & D. H. Saklofske (Eds.), *The SAGE handbook of personality theory and assessment, Vol 1:.Personality measurement and testing* (pp. 257–272). Thousand Oaks, CA, US: Sage Publications, Inc.

Boyle, G. J. (2008b). Critique of the five factor model of personality. In G. J. Boyle, G. Matthews, & D. H. Saklofske (Eds.), *The SAGE handbook of personality theory and assessment, Vol 1:.Personality measurement and testing* (pp. 295–312). Thousand Oaks, CA, US: Sage Publications, Inc.

Boyle, G. J., & Barton, K. (2008). Contribution of Cattellian personality instruments. In G. J. Boyle, G. Matthews, & D. H. Saklofske (Eds.), *The SAGE handbook of personality theory and assessment, Vol 2: Personality measurement and testing* (pp. 160–178). Thousand Oaks, CA, US: Sage Publications, Inc.

Boyle, G. J., Matthews, G. & Saklofske, D. H. (Eds). (2008a). *The SAGE handbook of personality theory and assessment, Vol 1: Personality theories and models*. Thousand Oaks, CA, US: Sage Publications, Inc.

Boyle, G. J., Matthews, G., & Saklofske, D.H. (Eds). (2008b). *The SAGE handbook of personality theory and assessment, Vol 2: Personality measurement and testing*. Thousand Oaks, CA, US: Sage Publications, Inc.

Boyle, G. J., & Start, K. B. (1988). A first delineation of higher-order factors in the Children's Motivation Analysis Test (CMAT). *Psycholoische Beitrage, 30,* 556–567.

Buss, A. (1989). Temperaments as personality traits. In G. A. Kohnstamm, J. E. Bates, & M. K. Rothbart (Eds.), *Temperament in childhood* (pp. 49–58). New York, NY: John Wiley & Sons Ltd.

Buss, A. H., & Plomin, R. (1975). *A temperament theory of personality development*. New York: John Wiley & Sons.

Buss, A. H., & Plomin, R. (1984). *Temperament: Early developing personality traits*. Hillsdale, New Jersey: Lawrence Erlbaum Associates, Publishers.

Callueng, C. M., Lee Hang, D. M., Gonzales, R. C., Ling-So'o, A. C., & Oakland, T. D. (2011). Temperament styles of children from Somoa and the United States. *Educational Measurement and Evaluation Review, 2,* 18–24.

Carlson, R., & Levy, N. (1973). Studies in Jungian typology: I. Memory, social perception, andsocial action. *Journal of Personality, 41*(4), 559–576.

Caspi, A., & Roberts, B. W. (2001). Target articles: Personality development across the life course: The argument for change and continuity. *Psychological Inquiry, 12,* 49–66.

Cattell, R. B., & Cattell, M. D. (1975). *Handbook for the Junior and Senior High School Personality Questionnaire*. Champaign, IL.: Institute for Personality and Ability Testing.

Cattell, H. E. P., & Mead, A. D. (2008). The Sixteen Personality Factor Questionnaire (16PF). In G. J. Boyle, G. Matthews, & D. H. Saklofske (Eds.), *The SAGE handbook of personality theory and assessment, Vol 2: Personality measurement and testing* (pp. 135–159). Thousand Oaks, CA, US: Sage Publications, Inc.

Cervone, D. (2008). Explanatory models of personality: Social-cognitive theories and the knowledge-appraisal model of personality architecture. In G. J. Boyle, G. Matthews, & D. H. Saklofske (Eds.), *The SAGE handbook of personality theory and assessment, Vol 2: Personality measurement and testing* (pp. 80–100). Thousand Oaks, CA, US: Sage Publications, Inc.

Chess, S., & Thomas, A. (1984). *Origins and Evolution of Behavior Disorders*. New York, NY: Brunner/Mazel.

Choca, J. P. (1999). Evolution of Millon's personality prototypes. *Journal of Personality Assessment, 72*(3), 353–364.

Coan, R.W., & Cattell, R. B. (1959). The development of the Early School Personality Questionnaire. *Journal of Experimental Education, 28*(3), 143–52.

Cohen, N. J., Gotlieb, H., Kershner, J., & Wehrspan, W. (1985). Concurrent validity of internalizing and externalizing profile patterns of the Achenbach Child Behavior Checklist. *Journal of Consulting and Clinical Psychology, 53,* 724–728.

Compas, B. E., Phares, V., Banez, G. A., & Howell, D. C. (1991). Correlates of internalizing and externalizing behavior problems: Perceived competence causal attributions, and parental symptoms. *Journal of Abnormal Child Psychology, 19,* 197–218.

Conners, C. K. (1969). A teacher rating scale for use in drug studies with children. *American Journal of Psychiatry, 126,* 884–888.

Conners, K. (2008). *Conners-3, Conners* (3rd ed.). San Antonio, TX: Pearson Assessments.

Costa, P. T., Jr., & McCrae, R. R. (1980). Still stable after all these years: Personality as a key to some issues in adulthood and old age. In P. B. Baltes & O. G. Brim, Jr. (Eds.), Life span development and behavior (Vol. 3, pp. 65–102). New York, NY: Academic Press.

Costa, P. T., Jr., & McCrae, R. R. (1985). *The NEO Personality Inventory manual*. Odessa, FL: Psychological Assessment Resources.

Costa, P. T., Jr., & McCrae, R. R. (1992). *Revised NEO Personality Inventory (NEO-PI-R) and NEO Five-Factor Inventory (NEOFFI) professional manual*. Odessa, FL: Psychological Assessment Resources, Inc.

Costa, P. T., Jr., & McCrae, R. R. (2001). A theoretical context for adult temperament. In T. D. Wachs, & G. A. Kohnstamm (Eds.), *Temperament in Context* (pp. 1–21). Mahwah, NJ: Lawrence Erlbaum Associates, Publishers.

Costa, P. T., & McCrae, R. R. (2008). The revised NEO Personality Inventory (NEO-PI-R0. In G. J. Boyle, G. Matthews, & D. H. Saklofske (Eds.), *The SAGE handbook of personality theory and assessment, Vol 2: Personality measurement and testing* (pp. 179–198). Thousand Oaks, CA, US: Sage Publications, Inc.

Digman, J. M., & Inouye, J. (1986). Further specification of the five robust factors of personality. *Journal of Personality and Social Psychology, 73*(6), 1246–56.

Dorr, D. (2006). Millon's Biosocial Learning perspective: Personologic psychotherapy. In F. Rotgers & M. Maniacci (Eds.), *Antisocial personality disorder: A practitioner's guide to comparative treatments* (pp. 63–90). New York, NY: Springer Publishing Company.

Dreger, R. M., Lichtenstein, D., & Cattell, R. B. (1995). Manual for the experimental edition of the Personality Questionnaire for Preschool Children Form A. *Journal of Social Behavior and Personality, 10 (suppl.),* 1–50.

Erikson, E. H. (1963). *Childhood and society* (2nd ed.). New York, NY: Norton

Erikson, E. H. (1982). *The life cycle completed: A review*. New York, NY: Norton.

Eysenck, H. J. (1947). *Dimensions of personality*. London, England: Routledge & Kegan Paul.

Eysenck, H. J. (1959). *The Maudsley Personality Inventory*. London, England: The University of London Press.

Eysenck, H. J. (1991). Dimensions of personality: 16, 5 or 3? Criteria for a taxonomic paradigm. *Personality and Individual Differences, 12*(8), 773–790.

Eysenck, H. J., & Eysenck, S. B. G. (1964). *Manual of the Eysenck Personality Inventory*. London, England: Hodder & Stoughton.

Eysenck, H. J., & Eysenck, S. B. G. (1976). *Psychoticism as a dimension of personality*. London, England: Hodder & Stoughton.

Eysenck, H. J., & Eysenck, S. B. G. (1991). *Manual of the Eysenck Personality Scales*. London, England: Hodder & Stoughton.

Eysenck, S. B., & Saklofske, D. H. (1983). A comparison of responses of Canadian and English children on the Junior

Eysenck Personality Questionnaire. *Canadian Journal of Behavioural Science/Revue canadienne des sciences du comportement. 15*(2), 121–130.

Fitts, W. H., & Warren, W. L. (1996). *Tennessee Self-Concept Scale.* Los Angeles, CA: Western Psychological Services.

Furnham, A., Eysenck, S. B. G., & Saklofske, D. H. (2008). The Eysenck personality measures: Fifty years of scale development. In G. J. Boyle, G. Matthews, & D. H. Saklofske (Eds.), *The SAGE handbook of personality theory and assessment, Vol 2: Personality measurement and testing* (pp. 199–218). Thousand Oaks, CA, US: Sage Publications, Inc.

Galen. (1916). *Galen on the natural forces.* (A. J. Brook, Trans.). Cambridge, MA: Harvard University Press. (Original work published date unknown)

Galen. (1992). *The art of cure-Extracts from Galen: Maimonides' medical writings.* (U.S. Barzel, Trans.). Haifa, Israel: Maimonides Research Institute. (Original work published date unknown)

Gjone, H., & Stevenson, J. (1997). The association between internalizing and externalizing behavior in childhood and early adolescence: Genetic or environmental common influences? *Journal of Abnormal Child Psychology, 25,* 277–286.

Goldberg, L.R. (1983). The magical number five, plus or minus two: Some considerations on the dimensionality of personality descriptors. Paper presented at a Research Seminar, Gerontology Research Center, Baltimore, MD.

Goldsmith, H. H., & Campos, J. J. (1986). Fundamental issues in the study of early temperament: The Denver twin temperament study. In M. E. Lamb, & A. L. Brown (Eds.), *Advances in developmental psychology* (pp. 231–283). Hillsdale, JH: Erlbaum.

Goldsmith, H. H., & Gottesman, I. I. (1981). Origins of variation in behavioral style: A longitudinal study of temperament in young twins. *Child Development, 52,* 91–103.

Greenbaum, P. E., & Dedrick, R. F. (1998). Hierarchical confirmatory factor analysis of the child behavior Checklist/4–18. *Psychological Assessment, 10,* 149–155.

Gresham, F. M., & Elliott, S. N. (2008). Social skills improvement system. Minneapolis, MN: Pearson Corporation.

Hartman, S. E., Hylton, J., & Sanders, R. F. (1997). The influence of hemispheric dominance on scores of the Myers-Briggs Type Indicator. *Educational and Psychological Measurement, 57*(2), 440–449.

Hippocrates. (1939). *Hippocrates, 1.* (W. H. S. Jones, Trans). Cambridge, MA: Harvard University Press. (Original work published date unknown).

Hippocrates. (1988). *Hippocrates, 5,* (P. Potter, Trans.). Cambridge, MA: Harvard University Press. (Original work published date unknown).

Hippocrates. (1994). *Hippocrates, 7,* (W. D. Smith, Trans.). Cambridge, MA: Harvard University Press. (Original work published date unknown).

Joyce, D. (2010). *Essentials of temperament assessment.* Hoboken, NJ: John Wiley & Sons.

Joyce, D., & Oakland T. (2005). Temperament differences among children with conduct disorder and oppositional defiant disorder. *California School Psychologist, 10,* 125–136.

Jung, C. G. (1971). *Psychological types.* (R. F. C. Hull, Revision of Trans. by H. G. Baynes). Princeton, NJ: Princeton University Press. (Original work published 1921).

Kagan, J. (2009). *The three cultures: Natural sciences, social sciences, and the humanities in the 21st century.* New York, NY: Cambridge University Press.

Kagan, J., & Snidman, N. (1991). Infant predictors of inhibited and uninhibited profiles. *Psychological Science, 2*(1), 40–43.

Kagan, J., & Snidman, N. (2004). *The long shadow of temperament.* Cambridge, MA: The Belknap Press of Harvard University Press.

Kamp, J., & Tringone, R. (2008). Development and validation of the Millon Pre-Adolescent Clinical Inventory (M-PACI). In T. Millon & C. Bloom (Eds.), *The Millon inventories: A practitioner's guide to personalized clinical assessment* (2nd ed, pp. 528–547). New York, NY: Guilford Press.

Kamphaus, R. W., & Frick, P. J. (2002). *Clinical assessment of child and adolescent personality and behavior* (2nd ed.). New York, NY: Springer.

Kamphaus, R. W., & Reynolds, C. R. (2007). *BASC-2 Behavior and Emotional Screening System.* San Antonio, TX: Pearson Assessments.

Keirsey, D. (1998). *The Keirsey Temperament Sorter—II.* Del Mar, CA: Prometheus Nemesis.

Kirby, L. K., & Barger, N. J. (1996). Multicultural applications. In A. L. Hammer (Ed.), *MBTI applications: A decade of research on the Myers-Briggs Type indicator* (pp. 167–196). Palo Alto, CA: Consulting Psychologists Press.

Lachar, D., & Gruber, C. F. (1995). *Personality Inventory for Youth.* Los Angeles, CA: Western Psychological Services.

Lachar, D., & Gruber, C. F. (2001). *Personality Inventory for Children* (2nd ed.). Los Angeles, CA: Western Psychological Services.

Lerner, R. M., Palermo, M., Spiro, A., & Nesselroade, J. R. (1982). Assessing the dimensions of temperament individuality across the life-span: The Dimensions of Temperament Survey (DOTS). *Child Development, 53,* 149–159.

Loehlin, J. C. (1982). Are personality traits differentially heritable? *Behavior Genetics, 12,* 417–428.

Martin, R. P., Hooper, S., & Snow, J. (1986). Behavior rating scale approaches to personality assessment in children and adolescents. In H. M. Knoff (Ed.). *Assessment of child and adolescent personality* (pp. 309–351). New York, NY: Guilford Press.

Maslow, A. (1943). A theory of human motivation. *Psychological Review, 50,* 370–396.

Maslow, A. (1954). *Motivation and personality.* New York, NY: Harper.

Massey, O. T., & Murphy, S. E. (1991). A study of the utility of the child behavior checklist with residentially placed children. *Evaluation and Program Planning, 14,* 319–324.

Matson, D. E., & Fischer, M. (1991). A comparison of internalizers, externalizers, and normals using the WISC-R and Wisconsin Card Sorting Test. *Journal of Psychoeducational Assessment, 9,* 140.

McCann, J. (2008). Using the Millon Adolescent Clinical Inventory (MACI) and Its Facet Scales. In T. Millon & C. Bloom (Eds.), *The Millon inventories: A practitioner's guide to personalized clinical assessment (2*nd ed., pp. 494–519). New York, NY, US: Guilford Press.

McConaughy, S. H., Achenbach, T. M., & Gent, C. L. (1988). Multiaxial empirically based assessment: Parent, teacher, observational, cognitive, and personality correlates of child behavior profile types for 6-to 11-year-old boys. *Journal of Abnormal Child Psychology, 16,* 485–509.

McCrae, R. R., & Costa, P. T. (2008). Empirical and theoretical status of the five-factor model of personality traits. In G. J. Boyle, G. Matthews, & D. H. Saklofske (Eds.), *The SAGE handbook of personality theory and assessment, Vol 1: Personality* theories and models (pp. 283–294). Thousand Oaks, CA, US: Sage Publications, Inc.

McGhee, R. L., Ehrler, D. J., & Buckhalt, J. A. (2007). *Five Factor Personality Inventory–Children*. Austin, TX: Pro-Ed Inc.

Mervielde, I., Buyst, V., & DeFruyt, F. (1995). The validity of the Big 5 as a model for teachers' ratings of individual differences among children aged 4–12 years. *Personality and Individual Differences, 18*, 525–534.

Millon, T. (1969). *Modern Psychopathology*. Philadelphia, PA: Saunders.

Millon, T. (1993). *Millon Adolescent Clinical Inventory manual*. Minneapolis, MN: National Computer Systems.

Millon, T., Millon, C., Davis, R., & Grossman, S. (2006). *Millon Adolescent Clinical Inventory (MACI) manual*. (2nd ed.). Minneapolis, MN: Pearson Assessments.

Millon, T. (2008). The Logic and Methodology of the Millon Inventories. In G. J. Boyle, G. Matthews, & D. H. Saklofske (Eds.), *The SAGE handbook of personality theory and assessment, Vol 2: Personality measurement and testing* (pp. 663– 683). Thousand Oaks, CA, US: Sage Publications, Inc.

Millon, T., & Bloom, C. (Eds.). (2008). *The Millon inventories: A practitioner's guide to personalized clinical assessment (2nd ed.)*. New York, NY, US: Guilford Press.

Millon, T., Millon, C., Davis, R., & Grossman, S. (2006). *MCMI-III Manual* (3rd ed.). Minneapolis, MN: Pearson Education.

Millon, T., Tringone, R., Millon, C., & Grossman, S. (2005). *Millon Pre-Adolescent Clinical Inventory (M-PACI) manual (2nd ed.)*. Minneapolis, MN: NCS Pearson.

Murphy, E., & Meisgeier, C. H. (2008). *A guide to the development and use of the Murphy-Meisgeier Type Indicator for Children*. Gainesville, FL: Center for Applications of Psychological Type.

Myers, I. B., McCaulley, M. H., Quenk, N. L., & Hammer, A. L. (1998). *MBTI Manual: A guide to the development and use of the Myers-Briggs Type Indicator* (3rd ed.). Palo Alto, CA: Consulting Psychologists Press.

Myers, I. B., & Myers, P. B. (1980). *Gifts differing: Understanding personality type*. Palo Alto, CA: Consulting Psychological Press.

Naglieri, J. A., LeBuffe, P. A., & Pfeiffer, S. I. (1994). *Devereux Scales of Mental Disorders*. San Antonio, TX: The Psychological Corporation.

National Association of State Directors of Special Education (2005). *Response to intervention*. Alexandria, VA: Author.

Norman, W.T. (1963). Toward and adequate taxonomy of personality attributes: Replicated factor structure in peer nomination personality ratings. *Journal of Abnormal and Social Psychology, (66)6*, 574–583.

Oakland, T., Callueng, C., Rizwan, & Aftab, S. (2011). Temperament styles of children from Pakistan and the United States. *School Psychology International, 33*, 207–222. doi: 10.1177/0143034311420358

Oakland, T., & Joyce, D. (2006). Temperament-based learning styles and school-based applications. *Canadian Journal of School Psychology, 19*, 59–74.

Oakland, T., Glutting, J. J., & Horton, C. B. (1996). *Student Styles Questionnaire: Star qualities in learning, relating, and working*. San Antonio, TX: The Psychological Corporation.

O'Connor, K. P. O. (2008). Eysenck's model of individual differences. In G. J. Boyle, G. Matthews, & D. H. Saklofske (Eds.), *The SAGE handbook of personality theory and assessment, Vol 1: Personality theories and models* (pp. 215–238). Thousand Oaks, CA, US: Sage Publications, Inc.

Ostrander, R., Weinfurt, K., Yarnold, P., & August, G. (1998). Diagnosing attention deficit disorders with the behavioral assessment system for children and the child behavior checklist: Test and construct validity analyses using optimal discriminant classification trees. *Journal of Consulting and Clinical Psychology, 66*, 660–672.

Piers, E. V., Harris, D. B., & Herzberg, D. S. (2002). *Piers-Harris Children's Self-Concept Scale* (2nd ed.). Los Angeles, CA: Western Psychological Services.

Porter, R. B., & Cattell, R. B. (1985). *Handbook for the Children's Personality Questionnaire*. Champaign, IL.: Institute for Personality and Ability Testing.

Prior, M., Sanson, A., Smart, D., & Oberklaid, F. (2000). *Pathways from infancy to adolescence: Australian temperament project 1983–2000*. Melbourne, Australia: Australian Institute of Family Studies.

Reynolds, C. R., & Kamphaus, R. W. (2009). *BASC-2 Behavior Progress Monitor*. San Antonio, TX: Pearson Assessments.

Quay, H. C., Morse, W. C., & Cutler, R. L. (1966). Personality patterns of pupils in special classes for the emotionally disturbed. *Exceptional Children, 32*, 297–301.

Quenk, N. L. (2000). *Essentials of Myers-Briggs Type Indicator assessment*. New York, NY: John Wiley & Sons.

Rawlings, D., & Dawe, S. (2008). Psychoticism and impulsivity. In G. J. Boyle, G. Matthews, & D. H. Saklofske (Eds.), *The SAGE handbook of personality theory and assessment, Vol 1: Personality theories and models* (pp. 215–238). Thousand Oaks, CA, US: Sage Publications, Inc.

Reynolds, W. M. (2001). *Reynolds Adolescent Adjustment Screening Inventory: Professional Manual*. Lutz, FL: Psychological Assessment Resources.

Reynolds, C. R., & Kamphaus, R. W. (2004). *Behavior Assessment System for Children—Second Edition*. Circle Pines, MN: American Guidance Service.

Reynolds, W. M. (1998). *Adolescent Psychopathology Scale: Psychometric and technical manual*. Odessa, FL: Psychological Assessment Resources.

Reynolds, W. M. (2000). *Adolescent Psychopathology Scale—Short Form*. Lutz, FL: Psychological Assessment Resources.

Roberts, B. W., & DelVecchio, W. F. (2000). The rank-order consistency of personality traits from childhood to old age: A quantitative review of longitudinal studies. *Psychological Bulletin, 126*(1), 3–25.

Rothbart, M. K., & Derryberry, D. (1981). Development of individual differences in temperament. In M. E. Lamb & A. L. Brown (Eds.), *Advances in developmental psychology: Volume I* (pp. 37–86). Hillsdale, NJ: Erlbaum.

Saklofske, D. H., Eysenck, H.J., Eysenck, S.B.G., Stelmack, R.M., & Revelle, W. (2012) Extraversion-introversion. In V.S. Ramachandran (Ed.). *Encyclopedia of Human Behavior—2nd Ed.* (pp. 150–159), San Diego, CA: Academic Press.

Saklofske, D.H., & Eysenck, S.B.G. (1998). *Individual differences in children and adolescents*. New Jersey: Transaction Press.

Salvia, J., & Ysseldyke, J. E., & Bolt, S. (2007). *Assessment in special and inclusive education (10th ed)*. New York: NY. Houghton Mifflin Company.

Sanson, A., Prior, M., Garino, E., Oberklaid, F., & Sewell, J. (1987). The structure of infant temperament: Factor analysis of the Revised Infant Temperament Questionnaire. *Infant Behavior and Development, 10*, 97–104.

Sattler, J. M., & Hoge, R. D. (2006). *Assessment of children: Behavioral, social, and clinical foundations.* La Mesa, CA: Jerome Sattler Publisher.

Scahill, L., Riddle, M. A., McSwiggin-Hardin, M., Ort, S. I., King, R. A., & Goodman, W. K., et al. (1997). Children's Yale-Brown obsessive-compulsive scale: reliability and validity. *Journal of the American Academy of Child and Adolescent Psychiatry, 36,* 844–852.

Shelton, J. (1996). Health, stress, and coping. In A. L. Hammer (Ed.), *MBTI applications: A decade of research on the Myers-Briggs Type Indicator* (pp. 197–215). Palo Alto, CA: Consulting Psychologists Press.

Stafford, M., & Oakland, T. (1996). Validity of temperament constructs using the Student Styles Questionnaire: Comparisons for three racial-ethnic groups. *Journal of Psychoeducational Assessment, 14,* 109–120.

Sternberg, G. (1990). *Brain and personality: Extraversion/introversion in relation to EEG, evoked potentials and cerebral blood flow.* Unpublished doctoral dissertation, University of Lund, Sweden.

Storch, E. A., Murphy, T. K., Bagner, D. M., Johns, N. B., Baumeister, A. L., Goodman, W. K., et al. (2006). Reliability and validity of the Child Behavior Checklist Obsessive-Compulsive Scale. *Journal of Anxiety Disorders, 20,* 473–485.

Strack, S. (2008). *Essentials of Millon inventories assessment (3rd ed.).* Hoboken, NJ, US: John Wiley & Sons Inc.

Strelau, J. (1983). *Temperament-personality-activity.* New York, NY: Academic Press.

Strelau, J., & Zawadzki, B (2008). Temperament from a psychometric perspective: Theory and measurement. In G. J. Boyle, G. Matthews, & D.H. Saklofske (Eds.), *The SAGE handbook of personality theory and assessment, Vol 2: Personality measurement and testing* (pp. 352–374). Thousand Oaks, CA, US: Sage Publications, Inc.

Thomas, A., & Chess, S. (1977). *Temperament and development.* New York, NY: Brunner/Mazel.

Thomas, A., & Chess, S. (1989). Temperament and personality. In G.A. Kohnstamm, J. E. Bates, & M. K. Rothbart (Eds.), *Temperament in childhood* (pp. 249–261). New York, NY: Wiley.

Thomas, A., Chess, S., & Birch, H. G. (1968). *Temperament and behavior disorders in children.* New York, NY: University Press.

van der Valk, J., van den Oord, E., Verhulst, F., & Boomsma, D. (2003). Using shared and unique parental views to study the etiology of 7-year-old twins' internalizing and externalizing problems. *Behavior Genetics, 33,* 409–420.

Walker, H. M., & Severson, H. H. (1992). *Systematic screening for behavior disorders, second edition.* Longmont, CO: Sopris West.

Wehr, G. (1971). *Portrait of Jung: An illustrated biography.* (W. A. Hargreaves, Trans.). New York: Herder and Herder. (Original work published 1969).

Weis, R., & Smenner, L. (2007). Construct validity of the Behavior Assessment System for Children (BASC) self-report of personality: Evidence from adolescents referred to residential treatment. *Journal of Psychoeducational Assessment, 25,* 111–121.

Wilson, M. A., & Languis, M. L. (1990). A topographic study of difference in the P300 between introverts and extraverts. *Brain Topography, 2*(4), 369–274.

Principles of Behavioral Assessment

Tanya L. Eckert *and* Benjamin J. Lovett

Abstract

The chapter defines behavioral assessment and covers its historical developments over the last century. A review of the theoretical foundations of behavioral assessment is provided, including materialism, determinism, and contextualism. The chapter also discusses the methodological foundations of behavioral assessment, which are influenced by psychometric principles and a particular conceptualization of causation and functional relationships. Five general behavioral assessment methods are reviewed (behavioral observation, behavioral interviewing, behavior rating scales, psychophysiological measurements, performance tasks) and three specific applications of behavioral assessment methodologies (functional assessment, intervention evaluation, diagnostic classification) are discussed.

Key Words: assessment, behavioral assessment

The psychological assessment of children and adolescents is a field full of controversies, where a certain assessment tool or approach can be dominant at one point in time and viewed poorly only a short time later. Behavioral assessment is an approach that has become more popular in recent years, but has always been acknowledged as an important part of clinical assessment. In this chapter, we focus on the theoretical principles that undergird behavioral assessment techniques, leaving other chapters to cover the practical details of each technique. We define behavioral assessment, cover its history and conceptual tenets, explore relevant psychometric principles, and briefly discuss specific techniques and applications.

What is Behavioral Assessment?

One challenge in defining behavioral assessment is that almost all assessment tools yield results that make reference, at least implicitly, to behavior. The administration of a standard IQ test typically leads

a child to engage in many behaviors, including responses to the task stimuli provided by the examiner. Similarly, an unstructured clinical interview will yield many verbal and nonverbal behaviors on the part of the interviewee. Although certain measures (e.g., behavioral observation systems) are more likely to be thought of as behavioral assessment tools than others (e.g., IQ tests), as we will see, behavioral assessment is more about an approach to interpreting information from assessment tools rather than the choice of the tools themselves.

This focus on a particular style of interpretation is important to keep in mind when examining common definitions of behavioral assessment, such as that given by Heiby and Haynes (2003):

> Behavioral assessment is a scientific approach to psychological assessment that emphasizes the use of minimally inferential measures, the use of measures that have been validated in ways appropriate for the assessment context, the assessment of functional

relations, and the derivation of judgments based on measurement in multiple situations, from multiple methods and sources, and across multiple times. (p. 7)

This definition serves as a useful foundation and deserves a thorough examination, provided that we emphasize the role of interpretation of assessment data in determining whether assessment is behavioral.

Heiby and Haynes (2003) list four emphases of behavioral assessment, beginning with "the use of minimally inferential measures." It would be more appropriate to say that behavioral assessment emphasizes minimal inferences from assessment data. For instance, if an adolescent girl referred for assessment tells an examiner that she has not been able to sleep through the night during the past month, inferring that the adolescent girl has been experiencing sleep problems recently requires only a minimal amount of inference. (Even this inference cannot be made with certainty, of course.) Inferring that the girl is anxious about something, based solely on her comment about sleep, incurs greater inferential risk. Inferring that she was severely traumatized one month ago would be an even riskier interpretation. A behavioral assessment approach would generally prefer those interpretations that require a minimal amount of inference. This preference does lead, albeit indirectly, to a preference for certain assessment tools—namely, those tools that require less inference to be useful. For instance, the data from a behavior rating scale completed by the mother of a seven-year-old boy referred for attention problems would generally require less inference than the data from a Rorschach inkblot test administered to the boy himself.

A second emphasis of behavioral assessment mentioned by Heiby and Haynes (2003) involves tools "validated in ways appropriate for the assessment context" (p. 7). For instance, if a school psychologist wishes to examine a child's anxiety in the classroom setting, a teacher-report rating scale may be superior to a parent-report rating scale, whereas the opposite may be true with regard to assessing anxiety at home. This logic is closely related to the principle of minimal inference, as using a teacher-report rating scale to assess anxiety at home requires an additional, risky inference that the child exhibits the same anxiety-related behavior at home and at school. As Messick (e.g., 1989) noted, measures themselves are never valid or invalid; instead, *interpretations* have more or less validation evidence, so interpretations about behavior at home from

teacher reports have less validation evidence than do interpretations about behavior at school. As such, we could modify Heiby and Haynes's characterization to say that behavioral assessment involves making interpretations that have validation evidence specific to the context that the measures cover.

Heiby and Haynes (2003) also mention that behavioral assessment emphasizes the assessment of functional relations—that is, the causal relationships between environmental events and behaviors. Behavioral assessment, then, goes beyond the description of behavior to encompass the explanation of behavior as well. Of course, other assessment paradigms make explanatory claims, but behavioral assessment uses principles of learning theory (discussed in detail below) to do so, and relies on direct evidence for these explanatory claims that require minimal inference from that evidence. For instance, a traditional clinical assessment of a preschool-aged boy referred for disruptive behavior may explain his behavior with reference to a neuropsychological condition such as attention-deficit/hyperactivity disorder (ADHD). Coming from a behavioral assessment perspective, the neuropsychological explanation might be viewed as incomplete (if not circular), and a behavioral approach to the assessment of this child would seek direct evidence of environmental variables (e.g., attention from peers) that are causing the disruptive behavior.

Finally, Heiby and Haynes (2003) note that behavioral assessment emphasizes measurements across different settings, sources, tools, and time periods. Although most best-practice recommendations for clinical assessment emphasize this as well, behavioral assessment again differs in its approach to interpretation. If two sources of assessment information (for instance, a referred child's mother and father) provide different, contradictory information, the behavioral assessment approach would not conclude that one or both of the sources is incorrect, but instead that the child may behave differently in the presence of the mother than in the presence of the father. Similarly, if assessments of the child's academic skills yield very different data one week from another week, the behavior assessment approach would be more likely to conclude that the child's skill levels had changed, and less likely to attribute the discrepancy to unreliability in the measurement tools. These interpretations are consistent with the principle of minimal inference, because assessing a child in many different ways, through different sources, and at various times in various settings lessen the inferential burden for any individual piece of assessment data. To summarize, then, behavioral assessment emphasizes direct measures of behavior and its environmental determinants, and minimal inferences from the data that these measures yield.

Historical Foundations of Behavioral Assessment

The history of behavioral assessment is bound up with the history of behavioral models of psychological disorders, and the history of scientific psychology generally (Ollendick, Alvarez, & Greene, 2003). Pioneers of scientific psychology such as Wilhelm Wundt emphasized the importance of careful measurement, and although mental processes were often inferred from experimental participants' behavior, direct quantifications of behavior such as reaction time were studied as well (Goodwin, 2008). After studying animal psychology, Watson (1913) formally founded behaviorism by suggesting that psychology study humans in the same way that we study other animals: by only making reference to observable behavior and eschewing all but the most minimal inferences about unobservable mental processes.

Slowly, behaviorism began to penetrate the realm of clinical psychology. After Watson used classical conditioning to induce a phobia (Watson & Rayner, 1920), one of Watson's students used classical conditioning to treat a phobia (Jones, 1924). Similarly, B. F. Skinner's student Ogden Lindsley applied operant conditioning techniques to treat individuals with severe mental illnesses (Reed & Luiselli, 2009). In each of these cases, the behaviors associated with psychological disorders were carefully described and measured, so that the dependent variables were clear and any change in behaviors could be assessed with precision.

Behavioral assessment came into its own in the 1960s and 1970s as behavior therapy flourished, and behavior therapists developed assessment methods that were especially useful in their own clinical contexts. When the *Journal of Behavioral Assessment* began in 1979, the first full article (Hartmann, Roper, & Bradford, 1979) emphasized the large differences between behavioral and traditional assessment, including the central idea that in behavioral assessment, behavior exhibited during assessment is viewed as merely a *sample* of the client's behavior more generally, rather than a *sign* of underlying traits. Since the blossoming of behavioral assessment, an important feature of the field has been an insistence on rigor and validity, while at the same time thoughtfully questioning whether the typical metrics for

these qualities are appropriate for behavioral assessments (e.g., Hayes, Nelson, & Jarrett, 1986).

Today, behavioral assessment is an indispensable part of the clinical assessment of children and adolescents. It is a rare child assessment protocol that does not include standardized behavior rating scales, even if clinicians insist on interpreting the scales as revealing an underlying diagnostic status. School districts across the country are using behavioral measures of academic skills as part of a comprehensive evaluation to determine whether a student has a learning disability (L. Fuchs, D. Fuchs, & Zumeta, 2008). At times, U. S. federal law even requires the use of behavioral assessments to determine whether problem behavior is due to environmental reinforcement (Barnhill, 2005). Even if the growth of these procedures has at times outpaced proper training, and enthusiasm has occasionally outrun prudence, it seems safe to say that in the context of child assessment, behavioral assessment is here to stay.

Theoretical Foundations of Behavioral Assessment
Materialism

The first broad theoretical perspective that undergirds behavioral assessment is materialism, often defined as the claim that all that exists is (physical) matter. Materialism rules out the existence of nonmaterial entities, including nonmaterial entities that are often thought to control behavior (for instance, minds, spirits, or souls). Human behavior, then, can be viewed as matter (human bodies) in motion, and we can usefully search for the causes of that motion. Scientific study of the patterns of human behavior identifies two observable sources of behavior. First, the brain and nervous system are the proximal (immediate) causes of behavior. Various types of research (electrical stimulation experiments, single cell recording, neurological case studies) have shown the precise, specific relationships between different parts of the brain and nervous system and different kinds of behaviors (Andrewes, 2001). Any time that behavior is observed, it should be viewed as an immediate consequence of the activity of the nervous system.

The nervous system is not, however, the ultimate cause of behavior, since it is always responding to the environment. Typically, the nervous system causes behavior in response to a stimulus—some environmental event. Stimuli are extremely variable, of course, and this variability is consistently related to variability in behavioral responses. Different stimuli, for instance, reliably lead to behavioral responses that we would interpret as anger, fear, or joy—that is, emotional responses. Behavioral assessment often involves the functional relations between stimuli and various behavioral responses, with the knowledge that these relations may be different for each person, although there is considerable similarity across people in these relations as well. For instance, behavioral assessment during family therapy may include observations of a fifteen-year-old boy interacting with his mother. If the boy's anger responses are consistently observed (seen 90% of the time) after the mother asks the boy a question, but they are not nearly as frequent (only seen 20% of the time) otherwise, hypotheses about the cause of the boy's anger can be generated.

Understanding that the environment is the ultimate cause of behavior relieves us of the burden of examining the nervous system directly. Although early behaviorists (e.g., Watson, 1930) spent considerable time describing the nervous system and its connections with muscles, in an effort to describe how individual "molecular" behaviors occur, later behaviorists (e.g., Skinner, 1974) placed the nervous system in the middle of a causal chain, between the environment and behavior, suggesting that neurological explanations of behavior beg the real question of what led the nervous system to respond in such a way. Therefore, behavioral assessment does not typically involve direct assessment of nervous system functioning, although as we review later in the chapter, certain physiological variables may be part of a behavioral assessment.

Determinism

Behavioral assessment also assumes determinism, the doctrine that all events (including occurrences of human behavior) are determined fully by prior events. There are many versions of determinism in academic philosophy, but determinism is often thought to be incompatible with free will, and is often viewed as a necessary assumption to be made if human behavior is to be studied scientifically. Behavioral models of psychology are not just deterministic in a general sense; they make very specific and testable claims about the exact processes by which environmental variables determine behavior. Many of these processes can be usefully classified under two groups: respondent conditioning and operant conditioning.

In respondent conditioning (also called classical conditioning or Pavlovian conditioning), an automatic, reflexive response to one stimulus becomes transferred to a second stimulus, after the two stimuli are paired repeatedly (Powell, Symbaluk, & Honey, 2009). In Pavlov's (1927) seminal experiments on classical conditioning, dogs began to salivate in response to such stimuli as the sound of a ticking metronome, after those stimuli had been paired with the presentation of food. Our understanding of the mechanisms underlying respondent conditioning continues to grow, and although early behavioral explanations of these mechanisms are no longer widely held (cf. Rescorla, 1988), we now can predict with great precision when the pairing of stimuli will lead to conditioning, and how strong a conditioned response will be.

Respondent conditioning has been implicated in many varieties of psychopathology (Plaud & Eifert, 1998), and behavioral assessment may involve detailing the nature of maladaptive behavior that follows respondent conditioning, describing the respondent conditioning situations that caused maladaptive behavior, or monitoring behavior change during the process of respondent conditioning-based therapy. Whenever behavioral assessment aims at explaining the origin of the behavior being analyzed, respondent conditioning is a likely explanation for behavior if an underlying reflex can be identified, and the unconditioned stimulus initiating the reflex has been paired with a second stimulus, to which the person now shows an unusual reaction (O'Donohue & Ferguson, 2003).

Operant conditioning is a second set of processes that determines behavior. Whereas respondent conditioning places emphasis on the stimuli that precede behavior, operant conditioning emphasizes the stimuli that function as behavioral consequences, namely reinforcement and punishment. Reinforcing stimuli increase the frequency of the behaviors that precede their presentation, whereas punishing stimuli decrease the frequency of behaviors that precede the punishment (Powell et al., 2009). Thorndike's (e.g., 1927) statement of the law of effect is often viewed as the first formal analysis of operant conditioning processes, but it was B. F. Skinner's work (e.g., Ferster & Skinner, 1957; Skinner, 1938, 1953, 1974) that first explored many of the details of operant conditioning, such as the presentation of reinforcing stimuli on various schedules, and the control that environmental cues acquire over reinforced behavior ("stimulus control"). Unlike respondent conditioning, which can only modify reflexive reactions that are already present, operant conditioning can lead to new behaviors through (for instance) the process of shaping, in which reinforcement is given for behaviors that come closer and closer to a target behavior (Miltenberger, 2008).

The role of operant conditioning in psychopathology is well established (Plaud & Eifert, 1998), and behavioral assessment techniques are often used to monitor changes in behavior in response to operant conditioning-based therapies. More recently, "functional behavioral assessments" have become common, in which behavioral assessment techniques are used to locate a hypothesized reinforcer that is responsible for maintaining maladaptive behavior. For instance, an eight-year-old boy referred for disruptive behavior may be disruptive every time that a math lesson begins in his classroom. A comprehensive assessment might find that the boy has very poor math skills, that he is sent to the school's main office whenever he is disruptive in the classroom, and that in the main office he is not asked to perform any tasks. This suggests the possibility that the boy is disruptive in order to escape task demands, and being sent to the main office serves as negative reinforcement for disruptive behavior.

Operationalism

A third theoretical perspective relevant to behavioral assessment, operationalism (also called *operationism*) is defined by Hung (1997) as the doctrine that "all terms should be operationally defined, and the meaning of a term is the set of the defining operations" (p. 226). Operational definitions define variables in terms of publicly observable operations performed to measure the variables, and so we might operationally define "hunger" as a person's rating of their feeling of hunger on a scale from 1 to 10, or as a certain number of hours having passed without eating. Operationalism has had a large influence on psychology, with behaviorists in particular embracing operational definitions (Zuriff, 1985). Skinner (1953) exemplified operationalism when he noted that in terms of publicly observable behavior, "a single set of facts is described by the two statements 'He eats' and 'He is hungry'" (p. 31).

Operationalism has particular relevance to assessment, since psychologists often assess traits that are in need of proper operational definitions. Whenever possible, behavioral assessment provides a statement of the publicly observable behavior itself rather than the trait name, since under operationalism, the two are functionally equivalent. Rather than describing a child as "highly intelligent" or "low in neuroticism," behavioral assessment describes exactly what behaviors might lead to a judgment of intelligence or neuroticism by observers. If, after all, the reason why an evaluator believes a nine-year-old boy to have a phobia of dogs is that he runs away whenever he sees a dog, the phobia label requires inferences that a simple description of behavior does not require. If a twelve-year-old girl is described as "hyperactive," but the only evidence for this is that she constantly fidgets in her seat in the classroom, the frequency of fidgets should be quantified and noted, rather than applying a label that might suggest other behaviors that have not yet been observed to be present or absent.

Because of its commitment to operationalism, behavioral assessment has generally been considered to be against formal diagnostic labels (Spiegler & Guevremont, 2003). Although some diagnostic classifications (for instance, those found in recent editions of the American Psychiatric Association's *Diagnostic and Statistical Manual of Mental Disorders*) emphasize observable behavioral features and can be reliably assessed, diagnostic labels always carry the danger that they will be viewed as more than a summary of behavior. This tendency to "reify" labels and assume that they refer to latent, internal characteristics of people that *produce* the behaviors being assessed leads many practitioners of behavioral assessment to de-emphasize diagnostic labels, and only provide labels when necessary for official purposes. To operationalists, a psychiatric diagnosis is, at best, equivalent to the observable symptoms of the disorder being diagnosed, with no additional meaning attaching to the diagnostic label (Lovett & Hood, 2011).

Methodological Foundations of Behavioral Assessment

Behavioral assessment is conceptualized as a psychological assessment methodology based on principles of scientific inquiry and inference (Heiby & Haynes, 2003). As a result, behavioral assessment methods are influenced by particular conceptions of causation and functional relationships as well as certain psychometric principles.

Causation and Functional Relationships

One of the central features of behavioral assessment is an emphasis on situational determinants of behavior across time and environments (Kenny, Alvarez, Donohue, & Winick, 2007). As a result, behaviors and environmental events are repeatedly measured in an effort to derive precise and minimally inferential results. The methods of behavioral assessment have been conceptualized as falling on a continuum ranging from direct assessment methods to indirect assessment methods (Cone, 1977, 1978). Many of the indirect behavior assessment methods rely on informant reports of behavior and events surrounding its occurrence to generate hypotheses regarding behavior-environmental relations (Gresham, Watson, & Skinner, 2001; McComas & Mace, 2000). Although these methods identify environmental events that influence behavior, this association reflects only a correlational relationship (Gresham et al., 2001; McComas & Mace, 2000). Interestingly, even the majority of direct behavior assessment methods (e.g., direct observation, performance tasks) reflect a correlational relationship when examined in relation to environmental events.

Determining causal factors in behavioral assessment is complex (Haynes, 1992; Kazdin & Kagan, 1994) and emphasizes temporally contiguous environmental events (i.e., antecedents and consequences), non-contemporaneous causes (e.g., family interactions) as well as the dimensions (e.g., magnitude, chronicity) of causal variables (Haynes, 2000). Haynes and colleagues (1993) identified five methods of inferring causal relationships from behavioral assessments: (a) empirical derivation from research findings; (b) causally focused self-report measures; (c) causal marker variables (e.g., physiological measures of arousal); (d) statistical analyses across time and behavior; and (e) manipulation of hypothesized causal variables. This last method, commonly referred to as experimental functional assessment, involves systematically manipulating antecedent and consequent events to verify functional relations between environmental events and behavior. Results from an experimental functional assessment identify one or more behavior-environment relations that maintain the problem behavior of children and youth (McComas & Mace, 2000). As noted by Carr (1993), the importance of identifying the functions of problem behavior cannot be overstated:

> Thus, knowing that a young boy diagnosed as autistic exhibits self-injury is, by itself, not very interesting. What is interesting is why the self-injury occurs (i.e., of what variables is it a function)...Topography (behavior) does not matter much; function (purpose) does. (p. 48)

Psychometric Principles

The psychometric models most appropriate to behavioral assessment approaches have created significant controversy, with some criticisms remaining unresolved (Dawes, 1994; Meehl & Rosen, 1955; Mischel, 1968; Peterson, 1968). Given the underlying assumptions of behavioral assessment, it has been argued by some that the application of classic psychometric principles is inappropriate (Hartmann et al., 1979; Suen, 1988). Others, however, have argued that basic psychometric concepts (e.g., reliability, validity) as well as alternative concepts (e.g., generalizability theory) should be applied to behavioral assessment methods (Bellack & Hersen, 1988; Cone, 1988; O'Leary, 1979).

Given that many behavioral assessment measures are designed for idiographic rather than nomothetic purposes, intraindividual changes are of interest, systematic error is relevant, and variance across participants does not exist (Suen, 1988). In contrast, in nomothetic assessment, individual performance is compared to group performance and variance across participants is considered true and meaningful. In behavioral assessment, however, it is the variance across points of observations that is considered true variance (Suen, 1988). Furthermore, whereas systematic error, such as observer error, is irrelevant and can be partitioned out in traditional assessment, systematic error can be extremely problematic in behavioral assessment. For example, an observer who systematically overestimates the occurrence of a behavior in traditional, nomothetic assessment will do so across all participants, maintaining the rank order and amount of variability across participants. However, if an observer overestimates the occurrence of a behavior in idiographic, behavioral assessment, the error will affect the relationship between the observed score and the criterion.

Conventional psychometric constructs clearly apply when behavioral assessment approaches include standardized measures such as behavior rating scales and checklists. Consistent with professional standards in psychology (Standard 9.02; American Psychological Association, 2002), core dimensions of reliability (i.e., test-retest, interrater, alternate-form, internal consistency, internal structure) and validity evidence (i.e., content, discriminative, concurrent, predictive) should be examined and considered in the selection of standardized behavioral assessment instruments (Bagner, Harwood, & Eyberg, 2006). However, other behavioral assessment strategies, such as direct observation, are associated with different psychometric conceptualizations that focus on behavior and its variation within individuals (Johnston & Pennypacker, 1993; Nelson, Hay, & Hay, 1977). Although information regarding the psychometric qualities of standardized observational codes is reported in manuals, other psychometric qualities, such as interobserver agreement, can only be determined after direct observations are conducted.

Recently, Hintze (2005) argued that reliability of direct observation procedures should be evaluated regarding the sensitivity to individual differences and the likelihood that similar results would be obtained across a variety of students and practice situations. In his work, Hintze argues that direct observation methods developed by practitioners should examine: (a) internal consistency reliability; (b) test-tetest reliability; (c) interobserver agreement; (d) content validity; (e) concurrent and convergent validity; (f) predictive validity; and (g) sensitivity to change. For those methods that are being used commercially or for research purposes, he argues that (a) interobserver agreement; (b) intraobserver reliability; (c) content validity; (d) concurrent and predictive validity; (e) convergent and discriminant validity; and (f) sensitivity to change should be formally evaluated. Moreover, one of the underlying assumptions of behavioral assessment is that decisions and the resulting consequences of these decisions (i.e., intervention development, diagnostic classifications) should be validated. This conceptualization includes producing socially significant outcomes, or social validation (Kazdin, 1977; Schwartz & Baer, 1991; Wolf, 1978) as well as valid treatment approaches (Messick, 1995). Thus, behavioral assessment strategies need to be considered within the context of a problem-solving and decision-making context (Barnett, Lentz, & Macmann, 2000), and the usefulness, or validity, of the behavioral assessment data obtained needs to be considered.

Behavioral Assessment Strategies

Although dozens of behavioral assessment techniques have been developed, behavioral assessment strategies are generally organized into five general categories: (a) behavioral observation, (b) behavior interviewing, (c) behavior rating scales, (d) psychophysiological measurements, and (e) performance tasks. In this next section of our chapter, we provide a broad overview of each of these techniques.

Behavioral Observation

Among the various behavioral assessment strategies developed, behavioral observation is considered the hallmark for measuring and recording behavior (Gresham et al., 2001; Steege, Davin, & Hathaway, 2001). Behavioral observation can be used in a variety of situational contexts (e.g., school, home) to identify behavior deficits and excesses of children and youth as well as identify the determining or controlling variables of problem behaviors (Cone

& Hawkins, 1977). In addition, objective features of behavior, such as frequency, temporality, and intensity, can be assessed using observation-based recording methods. When data collected from behavioral observation strategies are quantified, behavioral trends and variability can be readily examined (Barlow & Hersen, 1984; House, House, & Campbell, 1981; Shapiro & Skinner, 1990).

Systematic direct observation. Systematic direct observations are often used to quantify the behavior of children and youth (Hintze, Volpe, & Shapiro, 2003; Wilson & Reschly, 1996). They can be used within the context of a multi-method behavioral assessment to measure students' adaptive and maladaptive behaviors (Hops, Davis, & Longoria, 1995), and are often utilized as part of a functional assessment, discussed later in this chapter, to identify events that may serve to reinforce a behavior under specific conditions. As highlighted by Volpe and McConaughy (2005), systematic direct observations measure specific behaviors that have been operationally defined and follow standardized coding procedures. Unlike unsystematic direct observations, systematic direct observations provide quantitative data that are synchronized across children and youth, settings, and raters. The systematic nature of these instruments reduces common threats to the validity of observational measures, which include interobserver reliability, observer reactivity, and observer bias (Merrell, 1999).

A number of well-validated systematic direct observation instruments have been developed. Many of these measures have been developed for use in elementary classrooms. For example, Volpe, DiPerna, Hintze, and Shapiro (2005) provided a comprehensive review of a number of instruments including the Academic Engaged Time Code of the Systematic Screening for Behavior Disorders (AET-SSBD; Walker & Severson, 1990), the ADHD School Observation Code (ADHD-SOC; Gadow, Sprafkin, & Nolan, 1996), the Behavioral Observation of Students in Schools (BOSS; Shapiro, 2004), the Classroom Observation Code (COC; Abikoff & Gittelman, 1985), the Direct Observation Form (DOF; Achenbach, 1986), and the Student Observation System of the Behavioral Assessment System for Children-2 (SOS; Reynolds & Kamphaus, 2004). In addition, Leff and Lakin (2005) reviewed playground-based observational systems and identified two well-established systems: the Interpersonal Process Code (IPC; Rusby, Estes, & Dishion, 1991) and the Peer Social Behavior of the Systematic Screening for Behavior Disorders

(PSB of the SSBD; Walker & Severson, 1990). Finally, McConaughy (2005a) reviewed three standardized observational instruments for use during test sessions and child clinical interviews, the Guide to Assessment for Test Session Behavior (GATSB; Glutting & Oakland, 1993), the Test Observation Form (TOF; McConaughy & Achenbach, 2004), and the Observation Form for the Semistructured Clinical Interview for Children and Adolescents (SCICA; McConaughy & Achenbach, 2001).

Antecedent-Behavior-Consequence recording. A second form of direct observation, anecdotal observation, involves the written narrative of behaviors and environmental conditions under which the behaviors were emitted (Cooper, 1981). Information obtained from this type of observation not only provides a record of behavior within an environmental context, but also identifies events that happen before or after the behavior of interest (Cooper, Heron, & Heward, 1987). Commonly referred to as Antecedent-Behavior-Consequence recording (A-B-C; Bijou, Peterson, & Ault, 1968), this approach involves collecting data on the observable events preceding the target behavior ([A] antecedents of behavior), the target behavior [B], and the observable events following the target behavior ([C] consequences of behavior) (O'Neill, Horner, Albin, Storey, & Sprague, 1990). Following the completion of the observation, the data are reviewed to examine the relationship between the antecedents, behaviors, and consequences observed. The analysis of A-B-C recordings involves either visually analyzing or quantifying patterns in responding to identify the types of environmental events that either precede or follow the problem behavior (Sterling-Turner, Robinson, & Wilczynski, 2001). Temporal relations among behavior and events surrounding its occurrence can also be quantified from A-B-C recordings based on conditional probabilities. Conditional probability analysis requires the computation of proportions that reflect the likelihood that an antecedent or consequence is related to the occurrence of a target behavior (Eckert, Martens, & DiGennaro, 2005; Sterling-Turner et al., 2001).

Ecobehavioral classroom assessment. A more specialized form of direct observation, ecobehavioral classroom assessment, assesses classroom variables affecting the behavior of children and youth in school settings. This type of assessment is designed to assess the association between various environmental and instructional factors in the classroom (e.g., physical arrangement of classroom, teacher prompts) and the ensuing behaviors of children and youth

(Greenwood, Carta, Kamps, & Arreaga-Mayer, 1990). Ecobehavioral classroom assessment is based on Carroll's (1963) model of classroom learning as well as empirical research demonstrating that active student engagement is highly associated with student achievement and learning (e.g., Brophy & Good, 1986; Greenwood, 1991; Sindelar, Smith, Harriman, Hale, & Wilson, 1986).

Unlike systematic direct observations and A-B-C recording, the focus of ecobehavioral classroom assessments is to simultaneously measure classroom context, teacher instructional variables, and student responding. This results in standardized coding procedures that can be complex in the types of behaviors observed (e.g., child, peers, teacher) and time sampling procedures (e.g., momentary time sampling, partial interval, whole interval) employed. As summarized by Stichter and Lewis (2006), ecobehavioral classroom assessments serve four major purposes: (a) they describe the instructional context of the classroom; (b) they compare instructional contexts across classrooms; (c) they identify contextual variables associated with positive academic and behavioral student outcomes; and (d) they monitor changes in the instructional context of the classroom.

Based on the literature base examining classroom variables affecting student behavior and achievement, Stichter and Lewis (2006) developed a hierarchy of classroom assessment metrics common to ecobehavioral assessments. At the first level of this hierarchy, physical and structural classroom arrangements are measured. Examples of metrics assessed at this level include classroom traffic patterns, accessibility of classroom materials, and posting of classroom rules and daily classroom schedule. Inherent at this level are specific physical aspects (e.g., Where is the pencil sharpener located?) as well as procedural aspects (e.g., Are there standardized procedures for hand raising?) of the physical and structural arrangement of the classroom. The second level of the hierarchy focuses on assessing instructionally-specific contexts of the classroom, including types of instructional delivery (e.g., independent seatwork, transition activities) and student grouping techniques (e.g., small group, peer collaboration). The third level of the hierarchy examines the specific instructional techniques used by the teacher in the classroom. Examples of specific techniques assessed include instructional talk, wait time, downtime, previewing, organizational prompting, modeling, and providing instructional feedback. The final level of Stichter and Lewis's hierarchy assesses students' academic (e.g., work product accuracy) and behavioral (e.g., engagement) outcomes exhibited in the classroom.

A number of ecobehavioral assessment measures have been developed for use in classroom environments. Some of these measures, such as the Direct Instruction Observational System (DIOS; Englert & Sugai, 1981), focus primarily on teacher behaviors exhibited in the classroom. The majority of measures simultaneously measure teacher and student behaviors. These measures include the State-Event Classroom Observation System (SECOS; Saudargas & Creed, 1980), which assesses student and teacher behaviors; the Classroom Activity Recording Form (CARF; Sindelar et al.,1986), which assesses types of classroom instruction (i.e., direct instruction, independent work, non-instructional work) as well as student behaviors; the Teacher/Student Interaction Analysis (Sugai & Lewis, 1989), which assesses instructional behaviors and student responses; and the Setting Factors Assessment Tool (SFAT; Stichter, Lewis, Johnson, & Trussell, 2004), which assesses teacher and student behaviors across four levels (i.e., global classroom structural variables, nature of instructional content, specific teacher instructional cues, student behaviors). Furthermore, a number of computer-based ecobehavioral assessments have been developed including the Ecobehavioral Assessment Systems Software (E-BASS; Greenwood, Carta, Kamps, & Delquardi, 1993), the Mainstream Code for Instructional Structure and Student Academic Response (MS-CISSAR; Carta, Greenwood, Schulte, Arreaga-Mayer, & Terry, 1987), and the Ecobehavioral System for Complex Assessments of Preschool Environments (ESCAPE; Carta, Greenwood, & Atwater, 1985).

Interviews

Interviews are routinely used measures of behavioral assessment (Hughes & Baker, 1990), and provide detailed information from the perspectives of children, youth, and caregivers (McConaughy, 2003, 2005b). Behavioral assessment interviews are conceptualized as structured and quantitative measures that emphasize overt behavior, behavior-environment interactions, and situational sources of behavioral variation (Haynes, 2000). Ramsay, Reynolds, and Kamphaus (2002) identified six steps inherent in behavioral interviewing: (a) identify the problem behavior and specify target behaviors; (b) identify and analyze relevant environmental factors; (c) develop an intervention plan; (d) implement the intervention plan; (e) evaluate

outcomes associated with the intervention plan; and (f) modify the intervention plan as needed and reevaluate outcomes.

Although the accuracy and reliability of information obtained through this process requires verification, interviews afford the collection of an extensive amount of information that may be challenging to obtain using other types of behavioral assessment strategies. For example, some behaviors, such as those associated with anxiety and depression, may be difficult to capture using systematic direct observation methods. Interviews provide children, youth, and caregivers with the opportunity to articulate their perceptions of behavior and its consequences. It is important to note that the congruence of these multi-source interviews may be limited (Finch & Rogers, 1984) due to a number of errors associated with subjective reports, such as biases and memory errors (Haynes, 2000). However, there is some evidence to suggest that the perceptions of children and youth may be as important for behavior change as obtaining reliable and valid indices of the behavior itself (Ollendick & Hersen, 1984).

Two general categories of interviews have been developed: semi-structured interviews and structured interviews. Semi-structured interviews broadly assess children's perspectives on their functioning using a flexible interview format (McConaughy, 2003) and permit alterations in the wording and ordering of questions (Orvashel, 2006). The *Semistructured Clinical Interview for Children and Adolescents* (SCICA; McConaughy & Achenbach, 2001) is one example of a semi-structured interview for school-aged children that can be combined with data obtained from parent ratings on the *Child Behavior Checklist for Ages 6 to 18* (CBCL/6–18; Achenbach & Rescorla, 2001), teacher ratings on the *Teacher's Report Form* (TRF; Achenbach & Rescorla, 2001), youth self-ratings on the *Youth Self-Report* (YSR; Achenbach & Rescorla, 2001), and direct observations on the *Direct Observation Form* (DOF; Achenbach, 1986). The *Semistructured Clinical Interview for Children and Adolescents* protocol form provides instructions for introducing the interview, outlines samples of open-ended questions, and outlines topics in nine broad areas (e.g., family relations; self perceptions and feelings; parent- or teacher-reported problems). Profiles on seven syndrome scales (i.e., Anxious, Attention Problems, Language/Motor Problems, Self-Control Problems, Withdrawn/Depressed, Anxious/Depressed, Aggressive/Rule-Breaking) can be derived based on the informant's responses.

Structured interviews systematically assess a broad range of symptoms and specific diagnostic categories. However, unlike semi-structured interviews, the question format, rating responses, and ordering items are systematic and unvarying (Orvashel, 2006). Examples of highly structured interviews include the *Diagnostic Interview for Children and Adolescents-IV* (DICA-IV; Reich, 2000; Reich, Welner, Herjanic, & MHS Staff, 1999) and the *National Institutes of Mental Health's Diagnostic Interview Schedule for Children-Version IV* (NIMH DISC-IV; Shaffer, Fisher, Lucas, Dulcan, & Schwab-Stone, 2000). Both of these measures were developed to generate psychiatric diagnoses and cover the most common emotional and behavioral disorders of children and youth, including attention-deficit/hyperactivity disorder, conduct disorder, oppositional defiant disorder, major depression, dysthymia, and anxiety disorders. Admittedly, diagnoses such as these are not based solely on a child's observable behaviors. However, using structured interviews to make psychiatric diagnoses involves an equivalence between an informant's reports of symptoms and a psychiatric label, an equivalence that implies an operationalist conception of assessment (Lovett & Hood, 2011).

Behavior Rating Scales

Behavior rating scales rely on a retrospective assessment of a child or youth's behavior by others (e.g., caregivers, teachers) in order to provide a comprehensive assessment of behavior, including the identification of strengths and weaknesses that characterize the child or youth's behavior (Greene & Ollendick, 2000). Informants respond to a set of standardized, structured written statements pertaining to attitudes, beliefs, feelings, opinions, and physical states (Reynolds, 1993). This information can be compared with normative data to quantify the degree to which a behavior strength or weakness is manifested relative to that seen in the general population (Eckert, Dunn, Guiney, & Codding, 2000).

Administering behavior rating scales to multiple informants assesses the systemic influences that may affect a child or youth's behavior as well as measures the interrelationship among various individuals and environments (e.g., school, home) in a child or youth's life (Beaver & Busse, 2000). However, the limited association between responses on behavior rating scale across individuals, environments, and time has been acknowledged. Merrell (2000) summarized the major research findings regarding cross-informant correlations with child and youth

behavior rating scales and concluded: (a) correlations of behavior ratings made by all informants are statistically significant, but modest; (b) agreement among pairs of informants in similar roles is higher than agreement among informants in dissimilar roles; and (c) cross-informant ratings of externalizing problems is higher than ratings of internalizing problems.

Often behavior rating scales are organized into two separate categories, broad-band and narrow-band rating scales (Eckert, DuPaul, & Carson 2003). Broad-band behavior rating scales assess an extensive range of behaviors. The *Achenbach System of Empirically Based Assessment* (ASEBA; Achenbach & Rescorla, 2001) is the foremost example of a broad-band behavior rating scale that can be used to assess behavioral competencies, adaptive functioning, and behavior problems among school-age children and young adults. In addition, the *Behavior Assessment System for Children-2* (BASC-2; Reynolds & Kamphaus, 2004) represents a broad-band behavior rating scale that can be used for school-aged children to assess adaptive and problem behaviors exhibited in school and home settings. Both of these measures incorporate broad-band taxonomy of behaviors.

Narrow-band behavior rating scales focus exclusively on a single, specific construct such as hyperactivity, anxiety, or depression. Similar to broad-based behavior rating scales, narrow-band behavior measures can be administered to examine systemic influences on the behavior of children and youth. However, only one behavioral construct is typically examined in order to conduct an in-depth assessment (DuPaul, 1992). A significant number of narrow-based behavior rating scales have been developed to assess social and interpersonal relations (e.g., *Social Skills Rating System*; SSRS; Gresham & Elliott, 1990), self-concept (e.g., *Multidimensional Self Concept Scale*; MSCS; Bracken, 1992), depression (e.g., *Children's Depression Inventory*; CDI, Kovacs, 1992), anxiety (e.g., *Social Anxiety Scale for Children-Revised*; SASC-R; La Greca & Stone, 1993), and attention-deficit/hyperactivity disorder (e.g., *ADHD Rating Scale–IV*; DuPaul, Power, Anastopoulos, & Reid, 1998).

Psychophysiological Measurements

As the early behaviorists (e.g., Watson, 1930) pointed out long ago, behavior can be defined as the action of body parts, which are under the immediate control of the nervous and endocrine systems. Measures of muscle activity, as well as nervous and endocrine activity, can therefore be viewed as forms of behavioral assessment. Psychophysiological assessment is the term for these types of measures (Stern, Ray, & Quigley, 2000), and although the equipment needed for psychophysiological assessment is not available in every clinical setting, clinicians who work with children should consider its potential contributions to their practice. Indeed, Wilhelm, Schneider, and Friedman (2006) argue that psychophysiological assessment often provides information that other forms of behavioral assessment cannot provide. Specifically, people—and children in particular—cannot always keep track of their behavior well enough to answer interview questions or complete a rating scale accurately. Behavioral observation overcomes this problem but relies on subjective judgments of observers. Psychophysiological assessment bypasses both of these problems by providing direct *and* objective measures of behavior.

Electromyography (EMG) is the physiological measurement of muscle activity, and can be accomplished by placing EMG electrodes almost anywhere on the skin, although the most common placements are on the head, neck, arms and legs (Stern et al., 2000). Greater amplitude (height) of the waves shown on the EMG recording corresponds to more muscle contraction, and EMG is sufficiently sensitive that even very slight contraction can be detected. This is especially helpful when measuring activity in muscles whose contraction is not visible (for instance, in the head or neck), and where increased tension is associated with stress, anxiety, or other psychologically relevant variables (Wilhelm et al., 2006).

Eye movements are another frequently measured behavior in psychophysiology (electrooculography, or EOG), although rather than measuring activity in the muscles that control eye movements, EOG actually measures the electrical potential of the eyes directly (each eye is like a magnet, with the front part exhibiting a positive charge and the back exhibiting a negative charge; Stern et al., 2000). EOG can be used to detect interest in visual stimuli, by examining how long the eyes are moved to focus on a stimulus that was placed in the periphery of a child's visual field. Examining eye blinks is a related psychophysiological procedure, and possibly one with more clinical relevance, since blink frequency has been related to the presence of anxiety disorders and ADHD (Wilhelm et al., 2006).

Muscle contractions and eye movements are both classified as voluntary actions, since they cay often

be consciously controlled. These types of actions originate in the somatic nervous system (the system of nerves that innervate skeletal muscles), whereas involuntary actions (e.g., stomach contractions, the heartbeat, etc.) originate in the autonomic nervous system (Marieb & Hoehn, 2007). The autonomic nervous system has two divisions: the sympathetic branch prepares the body for quick action under conditions of stress, threat, or danger, by (for instance) dilating the pupils, increasing heart rate, and slowing digestive processes. The parasympathetic branch relaxes the body by reversing these and other processes. High levels of sympathetic activity are related to more intense experiences of stress and anxiety (Weems & Silverman, 2008), whereas low levels of sympathetic activity (e.g., pulse rate) have been found to relate to externalizing and antisocial behavior (Raine, 2002).

When determining whether to use psychophysiological procedures in clinical practice with children and adolescents, the core principles of behavioral assessment should be remembered: recall that behavioral assessment prefers data that require little inference to be meaningful. If there is reason to believe that tools such as behavior observation and interviews are yielding accurate information, psychophysiological assessment may be unnecessary. However, when observations and interviews are compromised in some way (e.g., through language barriers, unreliable informants, the covertness of the behaviors under examination), psychophysiological assessment techniques may be indicated, even if they are more cumbersome than other tools.

Performance Tasks

Performance tasks differ from many other forms of behavioral assessment in that they provide stimuli for the individual to respond to, rather than simply observing responses made in the presence of naturally occurring stimuli. The classification of performance tasks as *behavioral* assessment measures depends on whether those tasks satisfy our initial definition of behavioral assessment—that is, whether they are direct enough measures that they require little inference to be meaningful. Performance tasks used in this direct fashion have been developed for use with children and adolescents exhibiting academic and behavioral problems, and we discuss these tools separately.

Performance tasks measuring academic skills. A common criticism of many standardized tests of academic skills is that they are in some way "artificial," a vague criticism but one with a grain of truth in it. Certainly, many standardized tests of academic skills contain items different from those that students have seen during instruction, and many of the items are also unlike the real-world problems that students must one day solve using academic skills. The behavioral assessment of academic skills involves performance tasks that either directly map on to specific skills that are taught in the classroom, or that are used in everyday life outside classroom settings; either way, they link to stimuli that are not unique to the testing situation.

Measures that maximize the correspondence between test stimuli and stimuli presented during instruction are used in curriculum-based assessment (CBA; Hintze, 2009). There are several different models of CBA (e.g., curriculum-based measurement, curriculum-based evaluation), but they share many features, most importantly the construction of measures based on the academic curriculum that the student is exposed to. If a student's reading fluency is the skill under examination, the school's reading curriculum materials can be used to make a set of brief performance tasks, in which the student is asked to read passages aloud and the number of correctly read words per minute is recorded (for more details on construction, see Shapiro, 2004). The resulting score (the number of correctly read words per minute) is a portrait of behavioral assessment, since it has a much more direct interpretation than, for instance, a standard score obtained from a more typical reading achievement test.

Other performance tasks of academic skills maximize the correspondence between test stimuli and "real-world" tasks, and these measures are often referred to as "performance assessments" (Reynolds, Livingston, & Wilson, 2006). For instance, Gronlund and Waugh (2009) contrast several different ways of assessing a student's ability to apply math skills. One way would be to ask students how much change they would receive back if they paid one dollar for a toy that costs 69 cents. A more "authentic" performance assessment would involve asking students to serve as either customers or clerks in a mock "store." Many performance assessments do not have dichotomous, right-or-wrong answers, and require complex scoring rubrics to yield objective evaluations (Lane & Stone, 2006). For instance, a performance assessment of middle school students' science skills may involve the design of an experiment; the experiment will have many features, each of which could be assessed on many dimensions, and a rubric may be needed to direct examiners to focus on certain features and dimensions.

Importantly, both CBA and performance assessment have been plagued by psychometric concerns. For instance, Christ (2006) noted that many extraneous variables have been found to influence performance on CBA-type measures, and Christ and Hintze (2007) noted that even high reliability coefficients are not sufficient to show score replicability, since these coefficients assess whether the relative ranking of examinees change, and are insensitive to whether the examinees' mean scores change. Similarly, performance assessments have been criticized for showing low levels of agreement across different judges ever since Starch and Elliott's (e.g., 1912) classic studies of teachers' essay grading, and certain more recent evaluations of performance assessment programs (e.g., Koretz, McCaffrey, Klein, Bell, & Stecher, 1992) have reinforced these early conclusions. However, since these studies have generally been conducted using traditional psychometric theory, there is a need for newer evaluations incorporating a behavioral assessment perspective.

Performance tasks assessing psychopathology. Performance tasks can also be used in the clinical assessment of behavioral and emotional disorders. One such application is the continuous performance test (CPT), a measure of attention and impulsiveness used frequently in the assessment of ADHD (Gordon, Barkley, & Lovett, 2006). A typical CPT comprises several tasks; in one task, the child may be asked to press a key whenever he or she sees a particular stimulus ("X"), except when it follows another particular stimulus ("O"). Impulsivity is shown when the child responds to the X by pressing the key without first considering whether an O preceded the X. CPT scores differentiate children with and without psychopathology and are even sensitive to ADHD medication.

Another type of performance task is used in the assessment of anxiety disorders: the behavioral avoidance test (BAT; Southam-Gerow & Chorpita, 2007). In a BAT, the child is exposed to the feared stimulus and his or her reaction is carefully observed. Since children may have difficulty articulating the severity of their fear, or they may be unwilling to admit its true severity, a BAT can lead to a more accurate assessment, even if it is more unpleasant for most individuals than an interview or rating scale. Generally, BATs are conducted without a standardized procedure, but this is not necessarily a problem, as the BAT can be tailored to the client's desired outcome. For instance, a client who will merely need to be in the same room as a snake in a glass terrarium can be tested for his or her response to precisely that stimulus, whereas a client who will need to actually handle a snake can be tested for his or her response to having a snake put in his or her lap.

Behavioral Assessment Goals and Applications

In the beginning of our chapter, we reviewed many of the defining features of behavioral assessment that were discussed by Heiby and Haynes (2003). Based on these central features, the primary goals of behavioral assessment are to: (a) use direct measures of behavior and its environmental determinants across different settings, sources, tools and time periods; (b) emphasize the assessment of causal relationships between environmental events and behaviors; and (c) draw interpretations that have validation evidence specific to the measured contexts. Within the past two decades, advances have been made in the application of behavioral assessment methodologies that move the field closer towards achieving these primary goals. In the final section of our chapter, we will review three recent developments that address these goals: functional assessment, diagnostic classification, and intervention evaluation.

Functional Assessment

Functional assessment is a behavioral assessment methodology used to develop more effective and efficient interventions for children and youth (DuPaul & Ervin, 1996; Iwata, Dorsey, Slifer, Bauman, & Richman, 1982; Vollmer & Northup, 1996). Functional behavior assessment methods refer to a broad set of procedures that examine environmental and contextual events that maintain problem behaviors (Horner, 1994; Gresham et al., 2001; Witt, Daly, & Noell, 2000). These procedures can be used to identify antecedent and contextual factors as well as maintaining contingencies that directly influence behavior (Martens, Eckert, Bradley, & Ardoin, 1999). However, despite this widely accepted general definition, there is no consensus regarding the precise definition or the specific procedures that constitute a functional assessment (Ervin, Ehrhardt, & Poling, 2001; Ervin et al., 2001). Common procedures include many of the behavioral assessment methods previously reviewed in our chapter, including direct observation of problem behaviors and environmental events, as well as interviews with a variety of sources (e.g., student, parent, classroom teacher). More specialized procedures include systematically manipulating environmental events to examine the functional relationship between the child's problem behaviors and environmental events.

DuPaul, Eckert, and McGoey (1997) provided a broad guide to conducting functional assessments in school settings, which contained three steps: (a) conducting formal interviews to obtain descriptive information regarding the problem behaviors (i.e., What are the problem behaviors?); (b) completing behavioral observations of the problem behaviors in relation to environmental events in order to develop hypotheses regarding the function(s) of the problem behavior (i.e., What environmental variables set the occasion for the problem behavior?); and (c) experimentally manipulating environmental events to validate hypotheses regarding the function(s) of the problem behavior (i.e., What is the relationship between the problem behaviors and manipulated environmental events?). The experimental validation of hypotheses assists with the selection of interventions directly related to the function(s) of the problem behavior. For example, if it is determined that the function of a third-grade student's off-task behavior (e.g., talking to peers, moving around the classroom) is to avoid or escape task demands, then a number of interventions can be implemented to either alter classroom tasks (e.g., reduce assignment length) or make escape from task demands contingent on alternative behaviors (e.g., attention breaks contingent on task completion) (DuPaul & Ervin, 1996).

These methods, in particular Functional Behavior Assessment (FBA), have received substantial attention since the Individuals with Disabilities Education Act (IDEA) Amendments of 1997 (P.L. 105–17; IDEA '97), which require that a FBA must be conducted when a school district intends to: (a) remove students for more than 10 school days in a school year; (b) change students educational placements by removing them from school; or (c) place students in an interim alternative educational setting for a weapon or drug offense (Drasgow & Yell, 2001). In addition, the Individuals with Disabilities Improvement Act of 2004 (P.L. 108–446; IDEA '04) stipulated that if a student's problem behavior is determined to manifest from a disability, then a FBA should be conducted.

Diagnostic Classification

The most common diagnostic classification system for emotional and behavioral disorders is a categorical approach, which is used by the Diagnostic and Statistical Manual of Mental Disorders (DSM; American Psychiatric Association, 2000) and promoted by the Individuals with Disabilities Improvement Act of 2004 (P.L. 108–446; IDEA '04). One major limitation associated with categorical diagnostic classification systems is the limited treatment utility (Gresham & Gansle, 1992). Recently, an alternative system based on behavioral assessment techniques has been recommended. This approach integrates categorical classification and functional assessment models to address the needs of children and youth experiencing emotional and behavioral problems (Power & Ikeda, 1996; Zentall & Javorsky, 1995).

As outlined by Power and Eiraldi (2000), the integrated approach includes a multi-step diagnostic assessment model that is combined with a functional assessment model. In the diagnostic assessment model, the child or youth is first referred for an assessment. Next, the target behaviors are identified and record reviews are conducted. The third step of the diagnostic assessment model stipulates that a decision is made regarding the necessity of additional screening. If there is no need for additional screening, then a functional assessment is conducted, which includes developing an intervention plan, identifying outcome measures, and implementing the intervention. If it is determined that additional screening is warranted, the diagnostic assessment model continues. Once the screening has been completed, the fifth step of the diagnostic assessment model requires that a decision is made regarding whether the child or youth meets the screening criteria. If it is determined that the screening criteria are met, then a comprehensive evaluation is conducted, which includes conducting a functional assessment, to determine a diagnostic classification. However, if the screening criteria are not met, a functional assessment is still conducted, which includes developing and implementing an intervention. As part of the functional assessment model, the intervention is monitored closely and a maintenance plan is developed.

Intervention Evaluation

Both functional behavioral assessment and the integrated diagnostic classification model previously discussed (Power & Eiraldi, 2000) link assessment to intervention. Entrenched in this approach of linking behavioral assessment results to intervention selection is the evaluation of outcomes or data-based decision making. The use of data-based decision making evolved with the behavioral consultation approach developed by Bergan and Kratochwill (1990). A key component of this approach is to closely monitor

the effects of school-based interventions on the educational, behavioral, and mental health outcomes of children and youth while taking into considerations individual differences in responding to intervention components. This approach affords data-based judgments regarding intervention effectiveness and allows for intervention modifications when children and youth demonstrate inadequate progress.

An example of data-based decision making can be clearly illustrated using CBA (Shapiro, 2004; Shinn, 1998). For example, in order to evaluate the effects of an individualized reading intervention for a fourth-grade student experiencing oral reading fluency difficulties, CBA reading probes were administered twice a week over an eight-week period of time (i.e., progress monitoring data). Data are then graphed and compared to pre-determined goal and aim lines, which can be based on estimated performance, predicted performance, or mandated performance. Using this approach, progress monitoring data can be analyzed by comparing expected (i.e., goal line, aimline) and actual reading performance (i.e., CBM data points) (Shinn & Hubbard, 1992). An alternate method of analyzing progress monitoring data involves calculating a trend line for data collected over the course of an intervention. A trend line is computed to provide a statistical summary of student performance over time. Generally a line that represents the best fit to the data is drawn through the student's data. Based on the trend line, a slope value can be computed that allows for a mathematical analysis of student progress. In addition, weekly gain, or the number of words per minute the student has improved in one week, can be computed to provide a more meaningful index of student progress (Parker, Tindal, & Stein, 1992; Shinn, Good, & Stein, 1989).

Conclusion

Historical developments in the field of psychology have influenced the theoretical and conceptual foundations of behavioral assessment. Major theoretical perspectives (i.e., materialism, determinism, operationalism) have shaped behavioral assessment methods, which have also been influenced by psychometric foundations and the concepts of causation and functional relationships. A number of direct and indirect behavioral assessment techniques serve as the foundation of behavioral assessment methodologies, and recent advances in specific applications, including functional assessment, intervention evaluation, diagnostic classification, have permitted the evolution of behavioral assessment so that clinicians are better positioned to conduct comprehensive behavioral assessments of children and youth as well identify, select, and implement interventions.

Author Note

Correspondence concerning this chapter should be addressed to Tanya L. Eckert, Syracuse University, Department of Psychology, 430 Huntington Hall, Syracuse, NY 13244. Email: taeckert@syr.edu.

References

Abikoff, H. & Gittelman, R. (1985). Classroom Observation Code: A modification of the StonyBrook Code. *Psychopharmacology Bulletin, 21*, 901–909.

Achenbach, T. M. (1986). *The Direct Observation Form of the Child Behavior Checklist* (rev. ed.). Burlington, VT: University of Vermont, Department of Psychiatry.

Achenbach, T. M., & Rescorla, L. A. (2001). *Manual for the ASEBA School-Age Forms and Profiles*. Burlington: University of Vermont, Research Center for Children, Youth, and Families.

American Psychiatric Association. (2000). *Diagnostic and statistical manual of mental disorders* (4th ed., text rev.). Washington, DC: Author.

American Psychological Association. (2002). Ethical principles of psychologists and code of conduct. *American Psychologist, 57*, 1060–1073.

Andrewes, D. (2001). *Neuropsychology: From theory to practice*. Hove, UK: Psychology Press.

Bagner, D. M., Harwood, M. D. & Eyberg, S. E. (2006). Psychometric considerations. In M. Hersen (Ed.), *Clinician's handbook of behavioral assessment* (pp. 63–79). Burlington, MA: Elsevier Academic Press.

Barlow, D. H. & Hersen, M. (1984). *Single case experimental designs: Strategies for studying human behavior*. New York: Pergamon Press.

Barnett, D. W., Lentz, F. E. & Macmann, G. (2000). Psychometric qualities of professional practice. In E. S. Shapiro & T. R. Kratochwill (Eds.), *Behavioral assessment in schools: Theory, research, and clinical foundations* (2nd ed.) (pp. 355–386). New York: Guilford Press.

Barnhill, G. P. (2005). Functional behavioral assessment in schools. *Intervention in School and Clinic, 40*, 131–143.

Beaver, B. R., & Busse, R. T. (2000). Informant reports: Conceptual and research bases of interviews with parents and teachers. In E. S. Shapiro & T. R. Kratochwill (Eds.), *Behavioral assessment in schools: Theory, research, and clinical foundations* (2nd ed.) (pp. 257–287). New York: Guilford Press.

Bellack, A. S., & Hersen, M. (1988). *Behavioral assessment: A practical handbook* (3rd ed.). New York: Pergamon Press.

Bergan, J. R., & Kratochwill, T. R. (1990). *Behavioral consultation and therapy*. New York: Plenum.

Bijou, S. W., Peterson, R. F., & Ault, M. H. (1968). A method to integrate descriptive and experimental field studies at the level of data and empirical concepts. *Journal of Applied Behavior Analysis, 1*, 175–191

Bracken, B. A. (1992). *Multidimensional Self Concept Scale: Examiner's manual*. Austin, TX: RO-ED.

Brophy, J. H. & Good, T. (1986). Teacher behavior and student achievement. In M. C. Wittrock (Ed.), *Handbook of research in teaching* (3rd ed., pp. 328–375). New York: Macmillan.

Carr, E. (1993). Behavior analysis is not ultimately about behavior. *The Behavior Analyst, 16*, 47–49.

Carroll, J. B. (1963). A model of school learning. *Teachers College Record, 64*, 723–733.

Carta, J. J., Greenwood, C. R., & Atwater, J. (1985). *Ecobehavioral system for complex assessments of preschool environments (ESCAPE)*. Kansas City: Juniper Gardens Children's Project, Bureau of Child Research, University of Kansas.

Carta, J. J., Greenwood, C. R., Schulte, D., Arreaga-Mayer, C., & Terry, B. (1987). *The Mainstream Code for Instructional Structure and Student Academic Response (MS- CISSAR): Observer training manual*. Kansas City: Juniper Gardens Children's Project, Bureau of Child Research, University of Kansas.

Christ, T. J. (2006). Short term estimates of growth using curriculum-based measurement of oral reading fluency: Estimates of standard error of the slope to construct confidence intervals. *School Psychology Review, 35*, 128–133.

Christ, T. J., & Hintze, J. M. (2007). Psychometric considerations of reliability when evaluating response to intervention. In S. R. Jimmerson, A. M. VanderHayDen & M. K. Burns (Eds.), *Handbook of response to intervention* (pp. 93–105). New York: Springer.

Cone, J. D. (1977). The relevance of reliability and validity for behavioral assessment. *Behavior Therapy, 8*, 411–426.

Cone, J. D. (1978). The Behavioral Assessment Grid (BAG): A conceptual framework and a taxonomy. *Behavior Therapy, 9*, 882–888.

Cone, J. D. (1988). Psychometric considerations and the multiple models of behavioral assessment. In A. S. Bellack & M. Hersen (Eds.), *Behavioral assessment: A practical handbook* (3rd ed., pp. 42–66). New York: Pergamon.

Cone, J. D. & Hawkins, R. P. (Eds.). (1977). *Behavioral assessment: New directions in clinical psychology*. New York: Burner/Mazel.

Cooper, J. O. (1981). *Measuring behavior* (2nd ed.). Columbus, OH: Charles E. Merrill.

Cooper, J. O., Heron, T. E., & Heward, W. L. (1987). *Applied Behavior Analysis*. Columbus, OH: Merrill.

Dawes, R. M. (1994). Psychological measurement. *Psychological Review, 101*, 278–281.

Drasgow, E., & Yell, M. L (2001). Functional behavioral assessments: Legal requirements and challenges. *School Psychology Review, 30*, 239–251.

DuPaul, G. J. (1992). How to assess attention deficit hyperactivity disorder within school settings. *School Psychology Quarterly, 7*, 60–74.

DuPaul, G. J., Eckert, T. L., & McGoey, K. E. (1997). Interventions for students with Attention-Deficit/Hyperactivity Disorder: One size does not fit all. *School Psychology Review, 26*, 369–381.

DuPaul, G. J., & Ervin, R. A. (1996). Functional assessment of behaviors related to Attention—Deficit Hyperactivity Disorder: Linking assessment to intervention design. *Behavior Therapy, 27*, 601–622.

DuPaul, G. J., Power, T. J., Anastopoulos, A. D., & Reid, R. (1998). *ADHD Rating Scale-IV: Checklists, norms, and clinical interpretations*. New York: Guilford Press.

Eckert, T. L., Dunn, E. K., Guiney, K. M., & Codding, R. S. (2000). Self-reports: Theory and research in using rating scale measures. In E. S. Shapiro & T. R. Kratochwill (Eds.), *Behavioral assessment in schools: Theory, research, and clinical foundations* (2nd ed.) (pp.288–322). New York: Guilford Press.

Eckert, T. L., DuPaul, G. J., & Carson, P. M. (2003). Youth-completed and narrow-band child- behavior questionnaires. In M. Breen & C. Fielder (Eds.), *Behavioral approach to the assessment of youth with emotional/behavioral disorders: A handbook for school-based practitioners* (2nd ed.). (pp. 225–296). Austin, TX: PRO-ED.

Eckert, T. L., Martens, B. K., & DiGennaro, F. D. (2005). Describing antecedent-behavior- consequence relations using conditional probabilities and the general operant contingency space: A preliminary investigation. *School Psychology Review, 34,* 520–528.

Englert, C. S., & Sugai, G. (1981). *Direct Instruction Observation System (DIOS)*. Lexington: University of Kentucky.

Ervin, R. A., Ehrhardt, K. E., & Poling, A. (2001). Functional assessment: Old wine in new bottles. *School Psychology Review, 30,* 173–179.

Ervin, R. A., Radford, P. M., Bertsch, K., Piper, A. L., Ehrhardt, K. E., & Poling, A. (2001). A descriptive analysis and critique of the empirical literature on school-based functional assessment. *School Psychology Review, 30,* 193–210.

Ferster, C. B., & Skinner, B. F. (1957). *Schedules of reinforcement.* New York: Appleton-Century-Crofts.

Finch, A. J. & Rogers, T. R. (1984). Self-report instruments. In T. H. Ollendick & M. Hersen (Eds.), *Child behavioral assessment: Principles and procedures* (pp. 106–123). Elmsford, NY: Pergamon Press.

Fuchs, L. S., Fuchs, D., & Zumeta, R. O. (2008). Response to intervention: A strategy for the prevention and identification of learning disabilities. In E. L. Grigorenko (Ed.), *Educating individuals with disabilities: IDEIA 2004 and beyond* (pp. 115–135). New York: Springer.

Gadow, K. D., Sprafkin, J., & Nolan, E. E. (1996). *ADHD School Observation Code.* Stony Brook, NY: Checkmate Plus.

Glutting, J. J., & Oakland, T. (1993). *Manual for the Guide to the Assessment of Test Behavior.* San Antonio, TX: Psychological Corporation.

Goodwin, C. J. (2008). *A history of modern psychology* (3rd ed.). Hoboken, NJ: Wiley.

Gordon, M., Barkley, R. A., & Lovett, B. J. (2006). Tests and observational measures. In R. A. Barkley (Ed.), *Attention-Deficit Hyperactivity Disorder: A handbook for diagnosis and treatment* (3rd ed., pp. 369–388). New York: Guilford.

Greene, R. W., & Ollendick, T. H. (2000). Behavioral assessment of children. In G. Goldstein & M. Hersen (Eds.), *Handbook of psychological assessment* (pp. 453–470). New York: Pergamon.

Greenwood, C. R. (1991). Longitudinal analysis of time, engagement and achievement in at-risk vs. nonrisk students. *Exceptional Children, 57,* 521–535.

Greenwood, C. R., Carta, J. J., Kamps, D., & Arreaga-Mayer, C. (1990). Ecobehavioral analysis of classroom instruction. In S. Schroeder (Ed.), *Ecobehavioral analysis and developmental disabilities* (pp. 33–63). Baltimore: Paul H. Brookes.

Greenwood, C. R., Carta, J. J., Kamps, D., & Delquardi, J. (1993). *Ecobehavioral assessment systems software (EBASS): Observational instrumentation for school psychologists.* Kansas City: Juniper Gardens Children's Project, University of Kansas.

Gresham, F. M., & Elliott, S. N. (1990). *Social Skills Rating System manual.* Circle Pines, MN: American Guidance Service.

Gresham, F. M., & Gansle, K. A. (1992). Misguided assumptions of DSM-III-R: Implications for school psychological practice. *School Psychology Quarterly, 7,* 79–95.

Gresham, F. M., Watson, T. S., & Skinner, C. H. (2001). Functional behavior assessment: Principles, procedures, and future directions. *School Psychology Review, 30,* 156–172.

Gronlund, N. E., & Waugh, C. K. (2009). *Assessment of student achievement* (9th ed.). Upper Saddle River, NJ: Merrill.

Hartmann, D. P., Roper, B. L., & Bradford, D. C. (1979). Some relationships between behavioral and traditional assessment. *Journal of Behavioral Assessment, 1,* 3–21.

Haynes, S. N. (1992). *Models of causality in psychopathology: Toward synthetic, dynamic and nonlinear models of causality in psychopathology.* Des Moines, IA: Ayllon & Bacon.

Haynes, S. N. (2000). Behavioral assessment of adults. In G. Goldstein & M. Hersen (Eds.), *Handbook of psychological assessment* (pp. 471–502). New York: Pergamon.

Hayes, S. C., Nelson, R. O., & Jarrett, R. (1986). Evaluating the quality of behavioral assessment. In R. O. Nelson & S. C. Hayes (Eds.), *Conceptual foundations of behavioral assessment* (pp. 463–503). New York: Guilford.

Haynes, S. N., Uchigakiuchi, P., Meyer, K., Orimoto, B. D., & O'Brien, W. O. (1993). Functional analytic causal models and the design of treatment programs: Concepts and clinical applications with childhood behavior problems. *European Journal of Psychological Assessment, 9,* 189–205.

Heiby, E. M., & Haynes, S. N. (2003). Introduction to behavioral assessment. In S. P. Haynes & E. M. Heiby (Eds.), *Behavioral Assessment* (pp. 3–18). Hoboken, NJ: Wiley.

Hintze, J. M. (2005). Psychometrics of direct observation. *School Psychology Review, 34,* 507–519.

Hintze, J. M. (2009). Curriculum-based assessment. In T. B. Gutkin & C. R. Reynolds (Eds.), *Handbook of school psychology* (4th ed., pp. 397–409). Hoboken, NJ: Wiley.

Hintze, J. M., Volpe, R. J., & Shapiro, E. S. (2003). Best practices in the systematic direction observation of student behavior. In A. Thomas & J. Grimes (Eds.) (4th ed.), *Best practices in school psychology-IV* (pp. 993–1028). Silver Springs, MD: National Association of School Psychologists.

Hops, H., Davis, B., & Longoria, N. (1995). Methodological issues in direct observation: Illustrations with the Living in Familial Environments (LIFE) coding system. *Journal of Clinical Child Psychology, 24,* 193–203.

Horner, R. H. (1994). Functional assessment: Contributions and future directions. *Journal of Applied Behavior Analysis, 27,* 401–404.

House, A. E., House, B. J., & Campbell, M. B. (1981). Measures of interobserver agreement: Calculation formulas and distribution effects. *Journal of Behavioral Assessment, 3,* 37–58.

Hughes, J., & Baker, D. B. (1990). *The clinical child interview.* New York: Guilford.

Hung, E. H. C. (1997). *The nature of science: problems and perspectives.* Belmont, CA: Wadsworth.

Individuals with Disabilities Education Act Amendment of 1997 (PL 105–117). 20 USC Chapter 33, Sections 1400 et seq.

Individuals with Disabilities Education Improvement Act of 2004 (PL 108–446). 20 USC 1400 note.

Iwata, B. A., Dorsey, M. F., Slifer, K. J., Bauman, K. E., & Richman, G. S. (1982). Toward a functional analysis of self-injury. *Analysis and Intervention in Developmental Disabilities, 2,* 3–20.

Johnston, J. M. & Pennypacker, H. S. (1993). *Strategies and tactics of behavioral research.* Hillsdale, NJ: Erlbaum.

Jones, M. C. (1924). The elimination of children's fears. *Journal of Experimental Psychology, 7,* 382–390.

Kazdin, A. E. (1977). Assessing the clinical or applied importance of behavior change throughsocial validation. *Behavior Modification, 1,* 427–452.

Kazdin, A. E., & Kagan, J. (1994). Models of dysfunction in developmental psychopathology. *Clinical Psychology: Science and Practice, 1,* 35–52.

Kenny, M. C., Alvarez, K., Donohue, B. C., & Winick, C. B. (2007). Overview of behavioral assessment with adults. In M. Hersen & J. Rosqvist (Eds.), *Handbook of psychological assessment, case conceptualization, and treatment, volume 1, adults* (pp. 3–25). New York: Wiley.

Koretz, D., McCaffrey, D., Klein, S., Bell, R., & Stecher, B. (1992). *The reliability of scores from the 1992 Vermont portfolio assessment program: Interim report.* Los Angeles, CA: RAND Corporation.

Kovacs, M. (1992). *Children's Depression Inventory.* Pittsburgh, PA: University of PittsburghSchool of Medicine.

La Greca, A. M., & Stone, W. L. (1993). Social Anxiety Scale for Children-Revised: Factor structure and concurrent validity. *Journal of Clinical Child Psychology, 22,* 17–27.

Lane, S., & Stone, C. A. (2006). Performance assessment. In R. L. Brennan (Ed.), *Educational measurement* (4th ed., pp. 387–431). Westport, CT: Praeger.

Leff, S. S., & Lakin, R. (2005). Playground-based observational systems: A review and implications for practitioners and researchers. *School Psychology Review, 34,* 475–489.

Lovett, B. J., & Hood, S. B. (2011). Realism and operationism in psychiatric diagnosis. *Philosophical Psychology, 24,* 207–222.

Marieb, E. N., & Hoehn, K. (2007). *Human anatomy and physiology* (7th ed.). San Francisco, CA: Benjamin Cummings.

Martens, B. K., Eckert, T. L., Bradley, T. A., & Ardoin, S. P. (1999). Identifying effective treatments from a brief experimental analysis: Using single-case design elements to aid decision-making. *School Psychology Quarterly, 14,* 163–181.

McComas, J. J., & Mace, F. C. (2000). Theory and practice in conducting functional analysis. In E. S. Shapiro & T. R. Kratochwill (Eds.), *Behavioral assessment in schools: Theory, research, and clinical foundations* (2nd ed.) (pp. 78–104). New York: Guilford Press.

McConaughy, S. H. (2003). Interviewing children, parents, and teachers. In M. Breen & C. Fielder (Eds.), *Behavioral approach to the assessment of youth with emotional/behavioral disorders: A handbook for school-based practitioners* (2nd ed.). (pp. 123–169). Austin, TX: PRO-ED.

McConaughy, S. H. (2005a). *Clinical interviews for children and adolescents: Assessment to intervention.* New York: Guilford Press.

McConaughy, S. H. (2005b). Direct observational assessment during test sessions and child clinical interviews. *School Psychology Review, 34,* 490–506.

McConaughy, S. H., & Achenbach, T. M. (2001). *Manual for the Semistructured Clinical Interview for Children and Adolescents-Second Edition.* Burlington, VT: University of Vermont, Research Center for Children, Youth, and Families.

McConaughy, S. H., & Achenbach, T. M. (2004). *Manual for the Test Observation Form for Ages 2–18.* Burlington, VT: University of Vermont, Research Center for Children, Youth, and Families.

Meehl, P. E. & Rosen, A. (1955). Antecedent probability and the efficiency of psychometric signs, patterns, or cutting scores. *Psychological Bulletin, 52,* 194–216.

Merrell, K. W. (1999). *Behavioral, social, and emotional assessment of children and adolescents.* Mahwah, NJ: Lawrence Erlbaum Associates.

Merrell, K. W. (2000). Informant reports: Theory and research in using child behavior rating scales in school settings. In E. S. Shapiro & T. R. Kratochwill (Eds.), *Behavioral assessment in schools: Theory, research, and clinical foundations* (2nd ed.) (pp. 233–256). New York: Guilford Press.

Messick, S. A. (1989). Validity. In R. L. Linn (Ed.), *Educational measurement.* (3rd ed., pp. 13–103). New York: Macmillan.

Messick, S. (1995). Validity of psychological assessment: Validation of inferences from persons' responses and performances as scientific inquiry into score meaning. *American Psychologist, 50,* 741–749.

Miltenberger, R. G. (2008). *Behavior modification: Principles and procedures.* (4th ed.). Belmont, CA: Wadsworth.

Mischel, W. (1968). *Personality assessment.* New York: Wiley.

Nelson, R. O., Hay, L. R., & Hay, W. M. (1977). Comments on Cone's "The relevance of reliability and validity for behavioral assessment." *Behavior Therapy, 8,* 427–430.

O'Donohue, W. T., & Ferguson, K. E. (2003). Learning and applied behavior analysis: Foundations of behavioral assessment. In S. P. Haynes & E. M. Heiby (Eds.), *Behavioral Assessment* (pp. 57–68). Hoboken, NJ: Wiley.

O'Leary, K. D. (1979). Behavioral assessment. *Behavioral Assessment, 1,* 31–36.

O'Neill, R. E., Horner, R. H., Albin, R. W., Storey, K., & Sprague, J. R. (1990). *Functional analysis of problem behavior: A practical guide.* Sycamore, IL: Sycamore Publishing.

Ollendick, T. H., Alvarez, H. K., & Greene, R. W. (2003). Behavioral assessment: History of underlying concepts and methods. In S. P. Haynes & E. M. Heiby (Eds.), *Behavioral Assessment* (pp. 19–34). Hoboken, NJ: Wiley.

Ollendick, T. H., & Hersen, M. (1984) (Eds.). *Child behavioral assessment: Principles and procedures.* Elmsford, NY: Pergamon Press.

Orvaschel, H. (2006). Structured and semistructured interviews. In M. Hersen (Ed.), *Clinician's handbook of behavioral assessment* (pp. 159–179). Burlington, MA: Elsevier Academic Press.

Parker, R., Tindal, G., & Stein, S. (1992). Estimating trend in progress monitoring data: A comparison of simple line-fitting methods. *School Psychology Review, 21,* 300–312.

Pavlov, I. P. (1927). *Conditioned reflexes.* Oxford: Oxford University Press.

Peterson, D. R. (1968). *The clinical study of social behavior.* New York: Appleton-Century- Crofts.

Plaud, J. J., & Eifert, G. H. (Eds.). (1998). *From behavior theory to behavior therapy.* Needham Heights, MA: Allyn & Bacon.

Powell, R. A., Symbaluk, D. G., & Honey, P. L. (2009). *Introduction to learning and behavior* (3rd ed.). Belmont, CA: Wadsworth.

Power, T. J., & Ikeda, M. J. (1996). A clinic-school partnership in managing elementary school students with ADHD. In G. Stoner, (Chair), *Prevention and intervention for students with ADHD: Models for effective practice across levels of schooling.* Paper presented at the annual meeting of the National Association of School Psychologists, Atlanta.

Power, T. J., & Eiraldi, R. B. (2000). Educational and psychiatric classification systems. In E. S. Shapiro & T. R. Kratochwill (Eds.), *Behavioral assessment in schools: Theory, research, and clinical foundations* (2nd ed.) (pp. 464–488). New York: Guilford Press.

Ramsay, M. C., Reynolds, & Kamphaus, R. W. (2002). *The essentials of behavioral assessment*. New York: John Wiley & Sons.

Raine, A. (2002). The role of prefrontal deficits, low autonomic arousal, and early childhood health factors in the development of antisocial and aggressive behavior in children. *Journal of Child Psychology and Psychiatry, 43*, 417–434.

Reed, D. D., & Luiselli, J. K. (2009). Antecedents to a paradigm: Ogden Lindsley and B. F. Skinner's founding of "behavior therapy." *Behavior Therapist, 32*, 82–85.

Reich, W. (2000). Diagnostic Interview for Children and Adolescents. *Journal of the American Academy of Child and Adolescent Psychiatry, 39*, 59–66.

Reich, W., Welner, Z., Herjanic, B. & MHS Staff. (1999). *Diagnostic Interview for Children and Adolescents-IV*. North Tonawanda, NY: Multi-Health Systems.

Rescorla, R. A. (1988). Pavlovian conditioning: It's not what you think it is. *American Psychologist, 43*, 151–160.

Reynolds, C. R., & Kamphaus, R. W. (2004). *Behavior Assessment System for Children* (2nd ed.). Circle Pines, MN: American Guidance System Publishing.

Reynolds, C. R., Livingston, R. B., & Wilson, V. (2006). *Measurement and assessment in education*. Boston, MA: Allyn & Bacon.

Reynolds, W. M. (1993). Self-report methodology. In T. H. Ollendick & M. Hersen (Eds.), *Handbook of child and adolescent assessment* (pp. 98–123). Boston: Allyn & Bacon.

Rusby, J., Estes, A., & Dishion, T. (1991). *The Interpersonal Process Code*. Unpublished coding manual. Eugene, OR: Oregon Social Learning Center.

Schwartz, I. S. & Baer, D. M. (1991). Social validity assessments: Is current practice state of the art? *Journal of Applied Behavior Analysis, 24*, 189–204.

Saudargas, R. A., & Creed, V. (1980). *State-Event Classroom Observation System* (SECOS). Knoxville: Department of Tennessee, University of Tennessee.

Shaffer, D., Fisher, P., Lucas, C., Dulcan, M., & Schwab-Stone, M. E. (2000). NIMH Diagnostic Interview Schedule for Children Version, Version IV (NIMH DISC-IV): Description, differences from previous versions and reliability of some common diagnoses. *Journal of the American Academy of Child and Adolescent Psychiatry, 39*, 29–38.

Shapiro, E. S. (2004). *Academic skills problems: Direct assessment and intervention* (3rd ed.). New York: Guilford.

Shapiro, E. S., & Skinner, C. H. (1990). Best practices in observational/ecological assessment. In A. Thomas & J. Grimes (Eds.), *Best practices in school psychology-II* (pp. 507–518). Washington, DC: National Association of School Psychologists.

Shinn, M. R. (Ed.). (1998). *Advanced applications of curriculum-based measurement*. New York: Guilford Press.

Shinn, M. R., Good, R. H., & Stein, S. (1989). Summarizing trends in student achievement: A comparison of methods. *School Psychology Review, 18*, 356–370.

Shinn, M. R., & Hubbard, D. D. (1992). Curriculum-based measurement and problem-solving assessment: Basic procedures and outcomes. *Focus on Exceptional Children, 24*, 1–20.

Sindelar, P. T., Smith, M. A., Harriman, N. E., Hale, R. L., & Wilson, R. J. (1986). Teacher effectiveness in special education programs. *Journal of Special Education, 20*, 195–207.

Skinner, B. F. (1938). *The behavior of organisms*. New York: Appleton-Century-Crofts.

Skinner, B. F. (1953). *Science and human behavior*. New York: Macmillan.

Skinner, B. F. (1974). *About behaviorism*. New York: Vintage.

Southam-Gerow, M. A., & Chorpita, B. F. (2007). Anxiety in children and adolescents. In E. J. Mash & R. A. Barkley (Eds.), *Assessment of childhood disorders* (4th ed., pp. 347–397). New York: Guilford.

Spiegler, M. D., & Guevremont, D. C. (2003). *Contemporary behavior therapy* (4th ed.). Belmont, CA: Wadsworth.

Steege, M. W., Davin, T., & Hathaway, M. (2001). Reliability and accuracy of a performance- based behavioral recording procedure. *School Psychology Review, 30*, 252–261.

Starch, D., & Elliott, E. C. (1912). Reliability of the grading of high-school work in English. *School Review, 20*, 442–457.

Sterling-Turner, H. E., Robinson, S. L., & Wilczynski, S. M. (2001). Functional assessment of distracting and disruptive behaviors in the school setting. *School Psychology Review, 30*, 211–226.

Stern, R. M., Ray, W. J., & Quigley, K. S. (2000). *Psychophysiological recording* (2nd ed.). New York: Oxford University Press.

Stichter, J. P., & Lewis, T. J. (2006). Classroom assessment. In M. Hersen (Ed.), *Clinician's handbook of behavioral assessment* (pp. 569–585). Burlington, MA: Elsevier Academic Press.

Stichter, J. P., Lewis, T. J., Johnson, N., & Trussell, R. (2004). Toward a structural assessment: Analyzing the merits of an assessment tool for a student with E/BD. *Assessment for Effective Intervention, 30*, 25–40.

Suen, H. K. (1988). Agreement, reliability, accuracy, and validity: Toward a clarification. *Behavioral Assessment, 10*, 343–366.

Sugai. G., & Lewis, T. (1989). Teacher/student interaction analysis. *Teacher Education and Special Education, 12*, 131–138.

Thorndike, E. L. (1927). The law of effect. *American Journal of Psychology, 39*, 212–222.

Vollmer, T. R., & Northup, J. (1996). Some implications of functional analysis for school psychology. *School Psychology Quarterly, 11*, 76–92.

Volpe, R. J., DiPerna, J. C., Hintze, J. M., & Shapiro, E. S. (2005). Observing students in classroom settings: A review of seven coding schemes. *School Psychology Review, 34*, 454–474.

Volpe, R. J., & McConaughy, S. M. (2005). Observing students in classroom settings: A review of seven coding schemes. *School Psychology Review, 34*, 490–506.

Walker, H. M., & Severson, H. H. (1990). *Systematic Screening for Behavior Disorders: Users guide and administration manual*. Longmont, CO: Sopris West.

Watson, J. B. (1913). Psychology as the behaviorist views it. *Psychological Review, 20*, 158–177.

Watson, J. B. (1930). *Behaviorism* (2nd ed.). New York: Norton.

Watson, J. B., & Rayner, R. (1920). Conditioned emotional reactions. *Journal of Experimental Psychology, 3*, 1–14.

Weems, C., & Silverman, W. (2008). Anxiety disorders. In T. P. Beauchaine & S. P. Hinshaw (Eds.), *Child and adolescent psychopathology* (pp. 447–476). Hoboken, NJ: Wiley.

Wilhelm, F. H., Schneider, S., & Friedman, B. H. (2006). Psychophysiological assessment. In M. Hersen (Ed.), *Clinician's handbook of child behavioral assessment* (pp. 201–231). Amsterdam: Elsevier.

Wilson, M. S., & Reschly, D. J. (1996). Assessment in school psychology training and practice. *School Psychology Review, 25*, 9–23.

Witt, J. C., Daly, E. J. III, & Noell, G. (2000). *Functional assessment: A step-by-step guide to solving academic and behavior problems.* Longmont, CA: Sopris West.

Wolf, M. M. (1978). Social validity: The case for subjective measurement or how applied behavior analysis is finding its heart. *Journal of Applied Behavior Analysis, 11,* 203–214.

Zentall, S. S., & Javorsky, J. (1995). Functional and clinical assessment of ADHD: Implications of DSM-IV in the schools. *Journal of Psychoeducational Assessment: Special ADHD Issue,* 22–41.

Zuriff, G. E. (1985). *Behaviorism: A conceptual reconstruction.* New York: Columbia University Press.

Therapeutic Assessment with Adolescents and Their Parents: A Comprehensive Model

Deborah J. Tharinger, Lauren B. Gentry, *and* Stephen E. Finn

Abstract

The comprehensive model of Therapeutic Assessment (TA) as used with adolescents and their parents is introduced. TA is designed to answer specific questions parents and adolescents pose for the assessment, to form working alliances with parents and adolescents, to collaboratively engage adolescents and their parents in the assessment process, and to foster positive development in the adolescent and the family. TA uses a combination of assessment and intervention methods, is theoretically integrative and incorporates the unique tasks of adolescent development into the structure of the assessment itself. The goals and procedures for each step are provided and illustrated with a case study of an adolescent boy and his mother, along with effectiveness data. Finally, the application of TA across cultures, the use of selected steps of TA when the comprehensive model is not feasible, and the adaptation of TA to different settings and presenting problems are addressed.

Key Words: Therapeutic Assessment, adolescents, parents, collaborative

Psychological assessment and psychotherapy have traditionally been viewed as distinct endeavors. However, Therapeutic Assessment (TA) is a relatively new model of psychological assessment that has fused assessment and psychotherapy techniques. TA is a semi-structured form of collaborative assessment developed by Finn and colleagues (Finn, 1996, 2007; Finn & Tonsager, 1997). This model offers many of the benefits of a traditional assessment, while also serving as a short-term therapeutic intervention. Thus, with additional training and supervision, most psychologists could readily add TA to their repertoire by integrating their existing competencies in psychological assessment and clinical interventions.

Our primary goal in this chapter is to introduce TA to assessment psychologists, particularly as it applies to adolescents and their parents, and to encourage clinicians to consider how this model may be useful in their practices. A comprehensive discussion of TA with pre-adolescent children and their parents is available in Tharinger, Krumholz, Austin, and Matson (2011), along with an illustration of its use in school-based assessment practice. TA with pre-adolescent children is also discussed and illustrated in Hamilton et al., 2009; Tharinger, Finn, Austin et al., 2008; Tharinger, Finn, Gentry, et al., 2009; Tharinger, Finn, Wilkinson, and Schaber, 2007; and Tharinger, Matson, and Christopher (2011).

To explicate the TA model with adolescents, we will first briefly discuss the developmental changes of adolescence, as these inform the particular methods used in TA with teenagers and their parents (as compared to those used with children and their parents). Existing models of adolescent assessment have largely overlooked these developmental distinctions. Second, we will comment on the assumptions and goals of traditional models of psychological assessment. We will then introduce TA, and review its development and history, including its philosophical and theoretical underpinnings and core values. We will also summarize research findings on the efficacy of TA. In the latter sections of the chapter, we will turn to pragmatic issues. We discuss how to organize assessment findings so they are most likely to be therapeutic to clients. Next, we will delineate the comprehensive model of TA as used with adolescents, illustrating each step with the case of a 13-year-old boy and his mother. Finally, we will discuss the importance of evaluating the effectiveness of psychological assessment in both clinical practice and research endeavors.

Developmental Changes in Adolescence

Adolescence is a developmental period that spans, roughly, the ages of 12 to 18, and may extend into the early twenties. This life phase is characterized by intense neurological, biological, cognitive, social, and emotional evolution. Many formulations of adolescent development have focused predominantly on cognitive advances, recognizing that adolescents' budding intellectual capacities exceed those of younger children. For example, Piaget (1972) proposed that individuals transition from concrete operational thought to formal operational thought in early adolescence, with formal operations being characterized by the capacity to manipulate ideas and abstract concepts. Thus, teenagers are able to think in more relative terms and envision possibilities, rather than consider only what is concrete and observable. Further, Elkind (1978) asserted that it is during this developmental period that individuals also become capable of *metacognition*—that is, of thinking about their own thoughts and feelings.

More holistically, in addition to adolescents' burgeoning cognitive capabilities, they simultaneously face the challenges of personal and civic identity development, establishing a self-concept, building self-esteem, seeking autonomy, and cultivating a future orientation (Gibbons, 2000). Adolescence is a time wherein youth begin to explore different adult roles and grapple with developing a sense of self that is separate from their parents' view of them (Dusek, 1977; Holmbeck & Updegrove, 1995; Muus, 1988). More recently, some neuropsychological theories, fueled by an understanding of continued brain development, have framed change in adolescence as occurring within an interpersonal context. Within this context, a fundamental reorganization and individuation of the self occurs, and the neural mechanisms of self-regulation, memory consolidation, and motivation support the capacity for critical thinking that underlies abstract thought (Keating, 2004; Tucker & Moller, 2007).

Adolescence is often portrayed as a developmental period defined by awkwardness, turmoil, discord, and angst. In fact, most teenagers emerge from their adolescence unscathed, and the vast majority actually thrive. Nonetheless, unique vulnerabilities emerge during this period that have significant implications for the well-being of both teenagers and their families. Families with adolescents have been found to experience emotional distancing (Seiffge-Krenke, 1999) and a decline in marital satisfaction that may be precipitated by such separation (Steinberg & Silverberg, 1987). Given the emphasis on independence and autonomy during adolescence for both boys and girls (Seiffge-Krenke), much of this emotional distancing may be developmentally appropriate. However, the reasons for such decreases in family cohesion may also be due to more worrisome emotional changes in adolescence. For example, depressive symptoms have been found to increase markedly during adolescence, with such symptomatology being twice as likely in adolescent girls as in boys (Lau & Eley, 2008). Incidences of anxiety are also higher in adolescence (Kelley, Schochet, & Landry, 2004). Perhaps due to such affective disturbance—but also related to the increase in risk-taking and novelty-seeking behavior—alcohol and drug use and abuse, sexual activity, and eating disorders also increase during adolescence. In sum, multiple vulnerabilities during the developmental stage of adolescence can greatly affect the immediate and long-term health and welfare of teenagers and their families.

Thus, when negative developmental experiences do permeate the lives of adolescents and their families, they probably would benefit from psychological interventions that both honor the adolescent's growing independence and integrate family members into treatment. Fishman (1988) asserted that "the most powerful social therapeutic intervention for working with adolescents is family therapy" because the family is the "pivotal point" in every adolescent's life (p. 4). He further stated that "the very presence of a troubled adolescent in the family creates pressures that require the therapist to pay attention to the other family members. It is only ethical that the therapist address the problems of the context as a whole" (p. 5). Additionally, Fishman highlighted that it is often the family that has the most resources with which to mobilize and sustain change.

A number of other important considerations must also be kept in mind when working with adolescents. Teenagers are actively seeking to increase their autonomy as they work to successfully transition from childhood to adulthood. In an effort to maintain independence and self-consistency during this transition, they tend to resist people or situations that conflict with their developing self-concept (Meleddu & Guicciardi 1998; Muus, 1988). Thus, teenagers may be sensitive to situations where they feel their sovereignty is not being respected. This can create challenges within the family system as parents attempt to adapt to their child's new, and more autonomous, sense of self. Ideally, parents' relationships with their adolescents will begin to be characterized by cooperation and mutual respect rather than authority (Holmbeck & Updegrove, 1995). In combination with appropriate and consistent limits, new responsibilities and freedoms need to be given to teenagers in order to foster the development of a mature self-concept (Dusek, 1997). The need for a balance between giving adolescents privacy and autonomy, while still providing needed support and limits, can present a similar challenge in the context of psychological assessment. Some adolescents may feel as if seeking help or admitting a problem conflicts with their strivings for autonomy (Oetzel & Scherer, 2003). Thus, teenagers may enter into psychological assessment unwillingly (Fitzpatrick, & Irannejad, 2008; Keating & Cosgrave, 2006). Compounding this, assessment psychologists may initially be viewed as authority figures who might not respect adolescents' newfound autonomy.

Psychological Assessment with Adolescents

While a substantial literature exists on the psychological assessment of "children and adolescents" (e.g., Kamphaus & Frick, 2005; Kaufman & Kaufman, 2001; Knoff, 1986; Ollendick & Hersen, 1993; Smith & Handler, 2007), there is a dearth of information that directly addresses the subtleties of conducting psychological assessments specifically with adolescents. There are a few noteworthy exceptions, however. In his book entitled *Assessing Adolescents in Educational, Counseling, and Other Settings*, Hogue (1999) stated that adolescents "often [exhibit] characteristics and circumstances that set them apart from children and adults … these unique features mean that, in many cases, assessments and interventions appropriate for younger and older age groups may not be indicated" (p. 1). Hogue's book begins with a thorough review of various aspects of adolescent development as they pertain to psychologists' work. He then similarly reviews the basic concepts underlying psychological assessment,

ethical issues, and various measures of aptitude and achievement, personality, and behavior. However, outside of highlighting that conducting interviews with adolescents "often presents special challenges for the mental health professional" (p. 157), and identifying specific forms or versions of measures that are tailored for use with teenagers, Hogue does not clearly integrate these two bodies of literature in order to address the unique *process* of psychological assessment with adolescents.

Similarly, in their book entitled *Assessing Adolescents,* Oster, Caro, Eagen, and Lillo (1988) review general developmental considerations for working with adolescents, and present guidelines on how to sensitively approach the initial interview, given that "adolescents rarely refer themselves for treatment" (p. 16). The authors then review a variety of content areas about which it is useful to get information from adolescents in the interview (e.g., bodily concerns, friendships, sexual involvement, school problems). Furthermore, the authors suggest that adolescents have the opportunity to ask any questions that may arise during the interview process, and that assessors seek the adolescent's input surrounding the development of a cogent plan for intervention (Oster et al., 1988). The authors also briefly review the importance, and the process, of the adolescent and his or her family receiving assessment feedback. However, throughout the text, the major emphasis is placed on a review of appropriate psychometric instruments and tests that have been widely used in the assessment of adolescents, whereas the unique processes of assessment with adolescents are addressed only briefly.

In spite of the limitations of their respective books, both Hogue (1999) and Oster et al. (1988) address a notable gap in the literature base on psychological assessment. As is evidenced in the predominant content of these two texts, the literature on adolescent assessment generally focuses on the development and use of adolescent forms of well-known tests or measures specifically designed for adolescents. The value of these contributions must not be underestimated. Measures specifically tailored to adolescents inherently recognize such factors as (1) adolescents' increasing ability to understand more advanced language, (2) their ability to evaluate more complex psychological processes and emotions, (3) the inclusion of more mature content that has increasing pertinence to adolescents (e.g., drug use and sexual experiences), and (4) unique norms that account for the developmental, physical, and emotional differences that permeate the life stage of adolescence. However, as described earlier, there are additional considerations of great salience in conducting psychological assessments with adolescents. We will return to this topic after first reviewing traditional and collaborative models of assessment.

Traditional Psychological Assessment

The psychological assessment literature, education and training models, and the practice of assessment have been dominated by a natural science perspective that advocates "the use of standard techniques and rigid protocols to collect 'sterile' data" (Finn & Martin, 1997, p. 131). Given that "the hallmark of science [is] objectivity" (Fischer, 1985, p. 7), within this traditional perspective, testing is viewed as a tool through which to obtain an "accurate" classification of a client for the purposes of diagnosis, easier communication between professionals, treatment planning, and treatment evaluation (Finn, 2007). Typically, traditional evaluations end, as Fischer (1985) notes, with the client being represented "in terms of scores, bell-shaped curves, traits, psychodynamic forces, or diagnostic labels" (p. v). The assessor is viewed as "a scientist whose task [is] to identify the patient's traits, defenses, symptoms, and diseases through measurement" (Fischer, p. 7). Finn and Tonsager (1997) have called this the "information gathering" model of assessment. Handler and Meyer (1998) refer to this approach when applied to personality assessment as being executed by a "testing technician," rather than an "assessment technician" (p. 4).

In order to achieve the neutrality and accuracy that is the goal in the information-gathering model of assessment, threats to the objectivity of the testing need to be minimized. In this model, it is presumed that the assessor obtains knowledge and information about the client that the client does not have access to otherwise. The traditional paradigm of psychological assessment, then, does not consider testing to be a collaborative venture. It is, instead, an undertaking in which the client is the object of the psychologist's studied expertise (Riddle, Byers, & Grimesey, 2002).

The Development of Collaborative Assessment Models

Over the past several decades, psychologists working within a human science tradition have advocated a more accessible approach to assessment where the client and assessor work together to form a productive understanding of the client's situation (Fischer, 1985/1994). Over time, this model of psychological assessment has come to be called *collaborative assessment* (Fischer, 2000). This move to shift the intent of psychological assessment is somewhat surprising given that many humanistically oriented clinicians initially voiced strong objections to assessment, viewing it as "dehumanizing, reductionistic, artificial, and judgmental ... for clients" (Finn & Tonsager, 1997, p. 377). Thus, as a first step, key figures in the development of collaborative assessment, (e.g., Fischer, 1972, 1979, 2000; Handler, 1995, Purves, 2002) simply sought to make the assessment process more humane, respectful, and understandable to clients; they did not initially conceive of psychological assessment itself as a potentially therapeutic intervention. Fischer's (1979) conceptualization of psychological assessment was grounded in phenomenological psychology, with all knowledge being inextricably dependent upon the method of study and the mode of understanding. Because truth is intersubjective, she maintained, "objective" test data are best interpreted consensually with the client, and are fundamentally grounded in "historicity, situatedness, and perspectivity" (Fischer, 1979, p. 118). Each individual person simultaneously shapes, and is shaped by, the world while moving through it, and the goal of an assessment is to take a "snapshot" of this complex process.

Therefore, Fischer (1979, 2000) proposed that life events, rather than test scores, are the primary data within which assessment information should be contextualized. Collaborative assessors are urged to attend to narrative or idiographic information throughout the course of the assessment (including when providing oral feedback and consumer-friendly written reports, Fischer, 1985/1994). A collaborative assessment also requires clinicians to consider the interpersonal context in which an assessment takes place, evaluating the interactions and transactions that occur between client and assessor as a valuable source of additional information (Finn & Tonsager, 1997; Handler & Meyer, 1998). Thus, the more humanistic and phenomenological approaches to assessment sought to shift the assessor's focus from the integration of test scores back to understanding an individual's life. Through such practice, the assessor can ensure that "the mirror they hold up" (Handler & Meyer, 1998, p. 6) to the client is accurate, and avoid the client's feeling misunderstood, stigmatized or disrespected.

Collaborative assessment can be either loosely structured or semi-structured (Finn, 2007). Loosely structured techniques may use standardized testing materials in an unstandardized way, primarily as facilitators or therapeutic tools wherein a "valid" score is not obtained. For example, Fischer (2000) advocates for interrupting standardized testing procedures at "natural breaks" (p. 5) when it seems fruitful to further explore any content or process that was evoked by the testing stimuli. Conversely, Finn (2007) and his colleagues developed TA as a form of collaborative assessment that is semi-structured. In this model, assessment measures are administered using traditional standardized procedures, with possible idiographic inquiry following the standardized administration. Subsequently, the client and assessor discuss and interpret the testing experience together, which, in and of itself, may act as a therapeutic intervention (Finn & Tonsager, 1997).

Therapeutic Assessment

As in collaborative assessment, TA is based primarily on principles of phenomenological, intersubjective, and interpersonal psychological theories (Finn, 2002). This framework helps redefine aspects of psychological assessment, and delineate the different motivations that drive clients to seek assessments. Various theories of human change provide a lens for understanding three such underlying motivations: self-verification, self-enhancement, and self-efficacy/self-discovery (Finn & Tonsager, 1997). *Self-verification* concerns the well-known fact that people strive to maintain their self-views, and make every effort to discount conflicting information (Swann, 1996, 1997). This phenomenon was extensively discussed by Sullivan (1964), by Kohut (1977), and is recognized in intersubjectivity theory (Atwood & Stolorow, 1984). Accordingly, in psychological assessment, clients prefer to receive information that confirms their self-concept and aids them in maintaining a coherent view of themselves (Finn, 2007). Finn (2007) posits that clients often present, or are presented, for assessment when they are experiencing "disintegration anxiety," which is the uncomfortable (and possibly disorienting) feeling associated with receiving information that conflicts with an existing self-concept.

The second motivation, *self-enhancement*, is discussed within object-relations psychology as the need to feel loved and accepted by others, and to think highly of oneself (Fairbairn, 1952; Winnicott, 1957, 1975). Thus, clients participating in psychological assessments hope to receive praise and acceptance from the assessor and to internalize this experience (Finn & Tonsager, 1997). The third and final motivation, *self-efficacy/discovery*, initially posited by

self-efficacy theory and ego psychology, describes the need for humans to increase their knowledge of, and control over, themselves and their world (Freud, 1936; Hartmann, 1958; Hartmann, Kris, & Lowenstein, 1946; & Bandura, 1994). Through psychological assessments, then, clients seek to grow creatively, acquire self-knowledge, and obtain more control over their world.

Core Values of Therapeutic Assessment

TA is guided by a set of core values held by the assessor. These include collaboration, respect, humility, compassion, and openness/curiosity (Finn, 2009). We describe each in turn, as they are foundational to the practice of TA.

COLLABORATION

Assessors practicing TA believe that assessments are most useful, and the results most accurate, when clients are engaged as full collaborators. Clients are central in establishing the goals for their assessments; assisting in identifying relevant background information; aiding in deriving meaning from the test results, including tying them to real life examples; and providing input into recommendations. Clients also review and comment on any written documents that result from their assessment. Finally, assessors also collaborate with referring professionals and, when appropriate, with other important people in clients' lives, which may include family members, teachers, judges or employers.

RESPECT

TA seeks to respect clients' dignity; in so doing, assessors should treat clients as they would wish to be treated. Thus, clinicians practicing TA thoroughly explain assessment procedures so that clients may make an informed choice about whether or not to participate. Clients are also encouraged to provide input as the assessment unfolds, and to collaboratively construct recommendations at the end of the assessment. Clients are regarded as "experts on themselves" who work with assessors to better understand life impasses or dilemmas. TA is also suited to clients of different cultures in that assessment procedures are adapted to specific cultural contexts; clients are asked to help assessors understand how assessment findings relate to their unique cultural identities.

HUMILITY

Assessors practicing TA are acutely aware that they bring their own perspectives and biases into their work. They acknowledge that they can never fully understand another person's inner world. Assessors are also knowledgeable about the limitations of psychological tests, and do not view them as providing infallible "Truths" about clients. Test scores and interpretations are seen as starting points for discussions about clients' lives, and as tools for generating hypotheses that may assist clients in discovering new "self stories." Assessors trained in TA work to "find their own versions" of the struggles experienced by clients. They are humbled by how their clients' struggles mirror their own and are also acutely aware that all of us are growing, struggling human beings, generally doing the best we can given our respective backgrounds and resources.

COMPASSION

In TA, assessors integrate empathy and psychological testing to "feel into" their clients' lives, seeking to understand puzzles, behaviors, and patterns that are incomprehensible to others. This often results in clients' feeling more compassion for themselves, and receiving more acceptance and support from others in their lives. Often, as compassion increases and shame decreases, clients find that they are able to make needed changes that formerly eluded them.

OPENNESS/CURIOSITY

Assessors practicing TA aspire to conduct each assessment with openness to learning about themselves, the world, and the amazing resourcefulness of human beings to adapt and respond to challenging circumstances. They are genuinely curious about each person who presents for an assessment, and find that their curiosity often inspires clients to step back and view themselves and their life circumstances in new ways.

Research Findings

TA has been utilized with adults, couples, adolescents, and children and has shown great promise clinically. In controlled research with outpatient adults, TA has been shown to lead to decreases in symptomatology (Finn & Tonsager, 1992; Newman & Greenway, 1997), increases in self-esteem (Finn & Tonsager; Newman & Greenway; Allen, Montgomery, Tubman, & Escovar, 2003), and increases in hope (Finn & Tonsager). Compared to traditional information-gathering assessment, collaborative assessment has also been shown to lead to better compliance with treatment recommendations (Ackerman, Hilsenroth, Baity, & Blagys,

2000), and better alliance in subsequent psychotherapy (Hilsenroth, Peters, & Ackerman, 2004). With inpatient adults, a very brief (four-hour) TA resulted in better alliance, cooperation, and satisfaction with treatment; lower distress; and an increased sense of well being, as compared with a manualized, structured, supportive therapy or standard psychiatric treatment and milieu therapy (Little & Smith, 2008). A recent study with children under 13 and their families showed decreased symptomatology in children and mothers, decreased family conflict, and increased communication and cohesion following an eight-session TA. In addition, mothers had more positive and fewer negative feelings about their children after the assessment (Tharinger, Finn, Gentry, Hamilton, Fowler, & Matson, 2009).

Regarding adolescents, we are aware of two comparison studies. Newman (2004) compared distressed adolescents who received a brief (two-hour) TA ($N = 18$) to those receiving five hours of psychotherapy ($N = 18$). The group who received the TA showed significantly less symptomology and depression, and increased self-esteem, compared to the group receiving therapy. Ougrin, Ng, and Low (2008) compared TA with traditional, non-collaborative assessment in a group of 38 adolescents referred because they engaged in self-harm. Those receiving TA were much more likely to attend the first community follow-up appointment (75% vs. 40%) and to become engaged with services (62% vs. 30%); both factors have been associated with better psychosocial outcomes in this population of adolescents. In addition to controlled research, a number of case studies have been published on TA with adults (Finn, 1996a, 1996b, 2003, 2007; Finn & Martin, 1997; Finn & Kamphuis, 2006; Fischer, 1978; Fischer & Finn, 2008; Gorske, 2008; Peters, Handler, White, & Winkel, 2008; Wygant & Fleming, 2008); with children (Guerrero, Lipkind, & Rosenburg, 2011; Handler, 2006; Hamilton, et al., 2009, Haydel, Mercer, & Rosenblatt, 2011; Smith & Handler, 2009, Tharinger, Finn, Wilkinson, & Schaber, 2007; Tharinger & Roberts, in press); with couples (Finn, 2007); and with adolescents (Michel, 2002).

Principles for the Organization of Assessment Findings

In TA, assessors share aspects of their insights and interpretations with clients throughout the assessment process rather than waiting to share all their impressions at a closing feedback meeting (Riddle et al., 2002). In fact, Finn (2007) has re-conceptualized "feedback sessions," in which the assessor reports "data" obtained about the client, as "summary/discussion sessions," in which clients are invited to provide input as the assessment findings are interpreted. In these closing sessions of a TA, the assessor pays close attention to the order in which assessment findings are presented to ensure that clients are best able to internalize, and make use of, the assessment information (Finn & Tonsager, 2002).

Attending to the order of feedback is informed by the research on Swann and Read's (1981) *self-verification theory*. Their research indicates that individuals tend to accept feedback more readily when it is consistent with their self-views than when it is discrepant; this tendency persists whether people view themselves positively or negatively (e.g., Collins & Stukas, 2006; Finn, 2007; Giesler, Josephs, & Swann, 1996). Thus, Finn (1996a) recommended that the assessment findings that are congruent with how clients view themselves be discussed first (Level 1 findings). When working with adolescents and their families, it must also be considered whether assessment results are consistent with how parents view their son or daughter, as well as how parents view themselves in relation to their child. Presenting the most self-verifying information first serves to put adolescents and parents at ease, and supports their expectation that the assessment findings will be valid and useful.

Level 2 findings are those that reframe or amplify clients' typical ways of thinking about themselves or their families, and should be presented next. Although clients may be somewhat surprised by Level 2 feedback, and may not immediately accept it without question, it is expected that they will be able to integrate this new information into their self-views fairly easily. Ideally, the majority of the findings presented during the summary/discussion session should be Level 2 information (Tharinger, Finn, Hersh, et al., 2008); this is the information that is most likely to facilitate change in parents and adolescents.

Lastly, if the previous information is relatively well received, the assessor may go on to introduce Level 3 findings, which fundamentally conflict in some way with clients' self-views or the understandings of their family (Finn, 2007). Adolescents and parents are likely to become anxious upon hearing Level 3 information, and may initially challenge or reject these findings. Although parents or teenagers may be threatened by this higher-level feedback, within the context of a collaborative and supportive environment, and with the passage of time (e.g., weeks or months after the assessment is completed), they may come to understand and integrate these findings into the way they see themselves and their family. In addition, when their needs for self-verification and self-discovery are met through Level 1 and Level 2 feedback, many clients are quite open to receiving and integrating Level 3 feedback in the summary/discussion session.

The assessors' goal in the summary/discussion session is to help adolescents and parents accept and assimilate as many of the assessment results as possible. However, presenting too much new information may be overwhelming. Furthermore, some Level 3 feedback may be so threatening that it would not benefit clients to hear it for the first time in the summary/discussion session. For example, hearing that their adolescent suffers from significant depression may overwhelm parents if they have not been previously prepared for such a "bombshell." Furthermore, if the assessors know that clients are especially fearful of the word "depression," it is prudent to use phrases such as "lots of sadness" or "feeling really down" instead. If parents have, in some way, been exposed to Level 3 findings earlier in the assessment, and if the sequencing of information has been well executed and language mindfully used, clients are more likely to absorb and incorporate this higher level feedback into their existing views of themselves or their family. This then allows them to address their problems in living more effectively.

It is important to note that all of the assessment sessions should be executed with the intent of transforming Level 3 information into Level 2. When adolescents and parents have had the consistent experience of viewing themselves or their adolescent in a new way, hearing corresponding information from the assessor in the summary/discussion session is likely to be much easier. The practice of organizing feedback around clients' assessment questions also increases the likelihood that Level 3 findings will be accepted. If the information can be framed as an answer to a confounding question or an explanation for something that clients have long wondered about, they may be more motivated to process and consider the information rather than defensively reject it (Finn, 2007).

General Steps of Therapeutic Assessment

Finn (1996, 2007) has outlined a semi-structured, six-step, general model for TA. There is variation in the steps as applied to children, adolescents, adults, and couples. Each of the steps of TA, according to Finn, is important in its own right; additionally, however, in our experience, the whole is greater than the sum of the parts. The steps in the general model include: (1) the assessment question–gathering phase, (2) the standardized testing phase, (3) the intervention phase, (4) the summary/discussion phase, (5) the written communication phase, and (6) a follow-up phase. Finn acknowledges the reality that specifics of the client, setting, assessor, and resources available may preclude assessors' adoption of all six steps, and encourages assessors to adapt the model to their particular needs and circumstances.

The Model of Comprehensive TA with Adolescents

Figures 17.1 and 17.2 depict the comprehensive TA model as used with (1) children and their parents and (2) adolescents and their parents, respectively. The general steps of TA, as described above, are evident in both. As can be seen when comparing Figures 17.1 and 17.2, the major distinctions between TA with adolescents and TA with children is (1) the privacy and confidentiality afforded adolescents as compared to children, and (2) the direct work with adolescents in exploring and processing

their own testing findings, in contrast to the direct work with parents in exploring and processing the test findings of younger children. These distinctions are intended to reflect the differing developmental needs of children and adolescents discussed earlier. However, particularly in the age range of 11 to 13, a hybrid of the adolescent and child models may be used to fit the needs of individual children and families. As mentioned earlier, a comprehensive chapter on using TA with children and their parents also is available (Tharinger, Krumholz, Hall, & Matson, in press).

To grant adolescents some privacy and confidentiality, and with their parents' agreement, adolescents are allowed and encouraged to pose both shared and confidential assessment questions. In contrast, with pre-adolescent children, all their questions are disclosed to their parents. In addition, adolescents' testing sessions are not observed and processed by their parents, as they are in TA with children. Furthermore, adolescents often participate in an individual intervention session with the assessor, whereas children typically participate only in an intervention session in which their parents also

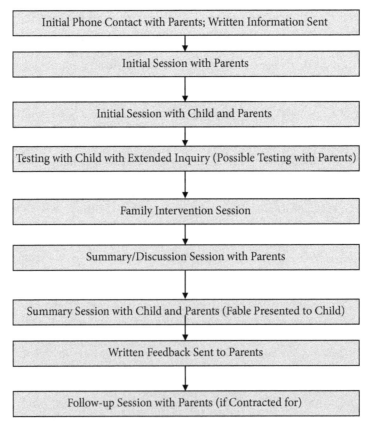

Initial Phone Contact with Parents; Written Information Sent

Initial Session with Parents

Initial Session with Child and Parents

Testing with Child with Extended Inquiry (Possible Testing with Parents)

Family Intervention Session

Summary/Discussion Session with Parents

Summary Session with Child and Parents (Fable Presented to Child)

Written Feedback Sent to Parents

Follow-up Session with Parents (if Contracted for)

Figure 17.1 TA with Children and Their Parents.

participate. Also, adolescents are provided with oral feedback addressing their private assessment questions prior to their parents' receiving oral feedback, which is not the case in the child model. Adolescents are also given a preview of the feedback their parents will receive, after which they may be given the option of attending their parents' feedback session, whereas children are not. In addition, adolescents receive a separate (and private) letter summarizing their specific feedback, while children's written feedback (usually in the form of a story or fable) is given to children and parents in a joint meeting. Thus, multiple steps in TA provide adolescents with privacy and confidentiality.

There is also a major distinction between adolescent and child TA with respect to the primary focus of clinician attention and intervention. In TA with children, the assessor works with the parents as they observe and process their child's test responses. The intent is to shift parents' "story" about the child, so that it is more coherent, accurate, compassionate, and useful (Tharinger et al., 2007). This is the main focus of attention because children respond readily to shifts in their environment, and their self-stories are not as "fixed" as are those of older clients. In contrast, in TA with adolescents, assessors work with the youth directly to further their insight into themselves. The extensive social and cognitive shifts that occur in this developmental stage allow adolescents to comprehend information derived from their cognitive and personality tests; they are able to scrutinize previously unexamined beliefs, behaviors, and values, and to observe themselves as the objects of their own thought (Elkind, 1978; Piaget, 1972). Thus, by affording privacy, confidentiality, and active processing of findings in the moment, the assessor invites adolescent clients to actively participate in their assessments as equal partners, which, in turn, allows them to feel that they are respected as valuable contributors throughout the intervention.

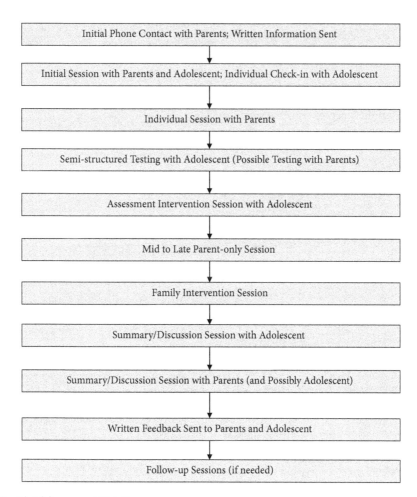

Figure 17.2 TA with Adolescents and Their Parents.

While this work with the adolescent is occurring, assessors also work with parents in a series of separate sessions, to facilitate and coordinate shifts in how they view their children, themselves, and their family.

We now describe and illustrate the goals and procedures for each step in the comprehensive TA model with adolescents and their parents. The majority of this material is abstracted from training materials designed by Finn and presented nationally and internationally over the past decade. We will illustrate each step with a recent case. The assessment presented herein was conducted as part of the Therapeutic Assessment Project (TAP) at the University of Texas. The assessment team consisted of the second author, Lauren Gentry, and Jamie Kuhlman, both doctoral students. The TA was supervised by Deborah Tharinger, licensed psychologist; and Pamela Schaber, licensed psychologist. Consultation was provided by Stephen Finn, licensed psychologist.

In TAP, we are studying the processes and outcomes of TA with children and adolescents. Variables of interest for potential change have included child symptomatology, family functioning, affective attitudes, and satisfaction with the assessment experience. Participants are recruited from the waiting list of a local outpatient community mental health clinic for children. If they meet entrance criteria, clients are offered a comprehensive TA, and, upon its completion, are placed at the beginning of the waiting list at the clinic, should they want additional services. The TAs are free of charge and take place at the university. Each assessment is conducted by an assessment team of two advanced graduate students in a doctoral-level professional psychology program, and supervised by licensed psychologists experienced in TA. In the TA model used in TAP, one assessment team member works primarily with the adolescent and the other with the parent(s). The assessment team comes together for all joint meetings with the family. The family members also work with independent research assistants to complete extensive pre- and post-assessment research measures and interviews, as well as brief interviews after each assessment session. Informed consent and assent is obtained from all family members prior to the start of the assessment. For the case illustrated in this chapter, both the mother and the adolescent boy gave their additional consent for us to write about them and their assessment experience in a published book.

TA with adolescents and their parents typically consists of 8 to 10 weekly sessions that take place over a two- to three-month period (although these sessions can be condensed into a shorter period if necessary). Meetings of an hour and a half are usually sufficient. We have found that weekly sessions allow time between sessions for adolescents and parents to process what they are learning, and to begin to construct a new story about themselves. This schedule similarly allows assessors time to absorb findings and thoroughly plan for the next session. This pacing, then, more closely resembles that of therapy or counseling than that of a traditional assessment.

Initial Phone Contact with Parents to Discuss Referral and Provide Information on TA

In the initial conversation with parents to explore the family's engaging in a TA, the assessor explicitly states that the assessment is intended to be a collaborative process, and stresses that parents' input is essential to the success of the TA. This assertion is then put into practice by asking parents to begin thinking about what questions they wish to address through the assessment, including those concerning their child, themselves, and their family. This invitation demonstrates from the beginning that parents will help to determine the course of the assessment. After the initial phone contact, more extensive information about the TA process is mailed to the parents, as is a separate information form designed specifically for adolescents. The intent of this separate information sheet is to support adolescents' individuation from the beginning, as well as to highlight the importance of their collaboration in the assessment process. The form for adolescents asks the following questions: "What is a Therapeutic Assessment?" "Why me, and what will this be like?" "What will I get out of this?" "What's the downside of this?" "Will you really tell me what you figure out?" "Who else will get the results of the assessment?" "Suppose I don't want to do the assessment?" and "What if I say yes, and then later I want to stop?"

For example, the information sheet answers "Why me and what will this be like?" as follows:

> Your parents have agreed that a psychological assessment with you could be useful to help them understand you better and help you understand yourself. Your parents will be invited to pose questions for the assessment that we will attempt to answer. In

our experience, parents ask questions such as, "Why is our son so angry all the time?" "Why is our daughter suddenly failing in school?" or "Why do we all fight all the time?" We will let you know the questions that your parents ask. We hope that you will work with us to figure out the answers to your parents' questions. We will also ask you, when we meet with you and your parents together, and when we meet with you privately, what questions you have about yourself and your life that you would like to ask. We will then work together to answer your questions as well. You can share your questions with your parents or you may keep them private. You might want to start thinking about questions you want the assessment to try to answer. Usually we can handle up to 4 or 5 different questions. Examples of questions teenagers have asked include, "Why don't my parents trust me like they should?" "Why do I get overwhelmed so easily?" "Why can't I get along with my parents any longer" "Why is school so hard for me now?" and "How come I'm having such problems with my friends?" After we settle on your and your parents' questions, we will be asking you to come for about 10 or so appointments. We will talk with you about your life, ask you to fill out some questionnaires, and ask you to do some psychological tests and talk with us about your experience. At the end of the assessment, we will meet with you privately to talk about the results of the assessment and answer your questions. Afterwards, we will meet with your parents to answer their questions. And at the end, we will write you a letter that tells you what we all figured out."

Initial Session with Parents and Adolescent

This first session is guided by multiple goals and procedures. The assessment team typically begins by meeting with the adolescent and parents together. This conjoint meeting may constitute one-half to two-thirds of the session, and is followed by a check-in with the adolescent alone. The session then closes with the parents rejoining the adolescent. In this initial meeting, the assessment team works hard to make connections with the multiple individuals involved, who often have long-standing conflicts or "feel stuck," which has led them to seek the assessment. For example, conflict between the parental subsystem and the adolescent is commonplace, as is disagreement within the parental subsystem. These conflicts are often exacerbated by the developmental tasks of adolescence discussed earlier. The competencies required of assessors in this first session are much like those used in therapy with adolescents and families: for example, listening, balancing, validating, summarizing, and exploring. We now discuss the goals and procedures of the first session, and illustrate by continuing our case example.

ESTABLISHING RELATIONSHIPS AND ALLIANCES

The first goal of the initial session is for assessors to begin establishing relationships and alliances with the adolescent and the parents. This includes helping the family to feel welcome, safe, accepted, and that they are truly valued as collaborators in the

---

Case material: Matt is a 13-year-old Caucasian male nearing completion of the eighth grade. He was referred for mental health services by his mother, Lisa, who reports that Matt is bright and mature beyond his years, but that he has recently been experimenting with an assortment of illicit and prescription drugs. Although Matt has yet to run into trouble with legal or school authorities, his mother is extremely concerned about his experimentation at this young age, as well as the influence that several of his friends have on his behavior. Lisa is a single mother who became pregnant with Matt when she was 16 years old and ended the relationship with Matt's father prior to his birth. Lisa describes her relationship with Matt as being close and open, but recently as more distant. Matt's contact with his biological father is sporadic at best, which has been upsetting for Matt throughout his life. Matt has a close relationship with Lisa's longtime boyfriend, Peter. Matt was diagnosed with Type 1 Diabetes at the age of seven and, although he is fairly responsible about managing his blood sugar, his health is an ongoing concern for Lisa. For example on one recent occasion, Matt had an overnight hospital stay after recreationally drinking a bottle of cough syrup. From the initial phone contact, we hypothesized that Lisa was probably struggling with letting her son individuate, as she described them as "best friends." We also felt that she genuinely had no understanding of why Matt was choosing to experiment with drugs.

Case material: In establishing relationships and alliances with Lisa and Matt, it was important for the assessment team to validate the concerns and experiences of each as they began to discuss their recent challenges. For example, the assessors normalized for Matt that it is developmentally appropriate for adolescents to distance from their parents as they work on their own identity formation, while they simultaneously validated how difficult this separation must be for Lisa. In further building rapport with Matt, it was invaluable for the assessor to engage him in a conversation about the things he liked, including music, sports, and leisure-time activities, rather than focusing exclusively on his recent problem behaviors. Both Matt and Lisa were highly personable, appeared to have a positive relationship with one another, and were willing participants in the assessment; as such, relational foundations were established with ease in this initial session.

assessment process, thus establishing a foundation of trust that will be further developed throughout the assessment. We have found the following steps to be especially useful:

(1) Warmly welcome everyone and explain the goals of the session;

(2) Introduce the session from a collaborative perspective;

(3) Ask if the adolescent or parents have any questions about the assessment at this point;

(4) Listen attentively, with interest and concern;

(5) Restate what you learned from talking to the parent over the phone and ask for clarification;

(6) Ask for any reactions to the information sheets that were sent home;

(7) Listen carefully and ask questions of each person present; give each family member the opportunity to state how he or she views the situation and, if there is disagreement, how each person feels about that.

It is also important to give the adolescent and parents permission to ask questions about you, the assessor, and any aspect of the assessment, as well as to discuss the limits of confidentiality. Additionally, in our experience, it is also very useful in this first session to ask about previous assessment experiences that the adolescent or the parents have had, and to listen for past hurts or disappointments, to accept and empathize with these, and to then offer an assessment contract that addresses the previous negative experience. Assessors should also encourage the family to alert them if they feel upset or poorly treated during any part of the TA. Finally, it is imperative that the assessor be attuned to interactions between family members during this session and throughout the assessment, gaining first hand experience of the family members' relationships and readiness for change.

NEGOTIATING SOME PRIVACY FOR THE ADOLESCENT

A second goal of the initial session is for the assessors to suggest and negotiate appropriate autonomy and privacy for the adolescent throughout the assessment. Typically, this involves securing the parents' permission for the adolescent to ask private assessment questions and to receive confidential feedback that addresses those questions. As most adolescents being assessed will be under the age of 18 and, thus, not *legally* entitled to confidentiality from their parents in relation to health and mental health care, this request is not made lightly and is understood not to be legally binding. The intention of seeking such privacy for adolescent clients is therapeutic. It acknowledges that most adolescents are beginning to individuate from their parents, and that, in our society, this is typically developmentally appropriate. Most adolescents appreciate this recognition, and thus are more likely to engage in the assessment. The request also encourages parents to accept this age-appropriate shift in their child, and to tolerate some expression of their son or daughter's autonomy. In many families, this request (and the subsequent negotiations) are, in and of themselves, an intervention, wherein boundaries are challenged and developmentally appropriate privacy needs explored. Such a request can also provide an opportunity to educate parents about the appropriate developmental needs of adolescents.

In our experience, most parents are very open to the request that their teenagers be able to pose private questions and receive individual feedback. Generally, parents appreciate their children's developmental changes and hope that their adolescents will confide in the assessor, obtaining needed help that they no longer seek from the parents. We have also found that some parents are not able to tolerate this request, or that one parent can but the other

Case material. Having normalized Matt's separation and individuation from his mother led relatively seamlessly into discussing Lisa's willingness for Matt to pose private questions for the assessment. Lisa readily agreed to honor such privacy for her son. However, the assessment team assured her (and informed Matt) that if Matt were to disclose any information in the course of the assessment that indicated a threat to his safety (particularly given that Matt's drug experimentation had previously resulted in a hospital stay), Lisa would be informed immediately. As is sometimes the case, in spite of Lisa's affording Matt the opportunity to pose confidential assessment questions, Matt chose to be continually open with his mother about his experience of the assessment.

cannot. When this is the case, more time is often needed to discuss the issue, and slowing the assessment process down until the matter can be satisfactorily resolved is generally good for everyone. We have also found that, by the end of the assessment, adolescents often choose to share their private questions and feedback with their parents, perhaps as a reflection of the paradox of trust.

OBTAINING ASSESSMENT QUESTIONS FROM PARENTS AND ADOLESCENT JOINTLY

The third goal of the initial session is to gather and co-construct assessment questions from the parents and the adolescent together, with the adolescent knowing that, if they are so negotiated, he or she will still have the opportunity to privately pose additional questions later. In our experience, most adolescents pose some questions with their parents present and some questions privately. In helping parents and adolescents frame questions to be explored through the assessment, it is important to use the clients' own words if possible, and to refine questions that are too broad or too narrow. It is also helpful to continually engage clients' curiosity, as this tends to suspend their emotional reactions, instead putting them in a role wherein they are more objectively exploring themselves. It can also be very useful for assessors to suggest implicit questions that they have heard with their "third ear" (i.e., queries that have been alluded to or implied, but not explicitly articulated), thus assisting the client in making the question explicit. If a client is struggling with posing questions, or insists that he or she has no questions, it may be useful to return to discussing the aims of collaborative assessment and the importance of its being guided by clients' curiosities about themselves or their families. In cases like these, it is possible that the relationship and trust are not adequately established and the process may need to be slowed down. In other cases, it may be that one of the participants, perhaps one of the parents, is not fully

on board with the assessment. In these cases, it is useful to comment on this and ask about the person's reservations so that the assessor may work to address these concerns.

In our experience, assessment questions are a crucial component of the collaborative assessment process. They serve to lower clients' anxiety by defining the contract for the assessment and, from the start, engage clients as active participants in the assessment process. Constructing questions also tends to engage clients' curiosity about themselves or their children, and very importantly, provide "open doors" to discuss difficult or awkward information. For the assessor, the constructed questions provide information about clients' current self-schemas/stories and indicate where those self-structures may be open to change. Finally, collecting assessment questions from clients sets the stage for them to "mentalize" (Allen, Fonagy, & Bateman, 2008) about their problems, which in itself can be therapeutic. Many clients report that they experience relief just from framing their persistent problems in the form of questions.

After the questions are formed, the assessor typically collects relevant background information to flesh out the history and context underlying each question. In collecting background information about each question, we have found queries such as the following to be very helpful: "What does the problem look like in daily life?" "If this problem were resolved today, what would be different about your life?" "If you had to answer the assessment question today, what would you say?" and "What would be the most difficult thing to hear at the end of the assessment?" In posing such follow-up questions, however, it is essential to respect the client's right to privacy at all times. Information-gathering questions should be connected to the client's agenda for the assessment in a face-valid way, which is exemplified by the client's assessment questions. If the assessor wishes to ask a follow-up question that does not appear to be related to the client's concerns, it

Case material. With minimal guidance, Lisa and Matt readily developed questions for the assessment. Lisa's questions were: (1) Why is Matt experimenting with drugs? (2) "Am I communicating with him in the right way?" and (3) "Why is Matt not motivated to reach his potential in school?" The question that Matt posed in his mother's presence was: "Why does my mind go blank in tests for algebra?" He subsequently alluded to the fact that he sometimes has difficulty putting his thoughts into words, but did not develop an additional question about this. While discussing Matt's recent history of drug experimentation (which had also included taking prescription stimulant medications and smoking marijuana), Lisa made a comment about how she was unable to relate to Matt's behavior because she had never experimented with drugs in her youth. Although it seemed somewhat uncomfortable for Matt to hear his mother talk with two relative strangers about his experimentation with drugs, he did not become defensive or withdrawn at any time. In fact, he only contradicted his mother on one occasion, saying that his experimentation with drugs had nothing to do with "peer pressure," and he remained engaged throughout the session.

is important that the assessor ask permission and explain why the question is relevant. In addition, it is important to allow clients to declare certain topics "off limits," even though the absence of the information may constrict the ability to fully address a particular assessment question.

In wrapping up the information gathering portion of the session, the assessor summarizes the assessment questions that have been agreed upon, invites both the parents and the adolescent to develop additional questions as the assessment unfolds, and reminds everyone that there will be ample opportunity to further discuss the questions as the TA progresses.

OBTAINING PRIVATE ASSESSMENT QUESTIONS FROM THE ADOLESCENT

The next goal of the initial session is to gauge how the adolescent is experiencing the process, and to invite him or her to meet individually to pose private questions. If so negotiated, the parents are asked to leave the room, and the assessor solicits reactions from the adolescent in response to the session so far. The assessor attempts to align with the adolescent, conveying genuine understanding of the difficulties that come with adolescence, including that relationships with parents can be challenging. The assessor continually encourages questions and reactions from the teen, seeks his or her explicit agreement to take part in the assessment, and highlights that the process will only be useful if the adolescent is on board and curious. If the teen is hesitant or unsure, the assessor may suggest that he or she take more time to think about it, and will support the adolescent in doing so. If, at any time, the adolescent decides not to participate, the assessor must respect this decision and agree to represent to the parents that this is not

the right time for a TA. If the teen agrees to participate collaboratively, the assessor then invites private assessment questions and again reviews the legal limits of confidentiality. The process of constructing questions and exploring their context is very similar to that described earlier for the joint session with the adolescent and the parents.

However, it should be mentioned that sometimes it is difficult to get adolescents to formulate individual questions to be answered through the assessment. This can happen for a number of reasons, including an underlying reluctance to participate in the assessment, distrust of the assessor, limited intellectual abilities, or, in some cases, an inability to "step back" and become curious about oneself. If an adolescent says he or she has no questions, but seems very willing to participate, it is best to proceed, keeping in mind that assessment questions may emerge in subsequent sessions. If the lack of questions seems to be a reflection of marginal motivation to participate (perhaps accompanied by a desire to mollify parents), the assessor should once again reassure the adolescent that it is not necessary to do the assessment, and that the assessor will back up the adolescent with his or her parents. Again, some adolescents will insist on proceeding and may generate questions once they develop more trust with the assessor.

REUNITING AND COMPLETING THE ASSESSMENT CONTRACT

The fourth goal involves reuniting the adolescent and parents to summarize what has happened in the first session, as well as discuss what is to come. We have found that meta-processing can be useful at this point. Questions such as: "What was it like to talk about these things today?" or "How are you feeling as you leave today?" may help

Case material. In his individual check-in, Matt was open to discussing his recent struggles, including his experimentation with drugs; he readily came up with private assessment questions. These included: (1) "Why do I feel distant from my friends sometimes even when I'm hanging out with them for hours on end?" (2) "Why did I take Adderall the second time without weighing the pros and the cons?" and (3) "Why do I smoke pot when I don't remember anything the next day?" When the assessor asked Matt what his best guess was about the answer to his final question, he said that, when he smokes marijuana, "it's an hour or two that I don't have to contain myself. It feels like nothing can, kinda, tear me down at all." The assessor then reiterated that smoking marijuana allows him to "let go," and asked if he felt like he had to "contain himself" during other times in his life. He said: "At school, I feel like I can't be myself. I can't wear what I want to wear. I have to be careful about jokes I make because I might offend someone." Matt also talked at length about all of the research he had done on the drugs he had used, including that he did not have the experience he was "supposed" to have when he drank the bottle of cough syrup. In fact, Matt was very forthright about his embarrassment at having ended up in the hospital following that incident. During this conversation, Matt also asserted that there are many drugs he would "never" try, including drugs like "meth, coke, PCP, and heroin."

solidify the experience and unite the family in their commitment to the assessment. The desired outcome at the end of the first session is for the family to leave feeling less shame, and more calm, understood, curious, and hopeful. Before ending the session, any additional details of completing the contract for the assessment are discussed, such as the projected number of sessions, ending date, procedures, and if any formal written feedback will be needed (although some details may be handled privately with the parents, such as cost, insurance, etc.). Releases to contact collateral professionals are also obtained from parents, and even though it is not legally necessary, we generally also ask for adolescents' permission to contact previous therapists, teachers, etc. Finally, the next session is scheduled, which typically involves a meeting with the parents to obtain family and developmental history. As addressed shortly, it is important for the assessor to explain to the adolescent the reasons for the upcoming meeting with the parents alone "e.g., we want to ask your parents questions about when you were little and we think it might be boring for you to sit there", and to address any questions or concerns he or she may have about such a plan.

REFLECTING ON THE SESSION AND INITIAL IMPRESSIONS/HYPOTHESES

The final goal of the initial session involves the assessor taking time to consolidate initial impressions and hypotheses, and to sort through any emotional reactions and anxieties that may be surfacing in relation to the clients. Such reflection underscores that the assessor and his or her reactions to, and relationships with, family members are a valuable source of information throughout the assessment process.

Session with Parents Only

The primary goal of this session is to further explore the parents' assessment questions by asking about relevant developmental and family history. This private session also allows the parents to share information that they might not have felt comfortable discussing in front of their child, or that would not have been appropriate for the teenager to hear (e.g., marital conflict, details about financial stress,

Case material. Upon coming back together, neither Lisa nor Matt expressed any lingering hesitations about participating in the assessment, and, in fact, both were very upbeat about their willingness to take part. Matt asked some brief questions about the kinds of assessment activities he would be doing in the ensuing weeks, but he had no concerns about the assessment team meeting with his mom individually the following week. Additionally, both Lisa and Matt appeared somewhat reenergized by the end of the first session.

Case material. Upon reflection, the assessment team noted that both Lisa and Matt were immediately likable. They were personable and seemed bright and open. They were both engaged and present throughout the session. In spite of the challenges their family was facing, they appeared to have a close and positive relationship with one another. The assessment team felt they had made a good connection and that the case would proceed well.

information about an absent parent, etc.). Parents may also have additional assessment questions that they were not comfortable posing in front of their adolescent. If this is so, the assessor works with the parents to formulate these additional assessment questions so they may be shared comfortably with the teen. For, while the adolescent may be allowed private assessment questions, all of the parents' questions for the assessment are shared with the adolescent—except in very rare instances. This session is also an opportunity for the assessor to strengthen the collaborative relationship with the parents, and to empathize with aspects of their lives, especially the difficulties of parenting and frustration with their adolescent. Additionally, it allows the assessor the opportunity to discern parents' readiness for change. In our experience, some parents need much of the session to complain about their adolescent in a scapegoating manner before they can begin to develop or resurrect empathy for their child. Other parents need time to express guilt for the challenges their child has had to endure, and to seek some "absolution" from the assessor before being able to move on. The assessor needs to be flexible and able to adjust to parents' specific needs, gathering information and offering support in ways that will facilitate the family's moving toward positive change.

It is also in the first parent-only session that the assessor typically introduces the idea of parents undergoing some psychological testing as well. This possibility is usually raised seamlessly if the parents have posed an assessment question that addresses their parenting style or how their personality fits with their adolescent. For example, a parent may have asked, "Are there ways that my reactions to Sam's behavior contribute to his withdrawal and secrecy?" or, "My guess is that my personality really clashes with Ellen's sometimes, resulting in a real firestorm between us. How can I get that under control?" If parents have provided such an opening, the assessor offers to do some testing with them with private feedback focused on the interface of their personality and parenting style and how these factors impact their adolescent. This parental

assessment feedback remains within the bounds of the goals established for the assessment. In the TAP project, if parents agree to be tested, we typically use the Minnesota Multiphasic Personality Inventory-2 (MMPI-2) with them, but depending on the parents' questions about themselves, any of a number of tests may be appropriate. Sometimes, adolescents are aware that their parents are engaging in testing of their own, and this can help them feel less scapegoated. Regardless, typically they are not privy to their parents' test results, unless their parents offer this information.

Testing Sessions with the Adolescent

Typically the standardized testing begins in the third session of a TA with an adolescent. Although the number of testing sessions varies by case, four or five is average. As Finn (2007) has recommended, it is of utmost importance to begin with assessment measures that clearly reflect the clients' central concerns. Commencing with tests that are tied in their face validity to the adolescents' and parents' goals communicates to clients that: (1) they are being taken seriously; (2) their concerns are the first priority; and (3) their questions will be addressed collaboratively from the start. The tests administered vary based on clients' presenting problems and assessment questions. Nonetheless, assessments often consist of: (1) cognitive testing, (2) academic achievement testing, (3) basic neuropsychological measures, (4) socio-emotional testing, which may include behavior rating scales like the Behavior Assessment System for Children, Second Edition (BASC-2), the Child Behavior Checklist (CBCL), (5) a self-report inventory, such as the Minnesota Multiphasic Personality Inventory for Adolescents (MMPI-A), and (6) performance-based personality measures such as the Rorschach, sentence completions, projective drawings, apperception tests. Again, depending on the issues to be explored, there are a number of other psychological assessment tools that may be useful in informing the assessment questions. Beginning with the first assessment measure and continuing for all remaining testing

Case material. Lisa needed no time to vent or disclose guilt. Rather, she began by discussing Matt's development chronologically, including willingly disclosing many of the details surrounding her teenage pregnancy. In so doing, Lisa matter-of-factly detailed her remarkable efforts to keep her life on track after finding out about her pregnancy. While continuing to attend high school, she also took night classes in order to complete her graduation requirements prior to giving birth. Lisa then spent the summer at her parents' home. That fall, when Matt was about four months old, Lisa began college, finishing her degree four years later. In discussing Matt's early life, Lisa also talked about the trauma and overwhelming feelings associated with Matt's diabetes diagnosis. It appeared that she had sought out positive ways for Matt to manage his illness. She arranged for him to give presentations to his classmates, involve his peers in his treatment, and attend a summer camp for diabetic children and their siblings annually. Nonetheless, Lisa did report feeling that Matt's diabetes had impacted him emotionally. Lisa also described Matt's relationship with his biological father as being characterized by unmet promises and infrequent contact, and highlighted how hurt and disappointed Matt continued to be by his father's failure to maintain a relationship with him. She also relayed how painful and angering this was for her. In spite of his father's absence, Lisa noted that Matt had positive relationships with her many close male friends, and that Matt also was extremely connected to her longtime boyfriend, who had been actively engaged in Matt's life since he was six.

In discussing developmental history, Lisa stated that Matt had been an easy child, notwithstanding his recent drug use, and that he was respectful and obedient. While Lisa emphasized her closeness with Matt, she also highlighted the importance of acting as a mother and not as a friend with her son when he needed to adhere to structure and limits. She also indicated that, although he had many friends, Matt appeared less confident with his age mates than with adults, and often allowed himself be "taken advantage of" by his peers. She suggested that many of his problem behaviors (like drug use) were due to his succumbing to peer pressure. When asked what she would be most afraid to learn through the assessment, Lisa stated that the worst thing she could find out would be that Matt wanted to commit suicide, and that he could be that depressed without her being aware of it.

Finally, while Lisa was obviously very concerned about Matt's drug use, she also recognized, and was troubled by, a shift in their relationship towards less open communication. Given the systemic nature of her question about whether she was communicating with Matt in the "right way," it seemed very appropriate for the assessors to explore her willingness to engage in testing of her own. Lisa readily agreed, stating that she was willing to do anything necessary to help her son.

activities, the assessor explains to adolescents, in an accessible way, how each test will address their (or their parents') agenda for the assessment. Following standardized administration of each task, the assessor then asks teenagers to expand, reflect upon, and discuss noteworthy responses or experiences as they completed the activity.

This exploration of the testing experience and particular responses may take the form of *extended inquiry* or *testing the limits*. In extended inquiry, the assessor seeks to further engage clients as collaborators by inviting them onto "an observation deck" where they can think about their own test responses more objectively (Finn, 2007; Handler, 2006). From this viewpoint, clients are encouraged to connect their test responses to their lives outside of the assessment room, as well as to access any painful affect that is revealed through the assessment

experience. Through such conjoint observation, clients can begin to collaboratively "weave a new story" about themselves that often relates to their assessment questions.

So, after completing a particular standardized test, the assessor simply inquires about clients experiences of the task ("What was that like for you?" or "What did you think of that?"). The assessor then asks follow-up questions on any observations that clients' have made, and encourages them to make connections to their outside lives, as well as to their assessment questions. After seeking clients' input, the assessor is then free to share relevant observations or thoughts; however, the assessor must do this tentatively, inviting clients' feedback and honoring their reactions to the assessor's suggestions or ideas.

Extended inquiry can take different forms, depending on the assessment tool with which it is being used, as well as the nature of the parents' or adolescent's questions for the assessment. For example, it may be useful for the assessor to inquire about a client's experience of the performance IQ tasks as compared to the verbal IQ activities, or to ask about their feelings about the timed versus untimed academic tasks. With the MMPI-A, it is often helpful to look at the critical items and follow-up with the adolescent on any items that were endorsed. Typically, there are at least a few surprising responses. It is important to remember that adolescents can have a multitude of reasons for endorsing a particular item, some of which may be more benign than they seem. These endorsements could be affecting elevations in the profile and it is important to fully understand the reasons underlying such responses. With the Rorschach, it can be useful to pose such queries as: "Does this response remind you of anything we've been talking about?" "Could you tell me a story about … ?" or "If this monster could talk, what would he say?" (Handler, 2006). The assessor can also ask clients to review their own responses and identify those that have personal significance. When engaging in extended inquiry, it is important for the assessor to assure clients that the only intent is to understand why they endorsed certain items, or gave particular responses.

Case material. When taken together, Matt's assessment data suggested that he was quite bright; he performed in the high average range of cognitive functioning, exhibiting a significantly stronger performance in tasks that were verbal as opposed to visual-spatial in nature. In his academic achievement testing, Matt's scores ranged from the low average range to the superior range. While he exhibited some difficulty with academic fluency, spelling, and reading novel words, his profile was not indicative of the presence of a learning disability in any area of academic functioning.

When Matt was completing the Woodcock-Johnson Tests of Cognitive Abilities, after he exhibited substantially more difficulty on the performance IQ tasks as compared to the verbal IQ activities, the assessor asked "Matt, if you had a choice between working on a puzzle or doing something that had to do with language or vocabulary, which would you choose?" Matt, not surprisingly, explained that he would prefer a language-based task. Similarly, when Matt completed the Woodcock-Johnson Tests of Achievement, the assessor inquired about his experience of the timed versus the untimed math tasks, and how these activities might have related to his tendency to "go blank" in algebra class. Matt's social-emotional-personality assessment results indicated that he was experiencing a great deal of negative emotionality, including depression and anxiety. Further, Matt appeared to engage in over-introspection and excessive rumination, and to be vulnerable to chronic feelings of insecurity, inadequacy, and sensitivity to criticism. Socially, Matt exhibited a tendency to withdraw and be passive in relationships, a propensity that led to his needs for interpersonal closeness not being met. Further, he indicated often feeling misunderstood by others, distant, lonely, and plagued with social anxiety.

Related to these feelings, we noted that Matt failed to give any full human responses during the standardized Rorschach administration. The assessor subsequently gained more information about Matt's ability to perceive humans and human connection through testing the limits with Matt in this activity. In so doing, the assessor chose the two Rorschach cards in which the human form is most readily recognizable (III and VII) and said, "A lot of people see humans in this card. Do you see where the people might be?" When Matt immediately said that he recognized the human figures, the assessor had him identify each part of the human form he saw in the inkblot in order to ensure that he was, in fact, seeing the popular response. In the event that Matt had been unable to accurately identify the human figures in these blots, the assessor would have used a scaffolding technique to help him recognize these more common percepts. For example, saying: "Most people see this as a face. Can you show me the different parts of that face?" Matt's success in seeing humans on the extended inquiry suggested that his initial failure to report such percepts was not due to some serious deficit in interpersonal perception. Instead, Matt seemed to "leave out" these percepts to focus on non-human content. To us, this suggested that Matt's feelings of social isolation were very real and may have been triggering a tendency to exercise poor judgement in decision-making; additionally, his risk-taking activities (like drug use) were possibly an attempt to cope with his loneliness.

In garnering more information about clients' assessment data, the assessor can also "test the limits," which is a process that seeks to establish if clients can give a better performance, or more common test response when provided with additional resources (time, encouragement, help, etc.). While widely utilized in traditional assessment, "testing the limits" in TA is practiced with the intent of collaborating with, "scaffolding," or emotionally supporting clients in such a way that they more capably perform the task at hand. So, for example, a client who has significant test anxiety in her math class may, following standardized administration, be given unlimited time on an alternate form of some math subtests to see if that testing context ameliorates her stress response. Such exercises can give the assessor a sense of which contextual variables are related to clients' problematic behaviors, and which variables could be changed to help them improve their performance. It is important to note that the additional information that is gleaned through extended inquiry and testing the limits in no way alters the standardized scoring of the assessment measures; however, this additional data can be used to more comprehensively interpret and derive meaning from the assessment results.

Adolescent Intervention Session

In addition to what the adolescent may learn through the testing and exploration through extended inquiry methods, an important component of TA with adolescents is an individual intervention session that provides an opportunity for the adolescent and assessor to experientially work together to provoke a salient problem and enact a more adaptive solution. This *in vivo* experience can shed light upon the reasons for teenagers' problems in living and provide them with an alternate experience that is, in some way, corrective or healing. Although increases in self-knowledge and understanding are valuable, they are not synonymous with behavior change. Thus, facilitating such experiential learning increases the likelihood that the TA will have an enduring impact on clients' lives. Intervention sessions are highly complex, and, as such, are conducted with an eye to a multitude of smaller goals. The assessor is seeking to engage clients in:

(1) exploring hypotheses derived from the testing,
(2) understanding aspects of the assessment findings,
(3) heightening awareness of findings that would otherwise probably be rejected,
(4) experiencing a "living example" of an assessment finding,
(5) independently discovering assessment findings,
(6) testing out possible interventions for managing clients' problems in living and experiencing more adaptive solutions, and
(7) preparing for the summary/discussion sessions.

See Finn (2007) for a more complete explanation of the goals and techniques of individual assessment intervention sessions.

Given these ambitious goals, extensive planning is needed. First, the assessor needs a clear understanding of the adolescent's problem behaviors and how he or she names, understands, and experiences them. The assessor must also be capable of aiding clients in drawing connections to experiences outside of the assessment room; that is, conjointly extrapolating how these problematic behaviors present themselves in clients' daily lives. Furthermore, the assessor needs a hypothesis regarding the factors that are necessary and sufficient to produce the problem behaviors, and must be prepared to engage clients in an exploration of the context of their problems in living. Such contextual understanding is imperative to enlisting clients in imagining (and experiencing) solutions to their challenges. The assessor must also have some idea as to how contexts might be altered in order to elicit more adaptive strategies from clients. It is these collaboratively generated possible solutions, then, that are tested *in vivo*. It is the hope that as this exploration unfolds, the client will have a more positive experience and will exhibit more adaptive behavior. If not, the assessor must continually revise the possible solutions until clients experience some success. Thus, adolescent intervention sessions can take a wide variety of forms, and are an opportunity for the assessor to be creative.

Once the adolescent has a new or more successful experience in the intervention session, the assessor then engages him or her in a discussion about how to implement and generalize the experienced solutions to life outside of the assessment room. In these discussions, it is also important for the assessor to consider and address the challenges that may be faced as adolescents attempt to broadly implement these new behaviors in their lives, as well as how these difficulties might be managed. The assessor then asks clients to report back at the following assessment session after they have reflected on the intervention experience, and have had the opportunity to try to apply it to contexts outside of the assessment.

Case material. The intervention session was introduced to Matt as an "experiment" during which he and the assessor would try to address some of his assessment questions in a more experiential way. As usual, the assessor assured Matt that his experience of the session would be discussed at the end, including how well the "experiment" had worked for him. As reviewed above, Matt had reported a tendency for his mind to "go blank" in various situations. Although this tendency may have been exacerbated in part by his diabetes, it was hypothesized on the basis of the standardized test findings that his "bottled up" emotions were "leaking out" at times, overwhelming his capacity to cope, and also contributing to this "blankness."

Thus, Matt's intervention session was planned as follows: he would begin the session by rating his "blankness" on a scale of 0 to 10, (with 0 being "totally blank/unable to express himself" and 10 being "completely clear/able to express himself perfectly"). Matt would then complete a memory-for-words task, followed by telling stories drawn from two to four thematic apperception test (TAT) cards. The first card was to be relatively benign in order to introduce him to the task, followed by progressively more emotionally evocative cards, with the intention of getting him emotionally aroused or "stirred up." In the event that his stories failed to be emotionally evocative, the assessor was going to prompt him to: "… tell a story that is emotional, sad, or worrisome in some way.…" Following this exercise, Matt would again be asked to rate his "blankness" and would then be administered an alternate memory-for-words list. It was hypothesized that his performance would worsen (due to his emotional arousal), at which point the assessor would provide him with various emotional regulation strategies, such as mindfulness techniques and/or muscle tensing and relaxing exercises in order to ameliorate his "blankness." After working through these coping strategies, Matt would then be given a third form of memory-for-words, at which point, it was hoped, his performance would improve. Lastly, he would be asked one final time for a rating of his "blankness," after which he and the assessor would discuss the experience.

In spite of the careful attention that went into the design of this session, as sometimes happens with assessment interventions, it did not unfold as planned. In fact, Matt did only negligibly worse on the second administration of the memory-for-words list, indicating that either: (1) the TAT stories did not sufficiently emotionally arouse him, or (2) it was not his emotional arousal that was precipitating his "blankness." So, after some impromptu consultation with the other assessor and a supervisor, the primary assessor abandoned the plan for the session and instead transparently talked with Matt about what the hypothesis had been for the session, what his thoughts were about that hypothesis, and about his general experience of the session. The assessor also began to "trickle in" some feedback from the assessment data to see how accepting Matt would be of it.

Although Matt had previously informed the assessor that he tended to "bottle up" his negative emotions for fear that they would threaten his interpersonal relationships, he had a very strong reaction to the assessor's suggestion that he was experiencing any negative affect at all. This fit with Lisa's presentation, for whom, the assessment team slowly learned, it was important to tirelessly present herself as a positive and strong person. Matt similarly insisted that he was "basically a happy person" and worked very hard to keep his negative feelings to himself. The assessor validated Matt's "content" self-presentation, and recognized his work to keep his negative emotions "in check." However, the assessor also sought to normalize, accept, and help Matt acknowledge and "sit with" his painful affect. Subsequently, Matt relayed that he had just told his mother during the past week that he tended to not express any of his negative feelings, but, instead, bottled them up and held them inside. The assessor was then able to tie this disclosure back to what Matt had said in his first session about being able to "let go" when he smoked marijuana. He acknowledged that smoking "weed" was the only time his bottled-up feelings went away. By the end of the intervention session, Matt was able to "name" his negative feelings as "sadness, anger, and frustration." The assessor was then able to validate Matt's feelings and compliment him on his insightfulness, given that much of the assessment data indicated that he was experiencing just those kinds of feelings. Thus, this case illustrates that, even when adolescent intervention sessions do not go as planned, they may still serve to offer clients a corrective emotional experience and a more integrated view of themselves.

In Matt's next meeting with the assessor, before the start of the family intervention session, he shared that he was still struggling with some of the assessment findings that had been discussed the week before. He said that he had thought a great deal about it, and he continued to believe that he did not exhibit any negative emotionality. In fact, he had talked with some friends about whether or not he came across as sad or angry, and they had confirmed that he did not. In response, the assessor validated that, in casual interaction, Matt did not come across as sad or angry. In that moment, Matt shared a realization that the activities he had completed throughout the assessment were not intended to get at the image he wanted to project, but at how he was really feeling. Compellingly, Matt was then able to recognize that he had "let out a little bit" of how he was really feeling in these activities. The assessor emphasized how much she appreciated and valued Matt's having shared himself with her. Matt was then able to disclose that he had told some of his friends about his negative emotions. The assessor then asked Matt if he had been satisfied with how his friends had responded to his inquiry about if he came across as sad or angry. He said that, while it felt good to be reassured that he did not come across as feeling mad or depressed, he had also wanted some of his friends to recognize his negative emotions, and was disappointed when they failed to do so. The assessor then talked with Matt about what it would be like for him to tell his friends that he sometimes wanted them to recognize and talk with him about his negative feelings. Matt seemed curious and open to undertaking this next step with his friends.

Mid to Late Parent-Only Session

Following the completion of the adolescent testing and intervention sessions, another parent-only meeting typically is scheduled. The goals of this session are as follows:

(1) Continuing to build and develop the relationship with the parents,

(2) Collecting additional background information that may shed light on some of what is being gleaned from the adolescent,

(3) Assessing how the parents and family have been functioning since the start of the assessment, and

(4) Beginning to tentatively provide and discuss some of the initial assessment findings, including feedback from the parents' own assessment (e.g., the MMPI-2).

In preparing for this session, several considerations are useful in guiding decision making. First, the assessor needs to evaluate whether the adolescent can tolerate the assessor meeting individually with his or her parents at this late point in the assessment. As the adolescent and assessor have met privately for the past many sessions, it is understandable that he or she could have concerns about what might be shared with the parents at this point, as well as how the parents may respond to any information that is divulged. It is important to let the adolescent know the plan and goals for the parent meeting, as well as to review and discuss any concerns the

adolescent may have. It is likely that the strong alliance and collaborative relationship that the assessor has developed with the adolescent, wherein respect for the teen's autonomy has been repeatedly demonstrated, will serve to allay any apprehension. If not, persistent concerns may be very useful in informing the remainder of the assessment.

Another question that is important to consider is, "Can the parents contain information without 'spilling it' to the adolescent?" This session usually involves "sprinkling in" some of the findings and assessing the parents' reactions in an effort to begin preparing them for the summary/discussion session. Therefore, if the assessor's experiences with the parents to date suggest that the parents would be highly reactive to a particular assessment finding, and would subsequently rush home and interrogate their child about his or her experience of this finding, the assessor would probably want to broach the topic conservatively at first. For example, the assessor might say: "I'm still bringing together and making meaning out of all of the assessment information, but one thing I wanted to do today is just get a little bit more information from you about the way you see John at home. Does it ever seem to you that he might feel a little sad or worried?" as opposed to, "The assessment information is indicating that John is severely depressed and anxious." If, however, the assessor judges that there are clear parental boundaries, and that the parents are more prepared for a given assessment finding, the assessor may feel safe being less tentative. For example, the assessor may say: "Many of the assessment results suggest that John is struggling with some pretty significant feelings of sadness and worry right now. Does this fit for you? How have you seen this come across at home?"

Similarly, it is useful to explicitly consider the question, "What findings might be most difficult for the parents to accept?" As reviewed previously, such information can be conceptualized as "Level 3 feedback"—assessment findings that are highly incongruent with how parents see themselves, their family, or their adolescent. Often, parents are unwilling or unable to readily accept such information, due to fear, shame, or a conflicting worldview. It may be the case that testing supports parents' worst fears about their child or their family. Often, parents may recognize on some level that their worst fears are well within the realm of possibility. As such, they actually may be more ready to accept the information than the parents who do not articulate such a possibility. Regardless, considering this question allows the assessor to "test the waters" by beginning to share pieces of findings that are expected to be difficult for parents to integrate, in order to see how they are received.

Giving parents feedback at this time allows the assessor to see how readily the parents can absorb personal feedback, as well as if they express curiosity about how their personalities and parenting styles are affecting their adolescent. Again, parents' openness is likely to be an accurate gauge of how they will approach final feedback, and is indicative of their openness to recommendations that may be more systemic in nature (e.g., a referral for family therapy). The assessor should be alert to the possibility of resistance or negativity, as some parents may be recognizing the complementarity that exists between their parenting style and their adolescent's challenges for the first time. Some parents may be relieved to have this insight, while others may be overwhelmed, initially dismissing the information, or responding with feelings of guilt and shame. In our experience, within the context of a strong collaborative relationship, the assessor can accept the parent's reaction and work with it in ways that offer potential for change.

Lastly, it is important for the assessor to be thinking about what can be learned in this session that would help in planning the family intervention session, which is coming up next. For example, if it is expected that parents are going to be highly resistant to a major finding of the assessment, it may be extremely useful to design the upcoming family intervention session around that finding (and the related assessment question), given that parents are likely to be more open to receiving unsettling feedback if they have recently experienced it *in vivo* with the emotional support of the assessor.

Case material. The assessment team began the session by checking in with Lisa about her week and asking if she had noticed any changes in Matt since the beginning of the assessment. She said that he had been more motivated to complete his schoolwork and had not, to her knowledge, used any illegal substances. She also reported a recent fight that she had had with her son wherein Matt had yelled at her, which he had never done before. Interestingly, Matt had just shared with the assessor that he was fearful of exhibiting any negative affect due to his belief that such expression would estrange his friends and family. The assessment team then inquired about how much Matt had shared with Lisa so far about his testing experiences. She said that typically they discussed the assessment only minimally, but that, in the last week, he had brought up his intervention session twice. As he did with some friends, Matt also told Lisa that he had been surprised to hear that the testing indicated that he was experiencing some sadness and worry. Lisa reported that she, similarly to Matt's friends, had assured Matt that she did not view him as being sad or worried. As Lisa relayed this story, it did not seem that she had entertained the possibility that Matt might have been checking in with her about this emotionally laden feedback to see if she could "handle" his being depressed or anxious. If only subtly, it appeared that Lisa had communicated that, in fact, she could not accept it.

The assessment team then reviewed Lisa's MMPI-2 feedback with her, sharing that her profile suggested that she was resilient, strong, optimistic, and a "superwoman." Lisa readily agreed with this feedback and related it to her life experiences. She said that, rather than viewing the trials and tribulations of life as hard, they were "just what life gave her." She further said that she has no need to "wallow"; problems just need to be fixed. She frequently referred to the metaphor that "sometimes you bite off more than you can chew, but you just have to chew faster." While she ultimately acknowledged that "everybody crawls into bed and cries for a half hour sometimes," she said that Peter, her long-term boyfriend, was the only person in her life who had seen her "break down." Lisa then said that, when she is upset, the best way for her to feel better was to help others, and that, in facing obstacles, thought and action are better than emotion. Lisa was able to discuss some of the negative aspects of her personality style as well. She acknowledged that she tried to avoid confrontation "at all costs." Similarly to Matt, Lisa said that she feared that, if she confronted others, they would get angry and leave her.

When the assessment team asked Lisa if she viewed Matt as having this same coping style, she readily recognized that he did not, at which point the assessment team validated this, but also emphasized that it often seemed that Matt tried to be this way. Lisa was then able to acknowledge that he may have learned this coping style from her. At this point, the assessment team began to "trickle in" the sadness and worry evidenced in Matt's testing responses. Lisa was able to appreciate that Matt's outside presentation might be different from his internal experiences. The assessment team then addressed Lisa's worst fear, assuring her that nowhere in Matt's testing was there any indication of suicidal ideation. Upon hearing this, Lisa was visibly relieved and said, "If he's sad, we can fix it." She then wanted to know what, specifically, was triggering Matt's negative emotional experiences. While the assessment team acknowledged that there was no way of knowing definitively, these feelings appeared to be long-standing and may have been related to issues like Matt's feelings of loss related to his relationship with his biological father, as well as to his chronic struggle with diabetes.

Lisa then began to talk about how Matt often said that he did not have friends, or had a hard time making friends. In response, Lisa reported that she told him that he did have friends and that he did make friends well. Similarly, Lisa brought up how Matt had only recently shared with her that he had been struggling with some long-standing sleep disturbance. In response, Lisa relayed that she promptly tried to "fix it" by bringing several sleep CDs home the following day. When the assessment team inquired about Matt's response to Lisa's problem-solving and "wondered aloud" if this was always what he needed, Lisa was able to recognize that Matt might not always want her to immediately try to fix things, but may just want her to empathize or to try to understand how he is feeling. The assessment team ended on a positive note, praising Lisa for her insights and telling her of Matt's many strengths, as well as what a pleasure it had been to work with him. Nonetheless, it became clear in this session that it would be important to integrate Lisa's tendency to gloss over Matt's emotionality by entering "problem-solving mode" into the family intervention session: Matt needed to have the corrective emotional experience of having his mother "sitting with him" in his sad and worried feelings in order to learn that such emotionality was acceptable and not shameful. Also, unless he could get this kind of support from his mother and others, he was destined to find other ways (e.g., drugs) to manage his negative emotions.

Family Intervention Session

Just as is the case in adolescent intervention sessions, the overarching goal of family intervention sessions is for the assessor to create an *in vivo* experience that allows the clients to grasp a systemic formulation of the youth's presenting problems (Tharinger et al., 2008). In family intervention sessions, the assessor has the opportunity to meet with the adolescent and family together, and, in so doing, can gain rich information about these interpersonal relationships. The family context is vastly influential to teenagers' development; as such, the assessor may gain some insight into the ways in which family dynamics contribute to adolescents' struggles, as well as any distortions adolescent clients may have about other family members. Working within the family context, the assessor is able to form and test systemic hypotheses. Simultaneously, the assessor encourages parents to develop more systemic views of their child's challenges, and experiment with potential solutions. Just as in adolescent intervention sessions, in family intervention sessions, the assessor seeks to give the family a positive, healing, and successful experience of managing family challenges. The development of a systemic perspective on adolescents' problems helps both teenagers and parents feel less blamed and more hopeful about managing problems conjointly, thus fostering more positive family relationships.

COMMON TECHNIQUES USED IN FAMILY INTERVENTION SESSIONS

There is a wide array of possible activities to consider when designing family intervention sessions (see Tharinger et al., 2008). We have found the Consensus TAT or the Consensus Rorschach to be especially useful in family sessions with adolescents. Family members are asked to work together to develop a story or a response to each stimulus card about which they all agree. They are to talk through the development of these responses aloud. These techniques, then, involve using projective assessment materials in a non-standardized way to help the family observe their own processes and interactions when completing a novel task (rather than obtaining responses that can be scored).

QUESTIONS TO CONSIDER IN PLANNING THE FAMILY INTERVENTION SESSION

Planning family intervention sessions can be quite complex. We have developed questions that are useful in the planning process. First, *Whom should I invite to attend?* Generally, it is desirable for all family members who reside in the adolescents' household to participate in this session. It may also be useful for family members who play a significant role in adolescents' lives, but do not live with the teenager, to participate as well. Sometimes, when parents are separated or divorced, it is necessary to have separate intervention sessions for each parent, including the adolescent in each. Also, if one wishes to target particular aspects of the family's functioning, one may restrict the session to only certain family members. Second, *What do I most want the parents to learn?* Ideally, in family intervention sessions, parents become aware of how they contribute to their child's problems through experiencing the way in which *their own behavior change* (in the area that is problematic for the teenager) ameliorates their child's challenges. Third, *What do I most want the adolescent to learn?* It is hoped that through participating in the family intervention session, teenagers will come to recognize that their parents are willing and able to help them with their difficulties, and that they do not have to "go it alone" in managing their problems in living. Also, teenagers may come to see how their own behavior elicits certain responses in their parents, and consider the possibility of acting differently. Fourth,

What are the most important assessment questions? Often the answer to this question readily comes to light throughout the course of the assessment. It may be that the most central assessment questions are those related to the issues that are creating the most distress in the adolescents' lives, those that are most systemically rooted, or those that are most amenable to change.

Another important question is, *How does the system work to create and maintain the adolescent/family problems?* Again, the answer to this question may become clear during the course of the assessment. If not, it is likely to become apparent as the family intervention session unfolds. It is often the case that a youth's problem behavior is symptomatic of a larger, systemic issue. For example, the adolescent's difficulties may be masking marital conflict, or the adolescent's depression might be distracting from a parent's own mental health challenges. Therefore, the moment the parents begin to fight, or a father's depressive symptoms begin to be unearthed, the adolescent's motivation to maintain his or her problematic behavior is powerfully renewed. The assessor must be very sensitive to these possibilities throughout the course of the assessment, as well as in planning for, and facilitating, the family intervention session. Another important question is, *What are more adaptive solutions?* It is hoped that through participating in the assessment and experiencing the family intervention session, adolescents learn that they are not responsible for shielding their parents from their own, "adult" problems in living; that, in fact, parents are capable of managing their own challenges *and* helping their children with theirs. Assessors further seek to ensure that families have a different, and more positive, experience in the family intervention session than they typically enact at home, allowing them to recognize that they can create this more adaptive solution conjointly.

It is also important to consider, *How much intensity can the family handle?* Family intervention sessions can be very intense (see Tharinger et al., 2008). Family patterns are often quite resistant to change; therefore, the experience of altering ingrained systemic patterns can be quite powerful. When adolescents' challenges are symptomatic of a larger, systemic issue, illuminating the "real" problem (such as the parents' marital conflict or a father's depression) can be highly threatening because the family is being stripped of the coping mechanism they were using to manage those difficulties, which are now exposed and vulnerable.

As such, assessors must carefully monitor the way family intervention sessions unfold, assessing each family member's response to it and tolerance for the experience. In the event that one or more family member appears "flooded," the assessor may pull back from the plan for the session and/or enlist an appropriate family member to support the distressed loved one. Seeing this interaction, then, can provide the assessor, and the family, with additional information from which to derive understanding and meaning. Most importantly, the assessor must provide the family with an alternate and more adaptive way in which to manage their problems.

It is always a good idea when planning this session to ask, *What could go wrong?* Just as in adolescent intervention sessions, family intervention sessions sometimes do not go as planned. For example, one or more family members may become overwhelmed; parents may demonstrate an unwillingness to alter their behavior in any way in order to better support their child; and the adolescent could be resistant to accepting a parent's new behavior, thus discouraging the parent from pursuing the more adaptive solution. Alternatively, family members may create an experience that is different from the one the assessor was planning, but one that is beneficial nonetheless. Such challenges and detours often cannot be anticipated fully. So the assessor must be adaptable, spontaneous, creative, and attuned to the family's experience and needs as the session unfolds.

Summary/Discussion Session with Adolescent

TAs with adolescents culminate in summary/discussion sessions; the assessor first has a session with the adolescent alone, and subsequently a session with the adolescent's parents, preferably that same day or a day or two after. Sometimes adolescents are invited to this latter meeting, and sometimes, even if invited, the adolescent declines to

---

Case material. In the family intervention session with Matt and Lisa, the assessment team presented this mother and son with two thematic apperception test cards and one adolescent apperception test card, in turn. The pair was instructed to conjointly develop a story to each card, which they subsequently shared with the assessors. The assessment team introduced this consensus story telling task as being directly related to Lisa's assessment question concerning whether or not she was communicating with her son in the "right way." In planning for the session, it was hypothesized that Matt would contribute sad content to the stories, and that Lisa would cheerily transform these themes into happy endings.

Prior to the start of the session, while checking in one-on-one with the parent assessment team member, Lisa indicated that she had thought a great deal about the feedback provided to her in the previous sessions, and shared her fear that her positive, optimistic coping style was making it difficult for her son to share any sad feelings he was experiencing with her. She relayed that, because Matt continually saw her engaging in active and positively framed problem solving, he might feel that he, too, had to be this way. She wondered if this personality difference was precipitating some of their communication problems. Matt similarly shared with the adolescent assessment team member while meeting one-on-one that, when he was feeling down, another's extreme happiness and positivity made him feel not understood, and ultimately worse, while having someone "sit with him" in his negative emotion led to his feeling more understood and, ultimately, better.

While executing the intervention task, Matt and his mother generally worked well together; they were receptive to one another's ideas, and Lisa asked for Matt's opinion frequently as they developed their conjoint stories. As was anticipated, however, Lisa did attempt to positively reframe any negativity Matt brought into their stories. When she was able to preserve themes of negative emotionality, she consistently attributed these bad feelings to a neutral source ("They're just mad because it's raining"), or gave the option of a neutral feeling rather than a negative emotion ("Do you think he's lonely, or just hungry?"). In response to the most emotionally evocative card in the intervention activity (which came third), Lisa took the lead in telling a very humorous story that kept her and Matt laughing. Interestingly, Lisa was aware of the fact that Matt had created a very sad story in response to this same card in his individual intervention session. Both she and Matt commented on the fact that her story was much less emotional than his had been. The assessment team then asked what kind of story Matt and Lisa thought most people told in response to this particular card. Matt acknowledged that most people probably told a sad story. The assessment team then asked Matt and Lisa to tell a story that was more similar to what they thought most people would tell. Again, Lisa appeared to shy away from negative emotionality through making jokes or attributing any negativity to neutral sources like having to "work in the fields." The assessment team then made the observation that it seemed much easier for Matt and Lisa to talk about the details of chores, for example, than a story character's feelings of loneliness. The assessment team went on to ask Matt and Lisa if the dynamics of this interaction related to their lives at all (with respect to it being more difficult for them to discuss negative emotions).

Ultimately, Matt was able to state that he thought "normal" people are supposed to be happy all the time, and that this was the way his mom acted. In response, the assessment team validated that Matt felt like an outsider when he had feelings that were not happy, and that it was really hard work for him to keep all of his negative emotions "bottled up." Lisa was then able to share with Matt that she did, in fact, get sad. She powerfully stated that, often, when she took a bubble bath in the evenings, it was because she had had a difficult day and she needed to cry. Matt said that he was surprised to hear this, but promptly shared with his mom that his equivalent is going to his room, turning off the lights, and listening to music. Lisa then explained that, while she wanted to protect Matt from her negative emotional experiences, she wanted him to feel free to share any negative feelings he had with her.

However, even after these powerful exchanges, there continued to be occasions throughout the remainder of the session wherein Lisa would try to put a positive spin on Matt's emotions and/or where she would enter "problem-solving mode," glossing over Matt's negative feelings. These occasions presented opportunities for the assessment team to model acknowledging and validating Matt's feelings, and to explain to Lisa that, while her inclination to comfort or problem solve for her son was very natural, it was not what he needed in order to feel heard and understood. In an effort to emphasize this point, the assessment team then asked Matt if he preferred it when his mom entered "problem-solving mode," or when she just listened and tried to understand his feelings. He said that, while it was "okay" when his mom tried to help him solve his problems, it felt better when she just listened and tried to understand how he was feeling. The resolution of the session was for Matt and Lisa to work together to "catch" Lisa when she entered problem-solving mode, and for Matt to tell her when he just needed her to listen. This family intervention session was central to creating a breakthrough experience for this mother and son. While they were both beginning to recognize their personality differences and how these dissimilarities affected their relationship, openly discussing and experiencing these differences in a concrete way opened the door to positive change for this family system.

participate. It usually is fairly clear from the topics to be discussed with the parents whether it is appropriate for the adolescent to attend the parental feedback. The goals of the adolescent summary/discussion session are:

(1) to answer adolescents' assessment questions and increase their self-knowledge;

(2) to present a more accurate/compassionate story through which to understand the adolescents' problems in living—for example, that they are depressed rather than being "lazy and unmotivated";

(3) to provide adolescents with the experience of being understood in an emotionally supportive environment;

(4) to promote systemic and contextual thinking rather than focusing on the adolescents in isolation; and

(5) to promote abstract thinking, which is developmentally appropriate, given adolescents' burgeoning cognitive capacities.

Lastly, it is important to note that adolescents are typically given individual feedback prior to their parents in an effort to promote individuation, which is also developmentally appropriate.

Ideally, by the time the assessor reaches this stage of a TA, all of the most poignant assessment findings have already been discussed with, or experienced by, the client. Nonetheless, this may not always be the case; it is also quite possible that even when the assessor has "trickled" certain findings into clients' sessions, they have been resisted in some way. Finally, even when each finding has been discussed in isolation, it is often a different experience for the client when the assessor "puts the pieces together" to form a whole picture, so summary/discussion sessions must be carefully planned.

First, the adolescent's questions must be considered. Reviewing teenagers' assessment questions often sheds light on what they are ready to hear. However, this consideration must also be attended to with all of the major assessment findings. Furthermore, it is important to note that what adolescents are open to hearing does not always map onto what their parents are prepared to hear. Therefore, the information that is shared with teenagers must, at times, be tailored according to what their parents are judged to be capable of taking in. In considering this, it is helpful to bear in mind how differentiated the adolescent seems to be from his or her parents. Regardless, it is important that assessors not put adolescents in the position of harboring "secret information" from their parents.

Similarly, the assessor must carefully consider what the adolescent's worst fears are and how much information the teenager can handle without becoming overwhelmed, as well as how the adolescent tends to behave when he or she is overwhelmed. In preparing for this session, the assessor also needs to carefully consider what language is accessible to the adolescent and how the various assessment findings can be presented in a way that is meaningful for the teenager. Finally, it is imperative that the assessor be mindful of incorporating knowledge of the adolescent's strengths into the feedback in addition to data related to their areas of difficulty. In so doing, however, the assessor must prepare for the fact that such strengths-based information must be sensitively delivered if it conflicts with the teenager's self-perception. For example, an adolescent who views herself as being "stupid" may be rejecting of feedback from the assessor that her cognitive abilities are higher than those of 87 percent of her peers; such information is likely to be Level 3 information and must be prepared accordingly.

CONDUCTING THE SUMMARY/DISCUSSION SESSION WITH THE ADOLESCENT

In beginning summary/discussion sessions with adolescents, it is often useful to review the purpose of the session. The assessor may then want to check in with teenagers about anything they feel anxious or worried about in beginning the session, or if there is any particular information they would prefer to review first. The assessor can then choose to begin with a discussion of assessment results as they relate to teenagers' assessment questions, or to summarize the assessment information first, followed by a review of "answers" to adolescents' assessment questions. The former format is typically preferable when the assessment information maps well onto the assessment questions; the latter approach may be better when the teenagers' questions differ significantly from the findings of the assessment. Regardless of the order in which the assessor presents the assessment results, it is crucial that teenagers' are continually asked for confirmation, examples, and any disagreements they have as findings are reviewed. Additionally, throughout the session, the assessor needs to stay carefully attuned to the teen's reactions to the assessment information. If the adolescent appears overwhelmed at any time, the assessor needs to "back off" and provide emotional support. Once all of the feedback is reviewed, it is nice for the assessor to end with something he or she appreciates about, or has learned from the adolescent.

Case material. Matt was highly receptive to all of the assessment information. Following his experience in his individual intervention session, as well as in the family intervention session with his mother, all of the assessment findings going into the summary/discussion session were conceptualized as being Level 1 or Level 2 information. Given that his questions were congruent with the assessment results in many ways, the assessor began Matt's feedback session with a discussion of his assessment questions. In fact, while reviewing Matt's assessment questions, the assessor was able to cover nearly all of the assessment findings, and was also able to integrate a discussion of what would be shared with Lisa given her assessment questions (which also fit very well with the findings and with Matt's questions for the assessment). Matt was consistently able to expand on the assessor's presentation of the assessment results by discussing how they related to his experience in the assessment, as well as to his broader life experiences.

Prior to ending the session, it is also quite useful to review with teenagers what will be said to their parents at their upcoming summary/discussion session, and address if the adolescent will be invited to attend. Once this has been decided, the assessor should specify if there will be future contacts, such as a follow-up session in several months.

Summary/Discussion Session with Parents

This is the final session of the TA process, with the exception of a follow-up that may be scheduled several months later. This meeting follows shortly after the summary/discussion session with the adolescent only. As mentioned earlier, often parents attend without the adolescent, but in some cases the decision is made to include the teenager. Although this is the culminating session of the TA (and in traditional assessment would be where parents are first informed about the findings), paradoxically, if all has gone well in earlier sessions, much of the information in the parents' summary/discussion sessions has already been shared. This meeting, then, can be viewed as "icing on the cake," tying together all of the pieces of the assessment experience, and looking forward to next steps. This is not to underestimate the potential impact of these sessions, however. For, even if all the pieces have been shared previously, it often is very powerful for parents to hear them put together into a coherent story.

The major goal of this session is to answer the questions the parents have posed for the assessment. Adhering to the collaborative underpinnings of the TA method, the assessor seeks parents' continued input throughout the session and strives to provide them with continued emotional support and an experience of being understood. This alliance, which has been developed throughout the course of the assessment, provides the framework that allows parents to continue to absorb the findings from the assessment, and to consider their role in resolving their adolescent's challenges. Just as is the case with adolescents, it is imperative that the assessor conceptualize and organize feedback to the parents according to the "Level" system described previously.

As the assessor addresses the parents' questions in this thoughtful manner, he or she is offering a more accurate and compassionate story about the teen that serves to reframe the parents' thinking and adjust their earlier misunderstandings or distortions without overwhelming or "flooding" them. In most cases, the new story is systemically framed, serving to help the parents view their adolescent within the context of the family, its history, and how that has

impacted their son's or daughter's development. An implicit aim is to encourage systemic rather than individual change (i.e., it is the family's obligation to work together to develop and enact solutions rather than it being the adolescent's job to change in isolation). Lastly, this session is geared towards promoting differentiation within the family, supporting the growing autonomy of the adolescent, and empowering him or her within the connectivity of the family unit; this is, in many ways, the heart of the adolescent TA model.

We have found that in-depth planning is essential for an effective summary/discussion session with parents. While reviewing the parents' questions in light of the assessment findings, the assessor is well served by considering what the parents seem ready to hear, what their worst fears are, and how much information they can handle at this time. These considerations about parents' readiness for various findings very much shape the plan for this session. The success of the mid to late parent-only session, where initial, tentative feedback was provided (in some cases from both from the adolescent's and the parents' test findings) is probably a useful gauge in anticipating the pace and depth of the summary/discussion session. It is also useful to review how the parents have responded in the past when they become psychologically overwhelmed, and to build this knowledge into planning for this session. Assessors also need to review what was told to the adolescent in his or her feedback session, how enmeshed or triangulated the parents are with their child, and whether it would be beneficial for the teenager to attend this session. As discussed below, adjustments are made to the session if the adolescent participates.

CONDUCTING THE SUMMARY/DISCUSSION SESSION WITH THE PARENTS

We recommend that the assessor begin the session by acknowledging that feedback meetings can be anxiety-producing, and checking in with the parents about their emotional state prior to starting the session. It is then a good idea to review the plan for the session, including explaining what will happen, and encouraging questions and collaboration. Before beginning the discussion of findings, we suggest that the assessor thank the parents for participating in the assessment, and in particular acknowledge any factors that may have been especially difficult for the parents. It can be very helpful at this point to show some empathy for the parents' struggles with or confusion about their child, perhaps by acknowledging that the assessor also struggled in putting all the pieces together, as their child is complex, and a thorough assessment was needed for understanding to be reached. The assessor then moves into answering the parents' assessment questions. In some cases (as is the case with giving adolescents feedback), it may be useful to provide an overview of the findings before moving into addressing the parents' questions. Regardless, because the assessor cannot accurately predict all of the parents' reactions to the feedback, parents' responses must be carefully monitored as the session unfolds. If parents appear to be experiencing overwhelming emotions, the assessor must modify the plan for the session and stop to provide emotional support whenever necessary.

In the event that parents disagree with the assessor about any assessment findings, it is imperative that the he or she avoid arguing with parents, and instead encourage them to share their own perspective. If necessary, the assessor can "agree to disagree" with the parents. Although recommendations may have been offered throughout the session, all recommendations are summarized at the end of the session. The parents are encouraged to discuss how feasible the recommendations may be, and whether they have any questions or concerns about how to implement them. The assessor then thanks the parents again, and shares genuine sentiments about what he or she appreciated about being involved with the family. Finally, just as was done with the adolescent, the assessor clarifies if there will be future contacts, such as a follow-up session within a few months.

There are some variations to this summary/discussion session if the adolescent does or does not attend, and advantages to each. If the adolescent does *not* attend, one additional step early in the session is to summarize the feedback session with the adolescent, being careful to respect the confidentiality afforded the adolescent. The assessor may ask the parents if their child shared anything with them from the earlier summary/discussion session, and what they took away from that discussion. In addition, if the adolescent does not attend, it is important that the assessor discuss with the parents what to say to their adolescent after their summary/discussion session. It is often beneficial for the parents to talk more fully and openly with their child about integrating and making meaning out of the assessment findings; if this is the case, the assessor should encourage and scaffold such a discussion. If it appears that the parents are uncomfortable with the idea of independently broaching this topic, the assessor can offer a family session to help with the integration of the assessment findings and recommendations.

If the adolescent *does* attend the session, it is often useful to empower the teenager to summarize his or her understanding of the test findings; if they so choose, they may also share information that relates to their private assessment questions at this time. Subsequently, as the assessor reviews the findings in relation to the parents' questions, probably in more depth, everyone in attendance has the opportunity to work collaboratively with their own understandings of the assessment findings, and to express their respective views of how to proceed. Thus, when the adolescent is in attendance at this final session, it becomes an amalgamation of feedback and family therapy, wherein healthy family interactions are facilitated. With some families, this model will prove to be very effective; in others, it is overly ambitious, asking the family to take too many steps at once. Thus it is important to carefully weigh the potential costs and benefits of including the adolescent. It is also useful to note that the adolescent himself or herself may have insight into

Case material. Matt was invited to, and did attend, Lisa's summary/discussion session. This decision seemed appropriate, given that much of Lisa's feedback overlapped significantly with Matt's, and that a goal was to enhance their communication with each other. We noted that Matt seemed quieter and less active in this session than he had been in his individual session. Lisa seemed very well prepared to hear and take in all of the findings, as they had been shared with her in her second parent-only session and reviewed both verbally and experientially in the family intervention session. Thus, the session went very smoothly. Lisa readily related the assessment findings to their lives, and demonstrated great openness to reflecting on how her personality and coping style had contributed to Matt's challenges; she exhibited notable readiness for change.

the appropriateness of attending (the teen may adamantly refuse to join the session, or, alternatively, may push to be present); the adolescent's wishes should carefully be considered.

Written Feedback for Adolescents and Parents

It is customary in TA with adolescents to compose a letter for the teenager that closely follows the presentation of their summary/discussion session, usually organized around his or her assessment questions. The letter is written in the first person with colloquial language and active voice, and incorporates comments, examples, or even disagreements that the adolescent offered during the summary/discussion session. The written feedback to

parents typically follows a similar framework; that is, a letter is written rather than a traditionally organized psychological report (Finn, 2007). However, a formal report may also be provided if it is needed for other purposes, such as documenting a diagnosis or a disability for school accommodations. As the format of the letters is typically very similar to the organization of oral feedback, the preparation time put into the oral feedback pays off greatly when it comes to producing the letter. The letters are typically mailed, and the adolescent receives a copy of both his or her letter and the parent letter, while the parents receive only their letter. As is often the case with teenagers' private feedback, in our experience, many adolescents also end up sharing their letter with their parents.

Case material. Here is an excerpt from our letter to Matt:

"'Why did I take Adderall the second time without weighing the pros and the cons?' First of all, it's normal in adolescence to experiment with lots of different kinds of new things, and sometimes drugs are a part of that experimentation. But, with you, it seems like the way you have used drugs has been a little bit different—the testing we did together showed that you're feeling quite a bit of stress right now that's overwhelming your coping resources (this makes a lot of sense given everything you're dealing with—school feels harder this year, your diabetes, your dad, not being at the same school as your closest friends … each one of those things is a lot, Matt—let alone all of them together).

"I know we talked a lot about how your mind goes blank sometimes—this 'blankness' is sometimes called 'dissociation' and may be related to being overwhelmed by feelings. This seems to happen to you more than it does to other people your age. When people feel overwhelmed like this, they sometimes don't have as much self-control, or are more impulsive in their decisions and behaviors (they don't carefully weigh pros and cons). It seems like trying different kinds of drugs is kind of an escape for you—it's a way to let go of all the hard feelings you're trying to keep bottled-up inside. This fits with an item you marked on [the MMPI-A] when you responded 'false' to 'talking over problems and worries with someone is often more helpful than taking drugs or medicines.' It seems like escaping your bad feelings might be more important than facing the consequences for experimenting with drugs. It might be that the more you are able to talk about and express the negative feelings you're bottling up, the less overwhelmed you'll feel and the less you'll need to escape them with drugs like Adderall."

And here is an excerpt from Lisa's letter:

"'Am I communicating to him in the right way?' We could really see how important open communication has been for you and that you have always felt close to Matt. A part of adolescence is trying to find some independence and autonomy. As a result, teenagers often distance themselves more from their parents and start to become closer to their peers. We think that some of this shift in communication is a natural part of growing up. However, there may also be some other reasons why your communication has slowed down.

"It is really evident how much you care about Matt, are concerned about him, and want him to be happy. One of the ways in which parents tend to show this to their kids is to try to reassure them that 'everything will be ok.' Just like we talked about, this is a completely natural reaction to when children seem worried or upset, and it is important to show them that they are safe. However, sometimes teenagers need to know that adults understand how they are feeling. We think that some of Matt's behaviors, like the drug use, may be his way of trying to let people know what is going on with him.

It's really important for teenagers that other people see how they are feeling, acknowledge it, and let them know that it isn't wrong to feel that way.

"Like we discussed in the family session, sometimes adolescents need to feel 'mirrored' and understood in their emotions. This helps them know that people understand them and see when they are in distress. It also lets them know that they are not 'bad' for having certain feelings. When adults communicate to teenagers that they see how they are feeling, and accept it, teenagers feel safer, more hopeful, and more protected. Just like you described that everyone sometimes need to cry and express negative emotions, Matt sometimes needs your help in doing this. Sometimes he may just need for you to let him be upset and talk about these emotions instead of having you try to 'fix it' right away. You did a great job doing this during the family session. It was really nice to see you listen to Matt as he admitted that sometimes he feels sad, and to open up to him about the feelings of sadness you experience sometimes. I think it was really important for him to learn that it is normal not to be happy all of the time. As we saw, this really made Matt feel better. Sometimes, all it takes to work through hard feelings is to have someone you love really listen to you.

"We know that this is very different from how you tend to approach problems. Like we discussed, your testing results showed that you are a very resilient, strong, and optimistic person. While you do allow yourself to be emotional at times, you tend to approach problems as things to overcome. However, you noted that Matt doesn't seem to have this same approach. You were really perceptive to notice that there may be aspects of your way of communicating and your coping style that might be preventing Matt from being open with you. As he shared, you being more open and willing to 'sit' with his painful emotions makes him want to communicate more with you."

Follow-up Session

If possible, it is highly recommended that a follow-up session occur one to three months after the TA has been completed with the adolescent and his or her parents. The assessor typically meets with the parents and the adolescent to discuss any progress the teen and family have made, as well as any difficulties they have encountered. Thus, the assessor has the opportunity to explore with the family any factors that may be promoting or hindering their progress, as well as to answer any questions that have arisen for the parents and/or the adolescent since the conclusion of the assessment. In the event that the family is experiencing some ongoing challenges, the assessor can assist the family in problem solving any difficulties that may be interfering with the implementation of recommendations. New events in the family's life, both positive and negative, may also be

Case material. Matt and his mom returned for a follow-up session approximately 10 weeks after the final summary/discussion session, which coincided with the end of Matt's summer vacation. Matt's summer had been divided into spending a few weeks with his grandparents, a few weeks at camp, and a few weeks at home with his mother. Matt indicated feeling that the assessment had facilitated some changes for him and his mom. He said that he was talking about his difficult feelings more with a friend. He also acknowledged that, although his mother still almost always acted happy, it continued to be comforting to him to know that, underneath, she, too, struggled with some hard feelings. Matt also relayed that he better understood his academic and cognitive strengths and weaknesses as a result of the assessment, which was helpful given that he was about to enter high school. He also revealed more about his drug use that occurred prior to the assessment, and proudly described how he had recently resisted the opportunity to use various drugs. Matt also said he was using new coping methods to manage his negative emotionality, including writing and planning a community volunteer project. Lisa shared that she felt as though Matt had seemed more confident and more mature over the summer, and that Matt had commented on feeling more mature as well. Lisa also shared that she had made an effort to approach their interactions differently, and provided an example that supported her assertion.

explored as to their impact on the adolescent and the family. In our experience, it is often most useful to divide the session into three parts: individual check-ins with the parents and adolescent, followed by a joint meeting with everyone.

Evaluating the Effectiveness of TA in Clinical Practice and Research

We recommend that assessors using TA in their practices systematically and efficiently collect information to help gauge the effectiveness of TA as an assessment process and as an intervention. The process can be as simple as asking the parents and adolescent to complete a short, open-ended satisfaction measure at the conclusion of the assessment, accompanied by some standard items that can be rated on a numerical scale. For example, clients can be asked to describe how the process was for them and then rate how well their assessment questions were addressed. This information can aid the clinician in becoming more effective at TA, and can help the clients know that their input—their collaboration in the process—is honored through to the end.

In addition, TAP is in the process of developing measures that can be utilized to assess the process of and satisfaction with psychological assessment. At this point, the Parents' Experience of Assessment Survey (PEAS; Finn, Tharinger, & Austin, 2008) has been developed, and is undergoing further study to address its length and psychometric properties. The PEAS has six subscales: Collaboration, Learning, Feelings about the Assessment, Assessor–Child Relationship, Assessor–Parent Relationship, and Family Involvement, and is filled out by parents at the end of their children's psychological assessments.

Case material. We were very pleased to see the research findings on this case. At pre-testing on the BASC-2, Matt had rated various clinical scales in the clinical range (Anxiety, Depression, Sense of Inadequacy, Internalizing Problems, and Emotional Symptoms Index). None of these scales was in the clinical range at post-testing, and the decrease across the previously elevated scales averaged a full standard deviation (e.g., Depression, 75 to 59; Anxiety, 73 to 62; Sense of Inadequacy, 79 to 69). Matt also evidenced much improvement on the adaptive scales of the BASC-2. His score on the Self-Esteem scale improved over one standard deviation (21 to 37); similarly, his score on the Interpersonal Relations scale increased almost one standard deviation (43 to 51). His overall Personal Adjustment score went from 34 to 43. On another measure developed for TAP, Matt reported a large decrease in his negative affect related to his future. Matt also indicated that his assessment questions had been addressed well.

Lisa's data told a bit of a different story, yet they fit well with her process throughout the TA. At pre-testing on the BASC-2, all of her ratings of Matt on both the clinical and adaptive scales were in the "normal" range. At post-testing, she rated Matt in the "at risk" range on the Anxiety scale (from 57 to 65), and noted improvement on Functional Communication scale (from 43 to 50). All other scales were in the normal range at post-testing. On another measure developed for TAP, Lisa also noted a substantial decrease in her negative feelings about Matt's future, as well as an increase in her positive feelings. Lisa reported feeling that her assessment questions had been extremely well addressed. On the PEAS, Lisa averaged a 4.5 out of 5.0 across the six scales, indicating a very high sense of satisfaction with the process and outcome of the TA. More specifically, Lisa indicated a 4.8 on the Collaboration subscale, a 4.9 on the Relationship between Assessor and Parent subscale, a 4.8 on the Relationship between Assessor and Child subscale, a 4.4 on the Learned New Things subscale, a 5.0 on the Feelings subscale, and a 3.8 on the Family Involvement subscale. Finally, on a measure of family functioning, both Matt and Lisa reported an increase in family cohesion.

In summary, both Matt and Lisa indicated high satisfaction with the TA and an enhanced sense of hope for the future. Matt perceived his internalizing symptoms as having decreased significantly, and his self-esteem and relationships with others as having improved greatly over the course of the TA. Lisa demonstrated a change in her "story" about her child that is illustrative of one of the primary goals of TAs conducted with youth and their families. Instead of minimizing or denying her son's distress (as she did before the TA began), at the end she was able to acknowledge his anxiety. She also perceived an enhanced parent–child relationship, which fit our observations. We certainly felt that our goals had been met in helping this family.

Similar instruments for children and for adolescents are also in development.

In TAP, as mentioned earlier, we are researching the processes and outcomes of TA with children and adolescents. We have focused on pre- and post-change in child symptomatology, family functioning, and parental affective attitudes, as well as satisfaction with the assessment experience, using the PEAS. The measures are well described in Tharinger, Finn, Gentry et al. (2009). We also have conducted brief interviews after each session with both the parents and the children. We briefly describe the findings of the case we have been following.

Conclusion

Our intention in this chapter has been to introduce TA and its use with adolescents and their parents to current and future assessment psychologists and, in turn, to encourage psychologists to consider how this model may be useful in their clinical work. We believe we have made three major contributions. The first is the explicit acknowledgement that adolescents (and families with adolescents) are unique clients with distinctive clinical needs. Current assessment models have only begun to address these needs, and primarily through the development of measures and norms specific to adolescents. The TA model we presented and illustrated herein demonstrates the importance of integrating the unique tasks of adolescent development into the structure of assessment itself.

The second contribution is the TA model itself. TA is a unique integration of theoretical frameworks, as well as a combination of assessment *and* intervention methods and techniques. The TA model can be used with a variety of clients across all ages and many concerns, and may be particularly suited to adolescents in that it attends to such fundamental issues such as teenagers' simultaneous need for autonomy and their continued reliance on their parents. As such, we described and illustrated the goals and procedures for each step in the comprehensive TA model as used with adolescents and their parents, and illustrated each step with a case study. It is hoped that this approach provided the reader with concurrently conceptual and clinical lenses through which to view the workings of TA with adolescents and their parents.

The third contribution of the present chapter is that it encourages practitioners to evaluate the process and outcomes of psychological assessment in both clinical practice and research endeavors. Assessment practice has been challenged in the past decade to demonstrate its usefulness. By providing clinical and research data that support its efficacy and effectiveness (thus building an evidence base), the practice of psychological assessment is more likely to be valued, advanced, and sought out by consumers and sites where psychological services are offered.

Future Directions

We close by raising issues about the ongoing development of therapeutic assessment with adolescents and their parents. These include TA's application across cultures, the use of selected steps of TA when the comprehensive model is not feasible, adapting TA in different settings and with different presenting problems, and education and training opportunities to establish competence in TA.

It is imperative to consider cultural differences in the practice and research on TA. In the case we followed in this chapter, Matt and Lisa were Caucasian. Lisa was a single mother who had given birth to Matt when she was a teenager. How did these cultural factors impact their respective experiences of the assessment? How would their experience of the TA been different if, for example, they were Hispanic and had presented as an "intact" family? If they were African American? Asian? Native American? Wealthy? Living in poverty? A single-father–headed household? Factors of cultural variability in TA are yet to be formally explored. Questions such as: "Are there differential effects or experiences of TA based on culture differences?" are essential given the ever-increasing multicultural nature of our clients.

Further, are there particular components of the assessment intervention described herein that are more or less effective in precipitating therapeutic changes in various clients? Thus, future research should include inquiries into: (1) the differential experiences of participants from various cultural groups, and (2) the acceptability and efficacy of individual components of the intervention across cultural groups, particularly cultures with differing norms and values about adolescent development (e.g., differential impact of seeking assessment questions from participants; collaborative approaches to test administration, interpretation, and application to real life experiences of the participant; and implementation of intervention sessions and summary/discussion sessions). TAs are complex and multifaceted and must be retrofitted to the individual client and his or her family and cultural system. Inquiry in this area would increase our understanding not only of how to adapt TA to different cultural groups, but also of the effective components of TA and how those interface with different contexts.

As briefly mentioned earlier, certain practitioners will find that it is not feasible to apply the comprehensive model of TA because of constraints (typically time and money) in their particular settings. Thus, a challenge for future research is to determine the relative effectiveness of components of TA. Tharinger and Finn have written elsewhere (Tharinger, et al., 2007) about the bare bones of TA that are required to deem that TA is being practiced and researched. In addition to adopting the core values described earlier, essential ingredients include:

(1) Embracing a collaborative orientation to assessment, which in itself will enhance the intervention potential of assessment;

(2) Co-constructing and addressing assessment questions from parents and children/adolescents;

(3) Organizing the findings around the assessment questions and tailoring feedback to parents, children/adolescents in ways that are meaningful to them;

(4) Adopting multi-theoretical orientations for integration and interpretation of assessment findings.

Questions remain about the added value of other steps. That is, what is the added benefit of intervention sessions? Follow-up sessions? Adolescent summary/discussion sessions? Data informing these questions could guide the psychologist in deciding which steps are essential and which are add-ons, but do not necessarily result in better outcomes. Anecdotally, the authors have noticed in TAs with *children* and their parents that some of the families appeared to benefit most from observing and subsequently processing the testing of the child; others, from the impact of the family intervention session; and still others, from the summary/discussion session. Thus, although future research should attempt to determine the moderators that might impact the efficacy of each step of TA, practitioners will need to thoroughly plan and flexibly adjust to meet the needs of individual clients—utilizing both clinical experience and research findings.

It is also important that TA with adolescents and their parents be conducted and studied across a wide range of settings, including psychiatric hospitals, pediatric hospitals, residential treatment centers, community mental health clinics, independent practices, and schools. Our research has been conducted at a university-based clinic,

and our practice has been conducted primarily in independent practice settings. We also have implemented components of TA with adolescents in the schools and have several other such projects underway. Others are using TA with children and adolescents in a community-based clinic that primarily serves economically disadvantaged children and their families (Mercer, 2011; Guerrero, Lipkind, & Rosenburg, 2011; Haydel, Mercer, & Rosenblatt, 2011). This work has shown that TA can be applied and is effective in such settings, but assessors must be acutely aware of the cultural context.

It is also our experience that careful determination of when TA will have the most payoff (e.g., in terms of adolescent and parental motivation and follow-through) will be wise, as the comprehensive TA model can be time-consuming and demands extensive competence from the psychologist. We recommend using TA with complex cases in which the adolescent and parents are stuck, and in their "stuckness," may be doing psychological harm to themselves or each other, or at least obstructing progress. Also TA may be particularly applicable to adolescents and families where previous treatment efforts have repeatedly failed. These points underscore one more constraint on the practice and research on TA at this time—the competence of the practicing psychologist or supervised students in training. As we mentioned in the introduction, it is our experience that psychologists with expertise in assessment and several schools of psychotherapy can add TA to their repertories by obtaining additional education, training, and supervised experience. Such opportunities are available and growing (cf. www.therapeuticassessment.com for a list of training workshops), and Finn and colleagues are currently exploring setting up a certification program in therapeutic assessment. In addition, it is important for faculty in professional psychology graduate programs to introduce and teach the basics of TA to their students to encourage their consideration of additional training. It is our experience that graduate students are extremely excited about learning and practicing TA, and some see it as the pinnacle integrative experience of their graduate training.

References

Ackerman, S. J., Hilsenroth, M. J., Baity, M. R., & Blagys, M. D. (2000). Interaction of therapeutic process and alliance during psychological assessment. *Journal of Personality Assessment, 75*, 82–109.

Allen, J. G., Fonagy, P., & Bateman, A. W. (2008). *Mentalizing in clinical practice*. Washington, DC: American Psychiatric Publishing.

Atwood, G. E., & Stolorow, R. D. (1984). *Structures of subjectivity: Explorations in psychoanalytic phenomenology*. Hillsdale, NJ: Analytic Press.

Collins, D. R., & Stukas, A. A. (2006). The effects of feedback self-consistency, therapist status, and attitude toward therapy on reaction to personality feedback. *The Journal of Social Psychology, 146*(4), 463–483.

Elkind, D. (1978). Understanding the young adolescent. *Adolescence, 13*(49), 127–134.

Finn, S. E. (1996a). *Using the MMPI-2 as a therapeutic intervention*. Minneapolis: University of Minnesota Press.

Finn, S. E. (1996b). Assessment feedback integrating MMPI-2 and Rorschach findings. *Journal of Personality Assessment, 67*, 543–557.

Finn, S. E. (2003). Therapeutic assessment of a man with "ADD." *Journal of Personality Assessment, 80*, 115–129.

Finn, S. E. (2007). *In our clients' shoes: Theory and techniques of therapeutic assessment*. Mahwah, NJ: Lawrence Erlbaum Associates.

Finn, S. E., & Kamphuis, J. H. (2006). Therapeutic assessment with the MMPI-2. In J. N. Butcher (Ed.), *MMPI-2: A practitioner's guide* (pp. 165–191). Washington, DC: APA Books.

Finn, S. E., & Martin, H. (1997). Therapeutic assessment with the MMPI-2 in managed health care. In J. N. Butcher (Ed.), *Personality assessment in managed health* (pp. 131–152). New York: Oxford University Press.

Finn, S. E., Tharinger, D. J., & Austin, C. (2008). Parent Experience of Assessment Survey (PEAS). Unpublished test (available from S. E. Finn).

Finn, S. E., & Tonsager, M. E. (1992). Therapeutic effects of providing MMPI-2 test feedback to college students awaiting therapy. *Psychological Assessment, 4*(3), 278–287.

Finn, S. E., & Tonsager, M. E. (1997). Information-gathering and therapeutic models of assessment: Complementary paradigms. *Psychological Assessment, 9*(4), 374–385.

Finn, S. E., & Tonsager, M. E. (2002). How therapeutic assessment became humanistic. *The Humanistic Psychologist, 30*(1–2), 10–22.

Fischer, C. T. (1972). Paradigm changes which allow sharing of results. *Professional Psychology*, Fall, 364–369.

Fischer, C. T. (1978). Collaborative psychological assessment. In C. T. Fischer & S. L. Brodsky (Eds.), *Client participation in human services* (pp. 41–61). New Brunswick, NJ: Transaction Books.

Fischer, C. T. (1979). Individualized assessment and phenomenological psychology. *Journal of Personality Assessment, 43*(2), 115–122.

Fischer, C. T. (1985). *Individualizing psychological assessment*. Monterey, CA: Brooks/Cole Publishing Company.

Fischer, C. T. (2000). Collaborative, individualized assessment. *Journal of Personality Assessment, 74*(1), 2–14.

Fischer, C. T., & Finn, S. E. (2008). Developing the life meaning of psychological test data: Collaborative and therapeutic approaches. In R. P. Archer & S. R. Smith (Eds.), *Personality assessment* (pp. 379–404). New York: Routledge.

Fishman, H. C. (1988). *Treating troubled adolescents: A family therapy approach*. New York: Basic Books, Publishers.

Fitzpatrick, M. R., & Irannejad, S. (2008). Adolescent readiness for change and the working alliance in counseling. *Journal of Counseling & Development, 86*(4), 438–445.

Gibbons, J. L. (2000). Personal and social development of adolescents: Integrating findings from preindustrial and modern industrialized societies. In A. L. Comunian & U. P. Gielen (Eds.), *International perspectives on human development* (pp. 403–429). Lengerich, Germany: Pabst Science Publishers.

Giesler, R. B., Josephs, R. A., & Swann, W. B. (1996). Self-verification in clinical depression: The desire for negative evaluation. *Journal of Abnormal Psychology, 105*(3), 358–368.

Gorske, T. T. (2008). Therapeutic neuropsychological assessment: A humanistic model and case example. *Journal of Humanistic Psychology, 48*, 320–339.

Guerrero, B., Lipkind, J., & Rosenberg, A. (2011). Why did she put nail polish in my drink? Applying the therapeutic assessment model with an African-American foster child in a community mental health setting. *Journal of Personality Assessment, 93*, 7–15.

Hamilton, A. M., Fowler, J. L., Hersh, B., Hall, C., Finn, S. E., Tharinger, D. J., et al. (2009). "Why won't my parents help me?" Therapeutic assessment of a child and her family. *Journal of Personality Assessment. 91*, 108–120.

Handler, L. (1995). The clinical use of figure drawings. In C. Newmark (Ed.), *Major psychological assessment instruments* (pp. 206–293). Boston, MA: Allyn & Bacon.

Handler, L. (2006). Therapeutic assessment with children and adolescents. In S. Smith & L. Handler (Eds.), *Clinical assessment of children and adolescents: A practitioner's guide* (pp. 53–72). Mahwah, NJ: Lawrence Erlbaum & Associates.

Handler, L., & Meyer, G. J. (1998). The importance of teaching and learning personality assessment. In L. Handler & M. J. Hilsenroth (Eds.), *Teaching and learning personality assessment* (pp. 3–30). Mahwah, NJ: Lawrence Erlbaum Associates, Publishers.

Haydel, M. E., Mercer, B. L., & Rosenblatt, E. (2011). Participant or observer: Training assessors to work with objective data and feelings. *Journal of Personality Assessment, 93*, 16–22.

Hilsenroth, M. J., Peters, E. J., & Ackerman, S. J. (2004). The development of therapeutic alliance during psychological assessment: Patient and therapist perspectives across treatment. *Journal of Personality Assessment, 83*(3), 332–344.

Kamphaus, R. W., & Frick, P. J. (2005). *Clinical assessment of child and adolescent personality and behavior* (2nd ed.). New York: Springer Science.

Kaufman, A. S., & Kaufman, N. L. (Eds.). (2001). *Specific learning disabilities and difficulties in children and adolescents: Psychological assessment and evaluation*. New York: Cambridge University Press.

Keating, D. P. (2004). Cognitive and brain development. In R. M. Lerner & L. Steinberg (Eds.), *Handbook of adolescent psychology* (2nd ed.; 45–84). Hoboken, NJ: John Wiley & Sons.

Keating, V., & Cosgrave, E. (2006). The first ten minutes: Clinicians' perspectives on engaging adolescents in therapy. *Australian Journal of Guidance & Counselling, 16*(2), 141–147.

Kelley, A. E., Schochet, T., & Landry, C. F. (2004). Risk taking and novelty seeking in adolescence: Introduction to Part I. In R. E. Dahl & L. P. Spear (Eds.), *Adolescent brain development: Vulnerabilities and opportunities* (pp. 27–32). New York: New York Academy of Sciences.

Knoff, H. M. (Ed). (1986). *The assessment of child and adolescent personality*. New York: Guilford Press.

Kohut, H. (1977). *The restoration of the self*. New York: International Universities Press.

Lau, J. Y. F., & Eley, T. C. (2008). Attributional style as a risk marker of genetic effects for adolescent depressive symptoms. *Journal of Abnormal Psychology*, *117*(4), 849–859.

Little, J. A., & Smith, S. R. (2008, March). *Collaborative assessment, supportive psychotherapy, or treatment a usual: An analysis of ultra-brief individualized intervention with psychiatric inpatients.* Paper presented at the annual meeting of the Society for Personality Assessment, Chicago, IL.

Mercer, B. L. (2011). Psychological assessment of children in a community mental health clinic. *Journal of Personality Assessment, 93*, 1–6.

Michel, D. M. (2002). Psychological assessment as a therapeutic intervention in patients hospitalized with eating disorders. *Professional Psychology: Research & Practice, 33*(5) 470–477.

Newman, M. L., & Greenway, P. (1997). Therapeutic effects of providing MMPI-2 test feedback to clients at a university counseling service: A collaborative approach. *Psychological Assessment, 9*(2) 122–131.

Oetzel, K. B., & Scherer, D. G. (2003). Therapeutic engagement with adolescents in psychotherapy. *Psychotherapy: Theory, Research, Practice, Training, 40*(3) 215–225.

Ollendick, T. H., & Hersen, M. (1993). *Handbook of child and adolescent assessment.* Needham Heights, MA: Allyn & Bacon.

Ougrin, D., Ng, A. V., & Low, J. (2008). Therapeutic assessment based on cognitive-analytic therapy for young people presenting with self-harm: Pilot study. *Psychiatric Bulletin, 32*, 423–426.

Oster, G. D., Caro, J. E., Eagen, D. R., & Lillo, M. A. (1988). *Assessing adolescents.* Oxford, UK: Pergamon Press.

Peters, E. J., Handler, L., White, K. G., & Winkel, J. D. (2008). "Am I going crazy, doc?" A self psychology approach to therapeutic assessment. *Journal of Personality Assessment, 90*, 421–434.

Piaget, J. (1972). Intellectual evolution from adolescence to adulthood. *Human Development, 15*(1), 1–12.

Purves, C. (2002). Collaborative assessment with involuntary populations: Foster children and their mothers. *The Humanistic Psychologist, 30*, 164–174.

Riddle, B. C., Byers, C. C., & Grimesey, J. L. (2002). Literature review of research and practice in collaborative assessment. *The Humanistic Psychologist, 30*(1–2), 33–48.

Seiffge-Krenke, I. (1999). Families with daughters, families with sons: Different challenges for family relationships and marital satisfaction? *Journal of Youth & Adolescence, 28*(3), 325–342.

Smith, S. R., &Handler, L. (Eds.). (2007). *The clinical assessment of children and adolescents.* Mahwah, NJ: Lawrence Erlbaum Associates.

Smith, J. D., & Handler, L. (2009). "Why do I get in trouble so much?" A family therapeutic assessment case study. *Journal of Personality Assessment, 91*, 197–210.

Steinberg, L., & Silverberg, S. B. (1987). Influences on marital satisfaction during the middle stages of the family life cycle. *Journal of Marriage & the Family, 49*(4), 751–760.

Sullivan, H. S. (1964). *The fusion of psychiatry and social science.* New York: W. W. Norton & Co.

Swann, W. B., & Read, S. J. (1981). Self-verification processes: How we sustain our self-conceptions. *Journal of Experimental Social Psychology, 17*(4), 351–372.

Tharinger, D. J., Finn, S. E., Austin, C., Gentry, L., Bailey, E., Parton, V., et al. (2008). Family sessions as part of child psychological assessment: Goals, techniques, clinical utility, and therapeutic value. *Journal of Personality Assessment, 90*, 547–558.

Tharinger, D. J., Finn, S. E., Gentry, L., Hamilton, A., Fowler, J., Matson, M., et al. (2009). Therapeutic assessment with children: A pilot study of treatment acceptability and outcome. *Journal of Personality Assessment, 91*(3), 238–244.

Tharinger, D. J., Finn, S. E., Hersh, B., Wilkinson, A., Christopher, G., & Tran, A. (2008). Assessment feedback with parents and pre-adolescent children: A collaborative approach. *Professional Psychology: Research & Practice, 39*, 600–609.

Tharinger, D. J., Finn, S. E, Wilkinson, A. D., & Schaber. P. M. (2007). Therapeutic assessment with a child as a family intervention: A clinical and research case study. *Psychology in the Schools, 44*, 293–309.

Tharinger, D. J., Krumholz, L. Austin, C., & Matson, M. (2011). The development and model of therapeutic assessment with children: Application to school-based assessment. In M. A. Bray & T. J. Kehle (Eds.), *Oxford University Press handbook of school psychology* (pp. 224–259). New York: Oxford University Press.

Tharinger, D. J., Matson, M., & Christopher, G. (2011). Play, creative expression, and playfulness in therapeutic assessment with children. In S. W. Russ & L. N. Niec (Eds.), *An evidence-based approach to play in intervention and prevention: integrating developmental and clinical science* (pp. 109–148). New York: Guilford.

Tharinger, D., & Roberts, M. (in press). Human figure drawings in therapeutic assessment with children: Process, product, life context, and systemic impact. In L. Handler (Ed.), *Projective techniques: Research, innovative techniques, and case studies.* Mahwah, NJ: Lawrence Erlbaum & Associates.

Tucker, D. M., & Moller, L. (2007). The metamorphosis: Individuation of the adolescent brain. In D. Romer & E. F. Walker (Eds.), *Adolescent psychopathology and the developing brain: Integrating brain and prevention science* (pp. 85–102). New York: Oxford University Press.

Wygant, D. B., & Fleming, K. P. (2008). Clinical utility of the MMPI-2 Restructured Clinical (RC) scales in a therapeutic assessment: A case study. *Journal of Personality Assessment, 90*, 110–118.

PART 3

The Practice of Psychological Assessment

History Taking, Clinical Interviewing, and the Mental Status Examination in Child Assessment

Mauricio A. Garcia-Barrera *and* William R. Moore

Abstract

Best assessment practices incorporate a multi-step and multi-method approach, as well as sensitivity to the client's cultural background, including their race, language, beliefs, and practices. In this context and emphasizing pediatric assessment, this chapter presents a review of some of the earlier steps in a psychological assessment process, including referral review and intake, review of records, history taking, clinical interviews, and mental status examination. Emphasis is placed on the relevance of the clinical assessment interview to the establishment of rapport and to gather information about the current functioning of the child. Information is significantly richer and more reliable if several sources are included; thus, background questionnaires, review of medical and academic records, interviews with teachers and others involved in the child's life, are recommended. Common methods of clinical interviewing are discussed, including unstructured, semi-structured, and structured formats. Finally, this chapter includes a review of the components of the child Mental Status Examination.

Key Words: clinical interview, history taking, semi-structured interview, structured interview, background questionnaire, mental status examination, rapport

Introduction

The clinical assessment of a child is staged in a multi-step process, in which each component serves as a pillar for the next, and in which both structure and flexibility play important roles. Although there is no fixed model for child assessment practice, knowledge of each one of these steps will certainly help the clinician to organize an assessment plan that would serve as an instrument to better understand the child. It is worth noting that in the context of this chapter, the word "child" is brief for "children and adolescents." When assessing a child, the clinician will most likely be dealing with several sources of information, including the referral source, parents, teachers, other clinicians, and of course, the child. Thus, a strategic, organized, and efficient assessment process facilitates communication between the clinician and the parties involved,

with the ultimate goal of making informed decisions about the child's needs.

Furthermore, a clinical assessment is not just an activity, it is a professional responsibility; subsequently, there are several stages of professional training that must take place before facing an evaluation. Most frequently, a clinician has completed supervised clinical practices or externships and an internship; in some cases, she or he has received post-doctoral training. Most likely, the professional conducting the evaluation has received a graduate degree in psychology and has obtained a professional license to practice. The clinician may be in advanced stages towards completion, in which case her or his assessments are conducted under the close supervision of a licensed psychologist. A professional license in psychology gives full privileges to clinicians to conduct independent evaluations in their area of expertise. Moreover, a pediatric clinical assessment requires an integration of several layers of knowledge, including areas such as normal and abnormal child development (e.g., psychopathology, neurodevelopmental disorders, personality theories), clinical practice (e.g., establishing rapport, ethics, diversity issues) and psychometrics (e.g., test mastery, statistics). In North America, the American Psychological Association (APA) and the Canadian Psychological Association (CPA) regulate the academic curricula of institutions offering a clinical degree in psychology, to assure that the necessary content areas are included in each program of studies.

Finally, a clinical assessment is not a process in isolation; each evaluation includes a series of recommendations that should provide parents, teachers, and other professionals involved with some tools to initiate both short-term and long-term intervention programs for the child. The psychological report, which summarizes the assessment and includes the recommendations, is a very important piece of the process. In several cases, this report initiates a progression of events in the life of the child, such as individual interventions and counseling, special education accommodations, and follow-up assessments including specialized medical examinations and pharmacological interventions; some of them with life-long repercussions. Due to the sensitive implications of psychological assessment, state and provincial psychology boards in North America regulate this activity.

Best assessment practices incorporate a multi-step and multi-method approach (e.g., Baron, 2003; Garcia-Barrera & Kamphaus, 2006; Kamphaus & Reynolds, 2003; Lezak, Howieson, & Loring, 2004; McConaughy, 2005; Sattler, 2008). Emphasizing pediatric assessment within this context, this chapter presents a review of some of the earlier steps in a psychological assessment process, including intake, history taking, initial clinical interviews, and mental status examination. Information in this chapter does not attempt to substitute the broad spectrum of experiences that only practice can provide clinicians with, nor does it cover the vast extent of information that several clinical graduate courses would. This chapter aims to complement those two sources of knowledge, while providing you with specific best practice guidelines to develop your own child assessment protocols. Figure 18.1 presents a flow chart summarizing the assessment steps to be discussed in this chapter.

Intake and Type of Assessment Identification

In most cases, a clinical evaluation process starts with an intake. This intake should be a formal step in the process and it is recommended that it follows the format of an interview. As is the case with any type of interview, the goal the clinician has in mind during the intake interview is to obtain as much information as possible about the referral in order to determine if it is appropriate for his/her area of expertise. In some cases, the appropriateness of the evaluation itself is also considered (Baron, 2003). Furthermore, the intake interview is an opportunity for those involved in the case (e.g., most likely, the guardian and the referral source) to better understand the characteristics of a pediatric psychological evaluation process, the nature of the questionnaires and tests that are usually administered, the potential goals and limits of the evaluation, and the type of assessment that best fits the needs of the child. Moreover, it could be the case that during this intake process the referral source will in turn be consulted with to clarify the referral question, to jointly formulate a strategy, and to obtain more information about the child, upon the guardian's consent. Communication about the case is facilitated by the creation of a common vocabulary with the referral source (Sattler, 2008). During the intake, the clinician clarifies his/her role in the process, along with the role that each player would perform; in other words, how much involvement may be required from parents, teachers, other informants, and the child.

The best case scenario for the intake interview is a personal one-to-one interaction, either in a visit to the clinician's office or in any other appropriate setting; however, in some cases a phone interview can be efficacious. Having the opportunity to meet personally with all parties involved in the process facilitates the early establishment of rapport. Regardless of how it is conducted, the intake interview should help all parties reach the final decision of whether the evaluation is appropriate, whether the evaluation goals and methods meet the clinician's qualifications, and whether the parties are compatible. It could be the case that the information provided during the intake is enough for the clinician to determine that a formal evaluation is not needed, and provided some interventions, the child's behavior may be consequently modified. However, if the evaluation is deemed appropriate, the next step in most cases is to obtain a written and signed consent from all parties involved. The written consent is a contract recording an agreement between the

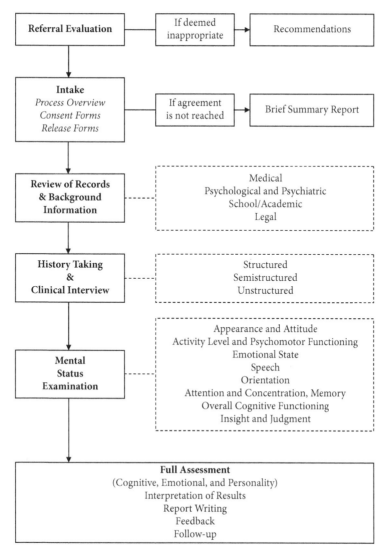

Figure 18.1 Flow chart of the initial steps in a multi-stage and multi-method psychological assessment of a child.

clinician and all parties, as well as documenting the authorization to initiate the process; certainly it is a document the clinician would like to keep. This agreement is crucial, as it establishes the extent of the expectations, goals for the evaluation, names and positions of the parties involved, permission to contact and discuss the case with them (e.g., teachers, other clinicians), and in some cases, future uses of the information collected (e.g., research purposes in academic settings, case presentations, court mandates).

Finally, the clinician may use the intake interview as an opportunity to create a list of records needed to better understand the case, have the guardian sign the appropriate release forms for these records,

and identify the most efficient way to locate them (e.g., school, pediatrician's office). At times, parents may have the belief that an uninformed, fresh start is better for the evaluation process, as they may fear that the records are going to bias the clinician's point of view (Baron, 2003). Rather than an obstacle, this common situation offers an opportunity to address the issue of individualization of the assessment process, and the importance of obtaining as much information as possible about the child's developmental background. After all, an assessment is conducted cross-sectionally rather than longitudinally; thus, the clinician's perception of the child's situation is biased by the most current presentation of the behaviors in question, and a more diverse range of information facilitates a better understanding of the child's behavior. Taking the time to have this discussion will most certainly assist the subsequent steps in the evaluation process.

Review of Records and Background Information

The review of any obtainable record is oftentimes a continuous process rather than a step in isolation, as the data may not be readily available to the clinician. Access to these records varies significantly between settings. For instance, a school psychologist may have an easy time locating a child's educational history, while finding it difficult to obtain medical records. In contrast, a psychologist in an inpatient medical unit may have easier access to such records but lacks access to school information. On occasion, the referral source sends valuable records to the psychologists in order to facilitate the intake process (e.g., copies of their own reports or notes). More often, parents provide clinicians with copies of previous reports, hospital and school records, and other supplementary information that aids the clinician's understanding of the case. In most instances, records are obtained upon guardian's authorization and via direct request to the original sources (e.g., school, pediatrician's office) as deemed necessary during intake and clinical interviews. In any psychological assessment, records play a crucial role in providing clinicians with information about the history, environment, and behaviors, not only about the child but also about his or her family and their dynamics. Records provide clinicians with a documented, multi-setting, and hopefully, multidimensional registry of variables that must be taken into account during the assessment process. Some of these variables include socio-economic conditions, familial mental health history, educational background and academic achievements, developmental milestones, child's strengths and weaknesses, physical health, relevant medical preconditions, interventions, and cultural background. Table 18.1

Table 18.1 List of Relevant Background Documents and Information to Review

Medical records	Birth history and developmental charts.
	Relevant pediatrician records.
	Recent or relevant hospitalization records.
	Medical treatment records.
School records	Academic achievement (e.g., marks and progress notes, awards, areas of strength and weaknesses).
	Teacher notes (special attention to records of early adjustment, changes in achievement, classroom conduct).
	Special education records (e.g., special education classification, services and placements, records of accommodations).
	School evaluations (history of behavioral problems in school, school activity/service participation).
Psychiatric records	Psychiatric evaluations (emphasis on consultation, onset and progression of symptoms, diagnosis and clinical recommendations).
	Medication intake records.
Psychological records	Reports from previous evaluations (diagnosis, areas assessed, instruments used, findings, observations, and any information that would allow identification of clinical change, symptom progression, relapse or remission).
	School psychologist or counselor records (as presented above, with special emphasis in history of learning and/or behavioral problems in school).
	Previous neuropsychological evaluations (as above, plus emphasis on history of head trauma, neurodevelopmental, inherited or congenital disorders, exposure to neurotoxins, neurosurgical evaluations, and notes on neuroimaging records and findings).
	Reports from psychological interventions (individual or group psychotherapy or neurorehabilitation).
Legal reports (if applicable)	Documented family legal issues involving the case (e.g., child custody, child abuse, social worker reports, foster care).
	Criminal records or charges (e.g., adolescent cases).

includes examples of relevant records to collect. This information can serve as a guideline during the clinical interview process and for the design of the assessment itself

Obtaining these records is only the initial part of the process. A skillful review of them requires training and practice. Having clarity about the relevant information one is looking for facilitates the process. At times, clinicians find themselves flooded with amassed pieces of information that may not be meaningful or pertinent to the assessment at hand; thus, there is skill in sorting them. When available, the records of any previous psychological or psychiatric assessments are highly desirable. Depending on the age of the child, educational records may be abundant, and some isolated pieces of information on them may be highly relevant to the case (e.g., marks, a teacher's note); or, in contrast, distracting to the assessment goals as they may lead to faulty interpretations. For example, a grade teacher may use descriptors, adjectives, or make rich comments about a child's performance and behavior based on isolated situations; or perhaps some of those notes tend to be similar to those made about most peers in the same class. Due to the multitude of possibilities, looking for patterns of behavior, consistent observations across raters and settings, and placing some emphasis on objective variables (e.g., composite scores or averages), becomes crucial during the review of records. At the same time, looking for salient and unique observations that may contribute to our understanding of the child's current behavior or situation is equally relevant. Thus, reviewing records is a very dynamic and ongoing process; a clinician may have to revisit them at different stages during the assessment process.

When reviewing these historical records, two approaches could be used: an exploratory or a guided approach. An *exploratory approach* includes a thorough review of all the materials collected, allowing the data to "speak" about possible patterns of behaviors, forgotten or potentially withheld information, and consistent observations. In this approach, there is no preconceived idea about the kind of information the clinician may find; it is simply an exploration. In contrast, a *guided approach* includes a search for a specific behavioral pattern, pieces of information or answers to *a priori* questions, and it is mostly confirmatory. Both approaches are complementary rather than exclusive, and some assessment protocols may require both or only one of them. An exploratory approach may facilitate an unbiased comprehension of a case in which there is not a clear consulting question (e.g., inconsistent concerns about the child's performance at school). A guided approach may be useful when the case is presented with a specific referral question: for instance, does this child classify for a diagnosis of learning disability? In synthesis, understanding the referral question at intake facilitates the subsequent review process.

History Taking and the Clinical Interview

One of the most important milestones in the assessment process is the completion of the clinical interview (McConaughy, 2005; Strauss, Sherman, & Spreen, 2006). Groth-Marnat (2009) stated that the interview is perhaps "the single most important means of data collection during psychological evaluation" (p. 65). Sattler (2008) includes clinical interviews as one of the core pillars of any psychological assessment, stating that "results of an assessment may be meaningless or inconclusive if you examine the child without interviewing those who play an important role in his or her life" (p. 6). Designed to complement our information about the case, the clinical interview is perhaps the most relevant scenario to establish rapport and obtain detailed information about the developmental history of the child and his or her family. As presented by Merrell (2008), "[i]n contrast to other methods of assessment that may be used for the same purposes, clinical interviewing is unique in its emphasis on direct face-to-face contact and interpersonal communication between the clinician and the client" (p. 133). During clinical interviews, there is a shared amount of verbal and nonverbal communication that becomes crucial in understanding the child's situation and for the child and his or her family to understand the clinician's evaluation methods and goals. The clinician usually controls this flow of communication as he or she plays the role of the interviewer. Therefore, interviewing is a highly demanding clinical skill, requiring training and experience, and further, it can potentially facilitate or impede the ease of the assessment process. The quality of the interviewer has an impact on the reliability of the background information recalled during the history taking process. A clinician's verbal and nonverbal communication during the interview process can signal personal biases, judgements, cultural differences, and other variables that may lead the clients to somewhat distort their valuable information.

Merrell (2008) pointed out several advantages of clinical interviewing as an assessment method: (a) it provides a great deal of flexibility that is lacking in other assessment methods; (b) it provides a structured context for behavioral observations during a social interaction; and (c) as it serves a medium for the establishment of rapport and trust, clinical interviews facilitate the bridge between assessment and intervention. One of the limitations of clinical assessment interviews, and perhaps the most worrisome of all, is its own vulnerability to an unreliable and inconsistent collection of data. Ironically, this particular disadvantage of this assessment method is derived from its flexible nature (McConaughy, 2005; Merrell, 2008). To compensate for this significant pitfall, obtaining data from several sources in addition to the interview becomes a crucial step in any assessment process; it is, in fact, the defining characteristic of the multi-method assessment approach. This method includes direct behavioral observations; rating scales from parents, teachers, and other relevant caregivers; self-reports; psychological tests; and other strategies deemed appropriate to the specifics of the evaluation. Examples of commercialized multi-method assessment approaches for child psychological assessment include the Behavioral Assessment System for Children–Second Edition (BASC-2; Reynolds & Kamphaus, 2004) and the Achenbach System of Empirically Based Assessment (ASEBA; Achenbach, 1986, 2001; Achenbach & Rescorla, 2000, 2001; McConaughy & Achenbach, 2001). Chapter 26 in this handbook provides more information on the combined utility of behavioral observations and rating scales. Furthermore, if the appropriate written consent forms have been received from the parents or guardians, interviewing teachers and consulting with other professionals involved in the case can serve as a valuable source of additional information.

Due to the relevance and sensitivity of clinical interviews, it does not come as a surprise that psychologists have classified them as the most used assessment method. A survey conducted on 412 active clinical psychologists demonstrated that 83 percent of them classified clinical interviewing as the assessment procedure they "always" used in their clinical practice. In the same study, "clinical interview" was ranked from 1 to 4 (out of 37 options) as the most frequently assessment method used across settings (e.g., private, university, medical; Watkins, Campbell, Nieberding, & Hallmark, 1995). Another study surveyed 162 child and adolescent psychologists across the United States, and in a range of settings, including private practice, hospitals and outpatient clinics, and schools,

clinical interviewing was ranked as the number-one social-emotional assessment procedure, used by 71 percent of the sample, followed by behavioral observations (ranked number two) used by 51.9 percent of their sample (Cashel, 2002). An earlier survey among the clinical psychology internships demonstrated that 53 percent of the training facilities with a pediatric emphasis have included child assessment interviews as a regular topic in their didactic seminars (Elbert & Holden, 1987).

Clinical Assessment Interview Methods

While there are shared commonalties among clinical interviewing methods in several contexts, clinical interviews in a multi-method assessment process significantly differ from those conducted under an intervention process (e.g., psychotherapy, counseling), and from those performed in some research and survey studies. As pointed out by McConaughy (2005), "[a] major goal of clinical assessment interviews is to obtain information" (p. 4), which explains why clinical interviews are often discussed in the context of history taking. For this reason, when conducting clinical assessment interviews, clinicians oftentimes resort to structured or semi-structured interviewing protocols to elicit the discussion of relevant pieces of information, to facilitate the cohesion and progression of the interview, and to make the process more efficient and effective. In some assessment situations, a skilled clinician may feel more comfortable using an unstructured, open-ended type of interview; however, their level of experience is not the main variable to consider when making the choice between interviewing formats. Several variables play an important role in this decision, such as the context of the interview (e.g., as part of a behavioral assessment versus neuropsychological assessment), intended aim (e.g., as a diagnostic tool versus historical background), and clinician's theoretical orientation (e.g., psychodynamic versus cognitive; Merrell, 2008). A discussion of unstructured, semi-structured, and structured methods follows.

UNSTRUCTURED INTERVIEWS

Flexibility is perhaps the most descriptive characteristic of this type of clinical interview. As the name implies, "unstructured" interviews are defined in terms of their open-ended, conversational format in which there is more demand put on the role of the interviewer as the director of the communicative flow, due to the lack of a preconceived structure. Analogous to a dance performed by a skillful ballerina, the art of the unstructured clinical interviewing arises in how effortlessly the clinician facilitates the communication between the parties involved. Moreover, this effortlessness also reflects how well the child and his or her caregivers' make use of the opportunity to express their thoughts, feelings, fears, and needs concerning the issues that brought them to the assessment, while divulging the relevant historical background and other diagnostic information.

There is no gold standard for the administration of an unstructured interview, and the format varies across different theoretical orientations. Some clinicians use the unstructured format to frame the interview while nevertheless maintaining full control over the questions that will be asked of the client. This control is exerted by moderating shifts in the direction of the interview, signaling and changing the flow at times, and deciding what could be considered a satisfying response or not. Others may consider this format too invasive, and furthermore, that it could leave the client unguided in expressing themselves without cues. A skillful clinician may be able to engage the child in either play (e.g., in the case of younger children) or conversation (e.g., in the case of teens and adolescents), allowing them to express themselves without an intrusive layout of questions. Because of the nature of this type of interview, the clinician must feel comfortable with letting the patient take charge, while making careful notes of a range of observations regarding symptoms (e.g., anxiety, inattention, speech problems, slowness of movement), emotions, and behaviors, in addition to recording the appropriate background information provided in their discourse (Greenspan & Greenspan, 2003).

It is worth noting that "unstructured" does not equal "aimless." An experienced clinician uses this conversation-like environment to facilitate gathering of the most valuable assessment information. Although it is recognized that one of the main benefits from this method is, ultimately, the facilitation of rapport with the client, there has been a growing concern among clinicians about the degree of reliability of the information gathered during this kind of interview (Kamphaus & Frick, 2002). This reliability issue can be aggravated by the clinician's personal biases and values, the client's perception of the clinician's assessment goals, the nature of the assessment situation, and the potential associated outcomes. Furthermore, the clinician's orientation has been identified as an important source of bias, having an impact on the clinician's perception of the case

and their clinical judgement, particularly in the case of junior clinicians (Houts, 1984). Research-based interviewing can be especially susceptible to these reliability limitations. Dougherty, Ebert, and Callender (1986) found that when interviewers are trained in specific strategies, intra-rater consistency rates decrease, but inter-rater reliability scores rise. Increasingly, research has demonstrated that adding structure to an interview format increases its validity and reliability indexes (Groth-Marnat, 2009). These consistent findings originated the development of a series of structured and semi-structured interview protocols, to aid not only clinical assessment in the context of research but also as a component of any multi-method assessment in the general psychology practice. Chapter 3 in this handbook offers a complete review of the measurement issues frequently observed in child assessment.

SEMI-STRUCTURED CLINICAL INTERVIEWS

As a general practice, established clinicians often times create or adapt their own assessment interviewing protocols following a semi-structured format. As the name entitles, a "semi-structured" clinical interview is somewhat flexible, yet it is also fairly contained within a set of questions that prompt dialogue and face-to-face interactions between the clinician and the child. Semi-structured interviews are often used to gather general information about the child and to obtain an overall appraisal of his or her current psychological and adaptive functioning. Due to their flexibility, they are easily adapted to different assessment needs, theoretical orientations, clinicians' styles, and settings. For these reasons, they are often referred to as "traditional" interview methods.

Different referral questions may prompt the clinician to make changes in a semi-structured interview protocol, making it relevant to emphasize some areas over others. For instance, a child who is brought to an assessment due to school adjustment issues may require extensive collection of information about his or her peer relationships, educational experiences, areas of academic strength and weakness, quality of relationship and interactions with teachers and school personnel, separation anxiety symptoms, and history of abuse. In contrast, a child who has been brought in to a consultation due to cognitive deficits following a traumatic brain injury would require a fairly different set of questions. Merrell (2008) recommends targeting at least five areas during an interview with children: (1) intrapersonal functioning, (2) family relationships, (3) peer relationships, (4) school adjustment, and (5) community involvement. Table 18.2 illustrates a few examples of the types of questions that can be used to gather information around those five areas.

There are relatively few valid and reliable semi-structured interviews available for pediatric clinical assessment. In this regard, the Semi-structured Clinical Interview for Children and Adolescents (SCICA; McConaughy & Achenbach, 1994) was made available earlier in the literature (e.g., Verhulst, 1995), and recently, it was formally introduced as a component of the ASEBA system. Examples of

Table 18.2 Typical Areas of Questioning Included in a Nonstandardized Semi-Structured Clinical Interview with a Child

Area of Questioning	Specific Issues to Address
Intrapersonal functioning	*Feelings and emotions* How does the child feel about him/herself? What kind of emotions are he/she expressing? How does the child feel about the issues that brought him/her to the consultation? Have there been any significant change/trauma/loss in this child's life? *Activities and well-being* How is a regular day for this child? Does he/she have any particular hobbies, interests, or activities? How independent and well-adjusted is the child? Is there any concern about his/her sleep hygiene/habits? *Development and mental health functioning* Is there any concern about this child's development? Is there report of any unusual experience?—including hearing or seeing things. Does the child seem oriented?
Family Relationships	Who are the members of this child's family? How are the relationships among them? Does the child get along with brothers and sisters? What is the child's role in this family? Does he/she have chores and responsibilities? Who lives in the house with the child? Is this child's family supportive of his/her needs? How is discipline implemented? Is there any concern about abuse or danger to the child?
Peer Relationships	How many close friends does the child have? Can he/she name them? In what kind of activities are they usually engaged? How easy does he/she make new friends? How easily does he/she cope with losing a friendship? Does the child feel like an outcast, an outsider? Is he/she a member of a social clique, club, band, team, or gang? Is he/she being victimized or bullied by peers?
School Adjustment	Does the child like school? Learning and studying? What are this child's academic strengths and weaknesses? Does the child go to school regularly? Is he/she home-schooled? How are his/her relationships with teachers? Is there a favorite? One he/she dislikes? Is he/she enrolled in extracurricular activities or school clubs? Has he/she been in trouble at school?
Community Involvement	Is the child part of a community group or activity (e.g., church, youth clubs, and sport teams)? Is he/she working part-time? Does he/she volunteer in any community services? Does he/she have friends not associated with his/her school? Are there concerns or complaints about this child's behavior in the neighborhood?

items included in the SCICA and some applied case examples are further described by McConaughy (2005). This instrument was designed for use with children and adolescents aged six to 18, and comprises two sections. During the first section, the clinician conducts a semi-structured interview using open-ended questions from a list of six areas: activities and interests, school and homework, friendship and relations, home situation and family relations, self-awareness and feelings, and adolescent issues. The second section includes the scoring of two forms, a child's self-report form (125 items) and an interviewer observations form (120 items) to rate the child's behavior during the interview using a four-point Likert scale. The ratings are further scored into a standardized system that yields profile information on five syndrome or behavioral scales: Anxious, Withdrawn/Depressed, Language/Motor Problems, Attention Problems, and Self-Control Problems; three more scales are derived from the child's self-report: Anxious/Depressed, Aggressive/Rule-Breaking, and Somatic Complaints (McConaughy, 2005). Merrell (2008) states that, although information on its psychometrical properties is still limited, "the SCICA is recommended as an innovative semi-structured interview tool for use with children and adolescents" (p. 166).

Semi-structured interviews are often used to aid a functional assessment of behavior, aiming at collecting information about the problem behaviors, factors that may elicit and maintain them, and potential reinforcers and mediators of the associations between behaviors and their consequences. Furthermore, there are semi-structured clinical interviews designed to serve the purpose of identification of specific symptomatology, ultimately aiming for diagnostic classification of childhood psychopathology (e.g., ADHD, conduct disorder, pervasive developmental disorder). For example, Angold & Costello (2000), used a construct-validation approach to develop the Child and Adolescent Psychiatric Assessment (CAPA), a semi-structured and flexible interview system that includes forms for children (aged 8–17) and their parents. For the scoring of the CAPA, a coding system is applied after the clinical interview, and, once entered into the software database, its algorithm generates diagnoses for DSM-III, DSM-IV and ICD-10. Test-retest reliability coefficients for the CAPA, available for child report forms only, range from 0.55 for conduct disorder to 1.0 for substance abuse/dependence (see Angold, Costello, & Egger, 2007), while the construct validity of the CAPA

has been strongly attested to by its creators (Angold & Costello, 2000). A preschool version of the CAPA has also been developed: the Preschool Age Psychiatric Assessment (PAPA; Egger & Angold, 2004), with test-retest reliability coefficients ranging from 0.36 for specific phobias to 0.74 for attention deficit/hyperactivity disorder (ADHD; see also Angold, Costello, & Egger, 2007).

Another example comes from Sherrill and Kovacs (2000), who reviewed a series of versions of the Interview Schedule for Children (ISC; Kovacs, 1985) and developed the Interview Schedule for Children and Adolescents (ISCA). This semi-structured, symptom-oriented psychiatric interview has been standardized for use in children aged eight to 17, and includes forms for children and their parents. It is composed of five sections: symptoms and signs, mental status, behavioral observations, clinician's impressions, and developmental milestones. It uses an open-ended questioning format, and responses and impressions are rated using a Likert scale, according to severity of symptoms. In contrast to the CAPA, the examiner inputs the ratings of the ISCA *during* the interview (Sherrill & Kovacs, 2000). These authors suggest that the inter-rater reliability of the ISCA is quite good, whereas more evidence is needed for the test-retest reliability. Moreover, research on the predictive validity of specific disorders diagnosed using the ISCA suggest it has high predictive utility (Phillips & Gross, 2010).

Although criticized for lacking sufficient reliability and validity data (Kamphaus & Frick, 2002), an interesting semi-structured *pictorial* interview system was introduced by Ernst, Cookus, and Moravec (2000), the Pictorial Instrument for Children and Adolescents (PICA-III-R). This interview system includes 137 simple, schematic, and neutral pictures (Ernst et al., 2000) representing DSM-III-R criteria for five diagnostic categories: anxiety disorders, mood disorders, psychotic disorders, disruptive behavior disorders, and substance abuse. The child is asked to rate on a five-point Likert scale how much he or she likes the person in the picture. Along with ranking, open-ended questions are provided to the interviewer to enhance the interactions with the child. However, some limitations of this interview are that the standardization data included only severely disturbed children and diagnostic classification is outdated.

Other commonly used semi-structured interviews include the Anxiety Diagnostic Interview for DSM-IV–Child and Parent versions (ADIS-C/P; Silverman & Albano, 1996) and the Schedule for Affective Disorders and Schizophrenia for School-Aged Children (K-SADS; Ambrosini, 2000). As reported by Rapport, Kofler, Bolden, and Sarver (2008), "the inter-rater reliability estimates for the K-SADS are among the highest of any semi-structured clinical interviews" (p. 394). However, even though both are used in the context of a clinical interview, the focus of these two schedules is too narrow for the present discussion. The following chapter (see Chapter 22) further reviews formal methods in assessing mood and affect in children and adolescents.

STRUCTURED CLINICAL INTERVIEWS

Structured interviews became popular among researchers interested in using reliable tools to collect their data. Due to its psychometric strength, this form of interview gained a relevant place in most clinician's assessment protocols (Kamphaus & Frick, 2002). Although structure yields reliability, these instruments are fallible to the periodic updates on the diagnostic criteria they are based on, the *Diagnostic and Statistical Manual* (DSM; Verhulst, 1995). Two of the best-known instruments in this category are the Diagnostic Interview for Children and Adolescents–Fourth Edition (DICA-IV; Herjanic & Reich, 1997; Reich, 2000) and the Diagnostic Interview Schedule for Children (DISC; Piacentini et al., 1993; Schwab-Stone et al., 1993; Shaffer et al., 1993).

The DICA (Herjanic & Reich, 1982; Reich, Herjanic, Welner, & Gandhy, 1982) was first introduced to "improve the extent and quality of information obtainable from children, particularly younger children," with later versions including separate forms for children and adolescents (Reich, 2000, p. 59). The current version, DICA-IV, can be administered to children aged 6–12 or adolescents aged 13–17, as well as their parents. As it closely follows diagnostic classifications such as the DSM-IV and ICD-10, this schedule is very extensive; it includes over 1,600 possible questions, yet, it is structured following an algorithm that allows systematic selection of questions within dimensions and diagnostic categories, minimizing the length. Completion of the DICA-IV can take about one to two hours, depending on the number of categories to be covered. A computerized version of this instrument facilitates data entry. Although it is still often classified as a highly structured interview schedule (e.g., Kamphaus & Frick, 2002; Merrell, 2008), authors' revisions enhanced the wording flexibility to the extent that they actually described it as

a semi-structured, polydiagnostic, glossary-based, and highly criteria-based tool (Reich, 2000). These characteristics have made the DICA a preferred instrument for research purposes; and subsequently, several studies have demonstrated moderate to high indices of inter-rater agreement (e.g., Ezpeleta et al., 1997), test-retest reliability (e.g., Boyle et al., 1993), parent–child agreement (e.g., Reich et al., 1982), and sensitivity to differentiate clinical from nonclinical samples (Merrell, 2008). Although efforts have been made to evaluate the clinical validity of this instrument (e.g., Welner, Reich, Herjanic, Jung, & Amado, 1987), caution about the minimal level of validity evidence available for the DICA has been also raised (e.g., Hodges, 1993; Kamphaus & Frick, 2002; Merrell, 2008).

The most recent version of the DISC, the DISC-IV (Shaffer, Fisher, Lucas, Dulcan, & Schwab-Stone, 2000), was produced by the National Institute of Mental Health (NIMH) and was based on both the DSM-IV and ICD-10 diagnostic classifications. It is described by its authors as "a highly structured diagnostic instrument designed for use by nonclinicians" (Shaffer et al., 2000, p. 28). It is this last characteristic (i.e., minimal training) that has made the DISC an appealing instrument for epidemiological and screening research studies. The DISC is composed of two forms: the DISC-P (parent of children 6–17) and the DISC-Y (children aged 9–17). It includes almost 3,000 possible questions, but only 358 are considered "stem" and are therefore included in every interview. About 1,300 questions are asked according to the positive or negative response to one of the stem questions; in this way, they are contingent to the initial responses collected. Similar to the DICA, the interviewer can use computerized software to facilitate the administration of the DISC. The time to complete the interview ranges from 70 minutes (in community samples) to 90 to 120 minutes for clinical cases. Authors acknowledged that this highly structured instrument can be limited in that it does not allow for documentation of atypical presentations, and it is vulnerable to undetectable mistakes in data entry (Shaffer et al., 2000). Furthermore, Verhulst (1995) pointed out that this level of structure and symptom dichotomous approach (presence/absence) dismisses the "extent of psychopathology that is just below or above the cutoff for diagnosis" (p. 205). Among its strengths, it is noted that the DISC is available in Spanish and English, only requires trained lay interviewers, and its psychometric properties (i.e., reliability and validity) are fairly strong (Kamphaus & Frick, 2002; Merrell, 2008; Shaffer et al., 2000).

Conducting Developmentally Appropriate Interviews

It is important to consider the developmental stage of the child when conducting a clinical interview. Knowledge of typical and atypical child development is crucial, including a thorough understanding of the range of cognitive, social, and emotional characteristics that underlie each stage. Equally relevant is the clinician's sensitivity toward the needs of the children at different developmental levels which facilitates the establishment of rapport (Morrison & Anders, 1999). A skilled clinician makes an effort to adapt the assessment protocol to these explicit or implicit needs, from the beginning to the end of the process. For instance, when selecting an interview format or method, a clinician may be inclined to use an unstructured and nondirective format for preschoolers; one that is full of flexibility, avoids questions when possible and uses declarative statements instead, such as, "It seems that you are angry" instead of "Are you angry with me?" (Greenspan & Greenspan, 2003, p. 179). Use of toys and props to elicit pretend play and communication is highly recommended. In contrast, a school-aged child or teenager may be able to communicate more concretely, answering direct and specific open-ended questions, expressing their opinions about familiar concrete situations (McConaughy, 2005), and demonstrating a better understating of their social circles (Merrell, 2008). They respond well to the introduction of humor to ease the conversation (Cepeda, 2010). The clinical interview with younger children may take place with the parents present; at least initially, as this will ease trust and rapport.

Adolescents may be able to handle a more structured interaction with the clinician, in which open-ended questions are presented and answered in an organized manner; yet, their sensitivity about feeling judged for their developing lifestyles, choices, and relationships, in combination with a growing sense of self-consciousness, make interviewing them equally challenging. Adolescents can provide a rich range of information during an interview, but they can easily feel intimidated or challenged by the clinician's interest in their developing identities, and rapidly disengage from the assessment. It is important to show respect for their opinions and feelings, as well as avoid signs of judgement and a condescending attitude. Developing trust is the most important feature of an interview with young adolescents, weighing heavily the acquisition of trustworthy data. Morrison and Anders (1999) recommend using statements such as: "Don't tell me what you don't want to, but don't lie. If you can't tell me the truth about something, just ask me to move on to another topic" (p. 71).

To facilitate the establishment of rapport and trust with a teenager or young adolescent, a clinician may have a two-section interview. During the first section, both the adolescent and the parents are welcomed to the office, where the parents are invited to present their concerns openly and transparently to the clinician. The clinician will then ask them to leave and will follow up during a second part in which the adolescent is left alone to further discuss his or her own insights into the issues (Cepeda, 2010). Some clinicians recommend the reverse order—the adolescent enters the interview first, and then both parents and adolescent together (Morrison & Anders, 1999). Independently of the method used, significant differences in their points of view may direct the examiner to talk about their relationships. It is recommended to carefully evaluate suicidal risk, which may not be included in the parents' concerns but may become apparent during the individual interview with the child. Table 18.3 includes a range of recommended strategies for the clinical assessment interview with children at different developmental stages.

Conducting Culturally Appropriate Interviews

In order to fully benefit from any clinical interviewing technique, the clinician must feel comfortable with managing cultural matters, language and communication, as well as any interpersonal issues that may interfere with the assessment's ultimate goal: obtaining reliable information about the child. Common barriers to effective communication during an interview are the cultural differences between the clinician and the child and his or her family. In a growingly pluralistic North American community, census data demonstrate increasing changes in the demographic distribution of countries such as the United States and Canada. These demographic shifts are characterized by an increasing representation of a diverse range of ethnical groups, and a reduction of the size of the mainstream Caucasian group. The American and Canadian Psychological Associations have all made efforts to increase our awareness of the professional and ethical importance of considering cultural differences when conducting psychological assessments, including child assessment. Despite these efforts, a

Table 18.3 Conducting a Developmentally Appropriate Interview

Developmental Group	Clinical Interview Strategies
Preschoolers (aged 3–5)	Make sure the space for the interview is adequate for a young child. Appropriate low-level table and chairs are recommended; be prepared to conduct the interview on the floor; a comfortable mat would make a difference. Involve the child in the interview as early as possible; for instance, initiating questions and interactions during the family interview. Early engagement and cooperation ease the clinical interview. Pretend play may facilitate interactions and child conversation. Allow the child to take control over the interview/play and use toys and props accordingly. If questions are asked, limit them to short, simple, and open-ended questions. Start with questions you know the child can answer. Avoid questions that can be answered with "yes/no." At times, using declarative statements may be more efficacious, "I think you are upset right now." Sentence completion may facilitate indirect expression of emotions and feelings. Use reassurance when appropriate, demonstrating interest. Positively phrased comments are also recommended; e.g., "it may be scary to feel out of control," instead of "I think you are scared." Take your time.
School-aged children (6–11)	Be as flexible as possible. You may want to go for a walk around the clinical setting, play a short video game on a computer, or draw together. Take your time establishing rapport and trust. Straightforward and simple communication with the child is recommended. Let the child initiate conversation and redirect if necessary. Avoid constant eye-contact; it can be intimidating for a child. Use concrete examples; refer to situations, contexts, or events that are very familiar to the child. Demonstrate deference to the child's feelings and expressions by avoiding any kind of judgement. An intellectually adept child may disengage when being asked questions with obvious answers. Be creative without being too abstract. Examples or choices may help. Sparse use of sensitive humor is always welcome. Direct questions may elicit too-concrete answers; e.g., "tell me about your family." Instead, a question such as, "How is a typical day at home?" or "What does your family do for fun?" may generate more information. Allow the child to express negative feelings. You may express assumptions that lead to it: "All children fight with their brothers and sisters at times" or "Many children would feel angry in a situation like that!" Talk about peer relationships: it can be an excellent way to gather information about the child's emotional and social development.
Adolescents (12–18)	Make an effort in establishing trust and rapport. Treat the adolescent with deference, but avoid being too distant. Offer a comfortable, private, and safe place to talk. Avoid physical contact. It is important not to pretend to be "cool" or too "hip." Adolescents would easily see through it. Establish the limits of confidentiality early on. Elicit conversation about their opinions on peer activities, social distress, and risk behaviors. Make sure to follow up on any indication of suicidal risk or harm to others. Avoid judgemental comments.

disproportionate representation of students from ethnic minorities in special education placement continues to be an issue (Rhodes, Ochoa, & Ortiz, 2005).

When language differences are evident, significant obstacles arise in communication and information gathering. At times, it may be recommended to refer the patient to a clinician that is proficient in the child's and his or her family's native language. Not being familiar with their first language would interfere not only with reliable data collection about the child but also with the establishment of rapport and trust. On occasion an interpreter may be needed; for instance, when relevant information from a caregiver is needed, but he or she does not speak fluent English. It is becoming increasingly common that the child is fluent in English (e.g., due to schooling) but his or her parents (and extended-family members) may not be fluent in the language, especially in the case of recently immigrated families or when elders are involved. In these instances, the clinician must be sensitive to their communication needs and make the appropriate accommodations. Under other necessary circumstances, the interview pace and format may be modified, keeping in mind that deference and courtesy would facilitate rapport. To enhance verbal communication in all contexts, it is recommended to avoid using slang, colloquial expressions with double meanings, or jargon. Clear communication is encouraged, while being mindful that there is a sensitive line between trying to communicate more clearly and being disrespectful to the client. Adolescents who have recently immigrated may be particularly sensitive and self-conscious about language barriers.

Furthermore, beyond language differences, and even in the absence of significant verbal barriers, there are several behavioral and nonverbal communication styles across cultures to take into account (McConaughy, 2005; Merrell, 2008; Rhodes et al., 2005; Sattler, 2008). Efforts to accommodate for cultural differences between the client and the examiner should start with active research into the child's cultural background, typical parenting and education styles accredited to their culture, health and healing practices, level of acculturation to the new dominant culture, and language proficiency. The clinician should also evaluate personal beliefs and expectations about the child's culture, as those may interfere with the quality and reliability of observations and, ultimately, interpretation of the data. Although any attempt to generalize patterns across cultures is cautioned against, an awareness of some typical characteristics of their nonverbal communication styles is relevant. In this regard, Sattler (2008) noted that significant differences arise in terms of quality of physical interactions (i.e., kinesics and proxemics) and paralanguage. *Kinesics* refers to the use of facial expressions, manual movements, and use of gestures during a communicative interaction. Hispanics and African Americans, for instance, tend to present a very expressive range of gestures and facial and hand movements; in contrast, Asians and Native Americans tend to exert more control over their expressions. There are also different values associated with these different expressions. What, in one culture, may mean character and confidence (e.g., smiling and gesturing for Hispanic cultures), in others may be a sign of immaturity and insecurity (e.g., Asian Americans). An inexpressive face creates mistrust among Latinos, while it may be an admirable sign for members of other cultures. *Proxemics* refers to the personal distance or space between the persons involved in the communication. In the case of an interview, the clinician should make an effort to arrange the seating in a manner that accommodates the child's and his or her family's needs (Sattler, 2008). For instance, some Asian cultures (e.g., Chinese) may prefer a side-by-side seating (avoiding direct eye contact) while a Caucasian "mainstream" American may feel uncomfortable with this seating arrangement during an interview. Distance and personal proximity may also vary according to status, age differences, or types of relationships. An African American child may distance him- or herself during the first stages of an evaluation and eventually allow some proximity later in the process; while a Hispanic child may maintain some proximity throughout the entire assessment process. In contrast, a Native American child may maintain some distance consistently throughout the assessment (McConaughy, 2005). Eye contact is an important behavior to monitor. Whites/Caucasians may feel comfortable with direct eye contact, while other cultures may avoid it as a sign of respect. Hispanics may lower eye contact if feeling punished or judged, whereas African Americans may prolong eye contact when speaking and lower it while listening (McConaughy, 2005; Merrell, 2008; Sattler, 2008). *Paralanguage* refers to the use of nonverbal communication cues such as tone of voice, pitch, and volume. Different cultures value pace, silent pauses, and voice volume differently. Asians and Native American children may use a soft voice to show respect. Hispanic children may be louder and more vivacious at times, with variations of this pattern being associated with their status and acculturation level.

To conclude, it is worth noting once again that there is no rule of thumb or specific behavioral characteristics that can be generalized to everyone within a group. Clinician's discretion is advised. Chapter 7 is recommended for a review of assessment of diverse populations. Furthermore, Rhodes, Ochoa, and Ortiz's (2005) book is highly recommended for a review of assessment practices with bilingual children.

Background Questionnaires

The clinical interview should be an opportunity to establish rapport, to get to know the child and his or her family, to interact with all members involved, and to gather as much information as possible about the child's current situation. A review of the child's records complements the information about the antecedents and relevant historic background of that child. An additional common source of information is the background questionnaire. Child questionnaires are often used to collect specific information regarding the development, medical/academic history, and current functioning (at home and at school) of the child being brought to the assessment (Baron, 2003; Strauss et al., 2006). As the main purpose of background questionnaires is to complement information gathered through the clinical interview and the records collected, most background questionnaires are highly structured and could be administered prior to, during, or after the clinical interview. Some clinicians may attach a developmental questionnaire to the consent and intake forms, getting as much information as possible in anticipation of the assessment and to aid in the planning of it. Other clinicians may prefer having the parents or guardians complete the form while they interview the child. Similarly, some clinicians prefer to develop their own structured or semi-structured questionnaires according to the needs of their typical clientele, their theoretical orientation, or assessment method preferences. Some research, academic, and institutional settings (e.g., schools and hospitals) have established a protocol that is systematically followed. Regardless of how questionnaires are used or administered, it is recommended that they not replace the clinical interview (Strauss et al., 2006).

There are several published examples of detailed background questionnaires (e.g., Baron, 2003, pp. 61–65; Strauss et al., 2006, pp. 68–74). For example, among some commercialized forms like the BASC-2 (Reynolds & Kamphaus, 2004), a structured developmental history (SDH) is included that provides a comprehensive and detailed review of medical, developmental, academic, social, psychological, and familial history of the child. Items that survey information about family configuration and

health and socioeconomic status are included in the SDH. Items of the developmental history include questions associated with prenatal, perinatal, and postnatal history, milestones in development, and level of maturation. In addition to the level of comprehensiveness of the SDH, one of its main strengths is its current availability in English and Spanish. Table 18.4 summarizes some of the typical areas covered in standard background questionnaires.

Child Mental Status Examination

The Mental Status Examination (MSE) is a common tool used to obtain an overall perspective about a person's general level of functioning, including his or her emotional state, perceptual functioning, flow and content of thought processes, overall intellectual functioning (language, memory, attention, concentration, and orientation), psychomotor speech, and general appearance (Aiken & Groth-Marnat, 2006; Lezak et al., 2004). The MSE was originally designed for neurological and psychiatric evaluations; accordingly, they were brief (about 20–30 minutes), semi-structured, and usually combined questioning with direct observations. This approach has been defined as a "method of organizing and evaluating clinical observations pertaining to mental status or mental condition" (Sommers-Flanagan & Sommers-Flanagan, 2003, p. 214). In 1902, Adolf Meyer introduced the MSE into American psychiatry (Groth-Marnat, 2009), and ever since, there have been many prototypes of the MSE, ranging from brief to comprehensive, and from fully structured to semi-structured. Despite its popularity among pediatricians, child psychiatrists, and clinical neurologists, the MSE is not typically used in child psychological evaluations; perhaps because the information provided by the MSE can be collected from pieces of the full assessment process. In most cases, the MSE is not used in isolation but rather as a component of a multi-stage assessment. Oftentimes it will be administered during the early clinical assessment interview to provide the clinician with some guidelines about the client's broad strengths and weaknesses, facilitating subsequent design of the full assessment protocol. This is frequently the case in neuropsychological assessments in which a more comprehensive and detailed evaluation of core cognitive areas will follow the initial interview (for a review, see chapters 14 and 20).

Though the MSE has its advantages, it should be used with caution. Similar to screening measures, the MSE could provide the clinician with a biased view, as well as potentially generate

Table 18.4 Sample of Areas Covered in a Child Background Questionnaire

Demographics	Name Date and country of birth Race /gender /primary language Grade at school Information about the person completing the form
Referral Information	Motive of consult Referral source Strengths and weaknesses Type of assessment requested
Family Information	Available information on biological parents Parents/guardians/caregivers Family and household configuration Who is the primary caretaker of the child? Family income/members' occupations Current family stressors
Pregnancy and Birth	Maternal pregnancy history/health problems/substance use or abuse/medications Type of delivery/labor conditions Neonatal conditions: Term, weight, size, APGAR scores, neonatal intensive care, hypoxia/anoxia, medical problems at discharge Perinatal problems
Developmental History	Developmental motor milestones Language development Toileting and adaptive/independent functioning Social behavior Cognitive development
Medical History	Sensory and perception (hearing, vision) Head injuries/accidents/loss of consciousness History of seizures History of surgery History of medical illnesses or chronic conditions Previous assessments
Educational History	Learning problems Areas of strengths and weaknesses Current educational placement Problems in any academic area Behavior at school Social adjustment
Family Health History	Learning disabilities Attention deficit hyperactivity disorder Mental health/psychiatric history Substance abuse Physical abuse Chronic illnesses (e.g., cancer, epilepsy, diabetes) Familial disease (e.g., Alzheimer's, Parkinson's)
Child's Current Functioning	Adaptive behavior Leisure activities/hobbies/sports Social interactions History of physical/sexual abuse Alcohol/drugs use/abuse Trouble with the law Distressing situations (e.g., illness, deaths, separations, accidents, significant changes, financial problems) and ability to cope Mental health concerns/features

initial false positive or negative classifications of the child's behavioral pattern. A common vulnerability of the brief MSE is cultural insensitivity (Sommers-Flanagan & Sommers-Flanagan, 2003). Cultural styles and beliefs could be easily misinterpreted in the context of a brief examination of thought processing; socioeconomic variables, parental neglect, or other environmental variables may be associated with disorganized or inappropriate physical appearance in the absence of psychopathology. Eye-contact–avoidance may be associated with cultural values of respect and hierarchy in the absence of developmental disorders. The most common MSE structure includes nine areas, which are discussed below in the context of child assessment. Table 18.5 contains a list of helpful indicators for each area, which are presented in the form of questions to the clinician.

Appearance and Attitude

There is a wealth of information in a client's appearance, which by itself may be less relevant than when placed in the context of a psychological assessment. Although a client's appearance is often a sign of his or her mental health (Wiger & Huntley, 2002), in the case of a pediatric evaluation, it may also indicate the parents' mental health, parenting quality and style, caregivers' attention to the child's needs, or the guardian's level of concern for the child's well-being.

The examiner should document his or her first impressions that the child evokes, while answering questions such as: "Is the child likeable?" or "Is there anything odd about this child?" (Cepeda, 2000). Furthermore, the examiner should note the physical characteristics of the child, including height and weight in relation to age, facial characteristics and expressions, eyewear, pupils' dilation and contraction, eye contact, unique body odors, hair and skin quality that may indicate nutritional status, and skin markings that may be signs of injuries or self-abusive behaviors. Several developmental genetic disorders include specific facial features as part of their phenotypic expression; thus, it is relevant to make note of the relevant features on the child's face and head, such as head size in relation to age, weight, and height; different irises' coloration; eyes' separation; and the shape of the forehead. The examiner should observe the child's grooming and general hygiene, the appropriateness of his or her attire for the assessment and the current weather conditions, footwear, presence of body piercings or tattoos, and make-up. All these observations should be placed in the context of the child's sex, age, race, and socioeconomic and ethnic background.

Moreover, the examiner takes notes about the child's manner in relating to the examiner, and the child's overall attitude toward the assessment and the clinician, including ease in separation from parents or guardian and the overall posture of

Table 18.5 Components of the Child Mental Status Examination

Mental Status Examination Components	Indicators
Physical Appearance and Attitude	Is this child likeable?
	What first impression do I have of his/her family?
	How easily did the child separate from his/her parents?
	Does this child look his/her age? His or her gender?
	Is the child too slim? Overweight? Is there presence of marked obesity?
	Does the child look tired and sleepy, or animated and energetic?
	What is the child wearing? Is this attire age-appropriate? Weather-appropriate? Clean?
	Is the child well groomed? Is there any marked body odor?
	Are there observable tattoos, piercings, body ornaments? (If not visible, ask the child).
	Are there signs of injuries or self-abusive behaviors? Are there noticeable scars?
	Is there any sign of any physical compulsive traits such as nail biting, licking, or hair pulling?
	Is there a physical disability?
	How are this child's facial features? Skin complexion? Do the skin and hair look healthy?
	How is the shape of the head?
	How would you qualify the child's attitude towards you and towards the assessment situation? Is the child aggressive? Impatient? Indifferent? Defiant? Cooperative?
	Is there any memorable aspect about this child?

(continued)

Table 18.5 (Continued)

Mental Status Examination Components	Indicators
Activity Level and Psychomotor Functioning	How is this child's gait? Is the child constantly changing postures, moving, or fidgeting? Is there any observable tic, mannerism, or eye-contact avoidance? Does the child smile? Is the child alert, awake? Is this child impulsive, agitated, or slow to respond? What kind of games does the child like? Does he/she help at home with chores? Which ones?
Emotional State	*Range*: Does the child express a full range of affect? Is affect restricted, expansive, or flat? *Intensity*: Is the intensity of the child's emotional expression normal? *Stability*: Is the affect stable or labile? *Appropriateness*: What is the predominant affect during the interview? Is it appropriate? Does the child become angry, frustrated, or impatient during the assessment? Does the child manifest anxiety? Does he/she fidget or is calm during the interview?
Speech	*Form*: Is the child's speech articulated? Is the volume of his/her speech loud? Soft? Normal? Is the pace of the speech fast, slow, or normal? Is the child talkative or reserved? Is there a delay in the response to questions or instructions? Are the child's speech tone and melody (prosody) monotonous or normal? *Content*: Is the child's speech full of details? Is it excessive? How is the child's vocabulary level? Appropriate for age, limited, or advanced? Is the content organized? Is it grammatically correct? Are words used appropriately? Does the child make sense? *Receptive language*: Does the child follow the instructions correctly? Does he/she require multiple repetitions and clarifications? Does the child seem to understand questions? Does he/she react to comments and feedback? *Expressive language*: Is the child verbally fluent? Can the child read aloud correctly? Can the child adequately describe a picture?
Thought Process	*Flow and form*: Is it logical and coherent? Spontaneous? Conversational? Pertinent? Is the language purposeful and goal-directed? *Content*: Is it selective? Obsessive? Distorted? Delusional? Is it inappropriate or bizarre for age level? Is the content indicative of harm risk for him/her or others? Is there any evidence of visual, auditory, or other kinds of hallucinations?

(continued)

Table 18.5 (Continued)

Mental Status Examination Components	Indicators
Orientation	Is the child oriented in person, time, place, and situation? Examples of typical questions about orientation include: *Person* "What is your name?" "What school do you go to?" *Time* "How old are you?" "When is your birthday?" "What time is it?" "What date is it?" "Is it morning or afternoon?" *Place* "Where do you live?" "Where are you now?" *Situation* "Why are you here?"
Attention and Concentration	Does the child sustain attention during the interview? Is the child able to shift the focus of his or her attention from one task to another? Is the child distractible during the examination?
Memory	Is the child able to repeat an instruction? Can the child repeat a series of letters or digits? Can the child recall names of people or places from his or her recent past? Can the child recall some recent past events?—e.g., the last weekend activities, last movie seen. Can the child recall events from his or her life history?—e.g., early school years, last year's Halloween, or vacations.
Overall Cognitive Functioning and Development	After interacting with the child and throughout the interview, does the child seem to behave and think at an appropriate age level? How is the child's general vocabulary level?—Advanced for his age, adequate, below expectations? What is your impression of this child's level of responsiveness? Can the child comprehend most of your instructions? (Have in mind cultural and language barriers.) What is your impression of this child's abstract thinking? (e.g., establishing similarities and differences between two objects). Can he or she point at a few body parts? In young children, how is this child's drawing of a person?—Advanced, mature, age-appropriate, immature? How is this child's academic performance in the school?
Insight and Judgement	Is the child aware of the situation or problems that brought him/her to the consultation? How easy or difficult is it for him/her to make decisions? What words does the child use to describe him/herself? Does the child recognize hazardous situations and risk-taking behaviors? Is the child aware of the consequences of his/her behaviors? Does the child have plans for the short and long-term future? How does the child relate past situations or events to his/her current difficulties?

the child. Carlat (2005) stated that "[d]escriptors of attitude are similar to descriptors of affect, but the emphasis is on words that describe a relationship toward someone" (p. 126). Sommers-Flanagan and Sommers-Flanagan (2003) defined some useful descriptors to characterize the overall attitude of a client towards the interviewer. Some examples include *aggressive* (e.g., attacking the examiner verbally or physically), *cooperative* (e.g., teamwork gathering information during the interview), *hostile* (e.g., the client uses sarcasm, irony, or other such gestures), *impatient* (e.g., Type A personality style), *indifferent* (e.g., lack of concern), *intense* (e.g., loud, inquisitive eye contact), *manipulative* (e.g., efforts to solicit agreement from the interviewer), *negative* (e.g., opposes examiner comments), *open* (e.g., actively engaged), *passive* (e.g., disconnected from interview), *seductive* (e.g., flirtatious or suggestive comments), and *suspicious* (e.g., remarks on examiner's notes; Sommers-Flanagan & Sommers-Flanagan, 2003, p. 219). Once again, it is important to evaluate these perceived attitudes in the context of the child's cultural background.

Activity Level and Psychomotor Functioning

When possible, it is recommended that the examiner walk the child into the interviewing room while observing his or her gait and coordination (Cepeda, 2000). Throughout the interview, the examiner pays close attention to the child's psychomotor activity and should register any sign of excessive or reduced motor activity, tics, muscle twitching, fidgeting, odd and repetitive movements, slowness of movement, clumsiness, and both gross and fine motor coordination. Any observable, atypical activity-level of a child should lead to further examination of his or her medical records, medications, mood, and affect (Wiger & Huntley, 2002). In the case of an adolescent, inquiries about substance abuse may be relevant. Psychomotor retardation and psychomotor agitation can be indicators of neurodevelopmental disorders, mood disorders, or medication side effects (e.g., akathisia produced by neuroleptics or serotonin reuptake inhibitors). The examiner should make an effort to identify if the motor activity exhibited by the child is goal-directed or if it should be characterized as aimless behavior. If suspecting mania, the examiner should pay attention to other manifestations (e.g., pressured speech, grandiosity; Cepeda, 2000).

In the context of a MSE, and in combination with the behavioral observations, a quick examination of psychomotor coordination can also include a few questions directed to the child and his or her parents (when appropriate) about the child's everyday activities, independence, playfulness, home management participation, adaptive skills, and self-care. It is worth noting that these observations are only meaningful if the developmental and cultural contexts of the child are taken into consideration.

Emotional State

This concerns the child's reported mood (emotional tone) and overall observable affect. There are some noteworthy differences in the evaluation of mood and affect. For instance, *mood* refers to a persistent emotional state over time; therefore, information about mood is often obtained by direct endorsement of the child (if developmentally appropriate) or via the parents' reports. When assessing *affect* in the context of the MSE, the examiner should pay close attention to the range, frequency, intensity, stability, and appropriateness of emotional expressions. Depending on their developmental stage, children may present some emotional characteristics more overtly (e.g., joyful or irritated), while anxiety and depressive symptoms may be covertly camouflaged by an adolescent. A tearful preschooler may not be considered "sad"; the stress associated with the assessment may create fear, and the novelty of the situation could have triggered their underdeveloped ability to cope with this stress (Goodman & Sours, 1967). In these cases, a skilled clinician pays attention to nonverbal clues about the child's feelings, and the consistency between their emotional display and verbal statements.

Speech

The child's speech is a crucial indicator of his or her thought processes; consequently, it should be observed throughout the assessment. Speech examination can include both *delivery* (rate, volume, tone quality, articulation, and amount) and *content* (age-inappropriate confusion of words, grammatical and syntactical errors, organization, and spontaneity). It is important to rule out the possibility of a developmental hearing impairment before drawing any definite conclusions about the child's language.

Receptive language abilities can be informally examined during the early stages of the clinical assessment interview. A child who is able to follow instructions and responds accordingly arouses no major concerns at this point. Children with receptive language difficulties may look very confused during the interview. A short formal assessment can include a series of questions and verbal commands. Zuckerman (2005) offered examples for the assessment of language comprehension in the context of conducting the MSE, such as, "The lion killed the tiger, which one is dead?" and commands such as, "Close your eyes. Open them. Raise an arm" (p. 29). Expressive language can be observed in the child's verbal fluency rate (spontaneous or if prompted), or by asking the child to describe an object or a picture. With a school-aged or older case, reading some sentences or a short paragraph, and describing a situation, should allow the clinician to build an overall appreciation of the individual's fluency and language expression.

The child's ability to communicate can be affected by neurodevelopmental disorders such as autism. To distinguish autism from other communication disorders, Cepeda (2000) recommended considering the following questions: "Is the patient attempting to communicate at all? Is the patient gesturing or attempting to use other nonverbal behavior? Is the patient capable of developing rapport? Is the patient attempting to connect with the examiner?" (p. 102). Carlat (2005) recommended using descriptors such as "normal, thoughtful, articulate, intelligent, continuous, rapid, rambling, pressured, loud, soft, slow, and halting" (p. 127) when noting the characteristics of the client's speech.

Thought Process

Wiger and Huntley (2002) stated that "[a] person's stream of consciousness is a measurement or indication of how one's speech reflects thought processes" (p. 172). Thus, the examiner should observe the flow and form of the child's thought process, as well as the content. Evaluation of thought content in children is challenging, and caution in making conclusive statements is advisable; delusions are rare in children, and while auditory and visual hallucinations could be identified during the clinical interview, they can also be easily confused with imaginary, fantasy, or play situations. Furthermore, severe language disorders can make it difficult to determine thought content.

In addition to form and content, during the brief screening of thought processing in the context of the MSE, it is recommended that the examiner pay attention to speech content involving risk of harm toward the child or others, including suicidal and homicidal ideation, involvement in violent actions, gangs, delinquent or antisocial risk behaviors, or obsessive thinking, among others.

Orientation

The examiner identifies if the child is oriented in person, place, time, and situation. Age-appropriate expectation of child's orientation is important; a younger child may only have a vague reference of the date (month, year) and may be confused about place or type of setting. Common questions to a child include, "What is your name? What school do you go to? Where do you live? How old are you? When is your birthday? What time is it? What date is it? Is it morning or afternoon? Where are you?" and "Why are you here?"

Attention, Concentration, and Memory

Attention and memory are fundamental functions for information processing and cognitive functioning. A distractible child who cannot concentrate during the interview and MSE may perform poorly during testing as well. Therefore, assessment of attention, concentration, and basic memory skills at this early stage of the assessment process is recommended. Morrison and Anders (1999) suggested a brief evaluation of these three areas using age-appropriate simple math such as counting backwards by ones, and other indicators of immediate (e.g., digits or visual objects), recent (e.g., "What did you have for breakfast this morning?"), and remote memory processing (e.g., information about people, things, or events). Observations collected during the brief assessment of attention and memory in the context of an MSE will help the clinician to further design and personalize the full cognitive assessment protocol. In some cases, referral to neuropsychological assessment may be appropriate.

Overall Cognitive Functioning and Development

One of the primary goals of the brief MSE is to provide the clinician with an overall initial appreciation of the child's cognitive capacity. The underlying question would be, "Does this child seem to behave and think at an appropriate age level?" With this in mind, the examiner can estimate the level of general mental ability of the child by observing his or her general vocabulary, responsiveness, comprehension of instructions, abstract thinking (e.g., establishing similarities and differences between two objects), identification of body parts, drawing a person, writing, and demonstration of age-appropriate ability to read or recognize graphemes, letters, or words. Information about the academic performance of the child can also facilitate the estimation of his or her overall intellectual functioning.

Insight and Judgement

Examination of this area varies greatly according to the age and developmental stage of the child. The clinician should aim to develop some appreciation of the child's awareness about his or her problems (e.g., "Why are you here today?"); make-believe situations can be posed to an older child in order to observe his or her position about them (e.g., "What would you do if...?"). Furthermore, an informal, yet skilled conversation with the child during the interview can provide the clinician with information about his or her abilities to think about their present and future plans, to make decisions; his or her awareness of consequences of one's behavior, self-image, insights into social situations, moral judgements, hobbies and favorite activities, risk-taking behaviors, and hazard recognition.

Groth-Marnat (2009) states that, "Adequate insight and judgement involves developing and testing hypotheses regarding their own behavior and the behavior of others" (p. 83). The examiner may propose questions that allow for an evaluation of the child's insights into his or her current situation, and how these insights may be related to past events, decisions made by the child or others, and any potential explanations the child may have for his or her problems.

References

Achenbach, T. M. (1986). *The Direct Observation form of the Child Behavior Checklist* (rev. ed.). Burlington, VT: University of Vermont, Research Center for Children, Youth, and Families.

Achenbach, T. M. (2001). *Youth self-report for ages 11–18.* Burlington, VT: University of Vermont, Research Center for Children, Youth, and Families.

Achenbach, T. M., & Rescorla, L. A. (2000). *Manual for the ASEBA preschool forms and profiles.* Burlington, VT: University of Vermont, Research Center for Children, Youth, and Families.

Achenbach, T. M., & Rescorla, L. A. (2001). *Manual for the ASEBA school age forms and profiles.* Burlington, VT: University of Vermont, Research Center for Children, Youth, and Families.

Aiken, L. R., & Groth-Marnat, G. (2006). *Psychological testing and assessment* (12th ed.). Boston, MA: Pearson, Allyn & Bacon.

Ambrosini, P. J. (2000). Historical development and present status of the Schedule for Affective Disorders and Schizophrenia for School-Age Children (K-SADS). *Journal of the American Academy of Child & Adolescent Psychiatry, 39,* 49–58.

Angold, A., & Costello, E. J. (2000). The Child and Adolescent Psychiatric Assessment (CAPA). *Journal of the American Academy of Child & Adolescent Psychiatry, 39,* 39–48.

Angold, A., Costello, E. J., Egger, H. (2007). Structured interviewing. In A. Martin, F. R. Volkman, & M. Lewis (Eds.), *Lewis's child and adolescent psychiatry* (4th ed., pp. 344–357). Philadelphia: Lippincott, Williams & Wilson.

Baron, I. S. (2003). *Neuropsychological evaluation of the child.* New York: Oxford University Press.

Boyle, M. H., Offord, D. R., Racine, Y., Sanford, M., Szatmari, P., Fleming, J. E., et al. (1993). Evaluation of the Diagnostic Interview for Children and Adolescents for use in general population samples. *Journal of Abnormal Child Psychology, 21,* 663–681.

Carlat, D. J. (2005). *The psychiatric interview: A practical guide* (2nd ed.). Philadelphia: Lippincott, Williams & Wilkins.

Cashel, M. L. (2002). Child and adolescent psychological assessment: Current clinical practices and the impact of managed care. *Professional Psychology: Research & Practice, 33,* 446–453.

Cepeda, C. (2000). *Concise guide to the Psychiatric Interview of Children and Adolescents.* Washington, DC: American Psychiatric Press.

Cepeda, C. (2010). *Clinical manual for the Psychiatric Interview of Children and Adolescents* (1st ed.). Washington, DC: American Psychiatric Pub.

Dougherty, T. W., Ebert, R. J., & Callender, J. C. (1986). Policy capturing in the employment interview. *Journal of Applied Psychology, 71,* 9–15.

Egger, H. L., & Angold, A. (2004). The Preschool Age Psychiatric Assessment (PAPA): A structured parent interview for diagnosing psychiatric disorders in preschool children. In R. DelCarmen-Wiggins & A. Carter (Eds.), *Handbook of infant, toddler, and preschool mental health assessment* (pp. 223–243). New York: Oxford University Press.

Elbert, J. C., & Holden, E. W. (1987). Child diagnostic assessment: Current training practices in clinical psychology internships. *Professional Psychology: Research & Practice, 18,* 587–596.

Ernst, M., Cookus, B. A., & Moravec, B. C. (2000). Pictorial Instrument for Children and Adolescents (PICA-III-R). *Journal of the American Academy of Child & Adolescent Psychiatry, 39,* 94–99.

Ezpeleta, L., de la Osa, N., Domenech, J. M., Navarro, J. B., Losilla, J. M., & Judez, J. (1997). Diagnostic agreement between clinicians and the Diagnostic Interview for Children and Adolescents—DICA-R—in an outpatient sample. *Journal of Child Psychology & Psychiatry & Allied Disciplines, 38,* 431–440.

Garcia-Barrera, M. A., & Kamphaus, R. W. (2006). Diagnosis of attention-deficit/hyperactivity disorder and its subtypes. In R. W. Kamphaus & J. M. Campbell (Eds.), *Psychodiagnostic assessment of children: Dimensional and categorical approaches* (pp. 319–355). Hoboken, NJ: John Wiley & Sons.

Goodman, J. D., & Sours, J. A. (1967). *The child mental status examination.* New York: Basic Books.

Greenspan, S. I., & Greenspan, N. T. (2003). *The clinical interview of the child* (3rd ed.). Washington, DC: American Psychiatric Pub.

Groth-Marnat, G. (2009). *Handbook of psychological assessment* (5th ed.). Hoboken, NJ: John Wiley & Sons.

Herjanic, B., & Reich, W. (1982). Development of a structured psychiatric interview for children: Agreement between child and parent on individual symptoms. *Journal of Abnormal Child Psychology, 10,* 307–324.

Herjanic, B., & Reich, W. (1997). Development of a structured psychiatric interview for children: Agreement between child and parent on individual symptoms. *Journal of Abnormal Child Psychology, 25,* 21–31.

Hodges, K. (1993). Structured interviews for assessing children. *Journal of Child Psychology & Psychiatry, 34,* 49–68.

Houts, A. C. (1984). Effects of clinician theoretical orientation and patient explanatory bias on initial clinical judgements. *Professional Psychology: Research & Practice, 15,* 284–293.

Kamphaus, R. W., & Frick, P. J. (2002). *Clinical assessment of child and adolescent personality and behavior* (2nd ed.). Boston, MA: Allyn and Bacon.

Kamphaus, R. W., & Reynolds, C. R. (2003). *Handbook of psychological and educational assessment of children: Personality, behavior, and context* (2nd ed.). New York: Guilford Press.

Kovacs, M. (1985). The Interview Schedule for Children (ISC). *Psychopharmacology Bulletin, 21,* 991–994.

Lezak, M. D., Howieson, D. B., & Loring, D. W. (2004). *Neuropsychological assessment.* New York: Oxford University Press.

McConaughy, S. H. (2005). *Clinical interviews for children and adolescents: Assessment to intervention.* New York: The Guilford Press.

McConaughy, S. H., & Achenbach, T. M. (1994). *Manual for the semi-structured clinical interview for children and adolescents.*

Burlington, VT: University of Vermont, Department of Psychiatry.

McConaughy, S. H., & Achenbach, T. M. (2001). *Manual for the semi-structured clinical interview for children and adolescents* (2nd ed.). Burlington, VT: University of Vermont, Research Center for Children, Youth, and Families.

Merrell, K. W. (2008). *Behavioral, social, and emotional assessment of children and adolescents* (3rd ed.). New York: Lawrence Erlbaum Associates.

Morrison, J. R., & Anders, T. F. (1999). *Interviewing children and adolescents: Skills and strategies for effective DSM-IV diagnosis*. New York: Guilford Press.

Phillips, M. A., & Gross, A. M. (2010). Children. In D. L. Segal & M. Hersen (Eds.), *Diagnostic interviewing* (pp. 423–441). New York: Springer.

Piacentini, J., Shaffer, D., Fisher, P., Schwab-Stone, M., Davies, M., & Gioia, P. (1993). The Diagnostic Interview Schedule for Children–Revised Version (DISC-R): III. Concurrent criterion validity. *Journal of the American Academy of Child & Adolescent Psychiatry, 32*, 658–665.

Rapport, M. D., Kofler, M. J., Bolden, J., & Sarver, D. E. (2008). Treatment research. In M. Hersen & A. M. Gross (Eds.), *Handbook of clinical psychology. Vol. 2: Children and adolescents* (pp. 386–396). Hoboken, NJ: John Wiley & Sons.

Reich, W. (2000). Diagnostic Interview for Children and Adolescents (DICA). *Journal of the American Academy of Child & Adolescent Psychiatry, 39*, 59–66.

Reich, W., Herjanic, B., Welner, Z., & Gandhy, P. R. (1982). Development of a structured psychiatric interview for children: Agreement on diagnosis comparing child and parent interviews. *Journal of Abnormal Child Psychology, 10*, 325–336.

Reynolds, C. R., & Kamphaus, R. W. (2004). *Behavior Assessment System for Children (2nd ed.) manual*. Circle Pines, MN: American Guidance Services (AGS).

Rhodes, R. L., Ochoa, S. H., & Ortiz, S. O. (2005). *Assessing culturally and linguistically diverse students: A practical guide*. New York: Guilford Press.

Sattler, J. M. (2008). *Assessment of children: Cognitive foundations* (5th ed.). San Diego: Jerome M. Sattler.

Schwab-Stone, M., Fisher, P., Piacentini, J., Shaffer, D., Davies, M., & Briggs, M. (1993). The Diagnostic Interview Schedule for Children-Revised Version (DISC-R): II. Test-retest reliability. *Journal of the American Academy of Child & Adolescent Psychiatry, 32*, 651–657.

Shaffer, D., Fisher, P., Lucas, C. P., Dulcan, M. K., & Schwab-Stone, M. E. (2000). NIMH Diagnostic Interview Schedule for Children Version IV (NIMH DISC-IV): Description, differences from previous versions, and reliability of some common diagnoses. *Journal of the American Academy of Child Adolescent Psychiatry, 39*, 28–38.

Shaffer, D., Schwab-Stone, M., Fisher, P., Cohen, P., Piacentini, J., Davies, M., et al. (1993). The Diagnostic Interview Schedule for Children-Revised Version (DISC-R): Preparation, field testing, inter-rater reliability, and acceptability. *Journal of the American Academy of Child & Adolescent Psychiatry, 32*, 643–650.

Sherrill, J. T., & Kovacs, M. (2000). Interview Schedule for Children and Adolescents (ISCA). *Journal of the American Academy of Child & Adolescent Psychiatry, 39*, 67–75.

Silverman, W. K., & Albano, A. M. (1996). *The Anxiety Disorder Interview Schedule for Children for DSM-IV: Child and parent versions*. San Antonio, TX: Psychological Corporation.

Sommers-Flanagan, J., & Sommers-Flanagan, R. (2003). *Clinical interviewing* (3rd ed.). New York: Wiley.

Strauss, E., Sherman, E. M. S., & Spreen, O. (2006). *A compendium of neuropsychological tests: Administration, norms, and commentary* (3rd ed.). New York: Oxford University Press.

Verhulst, F. C. (1995). Recent developments in the assessment and diagnosis of child psychopathology. *European Journal of Psychological Assessment, 11*, 203–212.

Watkins, C. E., Campbell, V. L., Nieberding, R., & Hallmark, R. (1995). Contemporary practice of psychological assessment by clinical psychologists. *Professional Psychology: Research & Practice, 26*, 54–60.

Welner, Z., Reich, W., Herjanic, B., Jung, K. G., & Amado, H. (1987). Reliability, validity, and parent–child agreement studies of the Diagnostic Interview for Children and Adolescents (DICA). *Journal of the American Academy of Child & Adolescent Psychiatry, 26*, 649–653.

Wiger, D. E., & Huntley, D. K. (2002). *Essentials of interviewing*. New York: Wiley.

Zuckerman, E. L. (2005). *Clinician's thesaurus: The guide to conducting interviews and writing psychological reports* (6th ed.). New York: Guilford Press.

Psychological Testing by Models of Cognitive Ability

A. Lynne Beal, John O. Willis, *and* Ron Dumont

Abstract

Intelligence has been conceptualized as both a general ability (*g*) and as multiple abilities. These two views have been the basis for several theories of cognitive abilities. Derived from those theories, models of cognitive functioning have formed the basis of recent tests of intelligence and component abilities. This chapter maps the CHC theory, Luria theory and Cross-Battery approaches and models of cognitive abilities onto the most recent tests of cognitive ability. By understanding the abilities measured by cognitive tests, practitioners can better appraise the strengths and needs of the clients they assess. Reviews of recent tests guide practitioners in choosing the most appropriate tests and subtests to measure their client's abilities as they relate to learning disabilities, giftedness, and intellectual disability.

Key Words: cognitive, ability, assessment, models, theory, learning disabilities, intelligence, gifted, mental retardation, review

Introduction

Knowledge about human cognitive abilities has evolved over the years based upon a variety of theories of cognitive functioning. With this knowledge have come the desire and then the need to actually assess those abilities thoroughly and accurately. This evolution from theory to practice is described from an historical perspective in the Greenberg, Lichtenberger, and Kaufman chapter (Chapter 2) in this book (2012). Willis, Dumont, and Kaufman (2011) traced the factor-analytic models of intelligence from their theoretical roots to the specific models upon which modern-day intelligence tests have been built. These two chapters provide excellent theoretical underpinnings to understanding how models of cognitive ability link to cognitive ability tests.

A large body of research literature shows that IQ scores predict many important variables, including academic achievement test scores, grades, job performance, occupation and social status, and income

(Brody, 1997; Jensen, 1998; Schmidt, 2002). Because results from a cognitive assessment are often required for the identification of individuals with intellectual disability (mental retardation), learning disabilities, or intellectual giftedness (American Psychiatric Association [APA], 2000; Individuals with Disabilities Education Act, 2004; National Research Council, 2002; Rosa's Law, 2010), intelligence test batteries are considered essential tools in the fields of psychology and education, and in particular in special education. They are among the most frequently used assessment instruments in clinics, schools, and forensic settings (Camara, Nathan & Puente, 2000; Rabin, Barr, & Burton, 2005; Ryba, Cooper, & Zapf, 2003). According to Belter and Piotrowski (2001), intelligence test batteries were considered by psychology training directors to be essential for practice.

The purpose of this chapter is to link various models of cognitive ability, described elsewhere in this volume, to several of the intelligence test batteries that are currently in use in psychological practice. Given the plethora of tests available, it is possible to include in this short chapter only a very few of actual tests available. As Floyd, Clark, and Shadish (2008) discovered when they searched the Buros Institute of Mental Measurements' *Test Reviews Online* website (http://www.unl.edu/buros) looking for tests that assessed "intelligence and general aptitude," there were no fewer than 250 published instruments to choose from.

The tests discussed in this chapter are those that seem most relevant and useful in the diagnosis of broad cognitive abilities and are commonly used by psychologists, school psychologists, and educational specialists. Some of the tests incorporate in their structure the major models described in this chapter. The chapter ends with short reviews of several individual tests of cognitive ability that are often used today. The historical roots and the derivations of the models underlying these tests will not be reiterated here. Our assumption is that, by understanding the various broad theories of cognitive functioning across the lifespan and the functional models—the actual tests—that are derived from those theories, practitioners and researchers can better understand the abilities and human functions that current cognitive ability tests measure. Indeed, as Flanagan, Ortiz, Alfonso, and Mascolo (2006) have suggested, application of theory to the assessment of learning disabilities (LD) is perhaps one of the most significant advances necessary if LD assessment is to improve and become more reliable and valid. This understanding enables practitioners and researchers to rely on the results of cognitive ability tests, to integrate the results of different tests, to combine those test results with other sources of information, and to draw conclusions about cognitive strengths and deficits, and their implications for education, careers and other daily activities of the people they assess.

The second purpose of this chapter is to link the current tests of cognitive abilities based on the various models to the practice of diagnosis and the determination of eligibility for special services. We will focus on the diagnosis and identification of learning disabilities using the definition of "learning disability" in the United States from the Individuals with Disabilities Education Act (IDEA; 2004), and in Canada using the Learning Disabilities Association of Canada definition (2003). We will focus on the diagnosis of developmental delay using the definition of "mental retardation" from the *Diagnostic*

and Statistical Manual IV-TR (American Psychiatric Association, 2000). We will focus on the identification of gifted students based on overall intellectual level. The significance of assessment as a means to identify and to develop interventions for children with disabilities is evident in the United States in the passage of multiple legislative acts safeguarding children's rights. One of the most important of those laws is the Individuals with Disabilities Education Act (IDEA, 2004), under which children with identified disabilities must be provided free appropriate public education (FAPE), often through direct services provided as special education. IDEA defines "special education" as specially designed instruction to meet the unique needs of children with disabilities at no cost to parents. To be eligible, children must demonstrate impairments in areas (e.g., academic, cognitive, physical, behavioral) that interfere with their ability to learn from the general education curriculum. IDEA thus mandates that states evaluate all children suspected of having a disability, including young children not yet enrolled in schools, to determine whether they are eligible to receive early intervention or special education services. According to the IDEA, "evaluation" means procedures used to determine eligibility for special education services. States are required to conduct multidisciplinary comprehensive assessments when determining eligibility for special education services under IDEA. There is, of course, a difference between the constraints and special considerations imposed by IDEA (2004) on *identification* of a disability when one is evaluating school-aged children and the guidelines for a *diagnosis* by, for example, the criteria of the *Diagnostic and Statistical Manual* (DSM-IV-TR) (American Psychiatric Association, 2000). While federal regulations provide general guidelines in regard to identification and classification, states have considerable flexibility in how they interpret and institute policies and practices in definitions, classification criteria, assessment processes, and other considerations (Bergeron, Floyd, & Shands, 2008; Reschly & Hosp, 2004).

In Canada, the definition of "learning disabilities" can vary greatly, depending upon whose definition one is working under. The definition offered by the Learning Disabilities Association of Canada (2003) has not been universally adopted by ministries of education within the various provinces. Ministries and advocacy groups promote their own consensus-based definitions within each province (Kozey & Siegel, 2008). Definitions within Canadian educational settings are often related more to the need for special education, rather than the specific diagnostic criteria for any disorder or disability. Nonetheless, the Ontario Ministry of Education, for example, has adopted the opinion of the Expert Panel on Literacy and Numeracy Instruction for Students with Special Education Needs that notes, "knowledge about a student's strengths and weaknesses in cognitive processing helps teachers provide appropriate instruction and accommodations for children in their classrooms" (Ministry of Education, 2005, retrieved from http://www.edu.gov.on.ca/eng/document/reports/speced/panel/speced.pdf)

A diagnosis of a specific learning disability or of intellectual disability is not always necessary to access special education services in schools because there are, at least in the United States, 13 categories of disability under which a child might be eligible, and under IDEA, a child does not have to be labeled with any particular disability, although most states require a specific identification. Nonetheless, cognitive ability tests are frequently used in assessments of students seeking services. We focus in this chapter on current tests of cognitive ability for children and adults, including promising developments in group tests of cognitive ability related to specific models.

Models of Intelligence and Component Abilities

Since scores on various intelligence tests are correlated with each other, people who do better than average on one test tend to do better than average on another. The same is true of school grades and many other measures of human performance. The idea that these correlations are due to a single "general factor of intelligence," which has come to be called g, was originally proposed by Charles Spearman at the turn of the twentieth century (Spearman, 1904, 1927). Researchers interested in human cognitive abilities responded to the difficulties of the one-general-factor theory (such as obviously disparate strengths and weaknesses in an individual) by developing models with *multiple* unobserved factors. In the multiple-factor models, the bulk of the correlations between tests are attributed to a leading common factor, still called g. However, the smaller but non-negligible correlations left after accounting for g are attributed to other, lesser factors. The reality and importance of g are retained because g accounts for so much of the correlations among the tests.

In contrast to the focus on g, L. L. Thurstone (viz., 1926, 1931), developed and applied techniques of factor analysis to emphasize several separate mental abilities established by clusters of subtests that correlated with each other in addition to correlating with the total, and more than they correlated with other subtests in other clusters. Thurstone's (1938) theory of *primary mental abilities* offered an alternative to Spearman's g.

Borrowing McKusick's (1969) terms, we can differentiate between these approaches by describing advocates of theories and models based on the concept of one overall level of "intelligence" or g as "lumpers"; and proponents of theories based on a set of several separate abilities as "splitters." Reference to g and correlations of the split-off, or component abilities, to the lump or general ability factor have been studied extensively, largely through factor-analytical studies. We will find in the models of cognitive ability and the more recent tests based on these models that splitting has become a more important feature, while retaining the importance of the lump, or measure of overall cognitive ability.

As for the separate abilities, Carroll (1993, p. 8) provides a thoughtful definition that is first dependent on the definition of *cognitive task* as "any task in which correct or appropriate processing of mental information is critical to successful performance." A *cognitive ability* is "any ability that concerns some class of cognitive tasks, so defined." Finally, he defines a *cognitive process* as "one in which mental contents are operated on in order to produce some response."

The history of intelligence testing can be characterized as a quest for two outcomes: (1) to provide reliable measures of g, or general intellectual ability; and (2) to catalogue and measure the critical cognitive abilities embodied within g. Greenberg et al. trace that history in Chapter 2 in this volume through the role of theory in psychological assessment. Willis et al. (2011) trace the history through factor-analytic models of intelligence. Over the years the varying theories and models have resulted in different numbers of cognitive abilities being identified and validated. John Carroll's (1993) landmark meta-analysis of factor-analytic studies is the best existing compilation and analysis of the cognitive abilities. He reanalyzed 461 data sets from a collection of about 1,500 studies using exploratory factor analysis to present extensive data in the domains of language, reasoning, memory and learning, visual perception, auditory reception, idea production, cognitive speed, knowledge and achievement, psychomotor abilities, miscellaneous domains of ability and personal characteristics, and higher-order factors of cognitive ability (1993, p. v). Raymond Cattell (e.g., 1941, 1963, 1987; Cattell & Horn, 1978) and his student and colleague, John Horn (e.g., 1988, 1991, 1994; Horn & Blankson, 2005), developed a theory of fluid (Gf) and crystallized (Gc) abilities, to which other abilities were later added. Carroll's work was remarkably congruent with that of Cattell and Horn, which provided the foundation for the development of the Cattell-Horn-Carroll (CHC) Theory of Cognitive Ability (Flanagan, McGrew, & Ortiz, 2000; McGrew, 2005; McGrew & Woodcock, 2001; Woodcock, 1990, 1993, 1997).

Constructs of cognitive abilities, cognitive processes, cognitive tasks, and g from psychological science have found their way into the nomenclature for the diagnosis of cognitive disorders and disabilities. The definition of *mental retardation* (American Psychiatric Association, 2000) refers to "significantly sub-average intellectual functioning." There must also be deficits in adaptive behavior and onset before adulthood. A wide range of subtest scores with some in the average range, despite a significantly sub-average total, is problematic, especially for splitters. The definition of *learning disability* in Canada (2002) refers to "average abilities essential for thinking and/or reasoning," and "global intellectual deficiency." It goes on to include "impairments in one or more processes related to perceiving, thinking, remembering or learning. These include, but are not limited to: language processing, phonological processing; visual spatial processing, processing speed; memory and attention; and executive functions (e.g. planning and decision-making)." In the United States, the definition of a *specific* learning disability in the 2004 Individuals with Disabilities Education Act (IDEA) statute, 20 USC 1401, Section 603 (3) is as follows:

(A) IN GENERAL.—The term "specific learning disability" means a disorder in 1 or more of the basic psychological processes involved in understanding or in using language, spoken or written, which disorder may manifest itself in the imperfect ability to listen, think, speak, read, write, spell, or do mathematical calculations. (B) DISORDERS INCLUDED.—Such term includes such conditions as perceptual disabilities, brain injury, minimal brain dysfunction, dyslexia, and developmental aphasia. (C) DISORDERS NOT INCLUDED.—Such term does not include a learning problem that is primarily the result of visual, hearing, or motor disabilities, of mental retardation, of emotional disturbance, or of environmental, cultural, or economic disadvantage.

Nowhere in the IDEA definitions and descriptions does it specifically name the "basic psychological processes" that might be impaired. Indeed a 1990 letter from the Office of Special Education Programs, quoted in McBride, Dumont & Willis, 2011 (pp. 89–90) indicates that the U.S. federal law and regulations do not require documentation of a processing disorder. Still, there is nothing in the final 2006 Regulations for the IDEA that would prohibit an evaluation team from requesting assessments of psychological processing,

Despite the lack of any clear definition, and no requirement to actually assess for the "disorder," states are allowed to impose their own understanding of these terms based on the congressional definition and to require adherence to those guidelines as an additional burden on eligibility groups. Models of intellectual abilities that include separate cognitive abilities seem to offer some candidates for processes to evaluate.

Flanagan and Mascolo (2005) present an operational definition of *learning disability* that includes "analysis of cognitive ability." Their rationale for the model includes the concept that a significant ability–achievement discrepancy need not be present to establish a learning disability (Siegel, 1999; Stanovich, 1999), primarily because different ability measures will result in different discrepancies (either significant or non-significant) for different reasons (p. 22).

Effective diagnosis of these disabilities as defined through cognitive abilities relies on tests that provide effective measures of these cognitive abilities and processes. Cognitive ability tests that have evolved along with theories and models of cognitive ability are integral to the diagnoses of these disorders. This chapter will focus on those models and their utility for understanding people's abilities and impairments, and diagnosing learning disabilities, and developmental delay. Current individual tests of cognitive ability will be evaluated within the models.

Intelligence as Overall Ability or g

According to Hale and Fiorello (2004) (who believe "that IQ overemphasis is one of the major problems in psychology practice" [p. 18]), researchers such as Jensen (1998), Gottfredson (1997), and Herrnstein and Murray (1994) have asserted that general intelligence (g) is the single most important predictor of important life outcomes such as academic success, job attainment, income level, and the likelihood of incarceration. Despite its importance, there is still a lack of an accepted definition for the construct of *intelligence*. Sattler (2008, p. 223) provides a list of

Table 19.1 Cognitive Ability Tests and the Name Given to the Global Score

Test	Name of Global Score
Cognitive Assessment System	Full Scale
Differential Ability Scales–II	General Conceptual Ability
Insight	Insight Ability Index
Kaufman Assessment Battery for Children–II	Fluid Crystallized or Mental Processing Index
Kaufman Brief Intelligence Test–II	IQ Composite
Leiter International Performance Scale–R	Full Scale Quotient
Reynolds Intelligence Assessment Scales	Composite Intelligence Index
Stanford Binet–5	Full Scale IQ
Wechsler Scales	Full Scale IQ
Woodcock-Johnson III	General Intellectual Ability

19 different definitions that have been suggested over the years by several of the major experts in the field of psychology. The lack of a single, accepted definition of intelligence has further contributed to many disagreements about how to actually assess intelligence (or intelligences, as the case may be). Without agreement on the definition of intelligence—and even on whether IQ exists—it is no wonder that there is little agreement on how to measure intelligence. For information about the major theories of intelligence that have influenced testing, see Anastasi and Urbina (1997); Carroll (1993); Eysenck vs. Kamin (1981); Flanagan, Genshaft, and Harrison, (1997); Gould (1981); Kaufman (2009), McGrew & Flanagan (1998, Chap. 1), Sattler (2008, Chap. 7); and Woodcock (1990), among many others.

As shown in Table 19.1, because there has not been a single, agreed-upon definition of intelligence, cognitive ability measures have themselves utilized many different names for the global constructs or abilities they purport to measure. The choice of a measure of intellectual functioning in a particular setting, such as school or clinic, and for a particular child, adolescent, or adult may have much to do with the individual evaluator's definition and understanding of intelligence or intellectual functioning. Consequently, it is important for the evaluator to adopt or develop an explicit theory of intellectual functioning and reflect on the possible consequences of that theory in evaluating and reaching conclusions about the client.

Many of the current cognitive ability tests have their roots primarily as measures of g. Examples include the

Stanford-Binet Intelligence Scale (e.g., Form L and M, Terman, 1960)); and the early Wechsler scales (WISC, Wechsler, 1949), and the Wechsler-Bellevue Intelligence Scale (Wechsler, 1939).

Several intellectual ability tests, such as the Reynolds Intellectual Assessment Scales (RIAS; Reynolds & Kamphaus, 2003, 2005), are explicitly designed to assess g; for example, "general intelligence and its two primary components, fluid and crystallized intelligence" (Reynolds & Kamphaus, 2003, p. iv). The RIAS would be ideal for the evaluator who believes that intellectual functioning is a matter of g, including only or primarily fluid (Gf) and crystallized (Gc) abilities (see, for example, Cattell & Horn, 1978). [The RIAS also includes a separate verbal and visual memory scale.]

Components of g as Multiple Abilities

Many current cognitive ability tests are structured on different conceptualizations of intellectual functioning, placing less emphasis on g and more emphasis on the multiple indexes tapping various levels of processing. For example, the Differential Ability Scales (DAS-II, Elliott, 2007a) includes only verbal ability, nonverbal (fluid) reasoning, and spatial ability in its total, general conceptual ability (GCA) score. Although other important abilities are assessed with the "diagnostic" subtests and clusters, these do not influence GCA score (Elliott, 2007b; Dumont, Willis, & Elliott, 2008). The fifth edition of the Stanford-Binet (SB5; Roid, 2003a,b) divides intellectual functioning into verbal and nonverbal domains, within which it assesses fluid reasoning, knowledge, quantitative reasoning, visual/spatial ability, and working memory (including nonverbal knowledge and verbal visual/spatial ability).

The Wechsler scales (WISC-IV; Wechsler, 2003; WPPSI-III; Wechsler, 2002; WAIS-IV; Wechsler, 2008) are based on Wechsler's famous definition of intelligence: "the capacity of the individual to act purposefully, to think rationally, and to deal effectively with his environment" (1944, p. 3). However, over the years, through various editions, these scales have gradually given greater emphasis to separate index scores, expanding from the original verbal and performance IQ scales to current verbal comprehension, perceptual reasoning, working memory, and processing speed index scores. Although the Wechsler scales are not explicitly based on CHC theory, these indices more or less correspond to the CHC broad abilities of crystallized ability, fluid reasoning and visual/spatial thinking, short-term memory, and processing speed, respectively.

Further cognitive ability tests have been developed based on cognitive theories that have multiple abilities in the model. They are discussed within the context of their models later in this chapter.

Table 19.2 provides a summary of the design characteristics of several cognitive assessment batteries. The table shows that an evaluator has many options for how to assess the concept of intelligence. The test batteries in Table 19.2 assess cognition using various numbers of measures (tests or subtests) that range from a single test like the TONI-4 to tests incorporating up to 31 tests or subtests like the WJ III, including the Diagnostic Supplement. The overall global scores (called different things by different tests, e.g., FSIQ, GIA, GAI, GCA, FCI, MPI), can include as few as one subtest or as many as 14 subtests.

Models of Intelligence as Multiple Abilities

The developments of many of the older cognitive ability tests and the more recently developed tests have largely moved toward models that describe intelligence as multiple abilities. For example, Wechsler (2008) describes the evolution of the Wechsler Adult Intelligence Scale–IV from its early roots considering intelligence to be a *global* entity characterizing behavior as a whole, as well as *specific* because it is composed of elements or abilities that are at least partly distinct from each other. More recent versions of the Wechsler intelligence scales have enhanced the measurement of more discrete domains of cognitive function. The author's evidence for support of a theoretical basis in the Wechsler scales is the appearance of the same or similar subtests in other measure of intelligence, as well as the high correlation of Wechsler Intelligence Scales with other measures of cognitive ability (Wechsler, 2008, pp. 2–4). Other tests, such as the Woodcock-Johnson Tests of Cognitive Ability, the Kaufman Assessment Battery for Children, and the Cognitive Assessment System have been developed through models of cognitive ability based on cognitive theory.

The next section presents the major theoretical models of cognitive ability and the tests developed within the models, including CHC theory and the Luria model. Cross-battery assessment (XBA) provides a framework for making optimal use of components of tests to assess the range of cognitive abilities subsumed by CHC theory. For each of the tests we describe the component abilities and revisit the overall *g* score as the composite or weighted average of the component abilities.

CHC Theory

"CHC" stands for "Cattell-Horn-Carroll," a synthesis of the research and theoretical model of Cattell and Horn with those of Carroll. CHC theory is one of the most widely recognized current theories of intellectual abilities (e.g., Alfonso, Flanagan, and Radwan, 2005; McGrew, 2005; Sternberg & Kaufman, 1998), although its application to test construction and interpretation is also subject to criticism (e.g., Frazier & Youngstrom, 2007). For a history of the development of CHC theory as it relates to theories and models of intelligence, see the Greenberg, Lichtenberger and Kaufman Chapter 2 in this volume; Flanagan, Ortiz, and Alfonso (2007); McGrew (2005); and Willis, Dumont, and Kaufman (2011).

CHC theory focuses on the measures of broad (stratum II) abilities as well as the narrow (stratum I) abilities within each broad ability. Carroll (1993, 1997/2005) strongly emphasized the importance of a third stratum (*g*) at the top of the hierarchy. Horn (1994; Horn & Blankson, 2005) emphatically did not. Assessments that utilize the CHC theory focus primarily on the broad abilities since they have been linked to the kinds of processing deficits that are integral to definitions of learning disabilities. The narrow abilities, while important in CHC theory, are described as individual subsets of the broad abilities, and thus less emphasis is placed upon them. Several books have been written that are useful in understanding how the individual subtests of many intelligence and achievement tests can be classified by the broad ability and even by narrow abilities they

Table 19.2 CHC Broad and Narrow Abilities and Cognitive Tests That Assess Them

The information in this table is provided only as a guide to the publications cited above and ***cannot stand alone***. You *must* use the essential references listed below to understand CHC theory and apply it to the McGrew, Flanagan, & Ortiz's Integrated Cattell-Horn-Carroll Cross-Battery Approach. Most of the examples of tests for various narrow abilities below are taken from those sources and from Mather & Woodcock (2001a; 2001b) and McGrew & Woodcock (2001). They are only a few examples of the many given in Alfonso's, Flanagan's, Mascolo's, Mather's, McGrew's, and Ortiz's cited texts. Tests in (parentheses) are secondary measures of the narrow ability and a primary measure of some other narrow ability. Tests or procedures marked with "?" are our guesses. The information on significant relationships between other CHC abilities and reading and math achievement are taken from Flanagan and Ortiz (2001, pp. 50–51); Flanagan, McGrew, and Ortiz (2000, p. 286), Flanagan, Ortiz, and Alfonso (2007), Flanagan, Ortiz, Alfonso, and Mascolo (2006), and McGrew and Flanagan (1998, p. 422), where there are also in-depth discussions of this issue, including the basis in research.

Broad Abilities	Narrow Abilities
Fluid Intelligence Gf Fluid reasoning. Problem-solving tasks that are not automatic. Often considered the essence of g. Glr and Gsm (MW) are probably essential components. I and RG "play a moderate role in reading comprehension.... [and] are consistently very important at all ages" in math achievement (Flanagan & Ortiz, 2000, p. 50). We suspect that first encounters with new, generally non-Gf tasks have a Gf component that wears off quickly.	*General Sequential Reasoning (RG)* (a.k.a. deductive reasoning) WJ III Analysis-Synthesis; (WJ III Planning); KAIT Logical Steps; LIPS-R Picture Context, Visual Coding; SB5 Nonverbal Fluid Reasoning & Verbal Fluid Reasoning. *Induction (I)* WJ III Concept Formation; LIPS-R, Classification, Design Analogies, Repeated Patterns, Sequential Order; Raven's & other matrix tests (DAS II Matrices, Wechsler Matrix Reasoning); WISC-IV & WPPSI-IV Picture Concepts; KABC-II Pattern Reasoning & Story Completion. *Quantitative Reasoning (RQ)* WJ III Applied Problems; (WJ III Quantitative Concepts); WJ III DS Number Matrices & Number Series; Wechsler Arithmetic; DAS II Seq., & Quant. Reasoning; SB:IV Equation Building, Number Series, Nonverbal Quant. Reasoning, & Verbal Quant. Reasoning *Speed of Reasoning (RE)* LIPS-R Attention Divided?
Crystallized Intelligence Gc Largely verbal intelligence; not only one's knowledge of one's culture, but also one's ability to apply that knowledge effectively. This *is* a *cognitive* ability. Most LD tests also measure VL and vice versa. Although most oral, verbal tests are classified under Gc, some clearly involve more reasoning (Gf?) than others. LD, VL, and LS are important [for reading and math achievement] at all ages. These abilities become increasingly … important with age" (Flanagan & Ortiz, 2001, p. 50). Obviously, Gc abilities are also very important for writing and for achievement in content-area subjects. Many Gc abilities are covered better by the tests used in speech and language evaluations that by those used in psychoeducational evaluations.	*Language Development (LD)* WJ III COG Verbal Comprehension; Wechsler Comprehension., Similarities; *Lexical Knowledge (VL) (vocabulary)* WJ III Verbal Comprehension; WJ III DS Bilingual Verbal Comp.; DAS-II Word Definitions, Naming Vocabulary; most vocabulary tests; KABC-II Expressive Vocabulary, Riddles, & Verbal Knowledge; SB5 Verbal Knowledge; Wechsler Similarities, Vocabulary, & Word Reasoning, WPPSI-IV Picture Naming & Receptive Vocabulary; *Listening Ability (LS)* General (verbal) Information (K0) WJ III COG General Information; Wechsler Information *Information about Culture (K2)* KAIT Famous Faces; K-ABC Faces & Places

(continued)

Table 19.2 (Continued)

Broad Abilities	Narrow Abilities
Visual Processing Gv Our favorite definition of Gv is Richard Woodcock's "fluent thinking with images that are visual in the mind's eye." Gv does include simple, perceptual, visual processing tasks, but it also includes higher-level cognitive reasoning and problem-solving. There might be some real merit to separating the two. Gv "may be important primarily for higher- level or advanced mathematics (e.g., geometry, calculus)" (Flanagan & Ortiz, p. 50). My experience is that students with much stronger Gv than Gc abilities use the Gv abilities in unexpected ways, sometimes maladaptively. Weaknesses in Gv can impair mental visualization (sometimes interfering with reading comprehension) and nonverbal communication. Visual Memory (MV) is a Gv narrow ability, not Gsm.	*Spatial Relations (SR)* WJ III COG Spatial Relations; Wechsler Block Design; DAS-II Pattern Construction; LIPS Figure Rotation; (WPPSI-IV Object Assembly); KABC-II Triangles; SB5 NV Visual-Spatial Processing; KM/R/NU Geometry
	Visual Memory (MV) DAS-II Recall of Designs, Recognition of Pictures; KAIT Memory for Block Designs; LIPS-R Immediate Recognition; Forward Memory; KABC-II Face Recognition; visual subtests in many memory batteries; WISC-IV Integrated Spatial Span?; WPPSI-IV Picture memory and Zoo Locations?
	Visualization (Vz) WJ III COG Spatial Relations; DAS-II Matching Letter-Like Forms; LIPS-R Matching, Form Completion; Paper Folding; (Wechsler Block Design; DAS-II Pattern Construction; LIPS Figure Rotation); KABC-II Block Counting, Conceptual Thinking, Pattern Reasoning, & Story Completion; SB5 Verbal Visual-Spatial; WJ III DS Block Rotation
	Closure Speed (CS) [target is not known in advance] WPPSI-IV Object Assembly; KABC-II Gestalt Closure; WJ III DS Visual Closure
	Flexibility of Closure (CF) [target is known in advance] LIPS-R Figure-Ground; Wechsler Picture completion
	Spatial Scanning (SS) WJ III COG Planning; KABC-II Rover; WISC-IV Integrated Elithorn Mazes
Auditory Processing Ga "Phonetic coding (PC) or 'phonological awareness/ processing' is very important [to reading development] during the elementary school years" (Flanagan & Ortiz, 2001, p. 50). Phonological abilities and Rapid Automatized Naming [Glr (NA)] are, of course, the hot topics in reading assessment. Even more fundamental sound discrimination and perception issues are important for neuropsychological assessment. The ability to hear clearly under less-than-ideal circumstances is very important for school functioning. See your friendly, local audiologist.	*Phonetic Coding: Analysis (PC:A)* WJ III COG Incomplete Words; DAS-II Phonological Processing
	Phonetic Coding: Synthesis (PC:S) WJ III COG Sound Blending; DAS-II Phonological Processing
	Speech Sound Discrimination (US) WJ III COG Auditory Attention; WJ III DS Sound Patterns-Music, & Sound Patterns-Voice
	Resistance to Auditory Stimulus Distortion (UR) WJ III COG Auditory Attention
	Musical Discrimination & Judgment (U1, U9) WJ III DS Sound Patterns-Music
Short-Term Memory Gsm Although this ability is very important in its own right and because of its contribution to Gf, I don't think it has been sorted out adequately. You note that visual memory is classified under Gv, not Gsm. MS "is	*Memory Span (MS)* DAS-II Recall of Digit Forward; WJ III COG Memory for Words; WJ III DS Memory for Sentences; Wechsler Digit Span forward; SB5 Nonverbal Working Memory & Verbal Working Memory; KABC-II Hand Movements, Number Recall, & Word Order; WISC-IV Integrated Spatial Span?

(continued)

Table 19.2 (Continued)

Broad Abilities	Narrow Abilities
important [for reading and math] especially when evaluated within the context of working memory" (Flanagan & Ortiz, 2001, p. 50). Weaknesses in working memory seem to be very significant for writing. It is an irony that those who need to memorize "math facts" or spelling rules because they cannot afford to be distracted while working are learning them.	*Working Memory (MW)* DAS-II Recall of Digit Backward, Recall of Sequential Order; Wechsler Digit Span backward; WJ III Numbers Reversed & Auditory Working Memory; Wechsler Letter-Number Sequencing; WISC-IV Arithmetic
	Learning Abilities (L1) (also in Glr) "A number of factors…specific to particular kinds of learning situations and memory ….Not clearly defined by existing research" (McGrew & Flanagan, 1998, p. 35). For example, speed of relearning material after other tasks, e.g., WJ III COG Visual-Auditory Learning-Delayed?
Long-Term Storage and Retrieval Glr The issue here is the storage *and* retrieval. Glr is how information gets into Gc. Glr seems to be very important for Gf. "Naming Facility (NA) or 'rapid automatic naming' is very important [for reading] during the elementary school years. Associative Memory (MA) may be somewhat important at select ages (e.g., age 6)" (Flanagan & Ortiz, 2001, p. 51). Weaknesses in both Ga (PC) and Glr (NA) constitute the "double-deficit" pattern of dyslexia that is receiving much current attention. The definition of NA seems to have shifted usefully from category naming to item naming. Lack of fluency in recalling "math facts" can be a serious hindrance to math achievement.	*Associative Memory (MA)* WJ III COG Visual-Auditory Learning & Visual-Auditory Learning-Delayed; WJ III DS Memory for Names & Memory for Names-Delayed; LIPS-R Delayed Recognition, Associated Pairs, Delayed Pairs; KABC-II Atlantis, Atlantis Delayed, Rebus & Rebus Delayed; KAIT Rebus and Rebus Delayed; various paired-associates learning tasks
	Meaningful Memory (MM) WJ III Visual-Auditory Learning & Visual-Auditory Learning-Delayed); (LIPS-R Associated Pairs, Delayed Pairs)
	Free Recall Memory (M6) DAS-II Recall of Objects
	Ideational Fluency (FI) WJ III COG Retrieval Fluency
	Associational Fluency (FA) WJ III COG Retrieval Fluency; KTEA-II Associational Fluency
	Naming Facility (NA) WJ III Rapid Picture Naming
	Sensitivity to Problems (SP) Wechsler Comprehension?
Processing Speed Gs "Attentive speediness" (McGrew & Flanagan, 1998, p. 44). Gs can be critical in allowing mental processes to be carried out within the limits of memory capacity. "Perceptual	*Perceptual Speed (P)* WJ III COG Visual Matching, Pair Cancellation; WJ III DS Cross Out; Wechsler Symbol Search; Wechsler Cancellation; LIPS-R Attention Sustained; DAS-II Speed of Info. Processing A, Rapid Naming

(continued)

Table 19.2 (Continued)

Broad Abilities	Narrow Abilities
speed(P) abilities are important [for reading and math] during all school years…"(Flanagan & Ortiz, p. 51).	*Rate of Test Taking (R9)* (WJ III Visual Matching); (WISC-IV Symbol Search); WAIS-IV Digit Symbol-Coding; Wechsler Coding; WPPSI-IV Bug Search; (LIPS-R Attention Sustained)
	Number Facility (N) WJ III Decision Speed; WJ III Math Fluency; DAS-II Speed of Information Processing B & C

Notes:

See Flanagan, Ortiz, and Alfonso (2007) for the most up-to-date advice on how to apply this information. When you simply average subtests, you get a different result than the total score for the same subtests from the norms of a test. There are two reasons for this: First, normative total scores are more extreme than the average of their parts, just as it is more unusual to excel (or do very poorly) at all ten events in the decathlon than at only one event. Second, when tests are combined, the one(s) with the largest standard deviation(s) carry more weight than the one(s) with the smaller standard deviation(s). People notice this effect most often on the WJ III because it uses standard scores for both (sub)tests and totals. However, you will see these effects on any test with subtests and total scores, not just the WJ III. If you are using only one test, you should, of course, use the total scores provided. If you are mixing tests, it might be best to be consistent and create your factor scores by averaging in every case, even when normative total scores are available from some groupings.

Flanagan, McGrew, and Ortiz (2000), Flanagan, Ortiz, and Alfonso (2007), and McGrew and Flanagan (1998) recommend translating all scores into standard scores with a mean of 100 and standard deviation of 15 [they, Sattler (2008), Willis & Dumont (2002), and others provide tables for this conversion, and there is a handy downloadable score-conversion program at http://alpha.fdu.edu/psychology/]. They recommend using a confidence band of ± 7 points for subtests and ± 5 points for totals. If the bands overlap, the total can probably be accepted as a reasonable summary of that ability for that examinee. If they do not overlap, the total is questionable. If the gap between confidence bands is wider than the narrowest band, the narrow abilities very probably cannot be summarized by the total [Flanagan, McGrew, & Ortiz (2000); Flanagan, Ortiz, & Alfonso (2007), and McGrew & Flanagan (1998)]. See also Elliott (2007b). However, scores may fluctuate for reasons other than genuine strengths and weaknesses and normal measurement error. Pay attention to reality! Consider test conditions, your observations, and the student's background when you make your interpretations (O'Neill, 1995).

This information is derived from detailed explanations in Appendix A in D. P. Flanagan, S. O. Ortiz, and V. C. Alfonso, (2007) *Essentials of cross-battery assessment* (2nd ed.) (New York: Wiley); from Table 2.1, pp. 32–41, in D. P. Flanagan, K. S. McGrew, and S. O. Ortiz (2000), The *Wechsler Intelligence Scales and Gf-Gc theory: A contemporary approach to interpretation* (Boston: Allyn & Bacon); and from Figure 1.1, p. 7, in D. P. Flanagan and S. O. Ortiz (2001) *Essentials of cross-battery assessment* (New York: Wiley) which were slightly changed from Table 1–1, pp. 15–19, in K. S. McGrew, and D. P. Flanagan (1998), The *Intelligence Test Desk Reference (ITDR): Gf-Gc cross-battery assessment* (Boston: Allyn & Bacon). "Most all definitions were derived from Carroll [J. B. Carroll (1993) *Human cognitive abilities: A survey of factor-analytic studies* (Cambridge, Eng.: Cambridge University Press)]. Two-letter factor codes (e.g., RG) are from Carroll (1993a). Information in this table was adapted from McGrew [K. S. McGrew (1997), Analysis of the major intelligence batteries according to a proposed comprehensive Gf-Gc framework. In D. P. Flanagan, J. L. Genshaft, & P. L. Harrison (1997), *Contemporary intellectual assessment: Theories, tests, and issues* (New York: The Guilford Press)] with permission from Guilford Press" (Flanagan, McGrew, & Ortiz, 2000, p. 41). See also Flanagan, Ortiz, Alphonso, and Mascolo, (2002) *Achievement Test Desk Reference (ATDR): Comprehensive assessment and learning disability* (Boston: Allyn & Bacon) and D. P. Flanagan, S. O. Ortiz, V. C. Alfonso, and J. T. Mascolo (2006) *Achievement Test Desk Reference (ATDR-II): A guide to learning disability identification* (2nd ed.) (Hoboken, NJ: Wiley).

tap (Flanagan and Harrison, 2005; Flanagan, Ortiz and Alfonso, 2007; Flanagan, Ortiz, Alfonso, and Mascolo, 2006; and McGrew and Flanagan, 1998). Some classifications were made by factor-analytic research, while others are made on the basis of surveys of expert opinion. The following definitions are brief summaries of syntheses compiled by Willis, Dumont, and Kaufman (2011) drawing very heavily on presentations in Carroll (1993); Flanagan and McGrew (1997); Flanagan, McGrew, and Ortiz (2000); Flanagan, Ortiz, and Alfonso, 2007; Flanagan, Ortiz, Alfonso, and Mascolo (2006); McGrew, 1997; and McGrew and Flanagan (1998).

Gf: fluid intelligence, refers to inductive, deductive, and quantitative reasoning with materials and processes that are new to the person doing the reasoning.

Gc: crystallized intelligence, refers to the application of acquired knowledge and learned skills to answering questions and solving problems presenting at least broadly familiar materials and processes.

Gv: or visual-spatial thinking, involves a range from fairly simple visual perceptual tasks to higher level, visual, cognitive processes.

Ga: auditory processing, involves tasks such as recognizing similarities and differences between sounds; recognizing degraded spoken words, such as words with sounds omitted or separated; and mentally manipulating sounds in spoken words.

G*s: processing speed* or *attentional speediness*, refers to measures of clerical speed and accuracy, especially when there is pressure to maintain focused attention and concentration.

G*t: decision/reaction time or speed*, reflects the immediacy (quickness) with which an individual can react to and make a decision about (decision speed) typically simple stimuli.

G*sm: short-term or immediate memory*, refers to the ability to take in and hold information in immediate memory and then to use it within a few seconds. Gsm is divided in current CHC formulations into memory span (MS) and working memory (MW) with a distinction between simple recall (MS) and mental manipulation of material held in short-term memory (MW).

G*lr: long-term storage and retrieval*, involves the efficiency of memory storage and retrieval over longer periods of time than Gsm.

G*rw: includes reading and writing.*

G*q: quantitative knowledge,* is distinct from the quantitative reasoning that is a narrow ability within G*f*.

For complete definitions and explanations, please see the above references, especially the most recent Flanagan, Ortiz, and Alfonso (2007) and Flanagan, Ortiz, Alfonso, and Mascolo (2006) and the Cross-Battery Assessment website (http://www.crossbattery.com/).

Those last two broad abilities (G*rw* and G*q*) in CHC theory challenge the traditional distinction between "academic achievement" and "intellectual ability," which is implicitly or explicitly a central component to many definitions of specific learning disability. Carroll (1993, p. 510) recommends that we "conceptualize a continuum that extends from the most general abilities to the most specialized types of knowledges." Flanagan, Ortiz, Alfonso, and Mascolo (2002, p. 21) quote both Carroll ("It is hard to draw the line between factors of cognitive abilities and factors of achievement. Some will argue that *all* cognitive abilities are in reality learned achievements of one kind or another" [emphasis in the original; 1993, p. 510]) and Horn ("Cognitive abilities are measures of achievements, and measures of achievements are just as surely measures of cognitive ability" [1988, p. 655]). Flanagan, Ortiz, Alfonso, and Mascolo similarly conclude, "Thus, rather than conceiving of cognitive abilities and academic achievements as mutually exclusive, they may be better thought of as lying on an ability continuum that has the most general types of abilities at one end and the most specialized types of knowledge at the other (Carroll, 1993)."

Given the various definitions of specific learning disabilities, and within those definitions specific language about "processing," researchers have attempted to show some logical link between a child's area of processing deficit and the deficits in areas of academic achievement. Tables summarizing the recent literature on the relationship between CHC cognitive abilities and specific academic abilities are provided in Flanagan and Mascolo (2005, p. 353) and are updated in Flanagan, Alfonso, Mascolo and Sotelo-Dynega (2012, pp. 656–662).

CHC theory is the basis for many instruments, or is at least acknowledged in the test manuals, Adherents to the Cattell-Horn-Carroll model of intelligence (Carroll, 1997, 2005; Flanagan, Ortiz, & Alfonso, 2007; Horn & Blankson, 2005; McGrew & Flanagan, 1998; Woodcock, 1990) would probably include in an assessment of intellectual functioning all stratum II broad abilities: fluid reasoning, crystallized ability, spatial thinking, long-term storage and retrieval, short-term memory, auditory processing, and processing speed. A single instrument designed to assess this wide array of abilities, such as the Woodcock-Johnson III (Woodcock, Schrank, McGrew, & Mather, 2007a) might be used, or the evaluator might choose to assemble a battery of tests and subtests to measure all of the desired abilities, performing the Cross-Battery Assessment developed by Kevin McGrew and Dawn Flanagan and still being expanded and refined by Dawn Flanagan, Samuel Ortiz, and Vincent Alfonso. The most recent formulations of the cross-battery approach may be found in Flanagan, Ortiz, and Alfonso (2007) and at the "official website of the CHC Cross-Battery approach" (http://www.crossbattery.com/). The cross-battery approach is a subject of lively debate: see, e.g., Floyd (2002); Ortiz and Flanagan (2002a, 2002b); Watkins, Glutting, and Youngstrom (2002); and Watkins, Youngstrom, and Glutting (2002).

Table 19.3 shows the CHC broad abilities measured in recent editions of the Wechsler Scales, the Woodcock-Johnson III Tests of Cognitive Ability and Diagnostic Supplement, the Stanford-Binet–V, the Differential Ability Scales–II, and the Kaufman Assessment Battery for Children–II. These charts show that not all of these tests measure all of the CHC abilities, and not all of the processing abilities within the definition of "learning disability" of the Learning Disabilities Association of Canada. In addition to these tests, CHC theory has been applied in the development of Insight (Beal, 2011),

Table 19.3 CHC Abilities as Measured by Frequently Used Individual Tests of Cognitive Ability

CHC Ability	WJ III	DAS II	Wechsler Scales	KABC-II	SB-V
Fluid Intelligence	Concept Formation	Matrices	Similarities	Pattern Reasoning	Object Series
(Gf)	Analysis Synthesis	Sequential & Quantitative Reasoning	Picture Concepts	Story Completion	Matrices
	Number Matrices	Picture Similarities	Matrix Reasoning		Early Reasoning
		Early Number Concepts	Figure Weights		Verbal Absurdities
					Verbal Analogies
Crystallized Intelligence	Verbal Comprehension	Verbal Comprehension	Vocabulary	Expressive Vocabulary	Procedural Knowledge
(Gc)	General Information	Word Definition	Comprehension	Riddles	Picture Absurdities
		Verbal Similarities	Information	Verbal Knowledge	Vocabulary
		Naming Vocabulary	Similarities		
			Receptive Vocabulary		
			Picture Naming		
			Word Reasoning		
Short-Term Memory	Numbers Reversed	Recall of Sequential Order	Digit Span	Number Recall	Delayed Response
(Gsm)	Memory for Words	Recall of Digits Backward	Letter-Number Sequencing	Word Order	Block Span
		Recall of Digits Forward	Arithmetic	Hand Movements	Memory for Sentences
					Last Word
Visual Processing	Spatial Relations	Copying	Block Design	Block Counting	Form Board
(Gv)	Picture Recognition	Recall of Designs	Picture Completion	Conceptual Thinking	Form Patterns
	Visual Closure	Pattern Construction	Object Assembly	Face Recognition	Position and Direction
	Block Rotation	Recognition of Pictures	Visual Puzzles	Rover	
		Matching Letter-Like Forms		Triangles	

(continued)

Table 19.3 (Continued)

				Gestalt Closure	
Auditory Processing	Sound Blending	Phonological Processing			
(Ga)	Auditory Attention				
	Sound Patterns—Voice				
	Sound Patterns—Music				
Long-Term Retrieval	Visual-Auditory Learning	Recall of Objects— Immediate	Vocabulary	Atlantis	
(Glr)	Retrieval Fluency	Recall of Objects— Delayed	Information	Rebus	
	Memory for Names			Atlantis Delayed	
				Rebus Delayed	
Processing Speed	Visual Matching	Rapid Naming	Coding		
(Gs)	Decision Speed	Speed of Information Processing	Symbol Search		
	Rapid Picture Naming		Cancellation		
	Pair Cancellation				
	Cross Out				
Quantitative Reasoning	Number Series		Arithmetic		Quantitative Reasoning
(Gq)	Number Matrices				

WJ III: Woodcock Johnson-III Tests of Cognitive Abilities classifications are from McGrew, R. W., Schrank, F. A., & Woodcock, R. W. (2007), *Technical manual. Woodcock-Johnson III normative update.* Rolling Meadows, IL: Riverside Publishing.

DAS II classifications are from Dumont, Willis, & Elliott (2008).

Wechsler classifications are from Alfonso, Flanagan, & Radwan (2005), Flanagan & Kaufman (2004), Lichtenberger & Kaufman (2009).

KABC-III classifications are from Kaufman, A. S., & Kaufman, N. L.. (2004), *KABC-II manual.* Circle Pines, MN: AGS Publishing.

SB-V classifications are from Nelson Education catalogue, available at http://www.assess.nelson.com/test-ind/stan-b5.html.

a group-administered cognitive abilities test for school-aged children, normed in Canada.

CHC theory works well within a diagnostic context. The general ability (stratum III) measure of *g* provides an overall level for establishing developmental delay. The CHC broad abilities map well onto the processing deficits linked to the diagnosis of "learning disability" as defined by the Learning Disability Association of Canada (2003). From their definition, phonological processing is measured by G*a*, auditory processing; memory and attention are measured by G*lr*, long-term storage and retrieval, and by G*sm*, short-term memory; processing speed is measured by G*s*, processing speed; language processing is measured by G*c*, crystallized ability; and visual-spatial processing is measured by G*v*, visual processing. Note that G*f*, fluid reasoning, is not considered to be a process, but stands alone as integral to establishing a learning disability, distinct from a more global developmental delay.

Further practical uses for the CHC model include linking cognitive strengths and weaknesses to skills integral to vocations and careers. While not exhaustive, the range of abilities measured provides a broad scope and a common language for discussing abilities.

Luria Theory

Alexander Luria presented his theory of brain organization and function in 1970. He described the basic building blocks of intelligence as *functional units*, which he believed were the basic cognitive processes that provide the "ability" to perform certain acts, each of which is distinctive in character. He postulated that the human brain can be considered to be made up of three main blocks incorporating basic functions. The first block regulates the energy level and tone of the cortex for organization of its various processes. Located particularly in the reticular formation, which controls wakefulness, it is responsible for selectivity of cortical actions and of normal discrimination of stimuli. These functions are referred to as arousal and attention. Block 2 plays a decisive role in the analysis, coding and storage of information. Located in the rear of the cortex, these areas include the occipital, parietal, and temporal lobes. Block 3 is involved in the formation of intentions and programs for behavior, referred to as executive functions of planning and programming behavior. Located in the frontal lobes, the functions serve primarily to activate the brain and regulate attention and concentration. Luria stressed that brain functions in the three blocks are integrated, and must work together for normal cognitive functioning. Yet, disruptions in each of the blocks will disrupt behavior in different ways. With this specificity, the Luria model is well suited as the basis for the development of cognitive ability tests for diagnostic purposes (Kaufman, Lichtenberger, Fletzer-Jantzen, & Kaufman, 2005; Kaufman & Kaufman, 2004; Luria, 1970).

The Kaufman Assessment Battery for Children (KABC (1983) and the Kaufman Assessment Battery for Children, Second Edition (KABC-II, 2004) operationalized the Luria model in tests of cognitive ability for children. Under the Luria model, the KABC-II examines four broad areas of cognitive ability: learning ability; sequential processing; simultaneous processing; and planning ability (Kaufman & Kaufman, 2004; Kaufman et al., 2005). When combined, these scales yield a total score called the Mental Processing Index. Note that crystallized knowledge is not a component of the Luria model.

Naglieri and Das developed the Planning, Attention, Simultaneous and Sequential theory of intelligence (PASS; e.g. Das, Kirby, & Jarman, 1979; Naglieri & Das, 2002; 2005). The theory proposes that planning, attention, simultaneous, and successive cognitive processes are the basic building blocks of human intellectual functioning. Within the Luria model, attention occurs within Block 1; simultaneous and successive processing occur within Block 2; and planning occurs within the executive functions of Block 3. The theory proposes that these four basic processes are interrelated and interact with person's knowledge base (Naglieri, 1999). While all PASS processes are involved in all human activities, sometimes one or more processes will dominate an activity. Naglieri and Das's (1997) Cognitive Assessment System (CAS) "is built strictly on the Planning, Attention, Simultaneous, and Successive (PASS) theory" (Naglieri, 2005, p. 441). Table 19.4 shows how the Luria model is operationalized in the KABC-II and the CAS for assessing children's cognitive abilities.

The KABC-II was also developed to fit within CHC theory (Kaufman & Kaufman, 2004). Under this model, the scales are called Short-Term Memory (G*sm*), Visual Processing (G*v*), Long-Term Storage and Retrieval (G*lr*), and Fluid Reasoning (G*f*), and a fifth scale (Knowledge or Crystallized Ability (G*c*) is added to complete the Fluid-Crystallized Index (Kaufman & Kaufman, 2004a, p. 2).

Since the KABC- II was developed to fit within both the Luria model and CHC theory (Kaufman & Kaufman, 2004), each subtest is classified by the block within the Luria model, and also by the broad ability within CHC theory. Subtests of other tests of cognitive ability might be mapped onto the Luria model, showing the block that each one measures through the linkage provided between the Luria model and CHC theory by Kaufman and Kaufman (2004). Subtests that are confirmed to measure G*lr* would measure Block 1, arousal and attention. Subtests that are confirmed to measure G*sm* would

Table 19.4 Processes of Luria Neuropsychological Model in the Kaufman Assessment Battery for Children–II and Cognitive Assessment System, Shown with CHC Classification.

			KABC-II	CAS
Block 1				
Arousal and Attention	**Learning Ability**	**Glr**	Atlantis	Expressive Attention
	Attention	**Long-Term Retrieval**	Rebus	Number Detection
		and Storage	Atlantis Delayed	Receptive Attention
			Rebus Delayed	
Block 2				
Use of Senses to	**Sequential**	**Gsm**		
Analyze, Code, and Store		**Short-Term Memory**	Number Recall	Word Series
Information			Word Order	Sentence Repetition
			Hand Movements	Speech Rate
				Sentence Questions
	Simultaneous	**Gv**	Block Counting	Nonverbal Matrices
		Visual Processing	Conceptual Thinking	Verbal-Spatial Relations
			Face Recognition	Figure Memory
			Rover	
			Triangles	
			Gestalt Closure	
Block 3				
Executive and Planning	**Planning**	**Gf**	Pattern Reasoning	Matching Numbers
Functions		**Fluid Reasoning**	Story Completion	Planned Codes
				Planned Connections
		Gc*	Expressive Vocabulary	
		Crystallized Knowledge	Riddles	
			Verbal Knowledge	

* The KABC-2 includes tests of crystallized knowledge that are not included in the Mental Processing Index for the Luria Model

measure sequential processing, and subtests that are confirmed to measure G*v* would measure simultaneous processing in Block 2, analyzing, coding and storing information. Subtests that are confirmed to measure G*f* would measure planning in Block 3, executive and planning functions.

Tests such as the KABC-II and the CAS, based on the Luria model, work well within a broader assessment battery for diagnostic purposes. The KABC-II was designed to be a clinical and psychological instrument, and to identify process integrities and deficits for assessment of individuals with specific learning disabilities (Kaufman, Kaufman, Kaufman-Singer, & Kaufman, 2005). The KABC-II's Mental Processing Index and the CAS's Full Scale each provide an overall measure of g that does not include G*c* crystallized knowledge. As such, they present less of a cultural demand than do *g* measures from cognitive ability tests that include G*c* and language abilities in their composite scores. Differences between scores of African-American and Euro-American students are notably smaller on the CAS (3.5 points' difference for Full Scale), and KABC-II (5 points' difference on the MPI and 6.5 points' difference on the FCI, even with the G*c* measure included) than on other comprehensive cognitive ability tests in current use (Kaufman & Kaufman, 2004; Kaufman et al, 2005; Naglieri & Das, 1997; Naglieri, 2005). This could be an important consideration for choosing the KABC-II MPI to assess an African American child in situations where the overall *g* level is important for determining eligibility for services. The KABC-II MPI or CAS Full Scale could also be a better measure of *g* for students with hearing impairments, who showed the lowest scores on the Knowledge/G*c* scale in a validation study (Kaufman et al., 2005). The same rationale would hold for the assessment of students with language impairment. This would have the effect of eliminating from the overall score an area of cognitive function that is reduced by the cultural difference or by the sensory disorder. Specific uses might be in qualification for gifted education or eligibility for programs for students with developmental disability.

For the diagnosis of learning disabilities, the Luria model measures processing deficits that are integral to the definitions of LD. For example, tests like math calculations may be heavily weighted toward planning functions, while reading decoding tasks may be heavily weighted toward successive processing (Naglieri, 1999). Children with reading disabilities generally evidenced average Planning, Attention and Simultaneous scores, but

low Successive scores (Naglieri, 2005). Research has revealed correlations between PASS measures and various aspects of educational achievement and has provided evidence that profiles of PASS abilities can be used for planning instruction (e.g., Naglieri & Johnson, 2000).

While LD definitions do not refer explicitly to Block 1, 2, and 3 processes, or specifically to sequential, simultaneous, and planning processes, these processes are easily linked through CHC theory to the processes in the definitions of LD. Processes that are not measured by the Luria model, such as G*c* crystallized knowledge and auditory phonemic awareness and processing speed, can be measured using other cognitive ability tests, under a cross-battery approach.

Further information on the applications of the Luria model for diagnostic purposes is provided in books and articles on interpreting the KABC-II and the CAS. Notably, *The Essentials of KABC-II Assessment* (Kaufman et al, 2005) has a chapter on clinical applications that addresses assessment of children with various characteristics and disabilities. *The Essentials of CAS Assessment* (Naglieri, 1999) also has a chapter on clinical applications.

Cross-Battery Assessment

In 1997, Flanagan and McGrew developed the CHC (Cattell-Horn-Carroll) Cross-Battery approach to intellectual testing. They stated that an intelligence battery ought to be able to measure the full range of broad cognitive abilities that define the structure of intelligence (McGrew & Flanagan, 1998, p. 356). While crossing or mixing tests in a neuropsychological or cognitive assessment was not a new concept, the cross-battery approach arose primarily out of the finding that none of the major intelligence batteries adequately measured the full range of important G*f*-G*c* abilities according to contemporary theory and research. The Woodcock-Johnson III (Woodcock, McGrew, & Mather, 2001a, 2007) was explicitly designed to assess all of the CHC abilities.

There are three "pillars" to this approach (Flanagan, & Ortiz, 2001; Flanagan, Ortiz & Alfonso, 2007, pp. 22–29; McGrew & Flanagan, 1998). Pillar 1 is the Cattell-Horn-Carroll Theory of Cognitive Ability, providing a relatively complete taxonomic framework for describing the structure and nature of cognitive abilities. Horn (1998) and others have likened this to a Periodic Table of the Elements for cognitive psychology. Pillar 2 is the CHC broad (stratum II) classifications of cognitive and achievement tests. Pillar 3 is the CHC narrow (stratum II) classifications of cognitive and achievement tests.

The classifications of current cognitive ability tests according to CHC theory have been published in various volumes (including Flanagan & Ortiz, 2001; Flanagan, Ortiz & Alfonso, 2007, and Flanagan, Ortiz, Alfonso & Mascolo, 2002; Flanagan, Ortiz, Alfonso & Mascolo, 2006; McGrew & Flanagan, 1998). Our updated summary, drawn from these sources, is in Table 19.3. Whether or not a practitioner or theorist agrees with CHC theory and the classifications, this approach represents a major step in linking cognitive ability subtests to a theory and model for more uniform interpretation.

The Cross-Battery Assessment model is implemented through a series of planned and sequential steps (Flanagan & Ortiz, 2001; Flanagan, Ortiz & Alfonso, 2007). Essentially, an examiner selects the primary intelligence battery for the assessment, notes the adequately represented CHC abilities and processes that are included; and then selects additional tests to measure the CHC abilities processes not measured by the primary battery. Guidelines are provided in the sources listed above and at the Cross-Battery Assessment website (http://www.crossbattery.com/) to assist the examiner in determining the adequacy of specific test's representation of the CHC abilities, and suggested testing procedures to utilize when measures of a broad ability are not consistent.

A similar template for crossing test batteries using Luria theory or any other theory of cognitive ability could be developed by classification of subtests according to that theory.

The cross-battery approach works well for the diagnosis of learning disabilities, particularly in Canada, where academic achievement deficits must be logically linked to deficits in underlying cognitive processes. This approach has also been linked to instructional, environmental, and assessment accommodations for students when underlying processing deficits are known to exist (Elementary Teachers' Federation of Ontario, 2007; Weiss, Beal, Saklofske, Packiam Alloway, & Prifitera, 2008).

The remainder of this chapter presents an updated review of several of the tests that assess the broad and narrow abilities within CHC theory.

Choosing the Model and Test to Best Assess the Client

Choosing the tests for a battery to assess a client should begin with the referral question. As discussed in this chapter, the model upon which the test is built, and the psychometric characteristics of the test for similar populations, will help guide the evaluator to an appropriate choice. The following test descriptions are meant to be a source of general information regarding each test to assist the evaluator in making a good choice for each client.

Cognitive Assessment System

The Cognitive Assessment System (CAS; Naglieri & Das, 1997a; see also Naglieri, 1999; Naglieri & Das, 1997b, 2005) is an individually administered test of cognitive ability for children ages 5 years through 17 years and 11 months. The test includes 12 subtests, and can be administered in two forms. The Standard battery consists of all 12 subtests, while the Basic battery is made up of 8 subtests. Standard scores are provided for all subtests, with a mean of 10 and a standard deviation of 3. The four scales, along with the Full Scale score, are reported as standard scores with a mean of 100 and a standard deviation of 15.

The CAS is based on the PASS model (Das, Kirby, & Jarman, 1975; Naglieri & Das, 2005), which is derived in part from Luria's theories (e.g., 1966, 1973, 1980). The model is represented by four scales representing Planning, Attention, Simultaneous, and Successive cognitive processes (PASS). *Planning* is the ability to conceptualize and then apply the proper strategies to successfully complete a novel task. The individual must be able to determine, select, and then use a strategy to efficiently solve a problem. *Attention* is a cognitive process by which an individual focuses on one cognitive process while excluding extraneous competing stimuli. *Simultaneous* processing is the integration of stimuli into a coherent whole. *Successive* processing involves organizing various things into a specific sequential order. A Full Scale score can also be obtained from the data.

Examiners who find Luria's theories especially helpful and examiners seeking a test structure and content different from Wechsler, Binet, and Cattell-Horn-Carroll formulations may find the CAS useful, especially when the PASS theory is most likely to answer the specific referral questions for a particular student.

Comprehensive Test of Nonverbal Intelligence

The Comprehensive Test of Nonverbal Intelligence (CTONI; Hamill, Pearson & Wiederholt, 1997) now in its second edition as CTONI-2 (Hammill, Pearson, & Wiederholt, 2009) measures nonverbal reasoning abilities of individuals aged 6 through 89. The CTONI-2 contains no oral responses, reading, writing, or object manipulation. There are six subtests in total. Three subtests use pictured objects and three use geometric designs. Examinees indicate their answers by pointing to alternative choices. The CTONI-2 provides three composite IQ scores: Nonverbal Intelligence Quotient, Pictorial Nonverbal Intelligence Quotient, and Geometric Nonverbal Intelligence Quotient.

The CTONI-2 offers the advantage of completely non-oral administration. The lack of verbal subtests is obviously helpful for testing children with limited oral language or English language abilities, but this omission also limits the scope of the assessment. The consistent multiple-choice format can be an asset for children who have difficulty learning or shifting between tasks; but this format again limits the scope of the assessment. See also the Test of Nonverbal Intelligence, 4th edition (TONI-4; Brown, Sherbenou, & Johnsen, 2010), which is a recently normed, non-oral multiple-choice test that offers two parallel forms.

Differential Ability Scales–Second Edition

The DAS-II (Elliott, 2007a, 2007b; see also Dumont, Willis, & Elliott, 2008; Elliott, 2005; Sattler, 2008) is an individually administered measure of cognitive ability designed to measure specific abilities and assist in determining strengths and weaknesses for children and adolescents aged 2 years, 6 months, through 17 years, 11 months.

At the Upper Early Years and School-Age levels, the DAS-II is composed of 10 "core" cognitive subtests and 10 "diagnostic" subtests. Four core subtests plus most of the diagnostic subtests are used at the Lower Early Years level. The core subtests are used to calculate a high-level composite score called the General Conceptual Ability (GCA) score, and three lower-level composite scores: Verbal Ability, Nonverbal (fluid) Reasoning Ability, and Spatial Ability cluster scores. The diagnostic subtests, which yield three cluster scores: Processing Speed, Working Memory, and School Readiness, are used predominantly to assess strengths and weaknesses and do not contribute to the composite scores.

The DAS-II uses standard scores (M = 100, SD = 15) for the composite scores and T scores (M = 50, SD = 10) for the 20 individual subtests. Overlapping age ranges for the Lower Early Years (with fewer subtests and clusters), Upper Early Years, and School-Age batteries and out-of-level norms allow considerable flexibility in standardized

testing of low- and high-scoring children. Examiners who agree with Elliott that verbal, fluid reasoning, and spatial abilities are core intellectual abilities and that other important cognitive functions with lower g loadings should be measured but not included in the total score will find the DAS-II especially appealing.

Kaufman Adolescent and Adult Intelligence Test

The Kaufman Adolescent and Adult Intelligence Test (KAIT, 1993; see also Lichtenberger, Broadbooks, & Kaufman, 2000) is an individually administered measure of general intellectual ability for use with persons between the ages of 11 and 85+ years. The KAIT consists of Crystallized and Fluid Scales that yield a Composite IQ score. The Crystallized Scale, a measure of knowledge acquired through education and sociocultural experience, includes Definitions, Auditory Comprehension, Double Meanings, and an alternate subtest—Famous Faces. The Fluid Scale, primarily a measure of problem-solving ability in novel situations, comprises Rebus Learning, Logical Steps, Mystery Codes and an alternate Memory for Block Designs subtest. In addition to the Core Battery subtests, the KAIT includes memory measures that allow for interpretation of immediate and delayed recall (Rebus Delayed Recall and Auditory Delayed Recall).

Subtests use scaled scores that have a mean of 10 and a standard deviation of 3. The Fluid, Crystallized, and Composite IQ scales yield scores with a mean of 100 and a standard deviation of 15.

While the Cattell-Horn concept of fluid (Gf) and crystallized (Gc) intelligence (1966, 1967) is the predominant theory on which the KAIT is founded, the test also draws upon neuropsychological and cognitive developmental models, specifically Golden's (1981) concept of planning ability as related to pre-frontal lobe development and Piaget's (1972) highest stage of cognitive development—formal operations.

Although old, the KAIT is a very useful measure of intelligence that can be used with a variety of populations. The use of fluid and crystallized scales is consistent with the multiple factor theory of intelligence and allows for administration to people with diverse backgrounds.

Kaufman Assessment Battery for Children–Second Edition

The KABC-II (Kaufman & Kaufman, 2004a; see also see also Kaufman, Lichtenberger,

Fletcher-Janzen, & Kaufman, 2005) contains a total of 18 subtests grouped into core or supplementary tests. Subtests not only combine to produce the Global Index scores (FCI or MPI) but also yield up to four (Luria model) or five (CHC model) Indexes. These Index scores represent sequential processing/short term memory (Gsm), simultaneous processing/visual processing (Gv), learning ability/long term storage and retrieval (Glr), planning ability/fluid reasoning (Gf), and crystallized ability (Gc). This last (crystallized ability) is represented only in the CHC model. The KABC-II uses standard scores (M = 100, SD = 15) for the five scales, and the three global indexes and scaled scores (M = 10, SD = 3) for the 18 individual subtests.

There are two interpretative models: the CHC (Carroll, 1997/2005; Flanagan, Ortiz, & Alfonso, 2007; Horn & Blankson, 2005) and the Luria (1966, 1973, 1980). The core subtests have individual scaled scores and are used to compute either the CHC Fluid-Crystallized Index (FCI) or Luria Mental Processing Index (MPI), while the supplementary subtests provide expanded coverage of the abilities measured by the core KABC-II subtests and allow for the computation of a Nonverbal Index (NVI). Some examiners will welcome the option of choosing either the Luria or the CHC interpretation and the availability of a nonverbal index.

Kaufman Brief Intelligence Test, Second Edition

The KBIT-2 (Kaufman & Kaufman, 2004b; see also Homack & Reynolds, 2007) is an individually administered test of verbal and nonverbal ability for persons aged 4 through 90. The KBIT-2 consists of two scales, verbal (crystallized or Gc) and nonverbal (fluid or Gf abilities). The verbal scale is composed of two parts: Verbal Knowledge and Riddles, and the nonverbal scale contains the subtest Matrices. For Verbal Knowledge, the individual is asked to point to one of six pictures to match a vocabulary word spoken by the examiner or to answer a question of general knowledge. Riddles requires the examinee to answer oral questions that require both knowledge and logical reasoning. Matrices is a nonverbal test in which the individual looks at a sequence or pattern and then selects the one of five or six alternative pictures or abstract designs that best completes the logical pattern. The KBIT-2 provides standard scores (M = 100, SD = 15) for both the subtests and the resulting IQ Composite.

The KBIT-2 is, as stated, a brief intelligence test. Brief tests are especially valuable when an assessment is directed at broader purposes and the examiner wants to check intellectual ability as one part of the assessment.

Leiter International Performance Scale–Revised

The Leiter International Performance Scale–Revised (Leiter-R; Roid & Miller, 1997; see also Braden & Athanasiou, 2005; McCallum, Bracken, & Wasserman, 2001) is an individually administered nonverbal test designed to assess intellectual ability, memory, and attention functions in children and adolescents ages 2 years to 20 years, 11 months. The Leiter-R requires no spoken language by either the examiner or the examinee. Instructions are given by pantomime, demonstration, and facial expression.

The Leiter-R consists of two groupings of subtests: the Visualization and Reasoning (VR) Battery, consisting of 10 subtests (4 reasoning and 6 visualization-spatial), and the Attention and Memory (AM) Battery, also consisting of 10 subtests (8 memory and 2 attention).

The subtests use scaled scores (mean 10, standard deviation 3) while Brief and Full Scale IQ scores are calculated using IQ standard scores (mean 100, standard deviation 15). Composite scores can also be obtained for fluid reasoning, fundamental visualization, spatial visualization, attention, and memory. The Leiter-R is obviously especially useful for assessment of children who have difficulty understanding or using spoken English. It taps a much wider variety of CHC abilities than do most non-oral, non-reading tests.

Reynolds Intellectual Assessment Scales

The RIAS (Reynolds & Kamphaus, 2003; see also Reynolds & Kamphaus, 2005) is an individually administered test of intelligence assessing two primary components of intelligence, verbal (crystallized or Gc) and nonverbal (fluid or Gf). Verbal intelligence is assessed with two tasks (Guess What and Verbal Reasoning). Nonverbal intelligence is assessed by visual fluid reasoning and spatial ability tasks (Odd-Item Out and What's Missing). The Verbal and Nonverbal scales combine to produce a Composite Intelligence Index (CIX). A Composite Memory Index (CMX) can be derived from two supplementary subtests: Verbal Memory and Nonverbal Memory. The subtests are reported as T scores and the Indexes as standard scores (M = 100, SD = 15).

In contrast to many existing measures of intelligence, the RIAS eliminates dependence on motor coordination, visual-motor speed, and reading skills. Examiners who wish to efficiently assess intelligence through only crystallized verbal and nonverbal (fluid reasoning and visual) measures and examiners who want an accurate assessment of intelligence for an examinee with motor coordination, motor speed, or reading challenges would find the RIAS valuable for this purpose.

Slosson Intelligence Test Revised–Third Edition

The Slosson Intelligence Test Revised–Third Edition for Children and Adults (SIT-R3, 2002 with 1998 calibrated norms) provides a quick and reliable individual screening test of crystallized verbal intelligence. The SIT-R3 has minimal performance items and features embossed materials, making it one of the few effective measures of intelligence not requiring special accommodations for the visually challenged population of both children and adults. The SIT-R3 is composed of the following subtests: Vocabulary, General Information, Similarities and Differences, Comprehension, Quantitative, and Auditory Memory.

Stanford-Binet Intelligence Scale, Fifth Edition

The SB5 (Roid, 2003; see also Roid & Barram, 2004; Roid & Pomplum, 2005) is an individually administered test of cognitive abilities for ages 2 to 85. The Full Scale IQ (FSIQ) is derived from the administration of ten subtests (five verbal and five nonverbal). Subtests are designed to measure five factors: fluid reasoning, knowledge, quantitative reasoning, visual-spatial processing, and working memory. The SB5 FSIQ and five factor scores have a mean of 100 and a standard deviation of 15. Individual subtests use scaled scores with a mean of 10 and a standard deviation of 3. Results are easily interpreted within CHC theory. On the basis of his factor analysis, Canivez (2008), recommends that "interpretation of the SB-5 should focus primarily, if not exclusively, on the general, Full Scale IQ" (p. 533).

The nonverbal subtests do involve some oral language; they are not purely non-oral like the Leiter-R, UNIT, CTONI-2, or TONI-4, for example. Examiners who wish to include crystallized ability, working memory, visual-spatial ability, and separate measures of fluid reasoning and quantitative reasoning (rather than subsuming quantitative reasoning under fluid reasoning) would find the SB5 appropriately structured for their needs.

Universal Nonverbal Intelligence Test

The UNIT (McCallum & Bracken, 1998; see also McCallum & Bracken, 2005; McCallum, Bracken, & Wasserman, 2001) is an individually administered instrument designed for use with children and adolescents from age 5 years 0 months through 17 years 11 months. The UNIT measures intelligence through six culture-reduced subtests that combine to form two primary scales (Reasoning and Memory), two secondary scales (Symbolic and Nonsymbolic), and a Full Scale (FSIQ). Each of the six subtests (Symbolic Memory, Cube Design, Spatial Memory, Analogic Reasoning, Object Memory, and Mazes) is administered using eight standardized hand and body gestures, demonstrations, sample items, corrective responses, and transitional checkpoint items to explain the tasks to the examinee. The entire process is nonverbal, but it does require motor skills for manipulatives, paper and pencil, and pointing. Half of the six subtests involve memory.

Three administrations are available for use depending on the reason for referral. These are an Abbreviated Battery, containing two subtests; the Standard Battery, containing four subtests; and the Extended Battery, containing six subtests.

Wechsler Abbreviated Scale of Intelligence–Second Edition

The Wechsler Abbreviated Scale of Intelligence–Second Edition (WASI-II; Wechsler, 2011; see also Homack & Reynolds, 2007) is an individually administered test designed for individuals between 6 and 90 years of age. The WASI-II consists of four subtests: Vocabulary, Similarities, Block Design, and Matrix Reasoning, which yield a Full Scale IQ score (FSIQ-4). An estimate of general intellectual ability can also be obtained from just a two-subtest administration that includes Vocabulary and Matrix Reasoning and provides only a FSIQ-2 score. Scores can also be split into the Verbal Comprehension Index (VCI) and the Perceptual Reasoning Index (PRI). The VCI is based on Vocabulary and Similarities, while the PRI is based on Matrix Reasoning, which measures nonverbal fluid ability, and Block Design, which measures visual-spatial thinking.

Wechsler Adult Intelligence Scale

The Wechsler Adult Intelligence Scale–Fourth Edition (WAIS-IV, 2008) is an individually administered measure of intellectual ability for ages 16 to 90. The WAIS-IV contains fifteen subtests, which provide four indexes: Verbal Comprehension (VCI), Perceptual Organization (POI), Working

Memory (WMI), and Processing Speed (PSI), and a global Full Scale IQ (FSIQ). Each of these scores is a standard score with a mean of 100 and a standard deviation of 15. Each of the 15 subtests is a scaled score with a mean of 10 and a standard deviation of 3.

The Verbal Comprehension Index is composed of three subtests (Similarities, Vocabulary, and Information), with Comprehension acting as a supplemental subtest. The Perceptual Organization Index is composed of three subtests (Block Design, Matrix Reasoning, and Visual Puzzles), with Figure Weights and Picture Completion provided as supplemental subtests. The Working Memory Index is composed of Digit Span and Arithmetic, with Letter-Number Sequencing serving as a supplementary subtest. Finally, the Processing Speed Index is composed of Symbol Search and Coding, with Cancellation being the single supplementary subtest.

The *WAIS-IV Technical and Interpretive Manual* provides evidence, based upon several confirmatory factor analyses, to support the four-factor structure. However, Lichtenberger and Kaufman (2009) report on CFA analyses done by Keith in which he compared several models, including the four-factor model of the WAIS-IV and a five-factor model in line with Cattell-Horn-Carroll (CHC) model. These analyses suggest that a CHC model, with separate Gf and Gv constructs, fits the data well.

Wechsler Intelligence Scale for Children–Fourth Edition

The WISC-IV (Wechsler, 2003; see also Flanagan & Kaufman, 2009; Prifitera, Saklofske, & Weiss, 2005, 2008; Weiss, Saklofske, Prifitera, & Holdnack, 2006) is an individually administered clinical instrument for assessing the cognitive ability of children of ages 6 years 0 months through 16 years 11 months. It includes 15 subtests (10 core and 5 supplemental). The test provides a composite score (Full Scale IQ) that represents general intellectual ability, as well as four factor index scores (verbal comprehension, perceptual reasoning, working memory, and processing speed). Each of the IQs and factor indexes is reported as a standard score with a mean of 100 and a standard score of 15. The subtests on the WISC-IV provide scaled scores with a mean of 10 and a standard deviation of 3.

Three subtests compose the Verbal Comprehension Index: Similarities, Vocabulary, and Comprehension. Two supplemental verbal subtests, Information and Word Reasoning, are also available.

These subtests assess verbal reasoning, comprehension, and conceptualization.

Three subtests compose the Perceptual Reasoning Index: Block Design, Picture, Concepts, and Matrix Reasoning. Picture Completion is a supplementary subtest. These subtests measure perceptual reasoning and organization.

There are two subtests in the Working Memory Index: Digit Span and Letter-Number Sequencing. Arithmetic is a supplementary subtest, These subtests measure attention, concentration, and working memory.

There are also two subtests in the Processing Speed Index: Coding and Symbol Search. Cancellation is a supplementary subtest. These subtests measure the speed of mental and graphomotor processing.

The WISC-IV is part of the long tradition of Wechsler scales, which allow examiners to draw on a wealth of research and interpretive opinions, including their own experience with various Wechsler scales. The theoretical model underlying the current development of this version is complex, and, while there is considerable overlap with CHC theory, which is discussed in the manual, CHC theory is not the basis for the WISC-IV.

Wechsler Preschool and Primary Scales of Intelligence–Fourth Edition

The Wechsler Preschool and Primary Scales of Intelligence–Fourth Edition (WPPSI-IV; Wechsler, 2012) is an individually administered instrument that assesses cognitive functioning and global intelligence for early childhood (ages 2:6 to 7:11). The instrument can provide information pertaining to a child's cognitive strengths and weaknesses related to language, visual-perceptual skills, visual-motor integration, reasoning, and memory. The test consists of fifteen subtests (not all used at all age) that combine into three or five Primary Index Scales and three to four Ancillary Index Scales. The primary indexes include Verbal Comprehension (VCI), Visual Spatial (VSI), Fluid Reasoning (FRI), Working memory (WMI), and Processing Speed (PSI). Ancillary indexes include Vocabulary Acquisition (VAI), Nonverbal (NVI), General Ability (GAI), and Cognitive Proficiency (CPI).

The FSIQ is a general measure of global intelligence reflecting performance across various subtests within several cognitive domains. In general, the VCI contains subtests that measure the general fund of information, verbal comprehension, and degree of abstract thinking. The VSI comprises subtests that collectively assess visual-motor integration and perceptual-organizational skills. The FRI measures the child's concept formation, while the WMI assesses working memory and attention span. PSI is a measure of speed of mental processing, nonverbal problem solving, and graphomotor ability. The composite standard scores have a mean of 100 and a standard deviation of 15. Subtest scaled scores have a mean of 10 and a standard deviation of 3.

The WPPSI-IV provides continuity of format and organization with the WISC-IV and WAIS-IV.

Wechsler Nonverbal Scale of Ability

The WNV (Wechsler & Naglieri, 2006; see also Brunnert, Naglieri, & Hardy-Braz, 2008) is a cognitive ability test with non-oral administration for ages 4 years 0 months through 21 years 11 months. There are six subtests, with four (Matrices, Coding, Object Assembly, and Recognition) used for the Full Scale at ages 4 years 0 months through 7 years 11 months; and Matrices, Coding, Spatial Span, and Picture Arrangement at ages 8 years 0 months through 21 years 11 months. There are also norms for a two-subtest battery at each age range. Subtests use T scores (M = 50, SD = 10) and the IQs are standard scores (M = 100, SD =15). Administration is normally accomplished with pictorial instructions and standardized gestures. Examiners are also permitted to use standardized verbal instructions provided in six languages, and they may use a qualified interpreter to translate the instructions into other languages in advance.

The WNV is an efficient nonverbal test. The four-subtest format, using mostly subtests similar to those on other Wechsler scales, is quicker than the Leiter-R, but provides fewer subtests and abilities to analyze. The flexibility of standardized pictorial, pantomime, and verbal instructions, with a provision for additional help as dictated by the examiner's judgement, makes the WNV especially useful. The lack of overlapping norms for low-scoring older students and high-scoring younger ones can be a limitation in rare cases.

Woodcock-Johnson III Tests of Cognitive Abilities and Diagnostic Supplement

The Woodcock-Johnson III Tests of Cognitive Abilities (WJ III COG; Woodcock, McGrew, and Mather, 2001a; Woodcock, Schrank, McGrew, & Mather, 2007; see also Mather & Jaffe, 2002; Schrank & Flanagan, 2003; Schrank, Miller, Wendling, & Woodcock, 2010) is an individually administered test of abilities appropriate for ages 2 to 90. The Diagnostic Supplement (Schrank, Mather, McGrew, & Woodcock, 2003) provides supplementary subtests. The WJ III COG Tests are explicitly designed to assess a person's abilities on many specific Cattell-Horn-Carroll Gf-Gc (CHC) "cognitive factors," not just a total score or a few factors. The General Intellectual Ability (GIA) score of the WJ III is based on a weighted combination of tests that best represents a common ability underlying all intellectual performance. Examiners can obtain a GIA (Standard) score (7 tests) or a GIA (Extended) score (14 tests). Additional tests from both the Tests of Cognitive Ability and Diagnostic Supplement (Woodcock, McGrew, & Mather, 2001) can be used to further explore CHC abilities and other factors. Each of the cognitive tests represents a different broad CHC factor.

Examiners are permitted to select the tests they need to assess abilities in which they are interested for a particular person. The WJ III Tests of Cognitive Abilities provide interpretive information from 20 tests, while the Diagnostic Supplement adds 11 more.

The WJ III provides raw scores that are converted, using age- or grade-based norms, to standard scores, percentile ranks, age and grade equivalents, Relative Proficiency Index (RPI) scores and W scores (Jaffe, 2009), instructional ranges, and Cognitive-Academic Language Proficiency (CALP) levels. All score transformation is performed through the use of the computer program (WJ III Compuscore).

The Current State and Possible Future Directions of the Science and Practice of Cognitive Assessment

In 1997 Mark Daniel surveyed the current status and trends in intelligence testing. He predicted that "tests based on the psychometric-ability model probably will continue to be prominent," partly because of its basis in "decades of empirical findings.... The model is well suited to the multiple-abilities perspective that is currently popular." Daniel stressed the need to "demonstrate the practical applications and benefits of abilities in educational, occupational, and clinical settings." Without such demonstrations, Daniel predicted that users of tests would "look for tests based on alternative models" (p. 1043). (See, for example, Braden & Niebling, 2005.)

Alan Kaufman, in the chapter, "The Future of IQ Tests" (2009, pp. 287–300), anticipates that current practices will continue with updates and improvements, but that computerized IQ testing will become common and will improve. Kaufman also contemplates research and development of the "test-teach-test paradigm" (p. 298) (see, for example, Feuerstein, Feuerstein, & Gross, 1997) and increased use of improved "neuroimaging techniques…in the psychologist's office, the classroom, or the local shopping mall" (Kaufman, 2009, p. 299).

In 1998, McGrew and Flanagan described Gf-Gc theory as "the most comprehensive and empirically supported psychometric theory of intelligence, and the theory around which intelligence tests should be interpreted" (1998, pp. 30–31.) They also predicted that the use of cross-battery assessment would foster a common language or nomenclature for what specific tests and subtests measure, thus dramatically increasing the likelihood of consistent interpretation by examiners of cognitive abilities (McGrew & Flanagan, 1998). Indeed, 14 years later, the authors of many new tests have incorporated CHC theory and the cross-battery classifications of abilities into the design and development for their tests, while others have adhered more loosely to the theory (Alfonso, Flanagan & Radwan, 2005). A good example is the Stanford-Binet 5, which was designed specifically to measure five of the ten CHC broad (stratum II) factors, within the verbal-nonverbal format of the Wechsler scales (Roid, 2003), a dramatic change in a test that was designed a century ago (Binet & Simon, 1916/1980) simply to measure g with only a single, total score, until its fourth edition (Thorndike, Hagen, & Sattler, 1986).

Many modern cognitive ability tests have embraced the CHC theory, if not in their design, then in their interpretations. Continuing to establish empirical links between the specific CHC cognitive abilities and academic and vocational functioning seems critical for those using cognitive ability tests as part of the evaluation of specific learning problems. The work of CHC researchers (e.g., Evans, Floyd, McGrew, & Leforgee, 2002; Flanagan, Ortiz, Alfonso, & Mascolo, 2006; Floyd, Bergeron, & Alfonso, 2006; Floyd, Evans, & McGrew, 2003; Proctor, Floyd, & Shaver, 2005) provides models for the work that needs to be done, and their preliminary endeavors offer some important understanding of links between cognition and specific learning successes or failures. Further refinements of CHC theory will need to strike a balance between the validation of broad abilities and their component narrow abilities. We predict that these developments will continue to lead practitioners to consistent interpretation of cognitive ability tests.

There are several important, current models of intelligence that we did not address in this chapter.

Two such models are Sternberg's Triarchic Theory (e.g., Sternberg, 1997, 1995, 1999, 2005) and Gardner's Multiple Intelligences (e.g., Gardner, 1983, 2006). To date, these theories have not been operationalized as practical, formal, standardized, normed tests in common use (see Chen & Gardner, 2005). However, continued research and validation of these theories may lead to their incorporation into a much broader model for the development of cognitive ability tests, a model acknowledging more facets of human cognitive abilities than do the theories discussed here.

One cautionary question about the incorporation of multiple models into one broad theory is, "How much is too much?" Alan Kaufman, in his *IQ Testing 101* (2009), described *size*, either too small or too big, as one of the problems associated with Guilford's Structure of the Intellect (SOI) model (Guilford, 1967, 1988; Meeker, 1969, 1975). Kaufman noted that SOI would not be the theory that would turn IQ testing into a theory-based profession. "On the most basic level, it suffered from a similar problem to the one that afflicted Spearman's g theory. If one ability was too few to build a theory on, then 120 was just as clearly too many. And Guilford did not stop at 120. He kept refining the theory, adding to its complexity" (p. 52). Guilford (1988) eventually described 180 separate mental ability factors. Acknowledging the merit of these theories and incorporating them into some broader model of cognition would move cognitive theorists more into the camp of "splitters," and maybe even into "micro-splitters," raising the question of how each of these abilities might contribute to the "lump," or overall intelligence, g.

Differential weightings of abilities as they contribute to g will probably become essential building blocks for cognitive measures. Most current tests convert subtest scores to standard scores, which are then summed and converted to standard scores for the total battery. This procedure assigns the same weight to each subtest. The KABC-II (Kaufman & Kaufman, 2004), however, permits use and interpretation of two different models, a four-factor Luria model or a five-factor CHC model, so each of the four Luria factors represents 25 percent of the total Mental Processing Index or 20 percent of the total Fluid-Crystallized Index, including a knowledge/Gc factor that is not part of the Luria model.

The WJ III General Intellectual Ability score (Woodcock, McGrew, & Mather, 2001) uses computer scoring to calculate a general intellectual ability score in which each of the seven CHC factors is weighted according to its loading on the overall *g* factor (McGrew, Schrank, & Woodcock, 2007). Similar complex procedures for differential weighting may become commonplace.

As the theories grow in size, there will still be the need to link the multitude of identified abilities to educational attainment and the selection and success of vocational pursuits (Daniel, 1997). Well-validated empirical links that provide an evidence-based foundation would be required in the development of any cognitive ability tests based on such theories. As Daniel warned, the failure to demonstrate such links would send practitioners in search of other models that offered more proven practical utility for educational and vocational planning.

Although we are predicting increased emphasis on measurement of discrete cognitive abilities, not just a total score, many authorities continue to discourage the interpretation of intelligence tests much beyond evaluation of overall *g*. Abilities other than *g* should, it is argued, be measured by specific, direct assessments, not by components of intelligence tests. See, for a few examples, Canivez (2008), Livingston, Jennings, Reynolds, and Gray (2003), McDermott, Fantuzzo, and Glutting (1990), and Watkins, Glutting, and Lei (2007).

The use of cognitive ability tests in the diagnosis of learning disabilities and developmental and intellectual disabilities and the identification of gifted functioning appears to be enshrined in current diagnostic definitions and legislation on disability entitlement in the United States and in Canada. It must be noted, however, that in the United States, with the increasing push toward Response to Intervention strategies and the IDEA guidelines allowing for the identification of learning disabilities to be done based on a lack of response to empirically based interventions as part of a comprehensive assessment, the use of, or reliance on cognitive ability testing is diminishing. This change may or may not be a good thing. The dramatic shift in the practice of school psychology has required school psychologists, ready or not, to master new skills, new approaches, and new roles for the parts of their jobs involving learning disabilities assessments. Willis and Dumont (2006) argued against a system of identification that was either/or (cognitive testing OR response to intervention) and for the integration of both approaches (cognitive testing AND response to intervention). Regardless of the reasons that a cognitive assessment is chosen, when it is, the ability to reliably interpret both a general ability factor, such as *g*, and specific abilities will continue to be an essential element expected for the use of cognitive ability tests. As the range of tests available for our use increases, it will be even more important to use a classification system that easily translates test and subtest scores into meaningful statements about the person's cognitive abilities. Theories of ability as they apply to models and design of tests will continue to make the linkage from score to understanding functioning.

It is likely that cognitive ability tests will continue to be influenced strongly by CHC theory and cross-battery classification. The benefit will be ease of comparing test scores across different tests, especially when a person is tested several times across their lifespan. Several major developments for future consideration are computerized assessments and group ability tests. In the future we do expect to see computerized cognitive ability tests that are developed, standardized, and normed specifically for that administrative procedure. One such attempt at this procedure is the Computer-Optimized Multimedia Intelligence Test (COMIT; Phelps & Martin, 2000; TechMicro, 1999). This interactive computer-administered measure of general intelligence has been standardized for ages of 6 through 18 and is composed of 12 subtests that assess associative reasoning, word knowledge, visual-spatial competencies, auditory and visual memory, hypothetical-deductive reasoning, general knowledge, processing speed, and social awareness. According to the manual (TechMicro, 1999), the design of the COMIT is explicitly based on the Gf-Gc and CHC models. The COMIT seems like a valuable and certainly interesting approach to computerized cognitive assessment

With regard to group-administered ability tests, CHC theory is the basis for a new test of cognitive ability called "Insight" (Beal, 2011), developed in Canada. Insight is the first group test of cognitive ability to be based specifically on a theory of cognitive ability. Subtests were classified by CHC ability through an expert consensus study early in its development. The test administration is through a DVD to ensure accuracy of administration. This format also frees up the examiner to observe the behavior of the students who are taking the test in a group format. Validation studies have been completed with WISC-IV Canadian norms and WJ III. This group test, which provides an overall ability score as well as cluster scores and individual subtest scores, can provide practitioners with a good starting point for forming hypotheses about possible processing deficits that would warrant further assessment for the purpose of diagnosing any disability. Insight provides clearer linkages between the abilities measured by this group test and by individual tests of cognitive ability since it is based on a current theory of cognitive ability. Further developments in group tests are likely to follow specific theories and models of cognitive ability.

Future cognitive ability tests will need to keep a focus on abilities that are logically linked to specific academic functions (for the purpose of diagnosing learning disabilities), and to specific vocational functions (for the purpose of career planning). Recently, Flanagan, Alfonso, Mascolo and Sotelo-Dynega (2012, pp. 653–662) have provided an updated summary of the logical and empirical links between CHC abilities and academic achievement. Continuing validation and research on these links will inform test developers on the importance of component abilities for the different areas of the academic curriculum. Clear linkages to intervention strategies have been developed, based on this research (Elementary Teachers' Federation of Ontario, 2007; Weiss, Beal, Saklofske, Packiam-Alloway & Prifitera, 2008). Research on the most important abilities in different vocational pursuits would be useful when using cognitive ability tests for career planning. These approaches all continue to take cognitive assessment more into the splitting approach than the lumping approach.

As Daniel (1997) cautioned, the usefulness of cognitive ability tests will continue to hinge on their predictive validity. The more we know about the abilities we are trying to predict and their relationship to specific cognitive abilities, the better the science will become in areas like compensation and remediation for deficit areas.

References

Alfonso, V. C., Flanagan, D. P., & Radwan, S. (2005). The impact of the Cattell-Horn-Carroll theory on test development and interpretation of cognitive and academic abilities. In D. P. Flanagan & P. L. Harrison (Eds.), *Contemporary intellectual assessment: Theories, tests, and issues* (2nd ed.; pp. 185–202). New York: The Guilford Press.

American Psychiatric Association. (2000). *Diagnostic and statistical manual of mental disorders* (4th ed., text revision). Washington, DC: APA.

Anastasi, A., & Urbina, S. (1997). *Psychological testing* (7th ed.). Upper Saddle River, NJ: Prentice Hall.

Beal, A. L. (2011). *Insight.* Toronto, ON: Canadian Test Centre.

Belter, R. W., & Piotrowski, C. (2001). Current status of doctoral-level training in psychological testing. *Journal of Clinical Psychology, 57,* 17–726.

Bergeron, R., Floyd, R. G., & Shands, E. I. (2008). States' eligibility guidelines for mental retardation: An update and consideration of part scores and unreliability of IQs. *Education & Training in Developmental Disabilities, 43*(1), 123–131.

Binet, A., & Simon, T. (1916/1980). *The development of intelligence in children,* with marginal notes by Lewis M. Terman and Preface by Lloyd M. Dunn. Translated by Elizabeth S. Kite with an introduction by Henry Goddard. Facsimile limited edition issued by Lloyd M. Dunn. Nashville, TN: Williams Printing Co.

Braden, J. P., & Athanasiou, M. S. (2005). A comparative review of nonverbal measures of intelligence. In D. P. Flanagan & P. L. Harrison (Eds.), *Contemporary intellectual assessment: Theories, tests, and issues* (2nd ed.; pp. 557–578). New York: Guilford Press.

Braden, J. P., & Niebling, B. C. (2005). Using the joint test standards to evaluate the validity evidence for intelligence tests. In D. P. Flanagan & P. L. Harrison (Eds.), *Contemporary intellectual assessment: Theories, tests, and issues* (2nd ed.; pp. 615–630). New York: Guilford Press.

Brody, N. (1997). Intelligence, schooling, and society. *American Psychologist, 52,* 1046–1050.

Brown, L, Sherbenou, R. J., & Johnsen, S. K. (2010). *Test of nonverbal intelligence* (4th ed.). Austin, TX: Pro-Ed.

Brunnert, K. J., Naglieri, J. A., & Hardy-Braz, S. T. (2008). *Essentials of WNV assessment.* Hoboken, NJ: Wiley.

Buros Institute of Mental Measurement's *Test Review Online* website. Retrieved from: http://www.unl.edu/buros.

Camara, W. J., Nathan, J. S., & Puente, A. E. (2000). Psychological test usage: Implications in professional psychology. *Professional Psychology: Research & Practice, 3,* 141–154.

Canivez, G. L. (2008). Orthogonal higher order factor structure of the Stanford-Binet Intelligence Scales–Fifth Edition for children and adolescents. *School Psychology Quarterly, 23*(4), 533–541.

Carroll, J. B. (1993). *Human cognitive abilities: A survey of factor-analytic studies.* Cambridge, England: Cambridge University Press.

Carroll, J. B. (1997/2005). The three-stratum theory of cognitive abilities. In D. P. Flanagan, J. L. Genshaft, & P. L. Harrison (Eds.), *Contemporary intellectual assessment: Theories, tests, and issues* (pp. 122–130). New York: Guilford Press. [Also in D. P. Flanagan & P. L. Harrison (Eds.), *Contemporary intellectual assessment: Theories, tests, and issues* (2nd ed.; pp. 41–68). New York: Guilford Press.]

Cattell, R. B. (1941). Some theoretical issues in adult intelligence testing. *Psychological Bulletin, 38,* 592.

Cattell, R. B. (1963). Theory of fluid and crystallized intelligence: A critical experiment. *Journal of Educational Psychology, 54,* 1–22.

Cattell, R. B. (1987). *Intelligence: Its structure, growth, and action.* Amsterdam, The Netherlands: North-Holland.

Cattell, R. B., & Horn, J. L. (1978). A check on the theory of fluid and crystallized intelligence with description of new subtest designs. *Journal of Educational Measurement, 15,* 139–164.

Chen, J-Q., & Gardner, H. (2005). Assessment based on multiple-intelligence theories. In D. P. Flanagan, J. L. Genshaft, & P. L. Harrison (Eds.), *Contemporary intellectual assessment: Theories, tests, and issues* (pp. 77–102). New York: Guilford.

Cross-Battery Assessment website. Retrieved from http://www.crossbattery.com/

Daniel, M. H. (1997). Intelligence testing: Status and trends. *American Psychologist, 52*(10), 1038–1045.

Das, J. P., Kirby, J. R., & Jarman, R. F. (1979). *Simultaneous and successive cognitive processes.* New York: Academic Press.

Dumont, R., Willis, J. O., & Elliott, C. D. (2008). *Essentials of DAS-II assessment.* Hoboken, NJ: Wiley.

Elementary Teachers' Federation of Ontario (2007). *Special education handbook.* Toronto: Elementary Teachers' Federation of Ontario.

Elliott, C. D. (2007a). *Differential Ability Scales–Second Edition: Administration and scoring manual.* San Antonio, TX: Harcourt Assessment.

Elliott, C. D. (2007b). *Differential Ability Scales–Second Edition: Introductory and technical handbook.* San Antonio, TX: Harcourt Assessment.

Evans, J. J., Floyd, R. G., McGrew, K. S., & Leforgee, M. H. (2002). The relations between measures of Cattell-Horn-Carroll (CHC) cognitive abilities and reading achievement during childhood and adolescence. *School Psychology Review*, 31(2), 246–262.

Eysenck, H. J., & Kamin, L. J. (1981). *The intelligence controversy.* Hoboken, NJ: Wiley-Interscience.

Feuerstein, R., Feuerstein, R., & Gross, S. (1997). The learning potential assessment device. In D. P. Flanagan, J. L. Genshaft, & P. L. Harrison (Eds.), *Contemporary intellectual assessment* (ch. 16; pp. 297–313). New York: Guilford Press.

Flanagan, D. P., Alfonso, V. C., Mascolo, J. U., & Sotelo-Dynega, M. (2012). Use of ability tests in the identification of specific learning disabilities within the context of an operational definition. In D. P. Flanagan & P. L. Harrison (Eds.), *Contemporary intellectual assessment: Theories, tests, and issues* (3rd ed., pp. 643–669). New York: Guilford Press.

Flanagan, D. P., Genshaft, J. L., & Harrison, P. L. (Eds.) (1997). *Contemporary intellectual assessment: Theories, tests, and issues.* New York: Guilford Press.

Flanagan, D. P., & Harrison, P. L. (Eds.) (2005). *Contemporary intellectual assessment: Theories, tests, and issues* (2nd ed.). New York: Guilford Press.

Flanagan, D. P., & Kaufman, A. S., (2009). *Essentials of WISC-IV assessment.* Hoboken, NJ: Wiley.

Flanagan, D. P., & Mascolo, J. T. (2005). Psychoeducational assessment and learning disability diagnosis. In D. P. Flanagan & P. L. Harrison (Eds.), *Contemporary intellectual assessment: Theories, tests and issues* (2nd ed.; pp. 521–544). New York: Guilford Press.

Flanagan, D. P., & McGrew, K. S. (1997). A cross-battery approach to assessing and interpreting cognitive abilities: Narrowing the gap between practice and cognitive science. In D. P. Flanagan, J. L. Genshaft, & P. L. Harrison (Eds.), *Contemporary intellectual assessment: Theories, tests, and issues* (pp. 314–325). New York: Guilford Press.

Flanagan, D. P., McGrew, K. S., & Ortiz, S. (2000). *The Wechsler intelligence scales and CHC theory: A contemporary approach to interpretation.* Boston, MA: Allyn & Bacon.

Flanagan, D. P., & Ortiz, S. (2001). *Essentials of cross-battery assessment.* Hoboken, NJ: Wiley.

Flanagan, D. P., Ortiz, S. O., & Alfonso, V. C. (2007). *Essentials of cross-battery assessment* (2nd ed.). Hoboken, NJ: Wiley.

Flanagan, D. P., Ortiz, S. O., Alfonso, V. C., & Mascolo, J. T. (2002). *The achievement test desk reference (ATDR): Comprehensive assessment and learning disabilities.* Boston, MA: Allyn & Bacon.

Flanagan, D. P., Ortiz, S. O., Alfonso, V. C., & Mascolo, J. T. (2006). *The achievement test desk reference (ATDR): A guide to learning disability identification* (2nd ed.). Hoboken, NJ: Wiley.

Floyd, R. G., Bergeron, R., & Alfonso, V. C. (2006). Cattell-Horn-Carroll cognitive ability profiles of poor comprehenders. *Reading & Writing*, 19(5), 427–456.

Floyd, R. G., Clark, M. H., & Shadish, W. R. (2008). The exchangeability of intelligent quotients: Implications for professional psychology. *Professional Psychology: Research & Practice*, 39, 414–423.

Floyd, R. G., Evans, J. J., & McGrew, K. S. (2003). Relations between measures of Cattell-Horn-Carroll (CHC) cognitive abilities and mathematics achievement across the school-age years. *Psychology in the Schools*, 60(2), 155–171.

Frazier, T. W., & Youngstrom, E. A. (2007). Historical increase in the number of factors measured by commercial tests of cognitive ability: Are we overfactoring? *Intelligence*, 35, 169–182.

Gardner, H. (1983). *Frames of mind: The theory of multiple intelligences.* New York: Basic Books.

Gardner, H. (2006). *Multiple intelligences: New horizons.* New York: Basic Books.

Golden, C. J. (1981). *Diagnosis and rehabilitation in clinical neuropsychology.* Springfield, Ill.: Charles C Thomas.

Gottfredson, L. S. (1997). Why g matters: The complexity of everyday life. *Intelligence*, 24(1), 79–132.

Gould, S. J. (1981). *The mismeasure of man.* New York: Norton.

Guilford, J. P. (1967). *The nature of human intelligence.* New York: McGraw-Hill.

Guilford, J. P. (1988). Some changes in the structure-of-intellect model. *Educational & Psychological Measurement*, 48, 1–4.

Hale, J. B., & Fiorello, C. A. (2004). *School neuropsychology: A practitioner's handbook.* New York: Guilford Press.

Hammill, D. D., Pearson, N. A., & Wiederholt, J. L. (1997). *Comprehensive test of nonverbal intelligence.* Austin, TX: Pro-Ed.

Hammill, D. D., Pearson, N. A., & Wiederholt, J. L. (2009). *Comprehensive test of nonverbal intelligence* (2nd edition). Austin, TX: Pro-Ed.

Herrnstein, R. J., & Murray, C. (1994). *The bell curve: Intelligence and class structure in American life.* New York: Free Press.

Homack, S. R., & Reynolds, C. R. (2007). *Essentials of assessment with brief intelligence tests.* Hoboken, NJ: Wiley.

Horn, J. L. (1988). Thinking about human abilities. In J. R. Nesselroade & R. B. Cattell (Eds.), *Handbook of multivariate experimental psychology* (2nd ed.; pp. 645–685). New York: Plenum.

Horn, J. L. (1991). Measurement of intellectual capabilities: A review of theory. In K. S. McGrew, J. K. Werder, & R. W. Woodcock (Eds.), *Technical manual, Woodcock-Johnson* (pp. 197–232). Chicago: Riverside.

Horn, J. L. (1994). The theory of fluid and crystallized intelligence. In R. J. Sternberg (Ed.), *The encyclopedia of human intelligence* (pp. 433–451). New York: Macmillan.

Horn, J. L. (1998). A basis for research on age differences in cognitive abilities. In J. J. McArdle & R. W. Woodcock (Eds.), *Human cognitive abilities in theory and practice* (pp. 57–92). Mahwah, NJ: Lawrence Erlbaum.

Horn, J. L., & Blankson, N. Foundations for better understanding of cognitive abilities. (2005). In D. P. Flanagan &

P. L. Harrison (Eds.), *Contemporary intellectual assessment: Theories, tests, and issues* (2nd ed.; pp. 41–68). New York: Guilford Press.

Individuals with Disabilities Education Act of 2004 (IDEA), P. L. 108–446 118 Stat. 2647 (2004).

Individuals with Disabilities Education Act (IDEA) P.L. 108–446 118 statute, 20 USC 1401, Section 603 (3) (2004).

Jaffe, L. (2009). *Development, interpretation and application of the W score and the relative proficiency index.* (Woodcock-Johnson III Assessment Service Bulletin No. 11). Rolling Meadows, IL: Riverside Publishing. Retrieved from http://riverpub.com/products/wjIIIComplete/pdf/WJ3_ASB_11.pdf.

Jensen, A. R. (1998). *The g factor: The science of mental ability.* Westport, CT: Praeger.

Kaufman, A. S. (2009). *IQ testing 101.* New York: Springer Publishing.

Kaufman, A. S., & Kaufman, N. L. (1983). *The Kaufman Assessment Battery for Children.* Circle Pines, MN: American Guidance Service.

Kaufman, A. S., & Kaufman, N. L. (1993). *Kaufman Adolescent and Adult Intelligence Test.* Circle Pines, MN: American Guidance Service.

Kaufman, A. S., & Kaufman, N. L. (2004). *The Kaufman Assessment Battery for Children* (2nd ed.). Circle Pines, MN: American Guidance Service.

Kaufman, A. S., & Kaufman, N. L. (2004). *KABC-II manual.* Circle Pines, MN: AGS Publishing.

Kaufman, A. S., & Kaufman, N. L. (2004b). *Kaufman Brief Intelligence Test* (2nd ed.).Upper Saddle River, NJ: Pearson.

Kaufman, J. C., Kaufman, A. S., Kaufman-Singer, J., & Kaufman, N. L. (2005). The Kaufman Assessment Battery for Children (2nd ed.). In D. P. Flanagan, & P. L. Harrison, (Eds.), *Contemporary intellectual assessment: Theories, tests, and issues* (2nd ed.; pp. 344–370). New York: Guilford Press.

Kaufman, A. S., Lichtenberger, E. O., Fletcher-Janzen, E., & Kaufman, N. L. (2005). *Essentials of KABC-II assessment.* Hoboken NJ: Wiley.

Kozey, M., & Siegel, L. S. (2008). Definitions of learning disabilities in Canadian provinces and territories. *Canadian Psychology/Psychologie Canadienne [Special Issue: Literacy Development in Canada],* 49(2), 162–171.

Learning Disabilities Association of Canada (2003). LD defined: Official definition of learning disabilities. Retrieved from http://www.ldac-acta.ca/learn-more/ld-defined/official-definition-of-learning-disabilities.html.

Lichtenberger, E. O., Broadbooks, D. Y., & Kaufman, A. S. (2000). *Essentials of cognitive assessment with KAIT and other Kaufman measures.* Hoboken, NJ: Wiley.

Lichtenberger, E. O., & Kaufman, A. S. (2009). *Essentials of WAIS-IV assessment.* Hoboken, NJ: Wiley.

Livingston, R. B., Jennings, E., Reynolds, C. R., & Gray, R. M. (2003). Multivariate analyses of the profile stability of intelligence tests: High for IQs, low to very low for subtest analyses. *Archives of Clinical Neuropsychology, 18,* 487–508.

Luria, A. R. (1966). *Human brain and psychological processes.* New York: Harper & Row.

Luria, A. R. (1970, March). The functional organization of the brain. *Scientific American, 222,* 66–78.

Luria, A. R. (1973). *The working brain.* New York: Basic Books.

Luria, A. R. (1980). *Higher cortical functions in man* (2nd ed.). New York: Basic Books.

Mather, N., & Jaffe, L. (2002). *Woodcock-Johnson III: Recommendations, reports, and strategies.* New York: Wiley.

Mather, N., & Woodcock, R. M. (2001a). Examiner's manual. *Woodcock-Johnson III Tests of Achievement.* Itasca, IL: Riverside Publishing.

McBride, M. M., Dumont, R., & Willis, J. O. (2011), *Essentials of IDEA for assessment professionals.* New York, NY: John Wiley & Sons.

McCallum, R. S., & Bracken, B. A. (1998). *The Universal Nonverbal Intelligence Test.* Chicago: Riverside.

McCallum, R. S., & Bracken, B. A. (2005). The Universal Nonverbal Intelligence Test, a multidimensional measure of intelligence. In D. P. Flanagan & P. L. Harrison, (Eds.), *Contemporary intellectual assessment: Theories, tests, and issues* (2nd ed.; pp. 425–440). New York: Guilford Press.

McCallum, R. S., Bracken, B. A., & Wasserman. J. (2001). *Essentials of nonverbal assessment.* New York: Wiley.

McDermott, P. A., Fantuzzo, J. W., & Glutting, J. J. (1990). Just say no to subtest analysis: A critique on Wechsler theory and practice. *Journal of Psychoeducational Assessment, 8,* 290–302.

McGrew, K. S. (1997). Analysis of the major intelligence batteries according to a proposed comprehensive Gf-Gc framework. In D. P. Flanagan, J. L. Genshaft, & P. L. Harrison (Eds.), *Contemporary intellectual assessment: Theories, tests, and issues* (pp. 151–180). New York: Guilford Press.

McGrew, K. S. (2005). The Cattell-Horn-Carroll theory of cognitive abilities. In D. P. Flanagan & P. L. Harrison (Eds.), *Contemporary intellectual assessment: Theories, tests, and issues* (2nd ed.; pp. 136–181). New York: Guilford Press.

McGrew, K. S. (n.d.) What does the WAIS-IV measure? CHC analysis and beyond. Available at http://www.slideshare.net/iapsuych/waisivchreport1. Accessed March, 2011.

McGrew, K. S., & Flanagan, D. P. (1998). *The intelligence test desk reference (ITDR) Gf-Gc cross-battery assessment.* Boston, MA: Allyn & Bacon.

McGrew, K. S., Schrank, R. A., & Woodcock, R. W. (2007). *Technical Manual. Woodcock-Johnson III Normative Update.* Rolling Meadows, IL: Riverside Publishing.

McGrew, K. S., & Woodcock, R. W. (2001). *Technical manual. Woodcock-Johnson III.* Itasca: IL: Riverside Publishing.

McKusick, V. A. (1969) On lumpers and splitters, or the nosology of genetic disease. *Perspectives in Biology & Medicine,* 12(2), 298–312.

Meeker, M. N. (1969). *The structure of intellect: Its interpretation and uses.* Columbus, OH: Charles E. Merrill.

Meeker, M. N. (1975). *Glossary for SOI definitions.* El Segundo, CA: SOI Institute.

Naglieri, J. A. (1999). *Essentials of CAS assessment.* Hoboken, NJ: Wiley.

Naglieri, J. A. (2005). The cognitive assessment system. In D. P. Flanagan & P. L. Harrison (Eds.), *Contemporary intellectual assessment: Theories, tests, and issues* (2nd ed.; pp. 441–460). New York: Guilford Press.

Naglieri, J. A., & Das, J. P. (1997a). *Cognitive Assessment System.* Itasca IL: Riverside.

Naglieri, J. A., & Das., J. P. (1997b) *CAS interpretive handbook.* Itasca IL: Riverside.

Naglieri, J. A, & Das, J. P. (2002). Practical implications of general intelligence and PASS cognitive processes. In R. J. Sternberg & E. L. Grigorenko (Eds.), *The general factor of intelligence: How general is it?* (pp. 855–884). New York: Erlbaum.

Naglieri, J. A, & Das, J. P. (2005). Planning, attention, simultaneous, successive (PASS) theory. In D. P. Flanagan, & P. L. Harrison (Eds.), *Contemporary intellectual assessment: Theories, tests, and issues* (2nd ed.; pp. 120–135). New York: Guilford Press.

Naglieri, J. A., & Johnson, D. (2000). Effectiveness of a cognitive strategy intervention to improve math calculation based on the PASS theory. *Journal of Learning Disabilities, 33,* 591–597.

National Research Council. (2002). *Mental retardation: Determining eligibility for Social Security benefits.* Washington, DC: National Academies Press.

Nelson Education website: Stanford-Binet Intelligence Scales, Fifth Edition. Retrieved from http://www.assess.nelson.com/test-ind/stan-b5.html.

Ontario Ministry of Education (2005). *Education for all: The report of the expert panel on literacy and numeracy instruction for students with special education needs, kindergarten to grade 6.* Retrieved from http://www.edu.gov.on.ca/eng/document/reports/speced/panel/speced.pdf.

Ortiz, S. O., & Flanagan, D. P. (2002a). Cross-battery assessment revisited: Some cautions concerning "Some Cautions" (Part I). *Communiqué, 30*(7), 32–34.

Ortiz, S. O., & Flanagan, D. P. (2002b). Cross-Battery Assessment revisited: Some cautions concerning "Some Cautions" (Part II). *Communiqué, 30*(8), 36–38.

Piaget, J. (1972). Intellectual evolution from adolescence to adulthood. *Human Development, 15*(1), 1–12.

Phelps, L., & Martin, N. (2000). *The Computer-Optimized Multimedia Intelligence Test technical manual* (COMIT). New York: TechMicro.

Prifitera, A., Saklofske, D. H., & Weiss, L. G. (2005). *WISC-IV clinical assessment and intervention.* Burlington, MA: Academic Press

Prifitera, A., Saklofske, D. H., & Weiss, L. G. (2008). *WISC-IV clinical assessment and intervention* (2nd ed.). San Diego, CA: Academic Press.

Proctor, B. E., Floyd, R. G., & Shaver, R. B. (2005). Cattell-Horn-Carroll broad cognitive ability profiles of low math achievers. *Psychology in the Schools, 42*(1), 1–12.

Rabin, L. A., Barr, W. B., & Burton, L. A. (2005). Assessment practices of clinical neuropsychologists in the United States and Canada: A survey of INS, NAN, and APA Division 40 members. *Archives of Clinical Neuropsychology, 20,* 33–65.

Reschly, D. J., & Hosp, J. L. (2004). State SLD identification policies and practices. *Learning Disabilities Quarterly, 27*(4), 197–213.

Reynolds, C. R., & Kamphaus, R. W. (2003). *Reynolds Intellectual Assessment Scales.* Lutz, FL: Psychological Assessment Resources.

Reynolds, C. R., & Kamphaus, R. W. (2005). Introduction to the Reynolds Intellectual Assessment Scales and the Reynolds Intellectual Screening Test. In D. P. Flanagan & P. L. Harrison (Eds.), *Contemporary intellectual assessment: Theories, tests, and issues* (2nd ed.; pp. 461–485). New York: Guilford Press.

Roid, G. H. (2003a). *Stanford-Binet Intelligence Scales* (5th ed.). Itasca, IL: Riverside Publishing.

Roid, G. H. (2003b). *Stanford-Binet Intelligence Scales, Fifth Edition, Interpretive Manual: Expanded guide to the interpretation of SB5 Test results.* Itasca, IL: Riverside Publishing.

Roid, G. H., & Barram, A. (2004). *Essentials of Stanford-Binet Intelligence Scales (SB5) assessment.* Hoboken, NJ: Wiley.

Roid, G. H., & Miller, L. J. (1997). *Leiter International Performance Scale—Revised.* Wood Dale, IL: Stoelting.

Roid, G. H., & Pomplun, M. (2005). Interpreting the Stanford-Binet Intelligence Scales, Fifth Edition. In D. P. Flanagan & P. L. Harrison (Eds.), *Contemporary intellectual assessment: Theories, tests, and issues* (2nd ed.; pp. 325–343). New York: Guilford Press.

Rosa's Law, U. S. Congress Public Law. No. 111–256, 124 Stat. 2643 (October 5, 2010). Retrieved March 30 2012 from http://www.gpo.gov/fdsys/pkg/BILLS-111s2781enr/pdf/BILLS-111s2781enr.pdf.

Ryba. N. L., Cooper, V. G., & Zapf. P. A. (2003). Juvenile competence to stand trial evaluations: A survey of current practices and test usage among psychologists. *Professional Psychology: Rh & Practice. 34,* 499–507.

Sattler, J. M. (2008). *Assessment of children: Cognitive foundations* (5th ed.). San Diego, CA: Jerome M. Sattler, Publisher.

Schmidt. F. L. (2002). The role of general cognitive ability and job performance: Why there cannot be a debate. *Human Performance. 15.* 187–211.

Schrank, F. A., & Flanagan, D. P. (2003). *WJ III Clinical Use and Interpretation: Scientist—Practitioner Perspectives.* San Diego, CA: Academic Press.

Schrank, F. A., Mather, N., McGrew, K. S., & Woodcock, R. W. (2003). *Manual. Woodcock-Johnson III Diagnostic Supplement to the Tests of Cognitive Abilities.* Itasca, IL: Riverside Publishing.

Schrank, F. A., Miller, D. C., Wendling, B. J., & Woodcock, R. W. (2010). *Essentials of WJ III Cognitive Abilities assessment* (2nd ed.). Hoboken, NJ: Wiley.

Siegel, L. S. (1999). Issues in the definition and diagnosis of learning disabilities: A perspective on *Guckenberger v. Boston University. Journal of Learning Disabilities, 32,* 304–319.

Slosson, R. L. ; revised by Nicholson, C. L., & Hibpshman, T. L. (2002). *Slosson Intelligence Test, Revised (SIT-R3).* Los Angeles: Western Psychological Services.

Spearman, C. (1904). "General intelligence," objectively determined and measured. *American Journal of Psychology, 15,* 201–293.

Spearman, C. (1927). *The abilities of man: Their nature and measurement.* New York: Macmillan.

Stanovich, K. E. (1999). The sociopsychometrics of learning disabilities. *Journal of Learning Disabilities, 32*(4), 350–361.

Sternberg, R. J. (1997). *Successful intelligence.* New York: Plume.

Sternberg, R. J. (1999). The theory of successful intelligence. *Review of General Psychology, 3,* 292–316.

Sternberg, R. J. (2005). *The triarchic theory of successful intelligence.* In D. P. Flanagan, & P. L. Harrison, P. L. (Eds.), *Contemporary intellectual assessment: Theories, tests and issues* (2nd ed.; pp. 103–119). New York: Guilford.

Sternberg, R. J., & Kaufman, J. C. (1998). Human abilities. *Annual Review of Psychology, 49,* 1134–1139.

TechMicro, Inc. (1999). *Computer-Optimized Multimedia Intelligence Test* (COMIT). New York: TechMicro.

Terman, L. M. (1916). *The measurement of intelligence.* Boston, MA: Houghton-Mifflin.

Terman, L. M., & Merrill, M. A. (1937). *Measuring intelligence.* Boston, MA: Houghton Mifflin.

Terman, L. M., & Merrill, M. A. (1960). *Stanford-Binet Intelligence Scale.* Boston, MA: Houghton Mifflin.

Thorndike, R. L., Hagen, E. P., & Sattler, J. M. (1986). *The Stanford-Binet Intelligence Scale: Fourth Edition.* Chicago: Riverside Publishing.

Thurstone, L. L. (1926). A method for scaling psychological and educational tests. *Journal of Educational Psychology*, *16*, 433–451.

Thurstone, L. L. (1931). Multiple factor analysis. *Psychological Review*, *38*, 406–427.

Thurstone, L. L. (1938). Primary mental abilities. *Psychometric Monographs*, No. 1. Watkins, M. W., Glutting, J. J., & Lei, P-W (2007). Validity of the Full-Scale IQ when there is significant variability among WISC-III and WISC-IV factor scores. *Applied Neuropsychology*, *14*(1), 13–20.

Watkins, M. W., Glutting, J., & Youngstrom. E. (2002). Cross-battery cognitive assessment: Still concerned. *Communiqué*, *31*(2), 42–44.

Watkins, M. W., Youngstrom, E. A., & Glutting, J. J. (2002). Some cautions regarding cross-battery assessment. *Communiqué*, *30*(5), 16–20.

Wechsler, D. (1939). *The measurement of adult intelligence*. Baltimore, MD: Williams & Wilkins.

Wechsler, D. (1944). *The measurement of adult intelligence* (3rd ed.). Baltimore, MD: Williams & Wilkins.

Wechsler, D. (1949). *Wechsler Intelligence Scale for Children*. New York: The Psychological Corporation.

Wechsler, D. (1999). *Wechsler Abbreviated Scale of Intelligence*. San Antonio, TX: The Psychological Corporation.

Wechsler, D. (2012). *Wechsler Preschool and Primary Scale of Intelligence–Fourth Edition*. San Antonio, TX: Pearson.

Wechsler, D. (2003). *Wechsler Intelligence Scale for Children–Fourth Edition: Administration and scoring manual*. San Antonio, TX: The Psychological Corporation.

Wechsler, D. (2008). *Wechsler Adult Intelligence Scale–Fourth Edition, Technical and interpretive manual*. San Antonio, TX: Pearson.

Wechsler, D. (2011). *Wechsler Abbreviated Scale of Intelligence – Second Edition*. San Antonio, TX: Pearson.

Wechsler, D., & Naglieri, J. A. (2006). *Wechsler Nonverbal Scale of Ability*. San Antonio, TX: Harcourt Assessment.

Weiss, L. G., Beal, A. L., Saklofske, D. H., Packiam Alloway, T., & Prifitera, A. (2008). Interpretation and intervention with WISC-IV in the clinical assessment context. In A. Prifitera, D. H. Saklofske, & L. G. Weiss, *WISC-IV clinical assessment and intervention* (2nd ed.; pp. 3–66). San Diego, CA: Academic Press.

Weiss, L. G., Saklofske, D. H., Prifitera, A., & Holdnack, J. A. (2006). *WISC-IV advanced clinical interpretation*. Burlington, MA: Academic Press.

Willis, J. O., & Dumont, R. P. (2002). *Guide to identification of learning disabilities* (3rd ed.). Peterborough, NH: authors (book available from johnzerowillis@yahoo.com, CD from Dumont@fdu.edu).

Willis, J. O., & Dumont, R. (2006). And never the twain shall meet: Can response to intervention and cognitive assessment be reconciled? *Psychology in the Schools*, *43*(8), 901–908.

Willis, J. O., Dumont, R., & Kaufman, A. S. (2011). Factor-analytic models of intelligence. In R. J. Sternberg & S. B. Kaufman (Eds.), *The Cambridge handbook of intelligence* (pp. 39–57). Cambridge, UK: Cambridge University Press.

Woodcock, R. W. (1990). Theoretical foundations of the WJ-R measures of cognitive ability. *Journal of Psychoeducational Assessment*, *8*(3), 231–258.

Woodcock, R. W. (1993). An information processing view of Gf-Gc theory. *Journal of Psychoeducational Assessment, Monograph Series: Advances in Psychoeducational Assessment: Woodcock-Johnson Psychoeducational Battery–Revised*, 80–102.

Woodcock, R. W. (1997). The Woodcock-Johnson Tests of Cognitive Ability–Revised. In D. P. Flanagan, J. L. Genshaft, & P. L. Harrison (Eds.), *Contemporary intellectual assessment: Theories, tests, and issues* (pp. 230–246). New York: Guilford Press

Woodcock, R. W., Mc Grew, K. S., & Mather. N. (2001). *Woodcock-Johnson III Tests of Cognitive Abilities*. Itasca, IL: Riverside Publishing.

Woodcock, R. W., Schrank, F. A., McGrew, K. S., & Mather, N. (2007). *Woodcock-Johnson III Tests of Cognitive Abilities: Normative update*. Rolling Meadows, IL: Riverside Publishing.

Methods of Neuropsychological Assessment

Susan Homack

Abstract

While the field of pediatric neuropsychology is young, neuropsychological assessment of children has much to offer toward understanding the functional systems of the brain and the mechanisms involved in learning. Child neuropsychology provides a theoretical framework for understanding patterns of strengths and weaknesses, and the extent to which patterns may remain stable over time. Once the clinician identifies the assessment needs of the individual child, he or she must make decisions regarding the appropriate assessment measures for exploring the dimensions of behavior. When an evaluation is complete, understanding the strengths and weaknesses of a child provides the neuropsychologist with needed information to recommended appropriate interventions. When communicating results, the clinician must remember that the audience includes caregivers who need straight-forward, easily understood information. Of paramount importance, clinicians must recognize that providing useful, scientifically supported conclusions that contribute to the treatment of the child is the ultimate purpose of assessment.

Key Words: neuropsychology, child assessment, test selection

Introduction

Neuropsychology is the study of brain–behavior relationships that uses the theories and methods of both neurology and psychology. The underlying premise of neuropsychological assessment is that different behaviors and abilities involve differing neurological structures or functional systems (Luria, 1980). Unlike CT or MRI scans, which show abnormalities in the structure of the brain, or EEG, which shows electrical abnormalities of the brain, neuropsychological assessment is used to show the ways in which a person can or cannot perform certain functions or tasks that are dependent upon brain activity. A neuropsychological evaluation typically involves assessment with a group of standardized tests that are sensitive to the effects of brain damage or differences in brain functioning. The standardized tests used in a neuropsychological evaluation typically assess functioning in the following areas: cognitive functioning, attention, memory, problem-solving, visual spatial functioning, language, and motor skills. Assessment of academic skills and emotional functioning are often assessed as well.

While neuropsychology has origins dating at least as far back as the 19th century, it is during the past 25 to 30 years that neuropsychology has been widely recognized and accepted as a formal professional specialty area (Hartlage & Long, 2009). The field of neuropsychology has rapidly matured since the early empirical work of Ralph M. Reitan (1955) and other important contributors (please see Fitzhugh-Bell, 1997, for a review of the early history of clinical neuropsychology). Historically, neuropsychology has been used for the assessment and diagnosis of adults with brain injury or other forms of central nervous system (CNS) dysfunction. Due to recent advances in neuroimaging techniques, the use of neuropsychological tests for the primary diagnosis of the presence or absence of CNS damage has declined (Mayfield, Reynolds, & Fletcher-Janzen, 2009). However, a rise in the use of neuropsychological testing has occurred for determining functional deficits. An assessment of strengths and weaknesses using a neuropsychological assessment is necessary because neuroimaging techniques cannot specify the true functional implications of any visualized abnormality or damage. As more became known about brain–behavior relationships, theories and findings also were applied to the understanding of learning and behavior problems in adults where brain injury was not evident.

With the increasing recognition that learning and other neuropsychological functions could be evaluated in adults, researchers and clinicians became interested in determining whether research gleamed from adults could be applied to children. The increased interest and emphasis in the application of neuropsychology to children may be due to a variety of factors, including: the development of neuropsychology as a specialty area, knowledge obtained from localized brain damage in childhood and adolescence, advances in technology (e.g., functional imaging) that are providing exciting new information regarding brain development and function, and continued research using neuropsychological assessment data to gain more information regarding specific problems encountered by children (Riccio & Reynolds, 1998).

Child neuropsychology provides a framework for understanding patterns of strengths and weaknesses and the extent to which these patterns remain stable or change over the course of development (Temple, 1997). Children in general have always posed special problems in clinical assessment due to their rapid and often uneven development in the areas of language and motor acquisition, attention, memory, and problem-solving. As the extent of disability increases, accurate assessment becomes more challenging (Reynolds & Mayfield, 1999). A minor variant of normal development need not be a cause for alarm; however, a significant problem should not be ignored.

An increased understanding of a child's strengths and weaknesses is useful for many reasons. Neuropsychological testing can help establish the presence of a cognitive disorder. In having a better understanding of the ways in which neurological conditions impact learning and behavior, clinicians are able to recommend compensatory strategies that

may be provided by the school, at home, or within the community. Children can be reevaluated over time to assess progress and determine whether there may be changing symptomatology. The effectiveness of interventions can be evaluated and altered as necessary based on the child's functioning.

As a result of the growing interest in child neuropsychology, the knowledge available regarding the developing brain has increased dramatically since the 1980s (Riccio & Reynolds, 1998). A great deal of information has been obtained regarding child development and neuropsychological functions (e.g., Miller & Vernon, 1996; Molfese, 1995). Furthermore, advances in educational areas have been made that facilitate the understanding of learning disabilities (Riccio, Gonzalez, and Hynd, 1994; Riccio & Hynd, 1996), traumatic brain injury (Dennis, Wilkinson, Koski, & Humphreys, 1995; Yeates & Taylor, 1997), the impact of cancer treatment on CNS function (Kerr, Smith, DaSilva, Hoffman, & Humphries, 1991; Seidel et al., 1994), and the sequelae in children with prenatal or perinatal difficulties (Aylward, 2002; Daniel, Lim, & Clark, 2003).

This chapter will provide an overview of the neuropsychological assessment process for children, both historically and in the context of current practices and future trends. Areas covered in this chapter include neurodevelopmental considerations and approaches to test selection in the assessment of children. An overview of the domains for assessment including examples of frequently used tests is provided. Finally, a description of the general organization of the neuropsychological assessment of children and adolescents is described.

Neurodevelopmental Considerations in the Assessment of Children

Due to the demand for neuropsychological testing of children and adolescents, traditional adult neuropsychological batteries such as the Halstead-Reitan Neuropsychological Battery (Reitan, 1955; Reitan & Davison, 1974) and the Luria-Nebraska Neuropsychological Battery (Golden, 1981; Plaisted, Gustavson, Wilkening, & Golden, 1983) were modified for use with children (Hartlage & Long, 1997). This involved altering or adding some tasks to the batteries that were more suitable for children. Another option involved collecting normative data on children for existing tests. Both of these attempts were based on the assumption that tasks for adults could measure the same constructs when used with children.

A pitfall of using adult tests with children results when neurodevelopmental differences that exist as a result of the age of the child are not taken into consideration. If one directly applies norms from adult tests to children, then one completely ignores what is known about changes in the functional organization of the brain of growing children. Rapid growth takes place during childhood and adolescence and occurs at different rates for individual children. Infancy and childhood are the times of the greatest breadth and depth of change throughout one's lifetime.

According to Luria (1980), neurodevelopment follows an ontogenetic course, with primary cortical zones generally maturing by birth, and secondary and tertiary areas continuing to develop after birth. Secondary and tertiary areas include systems involved in learning, memory, attention, emotion, cognition, language, and association. The association areas are the last of these areas to develop and myelinate (Goldman & Lewis, 1978). According to Spreen, Risser, and Edgell (1995), the developmental sequence for the formation of neural pathways and myelination of specific locations corresponding to specific behaviors have been identified; however, these sequences do not correspond directly to models of cognitive development.

Research suggests that traumatic brain injury (TBI) as well as other brain insults can disrupt the neurodevelopmental process of children, especially in young children (Kriel, Krach, & Panser, 1989). The impact of an injury is influenced by the child's age as well as by its location in the brain, and the nature of the injury. The theory of neural plasticity (Harris, 1957) has been used to explain the potential for recovery of function seen in children that is not observed in adults. It has been suggested that the young brain undergoes "reorganization" of brain function. For example, brain damage occurring in infants and toddlers may produce very different behavioral effects than in adults because early injury has also altered fundamental brain organization. The insult does not affect the function of only the brain areas that are damaged directly but also disrupts other neuroanatomical sites and circuitry that are dependent on intact structures (Kolb & Fantie, 2009).

Interestingly, researchers (Brink, Garrett, Hale, Woo-Sam, & Nickel, 1970; Kriel et al., 1989) found that children over 10 years of age at the time of brain insult were likely to have a better prognosis than those under age six, regardless of the injury's severity. According to Riccio & Reynolds (1999),

this may be due to the difference in neurodevelopmental status of children in these age groups. Alternatively, it may be because older children have spent more time in school, and many of the functions assessed by standard measures correlate highly with the number of years spent in school (Ryan, LaMarche, Barth, & Boll, 1996).

Evaluation of children and adolescents with acquired injury or neurodevelopmental disorders is complex because of the neurodevelopmental nature of abilities. When assessing these children, the evaluation not only evaluates skills that should already be acquired, but also requires follow-up evaluations to assess how well later-developing skills do indeed develop.

Approaches to Test Selection with Children
Nomothetic Approach

The fixed battery, or nomothetic approach, uses the same assessment battery for all children being assessed, regardless of their referral questions (Sweet, Moberg, & Westergaard, 1996). This approach may be either empirically or theoretically based. Using an empirical approach, the test battery is selected according to its ability to separate groups, while theoretically based batteries are founded on a theory of development as it relates to broad or narrow dimensions of behavior (Fennell & Bauer, 2009). Clinicians utilizing a fixed battery approach often use a published neuropsychological battery in conjunction with an IQ and achievement test. The published neuropsychological batteries most frequently used with school-aged children are the Luria Nebraska Neuropsychological Battery–Children's Revision (Golden, 1986) and the Halstead-Reitan Neuropsychological Test Batteries for Children (Reitan & Wolfson, 1985). The batteries contain numerous subtests that are considered crucial for understanding brain–behavior relationships in children and adolescents. Research has indicated that both batteries are effective in detecting the presence, lateralization, and localization of brain dysfunction (Bauer, 1994).

There are several advantages to using a fixed battery approach to assessment. A large number of functions are assessed using standardized procedures and objective measures and clinicians rely on cutoff scores for the determination of the presence of brain damage. In order to prevent the referral question from dictating the measures used, a "blind" assessment may be preferred (Goldstein, 1997). Additionally, by adhering to a fixed-battery approach, it is possible for clinicians to develop impressive research databases that provide interpretation of large numbers of clinical groups (Hartlage & Telzrow, 1986).

While there are advantages to using a fixed-battery approach, there are also disadvantages. A standardized battery may not take into account variables such as age, education, and other important idiopathic considerations. The standardized battery may not answer the referral question. Finally, while a certain number of functions need to be evaluated with any child, rarely do clinicians have the time to evaluate areas that do not appear compromised. The use of a fixed-battery approach to neuropsychological assessment appears to be declining (Sweet et al., 1996).

Idiopathic Approach

In contrast to the nomothetic or fixed-battery approach, the idiographic approach tailors the assessment battery to the referral question and the child's test performance on initial measures administered (Christensen, 1975, Luria, 1973). Rather than providing a comprehensive evaluation in all areas of functioning, this approach is intended to isolate the neurobehavioral mechanisms that underlie the difficulties of the individual being assessed. With the idiopathic approach, the primary goal is to answer the referral question, rather than provide a comprehensive assessment. With no uniformity across evaluations, this approach requires that the clinician have substantial clinical knowledge regarding brain–behavior functioning in order to determine the appropriate assessment tools necessary to meet this goal.

While this approach appears to be the most cost-effective of the methods described due to the small number of domains assessed (Goldstein, 1997), the major drawback of the idiopathic approach relies on the limited research base generated and the inability to study the efficacy of this method compared to the other approaches (Riccio & Reynolds, 1998). Furthermore, information regarding the neuropsychological functions and organization of behaviors in children and adolescents with various disorders is limited at this time (Baron, Fennell, & Voeller, 1995). As a result, the individualized approach is less frequently used than the other approaches (Fennell, 1994).

Flexible Approaches

The flexible battery involves choosing specific instruments based on the presenting issues or neurobehavioral mechanisms that underlie the difficulties of a child, rather than administering a predetermined neuropsychological battery. In order to meet this goal, the clinician administers a core set of standardized tests to all children in order to provide a comprehensive assessment. The clinician then supplements the battery with a selected set of additional tests designed to answer specific referral questions (Rourke et al., 1986) or to further examine potential areas of weakness that are detected while using the core battery (Bauer, 1994). Consistent with the fixed battery approach, the flexible battery approach may be either empirically or theoretically based. While the core set of tests may be empirically based, the components of the flexible battery often reflect the theoretical position of the clinician with regard to which behavioral performance reflects brain pathology (Bauer, 1994).

The major advantage of the flexible battery is that both a nomothetic and an ideographic approach to neuropsychological assessment are applied. This method allows for the assessment of a broad range of functions as well as specific areas related to the referral question. Clinicians generally agree that this approach more accurately identifies specific deficits. As such, the flexible approach is the method preferred by most neuropsychologists working with adult and child populations (Sweet & Moberg, 1990, Sweet et al., 1996).

The Boston Process Approach (Kaplan, 1988) is a good example of the use of the flexible battery. A core set of tests with low specificity is initially used to assess various neuropsychological constructs. In addition to core tests, several "satellite tests" are used to clarify particular problem areas and to confirm the hypotheses developed from observations of the individual. According to Milberg, Hebben, and Kaplan (1986), the only limits to the procedures that are employed are the examiner's knowledge of available tests of cognitive function and his or her ingenuity in creating new measures for particular deficit areas. With the Process Approach, there is less focus on the results of standardized testing and more focus on the presentation of symptoms, strategy used in task completion, and error analysis. The Process Approach uses standardized measures, experimental measures, and "testing the limits" that often involve procedural modifications in order to gain insight into brain–behavior relationships (Kaplan, 1988; Milberg, Hebben, & Kaplan, 1986). While the Boston Process Approach shows great promise, there is concern regarding the questionable reliability of scores obtained on measures where the standardized procedures have been compromised

(Rourke et al., 1986). In response to these concerns, the Wechsler Intelligence Scale for Children-Fourth Edition–Integrated (WISC-IV-Integrated; Wechsler et al., 2004) and Delis-Kaplan Executive Function System (D-KEFS; Delis, Kaplan, & Kramer, 2001) were designed so that changes to input modality were normed.

Domains for Assessment
Cognitive Functioning

A neuropsychological evaluation should include measures of the child's cognitive skills. To accomplish this task, a comprehensive IQ test is used to measure general intellectual ability (*g*). Using an intellectual test with a strong measure of *g* provides a solid baseline for the interpretation of other domains. However, interpretation of a child's performance on cognitive measures is complicated by the fact that no two tests conceive of intelligence in the same way. In fact, cognitive instruments that attest to measure the construct of intelligence can differ substantially from one another (Kamphaus, 2005).

The Wechsler Intelligence Scale for Children, Fourth Edition (WISC-IV; Wechsler, 2003) and the Kaufman Assessment Battery for Children, Second Edition (KABC-II; Kaufman & Kaufman, 2004) are two measures frequently used with children. The WISC measures are a downward extension of the Wechsler's adult measure, the Wechsler Adult Intelligence Scale. The most recent version, the WISC-IV was designed for use with children and adolescents six to 16 years old. According to Wechsler (2003), the neurocognitive models of information processing provide the basis for the structure of the WISC-IV. While the WISC-III adhered to the traditional verbal IQ/performance IQ dichotomy, the WISC-IV provides four index scores: Verbal Comprehension (VCI), Perceptual Reasoning (PRI), Working Memory (WMI), and Processing Speed (PSI). The full-scale IQ score is derived from the 10 subtests included in the four indices. Unlike previous versions of the WISC, the WISC-IV includes the working memory and processing speed subtests in calculating the full-scale IQ.

The Wechsler Intelligence Scale for Children, Fourth Edition–Integrated (WISC-IV-Integrated; Wechsler et al., 2004). is based on the Boston Process Approach and assists clinicians in better understanding the cognitive processes involved in the performance of core or supplemental WISC-IV subtests. While the WISC-IV-Integrated provides the same four indices and overall full-scale IQ score

as the WISC-IV, an extended array of 16 subtests is available to complete the core components of the WISC-IV. Based on the Boston Process Approach, the WISC-IV Integrated subtests use standardized approaches to modifying the input modality or item content in order to better understand the underlying cognitive processes that are involved in the performance of core or supplemental WISC-IV subtests.

The KABC-II was normed for children three to 18 years old and is composed of four required scales and one optional scale. The Simultaneous, Sequential, Planning, Learning, and Knowledge (optional) scales make up the Mental Processing Index, Fluid-Crystallized Index, and Nonverbal Index. The KABC-II was influenced by both the Lurian model and Cattell-Horn-Carroll (CHC) model. The Kaufmans define *simultaneous processing* as referring to the child's mental ability to integrate input simultaneously in order to a solve a problem correctly. *Sequential processing*, on the other hand, emphasizes the arrangement of stimuli in sequential or serial order for successful problem-solving (Kaufman & Kaufman, 1983). Sequential skills are tied to left-hemisphere, step-by-step logical analysis, while simultaneous skills were believed to assess right-hemisphere abilities. With an emphasis on processing rather than content, the KABC-II is far less dependent on prior learning and exposure to cultural experiences than many of the other mainstream intelligence measures.

Academic Achievement

Assessment of basic academic skills, including reading, mathematics, and written language, is important in determining the need for classroom modifications or special education support. A standardized battery such as the Woodcock-Johnson Psychoeducational Battery–Third Edition–Tests of Achievement (WJ-III; Woodcock, McGrew, & Mather, 2001) or the Wechsler Individual Achievement Test–Third Edition (WIAT-III; Wechsler, 2009) can provide information on the child's current functioning in major academic areas. According to Goldstein and Schwebach (2009), the WJ-III is the most comprehensive, well-developed assessment of academic skills. Subtest analysis of the WJ-III often reveals patterns of verbal, visual, rote, or conceptual weaknesses. Because one of the most common complaints of parents of children who have sustained a TBI is slowed processing speed, the WJ-III is the academic assessment tool of choice when evaluating children with TBI. The

WJ-III provides timed reading, math, and writing fluency subtests that evaluates a child's ability to work quickly and accurately.

In the absence of a comprehensive battery such as the WJ-III or the WIAT-III, a neuropsychologist may use other basic achievement data. In the area of reading, a measure should be used to assess phonetic skills, sight word reading, and comprehension. The Comprehensive Test of Phonological Processing (CTOPP; Wagner, Torgesen, & Rashotte, 1999) provides assessment of phonetic awareness, phonological memory, and rapid naming. The Gray Oral Reading Test–Fifth Edition (GORT-5; Wiederholt & Bryant, 2012) can provide clinicians with information regarding reading rate, accuracy, fluency, and comprehension. In the area of spelling, the Wide Range Achievement Test–Fourth Edition (WRAT-4; Wilkinson & Robertson, 2006) provides estimates of phonetic ability and sight word memory. The WRAT-4 measures an individual's ability to count, identify numbers, solve simple arithmetic problems, and calculate written math problems. In the area of written language, the Story Writing subtest of the Test of Written Language–Fourth Edition (TOWL-4; Hammill & Larsen, 2009) provides information regarding vocabulary, grammar, punctuation, sentence composition, and thematic organization.

Attention

Problems with attention are inherent in a multitude of disorders in children, including TBI, stroke, cancer, and developmental disorder, but they are most frequently noted in conjunction with attention-deficit/hyperactivity disorder (ADHD). Problems arising from symptoms of ADHD constitute the largest single source of referrals to mental health centers (Barkley, 1981); more recently, it has been suggested that children with ADHD may account for as many as 40 percent of referrals to child guidance clinics (Barkley, 1998). By definition, children with ADHD display difficulties with attention relative to normal children of the same age and sex. However, *attention* is a multidimensional construct that can refer to alertness, arousal, selective or focused attention, distractibility, and sustained attention, among others (Barkley, 1998; Mirsky, 1996). According to Douglas (1983), children with ADHD most likely have their greatest difficulties with sustaining attention to tasks, persistence to effort, and vigilance.

While a large number of children are referred to clinics, the development of a norm-referenced, psychometric assessment battery specifically designed to assess attention has been an elusive goal for clinicians (Goldstein, 1999). Computerized assessment of behaviors associated with attention problems represents an effort to incorporate reliable and objective assessment into evaluations. These techniques were born from concern about the degree to which diagnostic decisions were founded upon subjective measures and clinical judgment. Currently, the determination of attention problems is made primarily from anecdotal information from parents and teachers report. One problem with using scores from parents and teachers reports is the lack of congruence often found between these measures. As noted by Sattler (1990), a lack of reliability between these measures is primarily related to varying expectations and tolerance on the part of parents and teachers.

Computer-based measures allow the clinician to incorporate data into the assessment that is derived from a child's actual behavior. Unlike other clinical techniques, computer-based measures generate objective data about a child's ability to perform in situations tailored to assess the characteristic weaknesses of a child with attention problems (Gordon, 1986a). One venture for a computerized measure included the development of continuous performance tests (CPTs). The CPT is one group of paradigms used for the evaluation of attention and the response inhibition component of executive control. The CPTs are frequently used to obtain quantitative information regarding an individual's ability to sustain attention over time; the duration of the task varies, but is intended to be sufficient to measure sustained attention. The CPT involves selective attention or vigilance for an infrequently occurring target or relevant stimulus. The CPT paradigm is generally characterized by rapid presentation of continuously changing stimuli with a designated target stimulus or target pattern (Riccio, Reynolds, & Lowe, 2001).

The Gordon Diagnostic System (Gordon, 1983) was the first commercially available CPT and has probably been the most frequently used CPT in research studies (Riccio, Reynolds, & Lowe, 2001). The GDS is a microprocessor unit, as opposed to a computer software program, that generates 11 tasks. There are three basic paradigms: the delay task, the distractibility task, and the vigilance task. Of the three paradigms, the distractibility and vigilance tasks are CPTs. More than one version of the distractibility and vigilance tasks are available (Gordon, 1986a, 1986b; Gordon & Mettelman,

1988; Gordon Systems, Inc., 1991). The Gordon uses numbers as stimuli. The children's standard version of the vigilance task, for ages six to 16 years, lasts nine minutes and requires the child to press a button every time a two-number target combination (a 1 followed by a 9) is presented. The numerals for the children's version are displayed for 200 milliseconds, with a 1000-millisecond interstimulus interval (ISI). The distractibility task incorporates the two-number target presentation, but simultaneously includes the display of digits on either side of the target stimulus to assess whether the individual can selectively attend to the target stimuli (Gordon Systems, Inc., 1991). In addition to the vigilance and distractibility tasks, the GDS includes a delay task (lasting nine minutes) that is designed to measure impulse control. On this task, the child earns points for inhibiting a response.

Information provided in the technical manual (Gordon Systems, Inc., 1987) indicated that the GDS children's standard version provides moderate to high test-retest reliability for a clinical and non-clinical population. Test-retest reliability estimates for non-clinical population ranged from 0.67 to 0.85, while estimates for the clinical sample ranged from 0.68 to 0.94. Validity studies included in the 1987 manual supported the use of the GDS in the diagnosis of attention problems with approximately 70 percent agreement with parent and teacher ratings of children with ADHD depending on the age, the rater, and the scale.

The Conners' Continuous Performance Test (2nd ed.; CPT-II: Conners, 2000) is a visual paradigm used for the evaluation of attention as well as the response inhibition component of executive control. The standard version of the CPT-II can be administered to children six years of age and older and takes approximately 14 minutes to complete. Unlike traditional CPTs that require the individual to press a computer key after an X is presented, the CPT-II requires individuals to press the computer key immediately after every letter *except* the X. Conners (2000) asserted that this format ensured a greater number of responses and therefore decreased chance error. For four- and five-year-olds, the Conners' Kiddie CPT (K-CPT) may be used; this version is shorter in duration and uses pictures instead of letters as the stimuli. The updated version of the CPT-II (Conners, 2000) differs from previous versions of the CPT-II (Conners, 1992, 1995) in that it provides a validity test to identify invalid administrations, a confidence index (CI) score to assess the likelihood that the examinee's responses

fit those given by individuals with ADHD, new theory and methods for computing signal detection theory statistics, and new and expanded norms.

The CPT-II standard paradigm consists of six blocks, with each block divided into three subblocks. The targeted and non-targed stimuli (letters) are randomly shown for 250 milliseconds, with the interstimulus interval (ISI) varying within each block. For the three subblocks within a block, the ISI may be 1, 2, or 4 seconds; the order of the three difference ISIs subblocks varies from block to block (Conners, 2000). Examination of results by block allows for the assessment of vigilance. By varying the ISI, it is possible to assess the examinee's ability to adjust to changing tempo and task demands.

Conners (2000) provided reliability information obtained from the original standardization sample (Conners, 1994). Split-half reliabilities across variables appeared adequate and ranged from 0.66 and 0.95. Test- retest reliability estimates ranged from 0.05 to 0.92, indicating that some of the variables do not produce good consistency across administrations. In one validity study using the original standardization sample (Conners, 1994) the ADHD group responded more slowly, had greater variability of reaction times, made more omission and commission errors, and was more affected by changes in the ISI than the group with a variety of other clinical diagnoses. In a similar analysis using updated CPT-II data (Conners, 2000), no significant differences were observed between the ADHD and nonclinical groups on the commissions variable; for all other variables, a significant difference between the groups was evident, with the ADHD group performing more poorly on all variables.

The Test of Variables of Attention is an X-CPT available in separate visual (TOVA; Greenberg, 1988–1999) and auditory (TOVA-A; Greenberg, 1996–1999) versions. The TOVA is composed of both a clinical version and a preschool version. The TOVA and TOVA-A require an individual to press a microswitch every time the target stimulus is presented. The target stimulus consists of a colored square with a smaller square contained within and adjacent to the top edge of the larger square. In contrast, the non-target stimulus has a smaller inscribed square adjacent to the bottom edge of the larger square. For the TOVA-A, two audible tones are used as stimuli, one as the target and one as the non-target. Supporters of the TOVA and TOVA-A argue that by virtue of being non–language-based tests, these measures serve as "purer" measures of inattentiveness and executive control, compared to other CPT measures (Riccio, Reynolds, & Lowe, 2001). The clinical version of the TOVA and TOVA-A are approximately 22 minutes in duration.

For both the TOVA and TOVA-A, the target and non-target stimuli are presented randomly for 100 ms with an ISI of 2000 ms. The clinical versions are composed of four intervals. During the first half of the test (intervals 1 and 2), the target stimulus is randomly displayed on 22.5 percent of the trials. This condition is called the "stimulus-infrequent condition," and it is believed to create a situation in which an individual who is inattentive is less likely to respond and therefore will make omission errors. As such, the stimulus-infrequent state is used to assess the individual's attention. During the second half of the test (intervals 3 and 4), the target stimulus is shown on 77.5 percent of the trials. This stimulus-frequent condition creates a strong response set in which an individual who has an impulse control problem is more likely to respond and make commission errors. This stimulus-frequent condition is used to assess the individual's impulsivity (Greenberg & Crosby, 1992; Leark, Dupuy, Greenberg, Corman, & Kindschi, 1996).

Test-retest reliability studies indicated that the stability of performance across time (4 months) ranged from 0.51 to 0.82 (Llorente et al., 2000). Llorente and colleagues concluded that omission and commission error variables were the least stable, and reaction time and reaction time variability were the most stable. No test-retest study of the TOVA-A was found. Results of a factor analysis indicated a three-factor solution for the TOVA consistent with the premise that the task is measuring attention, disinhibition, and processing speed. For the TOVA-A, five factors emerged including the processing speed of the TOVA and separate attention and disinhibition factors for both the target-frequent and target-infrequent conditions. Results of a clinical validity study of children with ADHD and normal controls indicated that false positive rates of 80 and 90 percent were obtained, depending on the cutoff scores used (Leark, et al., 1996).

The Integrated (or Intermediate) Visual and Auditory Continuous Performance Test (IVA; Sandford & Turner, 1994–1999) is a 13-minute CPT that uses both auditory and visual stimuli within the same task. Of the CPTs discussed here, this is the only one that requires an individual to shift modalities within the same task. On the IVA, the individual is to press a mouse button in response to a visual or auditory target stimulus (the number

1) and to refrain from pressing the mouse button when the non-target stimulus (the number 2) is presented either visually or verbally. The target and non-target stimuli are presented in a random pattern with a 1500 ms ISI for 500 trials (Sandford & Turner, 1995). The IVA varies the frequency of the target. During the test, the IVA's target to non-target ratio is altered by blocks to elicit omission and commission errors. Under the frequent-target condition, a response set is created such that the dominant response is to press the mouse button. As such, an individual who is impulsive is more likely to make commission errors. During the infrequent-target condition, vigilance and response inhibition are assessed.

Test-retest reliability correlations across auditory and visual variables of the IVA ranged from a low of 0.18 to 0.88 (Sandford & Turner, 1995). These findings show that the temporal stability of some variables is adequate, whereas the stability of other variables is low. Results of a validity study using the IVA indicated that the IVA results were in agreement with group membership (ADHD or normal controls) in 92 percent of the cases.

In reviewing the above CPTs, it is important to point out that CPTs are not identical assessment tools. Different CPTs may measure different facets of attention and executive functioning. According to Conners (1992, 1995), CPTs are not a unitary measure, but rather a family of measures with differing parameters and scoring indices. Little is known about how the differences in measures affect diagnostic considerations.

Executive Functioning

Executive functions are a set of cognitive processes that guide goal-directed behaviors. They do not refer to an individual's knowledge or skills, but to the mental processes that direct whether and how these are applied to accomplish a goal. While a child may demonstrate an IQ and achievement abilities within the average range, he or she may struggle with executive functioning. Executive processes include control of attention, inhibition of impulses, cognitive flexibility, working memory, planning, organization, self-monitoring, and emotional regulation. From a brain–behavior relationship perspective, executive processes are related to the frontal and prefrontal areas. Because the frontal lobes constitute a complex neurological and functional system (Luria, 1966; Welsh & Pennington, 1988), both discreet and diffuse damage resulting from TBI can cause children to have difficulty with self regulation and problem-solving. Children with neurodevelopmental disorders (e.g., ADHD, autism spectrum disorder) also tend to have problems with executive functioning.

While the umbrella of executive functioning may include a variety of constructs, including attention, self-regulation, and working memory, the "executive" processes focus on strategic planning, effortful and flexible organization, and proactive reasoning (Denckla, 1994). Because the frontal and prefrontal areas continue to develop and mature throughout adolescence, it is difficult to assess executive functioning in children. Most executive function measures used with children are downward extensions of adult measures (Riccio & Reynolds, 1999), and many lack adequate normative data. Below is a review of measures used to assess executive functioning.

The Trail Making Test (TMT), parts A and B, is one of the most widely used screening instruments in current neuropsychological practice (Moses, 2004). It was originally developed by Partington in 1938 to serve as a model of "divided attention" (Partington & Leiter, 1949). While this test is an excellent global screening measure sensitive to the integrity of cognitive performance, it was not well normed, and there is not a set of current norms that matched the United States population.

In order to provide a revision and extension of the TMT, Reynolds (2002) developed the Comprehensive Trail Making Test (CTMT) that consists of five timed trials that are designed to highlight and isolate specific components of performance. On the first "trail," the examinee connects numbers in order. This task assesses sustained attention, as well as basic sequencing and visual-spatial scanning skills. On CTMT Trails 2 and 3, the examinee is again required to sequence numbers; however, simple empty circles (Trails 2) and complex, busy circles (Trails 3) are added to the visual array. The subject must sustain and focus attention despite the distracters. On the CTMT Trail 4, both numerical and lexical numbers are presented in a random alternating sequence. On the CTMT Trail 5, the examinee must connect numbers and letters in an alternating sequence, while also being presented with empty distracter circles.

The CTMT is appropriate for administration to individuals from age 11 years 0 months to age 74 years 11 months. More recently, Reynolds provided norms that extend to those aged 8 years 0 months to 11 years 0 months so that the test can be administered to younger children. In the areas of reliability and validity, the CTMT meets rigorous standards. All internal consistency values for the five CTMT trails meet or exceed a value of 0.70, and the reliability value of the Composite Index score is 0.92. Test-retest reliability values for the five trails of the CTMT range from 0.70 to 0.78, which are quite high for a speeded measure. Preliminary studies are provided in the manual that establish the test's construct, concurrent, and content validity. Results of a more recent study (Armstrong, Allen, Donohue, & Mayfield, 2008) indicated that the CTMT did a good job of correctly classifying adolescents with traumatic brain injury and controls; however, some variability in classification accuracy was present among various trails.

The Delis-Kaplan Executive Function System (D-KEFS; Delis, Kaplan, & Kramer, 2001) represents the first set of executive tests co-normed on a large and representative national sample and designed exclusively for the assessment of executive functions, including flexibility of thinking, inhibition, problem solving, planning, impulse control, concept formation, abstract thinking, and creativity. The D-KEFS is composed of nine tests that provide a standardized assessment of executive functions in children and adults between the ages of 8 and 89. Utilizing a "cognitive-process approach," the D-KEFS tests allow examiners to systematically generate and evaluate relevant clinical hypotheses on executive functioning of a given examinee by comparing and contrasting performance on multiple testing conditions and using contrast measure scores and error analyses. The D-KEFS is composed of the following nine stand-alone tests that can be individually or group administered: Trail Making Test; Verbal Fluency Test; Design Fluency Test; Color-Word Interference Test; Sorting Test; Twenty Questions Test; Word Context Test; Tower Test; and Proverb Test.

One of the important objectives of designing the D-KEFS was to provide psychologists with a large, comprehensive collection of executive-function tests for the assessment of complex and multifactorial domains of frontal lobe functioning. The authors noted that most of the existing executive-function tests were developed in the 1940s. As such, the authors indicated that the designs of these extant tests have not benefited from the knowledge that has accrued over the past 60 years of research and clinical practice. The authors sought to incorporate the principles and procedures from this extensive body of knowledge into a new set of executive-function tests by employing several unique approaches. By embracing a "cognitive-process approach," the component functions of higher-level cognitive tasks can be assessed. The authors indicate that most existing clinical instruments of higher-level cognitive functions yield a single score for each task, which is problematic because such tests typically tap a host of fundamental and higher-level cognitive skills. Several D-KEFS tests allow the examiner to assess the relative contributions of multiple fundamental and higher-level cognitive functions to overall performance on each executive-function test by using multiple testing conditions and providing "contrast measures." In using modifications of the traditional tests, it was possible to add features and testing conditions that would increase the sensitivity of the tests to mild brain damage.

Each D-KEFS test includes primary and optional measures and provides between six and 34 scores. In addition, five D-KEFS tests provide several primary or optional "contrast" measures. Some tasks measure similar cognitive functions but under somewhat different conditions. Separate normative scores are derived for each of the testing conditions. In addition, a total achievement score that reflects the examinee's ability at the task across the testing conditions is computed. The clinician can be flexible in terms of administering only some of the D-KEFS tests or conditions within a test. The selection of conditions or tests to be administered depends on the assessment needs of the specific examinee or the time constraints of the examiner.

Test developers presented correlations between the D-KEFS tests and other measures to provide evidence for adequate convergent and discriminant validity. Exploratory factor-analytic results were not provided, because factor scores derived from normative or mixed-clinical populations often mask critical cognitive distinctions, especially on process-oriented tests (Delis et al., 2003). Evidence of validity is provided in studies indicating that tests from the D-KEFS have reasonable sensitivity in distinguishing many different types of clinical groups (e.g., fetal alcohol exposure, focal frontal lesions, etc.) from controls. Many overall achievement scores of the tests have adequate to good reliability coefficients; however, some of the optional process measures have low reliability coefficients. A review of its administration, scoring and interpretation, test construction, standardization, and technical adequacy indicate that the D-KEFS holds much promise, not only as a clinical instrument, but also as a research tool for increasing knowledge of the frontal-lobe functions.

The NEPSY-II: A Developmental Neuropsychological Assessment (NEPSY-II: Korkman, Kirk, and Kemp, 2007) is the revision of the original NEPSY (Korkman, Kirk, and Kemp, 1998) and can be used with children three to 16 years of age. The NEPSY-II assesses six domains of functioning. In addition to the executive functioning/attention domain, the NEPSY-II also measures language, memory and learning, sensorimotor functioning, visuospatial processing, and social perception, the last of which is a new domain specific to the NEPSY-II. While the original NEPSY required a fixed administration of subtests to obtain domain scores, the NEPSY-II does not require a set administration of subtests and does not provide domain scores. Rather, the clinician is allowed to create a tailored assessment of subtests across the six domains and interpret individual subtest scores. The NEPSY-II also provides a greater array of subtests from which the examiner can select. The computerized scoring program provides an electronic "decision tree" that assists the clinician in selecting subtests based on the child's presenting history.

One of the greatest strengths of the NEPSY-II is the comprehensive standardization of the measure using 1200 children and adolescents, which closely approximates the demographics of the United States population based on 2003 census data. The NEPSY-II manual provided evidence that the NEPSY-II has good internal reliability; however, construct validity appears questionable in some areas. Although most subtests appear to have adequate reliability and validity, some of the subtests may not provide consistent and accurate scores. The Design Fluency, Oromotor Sequence, Manual Motor Series, and Route Finding subtests appear to have lower reliablity. Animal Sorting, Narrative Memory, and Visuomotor Precision subtests should be interpreted with care since they do not appear to measure the same construct as other subtests in these domains.

According to D'Amato and Hartlage (2008), there is general support for the clinical usefulness of the NEPSY-II in distinguishing between various neuropsychological disorders. Specific group studies by Korkman et al. (2007) reported lower functioning on subtests across all domains in groups of 23 autistic children. Severe deficits were evident in the areas of executive functioning, language, and memory. Children with Attention-Deficit/ Hyperactivity Disorder generally exhibit lower scores than control groups on Phonological Processing, Speeded Naming, Visuomotor Precision, Arrows, and

Geometric Puzzles subtests (Korkman, Kirk, & Kemp, 2007). Select subtests are particularly useful in diagnosing ADHD, autism spectrum disorder, and learning disabilities.

Learning and Memory

We rely on memory to carry out most daily activities (Reynolds & Bigler, 1997). Unfortunately, nearly every CNS disorder associated with disturbances of higher cognitive functions presents with some form of memory problems (Fletcher-Janzen & Reynolds, 2003; Lezak, Howieson, Loring, Hannay, & Fischer, 2004). Memory difficulties are the most common complaint in individuals with traumatic brain injury (D'Amato, Fletcher-Janzen, & Reynolds, 2005). According to Reynolds and Voress (2009), TBI produces the least predictable forms of memory loss, with the exception of increased forgetting curves. Furthermore, recovery of memory after a TBI is less predictable than improvement in general cognitive functioning and may be due to concurrent difficulties with attention. Some of the more frequently occurring disorders in which memory and learning are likely to be compromised in children include: attention deficit-hyperactivity disorder (ADHD), learning disabilities, mental retardation, autism and other developmental disorders, cancer and iatrogenic memory disorders (secondary to chemotherapy), cerebral palsy, Down syndrome, extremely low birthweight, fragile X chromosome, hydrocephalus, inborn errors of metabolism (e.g., PKU), *in utero* toxic exposure, meningitis, seizure disorders, and many more (Reynolds & Voress, 2009).

Surprisingly, the assessment of memory in children and adolescents has only recently become common practice for clinicians. As pointed out by Reynolds & Voress (2009), the major texts on child neuropsychology of the 1970s and 1980s do not discuss the assessment of memory in children. However, by 1995, assessment of memory function in children was routinely discussed in key textbooks.

The Wide Range Assessment of Memory and Learning (WRAML; Sheslow & Adams, 1990) was the first memory assessment tool designed for use with children. This test consisted of nine subtests that yielded a verbal memory and visual memory score with normative data from children ages five to 17 years. Delayed recall trials could be given for four of the subtests. Four summary indices were provided for interpretation, including the General Memory, Verbal Memory, Visual Memory, and Learning Index. The Verbal, Visual, and Learning Indices were composed of three subtests each and were derived on the supposition that the dimensions of memory as assessed by the WRAML. While subsequent studies supported the verbal and visual dichotomy as a valid subdivision of the WRAML, data supporting the Learning Factor were equivocal (Aylward, Gioia, Verhulst, & Bell, 1995; Gioia, 1998) with several studies questioning whether subtests may tap into attention/concentration (Burton, Mittenberg, Gold, & Drabman, 1999; Haut, Haut, Callahan, & Frazen, 1992).

The Wide Range Assessment of Memory and Learning–Second Edition (WRAML-2; Sheslow & Adams, 2003) now spans the age range of five to 85+ years. The WRAML-2 comprises six core subtests as well as optional subtests. The screening battery takes approximately 20 minutes to administer, while the administration of the full test to a child takes about 75 to 90 minutes (Hartman, 2007). Administration is flexible, as the authors did not develop the test with an expectation that the entire test would be used. In designing the test in this manner, the authors have satisfied clinicians who adhere to either the fixed or flexible battery (subtest-specific) approach to assessment. The WRAML-2 is composed of three factors: verbal, non-verbal, and attention/concentration. While scores on WRAML-2 subtests contain high reliability coefficients, scores continue to contain error variance. Small studies are cited in the WRAML-2 manual, involving learning-disabled children, suggesting that the WRAML-2 is sensitive to this influence.

The Test of Memory and Learning (TOMAL; Reynolds & Bigler, 1994) consisted of 10 core subtests (five verbal and five nonverbal) that yielded verbal and nonverbal memory scale scores in addition to a composite memory score. The delayed recall index was composed of both verbal and visual subtests. It was also possible to compare the student's learning curve with that of a standardized sample. While some of the subtests appeared similar to other memory measures, additional supplemental indices (e.g., sequential recall attention/concentration, and learning) were unique to this measure and provided useful information. Reynolds and Bigler (1996) examined the latent structure of the TOMAL and found that factor solutions were highly stable across age groups. Interestingly, none of the solutions obtained matched a verbal/nonverbal dichotomy usually represented by the two scales of the TOMAL. Instead, what emerged were components representing various levels of complexity in memory tasks and processing demands that cut across modalities. Alternative methods of interpretation based on factor-analytic results were provided (Reynolds & Bigler, 1996). In contrast to many neuropsychological measures that combine the forward and backward recall measures, the TOMAL provided separate scores for forward and backward digit and letter recall. The TOMAL included studies of ethnic and gender bias, and items showing cultural bias were eliminated.

The TOMAL-2 (Reynolds and Voress, 2007) is the revised edition of the original TOMAL. The TOMAL-2 can be administered to individuals aged five to 59. For adults ages 55–89, a shorter battery is available. Demographics of the normative sample correspond to 2002 Census Bureau statistics to provide the most updated comparison with the U.S. population. The TOMAL-2 has the broadest range of memory tasks available in a standardized memory battery (Hartman, 2007). The TOMAL-2 consists of eight core and six supplementary subtests. There are two subtests that evaluate delayed verbal memory. There is no index of nonverbal delayed recall; nonverbal recall indices could not be computed due to lower reliability and restriction of range (Reynold and Voress, 2007). The TOMAL-2 reportedly takes less time to administer than the original TOMAL, and the core battery can be given within 30 minutes for most examinees. Results of factor structure studies indicated that there is a clear congruence across the TOMAL and the TOMAL-2, demonstrating the factorial equivalence of the two editions of the TOMAL (Reynolds & Voress, 2009). Results suggested that memory as assessed by the TOMAL and TOMAL-2 is more process-driven than content-driven. Consistently with the original TOMAL, care was taken to control for cultural bias. Following positive feedback from the original TOMAL, forward and backward digit and letter recall scores are computed separately.

The Children's Memory Scale (CMS, Cohen 1997) was developed with connections to the Wechsler Intelligence Scale for Children–Third Edition (WISC-III) built into the standardization process. The CMS consists of six core subtests representing verbal memory, attention/concentration, and visual memory, as well as three supplemental subtests. Subtests allow for evaluation of a student's immediate and delayed recall in both verbal and visual areas. There is a total of seven index scores calculated to examine the differences between immediate/delayed recall, verbal/visual memory, learning, recognition, and attention/concentration. Results of factor-analytic studies of the standardization sample indicated that a three-factor solution (attention/concentration, verbal memory, and visual memory) provided the "best fit" (Cohen, 1997). To date, the Children's Memory Scale has not been revised.

Language/Communication Abilities

Language depends on the integrity of the association cortex of both cerebral hemispheres; however, the main language areas are generally located in the left hemisphere for most humans. Broca's area is primarily responsible for planning speech (expressive language) and is located in the inferior temporal lobe. Wernicke's area is involved in representing and recognizing sound patterns of words (receptive language) and resides in the superior temporal lobe. When evaluating the integrity of brain–behavior functioning, both regions should be assessed. While cognitive measures provide language-based measures of general intelligence, information obtained does not provide an adequate measure of listening comprehension that is independent of verbal expression. For this reason, it is imperative to include a measure of receptive vocabulary as part of the neuropsychological evaluation. If language issues appear problematic, a measure of expressive vocabulary may also provide additional useful information.

The Peabody Picture Vocabulary Test–Fourth Edition (PPVT-IV: Dunn & Dunn, 2007) is designed to assess receptive vocabulary by having the examinee select one of four pictures that best represents a target word. The test is untimed and does not require reading ability. The starting and stopping points for the PPVT-IV are determined by the individual's chronological age and basal and ceiling rules. The PPVT-IV is appropriate for individuals ages 2½ to over 90 years of age. The PPVT-IV is the first release that includes color-illustrated pictures. There are two parallel forms of the PPVT-IV. Although the PPVT-IV is limited to the assessment of receptive vocabulary, it is useful in establishing the level of verbal comprehension when expressive communication is not required. The PPVT-IV is co-normed with the Expressive Vocabulary Test–Second Edition (EVT-II: Williams, 2007). The EVT-II evaluates expressive vocabulary and word retrieval in English-speaking individuals age 2½ to over 90 years. Reliability and validity scores reported in the examination manuals ranged from the .80s to .90s.

The Oral and Written Language Scales- Second Edition (OWLS-II: Carrow-Woolfolk, 2011) is an individually administered assessment of receptive and expressive (oral and written) language for individuals aged three through 21 years old. The OWLS-II consists of four scales: Listening Comprehension, Oral Expression, Reading Comprehension, and Written Expression, which assess listening, speaking, and writing skills, respectively. The Listening Comprehension Scale is designed to measure one's understanding of spoken language. The examinee is required to look at four colorful pictures and select the picture that best depicts the verbal stimulus. The test is untimed, does not require reading ability, and the starting and stopping points are determined by the individual's chronological age and basal and ceiling rules. As the task becomes more difficult, items increase in length, linguistic complexity, and semantic content. Verbal logic, humor, and figurative language are also introduced into items.

To administer the Oral Expression Scale of the OWLS-II, the examinee answers questions, finishes sentences, and generates sentences in response to visual or oral prompts. Due to the recency of the OWLS-II publication, limited research is available; however, the OWLS-II is similar to the original OWLS that exhibited sound psychometric properties.

Perceptual/Sensory and Motor Functioning

Visual perception and motor functions are complex processes involving many different aspects of brain functioning. The assessment of visual perception is useful in determining the extent to which visual and tactile-kinesthetic information is received and integrated. When clinicians evaluate a child's motor functioning, they usually assess fine motor control and dexterity. The following measures are examples of tests that evaluate visual perception and motor functions.

The Beery-Buktenica Developmental Test of Visual-Motor Integration–6th Edition (VMI; Beery & Beery, 2010) involves copying a sequence of 24 increasingly complex geometric figures. This measure is normed for individuals age two to 100 years old, and takes approximately five to 15 minutes to administer. The VMI measures the extent to which an individual can integrate visual and motor abilities; however, if an individual has difficulties on this measure, it is not possible to ascertain whether it was due to visual, motor, or visual-motor integration problems. As such, if it is determined that further testing is warranted, optional visual perception and motor coordination subtests are available and help compare relatively pure visual and motor performance.

The Developmental Test of Visual Perception–Second Edition (DTVP-2; Hammill, Pearson, & Voress, 1993) and the Developmental Test of Visual Perception–Adolescent and Adult (DTVP-A; Reynolds, Pearson, and Voress, 2002) are comprehensive measures of visual perception that reliably differentiate visual perception problems from visual-motor integration difficulties. The DTVP-2 is designed to be used with children ages four to 10 years and consists of seven subtests, including Visual-Motor Speed, Position in Space, Eye–Hand Coordination, Copying Spatial Relations, Figure-Ground, Visual Closure, and Form Constancy. Subtests are grouped into either the Motor-Reduced Visual Index or the Visual-Motor Integration Index. A General Visual Perception Quotient is also generated. The DTVP-A may be used with individuals 11 to 74 years old and consists of six subtests: Copying, Figure-Ground, Visual-Motor Search, Visual Closure, Visual-Motor Speed, and Form Constancy. Consistent with the DTVP-2, Motor-Reduced Visual, Visual-Motor Integration, and General Visual Perception Index scores are obtained. The DTVP-2 and DTVP-A are especially useful in the evaluation of children and adolescents who have suffered a TBI or stroke where right hemisphere function may be compromised. These measures are well normed and have good internal consistency and validity.

The Children's Halstead-Reitan Neuropsychological Battery (CHRNB; Reitan & Wolfson, 1992) for children nine to 14 years, and the Reitan-Indiana Test Battery (RINB; Reitan, 1969) for children ages five to eight are two children's batteries based on the adult version of the Halstead-Reitan Neuropsychological Battery (Halstead, 1947; Reitan & Wolfson, 1985). These batteries contain numerous measures necessary for understanding brain behavior relationships, including assessment of sensory abilities, motor speed, and dexterity. In addition, abilities in the areas of concept formation, attention/concentration, verbal abilities, and memory are evaluated. Both the CHRNB and the RINB provide examination of overall performance, patterns of performance, right-left differences, and pathognomic signs (Reitan, 1986, 1987). The Luria Nebraska Neuropsychological Battery–Children's Revision (LNNB-CR: Golden, 1984) was developed according to neurodevelopmental stages and provides information specific to motor, rhythm, tactile, visual, verbal (receptive and expressive) and memory functioning. Interpretation of the LNNB-CR focuses predominantly on scale patterns as opposed to levels of performance or pathognomonic signs.

Emotional/Behavioral Functioning

Children who present with compromised CNS functioning or neurodevelopmental disorders often exhibit problems with emotional or behavior status. In order to adequately provide recommendations in regard to intervention planning, parent and teacher rating scales are often completed that provide information regarding functioning at home and school in a variety of areas. The assessment of emotional and behavior status has lagged behind the methods available for assessing other domains of functioning (Martin, 1988). However, during recent years, the publication of new instruments with improved psychometric properties has emerged.

The Conners' Rating Scale-Third Edition (CRS-3: Conners, 2008) is a widely used behavior rating scale used to assess children aged six to 18 years. The CRS-III was redefined with a focus on ADHD in school-aged children and a strengthened connection with the Diagnostic and Statistical Manual-Fourth Edition- Text Revision (DSM-IV-TR). Parent, teacher, and self-report measures are available. The self-report measure can be used with adolescents aged eight to 18 years. There are short and long forms available for each of the three rating scales. The long form consists of the following scales: general psychopathology, inattention, hyperactivity/ impulsivity, learning problems, executive functioning, aggression, peer relations, family relations, ADHD- Inattentive, ADHD Hyperactive-Impulsive, ADHD Combined, oppositional defiant disorder, and conduct disorder. The Conners 3 Global Index is a measure of general psychopathology. The Conners' ADHD Index 10-item index may be used for screening large groups of children to see if further assessment of ADHD is warranted.

The Behavior Assessment System for Children– Second Edition (BASC-II: Reynolds & Kamphaus, 2004) includes not only teacher and parent forms that can be used from ages two to 25, but also offers a structured observation system (SOS), and for children eight years old and older, a self-report measure that can effectively assess emotional and behavioral status. The primary scales assessed using the Parent and Teacher rating scale include: Adaptability, Activities Of Daily Living, Aggression, Anxiety, Attention Problems, Atypicality, Conduct Problems, Depression, Functional Communication, Hyperactivity, Leadership, Learning Problems,

Social Skills, Somatization, Study Skills, and Withdrawal. Composite score indices are presented for the following: Emotional Symptoms, Inattention/Hyperactivity, Internalizing Problems, Personal Adjustment, and School Problems. The SOS can be used with direct observation that may be more appropriate for monitoring small and gradual changes. Direct observation also provides an objective measure without the potential bias of raters, and can be especially useful when raters (e.g., parents and teacher) disagree in their portrayals of the child. The BASC-2 revision included many improvements from the original BASC that was published in 1992, including improved reliability and standardization the addition of more scales, updated norms, and the age range was expanded to use up through age 21. The BASC-2 also was designed to facilitate differential diagnoses. When adaptive behavior is an identified concern, completion of an adaptive behavior scale such as the Vineland Adaptive Behavior Scales (VABS-II: Sparrow, Cicchetti, & Balla, 2005) or the Adaptive Behavior Assessment System–Second Edition (ABAS: Harrison & Oakland, 2003), may be particularly helpful for intervention planning.

General Organization of the Neuropsychological Assessment of the Child

The neuropsychological evaluation of a child focuses more directly on CNS functioning, rather than on the identification of strictly neurological disorders. However, assessment can be useful in the diagnosis and identification of subtler conditions (e.g., ADHD, learning disabilities). A neuropsychological assessment of a child differs from that of an adult in that educational considerations are of paramount importance. Furthermore, information obtained from parent and teacher report often provides useful information regarding behavioral functioning.

A thorough history is an important part of a child neuropsychological evaluation. Information about gestation, delivery, postnatal period, and early speech and motor development are important. The length of time and functional changes since the trauma or the disease onset, premorbid levels of functioning, and family history of related problems provide information that will affect how information is interpreted. A review of school records including any special education records, standardized test scores, grades, and information regarding behavioral difficulties will provide additional useful information. If a child has had a previous psychological evaluation, the neuropsychologist must obtain a copy of that assessment if possible. Once information is obtained from a thorough clinical interview with a parent and school records are reviewed, there are nine guidelines, derived from a variety of sources (Reynolds & Mayfield, 1999; Riccio & Reynolds, 1998; Rourke, Bakker, Fisk, and Strang, 1983), that should be considered in the organization of a neuropsychological assessment.

1. *It is crucial to assess all, or at least a significant majority, of the child's educationally relevant cognitive skills or higher-order information processing skills.* General intellectual functioning via a comprehensive IQ test such as the Wechsler Individual Assessment of Children–Fourth Edition (WISC-IV; Wechsler, 2003) or Kaufman Assessment Battery for Children-Second Edition (KABC-II; Kaufman & Kaufman, 2004) is necessary. Strong measures of *g* that evaluate the efficiency of mental processing provide a baseline for interpreting all other aspects of the assessment (Riccio & Reynolds, 1998). Other areas to be assessed include memory, attention, concentration, and new learning as these are the most common of all complaints following any CNS compromise as well as neurodevelopmental disorders (e.g., ADHD, learning disabilities). Assessment of basic academic skills including reading, mathematics, and written language provide a performance-based measure of learning.

2. *Testing should assess the efficiency of the right and left hemispheres of the brain.* Different brain systems that impact treatment are involved in each hemisphere. In the right-handed majority, language-related processes are usually left-lateralized. The left hemisphere processes rapid sequential recognition, recall and recognition of order information, and the planning of motor and conceptual action skills. Visual-spatial processes, including facial recognition, arousal, and emotional perception, are right-hemisphere functions. Comprehending inferences, metaphors, and humor are also right-hemisphere abilities (Kinsbourne, 2009). Neuropsychological tests, including the Children's Halstead-Reitan Neuropsychological Test Battery (Reitan & Davison, 1974; Reitan & Wolfson, 1992), Reitan-Indiana Test Battery (Reitan, 1969; Reitan & Davison, 1974), and the Luria-Nebraska Neuropsychological Children's Battery (Golden, 1986) are useful in the assessment of brain systems.

3. *Testing should assess both anterior and posterior regions of brain function.* The anterior portion of the brain is generative and regulatory, while the posterior region is principally receptive (Riccio & Reynolds,

1998). Sensory perception should be evaluated. In the area of language, receptive and expressive vocabulary tests may evaluate the posterior and anterior regions, respectively. When care is taken to systematically evaluate both hemispheres as well as anterior and posterior regions, information can be gleamed from all major quadrants of the neocortex.

4. *Testing should determine the presence of specific deficits.* In contrast to many psychological tests, neuropsychological tests tend to be less *g*-loaded and have greater specificity of measurement. This is beneficial when the goal is to determine whether specific functional problems exist. In working with children and adolescents with traumatic brain injury (TBI), strokes, tumors, seizures, or chronic medical disorders, very specific changes in neocortical function are sometimes best addressed by a neuropsychological assessment.

5. *Determine the acuteness versus the chronicity of any present weaknesses.* The duration of a problem is important when formulating a diagnosis and planning treatment interventions. Following an evaluation of a child, a neuropsychologist is called to the task of integrating information from the clinical interview, school records, behavior observations, and testing data. When a comprehensive evaluation is undertaken, it is possible to distinguish chronic neurodevelopmental disorders (e.g., learning disabilities, ADHD) from acute problems resulting from trauma, stroke, or disease with reasonable certainty. The age of the child and the acuteness or chronicity of the problem are important factors to consider when planning treatment or rehabilitation strategies.

6. *The evaluation should locate intact complex functional systems.* While it is imperative in the assessment process to locate weaknesses that are likely to represent permanent or chronic difficulties in functioning, it is even more important to locate the strengths or intact systems of a child. In doing so, it is possible to enhance the probability of designing successful treatments. By identifying intact systems, parents and teachers are provided with useful information to help a child, rather than fostering low expectations. For example, if a child exhibits a weakness with verbal memory but her visual memory is fairly intact, the neuropsychologist can recommend strategies to use in the classroom that draw on her area of strength.

7. *Testing should assess mood, personality, and behavioral functioning.* Neuropsychologists need to be careful not to ignore changes in mood, personality, and behavior that affect a child or adolescent's

functioning. Some of these changes will be temporary, while others will be more permanent. Changes can be directly a result of the CNS compromise at the cellular and systematic levels and others will be more indirect (i.e., the reaction to a loss or change in function, or to how others respond to and interact with the individual). A thorough history can assist in determining direct versus indirect effects. At times, it will likely be an interaction between direct and indirect effects that cause mood disturbances. In adolescents with TBI, anger, and emotional lability are common complaints from six months to a year post-injury. Changes in frontal lobe functioning as a result of the injury, coupled with academic difficulties, social problems, and safety restrictions (i.e., no sports, no driving), collaboratively have an impact on mood and behavioral functioning.

The Behavior Assessment System for Children–Second Edition (BASC-2; 2004) or the Conners' Rating Scales–Third Edition (CRS-3; 2008) contain behavior rating scales and personality inventories that are useful in planning interventions. When planning interventions, it will be necessary to determine whether behavior changes are a direct or indirect result of brain insult or whether premorbid behaviors were evident (Reynolds & Mayfield, 1999).

8. *Evaluations should be written with the primary audience, the school setting, in mind.* Children and adolescents need to be able to function within a school or educational setting, regardless of whether they exhibit a neurodevelopmental disorder or have sustained a brain insult. Results of an evaluation should be presented so that academic and behavior concerns are addressed, as these are primary concerns for educators. Recommendations should provide guidance in determining appropriate services (i.e., special education, content mastery, or a 504 Accommodation Plan) necessary for them to successfully learn. Specific, simple recommendations regarding teaching to a child's strengths through the utilization of intact functional systems will be useful. If behavioral problems are evident, the clinician will need to explain how to best anticipate and diffuse negative situations. A behavior-management plan is often recommended in order to provide positive reinforcement for favorable behavior. Many educators have not had previous experiences with a child who has sustained a TBI, stroke, or other neurological insult. It is the neuropsychologist's role to explain academic and behavioral sequelae so that educators can better understand how to teach these children. For a child with TBI, rapid recovery takes place during the first six months post-injury, with slower, subtler improvements noted up to two years following insult. Neuropsychologists need to explain this rapid improvement and the need for schools to wait six months before conducting an assessment. It is also necessary to explain that children may not show deficits immediately following their injury but may develop difficulties over time as the demand for new skills emerges (Gronwall, Wrightson, & McGinn, 1997; Taylor & Alden, 1997).

9. *When working directly with the school, the evaluation processes should be efficient.* School districts often do not have a neuropsychologist on staff. Furthermore, they rarely have the time, assessment measures, or funding to provide a comprehensive neuropsychological evaluation. If a neuropsychologist is used to consult with a school to evaluate a child, care should be taken to conduct an evaluation in an efficient manner. The school, with permission from the parents, can provide school records and access to any prior evaluations. Recent intellectual and academic testing by the school district can be incorporated with neuropsychological findings. Behavior rating forms or classroom observations provided by the school may also be obtained and interpreted by the clinician.

Conclusions

While the field of pediatric neuropsychology is relatively young, neuropsychological assessment of children and adolescents has much to offer toward understanding the functional systems of the brain and the mechanisms involved in learning. Child neuropsychology provides a theoretical framework for understanding patterns of strengths and weaknesses, and the extent to which these patterns may remain stable or change over time (Temple, 1997). Once the clinician identifies the assessment needs of the individual child, he or she must make decisions regarding the most appropriate assessment measures for exploring the dimensions of behavior. In choosing appropriate measures, neurodevelopmental considerations and psychometric properties must be considered. Once an evaluation is completed, understanding the strengths and weaknesses of a child provides the neuropsychologist with needed information to recommended appropriate school modifications and community intervention. When writing neuropsychological reports, the clinician must remember that the audience includes parents, teachers, and other medical professions who are in need of straightforward information that is easily understood and applied. Of paramount importance is that clinicians must recognize that providing useful, scientifically supported conclusions that contribute to the treatment of the child is the ultimate purpose of assessment. The goal of this chapter is to provide the clinician with the knowledge necessary to make informed choices when evaluating children.

References

Armstrong, C. M., Allen, D. N., Donohue, B. & Mayfield, J. (2008). Sensitivity of the comprehensive trail making test to traumatic brain injury in adolescents. *Archives of Clinical Neuropsychology, 23*, 351–358.

Aylward, G. P. (2002). Cognitive and neuropsychological outcomes: More than IQ scores. *Mental Retardation & Developmental Disabilities Research Reviews, 8*, 234–240.

Aylward, G. P., Gioia, G., Verhulst, S. J., & Bell, S. (1995). Factor structure of the Wide Range Assessment of Memory and Learning in a clinical population. *Journal of Psychoeducational Assessment, 13*, 132–142.

Barkley, R. A. (1981). *Hyperactive children: A handbook for diagnosis and treatment.* New York: Guilford Press.

Barkley, R. A. (1998). *Attention-deficit hyperactivity disorder: A handbook for diagnosis and treatment (2nd ed.).* New York: Guilford Press.

Baron, I. S., Fennell, E. B., & Voeller, K. J. K. (1995). *Pediatric neuropsychology in a medical setting.* London: Oxford University Press.

Bauer, R. M. (1994). The flexible battery approach to neuropsychological assessment. In R. D. Vanderploeg (Ed.), *Clinician's guide to neuropsychological assessment* (pp. 259–290). Hillsdale, NJ: Lawrence Erlbaum Associates.

Beery, K. E., & Beery, N. A. (2010). *The Beery-Buktenica Developmental Test of Visual-Motor Integration–Sixth Edition.* Minneapolis, MN: Pearson Assessments.

Brink, J. D., Garrett, A. L., Hale, W. R., Woo-Sam, J., & Nickel, V. C. (1970). Recovery of motor and intellectual function in children sustaining severe head injuries. *Developmental Medicine & Child Neurology, 12*, 545–571.

Burton, D. B., Mittenberg, W., Gold, S., & Drabman, R. (1999). A structural equation analysis of the Wide Range Assessment of Memory and Learning in a clinical sample. *Child Neuropsychology, 5*(1), 34–40.

Carrow-Woolfolk, E. (2011). *Oral and written language scales-second edition.* Los Angeles, CA: Western Psychological Services.

Christensen, A. J. (1975). *Luria's neuropsychological investigation.* New York: Spectrum.

Cohen, M. (1997). *Children's memory scale.* San Antonio, TX: The Psychological Corporation.

Conners, C. K. (1992). *Conners' Continuous Performance Test user's manual.* Toronto, Canada: Multi-Health Systems.

Conners, C. K. (1994). *Conners' Continuous Performance Test* (Version 3.0) [Computer software]. Toronto, Canada; Multi-Health Systems.

Conners, C. K. (1995). *Conners' Continuous Performance Test user's manual.* Toronto, Canada; Multi-Health Systems.

Conners, C. K. (2000). *Conners' Continuous Performance Test user's manual.* Toronto, Canada: Multi-Health Systems.

Conners, C. K. (2008). *Conners' rating scales.* Toronto: Multi-Health Systems.

D'Amato, R. C., & Hartlage, L. C. (2008). *Essentials of neuropsychological assessment-Second edition.* New York: Springer Publishing Company.

D'Amato, R. C., Fletcher-Janzen, E., & Reynolds, C. R. (Eds.). (2005). *Handbook of school neuropsychology.* New York: Wiley.

Daniel, L. M., Lim, S. B., & Clark, L. (2003). Eight-year outcome of very-low-birth-weight infants born in KK Hospital. *Annals, Academy of Medicine, Singapore, 32*, 354–361.

Delis, D. C., Jacobson, M., Bondi, M. W., Hamilton, J. M., & Salmon, D. P. (2003). The myth of testing construct validity using shared variance techniques with normal or mixed clinical populations: Lessons from memory assessment. *Journal of the International Neuropsychological Society, 9*, 936–946.

Delis, D. C., Kaplan, E., & Kramer, J. (2001). *Delis Kaplan Executive Function System.* San Antonio, TX: The Psychological Corporation.

Denckla, M. B. (1994). Measurement of executive function. In G. R. Lyon (Ed.), *Frames of reference of the assessment of learning disabilities: New views on measurement issues* (pp. 117–142). Baltimore, MD: Brookes.

Dennis, M., Wilkinson, M., Koski, L., & Humphreys, R. (1995). Attention deficits in the long term after childhood head injury. In S.H. Broman & M. E. Michel (Eds.), *Traumatic brain injury in children* (pp. 165–187). New York: Oxford University Press.

Douglas, V. I. (1983). Attention and cognitive problems. In M. Rutter (Ed.), *Developmental neuropsychiatry* (pp. 280–329). New York: Guilford Press.

Dunn, L. M., & Dunn, D. M. (2007). *Peabody Picture Vocabulary Test–Fourth Edition.* Circle Pines, MN: American Guidance Service.

Fennell, E. B. (1994). Issues in child neuropsychological assessment. In R. Vanderploeg (Ed.), *Clinician's guide to neuropsychological assessment* (pp. 165–184). Hillsdale, NJ: Lawrence Erlbaum.

Fennell, E. B., & Bauer, R. M. (2009). Models of inference in evaluating brain–behavior relationships in children. In C. R. Reynolds & E. Fletcher-Janzen (Eds.), *Handbook of clinical child neuropsychology* (3rd ed.; pp. 231–243), New York: Springer.

Fitzhugh-Bell, K. (1997). Historical antecedents of clinical neuropsychology. In A. M. Horton, D. Wedding, & J. Webster (Eds.), *The neuropsychology handbook* (pp. 67–90). New York: Springer.

Fletcher-Janzen, E., & Reynolds, C. R. (2003). *Childhood disorders diagnostic desk reference.* New York: Wiley.

Gioia, G. A. (1998). Re-examining the factor structure of the Wide Range Assessment of Memory and Learning: Implications for clinical interpretation. *Assessment, 5*(2), 127–139.

Golden, C. J. (1981). The Luria-Nebraska children's battery: Theory and formulation. In G. W. Hynd & J. E. Obrzut (Eds.), *Neuropsychological assessment and the school-age child: Issues and procedures* (pp. 277–302). New York: Grune & Stratton.

Golden, C. J. (1984). *Luria-Nebraska Neuropsychological Battery: Children's revision.* Loss Angeles: Western Psychological Services.

Golden, C. J. (1986). *The Luria-Nebraska Neuropsychological Battery: Children's revision.* Los Angeles: Western Psychological Services.

Goldman, P. S., & Lewis, M. E. (1978). Developmental biology of brain damage and experience. In C. W. Cotman (Ed.), *Neuronal plasticity.* New York: Raven.

Goldstein, G. (1997). The clinical utility of standardized or flexible battery approaches to neuropsychological assessment. In G. Goldstein & T. M. Incagnoli (Eds.), *Contemporary approaches to neuropsychological assessment* (pp. 67–92), New York: Plenum.

Goldstein, S. (1999). Attention-deficit/hyperactivity disorder. In S. Goldstein & C. R. Reynolds (Eds.), *Handbook of neurodevelopment and genetic disorders in children* (pp. 154–184), New York: Guilford Press.

Goldstein, S., & Schwebach, A. (2009). Neuropsychological basis of leraning disabilities. In C. R. Reynolds & E. Fletcher-Janzen (Eds.), *Handbook of clinical child neuropsychology* (3rd ed.; pp. 187–202), New York: Springer.

Gordon, M. (1983). *The Gordon Diagnostic System.* DeWitt, NY: Gordon Systems.

Gordon, M. (1986a). How is a computerized attention test used in the diagnosis of attention deficit disorder? *Journal of Children in Contemporary Society, 19*, 53–64.

Gordon, M. (1986b). Microprocessor-based assessment of attention deficit disorders. *Psychopharmacology Bulletin, 22*, 288–290.

Gordon, M., & Mettelman, B. B. (1988). The assessment of attention: I. Standardization and reliability of a behavior-based measure. *Journal of Clinical Psychology, 44*, 682–690.

Gordon Systems, Inc. (1991). *Administration manual for the Gordon Diagnostic System.* DeWitt, NY: Gordon Systems, Inc. Greenberg, L. M. (1988–1999). *The Test of Variables of Attention (TOVA).* Los Alamitos, CA: Universal Attention Disorders.

Greenberg, L. M. (1996–1999). *The Test of Variable of Attention–Auditory (TOVA-A).* Los Alamitos, CA: Universal Attention Disorders.

Greenberg, L. M., & Crosby, R. D. (1992). Specificity and sensitivity of the Test of Variables of Attention (TOVA). Unpublished manuscript. Available from Universal Attention Disorders, Los Alamitos, CA.

Gronwall, D., Wrightson, P., & McGinn, V. (1997). Effects of mild head injury during the preschool years. *Journal of the International Neuropsychological Society, 3*(6), 592–597.

Halstead, W. C. (1947). *Brain and intelligence: A quantitative study of the frontal lobes.* Chicago: University of Chicago Press.

Hammill, D. D., & Larsen, S. C. (2009). *Test of written language* (4th ed.) (TOWL-4). Austin, TX: PRO-ED.

Hammill, D. D., Pearson, N. A., & Voress, J. K. (1993). *Developmental Test of Visual Perception–Second Edition.* Austin, TX: PRO-ED.

Harris, P. (1957). Head injuries in childhood. *Archives of Diseases in Childhood, 6*, 488–491.

Harrison, P., & Oakland, T. (2003). *Adaptive Behavior Assessment System–Second Edition.* Los Angeles, CA: Western Psychological Services.

Hartlage, L. C., & Long, C. J. (1997). Development of neuropsychology as a professional specialty: History, training, and credentialing. In C. R. Reynolds & E. Fletcher-Janzen (Eds.), *Handbook of clinical child neuropsychology* (2nd ed.; pp. 3–16), New York: Plenum.

Hartlage, L. C., & Long, C. J. (2009). Development of neuropsychology as a professional psychological specialty: History, training, and credentialing. In C. R. Reynolds & E. Fletcher-Janzen (Eds.), *Handbook of clinical child neuropsychology* (pp. 3–18). New York: Springer.

Hartlage, L. C., & Telzrow, C. F. (1986). *Neuropsychological assessment and intervention with children and adolescents.* Sarasota, FL: Professional Resource Exchange.

Hartman, D. E. (2007). Test Review: Wide Range Assessment of Memory and Learning–2 (WRAML-2): WRedsigned and WReally Improved. *Applied Neuropsychology, 14*(2), 138–140.

Haut, J. S., Haut, M. W., Callahan, T. S., & Franzen M. D. (1992, November). *Factor analysis of the Wide Range Assessment of Memory and Learning (WRAML) scores in a clinical sample.* Paper presented at the 12th annual meeting of the National Academy of Neuropsychology; Pittsburg, PA.

Kamphaus, R. W. (2005). *Clinical assessment of child and adolescent intelligence.* Boston, MA: Allyn & Bacon.

Kaplan, E. (1988). A process approach to neuropsychological assessment. In T. Boll & B. K. Bryant (Eds.), *Clinical neuropsychology and brain function* (pp. 125–167). Washington, DC: American Psychological Association.

Kaufman, A., & Kaufman, N. L. (1983) *K-ABC interpretation manual.* Circle Pines, MN: American Guidance Services.

Kaufman, A., & Kaufman, N. L. (2004). *Kaufman Assessment Battery for Children–Second Edition.* Circle Pines, MN: American Guidance Service.

Kerr, E. N., Smith, M. L., DaSilva, M., Hoffman, H. J., & Humphries, R. P. (1991). Neuropsychological effects of craniopharyngioma treated by microsurgery. Abstracts of the 19th annual INS meeting. San Antonio, Texas. *Journal of Clinical & Experimental Neuropsychology, 13*, 57.

Kinsbourne, M. (2009). Development of cerebral lateralization in children. In C. R. Reynolds & E. Fletcher-Janzen (Eds.), *Handbook of clinical child neuropsychology-third edition* (pp. 47–66), New York: Springer.

Kolb, B., & Fantie, B. D. (2009). Development of the child's brain and behavior. In C. R. Reynolds & E. Fletcher-Janzen (Eds.), *Handbook of clinical child neuropsychology-third edition* (pp. 19–46), New York: Springer.

Korkman, M., Kirk, U., & Kemp, S. (1998). *NEPSY–A developmental neuropsychological assessment.* San Antonio, TX: The Psychological Corporation.

Korkman, M., Kirk, U., & Kemp, S. (2007). *NEPSY-II–A developmental neuropsychological assessment–Second Edition.* San Antonio, TX: The Psychological Corporation.

Kriel, R., Krach, L., & Panser, L. (1989). Closed head injury: Comparison of children younger and older than six years of age. *Pediatric Neurology, 5*(5), 296–300.

Leark, R. A., Dupuy, T. R., Greenberg, L. M., Corman, C. L., & Kindschi, C. L. (1996). *TOVA Test of Variables of Attention: Professional manual, version 7.0.* Los Alamitos, CA: Universal Attention Disorders.

Lezak, M. D., Howieson, D. B., Loring, D. W., Hannay, H. J., & Fischer, J. S. (2004). *Neuropsychological assessment* (4th ed.). London: Oxford University Press.

Llorente, A. M., Amado, A. J., Voigt, R. G., Berretta, M. C., Fraley, J. K., Jenson, C. L., & Heird, W. C. (2000). Internal consistency, temporal stability, and reproducibility of individual index scores on the Tests of Variables of Attention (TOVA) in children with attention-deficit/hyperactivity disorder (AD/HD). *Archives of Clinical Neuropsychology, 15*, 1–12.

Luria, A. R. (1966). *Higher cortical functions in man.* New York: Basic Books.

Luria, A. R. (1973). *The working brain.* New York: Basic Books.

Luria, A. R. (1980). *Higher cortical functions in man.* New York: Basic Books.

Martin, R. P. (1988). *Personality and behavior assessment.* New York: Guilford Press.

Mayfield, J. W., Reynolds, C. R., & Fletcher-Janzen, E. (2009). Neuropsychological assessments in the school. In T. B. Gutkin & C. R. Reynolds (Eds.), *The handbook of school psychology* (Vol. 4; pp. 307–331). Hoboken, NJ: John Wiley and Sons.

Milberg, W. B., Hebben, N., & Kaplan, E. (1986). The Boston Process Approach to neuropsychological assessment. In I. Grant & K. M. Adams (Eds.), *Neuropsychological assessment and neuropsychiatric disorders* (2nd ed., pp. 58–80). New York: Oxford University Press.

Miller, L. T., & Vernon, P. A. (1996). Intelligence, reaction time, and working memory in 4- to 6-year-old children. *Intelligence, 22*, 155–190.

Mirsky, A. F. (1996). Disorders of attention: A neuropsychological perspective. In R. G. Lyon & N. A. Krasnegor (Eds.), *Attention, memory, and executive function* (pp. 71–96). Baltimore: Paul H. Brookes.

Molfese, D. L. (1995). Electrophysiological responses obtained during infancy and their relation to later language development: Further findings. In M. G. Tramontana & S. R. Hooper (Eds.), *Advances in child neuropsychology* (Vol. 3; pp. 1–11). New York: Springer-Verlag.

Moses, J. A. (2004). Test review: Comprehensive Trail Making Test (CTMT). *Archives of Clinical Neuropsychology, 19*, 703–708.

Partington, J. E. & Leiter, R. G. (1949). Partington's Pathway Test. *The Psychological Service Center Bulletin, 1*, 9–20.

Plaisted, J. R., Gustavson, J. C., Wilkening, G. N., & Golden, C. J. (1983). The Luria Nebraska Neuropsychological Battery–Children's revision: Theory and current research findings. *Journal of Clinical Child Psychology, 12*, 13–21.

Reitan, R. M. (1955). The relation of the Trail Making Test to organic brain damage. *Journal of Consulting Psychology, 19*, 393–394.

Reitan, R. M. (1969). *Manual for administration of neuropsychological test batteries for adults and children.* Indianapolis, IN: Author.

Reitan, R. M. (1986). *Theoretical and methodological bases of the Halstead-Reitan Neuropsychological Test Battery.* Tucson, AZ: Neuropsychological Press.

Reitan, R. M. (1987). *Neuropsychological evaluation of children.* Tucson, AZ: Neuropsychological Press.

Reitan, R. M., & Davison, L. A. (1974). *Clinical neuropsychology: Current status and applications.* Washington, DC: Winston.

Reitan, R. M., & Wolfson, D. (1985). *The Halstead-Reitan Neuropsychological Battery. Theory and clinical interpretation.* Tucson, AZ; Neuropsychological Press.

Reitan, R. M., & Wolfson, D. (1992). *Neuropsychological evaluation of older children.* Tucson, AZ: Neuropsychology Press.

Reynolds, C. R. (2002). *Comprehensive Trail Making Test: Examiner's manual.* Austin, Texas: PRO-ED.

Reynolds, C. R., & Bigler, E. D. (1994). *Test of memory and learning.* TX: Pro-Ed.

Reynolds, C. R. & Bigler, E. D. (1996). Factor structure, factor indexes, and other useful statistics for interpretation of the Test of Memory and Learning (TOMAL). *Archives of Clinical Neuropsychology, 11*(1), 29–43.

Reynolds, C. R., & Bigler, E. D. (1997). Clinical neuropsychological assessment of child and adolescent memory with the Test of Memory and Learning. In C.R. Reynolds & E. Fletcher-Janzen (Eds.), *Handbook of clinical child neuropsychology, 11*, 29–43. New York: Plenum Press.

Reynolds, C. R., & Kamphaus, R. W. (2004). *Behavior Assessment System for Children–Second Edition (BASC-2).* Circle Pines, MN: AGS.

Reynolds, C. R., & Mayfield, J. W. (1999). Neuropsychological assessment in genetically linked neurodevelopmental disorders. In S. Goldstein & C. R. Reynolds (Eds.), *Handbook of neurodevelopmental and genetic disorders in children* (pp. 9–37), New York: Guilford Press.

Reynolds, C. R., Pearson, N. A., & Voress, J. K. (2002). *Developmental Test of Visual Perception–adolescent and adult.* Austin, TX: Pro-Ed.

Reynolds. C. R., & Voress, J. K. (2007). *Test of memory and learning–Second Edition.* Austin, TX: PRO-ED.

Reynolds, C. R., & Voress, J. K. (2009). Clinical neuropsychological assessment with the Test of Memory and Learning, Second Edition. In C. R. Reynolds & E. Fletcher-Janzen (Eds.), *Handbook of clinical child neuropsychology* (3rd ed.; pp. 297–319). New York: Springer.

Riccio, C. A., Gonzalez, J. J., & Hynd, G. W. (1994). Attention-deficit hyperactivity disorder (ADHD) and learning disabilities. *Learning Disability Quarterly, 17*, 311–322.

Riccio, C. A., & Hynd, G. W. (1996). Neuroanatomical and neurophysiological aspects of dyslexia. *Topics in Language Disorders, 16*(2), 1–13.

Riccio, C. A. & Reynolds, C. R. (1998). Neuropsychological assessment of children. In M. Hersen & A. Bellack (Series Eds.) & C. R. Reynolds (Vol. Ed.), *Comprehensive clinical psychology. Vol. 4: Assessment* (pp. 267–301). New York: Elsevier.

Riccio, C.A., & Reynolds, C. R. (1999). Assessment of mild traumatic brain injury in children for neuropsychological rehabilitation. In M. J. Raymond, T. L. Bennett, L. C. Hartlage, and C. M. Cullum (Eds.), *Mild traumatic brain injury: A clinician's guide* (pp. 77–116). Austin, TX: PRO-ED.

Riccio, C. A., Reynolds, C. R., & Lowe, P. A. (2001). *Clinical applications of continuous performance tests.* New York: John Wiley & Sons.

Rourke, B. P., Bakker, D. J., Fisk, J. L., & Strang, J. D. (1983). *Child neuropsychology.* New York: Guilford Press.

Rourke, B. P., Bakker, D. J., Fisk, J. L., & Strang, J. D. (1986). *Neuropsychological assessment of children: A treatment oriented approach.* New York: Guilford Press.

Ryan, T. V., La Marche, J. A., Barth, J. T., & Boll. T. J. (1996). Neuropsychological consequences and treatment of pediatric head trauma. In E. S. Batchelor & R. S. Dean (Eds.), *Pediatric neuropsychology* (pp. 117–137). New York: Pergamon.

Sandford, J. A. & Turner, A. (1994–1999). *Integrated Visual and Auditory (IVA) continuous performance test.* Richmond, VA: BrainTrain.

Sandford, J. A., & Turner, A. (1995). *Manual for the Integrated Visual and Auditory (IVA) continuous performance test.* Richmond, VA: BrainTrain.

Sattler, J. M. (1990). *Assessment of children* (3rd ed.). San Diego, CA: Jerome M. Sattler.

Sattler, J. M., & Hoge, R. D. (2006). *Assessment of children: Behavioral, social, and clinical foundations.* La Mesa, CA: Sattler Publishing, Inc.

Seidel, W. T., Mitchell, W. G., Bell, T. S., Epport, K. L., Fodera, C., & Zelter, P. M. (1994). Developmental outcome in very young children treated for brain tumors. Abstracts of the Division of Clinical Neuropsychology, American Psychological Association Annual meeting, Boston. *The Clinical Neuropsychologist, 4*, 272.

Sheslow, D., & Adams, W. (1990). *Wide Range Assessment of Memory and Learning.* Wilmington, DE: Jastak Associates.

Sheslow, D., & Adams, W. (2003). Wide range Assessment of Memory and Learning Second Edition administration and technical manual. Lutz, FL: Psychological Assessment Resources.

Sparrow, S. S., Cicchetti, D. V., & Balla, D. A. (2005). *Vineland Adaptive Behavior Scales* (2nd ed.). Bloomington, MN: Pearson Publishing.

Spreen, O., Risser, A. H., & Edgell, D. (1995). *Developmental neuropsychology*. London: Oxford University Press.

Sweet, J. J., & Moberg, P. (1990). A survey of practices and beliefs among ABPP and non-ABPP clinical neuropsychologists. *The Clinical Neuropsychologist, 4*, 101–120.

Sweet, J. J., Moberg, P., & Westergaard, C. K. (1996). Five-year follow-up survey of practices and beliefs of clinical neuropsychologists. *The Clinical Neuropsychologist, 10*, 202–221.

Taylor, H. G., & Alden, J. (1997). Age-related differences in outcomes following childhood brain insults: An introduction and overview. *Journal of the International Neuropsychological Society, 3*(6), 555–567.

Temple, C. M. (1997). Cognitive neuropsychology and its application to children. *Journal of Child Psychology, Psychiatry, & Allied Disciplines, 38*, 27–52.

Wagner, R. K., Torgesen, J. K., & Rashotte, C. A. (1999). *Comprehensive Test of Phonological Processing*. Austin, TX: PRO-ED.

Wechsler, D. (2009). *Wechsler Individual Achievement Test-Third Edition*. San Antonio, TX: The Psychological Corporation.

Wechsler, D. (2003). *Wechsler Intelligence Scale for Children–Fourth Edition*. San Antonio, TX: Harcourt Assessment, Inc.

Wechsler, D., Kaplan, E., Fein, D., Kramer, J., Delis, D., & Morris, R., & Maerlender, A. (2004). *Wechsler Intelligence Scale for Children–Fourth Edition–Integrated*. San Antonio, TX: Harcourt Assessment, Inc.

Welsh, M. C., & Pennington, B. F. (1988). Assessing frontal lobe functioning in children; Views from developmental psychology. *Developmental Neuropsychology, 4*, 199–230.

Wiederholt, J. L., & Bryant, B. R. (2012). *Gray Oral Reading Tests* (5th ed.) (GORT-5). Austin, TX: PRO-ED.

Williams, K. (2007). *Expressive Vocabulary Test–Second Edition*. Circle Pines, MN. AGS.

Wilkinson, G. S., & Robertson, G. J. (2006). *Wide Range Achievement Test* (4th ed.) (WRAT-4). Lutz, FL: Psychologicla Assessment Resources.

Woodcock, R. W., McGrew, K. S., & Mather, N. (2001). *Woodcock-Johnson III Tests of Achievement: Examiner's manual*. Itasca, IL: Riverside Publishing.

Yeates, K. O., & Taylor, H. G. (1997). Predicting premorbid neuropsychological functioning following pediatric traumatic brain injury. *Journal of Clinical & Experimental Neuropsychology, 19*, 825–837.

Memory Assessment

Wayne Adams

Abstract

The chapter provides an overview of memory assessment of children and adolescents. The importance of memory to a developing organism is noted, and developmental trajectories of verbal and visual memory abilities are described. The relationship of memory with IQ is discussed, along with the additional background that is important for a clinician to understand when undertaking the assessment of memory. Historical roots are summarized, noting the empirical background reflected in contemporary memory tests. After touching on several assumptions made in memory assessment and describing types of memory that are assessed and the model assumed by most tests, five major instruments commonly used with children and teenagers are described in detail, including the WRAML2, TOMAL-2, the CMS, CVLT-C and NEPSY-II.

Key Words: memory, assessment, pediatric, children, WRAML2, TOMAL-2, CMS, CVLT-C, NEPSY-II

Memory is fundamental for most human cognitive and emotional functioning, and thus is represented in nearly all day-to-day activities, including intellectual, emotional, academic, social, self-care, vocational, and recreational domains. Memory contributes substantially to who we are and how we perceive ourselves and the world around us. Memory allows us to acquire and later find and utilize skills, feelings and knowledge, so it is an essential ingredient for most of cognitive and emotional developmental change. Simply stated, memory—the ability to acquire and recall information—is ubiquitous in the challenges and delights in the daily lives of infants, children and adolescents. This is true whether we focus on normal or atypical development.

Memory complaints are said to be the most common reason for referral with adults (Lezak, Howieson, Bigler, & Tranel, 2012). It was once thought that a child demonstrating a marked inability to acquire new information and having experienced no acute traumatic event, was likely to be suffering from an overall cognitive delay. Now it is recognized that there can be discrete to pervasive memory deficits that can range from mild to severe. Table 21.1 is adapted from Reynolds and Voress (2009) and includes a listing of common congenital childhood disorders in which learning and memory, in some form, are probably compromised. Accordingly, psychologists who are referred children for evaluation with any of these conditions, would normally include some kind of evaluation of memory.

While memory is a central cognitive process, it also is a very vulnerable brain function. Various traumas, whether minor or devastating, often affect the efficiency of the brain's laying down of new memories, and/or retrieval of those already stored. Generally speaking, if there is going to be some cognitive compromise resulting from a brain insult, it is most likely that memory will be among those processes negatively affected (Lezak, et al., 2012). Difficulties with memory and attention are the two most common complaints following even mild

Table 21.1 Chronic and Acute Childhood Disorders or Conditions for Which Compromise in One or More Memory Functions Is Likely

ADHD
Anoxia and sustained hypoxia
Attention-deficit-hyperactivity disorder
Autism
Cancer, especially brain tumors treated by radiation
Cerebral palsy
Down syndrome
Extremely low birthweight
Fragile X and related syndromes
Hydrocephalus
Intellectual disability
Kleinfelter syndrome, XXYY, etc.
Learning disability
Lesch-Nyhan disease
Meningitis
Neurodevelopmental abnormalities (e.g., callosal dysgenesis)
Neurofibromatosis
Prader-Willi syndrome
Seizure disorder
Teratogen exposure (e.g., alcohol, lead)
Traumatic brain injury (abuse, falls, motor vehicle accidents, etc.)
Tourette syndrome
Williams syndrome

head trauma (Levin, Eisenberg, & Benton, 1989). Furthermore, it seems that memory is susceptible to congenital insult as well. In fact, contrary to commonly heard assertions, Hebb's (1942) "vulnerability hypothesis" (that early neural insult is more devastating than later) has generally been supported, especially with larger lesions and those affecting white matter tissues (Aram & Eisele, 1992). Other than for more severe acute infection (e.g., encephalitis) and traumatic brain injury from events such

as motor vehicle accidents or falls, amnesias in children are rare (Mattis, 1992).

The importance of memory in estimating overall cognitive ability was assumed by pioneers in cognitive assessment. For example, several memory tasks appeared in the original scale developed by Binet and Simon that was published in 1905, and considered by many as the first test of intelligence (Sattler, 2008). While in one sense, all of the 30 items appearing on that scale required memory, eight made overt memory demands, and are described in Table 21.2. You can see that several have proven their worth, and adaptations of several continue to be included on contemporary IQ and memory tests.

Various assumptions are made when testing memory. First, it is assumed that, like intelligence, memory abilities differ across individuals, and that such variation is normally distributed. Furthermore, based upon research findings related to intelligence, memory is also assumed to gradually increase, in a developmentally linear manner, from birth to adolescence, asymptote in early adulthood, and then begin a decline that is inversely related to age. Also assumed is that the trajectory of developmental change is more rapid in childhood than adulthood, and fairly similar across various memory systems. Some might argue that these are not assumptions, but notions that have empirical grounding based on memory measures. However, it should be remembered that memory tests themselves are substantially created to be consistent with our assumptions (memory is what memory tests measure!). Figures 21.1–21.3 show performance trajectories of individual subtests found on the Wide Range Assessment of Memory and Learning, Second Edition (WRAML2), a memory battery to be discussed later in this chapter. These figures show developmental performance paths for immediate memory in both verbal and visual modalities; sample size for each age grouping is 80. Each point on a given plot represents the total raw score achieved by a given age band, expressed as a percentage of the highest performance achieved across age bands on that subtest. Therefore, the left-most square in Figure 21.1 shown for the Sentence Memory subtest indicates that performance on this subtest by children 5 years 0 months through 5 years 5 months is about 55 percent of the maximum performance on this subtest, that is shown will be achieved around 25 to 30 years of age. (The Sentence Memory subtest is a verbal, immediate memory subtest that requires the client to repeat, verbatim, sentences of increasing length.) At first glance, the plots found

Table 21.2 Items with Significant Memory Demands Included Within the 1905 Version of Binet and Simon's Measure of Cognitive Ability

Item Number	Task Name and Requirement
#6	Execution of Simple Orders and Imitation of Gestures. Follow verbal commands and imitate examiner movements.
#7	Verbal Knowledge of Objects. Follow verbal commands to touch specified body parts and find a object among many after a short delay.
#11	Repetition of Digits. Repeat three digits.
#15	Repetition of Sentences. Repeat 15-word sentences.
#17	Memory for Pictures. Shown pictures and then asked to recall their names.
#18	Drawing a Design from Memory. Shown two designs and then asked to reproduce them from memory.
#26	Three Words, One Sentence. Make up a sentence using three words (Paris, gutter, fortune).
#28	Reversal of Clock Hands. State the time if the large and small hands of pictured clock were reversed.

in Figures 21.1–21.3 seem to suggest that memory peaks at about the same age as intelligence, and like intelligence, the verbal modality seems to hold up better than the visual or nonverbal modality.

Inspection of the three figures also indicates several findings that question assumptions often made about memory in childhood and adolescence. First, memory skills do not seem to develop uniformly. For example, Sentence Memory performance gradually improves in a fairly uniform, incremental manner from five to 30 years of age. In contrast, for the Picture Memory subtest (which assesses visual immediate memory of the content within meaningful scenes), more than 70 percent of the maximum competency in this visual memory task is in place at age five years, and peak performance will occur around 16 to 17 years of age. Yet a different pattern is seen with another visual memory task (the Design Memory subtest requires drawing a pattern of simple shapes from memory). Figure 21.1 indicates that this kind of visual memory is poorly developed at five years (i.e., 30% of the maximum ability that is

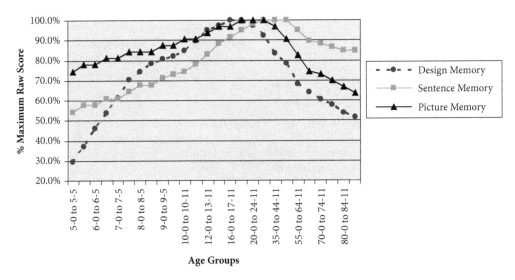

Figure 21.1 Differing developmental trajectories of performance on three WRAML2 subtests from 5–90 years of age. Design Memory and Picture Memory subtests are measures of immediate visual memory; the Sentence Memory subtest is a measure of immediate verbal memory.

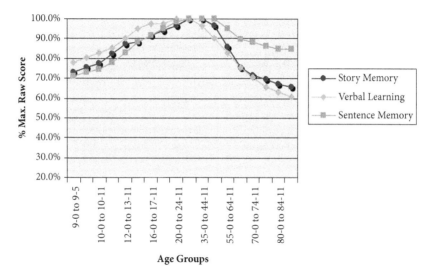

Figure 21.2 Developmental trajectories of three WRAML2 verbal immediate memory tasks. Story Memory measures highly meaningful verbal material; Sentence Memory measures recall using a less meaningful verbal material; and Verbal Learning is a list-learning task tapping more rote immediate verbal recall.

typically observed around 18–19 years of age), and the growth trajectory is rather steep until age eight, when it then resembles the developmental pace of the Sentence Memory task.

Figure 21.2 shows performance starting at age nine since the two subtests shown (Story Memory and Verbal Learning) use different (easier) items for five- to eight-year olds; therefore, comparison with maximum performance necessitates moving to nine years, at which age the subtest task items are equivalent into the adult years. Sentence Memory performance is again included to serve as a basis of comparison across figures. What is apparent when comparing Figures 21.1 and 21.2 is the relative consistency in acquisition rates across immediate verbal memory tasks, but relative inconsistency in the decay rates. As reported by many older adults, memory decline seems to begin sooner and drops more dramatically than has been shown with IQ performance. You may remember (!) that the results of the still ongoing Seattle Longitudinal Study (Schaie, 1996) suggested that verbal intellectual skills tend to hold up pretty well, with a decline starting at about age 60. Similar to memory, spatial intellectual skills begin to decline a bit earlier than verbal. However, visual memory shows a more precipitous

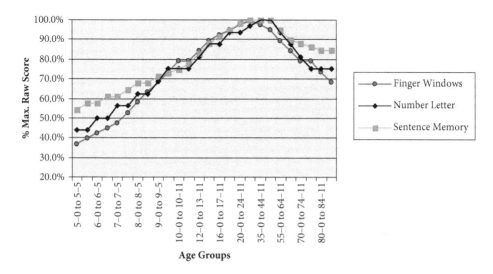

Figure 21.3 Developmental trajectories of two WRAML2 rote, immediate memory tasks, one of which is auditory (Number/Letter) and the other is visual (Finger Windows). Sentence Memory is included for comparison purposes across Figures 21.1–21.3.

drop. Therefore, while verbal memory shows greater resilience than visual, the downward trajectory for each starts considerably sooner than for IQ.

Figure 21.3 provides the performance plots for two WRAML2 subtests demanding rote immediate memory ability (low in meaning) as well as sequencing. The trajectories for these two tasks are rather similar, even though they ostensibly make rather dissimilar immediate-recall demands: one task is aural/oral (hearing and repeating unrelated numbers and letters) and the other is visual/motor (watching and then pointing out demonstrated sequences). While modality-specific memory is a generally accepted concept (Kolb & Whishaw, 2008), it appears that even within a given sensory modality, there are different "subclasses" of memory ability that have developmentally distinctive qualities from each other. Therefore, using tests that assess memory, findings would indicate that memory subsystems develop at different rates, within and across sense modalities. Furthermore, these different kinds of memory abilities peak at different ages that span more than two decades. This kind of variability often gets lost when clinicians are asked questions like, "How's his memory?" and when those same clinicians try to answer that question using too narrow a range of memory measures. Similarly, when assessing memory in a child who has sustained an acute brain insult, the child may ultimately be differentially impacted in memory, given where that system itself is in its development. That is, a five-year-old sustaining a significant brain injury would more likely demonstrate long-term deficits in those memory processes that are only 30 percent developed compared to other memory functions that are 75 percent developed. Once intelligence was thought to be a unitary trait, then consisting of verbal and nonverbal (or "Performance") components, and most recently, as something comprising multiple kinds of "intelligences" many of which are quite different from earlier variables that defined IQ. It seems reasonable to expect that our understanding of memory will evolve similarly and our assessment instruments will reflect an increasing sophistication resulting from that evolution.

Memory and Intelligence

While we would expect memory performance to be related to intelligence, we would not expect it to correlate as highly as intelligence measures inter-correlate. Generally, IQ measures show correlations > .70 with each other. Table 21.3 shows the correlations of scores from the three existing pediatric memory batteries with the Wechsler Intelligence Scale for Children (versions differ depending on when the research was completed). The WRAML2 has low to moderate correlations with intelligence, with the Test of Memory and Learning–Second Edition (TOMAL-2; Reynolds & Vorees, 2007) and the Children's Memory Scale (CMS, Cohen 1997) having correlations that are a bit higher, but below the usual range seen for IQ test inter-correlations. The reader should remember that, depending on the edition being considered, the Wechsler Intelligence Scale has at least one memory subtest (such as Information, Digit Span, or Arithmetic) contributing to the FSIQ score. Therefore, the degree of inter-correlation between memory and IQ measures is inflated somewhat because those creating IQ tests believe that short-term memory is an ingredient of intelligence.

It is interesting to note, though, that there is apparently a conceptual wrestling over how much to use memory processes to define intelligence. That is, with the WISC-III (Wechsler, 1991), *intelligence* (as defined by FSIQ) was operationalized as consisting 20 percent of memory (Information and Arithmetic subtests contributed, and Digit Span was non-contributory). With the WISC-IV (Wechsler, 2003), a Working Memory Index appears, as do four memory subtests, although still 20 percent of the FSIQ is derived from memory subtests (but they are different subtests—Digit Span and Letter-Number Sequencing) than contributed to the WISC-III FSIQ. In the most recent adult Wechsler IQ test revision (WAIS-IV; Wechsler, 2008), which may portend changes that will be seen on the WISC-V, Digit Span (in an expanded form), Arithmetic and Information all get the nod to contribute to the FSIQ (now 30 percent comprised of memory—a 50 percent increase!); Letter-Number Sequencing was exiled to supplemental status. So the trend in at least one highly regarded test-development camp accords memory greater involvement in defining IQ than in the past. Nevertheless, as we have already seen, memory is a complex and multifaceted construct, and therefore still demands assessment beyond how it is defined on contemporary measures of intelligence.

Finally, it should be mentioned that there are classifications of functioning assigned to intelligence. *Superior, impaired* or *average* levels of intellectual functioning are well defined. Such is not the case for memory. While one can use the same classification system for memory as for intelligence, it must be done by mapping onto an IQ framework

Table 21.3 Correlations of WRAML2, TOMAL-2 and CMS Core Indexes with the Wechsler Intelligence Scale for Children[1]

IQ Measure	WRAML2 (N = 29)				TOMAL-2 (N = 22)			CMS (N=126)			
WISC[1]	GMI	VMI	ViMI	A/CI	CMI	VMI	NVMI	GMI	VMI	ViMI	A/CI
Verbal IQ (or VCI)	.54	.29	.36	.42	.65	.53	.66	.54	.55	.23	.58
Performance IQ (or PRI)	.37	.14	.30	.28	.51	.51	.29	.46	.36	.29	.55
FSIQ	.44	.25	.33	.31	.66	.56	.65	.61	.56	.34	.72

[1]The third edition of the WISC was used for inter-correlations with the WRAML2; the second edition of the WISC for the TOMAL-2, and the WISC-IV for the CMS. The source for these data was the respective tests' manual, except for the CMS, for which the *WISC-IV Technical Manual* was used. Correlations corrected for reliability are used throughout. WISC = Wechsler Intelligence Scale for Children; VCI = Verbal Comprehension Index; PRI = Perceptual Organization Index; FSIQ = Full Scale IQ. WRAML2 = Wide Range Assessment of Memory and Learning, second edition; GMI = General Memory Index; VMI = Verbal Memory Index; ViMI = Visual Memory Index; A/CI = Attention/Concentration Index. TOMAL-2 = Test of Memory and Learning, second edition. CMI = Composite Memory Index; NVMI = Nonverbal Memory Index. CMS = Children's Memory Scale.

of conventional categories. Furthermore, using such classifications of intelligence has clinical utility, since, for example, IQ scores are endowed with meaning by DSM (American Psychiatric Association, 2013) when considering a diagnostic formulation. No equivalent exists for memory scores, especially not within a pediatric population. "Memory" is not even an entry in the index of the DSM (DSM-IV and DSM-V do list "Amnestic Disorders")! Technically, it is not possible to have a learning disability or be otherwise impaired based on a memory deficit, according to existing diagnostic systems, although I am sure such children exist. True, there is "Cognitive Disorder, not otherwise specified (NOS)," but as for most "NOS" appendages, Cognitive Disorder, NOS, is a very broad, ill-defined category that is not very helpful in focusing on memory impairment per se, and it implies an acute, not congenital etiology. It is hoped that future research efforts in pediatric memory will help us solve such dilemmas, as it has done in contributing a solid foundation for clinical application in the past.

Historical Roots

A full historical review of memory is beyond the scope of this chapter, but it is important to at least touch on major highlights, since probably more so than most areas assessed by psychological tests, memory had a significant advantage of having a rich legacy of empirical and clinical contributions to inform test content and interpretation. Comprehensive historical reviews of memory and

other cognitive processes are available (see Samuel, 1999; Bower, 2000; Finger, 2000; Finger, 2001; Squire, L., 2004).

While acknowledging the contributions of ancient China or Greece is the typical starting place for most historical overviews of anything, that is not the case for memory (or any brain functioning). One exception was the practice of Hippocratic adherents in the fifth century B.C., who associated epilepsy with the brain. However, this promising start was scuttled by Aristotle, who thought the brain was nearly inconsequential to thinking. Thanks to casualties from the Roman games, the physician Galen (c. A.D. 200) was able to gather evidence supporting his contention that the brain was central to thinking and motor coordination. Unfortunately, he concluded that the ventricles were the structures of greatest importance, a view that continued until the fifteenth century, when Leonardo da Vinci pointed out that ventricles of animals did not vary much in their relative size across species, despite the obviously extreme range of intellectual abilities exhibited (Samuel, 1999).

In the 1880s, Hans Ebbinghaus was the first to systematically study and record his observations of experimental findings with memory in humans (Ebbinghaus, 1913). Almost every introductory psychology text mentions Ebbinghaus and shows a curve similar to that seen in Figure 21.4. Even though these data were primarily based on results from memory tasks he administered to himself and/or his wife, replication using more credible samples

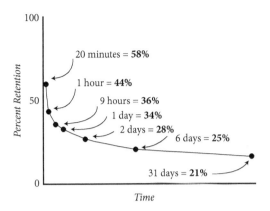

100

Percent Retention

20 minutes = **58%**

1 hour = **44%**

50

9 hours = **36%**

1 day = **34%**

2 days = **28%**

6 days = **25%**

31 days = **21%**

0

Time

Figure 21.4 Ebbinghaus' classic learning curve. There is a dramatic loss of learned information within the first hour, after which forgetting occurs at slower and slower rates. Adapted from: www.psych.purdue.edu/~ben/285su2001/notes/figures/5-forgettingcurve.htm.

substantiated his assertions. The findings represented by the "Ebbinghaus forgetting curve" (i.e., Figure 21.4) immediately suggest clinical applications, such as the appropriateness of testing recall of new learning after a 20- to 30-minute delay, since during this relatively brief interval, more "forgetting" occurs than at any other subsequent interval. This is but one example of how empirical findings from more than a century of research were available to memory-test developers.

Ebbinghaus notwithstanding, it was the twentieth century that witnessed a burgeoning of experimental and clinical evidence that gradually contributed to a modern understanding of memory. Those in the memory "Hall of Fame" include Sherrington (British neurophysiologist who in the 1920s posited an "enchanted loom" composed of bioelectric currents in the brain; he also gave us the term *synapse*); Ribot (around 1910, he wrote about three stages of memory that today we would call *encoding, storage* and *retrieval*); Freud (who started in neuroscience research, and whose debated theory of psychopathology in the 1920s heavily relied upon memory processes); Pavlov (investigating primitive levels of learning and memory); Luria (generating over several decades a still-influential theory of embedded brain systems, using what he learned from injured war victims; he also carefully documented the case of "S," a man with apparently limitless recall capabilities); William James (in 1890, James noted that recall consisted of what we now call *short-* and *long-term memory* components); Penfield, in the 1930s, was the first to "map" functional regions of the brain using an electric probe

in epilepsy patients; and Scovile (US neurosurgeon) with "HM" (the patient upon whom Scovile operated in 1953, and who dramatically demonstrated the existence of a brain structure essential for the creation of new memories). Other important contributors include Hebb (Canadian theorist and experimenter who defined the substance of memory in terms of "cell assemblies," which themselves are established by neural paths that are frequently and regularly "fired" in temporal contiguity); Lashley (U.S. psychologist demonstrating that long-term memory is not localized but distributed throughout a very interactive brain); and ending our historical march we should mention those inventing and using magnetic resonance imaging, which today allows us to actually witness real-time memory activity using computerized estimates of brain metabolism (Rosler, Ranganath, Roder, & Kluwe, 2009). Because of this rich historical legacy, a vocabulary related to memory gradually developed, is generally accepted, and comprises a required knowledge-base for professionals evaluating clients for memory disorders. Table 21.4 lists common terms related to memory phenomena, most of which were generated through research efforts, and most of which can be found today on tests of memory. A solid knowledge of these concepts is important for those engaged in the understanding and interpretation of memory assessment. Detailed discussions of these terms and how they were derived can be found in many advanced texts on cognition (e.g., Leahey & Harris, 2001; Radvansky, 2005), in more clinically oriented volumes (e.g., Reeves & Wedding, 1994; Haberlandt, K., 1999), or in a text dedicated to discussing memory terminology (Dudai, 2004).

Despite impressive growth in understanding many aspects of memory over the last century, the focus of these efforts was primarily on adults; other than studies using infants, few memory investigations focused on a pediatric population. Amazingly, "memory" does not appear as an entry in *Child Development Abstracts and Bibliography* until 1965. Even today, it is assumed that the phenomena and the associated mechanisms related to adult memory processing are similar or identical to that found in children (a variant on the idea that "children are just little adults"). Some memory phenomena clearly are not the same in children as adults, such as Miller's (1956) "magic number" of 7 ± 2. Those working with children know, as did Binet a century ago, that most "normal" seven-year-olds cannot repeat seven digits; their magic number is five (and probably not ± 2). Similarly, it is assumed that executive

Table 21.4 Vocabulary of Memory: Terms in Use That Emerged from Research, Are Common Terms in Current Clinical or Research Efforts with Memory Impairment, and Describe Components Found in Memory Test Batteries

Memory Term	Phenomenon Described
Anterograde Amnesia	Impaired ability to remember information *following* the onset of memory difficulties
Consolidation	Strengthening of the informational "engram" while it is stored
Declarative (Explicit) Memory ("knowing what")	Memory that is available to the conscious self (including episodic and semantic memory)
Episodic Memory	Autobiographical memory for events, including content, place, and temporal aspects (the "what," "when" and "where" of an event)
Learning/ Forgetting Curve	A plotted measure representing degree of recall of a set of material over a series of equivalent learning episodes (usually multiple "teaching" sessions or "trials" with that material); conversely, a plotted measure representing loss of material once learned, obtained by assessment periodically over time, is a forgetting curve
Long-term (Delayed) Memory	Storage of information after hours or days, with seemingly unlimited capacity, and a slow rate of decay. Presumably all information in long-term memory started as part of short-term memory and was "transferred" into storage
Primacy/Recency Effect	When learning new information (especially of a relatively rote nature), the material at the beginning and end of the learned material is retained best, with the end material (most recent exposure) being retained better than that found at the beginning; material in the middle is least well retained
Procedural memory ("knowing how")	Remembering focused skill sets, usually learned though much practice, and upon mastery are relatively automatic (non-conscious)
Recognition Memory vs. Retrieval	The ability to correctly recognize information previously encountered vs. being able to retrieve that information volitionally. Evidence of recognition suggests the information is stored, even if not retrievable
Retrograde Amnesia	Impaired ability to remember information *prior* to the onset of memory difficulties (often resulting from an acute brain insult)
Rote vs. Meaningful Memory	Remembering rote material (relatively meaningless to the learner, such as a foreign word or unfamiliar term) is more difficult than remembering meaningful material (a concept, sentence, story)
Semantic Memory	Knowledge of the world, like facts, concepts, and vocabulary (content is preserved but without a temporal marker (when it was learned)
Short-term (Immediate) Memory	Limited-capacity storage for a brief period (seconds) with rapid decay
Working Memory	Capacity to briefly utilize information in short-term storage without disrupting that information while working with it

functions are involved with working memory and learning over trials, and yet we are aware that frontal lobe myelination is relatively slow in development, continuing even into young adulthood (Giedd et al., 1996). Nevertheless, the impact of frontal lobe immaturity on memory performance has not been methodically explored. Despite these gaps in our knowledge of memory in children, results from existing memory batteries provide reasonable proof that memory phenomena found in adults can also be documented in children, and is probably one reason that child and adult memory tests are more alike than different.

Table 21.5 provides an abbreviated chronology of major memory tests. While parts of various adult memory procedures were adapted for use

Table 21.5 Chronology of the Emergence of Memory Tests

Year Introduced	Test Name and Author
1941	Complex Figure Test (Rey)
1945	Wechsler Memory Scale
1987	—2nd Edition
1997	—3rd Edition
2009	—4th Edition
1946	Benton Visual Retention Task
1963	Recurring Figures Test (Kimura)
1964	Rey Auditory-Verbal Learning Test
1974	Selective Reminding Task (Buschke)
1978	Judgment of Line Orientation Test (Benton, Varney, & Hamsher)
1991	Rivermead Behavioural Memory Test for Children (Wilson, Ivani-Chalian, & Adrich)
1987	California Verbal Learning Test (Delis,
2000	Kramer, Kaplan & Ober)
	—2nd Edition
1990	Wide Range Assessment of Memory
2003	and Learning (Sheslow & Adams)
	—2nd Edition
1994	Test of Memory and Learning
2007	(Reynolds & Bigler)
	—2nd Edition (Reynolds & Voress)
1994	California Verbal Learning Test– Children's Version (Delis, Kramer, Kaplan, Ober)
1997	Children's Memory Scale (Cohen)

with children, no set of memory tasks designed for children and co-normed using a pediatric sample existed until 1990 when the Wide Range Assessment of Memory and Learning (Sheslow & Adams, 1990) was released. Since then, two other child-focused memory batteries have been introduced, including the Test of Memory and Learning (Reynolds & Bigler, 1994) and the Children's Memory Scale (Cohen, 1997). Also, in 1994, the California Verbal Learning Test–Children's Version (Delis, Kramer, Kaplan, & Ober, 1994) was made available. These tests and others that are commonly used and/or psychometrically sound will be discussed later in this chapter.

Models of Memory

While numerous models of human memory have been proposed and have generated enthusiastic debate emphasizing disparities, generally there is more similarity than difference across models. The tests described later in this chapter generally understand memory in a manner characterized by Figure 21.5, which is reminiscent of a long-standing model of remembering originally advanced by Atkinson and Shiffrin (1968). Each memory test assumes an external world that impinges upon human sensory systems. Through selective attention, which itself is a function of evolving cognitive schemas, environmental stimulation is, usually, incompletely taken in. The incomplete encoding of information in one or more sensory systems is available (i.e., the person is aware of it) for a brief interval (short-term memory) of several seconds. Again, because of incomplete processing, a portion of that perceived information is stored in long-term memory, depending on many variables, including prior information stored, conscious effort of the learner to remember (e.g., rehearsal), and state of alertness. Longer-term memory storage is less evanescent than short-term, but still, as Ebbinghaus demonstrated, there is

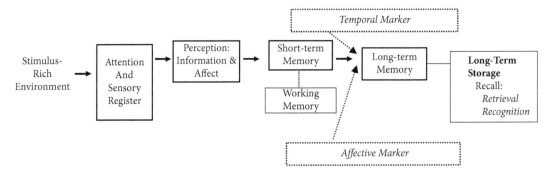

Figure 21.5 A common model used to conceptualize the human memory system (adapted from Atkinson and Shiffrin (1968)).

significant information loss with normal learning. Frequent and/or "emotionally strong" exposure to that and related information establishes a trace or *engram,* which should allow conscious (intentional) retrieval of that information at a later time (via semantic and episodic memory). The information seems to be stored in primary (probably related to the sensory system[s] perceiving the information) as well as secondary locations. In addition to the content of the information that gets stored, an affective valence is often stored as well, allowing the person to obtain an emotional weighting of the information along with the content being retrieved. For most events, a temporal marker is also stored with the informational and affective content allowing memories of events to be distinguished from each other using an internal calendar. Normally, with enough exposure (which can vary from one or more exposures), the information is stored or "laid down" in a relatively robust "memory bank." More vulnerable and/or inefficient is the retrieval mechanism, a conscious (i.e., intentional) memory component used to find the stored information when needed. Even if retrieval is not successful, the person can still, through a different and more basic memory system mechanism, recognize the information being sought if it or aspects of it are made available. Accessing the information successfully (i.e., remembering it) may or may not result in any observable output by the person.

While it is a oversimplification, the heuristic value of this model allows one to understand that a breakdown anywhere along the path can create recall problems. So, for example, either blindness or hearing impairment would lead to deficits in the sensory register that, in turn, would create distortions or omissions in the information being passed along, well before it gets to the actual memory processing devices. Likewise, at the other end of the route, deficits in short-term memory may contribute to the relaying of incomplete or faulty information into long-term storage. Weaknesses in long-term storage can exist because information was "misfiled," or filed but then lost partially or completely.

Therefore, memory assessment consists of evaluating the efficiency of various parts of this kind of system, using history, client report, observer report, the examiner's observations, as well as test results to assess functioning everywhere along the route just described. Medical status including sensory defects and/or knowledge of medications (taken or not), may be as important in this sequential process as are the memory test results—perhaps more so in some conditions, such as hypothyroidism. Likewise, through test results, identifying isolated problems with short- or longer-term memory can be very helpful in developing an effective remediation plan for the client.

It should be mentioned that it is common to establish a level of memory expectation based upon intellectual functioning. So, if a client is functioning in an extreme range, it is reasonable to expect memory skills to also reflect a similar extreme level, and for the examiner to form impressions of "atypical" based upon the degree of discrepancy based on this expectation. As noted earlier, memory and IQ are only moderately related, so exceptions are common, and therein is the justification for memory testing. However, if, for example, a child is functioning in the mildly impaired range of intelligence, and has memory test results falling within this same range, that child would not be considered having a memory deficit per se, since memory performance is consistent with his/her overall cognitive level.

Requisites for Clinicians Measuring Memory in Children

Most clinical training programs prepare students in individual assessment, especially intellectual assessment. Knowledge of and experience with intelligence testing provide an important foundation upon which one builds broader evaluation competencies including memory assessment. Important skill sets that should readily generalize include efficiently obtaining a thorough and focused history, establishing and maintaining rapport, being alert to make keen observations, adhering to standardized test administration and scoring details, being able to integrate information from a variety of sources, applying multicultural awareness and sensitivity to a given client and/or presenting problem, and providing informed feedback in an effective but caring manner. In addition, a clear understanding of the psychometric aspects related to item measurement, standardization, sampling, bias, reliability, and validity, are essential for test selection and interpretation. Furthermore, knowing what tests are available and their relative strengths and weaknesses for common referral or research questions are central to assessment mastery. While all of these assessment skills are important for any cognitive testing, there are some unique competencies important for memory assessment generally, and for assessing memory in children and teenagers, specifically.

Neuroanatomical Understanding of Memory

There have been major advances in our understanding of the neuroanatomical substrates involved with forming and laying down new memories, as well as retrieving and forgetting them. Almost monthly, findings from functional magnetic resonance imaging (fMRI) and related imaging techniques enhance our understanding of brain–behavior functions, with memory commonly a focus. An appropriate treatment of the neuroanatomy of memory is well beyond the scope of this chapter, but excellent reviews exist (e.g., Squire & Schacter, 2002; Kolb & Whishaw, 2008; Moscovitch et al., 2005). Those working with memory assessment and clients with memory disorders should remain knowledgeable of neuroscientific developments, since client understanding and test interpretation are becoming increasingly more informed by neuroanatomical findings related to remembering and forgetting, as well as cognition and emotion in general (e.g., Stark & Squire, 2000; Smith & Squire, 2009).

Psychological Understanding of Memory and Learning

There is an extensive literature that focuses on how humans (and animals) learn and remember. Courses entitled "Cognition" or "Learning and Memory" are found in most undergraduate and graduate psychology curricula, and use texts that provide excellent discussions of the terms listed in Table 21.4. Many aspects related to these descriptors of "normal" memory and learning phenomena are found within tests of memory abilities, therefore the examiner working with memory assessment should be knowledgeable about phenomena such as those listed in the table. Having a developmental appreciation of the client vis-à-vis expected memory change is also a real asset in relating to and understanding the client being evaluated.

Clinical Understanding of Common Referral Problems

Memory assessment tends to be especially important with certain conditions, many of which are listed in Table 21.1. Those to whom such referrals are made clinically, or those using a memory measure for research purposes, should directly or through a supervisor have an informed background of the clinical condition and its likely impact on cognition generally, and memory specifically. Knowing when there is no associated cognitive "profile" is important as well. Such background often requires some knowledge outside of the traditional domains

associated with psychology, pushing the minimum competency boundary into other fields such as language pathology, endocrinology, genetics, occupational therapy, nuclear imaging, or pharmacology. To make an accurate interpretation of test results, those working with children must be able to rule out conditions that can confound memory scores. More so in childhood than adulthood, these confounding conditions may not have been identified yet, such as expressive language impairment, ADHD, and peripheral acuity or hearing deficits, and so require greater examiner vigilance and diagnostic acumen.

Also, in contrast to those working with adults, psychologists working with children tend to omit specific memory inquiries when obtaining a comprehensive history. Accordingly, parent (and child) interviews or history questionnaires should invite responses to questions such as the ones that follow: Does your child:

(1) need reminders to do things and seems frustrated with him/herself because they were left undone?

(2) have the ability to be sent into another room and be asked to return with several things from that room?

(3) remember to bring home the correct materials for homework assignments? (or frequently need to phone or text friends to get a homework assignment?)

(4) easily memorize sets of facts like state capitals or new scientific terms? Are those still remembered a week or two later?

(5) usually locate his/her own belongings around the house?

(6) forget to take things to or bring things home from school (or a friend's house) even when he/she wants to?

(7) forget things important to him/her, such as invitation to a party or sports event?

(8) get temporarily lost, like in a store or when biking to a nearby friend's neighborhood?

(9) remember the rules of new games?

(10) remember the names of teachers from prior years or prior vacation spots?

(11) demonstrate impressive remembering, like being able to direct you to a location you have both driven to once or twice before?

(12) show the ability to repeat stories they read or have been read?

(13) have problems participating in sports because your child forgets things related to the game being played?

Note how, unlike in clinical work with adults, the professional working with children needs to make various developmental adjustments in expectations when asking and interpreting parents' responses to these questions. The relatively modest relationship between memory and academic achievement (Dehn, 2008) causes one to question whether obtaining teacher ratings on memory while at school supplies misleading information that is confounded by the many other factors required for school performance. Likewise, it is important to focus on memory facets embedded within tasks. Memory is involved in almost any task, but its importance on overall level of performance can vary considerably. For example, remembering a short list of afternoon chores or the details of a homework assignment each has memory demands, but only taking a history carefully can tease out whether the deficit in performing this multidimensional tasks is, in fact, memory-related, and/or more related to motivation, overall intellectual level, executive functioning, parental or sibling

involvement, distractibility, and unique aspects associated with task demands. Table 21.6 lists examples of "everyday procedures" that commonly make memory demands on children and teens, and may be useful to include during history-taking when assessing for memory deficits.

Psychometric Expectations

As noted at the outset of this section, a solid psychometric understanding of what makes a test a "good" test is important for any psychologist involved in assessment. And while an appreciation of what constitutes psychometric integrity of a given instrument is important in assessment generally, there are some ways memory assessment is unique. For example, it is not unusual in reading reviews of memory tests to see it pointed out that test-retest reliability is lower than "levels normally acceptable" for cognitive tests. Sometimes reviewers seem to forget that by their very nature, memory assessment involving new learning (which is a part of most all

Table 21.6 Examples of Everyday Tasks Involving Memory Components and Meriting Focus When Obtaining a Child's or Adolescent's History

Compared to Age Mates, Does the Child/Teen Remember:	
Names of familiar people? new acquaintances?	Math tables?
Phone number(s), street address, locker combination?	Spelling words past the weekly test?
How to find somewhat new places in the neighborhood or at school?	What was for supper last night?
Remember where things are located (e.g., can opener, batteries supply, soap replacement)?	A series of two or three directions related to a novel request? Or a homework assignment?
Parts of new chore assignments (utensil positions when setting the table)?	A phone message with reasonable accuracy?
The time and day of a favorite TV show?	The name for new object whose label has been given once or twice before?
Jokes or stories heard at school, at a party, etc.?	The rules and terms related to a relatively new game?
Things the parents forgot?	The plot and details of a novel story heard or read?
How to operate a new gadget after one or two interactions with it?	Poetry assignments? Memorizing lines of a play or speech?
Time and day of a social date, party or other "appointments" like meeting after school?	A few items to obtain while shopping in a store?
Lists of facts after originally mastered (e.g., state capitals, list of presidents, etc.)?	factual information, rather than looking to a parent or older sibling to provide the information?
Where important possessions are stored at home or school?	To which team he/she has been assigned during a daily or weekly phys. ed. class or intramural sports team?

memory measures) cannot be readministered to establish reliability. The task being used is different at the second test administration than it was for the first. The variable it is attempting to measure (i.e., memory) may, in fact, lower the test-retest reliability if the test is valid! Instead, what may be a better index of reliability are "person separation" and "item separation" statistics derived from Rasch item analysis (Wright & Stone, 1979). While some psychometrics courses include this within their syllabi, many do not, and for those that do, most students have forgotten this background by graduation.

Another example of the need for some psychometric adjustment in one's thinking about memory measures is found in maintaining an exacting demand for a full range of normed scores across the ability spectrum. For some tests, such as those measuring intelligence, detecting strength is often important. For other tests, however, measurement of strength is less important, or not really meaningful. For example, personality tests are not expected to have enough sensitivity to detect those whose positive self-esteem is at the 95th percentile. Generally, low self-esteem is the clinical interest and focus. Likewise, for some aspects of memory assessment, sensitivity to strength is often unimportant. For example, recognition memory is so robust in healthy individuals that sensitivity in detecting strengths in this area is very difficult, because few participants miss recognition items. As with some personality constructs, demanding test sensitivity to detect average, above average, and superior recognition memory probably has little clinical meaning or worth. While it is possible that tasks could be devised to achieve such discrimination, the expense and effort would not be deemed justified by an investing publisher, given the limited usefulness of the resulting data. While some components of memory tests do require a wide range of psychometric sensitivity (e.g., comparing visual vs. verbal memory abilities in the same child), generally, the focus is on sensitivity to weakness. That is where high psychometric sensitivity should normally be expected of a given instrument: "How good is the floor of the scale?" Seldom, if ever, has a referral been received to determine if a child is memory-gifted! The point being made is that assessing psychometric integrity of memory measures will at times require some adjustment in the traditional demands made for demonstrating psychometric adequacy. An otherwise useful tool might be erroneously dismissed because of inappropriate psychometric expectations.

Choosing an Instrument

Knowing the tools available to address a specific diagnostic focus is an essential competency for any psychologist doing comprehensive assessments. This is especially so for those undertaking an evaluation of memory deficits. It is typical to add memory tasks to supplement other "key" tests of a comprehensive assessment, such as intelligence, academic achievement, and/or personality. And while entire memory batteries are often administered, it is also common in today's managed healthcare environment for psychologists to choose how to fill an extra half hour that has been salvaged in order to screen for memory deficits. Many of the most common tests used to assess memory in children are listed in Table 21.7. The list is far shorter than what would appear for assessing memory in adults. The section that follows is intended to provide a useful examination of testing options for those wanting to develop a more thorough knowledge of those memory assessment tools available when working with children and teens. Measures that were created for use with adults and then imposed downward extensions to accommodate older children have not been included. The majority of such measures have task expectations, scoring modifications, directions, and/or norms that result in inadequate measurement precision to detect any but those children with gross memory impairments. Instead, particular attention will be given to the three comprehensive memory batteries that were specifically designed for use with a pediatric age group, plus a few additional measures that clinicians may want to consider having available on the memory shelf of their "test pantry."

Generally speaking, most global memory measures assess verbal and/or visual memory modalities, and such is the case with the three batteries receiving attention below. The focus, structure and contents of each battery will be examined along with a look at the psychometric grounding of each. In some ways, there is considerable similarity across the batteries; for example, each uses the recall of stories and a list-learning task to assess verbal memory. The batteries are also fairly comparable in terms of administration time. But there are also differences across the measures, and these are usually found in how visual memory is assessed as well as how various supplemental tasks provide the means to achieve greater diagnostic clarity. This section should be especially helpful to those new to memory assessment as well as to those who want to compare their current methods with what else is available for evaluating the domain of memory in their pediatric clients.

Table 21.7 Common Tests Used to Assess Memory in a Pediatric Population

Test	Age Range (yrs.)	Scope of Memory Measurement	Administration Time
Benton Visual Retention Test, 5th Edition (Sivan, 1991)	8 and up	Visual Memory: (drawing) copy, recall, and recognition	15–20 minutes
Buschke Selective Reminding Task (Buschke, 1973)	5–15	Verbal memory (list learning) recall, and recognition	10–15 minutes
California Verbal Learning Test; Children's Edition (Delis et al., 1994)	4–16	Verbal Memory (list learning) Immediate, delayed, and recognition	15–20 minutes
Children's Memory Scale (Cohen, 1997)	5–16	Verbal memory, Visual Memory; Immediate, delayed recall, and recognition.	30–60 minutes
NEPSY-II (Korkman, Kirk, & Kemp, 2007)	3–16	Verbal Memory, Visual Memory, Immediate Memory, Delayed Memory (4 tasks), Cued Recall (1 task)	15–30 minutes (age dependent)
Rivermead Behavioural Memory Test, Children's Edition (Wilson et al., 1991)	5–10	Tasks intended to mimic everyday memory demands; Verbal Memory, Visual Memory Immediate memory, delayed (2 tasks)	25–30 minutes
Test of Memory and Learning, 2nd Edition (Reynolds & Voress, 2007)	5–59	Verbal memory, Non-Verbal Memory Immediate and delayed; rote and meaningful	30–40 minutes
Wide Range Assessment of Memory and Learning, 2nd Edition (Sheslow & Adams, 2003)	5–85+	Verbal Memory, Visual Memory Immediate, delayed, and recognition memory; rote and meaningful	20–25 minutes for screening; 40–60 for full battery

Memory Measures
Wide Range Assessment of Memory and Learning, Second Edition (WRAML2)
OVERVIEW

The WRAML (Sheslow & Adams, 1990) was released in 1990 and was the first standardized and well-normed memory battery for children (ages 5–17 years of age). A second edition became available (Sheslow & Adams, 2003) containing significant revisions, chief of which was a significant extension of the age range (5–85+ yrs. vs. 5–17 yrs). Reviews of the test have been completed (e.g., Strauss, Sherman, & Spreen, 2006; Hartman, 2007a) and most include a discussion of the changes between the original and second edition. Given the child/adolescent focus of this volume, this chapter will focus primarily on child and adolescent aspects and applications of this measure.

Core Indexes/Subtests. As shown in Figure 21.6, the "core" components of the WRAML2 are its three memory indexes (Verbal, Visual and Attention/Concentration). Combined, these three indexes form the General Memory Index, which is a composite estimate of immediate memory ability. Each of the core indexes is formed by two core subtests. Therefore, administering six subtests yields the three core indexes and an overall memory composite score. All of the core indexes contain subtests that assess immediate memory, and together take 30 to 40 minutes to administer, depending on the child's age and the examiner's familiarity with the instrument. The Verbal Memory Index assesses immediate recall of verbal information, with one subtest focusing on retention of meaningful material (as found in real world conversations or brief stories) and the other focusing on less meaningful material (as found in remembering the names of the seven dwarfs or the 13 original colonies). The Visual Memory Index assesses immediate retention of visual information, with one subtest focusing on retention of

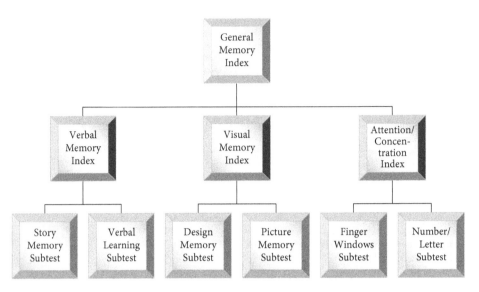

Figure 21.6 WRAML2 Core Indexes and Core Subtests.

contextually meaningful material (like a classroom photograph) and the other focusing on less meaningful material (like remembering a diagram from a workbook). Lastly, the Attention/Concentration Index assesses immediate retention of relatively meaningless information that is visual (like remembering a rote pattern on a map) and auditory (like retaining a phone number). More detailed information related to each of the core subtests is found in Table 21.8. Indexes use the familiar units of a mean of 100 and SD of 15; likewise, subtests have a mean of 10 and SD of 3. Percentiles and confidence intervals are also available.

Optional Subtests. In addition to the WRAML2 core components, there are 11 optional subtests, which are designed to complement and extend the interpretive value of the core subtest findings. Figure 21.7 shows various "sets" of these optional subtests. One set allows examination of performance on tasks emphasizing working memory. The Working Memory Index subtests allow the clinician to compare performance on, for example, a rote repetition task (sometimes mistakenly labeled "working memory") such as found with a subtest like Number Letter, with the more demanding Verbal Working Memory subtest. For example, on the latter subtest, the examiner asks a client to listen to a list of nouns which consist of an assortment of animals and non-animals. The client is asked to first report the animals in order of their sizes, followed by the non-animals also in order of size. Sometimes, children who do adequately with Number Letter rote recall do very poorly with the rote task when

the manipulation of information component that defines working memory is added. This may have important clinical implications as one considers the task demands of a classroom discussion or a reading assignment.

Another set of important optional subtests are the Delay and Recognition subtests. The former allows for assessment of retention of Core subtest material after a 10- to 15-minute delay. The Recognition subtests allow the examiner to assess memory recognition (vs. retrieval using the Delay subtests). Comparing immediate (core) with delay performance allows for examination of storage of newly learned information. Comparing delay with recognition performance allows for evaluation of retrieval. An example may make this clearer. A child who is read two short stories (i.e., the Story Memory subtest) is asked to recall each, thus providing a measure of immediate memory of meaningful verbal information. The examiner can then evaluate a longer-term recall (following a 10–15 minute delay) to assess forgetting of the material. If, compared to age mates, the client does more poorly on the longer-term free recall task than with the immediate free-recall task, recognition components can be used to distinguish between difficulty retrieving the information vs. difficulty storing the information. Retrieval is assessed by the examiner's asking about various aspects of the story, each of which is followed by three options from which the child can choose. If the information cannot be retrieved but is stored, performance, using this multiple-choice recognition format, should be done well above chance

Table 21.8 Description of WRAML2 Core Index and Subtest Components

Core Index	Core Subtest[1]	Subtest Description	Administration Time
Verbal Memory Index (Immediate, Delayed and Recognition components exist for each subtest of this index)	Story Memory (1)	After each of 2 stories is read, client repeats as much of the story as can be remembered.	7–10 minutes
	Verbal Learning (3)	A list of unrelated nouns is read; client repeats as many as can be remembered. This is repeated 3 more times, resulting in a learning acquisition curve.	6–8 minutes
Visual Memory Index (Immediate and Recognition components exist for each subtest of this index)	Design Memory (2)	Client looks at a configuration of simple geometric shapes for 5-sec, and must then draw what is remembered. Five configurations are included.	6–8 minutes
	Picture Memory (4)	Client looks at a colorful everyday scene for 10-sec and then inspects a facsimile trying to identify elements that have been "changed, moved or added." Four scenes are used.	5–8 minutes
Attention/ Concentration Index	Finger Windows (5)	The examiner places a pencil through holes found on a vertical board, and client is asked to replicate the pattern.	5–8 minutes
	Number Letter (6)	A series of digits and letters is read and the client is asked to repeat the span.	4–6 minutes

[1]Order in the administration sequence appears in parentheses.

levels of performance (i.e., 33%). However, if there is a problem with storage, both the delay and the recognition tasks will be performed poorly. In this way, use of the optional subtests can provide diagnostic clarity when compared to performance on the core subtests. Details related to these many core-optional interpretive comparisons can be found in a recent volume by Adams and Reynolds (2009). There are also numerous "qualitative" observations that can be meaningfully interpreted, because each can be given quantitative meaning in supplementary tables provided, such as comparing relative level of performance on the first story vs. the second (e.g., to assess relative consistency of performance), or comparing

performance in retaining the gist of the stories vs. specific details.

Memory Screening Index. Because of time constraints, a clinician may want to screen a client's memory skills in order to decide if more in-depth assessment is needed. For such instances, scores from the WRAML2's first four subtests can be combined to derive a Memory Screening Index (MSI). Performance on the MSI subtests alone is also tabled with a mean of 100 and an SD of 15. The four contributing subtests allow two samplings each of verbal and visual memory abilities. In addition, Verbal and Visual Memory Indexes can also be obtained. The two Attention/Concentration

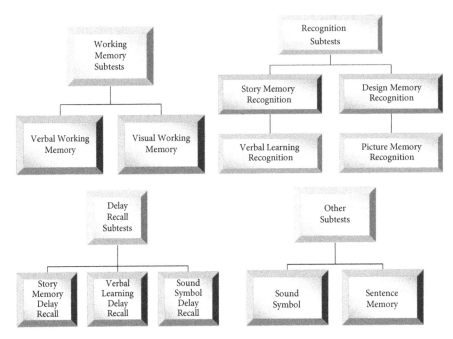

Figure 21.7 Optional WRAML2 subtests in domains of Working Memory, Recognition, Delay, and Other.

subtests are omitted, but some of this rote recall information has sometimes already been obtained, such as from a digit span task from an IQ test. By omitting the Attention/Concentration component of the WRAML2, the examiner saves about 10 minutes. The psychometric integrity of the MSI is strong since, the entire standardization sample was used in its creation (i.e., the first four subtests of the complete core WRAML2 administration). The MSI correlates .92 with the General Memory Index, and the average mean difference between the GMI and MSI is less than one standard score point (100.01 MSI vs. 99.98 GMI).

Technical Information. The standardization of the WRAML2 was based on the 2000 U.S. census and used a sample of 1,200 persons, stratified by age (15 age groups, each with 80 participants), gender, ethnicity (African-American, Hispanic, Caucasian, and other), educational attainment (four levels), and U.S. region of residence (four regions). The reliability statistics using Person and Item Separation coefficients range from .85 to .94 for core subtests, and those for the other subtests are similarly high other than for the recognition subtests, which, like all recognition formats, tend to have little variability because most persons do very well. Coefficient alphas (a measure of internal consistency) are also provided for the Indexes (ranging from .86 to .93), core subtests (.81 to .92) and optional subtests (.80 to .92, other than for the Recognition subtests, for

the reason just mentioned). As noted earlier in this chapter, a test-retest stability coefficient can be a misleading statistic for a memory test. Nevertheless, a subsample of 142 individuals ranging in age from 5 to 84 years was chosen and readministered the WRAML2 with a test-retest median interval of 49 days. Test-retest correlations ranged from .53 to .85. Of greater clinical relevance are the gains noted in Index and subtest performance, and reported in the WRAML2 *Manual.* One often hears the question, "When can the test be readministered without significant practice effects being encountered?" Practice effects may be more of an issue for IQ tests than for memory tests. Generally, clinicians are using memory tests to detect memory impairment (vs. strengths). That being the case, if one obtains no practice effect after a reevaluation a month or two following the original session, that may be diagnostic, since Index gains for the interval are reported as 6.3, 7.2, and 1.7 points (in a nonclinical sample) for Verbal, Visual, and Attention/Concentration Indexes, respectively. Documenting a practice effect is, in fact, strong evidence that information is being remembered for long-term retrieval, which is often the purpose of administering the battery in the first place! Likewise, finding no improvement (or lower performance) in a readministration a month or two later may be diagnostic evidence of memory impairment.

With respect to validity, the usual subtest and index inter-correlations are provided in the *Manual,* along with results from both Exploratory and Confirmatory factor analyses. A three-factor solution was found (Verbal, Visual, and Attention/Concentration) with the expected core subtests contributing mostly to their respective Indexes. Factor loadings are provided for five different age sub-groupings, as well as for the entire sample. Goodness-of-fit analyses are also described. Overall, there is strong support for the factor structure of the battery.

Especially important to test users is a presentation of Item Bias data using DIF (differential item functioning) analyses, correlating item calibrations from Rasch analyses for gender and ethnicity (African-American and Hispanic subgroupings). DIF analyses are provided for each core subtest. From the discussion found in the *Manual*, it should be reassuring to know that the WRAML2 shows little bias in item calibrations for both the ethnic and gender subgroups analyzed across all core subtests.

Convergent validity data are provided with comparisons with the following tests: Wechsler Memory Scale–III, Test of Memory and Learning, Children's Memory Scale, California Verbal Learning Test–II, Wechsler Adult Intelligence Test–III, Wechsler Intelligence Scale for Children–III, Wide Range Achievement Test–3, and the Woodcock-Johnson Tests of Achievement–III. Clinical studies of WRAML2 performance are provided for samples that included alcohol abuse, Alzheimer's disease, Parkinson's disease, traumatic brain injury, and learning disability. For each of these clinical groups, means and SDs are provided on WRAML2 Index and subtest performance, as well as indications of statistical difference and effect sizes.

Subsequent to the release of the WRAML2, an interesting study was conducted by Weniger (Weniger & Adams, 2006) using children with reading disorder; attention deficit-hyperactivity disorder, combined type; children with both disorders; and a fourth group of children chosen randomly from the standardization sample, after being matched for age and gender. Because these diagnoses are very common referrals to those working with children, details of that study are provided here.

Table 21.9 provides relevant identifying information about the three clinical groups. Table 21.10 includes the WRAML2 Index scores for those groups along with the matched non-clinical contrast group; indicators of statistical significance are provided. Figure 21.8 provides a corresponding bar graph of index performance for the four groups. It can be noted that children with ADHD generally resembled the standardization sample more than the samples with reading problems. Across most indexes, children with reading problems tended to show immediate memory impairment, whereas children with ADHD did not. One exception to this generalization was the performance of the ADHD group on Working Memory tasks. In this case, it seemed that the concentration demands and greater immediate memory load became too great for children with ADHD to adequately compensate. What is also striking is that children with both attention and reading disorders, generally estimated to be about half of those with ADHD (Barkley, 1998; Lyon, Fletcher, Fuchs, & Chharba, 2006), achieved the lowest memory scores, regardless of index—generally .65 SD lower than IQ would predict. So, from a memory processing perspective, reading disorder

Table 21.9 Characteristics of Subgroups of Children with ADHD and Reading Disorder

Variable	ADHD Group (n = 23)	Reading Disorder Group (n = 24)	ADHD + Reading Disorder Group (n = 23)
T-score Mean (and SD), Connors Rating Scale, Inattention Index	74.1 (11.2)	54.1 (5.6)	74.6 (8.1)
T-score Mean (and SD), Connors Rating Scale, ADHD Index	76.8 (10.9)	55.1 (5.3)	75.5 (8.8)
Reading standard score	88.1 (3.48)	78.9 (9.2)	70.8 (7.3)
Intelligence Quotient	95.6 (8.8)	95.9 (8.5)	92.5 (6.1)

Note. ADHD = Attention Deficit-Hyperactivity Disorder

Table 21.10 WRAML2 Index Means and (SDs) of Children with ADHD, Reading Disorder, Both Disorders, and a Non-Clinical Group

	ADHD	Reading Disorder	ADHD & Reading Disorder	Non-Clinical
Verbal Memory Index	102.5 (12.0) *b*	92.0 (8.0) *a*	86.2 (11.1) *a*	102.5 (12.7) *b*
Visual Memory Index	97.8 (13.9) *b*	92.4 (11.9) *a*	91.0 (10.9) *a*	100.4 (11.7) *b*
Attention/ Concentration Index	94.3 (11.6) *a*	94.1 (10.6) *a*	85.2 (10.6) *b*	99.7 (13.7) *a*
General Memory Index	97.4 (12.0) *b c*	90.0 (8.9) *a b*	84.3 (9.5) *a*	101.0 (12.9) *c*
Working Memory Index	92.9 (13.6) *a*	90.8 (12.4) *a*	82.7 (11.9) *a b*	102.9 (15.1) *c*
General Recognition Index	106.0 (13.7) *b*	90.8 (12.3) *a*	89.7 (8.9) *a*	99.9 (15.9) *b*

Note: ADHD = Attention-Deficit Hyperactivity Disorder. Means within a row with different italicized letter subscripts are statistically different from one another, $p \leq .05$.

is associated with greater deficit than ADHD, and having both disorders is associated with even greater memory deficit than having only one. An additional interesting finding was performance on the recognition tasks. Overall, children with ADHD have recognition scores equivalent to or slightly higher than the non-clinical sample, suggesting that children with ADHD struggle more with retrieval, whereas children with reading problems seem to have more difficulty with the storage component (or storage and retrieval). The WRAML2's Verbal Recognition Index was alone shown to be a reliable predictor of group membership, accurately classifying 82 percent of children with reading disorders and 80 percent of children with ADHD.

Figure 21.9 illustrates the study's findings at the subtest level. Only one of the core subtests fell significantly below average for children with ADHD; namely, Number Letter (ADHD group scaled score = 8.6). (Performance on the Number Letter subtest contributed to the Attention/Concentration Index appearing to be lower; the other subtest contributing to the Index, Finger Windows, was performed as well as the non-clinical sample, possibly because of

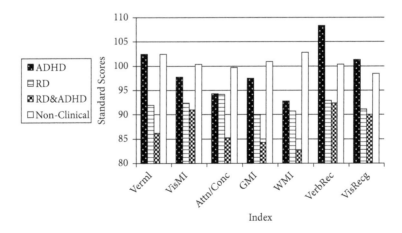

Figure 21.8 WRAML2 Index performance by children with ADHD, Reading Disorder, both disorders, and a non-clinical sample.

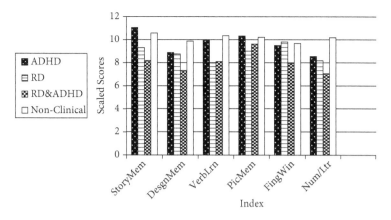

Figure 21.9 WRAML2 core subtest, scaled score performance by children with ADHD, Reading Disorder, both disorders, and a non-clinical sample.

its apparent novelty.) Design Memory performance tended toward significance (scaled score = 8.9) although the effect size for this difference was relatively small. However, slight delays in tasks making perceptual-motor demands are a common finding for children with ADHD (Litton, 2003; Yochman, Ornoy, & Parush, 2006). Therefore, taken overall, children presenting with lower Number Letter and Design Memory subtest scores as well as lower Working Memory Index scores, but with "normal" performance in the other Core subtests and all recognition memory tasks, are far more likely to be children with ADHD than reading disorder. This becomes even more probable if performance on the Verbal Learning subtest tends to be average, since that subtest was consistently poorly performed by children with reading disorder (average scaled score = 8.0). Subgroup placement sensitivity and specificity using these criteria each approached 80 percent.

The reader should not infer from this discussion that the WRAML2 can be used as a means to diagnose ADHD. However, when used with other well-chosen measures, WRAML2 results can provide additional useful information in the overall formulation of that diagnosis. Clearly, more research is needed in examining memory inefficiencies in children with various learning, emotional, and attention deficits.

Test of Memory and Learning, Second Edition (TOMAL-2)

OVERVIEW

The TOMAL-2 (Reynolds & Voress, 2007) was released as a revision of the original battery, TOMAL (Reynolds & Bigler, 1994). Like the WRAML2, the TOMAL revision extended its age range (5 to 59

years), although, unlike the WRAML2, there was little change in the structure or items of the battery. An extra story was added to the Memory for Stories subtest in order to better span the adult range. Reviews of the test have been completed: a brief though lively analysis by Hartman (2007b), and another that is more in-depth by Schmitt & Decker (2009). Also, an extended discussion of TOMAL-2 procedures and interpretation is also available (Adams & Reynolds, 2009).

Core Indexes/Subtests. There are eight core subtests, taking 30 to 40 minutes to administer. Four subtests contribute to each of the two core indexes, which themselves combine to define the overall Composite Memory Index, as shown in Figure 21.10. All of the core subtests assess immediate memory and each is described in Table 21.11 along with time estimates for administration. The Verbal Memory Index assesses immediate recall of meaningful verbal information (words) and comprises four subtests. The Non-Verbal Index is also composed of four subtests requiring immediate recall of visual material, some of which is meaningful (faces); some of which relatively non-meaningful (non-familiar abstract designs); and some of which is spatial.

Supplementary Subtests. In addition to the core components, there are eight optional subtests designed to complement and extend the interpretive value of the core findings. They are identified in Figure 21.11, and the name of each amply describes its content. The Visual Selective Reminding subtest is intended to parallel the Verbal Selective Reminding Task found within the Core subtests section, using visual materials. The examiner touches a grouping of dots found within each area of a 2 x 3 (5- to 8-year-olds) or 2 x 4

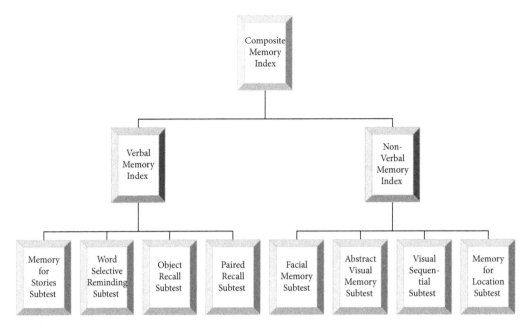

Figure 21.10 TOMAL-2 Core Indexes and their subtests.

(9 years and older) grid. Similar to the procedure in its verbal counterpart, the examiner informs the client of the dots that were omitted, ignoring the dots touched in error. A maximum of five learning trials are administered. The remaining supplementary subtest is Manual Imitation, which resembles a task found on other tests in which the examiner demonstrates various hand sequences (palm down, fist, palm up, side of hand), ranging from two identical hand positions to a series of eight varied positions.

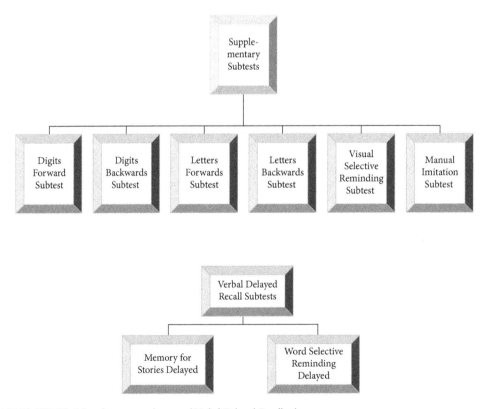

Figure 21.11 TOMAL-2 Supplementary subtests and Verbal Delayed-Recall subtests.

Table 21.11 Description of TOMAL-2 Core Index and Subtest Components

Core Index	Core[1] Subtest	Subtest Description	Administration Time
Verbal Memory Index (An Immediate component exists for each subtest of this index)	Memory for Stories (1)	After each of two 1-paragraph stories is read, client repeats as much of the story as can be remembered.	3–6 minutes
	Word Selective Reminding (3)	Client is asked to repeat a list of words (8 for 5–89 year olds; 12 for 9 years old and older). Only the words not recalled are repeated to the client. Six such learning trials are administered or until client succeeds with the entire list.	3–7 minutes
	Object Recall (5)	On a single page, pictures of 15 common objects are labeled. The page is removed, and the client is asked to recall the verbal labels. Five such exposures are administered or until the client recalls all the labels.	3–7 minutes
	Paired Recall (7)	A paired associate task with 6 (5–8 years old) or 8 (9 years and older) pairs to be learned. Up to four trials are allowed. For each trial, the examiner reads all word pairs, and then, using a different order, tests by giving the first word of each pair. Half the pairings are "easy;" half are "hard." Errors are corrected.	3–6 minutes
Non-Verbal Memory Index (An Immediate component exists for each subtest of this index)	Facial Memory (2)	Client looks for a set time at a stimulus page showing 2–12 black and white faces (children and adults of both genders and differing ethnicities), and then is shown a response page with 2–3 times as many foils. The client is asked to identify the stimulus faces.	4–7 minutes
	Abstract Visual Memory (4)	One abstract design is displayed on the stimulus page for 5 sec., after which the client is to find it on a response page amongst 5 foils.	4–8 minutes
	Visual Sequential Memory (6)	2 to 7 abstract shapes are viewed for 5 sec. on a stimulus page. Then on a response page the client is to point to the designs in the same order as they appeared on the stimulus page.	3–7 minutes
	Memory for Location (8)	For 5 sec. the client views an 8 x 11 inch page on which appears a large square or rectangle within which there is one or more large black dots. The page is turned, dots are gone, but a grid work appears within the square or rectangle. The client is asked to identify the location of the dot(s) by placing circular plastic chips within the grid work. Grids range from 3 x 3 (9 locations) to 4 x 4 (16 locations).	6–10 minutes

[1]Order in the administration sequence appears in parentheses.

In addition, two memory-delayed subtests are provided, to be administered approximately 30 minutes after their immediate recall exposure. Memory for Stories Delayed has clients repeat the two stories they heard earlier in the session. Word Selective Reminding Delayed asks the client to repeat all the words that can be remembered from the original list presented earlier. No recognition measures are part of the TOMAL-2. However, use of various supplemental subtests, by themselves or with core subtests, allows the derivation of several additional indexes: Attention/Concentration, Sequential Recall, Free Recall, Associative Recall, and Learning. As would be expected, all indexes have a mean of 100 (SD = 15) and subtests have a mean of 10 (SD = 3). Percentiles and age equivalents up to 14 years are also provided.

Technical Information. The standardization sample for the TOMAL-2 consisted of data gathered from the TOMAL and a supplemental sample (n = 579) that allowed an updating of the child subgroups, so their demographics were comparable to the 2002 U.S. census data, and as well, provided norms for the new adult subgroups. The resulting combined sample numbered 1,961 and was stratified based upon geographic area, gender, race (Black, White, Other), family income, educational attainment, and age. Coefficient alphas are reported for subtests and indexes. Median subtest alphas across age groups ranged from .67 to .96; median index alphas across age groups ranged from .90 to .98. Test-retest stability is reported for both a pediatric (n = 47) and an adult subsample (n = 35), based upon testing separated by one to three weeks. For children (ages 5–18 years), core subtest scaled score test-retest correlation coefficients ranged from

.63 to .82; core index standard score correlations ranged from .71 to .83. The obtained index scores for children differed by 11 standard score points for the Verbal Memory Index, and by 4 points for the Nonverbal Memory Index. With respect to validity, while no subtest or index inter-correlation tables are provided, a table of standard errors of measurement is. Findings from a factor analysis were discussed, using the entire sample, although the manual states that "the factor solutions were stable across the four age groupings studied." Results from two- vs. four-factor solutions are reported, with the four-factor solution found to be superior; the factors were described as General Memory, Spatial, Sequential Recall and Attention, and a Digits Forward vs. Backward separator. Percentages of the explained variance were not reported. Of interest, Alexander and Mayfield (2005) factor-analyzed TOMAL performance using a large sample of children who had sustained traumatic brain injury. A two-factor model provided a better fit than did the four-factor model; a large general factor was found along with a smaller but stable factor that was thought to capture sequential memory processing.

In the *Manual*, TOMAL-2 performance is compared to performance on several other measures including reading fluency tests, tests of expressive and receptive vocabulary, the WISC-R (Wechsler, 1974), the Test of Nonverbal Intelligence–3 (Brown, Sherbenou, & Johnsen, 1997), and the WRAML2, but the WRAML2 comparison used adults. Table 21.12 reports the degree of similarity between performance on the WRAML2 Core Index scores and those of the TOMAL, using a pediatric sample with learning disabilities (mean age = 9.3 years), and reported in the WRAML2 *Manual*

Table 21.12 Comparison Between WRAML2 and TOMAL Performance (N = 50)

WRAML2 Indexes	WRAML2 Means (SDs)	TOMAL Indexes[1]		
		CMI	VMI	NVMI
Verbal Memory	92.6 (17.0)	.50	.50	.34
Visual Memory	87.4 (18.0)	.46	.26	.58
Attention/Concentration	80.7 (16.6)	.50	.61	.24
General Memory Composite	80.6 (17.9)	.69	.62	.58
TOMAL Index Means (SDs)		86.7 (12.0)	83.3 (13.3)	90.8 (12.4)

[1]Corrected for reliability. WRAML2 = Wide Range Assessment of Memory and Learning, Second Edition; TOMAL= Test of Memory and Learning; CMI = Composite Memory Index; VMI = Verbal Memory Index; NVMI = Nonverbal Memory Index.

(Sheslow & Adams, 2003). As can be seen, the two memory measures yield standard scores that are near a half SD of each other, but with correlations of only moderate strength. The correlations using an adult sample and reported in the TOMAL-2 *Manual* are noticeably higher (Reynolds & Voress, 2007). Therefore, with a pediatric sample, it appears that the TOMAL-2 and WRAML2 are measuring somewhat different constructs.

Like the WRAML2, the TOMAL-2 reports analyses of potential item-bias by gender and ethnicity. No item bias was demonstrated for male vs. female, White vs. Non-White, or Anglo vs. Non-Anglo.

No new clinical studies are included in the TOMAL-2 *Manual*, although several studies that used the TOMAL are briefly mentioned. The TOMAL-2 authors felt that since there was little difference in content between the TOMAL and TOMAL-2, all prior study findings can be assumed to generalize to the new version. A study by Lowther & Mayfield (2004) is cited as showing children and adolescents who had sustained brain injury perform almost a standard deviation lower on the TOMAL than a sample of non-injured children. Children with various learning disabilities were reported in the TOMAL manual (Reynolds & Bigler, 1994) to perform less well on all of the subtests but one. Lowest performance was found on the Attention/Concentration

Index and Sequential Recall Index. The TOMAL-2 *Manual* cites an investigation using children with reading disabilities. Compared to a control group matched for age and IQ, those with reading problems scored lower than controls on all TOMAL subtests (Howes, Bigler, Lawson, & Burlingame, 1999). A study of children with 22q11.2 Deletion Syndrome (known as "velocardiofacial syndrome") using the TOMAL showed higher verbal than nonverbal memory abilities and a particular weakness, as found in children with autism, on the Facial Memory subtest (Lajiness-O'Neill, Beaulieu, Titus, Asamoah, Bigler, Bawle, & Pollack, 2005).

Children's Memory Scale (CMS)
Overview

The Children's Memory Scale (Cohen, 1997) is a third comprehensive memory battery developed for children and available to clinicians. Good reviews of the test are available (e.g., Skaalid, Dunham, & Anstey, 1999; Hildebran & Ledbetter, 2001; Monahan & Fennell, 2001). The age range is five through 16 years, and in many ways the scale is a downward extension of the subtests found on the Wechsler Memory Scale–III (Wechsler, 1997). The structure of the CMS is similar to that found on the WRAML2 and TOMAL-2, and is illustrated in Figure 21.12.

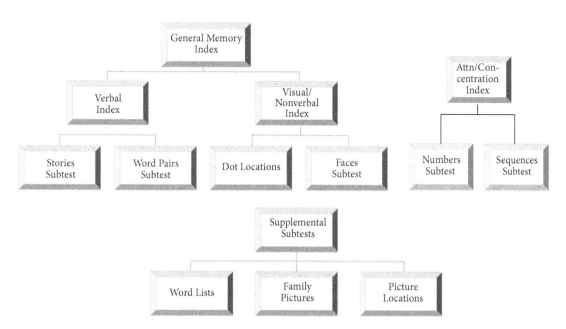

Figure 21.12 Structure of the Children's Memory Scale. The Verbal and Visual/Nonverbal Indexes are composed of both Immediate and Delayed Indexes generated from immediate and delayed components of their respective subtests. Verbal and Visual Indexes combine to form the General Memory Index. Supplemental tests are intended to map on to Verbal, Visual, and Attention /Concentration Index subtests.

The GMI is a composite statistic derived from immediate and delayed memory aspects of the subtests comprising the Verbal and Visual/Nonverbal Indexes. The subtests associated with the Verbal and Visual/Nonverbal Indexes each have Immediate and Delayed components. The verbal subtests also have Delayed Recognition components. The Attention/Concentration subtests have only an Immediate/Working Memory component. Consequently, there are eight Index scores: Verbal Immediate, Verbal Delayed, Visual Immediate, Visual Delayed, General Memory, Attention/Concentration, Learning, and Delayed Recognition. The six core immediate memory subtests take 30 to 40 minutes to administer. The four delayed and two recognition subtests add 10 to 20 minutes more and should follow the immediate presentations by about 30 minutes, which is expected to be filled with other assessment tasks if the examiner chooses not to administer the entire core battery in the recommended sequence. There are two record forms (5–8 and 9–16 years). The traditional conversion of raw scores to scaled scores with means of 10 (SD = 3) is utilized; raw scores are also used to derive memory indexes with

a mean of 100 (SD = 15). Percentiles are also provided. Scoring software is available. A description of each subtest appears in Table 21.13.

TECHNICAL INFORMATION

The normative sample includes 1,000 children, 100 in each of 10 age groups ranging in age from five through 16 years. The sample was stratified, based on 1995 U.S. census data, according to race/ethnicity (White, African American, Hispanic and Other), four U.S. geographic regions, and five parent-education levels. An equal number of each gender was used. Unique to the CMS, the scale was linked with the WISC-III and WPPSI-R, providing, an empirically grounded basis for predicting level of memory performance from IQ; with the subsequent release of newer Wechsler editions, this asset is less relevant.

Split-half reliability, across all age groups, for the eight Index scores ranged from .76, to .91. Internal consistency statistics for core subtests ranged from .71 to .91; supplemental subtest coefficients ranged from .54 to .86. Using a two-month average interval, test-retest reliabilities are reported, ranging from .29 to .89 across the age groups; the CMS *Manual*

Table 21.13 Description of CMS Core Index and Subtest Components

Core Index	Core Subtest	Subtest Description	Administration Time
Verbal Memory Index (Immediate, Delayed, and Recognition components exist for each subtest of this index)	Stories	Two of three stories (age-dependent) are read, immediately after which client repeats as much of the story as can be remembered.	6–10 minutes
	Word Pairs	A list of 10 or 14 (age-dependent) related and unrelated word-pairs are read; thereafter the stem is read and client recalls the associate. Three learning trials are administered.	5–8 minutes
Visual/Non-Verbal Memory Index (Immediate, Delayed, and Recognition components exist for each subtest of this index)	Dot Locations	Child is shown dots located in an empty rectangle. This page is replaced by a 3 x 4 or 4 x 4 (depending on age) rectangular grid and dot positions are to be indicated by client by placing circular chips. Three learning trials administered.	5–8 minutes
	Faces	16 (9- to 16-yr-old) human faces are displayed followed by 48 test photos by which immediate recognition is assessed.	5–8 minutes
Attention/ Concentration Index	Numbers	A digit span forward and backwards task (identical to the WISC-III subtest).	4–6 minutes
	Sequences	12 series of orally presented numbers and months of the year must be properly sequenced. Accuracy and speed earn points.	5–7 minutes

does caution about practice effects, with readministration "practice effects" that approach a standard deviation in magnitude on some of the subtests (Cohen, 1997). The Dot Locations and Faces subtests may be problematic with the youngest children because of an insufficient floor to discriminate between deficits of varying severity.

With respect to validity, the results of confirmatory factor-analysis yielded a three-factor solution consisting of verbal memory, visual/nonverbal memory, and attention/concentration. Performance on both the CMS and WRAML2 is reported in the latter test's Examiner's *Manual* (Sheslow & Adams, 2003), and shows a correlation of .49 between general memory indexes. While there was a low moderate correlation between the Verbal Memory (Immediate) Indexes (.36) as well as the Visual and Visual/Non-Verbal (Immediate) Indexes (.37), the Attention/Concentration Indexes correlated at a noticeably higher level (.58). Overall, the two tests seem to measure somewhat different aspects of memory and appear to be less related than the TOMAL-2 and WRAML2 (e.g., the general composite indexes between these tests are reported to correlate .76, and the range of correlations across core subtests is .34 to .82 (Reynolds & Voress, 2007). Inter-correlations with a number of intellectual, executive, linguistic, memory, and achievement test measures are included in the CMS *Manual*. Also, mean performance scores are provided for a number of small clinical samples, including children with ADHD (inattentive and combined types), learning disability (combined reading and mathematics disorder), language impairment, temporal lobe epilepsy, traumatic brain injury, and brain tumor.

California Verbal learning Test–Children's Version (CVLT-C)

The CVLT-C (Delis, Kramer, Kaplan, & Ober, 1994) is a memory task that provides the clinician a means of evaluating various components of verbal-auditory learning, recall, and recognition. Its structure is similar to the California Verbal Learning Test (CVLT; Delis, Kramer, Kaplan, & Ober, 1987) and its predecessor, the Rey Auditory Verbal Learning Test (Rey, 1964). The CVLT-C is appropriate for children five to 16 years of age. A Spanish version has also been developed (Rosselli et al., 2001). An extensive review of the CVLT-C was written by Strauss, Sherman, and Spreen (2006).

In administering the CVLT-C, the child initially hears and is asked to repeat, in free-recall format, a list of 15 words. The child's responses are recorded, and the recitation-recall procedure is repeated four additional learning/recall trials. Although not mentioned to the child, the words can be sorted into three categories: clothes, fruits, and toys, with an equal number of words associated with each category.

Following administration of the first list of words (List A, the "Monday list"), a second list of words is then presented (List B, the "Tuesday list"). The second list consists of 15 different words that can be sorted into the categories of furniture, fruits, and desserts (fruits being an overlapping category, desserts a partially overlapping category). Following a single learning/recall trial using the second list, the child is again asked to repeat the *first* shopping list. At this point, the child is told the three categories into which the words of the first list could be grouped. With this cue available, recall for each category is then elicited.

A 20-minute interval then elapses during which other nonverbal testing should be completed. At the end of this interval, the child is again given a free-recall trial of the first list, followed by a cued-recall trial. Finally, the child is asked to listen to a list of words that includes items from both learning lists as well as distracter words. The child is asked to identify those words from the first shopping list. The entire procedure requires approximately 30 minutes to complete, not including the 20-minute delay.

Care was exercised in determining item inclusion. The words chosen for the shopping lists were selected based on their frequency of occurrence in the English language as well as by how often they were reported by children. To address the possibility that children would only report the most common words in a category rather than those learned from the list, the three most commonly used words for each category were excluded. The two words lists were designed to be comparable in difficulty.

Perhaps the greatest strength of the test is that it allows a detailed examination of learning strategies. About two dozen age-normed scores can be generated from a child's performance. Examples of scores available include variables such as total recall, performance for trials 1 and 5 of List A, semantic clustering, serial clustering, primacy/recency recall, learning slope (the average number of new words recalled per learning trials), intrusion errors (reporting of words not on the list), short-term and long-term recall, and recognition. For ease of comparison, most of these scores are provided as z scores. Some of the variables are only meaningful at older ages; for example, semantic clustering is not typically observed until about nine to 10 years of age. While hand scoring is possible for most of the scores, because of the number of variables generated, use of available scoring software is desirable, plus it provides normative data for all the variables. Donders (1999a) has provided data on four additional variables: proactive interference, retroactive interference, rapid forgetting, and retrieval problems.

Technical Information

The CVLT-C used the 1988 U.S. Census to guide subject-inclusion. A sample of 920 children was stratified by age (12 subgroups), gender, ethnicity (White, African American, Hispanic and Other), geographic region (four) and parent education (four levels). Details of the standardization, including sampling statistics, are found in the CVLT-C Manual (Delis et al., 1994). Norms for four-year-olds were subsequently provided by Goodman, Delis, and Mattson (1999).

Reliability calculations for the CVLT-C are reported as measures of internal consistency, as well as test-retest reliability. Across the five trials for the first shopping list, the average internal consistency correlation is .88 with a range from .84 to .91. Reliability across categories yields an average internal consistency coefficient of .72 across all age groups. Test-retest measures were obtained from 106 8-, 12-, and 16-year-olds. The interval between test periods averaged 28 days. Total recall performance on the second CVLT-C administration increased by 5, 6, and 9 words for the 8-, 12-, and 16-year-olds, respectively. Reliability coefficients derived from the first and second administration scores ranged from .31 to .90, which the authors considered acceptable for the nature of this auditory-verbal memory assessment tool, especially given the contamination introduced into the readministration by giving the child the organizing strategy of categories during the first testing.

With respect to validity, an exploratory principal component analysis is reported in the test's Manual. Given that entire test batteries generally have fewer than three or four factors, the analysis with the CVLT-C surprisingly yielded a six-component solution, a result similar to the adult version of the measure. Donders (1999b) reanalyzed the standardization data and reported a five-factor solution. Also surprising is the apparent lack of concurrent validation data comparing the CVLT-C with other memory measures. The WRAML2 (Sheslow &

Adams, 2003) only reports correlations with the CVLT (Delis et al., 1987) and CVLT-II (Delis, Kramer, Kaplan, & Ober, 2000). The WRAML2 Verbal Memory Index score was found to correlate .68 with the CVLT-II Trials 1–5 Total score (vs. .03 with the Visual Memory Index). When compared to the WISC-III, using a psychiatric outpatient sample, the greatest amount of unique variance was found shared with the Perceptual Organization Index and CVLT-C short- and long-delay free recall; the Verbal Comprehension Index was a poor predictor explaining only 1.5%–4.5% of the variance) (O'Jile, Schrimsher, & O'Bryant, 2005).

There has been extensive reporting of CVLT-C use with various clinical populations, and these studies are nicely reviewed by Strauss, Sherman, & Spreen (2006) who cite investigations with samples as varied as those with head injuries, spina bifida, phenylketonuria, dyslexia, leukemia, epilepsy, stroke, and low birth weight. Because there are so many variables to examine, it is hard to easily summarize the results, although, in general, the principal CVLT-C variables indicated deficits compared to non-clinical groups. Surprisingly, while performing less well than controls, no lateralized differences were found when the CVLT-C was used with stroke victims with predominantly right- vs. left-hemisphere insults (Lansing, Max, Delis, Fox, et al., 2004). Overall, however, using a relatively simple format, the authors of the CVLT-C have deeply mined traditional and nontraditional learning and memory variables in a remarkable way that has demonstrated valuable clinical utility.

NEPSY-II

While the NEPSY-II (Korkman, Kirk, & Kemp, 2007) is a more general, pediatric-focused neuropsychological assessment battery, nonetheless, a substantial portion of the battery consists of memory subtests. Because many psychologists performing assessments supplement a basic set of measures with additional subtests dictated by the referral question and initial test findings, the memory components of the NEPSY-II are included here as another option that is available.

Overview

The NEPSY-II is a neuropsychological battery appropriate for children from age three to 16 years of age. Of its 32 stand-alone subtests, six are identified as memory subtests, and are described in Table 21.14. All the subtests were part of the original NEPSY other than Memory for Designs and Word List Interference, which are new to the revision; however, modifications in administration, scoring, and/or item content were undertaken for most of the tasks. The tasks include both verbal and visual memory demands, and most have both immediate and delayed recall components. The normative sample includes 1,200 children, 100 in each of 12 age groups ranging in age from 3 through 16 years. The sample was stratified, based on 2003 U.S. census data, according to race/ethnicity (White, African American, Hispanic and Other), four U.S. geographic regions, and four parent-education levels. Equal numbers of each gender were included. Starting and stopping points, along with discontinue rules, were empirically derived and are used to make the testing more streamlined and less burdensome for both client and examiner. The traditional conversion of raw scores to scaled scores with means of 10 (SD = 3) is utilized, but no overall memory score or verbal/visual composites are provided. Base rates, cutoffs, and other data grouping techniques are provided for numerous "Process Scores" that provide a normative basis for qualitative observations often made. Test-retest reliabilities for the memory subtests listed in Table 21.14 were determined using six sub-samples differing in age, each group consisting of about 30 children; correlations (corrected) generally ranged from .50 to .86 with the difference between first and second test (separated by about 3 weeks) differing by one to three scaled score points. Mean performance scores are provided for a number of clinical groups, including children with ADHD, Reading Disorder, Mathematics Disorder, Language Disorder, Mild Intellectual Disability, Autistic Disorder, Asperger's Disorder, and Hearing Impairment. Strangely, a group of only 10 children with TBI were evaluated, and because of the variability within that sample, no performance data were reported. Hand scoring templates as well as Scoring and Interpretive software are available for the entire battery.

Concluding Comment

Given what was available to evaluate memory in children twenty-five years ago, we have made enormous strides in the ensuing years. Specific tests and entire batteries are now available for clinicians, and most of these measures have reasonable psychometric integrity and reflect the growing sophistication in the neuroscience of memory. A literature examining the technical merits and clinical utility of these measures is gradually growing. One aspect that seems to have been overlooked, though, is tests' "ecological validity." That is, if a child does poorly or well on a given task or set of tasks, what does that mean in terms of real-world performance? This lack of careful mapping between our tests and a client's everyday world is not unique to memory assessment. Even though tasks like block design or digit span have been around for more than 70 years, do we really know what it means "in the real world" if a child or teenager does well or poorly on these tasks? Often in the Recommendations sections of our reports, we write like we know. However, there is scant research that gives clinicians a reasonable empirical foundation for interpreting a subtest's uncovered deficit (or strength), let alone for justifying diagnostic pronouncements or well-intentioned recommendations.

There have been attempts to bridge the gap between test findings and everyday functioning, such as the Rivermead Behavioural Memory Test for Children (RBMT-C; Wilson, Ivani-Chalian, & Aldrich, 1991). The RBMT-C is designed for children five through 10 years of age and takes about a half hour to complete; children generally like its tasks. Children are asked to perform "everyday memory" requests, such as remembering the first and last name of an unfamiliar person in a picture, remembering what to do when reminded later in the session, and finding an object hidden earlier in the session. Despite its generating a relatively truncated range of scores, its questionably appropriate British norms when applied to American children, and its marginal reliability (Aldrich & Wilson, 1991), this measure clearly has more face-validity to support claims that it is related to real-world memory demands. However, there does not seem to be much of a research basis upon which to support any such ecological claims more than the more traditional tests that purposely steer clear of tasks that might have been differentially practiced by children coming to be evaluated. The RBMT-C has shown clinical utility with children with more pronounced impairment, but has not fared so well with children with subtler deficits. Nevertheless, the RBMT-C test authors are to be applauded for attempting to create a more ecologically grounded instrument.

Perhaps one reason findings from memory measures do not have a clearer connection with the "real world" is because we are not altogether sure what the comprehensive memory demands are in children's everyday lives. There have been several instruments designed to provide something like a task analysis of "typical" memory demands made of children, employing a survey format (Hickox

Table 21.14 NEPSY-II Memory and Learning Subtests

NEPSY-II Subtest (and Administration Time Estimate)	Age Range (yrs.)	Subtest Description
List Memory (7 minutes)	7–12	A list-learning task using 15 common nouns, and 5 learning trials. A different 15-noun interference trial is then administered with recall, after which recall of the original list is requested. Several "Process Scores" are normed (e.g., number of non-list word intrusions).
List Memory Delayed (1 minute)		Recall of original list is asked after 25–35 minutes' delay.
Memory for Designs (10–15 minutes)	5–16	Spatial memory for novel visual content is assessed. A grid with 4–10 designs is displayed for 10 seconds, and immediately followed with a set of 1 x 2-inch cards from which the child selects the designs just viewed, placing them in the proper grid location. Both content and spatial criteria contribute to the scoring.
Memory for Designs Delayed (3–4 minutes)		Recall of original designs and their positions on the last page seen are assessed 15–25 minutes following initial task.
Memory for Faces (4–5 minutes)	5–16	Facial Recognition task. 5-sec. exposure to each of 16 single target faces (photographs), followed by 16 3-picture groupings, each of which contains a previous target face to be identified.
Memory for Faces Delayed (2–3 minutes)		The 16 3-picture groupings are again shown, and the one target face is to be identified in each.
Memory for Names (6 minutes)	5–16	6–8 2 x 3-inch cards of line drawings of children's faces are presented along with the child's name. The client is to remember which name goes with which face. Three paired-associate learning trials are administered. The presentation order remains invariant.
Memory for Names Delayed (2 minutes)		After a delay of 25–35 minutes, the cards are again presented and recall of each name requested.
Narrative Memory (6–11 minutes)	3–16	A single story is read (selection determined by age) and is immediately followed by a recall trial, and then a cued recall trial for any omitted content. A binary choice recognition task concludes this subtest for those under 11 years of age.
Sentence Repetition (4 minutes)	3–6	Single sentences are read and the child repeats each.
Word List Interference (6–8 minutes)	7–16	A verbal working memory task. One to three words are said and then repeated by the child. A second series of the same number of different words is said and repeated. Then the child is asked to repeat the first series, and then the second. The child's ability to repeat the words is contrasted with his/her ability to recall the words.

& Sunderlund, 1992). Unfortunately, the results have not been encouraging, psychometrically or ecologically. Accordingly, should not psychologists be somewhat less focused on pathology, and instead include wellness within our research interests, such as characterizes the "positive psychology" movement (Compton, 2005)? It would be interesting to explore whether our memory measures can discriminate among those who can and cannot perform impressive "everyday" memory feats such as easily memorizing theater lines, quickly learning a new piece of piano music, and winning spelling or geography bees. Working with strengths as well as deficits might allow us to better evaluate our assumptions related to good or bad scores on a particular memory subtest or index.

At the same time, we must continue to learn about the effects on memory from not-so-positive happenings, like traumatic brain insults from car accidents, strokes, and tumors. Hopefully, in two more decades we will have even better memory tools that will allow us to correctly identify and functionally map corresponding memory deficits in children who deserve more than another page of test scores enlarging their medical records. Instead, we hope that our tests will become more useful in generating diagnostic insight and effective recommendations that will prove valuable to children and their families, as well as assist those engaged in research trying to understand this nearly magical cognitive process.

References

Adams, W. V., & Reynolds, C. R. (2009). *Essentials of WRAML2 and TOMAL-2 assessment*. New York: Wiley & Sons.

Alexander, A. I., & Mayfield, J. (2005). Latent factor structure of the Test of Memory and Learning in a pediatric traumatic brain injured sample: Support for a general memory construct. *Archives of Clinical Neuropsychology, 20*, 587–598.

Aldrich, F. K., & Wilson, B. (1991). Rivermead Behavioural Memory Test for Children (RBMT-C): A preliminary evaluation. *British Journal of Clinical Psychology, 30*, 161–168.

American Psychiatric Association. (2013). *Diagnostic and statistical manual of mental disorders* (5th ed.). Washington, DC: APA.

Aram, D. M., & Eisele, J. A. (1992). Plasticity and recovery of higher cognitive functions following early brain injury. In I. Rapin & S. J. Segalowitz (Eds.), *Handbook of neuropsychology: Child neuropsychology (Part 1), Vol. 6* (pp. 73–92). New York: Elsevier.

Atkinson, R., & Shiffrin, R. (1968). Human memory: A proposed system and its control processes. In K. W. Spence & J. T. Spence (Eds.), *The psychology of learning and motivation* (Vol. 2; pp. 90–197). New York: Academic Press.

Barkley, R. (1998). *Attention-deficit hyperactivity disorder: A handbook for diagnosis and treatment*. New York: Guilford.

Bower, G. (2000). A brief history of memory research. In Tulving, E. & Craik, F. (Eds.), *The Oxford handbook of memory* (pp. 3–32). New York: Oxford University Press.

Brown, L., Sherbenou, R. J., & Johnsen, L. K. (1997). *Test of Nonverbal Intelligence (3rd ed.)*. Austin, TX: Pro-Ed.

Buschke, H. (1973). Selective reminding for analysis of memory and learning. *Journal of Verbal Learning & Verbal Behavior, 12*, 543–550.

Cohen, M. (1997). *Children's Memory Scale*. San Antonio, TX: Psychological Corporation.

Compton, W. C. (2005). *An introduction to positive psychology*. New York: Wadsworth Publishing.

Dehn, M. J. (2008). *Working memory and academic learning: Assessment and intervention*. Hoboken, NJ: Wiley & Sons.

Delis, D. C., Kramer, J. H., Kaplan, E.., & Ober, B. A. (1987). *California Verbal Learning Test*. San Antonio, TX: Psychological Corporation.

Delis, D. C., Kramer, J. H., Kaplan, E., & Ober, B. A. (1994). *California Verbal Learning Test, Children's version*. San Antonio, TX: Psychological Corporation.

Delis, D. C., Kramer, J. H., Kaplan, E., & Ober, B. A. (2000). *California Verbal learning Test* (2nd ed.). San Antonio, TX: Psychological Corporation.

Donders, J. (1999a). Performance discrepancies on the California Verbal learning Test–Children's version. *Developmental Neuropsychology, 16*(2), 163–175.

Donders, J. (1999b). Structural equation analysis of the California Verbal learning Test–Children's version in the standardization sample. *Developmental Neuropsychology, 15*(3), 395–406.

Dudai, Y. (2004). *Memory from A to Z: Keywords, concepts and beyond*. New York: Oxford University Press.

Ebbinghaus, H. (1913). *Memory: A contribution to experimental psychology* (H. A. Ruger & C. E. Bussenius, Trans.). New York: Teachers College, Columbia University. (Original work published 1885.)

Finger, S. (2000). *Minds behind the brain: A history of the pioneers and their discoveries*. New York: Oxford University Press.

Finger, S. (2001). *Origins of neuroscience: A history of explorations into brain function*. New York: Oxford University Press.

Giedd, J. N., Rumsey, J. M., Castellanos, F. X., Rajapakse, J., C., Kaysen, D., Vaituzis, A. C., et al. (1996). A quantitative MRI study of the corpus callosum in children and adolescents. *Development Brain Research, 91*, 274–280.

Goodman, A. M., Delis, D. C., & Mattson, S. N. (1999). Normative data for 4-year-old children on the California Verbal Learning Test–Children's Version. *The Clinical Neuropsychologist, 13*, 274–282.

Haberlandt, K. (1999). *Human memory: Exploration and application*. Boston, MA: Allyn Bacon.

Hartman, D. E. (2007a). Test review: Wide Range Assessment of Memory and Learning–2 (WRAML-2): WRedesigned and WReally improved. *Applied Neuropsychology, 14*, 138–140.

Hartman, D. E. (2007b). Test review: Psst! Wanna buy a good new memory test—cheap? The Test of Memory and Learning–2. *Applied Neuropsychology, 14*, 307–309.

Hebb, D. O. (1942). The effect of early and late brain injury upon test scores, and the nature of normal adult intelligence. *Proceedings of the American Philosophical Society, 85*(3), 275–292.

Hickox, A., & Sunderlund, A. (1992). Questionnaire and checklist approaches to assessment of everyday memory problems. In J. R. Crawford, D. M. Parker, & W. W. McKinlay (Eds.),

A handbook of neuropsychological assessment (pp. 103–112). East Sussex, England: Erlbaum Publishers.

Hildebran, D. K., & Ledbetter, M. F. (2001). Assessing children's intelligence and memory: The Wechsler Intelligence Scale for Children–Third Edition and the Children's Memory Scale. In J. Andrews, D. Saklofske, H. Janzen, & G. Phye (Eds.), *Handbook of psychoeducational assessment* (pp. 13–32). New York: Academic Press.

Howes, N. L., Bigler, E. D., Lawson, J. S., & Burlingame, G. M. (1999). Reading disability subtypes and the Test of Memory and Learning. *Archives of Clinical Neuropsychology, 14*, 317–339.

Kolb, B., & Whishaw, I. Q. (2008). *Fundamentals of human neuropsychology* (6th ed.). New York: Worth Publishers.

Korkman, M., Kirk, U., Kemp, S. (2007). *NEPSY-II* (2nd ed.). San Antonio, TX: Psychological Corporation.

Lajiness-O'Neill, R. R., Beaulieu, I., Titus, J. B., Asamoah, A., Bigler, E. D., Bawle, E. V., & Pollack, R. (2005). Memory and learning in children with 22q11.2 Deletion Syndrome: Evidence for ventral and dorsal stream disruption? *Child Neuropsychology, 11*(1), 55–71.

Lansing, A. E., Max, J. E., Delis, D. C., Fox, P. T., Lancaster, J., Manes, F. F., & Schatz, A. (2004). Verbal learning and memory after childhood stroke. *Journal of the International Neuropsychological Society, 10*, 742–752.

Leahey, T. H., & Harris, R. J. (2001). *Learning and cognition.* Upper Saddle River, NJ: Prentice Hall.

Lezak, M. D., Howieson, D. B., Bigler, E. D., & Tranel, D. (2012). *Neuropsychological assessment* (5th ed.). New York: Oxford University Press.

Levin, H., Eisenberg, H. M., & Benton, A. L. (1989). *Mild head injury.* New York: Oxford University Press.

Litton, M. B. (2003). Motor control in children with and without attention deficit hyperactivity disorder: A neuropsychological investigation. *Dissertation Abstracts International: The Sciences & Engineering, 63* (11-B), 5526.

Lowther, J. L., & Mayfield, J. (2004). Memory functioning in children with traumatic brain injuries: A TOMAL validity study. *Archives of Clinical Neuropsychology, 19*, 105–118.

Lyon, R. G., Fletcher, J. M., Fuchs, L. S., & Chhabra, Vinita. (2006). Learning disabilities. In D. Mash & R. Barkley (Eds.), *Treatment of childhood disorders* (3rd ed.; pp. 512–591). New York: Guilford.

Mattis, S. (1992). Neuropsychological assessment of school-aged children. In I. Rapin & S. J. Segalowitz (Eds.), *Handbook of neuropsychology* (pp. 395–418). New York: Elsevier.

Miller, George. (1956). The magical number seven, plus or minus two: Some limits on our capacity for processing information. *Psychological Review, 63*, 81–97.

Monahan, M. C., & Fennell, E. B. (2001). Book and test review: Children's Memory Scale. *Archives of Clinical Neuropsychology, 16*, 193–198.

Moscovitch, M., Westmacott, R., Gilboa, A., Addis, D. R., Rosenbaum, S., Viskontas, I., et al. (2005). Hippocampal complex contribution to retention and retrieval of recent and remote episodic and semantic memories: Evidence from behavioral and neuroimaging studies of health and brain-damaged people. In N. Ohta, C. M. McLeod, & B. Uttl (Eds.), *Dynamic cognitive processes* (pp. 333–380). Tokyo: Springer-Verlag.

O' Jile, J. R., Schrimsher, G. W., O'Bryant, S. E. (2005). The California Verbal Learning Test–Children's Version: Relation to factor indices of the Wechsler Intelligence Scale for Children (3rd ed.). *Journal of Clinical & Experimental Neuropsychology, 27*(7), 815–822.

Radvansky, G. A. (2005). *Human memory.* Boston, MA: Allyn Bacon.

Rey, A. (1964). *L'examen clinique en psychologie.* Paris: Presses Universitaires de France.

Reeves, D., & Wedding, D. (1994). *The clinical assessment of memory: A practical guide.* New York: Springer Publishing.

Reynolds, C. R., & Bigler, E. D. (1994). *Test of Memory and Learning.* Austin, TX: Pro-Ed.

Reynolds, C. R., & Voress, J. K. (2007). *Test of Memory and Learning* (2nd ed.). Austin, TX: Pro-Ed.

Reynolds, C. R., & Voress, J. K. (2009). Clinical neuropsychological assessment with the Test of Memory and Learning, Second Edition. In C. R. Reynolds & E. Fletcher-Janzen (Eds.), *Handbook of clinical child neuropsychology* (3rd ed.; pp. 297–319). New York: Springer.

Rosler, F., Ranganath, C., Roder, B., Kluwe, R. (Eds.). (2009). *Neuroimaging in human memory: Linking cognitive processes to neural systems.* New York: Oxford University Press.

Rosselli, M., Ardila, A., Bateman, J. R., & Guzman, M. (2001). Neuropsychological test scores, academic performance and developmental disorders in Spanish-speaking children. *Developmental Neuropsychology, 20*(1), 355–373.

Samuel, D. (1999). *Memory: How we use it, lose it and can improve it.* New York: New York University Press.

Sattler, J. M. (2008). *Assessment of children: Cognitive foundations (5th ed.).* San Diego, CA: Author.

Schaie, K. W. (1996). *Intellectual development in adulthood: The Seattle longitudinal study.* New York: Cambridge University Press.

Schmitt, A. J., & Decker, S. L. (2009). Review of Test of Memory and Learning: Second edition. *Journal of Psychoeducational Assessment, 27*(2), 157–166.

Sheslow, D. V., & Adams, W. V. (1990). *Wide Range Assessment of Memory and Learning.* Wilmington, DE: Wide Range, Inc.

Sheslow, D. V., & Adams, W. V. (2003). *Wide Range Assessment of Memory and Learning (2nd ed.).* Wilmington, DE: Wide Range, Inc.

Sivan, A. B. (1991). *Benton Visual Retention Test (5th ed.).* San Antonio, TX: Psychological Corporation.

Skaalid, C., Dunham, P., & Anstey, B. (1999). Test review: The Children's Memory Scale. *Canadian Journal of School Psychology, 14*, 59–65.

Smith, C. N., & Squire, L. R. (2009). Medial temporal lobe activity during retrieval of semantic memory is related to the age of the memory. *Journal of Neuroscience, 29*(4), 930–938.

Stark, C. E.., & Squire, L. R. (2000). Functional magnetic resonance imaging (fMRI) activity in the hippocampal region during recognition memory. *Journal of Neuroscience, 20*(20), 7776–7781.

Squire, L. R. (2004). Memory systems of the brain: A brief history and current perspective. *Neurobiology of Learning and Memory, 82,* 171–177.

Squire, L. R., & Schacter, D. L. (Eds.). (2002). *Neuropsychology of memory.* New York: Oxford University Press.

Strauss, E., Sherman, E. M., & Spreen, O. (2006). *A compendium of neuropsychological tests: Administration, norms and commentary* (3rd ed.). New York: Oxford University Press.

Wechsler, D. (1974). *Wechsler Intelligence Scale for Children, Revised Edition.* San Antonio: Psychological Corporation.

Wechsler, D. (1991). *Wechsler Intelligence Scale for Children* (3rd ed.). San Antonio: Psychological Corporation.

Wechsler, D. (1997). *Wechsler Memory Scale (3rd ed.)*. San Antonio: Psychological Corporation.

Wechsler, D. (2003). *Wechsler Intelligence Scale for Children* (4th ed.). San Antonio: Psychological Corporation.

Wechsler, D. (2008). *Wechsler Adult Intelligence Scale* (4th ed.). San Antonio: Psychological Corporation.

Weniger, R. A., & Adams, W. V. (2006, Nov). *Differences in performance on the WRAML2 for children with ADHD and reading disorder*. National Academy of Neuropsychology annual meeting, Tampa, FL.

Wilson, B. A., Ivani-Chalian, R., & Aldrich, F. (1991). *Rivermead Behavioural Memory Test for Children*. San Antonio, TX: Psychological Corporation.

Wright, B. D., & Stone, M. (1979). *Best test design*. Chicago: MESA Press.

Yochman, A., Ornoy, A., & Parush, S. (2006). Perceptuomotor functioning in preschool children with symptoms of attention deficit hyperactivity disorder. *Perceptual & Motor Skills, 102*(1), 175–186.

Formal Methods in Assessing Child and Adolescent Personality and Affect

Patricia A. Lowe, Erik L. Fister, Susan M. Unruh, Jennifer M. Raad, Justin P. Allen, Tiffany L. Arrington, Skylar A. Bellinger, Liesl J. Edwards, Belinda N. Kathurima, Jeaveen M. Neaderhiser, Christopher R. Niileksela, Jessica Oeth Schuttler, Matthew J. Grumbein, *and* Stephen W. Loke

Abstract

This chapter reviews established, newly developed, and updated structured personality inventories broad and narrow in scope used to assess children and adolescents' personality and affect. The psychometric properties of these structured personality inventories are discussed as well as their strengths and limitations. In addition to the structured personality inventories, informal methods, including clinical interviews and observations, used to assess children and adolescents' affect are discussed.

Key Words: structured personality inventories, norms, reliability, validity, clinical interviews, observations, children, adolescents

In an effort to develop a comprehensive definition of personality, scientists and researchers have defined personality in many different ways over time. These numerous definitions have led to the development of multiple assessment instruments that measure different aspects of personality. Personality inventories consist of objective or structured personality inventories, projectives, and other techniques (Drummond & Jones, 2010). For the purpose of this chapter, structured personality inventories will be reviewed.

Structured personality inventories are usually standardized, self-report measures with a selected response format that facilitates quick responding to the items, quick and reliable scoring, and accurate and efficient interpretation. Structured personality inventories may be broad in scope and assess multiple dimensions of personality or they may be narrow in scope and measure specific aspects of personality. Measures that are broad in scope tend to be comprehensive, consist of many items, are time-consuming to complete, and provide multiple scores on different scales and subscales. In contrast, measures that

are narrow in scope tend to be brief, address specific symptoms, take less time to complete, provide fewer scores to interpret, serve as screeners, and may prove invaluable in monitoring client progress and evaluating treatment outcomes (Drummond & Jones, 2010).

This chapter will review established, newly developed, and updated structured personality inventories broad and narrow in scope used in the assessment of children and adolescents, followed by a review of less formal methods or techniques, including clinical interviews and observations, used to assess children and adolescents' affect.

Structured Personality Inventories

Structured personality inventories broad in scope provide a global assessment of children and adolescents' personality and affect. Comprehensive self-report measures are generally well standardized and yield reliable and valid scores. These measures assist clinicians in identifying those children and adolescents who are at risk or may have a diagnosable disorder. In this section of the book chapter, selected established, newly developed, and updated structured personality inventories broad in scope will be introduced and discussed.

Adolescent Psychopathology Scale

The Adolescent Psychopathology Scale (APS; W. M. Reynolds, 1998a) is an innovative, comprehensive measure based on Achenbach and McConaughy's (1992) and W. M. Reynolds' (1992) conceptual distinction between externalizing and internalizing symptom presentation. The APS is a 346 item, multidimensional self-report measure and was developed to assess psychopathology, personality, and socio-emotional problems and competencies in adolescents, ages 12 to 19. The APS consists of three broad factors (Externalizing, Internalizing, and Personality Disorder) and 40 scales. The 40 scales include 20 Clinical Disorder scales and five Personality Disorder scales consistent with symptom specification of 20 Diagnostic and Statistical Manual of Mental Disorders-Fourth Edition (DSM-IV, American Psychiatric Association, 1994) Axis I clinical disorders and five DSM-IV personality disorders, respectively, 11 Psychosocial Problem Content scales, and four Response Style Indicators. The Psychosocial Problem Content scales assess social and emotional adjustment in adolescents, and the Response Style Indicators measure inconsistent and truthful responding as well as endorsement of low frequency or unusual behaviors, and significant symptoms and problems. The Diagnostic and Statistical Manual of Mental Disorders-Third Edition-Revised (DSM-III-R; American Psychiatric Association, 1987) served as the conceptual basis for the development of the APS items and scales, and these items and scales were re-evaluated and modified when the DSM-IV was published in order for the items and scales to be consistent with the most current version of the DSM diagnostic criteria. The APS items were written at a third grade reading level. Multiple response formats are used on the APS, and these response formats were developed with the DSM-IV symptom criteria in mind. Multiple response formats are used on the APS to best understand the nature of each symptom or each problem being evaluated. The response formats used include a true/false format, general frequency or general duration format, specific frequency format, and frequency of use format. The multiple response formats also allow clinicians to evaluate symptoms across different time periods. The multiple response formats are a unique feature of the APS. The

administration of the APS is straightforward and a test administrator reads the instructions aloud to one or more examinees. Test administrators should be trained in the administration of self-reports to individuals and groups in order to administer the APS. However, those who are not qualified professionals should be under supervision when they administer the APS to an individual or a group of individuals. Once test administrators complete reading the instructions, examinees read each item and record their responses in a 12-page booklet. The APS takes approximately 45 to 60 minutes to complete. APS scoring is accomplished through the use of a computerized scoring program. Interpretation of the APS involves a seven-step process clearly articulated in the administration and interpretation manual, but the interpretation should be done by a qualified professional. The administration and interpretation manual along with the technical manual are clearly written and well organized. The APS should be used to obtain information on the severity of symptoms associated with the DSM-IV clinical and personality disorders, but it should not be used to provide any formal diagnoses (W. M. Reynolds, 1998b).

The final standardization sample for the APS consisted of 1,827 adolescents (900 males and 927 females), 12 to 19 years of age ($M = 14.96$, $SD = 1.66$), in grades 7 through 12. The socioeconomic status (SES) of the sample was described as heterogeneous with a mean SES value of 8.16 ($SD = 2.91$) on the Hollingshead (1975) Occupational Index, indicating that the sample's SES was in the lower-middle class range. Racial/ethnic composition of the sample was 73.6% Caucasian, 18.6% African American, 5.4% Hispanic, 1.0% Asian, and 1.4% Other. The majority of the adolescents in the standardization sample were living with both parents (61.8%) and residing in suburban locations (74.5%). The demographic characteristics reported for the standardization sample are quite detailed and approximate the 1990 U.S. Census for gender, race/ethnicity, and age. The APS also has a clinical sample consisting of 506 adolescents (293 males, 211 females, and 2 individuals' gender was not reported), with a mean age of 15.57 years ($SD = 1.41$), which is slightly higher than the standardization sample. Grade in school for the clinical sample ranged from 7 to 12th grade. However, 10.1% of the sample reported not being in school. Racial/ethnic composition of the sample included 81.6% Caucasian, 6.4% African American, 5.8% Hispanic, 1.0% Asian, and 5.2% Other. The majority of the clinical sample (87%) was diagnosed with a Conduct Disorder based on the DSM-III-R diagnostic criteria. The adolescents in the clinical sample were recruited from 31 clinical sites in 22 states (W. M. Reynolds, 1998b).

Extensive work has been conducted to examine the reliability and validity of the APS scores. The majority of internal consistency reliability estimates for the standardization and clinical samples for the scores of the APS clinical, personality, and psychosocial scales were .80 or higher. Also, the majority of the test score stability coefficients for the scores of these same scales over a 14 day test-retest interval were .80 or higher (W. M. Reynolds, 1998c). These findings suggest that the item content on the different APS Clinical Disorder, Personality Disorder, and Psychosocial Problem Content scales are relatively homogeneous in content, and the scale scores show consistency over a relatively short period of time.

Evidence supporting the validity of the APS scores was examined through content analysis, concurrent validity studies, contrasted group studies, and factor analyses (W. M. Reynolds, 1998c). This information is reported in the technical manual. The content validity of the APS was ensured with the inclusion of items representing symptom descriptions of psychopathology, personality disorders, and social and emotional adjustment difficulties supported in the DSM-IV. Different APS clinical, personality, and psychosocial scale scores showed good convergent validity with the scores of the Minnesota Multiphasic Personality Inventory (MMPI; Hathaway & McKinley, 1943) and the scores of other established measures of anxiety, depression and self-esteem. In addition, the APS clinical, personality, and psychosocial scale scores demonstrated good divergent validity with the scores of measures of cognitive ability and social desirability. Results of a contrasted group study comparing the scores of the standardization group and the clinical group on the 40 APS scales with age and gender serving as covariates also provide support for the discriminant validity of the APS scores. Finally, a series of principal component analyses were performed, and the findings from these analyses provide support overall for the factor structure of the APS.

In sum, the APS is an innovative, multidimensional self-report measure designed to assess psychopathology, personality, and socio-emotional problems and competencies in adolescents. The APS is a comprehensive measure and it was designed specifically to assess psychopathology in adolescents. These are two of the many strengths of the measure. Other strengths include the extensive evidence

supporting the technical adequacy of the measure, well written and detailed manuals, clear seven-step process to interpret the APS scores and profiles, and multiple response formats to better understand the symptoms and problems being evaluated. In contrast, several weaknesses or limitations of the APS include the length of the measure (however, a short form has been developed), representation of the clinical sample (a large majority of the clinical sample had been diagnosed with a conduct disorder), and research on the specificity and sensitivity of the measure (more information is needed in this area).

Behavior Assessment System for Children, Self-Report of Personality

The Behavior Assessment System for Children-Self-Report of Personality (BASC-2-SRP; C. R. Reynolds & Kamphaus, 2004a) is a multidimensional self-report measure designed for use with children, adolescents, and college students, ages 6 to 25. The BASC-2-SRP is designed to elicit an individual's perceptions of his or her own behavioral and emotional functioning across several domains, as well as identify specific areas in which the individual exhibits strengths and weaknesses. According to the manual, the results of the BASC-2-SRP are intended to help identify emotional and behavioral difficulties, as well as guide intervention and treatment plans. However, the authors also list several other possible uses of the BASC-2 rating system, including educational classification, manifest determination, program evaluation, forensic/legal proceedings, and research (C. R. Reynolds & Kamphaus, 2004b).

According to C. R. Reynolds and Kamphaus (2004b), the BASC-2 composite scales were based on the factor structure of the original Behavior Assessment System for Children (BASC; C. R. Reynolds & Kamphaus, 1992) then modified to reflect the results of exploratory and confirmatory factor analyses. The item content of the composite scales and individual scales reflect the diagnostic criteria from the DSM-IV-TR (American Psychiatric Association, 2000), as well as information gathered from teachers, parents, children, and mental health professionals (C. R. Reynolds & Kamphaus, 2004b). Several versions of the BASC-2-SRP are available, a child form, the BASC-2-SRP-C, an adolescent form, the BASC-2-SRP-A, and the college form, the BASC-2-SRP-COL. However, the focus of this review will be on the child and adolescent forms. Detailed information about the college form can be found in the BASC-2 manual. The BASC-2 child and adolescent forms contain several validity scales to identify inaccuracies, inconsistencies, biases, and otherwise invalid responses. Each version is written at a third grade reading level, and can be completed in approximately 20 to 30 minutes. The BASC-2-SRP may be hand-scored or computer-scored (C. R. Reynolds & Kamphaus, 2004b).

Normative data were gathered for the BASC-2-SRP between 2002 and 2004 (C. R. Reynolds & Kamphaus, 2004b). Data were collected from 375 sites across the U.S., and included 3,400 children and adolescents, ages 8 to 18. The authors controlled for gender, race/ethnicity, geographic region, socioeconomic status, and inclusion of special populations in the normative sample, in an effort to reflect the 2001 U.S. population. Clinical norms were also gathered from a group of 1,572 children, ages 8 to 21, identified as having a clinical diagnosis or special education classification. The clinical group was not considered a random stratified sample, and therefore demographic characteristics were not controlled (C. R. Reynolds & Kamphaus, 2004b).

Extensive reliability and validity studies have been conducted with the BASC-2 scores. Test score stability was examined, with intervals ranging from 13 to 66 days (C. R. Reynolds & Kamphaus, 2004b). In addition, the convergent and discriminant validity of the BASC-2-SRP scores were assessed in comparison to the scores of several other behavioral and emotional scales. Specific reliability and validity estimates for the BASC-2 scores for the different forms based on the general normative group are discussed below. In addition, information on a supplementary form to the child form, the BASC-2-SRP-Interview is also discussed.

Self-Report of Personality—Interview (SRP-I). The Self-Report of Personality-Interview (SRP-I) is available for children, ages 6 to 7. The SRP-I consists of 64 items read aloud by an examiner, to which children respond in a yes/no format. The SRP-I contains one composite scale: the Emotional Symptoms Index, as well as the following individual scales: Anxiety, Attitude to School, Attitude to Teachers, Atypicality, Depression, Interpersonal Relations, and Social Stress (C. R. Reynolds & Kamphaus, 2005).

Based on the normative group of 250 children, the SRP-I scores demonstrated strong to very strong internal consistency reliability for the composite scale scores ($\alpha = .94$) as well as the individual scale scores (αs = .72 –.82). The SRP-I also exhibited moderate to strong test score stability for the composite scores ($r = .85$) and the individual scale

scores (rs = .56 –.79) over a three-week test-retest interval. These reliability estimates were adjusted for restriction of range (C. R. Reynolds & Kamphaus, 2005). Exploratory and confirmatory factor analyses were also performed on a sample of 315 children, and the results of these analyses supported a one-factor solution/model for the SRP-I. A moderate correlation of .53 was found between the SRP-I Anxiety scores and the Revised Children Manifest Anxiety Scale (RCMAS; C. R. Reynolds & Richmond, 1978) Total Anxiety scores, supporting the convergent validity of the SRP-I scores. In contrast, overall the correlations between the scores of comparable scales on the SRP-I and the scores of the BASC-2-TRS and BASC-2-PRS were relatively weak (C.R. Reynolds & Kamphaus, 2005). According to Reynolds and Kamphaus, additional studies are needed to assess the validity of the SRP-I scores.

Self-Report of Personality—Child Form (SRP-C). The SRP-C is designed for use with children, ages 8–11. The SRP-C contains a total of 139 items. Fifty-one items are presented in a true/false format, while 88 items are answered using a 4-point Likert scale, ranging from 1 (*never*) to 4 (*almost always*). The SRP-C includes five composite scales: Inattention/Hyperactivity, Internalizing Problems, Personal Adjustment, School Problems, and the Emotional Symptoms Index. In addition, each composite scale contains a number of individual scales. The SRP-C includes the following individual scales: Anxiety, Attention Problems, Attitude to School, Attitude to Teachers, Atypicality, Depression, Hyperactivity, Interpersonal Relations, Locus of Control, Relationship with Parents, Self-Esteem, Self-Reliance, Sense of Inadequacy, and Social Stress (C. R. Reynolds & Kamphaus, 2004b).

The SRP-C normative group included 1,500 children, ages 8 to 11. Based on the general normative group, the SRP-C exhibited strong to very strong internal consistency reliability for the composite scale scores (αs = .85 –.96) as well as the individual scale scores (αs = .71 –.86). Test score stability was assessed in a sample of 113 children, with a median test-retest interval period of 25 days. The SRP-C demonstrated moderate to strong test score stability for the composite scale scores (rs = .75 –.83) and the individual scale scores (rs = .63 –.82; C. R. Reynolds & Kamphaus, 2004b). Convergent and discriminant validity have also been examined between the scores of the SRP-C and the scores of established self-report measures, such as the Children's Depression Inventory (CDI; Kovacs,

1992), the RCMAS and the original child form of the BASC-SRP.

Self-Report of Personality-Adolescent Form (SRP-A). The SRP-A is designed for use with adolescents, ages 12 to 21. The SRP-A contains a total of 176 items. Sixty-nine items are presented in a true/false format, while 107 items are answered using a 4-point Likert scale, ranging from 1 (*never*) to 4 (*almost always*). The SRP-A contains the same composite scores as the SRP-C. However, the SRP-A also includes individual scales relating to Sensation Seeking and Somatization (C. R. Reynolds & Kamphaus, 2004b).

The SRP-A normative group included 1,900 adolescents, ages 12 to 18. Based on the normative group, the SRP-A exhibits strong to very strong internal consistency reliability for the composite scale scores (αs = .83 –.96) and moderate to strong internal consistency reliability for the individual scale scores (αs = .67 –.88). Test score stability was assessed in a sample of 107 adolescents, with a median test-retest interval time of 20 days. The SRP-A demonstrated moderate to strong test score stability for the composite scale score (rs = .74 –.84) and the individual scale score (rs = .61 –.84; C. R. Reynolds & Kamphaus, 2004b). With regard to validity, strong correlations were reported between the scores of the SRP-A scales and the scores of conceptually-similar scales on the Youth Self-Report of the Achenbach System of Empirically-Based Assessment (ASEBA; Achenbach & Rescorla, 2001d). Specifically, strong correlations were found among the inattention (r = .76), internalizing (r = .80), and overall emotional functioning (r = .75) scores of the ASEBA and the SRP-A. Evidence supporting the discriminant validity of the SRP-A scores with conceptually-dissimilar ASEBA scale scores is noted in the BASC-2 manual (C. R. Reynolds & Kamphaus, 2004b). Evidence supporting the convergent and discriminant validity of the SRP-A scores and the scores of other established self-report measures, including the CDI, the RCMAS, and the adolescent form of the original BASC is also reported in the manual (C. R. Reynolds & Kamphaus, 2004b).

The BASC-2-SRP is a widely-used and respected instrument, and is supported by a wealth of research data. The normative sample and procedures for the BASC-2-SRP represents a clear strength. The general normative group consists of a large sample, collected from many sites across the U.S., and appears representative of the general population. In addition, although the clinical sample is smaller than the normative sample, the inclusion of several clinical groups increases the utility and applicability of the instrument to diverse populations. As with the inclusion of a clinical sample, the expanded age range of the BASC-2-SRP (ages 6 to 25) increases the instrument's utility from a developmental perspective, and allows for its use among a wide age range. Similarly, the availability of Spanish versions of each of the BASC-2-SRP forms establishes the BASC-2-SRP as a useful tool when working with populations of increasing diversity. In addition, the inclusion of a 4-point Likert response format within the BASC-2-SRP improves upon the previous version, which relied solely on true/false responses. The expanded response range allows for greater sensitivity and specificity of responses and interpretation.

Limitations of the BASC-2-SRP include the relatively lower internal consistency reliability estimates of the individual scale scores in comparison to the composite scores. However, this is not unexpected, as reliability estimates often improve with the addition of items on scales. Therefore, the scores of the composite scales (based on multiple scales) appear to be a more reliable indicator of an individual's strengths and needs, and caution should be exercised when interpreting or making decisions based on individual scale results.

Minnesota Multiphasic Personality Inventory-Adolescent

The Minnesota Multiphasic Personality Inventory—Adolescent (MMPI-A; Butcher, Williams, Graham, Kaemmer, et al., 1992), designed for use with adolescents between the ages of 14 and 18, provides an estimate of psychopathology and adjustment in youth populations (Butcher, Williams, Graham, Archer, et al., 1992). The MMPI-A is a downward extension of the MMPI and the MMPI-2 (Butcher, Dahlstrom, Graham, Tellegen, & Kaemmer 1989); however, the MMPI-A underwent item revision, testing format redesign, and norming procedures with the adolescent population in mind (Conoley & Impara, 1995). In accordance with the MMPI's history of empirical test development, the MMPI-A continues this tradition. The MMPI-A consists of 478 items and 10 clinical scales (Hypochondriasis, Depression, Hysteria, Psychopathic Deviate, Masculinity-Femininity, Paranoia, Psychasthenia, Schizophrenia, Hypomania, and Social Introversion), three broad validity scales (Lie, Infrequency, and

Defensiveness), and four validity subscales (two Infrequency, Variable Response Inconsistency, and True Response Inconsistency). In addition to these scales and subscales, there are 15 adolescent content scales, six supplementary scales, 28 Harris-Lingoes subscales, and three social introversion subscales (Butcher, Williams, Graham, Archer, et al., 1992).

Test administration of the MMPI-A takes approximately 1–1/2 hours to complete. The MMPI-A assessment comes in three formats: a standard booklet format, computer-assisted format (which facilitates scoring), and audio administration format for the visually impaired. Adolescents respond to the statements on the MMPI-A using a true/false format. The complexity of the questions on the MMPI-A requires respondents to have at least a fifth to seventh grade reading level (Butcher, Williams, Graham, Archer, et al., 1992). The MMPI-A testing format allows respondents to complete the assessment in more than one administration period.

Scoring of the MMPI-A is rather easy. Practitioners completing hand-scored assessments do so by summing responses identified using the provided templates that match the appropriate items with the identified scale. Once scale scores are summed, the practitioner then transfers the scores to a profile sheet. However, interpretation of the MMPI-A is somewhat complex. Practitioners must be familiar with the various scale descriptors, as well as the number of interplays of profile representations before they attempt to interpret the measure for their clients.

The normative sample for the MMPI-A consisted of 1,620 adolescents (805 males and 815 females), ages 14 to 18. The adolescents were recruited from eight states. These states were selected to provide a balance in the demographic characteristics of the sample with regards to race/ethnicity, geographic region, and urban and rural settings (Butcher, Williams, Graham, Archer, et al., 1992). The normative sample was fairly representative of the U.S. population of adolescents in 1980, with a few exceptions. These exceptions include under-representation of Hispanics, SES distribution skewed toward the higher SES levels, fewer individuals in the higher age groups, and under-representation of school dropouts (Butcher, Williams, Graham, Archer, et al., 1992; Kamphaus & Frick, 2002; Rowe, 2003). In addition to the normative sample, a clinical sample of 713 adolescents (420 males and 293 females), ages 14 to 18, were recruited from treatment facilities in the Minneapolis area (Butcher, Williams, Graham, Archer, et al., 1992).

Studies have been conducted to examine the reliability and validity of the MMPI-A scores. Butcher, Williams, Graham, Archer, et al. (1992) reported test score stability coefficients for the scores of the validity scales and subscales and the clinical scales over a one-week test-retest interval. Reliability estimates for the scores of the validity scales and subscales ranged from .49 to .75, and test score stability coefficients for the scores of the clinical scales ranged from .65 to .84. Internal consistency reliability estimates for the scores of the validity scales and subscales and clinical scales ranged from .35 to .91. These reliability estimates are in the moderate to very strong range.

Evidence supporting the validity of the MMPI-A scores has been found. Butcher, Williams, Graham, Archer, et al. (1992) conducted a factor analytic study of the responses of adolescents to the validity and clinical scale items on the MMPI-A. Results of the factor analysis indicated a four-factor solution provided the best fit for the data. These factors were named General Maladjustment, Overcontrol, Social Introversion, and Masculinity-Femininity. However, follow-up factor analytic studies reported different factor structures for the MMPI-A (Archer, Belevich, & Elkins, 1994; Archer, Bolinskey, Morton, & Farris, 2002; Bolinskey, Arnau, Archer, & Handel, 2004). Similarly, some studies have demonstrated evidence of predictive validity for the content scale scores over the basic clinical scale scores (e.g. Forbey & Ben-Porath, 2003; McGrath, Pogge, & Stokes, 2002). While other researchers (e.g. Rinaldo & Baer, 2003) found that the clinical and content scale scores were both useful in predicting clinical and non-clinical group membership. Interestingly, recent studies (Hand, Archer, Handel, & Forbey, 2007; Hilts & Moore, 2003) have demonstrated that the MMPI-A produces normal profiles among some adolescents who experience significant psychological distress. In examining sensitivity and specificity rates, Fontaine, Archer, Elkins, and Johansen (2001) discovered that the accuracy of the MMPI-A classification rates improve when the cut score is raised from a T score of 60 to a T score of 65, thus arguing that a grey area of classification exists. Furthermore, convergent and discriminant validity studies found that the MMPI-A scores demonstrate adequate validity when compared to scores of other scales that purport to measure similar and dissimilar constructs (Arita & Baer, 1998).

Even among current assessment systems, the MMPI-A remains a peerless assessment system. Years of empirical research continue to support its effectiveness and refined administration and interpretation procedures. Yet the original MMPI, of which the MMPI-A is based, was developed using the same test development methods that were continued in the development of the MMPI-A. Thus, while the assessment remains useful, the MMPI-A is not as psychometrically sophisticated as it once was (Lanyon, 1995). For example, many test items overlap on a number of scales and this redundancy reduces the amount of unique variance the scores of each scale contributes to the overall assessment (Kamphaus & Frick, 2002). Additionally, the convergence of items across scales brings the results from factor-analytic studies into question (Kamphaus & Frick, 2002). Though maintaining fidelity to the original MMPI and MMPI-2 is commendatory in many respects, revising some of the scales and subsequent scale names would have proved useful. For example, the superannuated Psychasthenia and the sensational Psychopathic Deviate scales would have benefited from such revisions, reducing confusion and shock among practitioners and clients alike (Claiborn, 1995). While certain scales would have benefited from revisions, the overall assessment would have benefited from the removal of the Masculinity-Femininity scale. It is unclear why Butcher, Williams, Graham, Kaemmer, et al. (1992) maintained this scale. The Masculinity-Femininity scale provides a poor measure if presented as an assessment of interests and the contribution of this scale to the overall assessment remains questionable at best (Claiborn, 1995). The MMPI-A paper-and-pencil format allows practitioners to access a broader view of their clients; however, administration is rather long for adolescents. To counter this, practitioners must either utilize the computer adaptive assessment or remain cognizant of client fatigue in cases where it may affect the quality of responses. The low internal consistency reliability estimates and instability of some of the clinical scale scores are also of concern and suggest the need to interpret some MMPI-A scale scores with caution (Kamphaus & Frick, 2002).

Personality Assessment Inventory-Adolescent

The Personality Assessment Inventory-Adolescent (PAI-A; Morey, 2007a) is a 264-item, self-report measure designed to assess personality and psychopathology in adolescents, ages 12 to 18. The PAI-A consists of 22 non-overlapping scales, 11 clinical scales (Alcohol Problems, Antisocial Features, Anxiety, Anxiety-Related Disorders, Borderline Features, Depression, Drug Problems,

Mania, Paranoia, Schizophrenia, and Somatic Complaints), five treatment consideration scales (Aggression, Suicidal Ideation, Stress, Nonsupport, and Treatment Rejection), two interpersonal scales (Dominance and Warmth), and four validity scales (Inconsistency, Infrequency, Negative Impression, and Positive Impression). In addition, most of the clinical scales of the PAI-A have three conceptually driven subscales each, with the exception of the Alcohol Problems and the Drug Problems scales, which have no subscales, and the Borderline Features scale, which has four subscales, designed to provide full coverage of the clinical constructs assessed on the PAI-A and to assist in clinical interpretation. The clinical syndromes assessed by the PAI-A were chosen based on current views of nosology and diagnostic practice. The PAI-A parallels closely the adult version of the scale, the Personality Assessment Inventory (PAI; Morey, 1991). The structure of the PAI-A is similar to the PAI, and most of the items developed for the PAI were retained on the PAI-A; however, the items were modified to make them more applicable to adolescents and their experiences. Items were written at a fourth grade reading level. The instrument can be administered on an individual basis or in a group setting in either a paper-and-pencil format or on a computer. Minimal differences have been found when measures have been administered in these two different formats (Finger & Ones, 1999). Administration time for the paper-and-pencil and the computer versions of the PAI-A is approximately 30 to 45 minutes (Morey, 2007b).

The standardization sample for the PAI-A consists of two groups, a community-based sample and a clinical sample. The community-based sample consisted of 707 adolescents (361 males and 346 females), ages 12 to 18, with a mean age of 15.00 years ($SD = 2.00$). Racial/ethnic composition of the sample included 61.5% Caucasian, 15.4% African American, 16.3% Hispanic, and 6.8% Other. The adolescents were recruited from urban and rural settings in 21 states in the U. S. The sample was comparable to the 2003 U.S. adolescent population with regards to age, gender, and race/ethnicity. The clinical sample included 1,160 youths, 58.4% males and 41.6% females, seen in 78 different clinical sites in the U.S. The mean age of the clinical sample was slightly higher than the community-based sample ($M = 15.29$ years, $SD = 1.59$). Racial/ethnic composition of the clinical sample consisted of 72.3% Caucasian, 19.8% African American, 4.5% Hispanic, and 4.4% Other. Approximately half (49.7%) of the clinical sample was assessed in outpatient facilities, with the majority of the adolescents having a primary diagnosis of conduct disorder (23.6%), drug/alcohol abuse or dependence (19.3%), attention-deficit/hyperactivity disorder (18.8%), major depressive episode (15.9%), or oppositional defiant disorder (13.4%; Morey, 2007b).

Detailed information is provided in the PAI-A manual on the reliability and validity of the PAI-A scores. Internal consistency reliability estimates for the scores of the PAI-A clinical scales, validity scales, treatment consideration scales, and interpersonal scales ranged from .70 to .90 and .63 to .90 for the total community-based and clinical samples, respectively. Only one reliability estimate fell below .70 in the clinical sample. Coefficient alphas for the clinical subscale scores ranged from .47 to .80 and .47 to .85 for the total community-based and clinical samples, respectively. Test score stability coefficients for the scores of the PAI clinical scales, validity scales, treatment consideration scales, and interpersonal scales for a sample of 100 adolescents from the community-based standardization sample ranged from .65 to .89 over a 9 to 35 day test-retest interval. For the clinical subscale scores, test score stability coefficients over the same test-retest period with the same adolescents from the community-based standardization sample ranged from .59 to .88 (Morey, 2007b).

Internal structure of the PAI-A scores was examined through principal component and confirmatory factor analyses. Principal component analyses were performed separately on the responses of the community-based and clinical samples. Results of the principal component analysis indicated that a four-factor structure provided the best fit for the data for the community-based and clinical samples. The four factors appeared to assess subjective distress and affective disruption, egocentricity and exploitation in interpersonal relationships, substance involvement and abuse, and interpersonal detachment and alienation. In addition, confirmatory factor analyses were performed to examine the hypothesized conceptual subscale structures in relation to the actual subscale structures. Results indicated acceptable fit for all subscale structures. However, the fit was not as good for the PAI-A in comparison to the PAI. Morey indicated that the difference in the findings may be due to fewer indicators for each factor on the PAI-A in comparison to the PAI or the structure of these constructs is not as distinct in the adolescent population. Overall, strong evidence supporting the convergent and discriminant validity of the PAI-A scores is provided in the manual. The PAI-A scores were compared to scores of appropriate scales that measure similar and dissimilar constructs on the MMPI-A, the APS, the Personality Inventory for Youth (PIY; Lachar & Gruber, 1995a), the NEO Five Factor Inventory (NEO-FFI; Costa & McCrae, 1989), the Symptom Assessment-45 (SA-45; Davison et al, 1997), the College Adjustment Scale (CAS; Anton & Reed, 1990), the Clinical Assessment of Depression (CAD; Bracken & Howell, 2004a), the Adolescent Anger Rating Scale (AARS; Burney, 2001), the Conners' Adult ADHD Rating Scale (CAARS; Conners, Erhardt, & Sparrow, 1999), the Beck Depression Inventory (BDI; Beck et al., 1996a), and the State-Trait Anxiety Inventory (STAI; Spielberger, 1983) (Morey, 2007b).

The PAI-A is a promising new measure designed to assess personality and psychopathology in the adolescent population. Strengths of the PAI-A include its comprehensiveness, ease of administration, well organized and well-written manual, and detailed information in the manual on the psychometric properties and technical characteristics of the measure. Limitations of the PAI-A include its newness, the need for more independent studies to examine the reliability and validity of the PAI-A scores, moderate reliability estimates for the subscale scores, suggesting these scores should be interpreted with caution, and the length of time to complete the measure. Although there are some limitations associated with the PAI-A, it has the potential to become a major rival of the MMPI-A in the future.

Personality Inventory for Youth

The Personality Inventory for Youth (PIY) is a comprehensive, multidimensional, self-report measure used to assess behavioral and emotional adjustment, family interactions, school adjustment, and academic ability in children and adolescents, ages 9 to 18. The PIY consists of 270 items or true-false statements (Lachar & Gruber, 1995b). The items for the PIY were adapted from the Personality Inventory for Children-Revised (PIC-R; Lachar, 1982), with the majority of the items reworded to be age appropriate and rewritten in the first person. The PIY items were written at about a third grade reading level. An audio recording of the statements is also available for students who may have difficulty reading the items. Administration of the PIY takes 30 to 60 minutes and is completed independently with appropriate supervision. Group administration of the PIY is also possible. A shorter screening assessment called the Classroom Screening (CLASS) can also be administered using the first 80 items of the PIY and provides a general measure of adjustment (Lachar & Gruber, 1995b).

The PIY consists of nine clinical scales as well as four validity scales. The nine clinical scales are Cognitive Impairment, Impulsivity and Distractibility, Delinquency, Family Dysfunction, Reality Distortion, Somatic Concern, Psychological Discomfort, Social Withdrawal, and Social Skills Deficits. Each scale is comprised of two or three subscales, resulting in 24 subscales that provide more detailed information. The validity scales are Inconsistency, Validity, Dissimulation, and Defensiveness, which are designed to indicate whether the PIY results of children and adolescents are inaccurate or atypical. Both hand-scoring and computer-scoring are available for the PIY. However, due to the complexity in transferring clusters of item responses from the response sheet to the profile form, computer scoring is recommended for accuracy and efficiency. Standard scores (i.e. T scores) are reported for the different scales and subscales. Interpretation of the PIY scores involves a five-step process (Lachar & Gruber, 1995b).

The standardization sample of the PIY consisted of 2,347 children and adolescents, ages 9 to 18. The students were all in regular education in 13 public school districts across five states. In addition, a sample of 1,178 clinically-referred students was assessed to establish a clinical research base for the PIY (Lachar & Gruber, 1995b). While the demographics of the standardization sample did differ from those of the general U.S. population, according to the authors a study of a demographically representative subsample of 709 children and adolescents from the normative sample indicated it was unlikely that the differences in demographic characteristics reported significantly affected the test scores (Destefano, 2001).

The PIY includes a technical guide which provides extensive information regarding the reliability and validity of its scores (Lachar & Gruber, 1995c). The median internal consistency reliability coefficient for the PIY clinical scale scores was .82 for the regular education sample and 85 for the clinical sample. Median internal consistency reliability coefficients for the subscale scores were .70 for the regular education sample and .73 for the clinical sample (Merrell, 2008). Test score stability coefficients for the clinical scale scores ranged from .80 to .91 for the regular education sample and from .76 to .84 for the clinical sample over a 7- to 10-day test-retest interval. For the subscale scores, test score stability coefficients ranged from .66 to .90 for the regular education sample and .59 to .88 for the clinical sample over the same test-retest interval (Lachar & Gruber, 1995c).

Results of factor analyses support the structure and design of the PIY (Lachar & Gruber, 1995c). Evidence supporting the convergent and discriminant validity of the PIY scores was demonstrated through correlations with the scores of such measures as the PIC-R, the MMPI, and the Peabody Picture Vocabulary Test-Revised (PPVT-R; Dunn & Dunn, 1981) (Lachar & Gruber, 1995c). The PIY scores have also shown adequate sensitivity in distinguishing between clinical and non-clinical samples of children and adolescents (Merrell, 2008). Lachar, Harper, Green, Morgan, and Wheeler (1996) conducted a contrasted group study and found that the PIY scores were able to differentiate children with a major depressive disorder from children with a conduct disorder. These findings provide additional support for the discriminant validity of the PIY scores.

The PIY has the potential to make significant contributions in both research and clinical practice. Because the PIY was developed from the PIC-R, which is a well-established measure, the PIY has a significant theoretical and statistical base. The PIY allows for children and adolescents to supply information from their perspective. Due to its length, which can be a hindrance, the PIY may not be suitable as a general screening instrument; however, the abbreviated 80-item format may be useful for large-scale administrations (Marchant & Ridenour, 2001). Although the authors conducted a special study using the normative sample and a demographically representative subsample and reported that differences in the demographic characteristics were unlikely to affect the test scores, the authors did proceed and did create separate norms for males and females (Destefano, 2001). Additional research is needed in this area to examine issues of potential test bias. Overall, the research evidence supports the reliability and the validity of the PIY scale scores; however, lower reliability estimates reported for the PIY subscale scores suggest these scores should be interpreted with caution (Marchant & Ridenour, 2001).

Youth Self-Report

The Youth Self-Report (YSR; Achenbach & Rescorla, 2001d) is one component of the Achenbach System of Empirically Based Assessment

(ASEBA; Achenbach & Rescorla, 2001a) aimed at assessing competencies and problematic behaviors in adolescents. The YSR is a comprehensive self-report measure intended for adolescents, ages 11 to 18. This latest version is a revision of the popular and widely used 1991 YSR (Achenbach, 1991) and 1987 YSR (Achenbach & Edelbrock, 1987). Under ideal circumstances, the YSR is administered along with the Child Behavior Checklist (CBCL; Achenbach & Rescorla, 2001a) and the Teacher's Report Form (TRF; Achenbach & Rescorla, 2001c) of the ASEBA to acquire multiple raters' perceptions of an adolescent's problematic behaviors and competencies/adaptive functioning. The ASEBA consists of eight syndrome scales (Anxious/Depressed, Withdrawn/Depressed, Somatic Complaints, Social Problems, Thought Problems, Attention Problems, Rule-Breaking Behavior, and Aggressive Behavior). The raw scores from these various syndrome scales are summed together in different combinations to obtain an Internalizing Problems score and an Externalizing Problems score. The ASEBA also has a Total Problems score, computed by summing the raw scores from the Internalizing Problems, Externalizing Problems, Social Problems, Thought Problems, Attention Problems, and Other Problems scales. The Total Problems score provides an overall measure of problematic behavior. In addition, there are two competence scales on the YSR – the Activities and Social scales. The raw scores of these two scales are summed and added together to obtain a Total Competence score, which provides a measure of overall competence. A new feature of the latest YSR is the six DSM-oriented scales (Affective Problems, Anxiety Problems, Somatic Problems, Attention Deficit/Hyperactivity Problems, Oppositional Defiant Problems, and Conduct Problems). These scales consist of items developed to assess problematic behaviors found on the syndrome scales. The YSR protocol requires adolescents to complete demographic information, provide information on competencies in six categories, and respond to open-ended questions regarding strengths and concerns. In addition, the adolescent responds to 112 statements that describe his or her behavior in the past six months. Each statement is rated on a 3-point Likert scale, ranging from 0 (*not true*) to 2 (*very true or often true*). The items on the ASEBA were written at or above a fifth grade reading level. The YSR can typically be completed in 15 to 20 minutes. The measure can be either hand- (provided in detail in the manual's appendix) or computer-scored. If hand-scored, raw scores are summed on the different scales and converted to standard scores (i.e. T-scores) and percentiles (Achenbach & Rescorla, 2001b).

The YSR was standardized on two samples to create norms for the competence and syndrome scales. Representative of the 1999 U.S. population, the standardization sample for the competence scales consisted of 1,057 adolescents, ages 11 to 18. The standardization sample was comprised of 52% males. Ethnic/racial composition of the sample was 60% NonLatino White, 20% African American, 8% Latino, and 11% Mixed or Other. Regional characteristics included adolescents from 40 states and the District of Columbia, with 17% from the Northeast, 19% from the Midwest, 41% from the South, and 23% from the West. Socioeconomic status of the normative sample consisted of 32% upper SES, 53% middle SES, and 16% lower SES. This sample consisted of non-referred adolescents (Achenbach & Rescorla, 2001b).

The standardization sample for the syndrome scales consisted of 1,057 adolescents from the norming sample for the competence scales and 1,494 adolescents who were receiving treatment in inpatient and outpatient facilities. These 2,551 adolescents (1,429 males and 1,122 females) were from 40 states, the District of Columbia, one Australian state, and England. Ethnic/racial composition of this sample was 47% NonLatino White, 23% African descent, 17% Latino, and 13% Mixed or Other. The SES of this normative sample was described as middle class (Achenbach & Rescorla, 2001b).

Evidence supporting the reliability and validity of the ASEBA scores has been found. Internal consistency reliability estimates for the Total Problems, Internalizing and Externalizing Problems, and syndrome scale scores ranged from .71 to .95. For the DSM-oriented scale scores, coefficient alphas ranged from .67 to .83 and for the Total Competence, Activities, and Social scale scores, coefficient alphas ranged from .55 to .75. A sample of 1,938 referred and non-referred individuals were assessed in determining these reliability estimates. Temporal stability coefficients of the YSR scores were examined over an 8-day test-retest interval with a sample of 89 adolescents. Test score stability coefficients ranged from .67 to .89 for the YSR scores. Temporal stability of the YSR scores was also assessed over a 7-month test-retest interval in a sample of 144 adolescents, ages 11 to 14. As one would expect, test score stability coefficients across all scales tended to decrease and ranged from .34 to .63 (Achenbach & Rescorla, 2001b).

Evidence supporting the construct validity of the YSR scores has been reported. A principal component analysis was performed on the responses of the 2,551 adolescents in the norming sample for the YSR syndrome scales, and the analysis produced an eight factor solution. An eight factor solution was also determined to be the best fit for the YSR data drawn from another sample of adolescents using confirmatory factor analysis (Achenbach & Rescorla, 2001b). These findings were comparable to the factor analytic results reported for the 1991 version of the YSR (Achenbach, 1991). Correlations reported between the scores of the YSR syndrome scales and the scores of the adolescent form of the BASC-2 clinical scales support the convergent validity of the YSR scores. Reynolds and Kamphaus (2004b) reported moderate to strong correlations between the scores of conceptually similar scales on the YSR and BASC-2. Correlations were also examined between the YSR scores and the CBCL scores and were found to be moderate (rs = .37 to .60; Achenbach & Rescorla, 2001b). Discriminant analyses were also performed to determine whether the YSR scores could differentiate adolescents who were referred from adolescents who were not referred. Using unweighted combinations of scale scores, the average percentage of correctly classified adolescents ranged from 68% for the syndrome scale scores to 83% for the scores of the competence and problem behavior items combined (Achenbach & Rescorla, 2001b). These findings support the discriminant validity of the YSR scores.

The YSR is an excellent self-report measure that has been extensively studied and well reviewed (Flanagan, 2005; Watson, 2005). Used in conjunction with the CBCL and TRF, the YSR is on a short list of measures able to provide valuable multi-rater information. The psychometric properties have proven to be strong overall throughout the years and the accompanying manual is meticulously written and user friendly. Considering its length in comparison to other structured personality inventories, the YSR is a cost effective measure that provides a global assessment of the behavioral, emotional, and social functioning of adolescents.

Besides comprehensive measures, structured personality inventories may be narrow in scope. Although these measures do not provide a global assessment of children and adolescents' behaviors, they assess specific aspects of individuals' personality and affect. In this section of the book chapter, selected established, newly developed, and updated structured personality inventories narrow in scope will be reviewed.

Beck Depression Inventory-Second Edition

The Beck Depression Inventory-Second Edition (BDI-II; Beck, Steer, & Brown, 1996a) is a 21 item, self-report measure used to assess the severity of depressive symptoms in adolescents and adults, ages 13 and older. The BDI-II's predecessors, the Beck Depression Inventory—Amended (BDI-IA; Beck, Rush, Shaw, & Emery, 1979), and the original Beck Depression Inventory (BDI; Beck, Ward, Mendelson, Mock, & Erbaugh, 1961) have been the most popular and widely used instruments for detecting depression in non-referred populations over the past 35 years. The BDI-II was developed to be consistent with the diagnostic criteria in the most recent edition of the DSM, the DSM-IV (Beck et al., 1996b). A Spanish version of the BDI-II is also available.

Administration of the BDI-II takes five to ten minutes to complete. However, individuals with severe depression or obsessive symptoms may take longer to complete the instrument. Individuals are required to read each statement and select the best statement out of a group of four statements for each item that describes how they have felt over the last two weeks. Items may be read aloud to accommodate non-readers or those with reading difficulties. The response options for each item on the BDI-II are arranged on a 4-point Likert scale, ranging from 0 (symptom is absent) to 3 (symptom is most severe or is most frequent). Item 16, which pertains to sleep patterns, and Item 18, which pertains to appetite changes, both have unique options (i.e. for each statement within the group of four statements, there are two options). Although the BDI-II can be administered by individuals who have received little training, interpretation is reserved for trained professionals (Beck et al., 1996b).

Scoring of the BDI-II involves summing the weights of the 21 items to obtain a Total score. Possible BDI-II Total scores are grouped by levels of severity– 0–13, 14–19, 20–28, and 29–63, which correspond to minimal, mild, moderate, and severe levels of depression, respectively. Cut scores for these ranges were derived by receiver operating characteristic curves (ROC) that differed across four groups of mild, moderate, severe and non-depressed responders. The cut scores were designed to be sensitive to depression while reducing the number of false positives. Researchers in need of a "true" depression score are encouraged to use a raw score of 17 as their cut score. A cut score of 17 was the score in the BDI-II clinical sample that yielded a 93% positive and 17% false positive rate (Beck et al., 1996b).

A college student sample (n = 120) and a psychiatric outpatient sample (n = 500) were used to examine the psychometric properties of the BDI-II. The demographic characteristics reported for these two samples are lacking in detail. The mean age of the student sample was 19.58 years (SD = 1.84) and the mean age of the psychiatric outpatient sample was 37.20 years (SD = 15.91; range 13–86 years). Sixty-three percent of the psychiatric outpatient sample and 56% of the college student sample was female. Racial/ethnic composition of the psychiatric outpatient and college student samples was predominately White (Beck et al., 1996b).

The manual reports on the alpha levels for the BDI-II Total scores for the psychiatric outpatient (α = .92) and college student (α = .93) samples. In addition, corrected item-total correlations for the outpatient and college student samples ranged from .39 to .70 and .27 to .74, respectively. All corrected item-total correlations were statistically significant. Test score stability for the BDI-II scores was established with a subsample of psychiatric outpatients (n = 26) during their first and second therapy sessions, one week apart. A strong test score stability coefficient of .93 was found (Beck et al., 1996b).

Validity of the BDI-II scores was established on several fronts. Support for the content validity of the BDI-II came through the writing of items that captured the diagnostic criteria for depressive disorders in the DSM-IV. New items were added and nearly all items were reworded to reflect the latest criteria. Convergent validity was assessed by comparing the BDI-II scores with the scores of the Beck Hopelessness Scale (BHS; Beck, 1988; r = .68), the Scale for Suicide Ideation (SSI; Beck, Kovacs, & Weissman, 1979; r = .37), the Hamilton Psychiatric Rating Scale for Depression–Revised (HRSD-R; Riskind, Beck, Brown & Steer, 1987; r = .71), and the Hamilton Anxiety Rating Scale-Revised (HARS-R; Hamilton, 1959; r = .47) in psychiatric outpatient samples of various sizes. In contrast, discriminant validity of the BDI-II scores was supported based on the difference between the strong correlation of the BDI-II scores with the HRSD-R scores and the moderate correlation of the BDI-II scores with the HARS-R scores (Beck et al., 1996b).

Results of factor analyses for the responses of the psychiatric outpatient sample and college student sample to the BDI-II items differed across samples. Both factor analyses produced a two-factor solution for the BDI-II items, but the dimensions and the number of items loading on those dimensions were different. In the outpatient sample, the two factors were named Somatic-Affective and Cognitive. Twelve items loaded on the Somatic–Affective dimension while the remaining 9 items loaded on the Cognitive dimension. In the college student sample, the two factors were named Cognitive-Affective and Somatic. Fourteen items loaded on the Cognitive–Affective dimension and five items loaded on the Somatic dimension (Beck et al., 1996b). Independent studies have also reported variations in the BDI-II factor structure (e.g. Buckley, Parker, & Heggie, 2000).

Criticisms of the BDI-II include absence of ROC development procedures in the BDI-II manual, inconsistent findings in the factor structure across populations, and optimal information on the research samples used to examine the psychometric properties of the BDI-II (Farmer, 2001). Farmer's review of the BDI-II highlights the lack of detailed information on the samples in the manual, including missing information on the education level, geographic patterns, and family income of the responders. Strengths of the BDI-II include a strong empirical foundation, innovative methods to determine cut scores (Farmer, 2001), excellent reliability, and ease of administration, scoring, and interpretability. Based on these strengths, the BDI-II remains a popular instrument among many clinicians and researchers.

Beck Youth Inventories-Second Edition

The Beck Youth Inventories-Second Edition (BYI-II; Beck, Beck, Jolly, & Steer, 2005a) is a measure designed to assess socio-emotional functioning in children and adolescents, ages 7 to 18. The BYI-II is composed of five scales or inventories (Beck Depression Inventory for Youth (BDI-Y), Beck Anxiety Inventory for Youth (BAI-Y), Beck Disruptive Behavior Inventory for Youth (BDBI-Y), Beck Self-Concept Inventory for Youth (BSCI-Y), and Beck Anger Inventory for Youth (BANI-Y)) that can be completed independently or in aggregate in the combination booklet. Each scale is composed of 20 items. The items were constructed based on the DSM-IV-TR criteria. Respondents self-report using a 4-point Likert scale, ranging from 0 (*never*) to 3 (*always*) regarding the frequency of various behaviors and feelings experienced. The time to complete the entire BYI-II is 30 to 60 minutes (5 to 10 minutes per scale). Once completed, raw scores for each BYI-II scale are tallied, converted to T-scores, and plotted on a profile (Beck, Beck, Jolly, & Steer, 2005b).

Norming and development of the BYI-II was accomplished in two phases. In the first phase, data were collected from a community sample of youth, ages 7 to 14, and analyzed for the first edition of the Beck Youth Inventories of Emotional and Social Impairment (Beck, Beck, & Jolly, 2001). The second phase focused on obtaining data from a community-based sample of adolescents, ages 15 to 18, and this data and the data from the first edition of the BYI were combined in the second edition. In both phases, data from clinical samples were also collected (Beck et al., 2005b).

The community-based sample of children and adolescents, ages 7 to 14, consisted of 1,100 individuals living in the four major geographic regions of the U.S. The children and adolescents were recruited through churches, community groups, public and private schools, and national mailing lists. For the standardization sample, 800 children and adolescents were selected from the community-based sample, stratified to match the 1999 U. S. Census data by race/ethnicity and parent education level. Age-by-gender norms were developed for the standardization sample based on the analyses of age and gender effects. A special education sample was also identified, comprised of 89 children between the ages of 8 and 12. The clinical sample included 107 children who were receiving outpatient mental health services in a state in the Northeastern region of the U.S. (Beck et al., 2005b).

The community-based sample of adolescents, ages 15 to 18, included 252 adolescents from the four major geographic regions in the U.S. The sample was recruited through advertising, school districts, and professionals who conduct evaluations. For the standardization sample, 200 individuals were selected from the community-based sample to match the 2002 U.S. Census data for age, gender, ethnicity, and parent education level. Adolescents were excluded from the standardization sample if there were any indication they were currently receiving psychiatric services. The clinical sample of adolescents, ages 15 to 18, consisted of 178 individuals (Beck et al., 2005b).

Overall, the reliability and validity of the BYI-II scores are solid. Internal consistency reliability estimates for the scores of the five inventories for the norming sample ranged from .86 to .96. Standard errors of measurement ranged from 2.04 to 3.00 for the norming sample across inventories. Test score stability coefficients based on a sample of 170 children and adolescents ranged from .74 to .93 for the scores of the BYI-II Inventories (Beck et al., 2005b). Principal components factor analysis indicated the presence of an underlying negative affect principal factor, as well as factors for negative self-concept and negative behavior. Convergent and discriminant validity studies for the BYI-II scores were conducted with the scores of the CDI, the RCMAS, the Reynolds Bullying and Victimization Scales for Schools (RBVSS; Reynolds, 2003), the Conners-Wells Scales (CASS:S; Conners, 1997), and the Piers-Harris Children's Self-Concept Scale (PHCSCS; Piers, 2002). Relationships were found among the expected scale scores in the expected directions, supporting convergent and discriminant validity, with stronger relationships for the adolescent sample. Convergent validity for the BDI-Y scores and the scores of the CDI was indicated by a strong validity coefficient of .72 for a sample of 128 children, ages 11 to 14. The BDI-Y scores and the CDI scores were moderately correlated ($r = .67$) in a sample of 26 adolescents. The BAI-Y scores were moderately to strongly correlated with the RCMAS anxiety scores for children and adolescents ($r = .70$; $r = .64$, respectively), while the scores of the RCMAS anxiety scores did not correlate as highly with the BDBI-Y ($r = .21$) and BANI-Y ($r = .36$) scores for adolescents, providing some support for the discriminant validity of some of the BYI-II scale scores. The BAI-Y scores also correlated strongly with the RBVSS Bully Victimization Distress Internalizing scores ($r = .72$) for a sample of 111 children. Moderate to strong correlations ($r = .69$, n = 108 children, and $r = .76$, n = 89 adolescents) between the BDBI-Y scores and the CASS:S Conduct Problems scale scores were found. For adolescents, the BDI-Y scores were most strongly correlated with the RCMAS anxiety scores ($r = .70$; Beck et al., 2005b), suggesting a strong overlap between the two constructs in the area of negative affectivity (Watson & Clark, 1984). The BDBI-Y scores were strongly correlated with the CASS:S Conduct Problems scores for a sample of 108 children, ages 7 to 14 ($r = .69$) and for a sample of 108 adolescents, ages of 12 to 14 ($r = .76$). Moderate to strong correlations between the BANI-Y scores and the CASS:S ADHD Index scores ($r = .73$) and the Hyperactive Impulsive scores ($r = .68$) for children were reported, suggesting that the BANI-Y scores may be sensitive to the externalizing characteristics of ADHD. The BSCI-Y scores were moderately to strongly correlated with the PHCSCS Total scores ($r = .61$ for children and

$r = .77$ for adolescents; Beck et al., 2005b). Group differences were also evaluated using a sample of children receiving special education services and a sample of children presenting for treatment at an outpatient mental health clinic compared to a sample of matched controls. Students receiving special education services scored statistically significantly higher on the BDI-Y, BAI-Y, BDBI-Y, and BANI-Y scales and significantly lower on the BSCI-Y scale than children not identified. For the clinical sample, statistically significant differences between the outpatient sample and the matched controls were found for the scores of three of the five inventories: BSCI-Y, BDBI-Y, and BANI-Y, with the BSCI-Y scores showing the largest differentiation between the groups (Beck et al., 2005b).

Beck and colleagues (2005b) outlined four reasons for evaluators to use the BYI-II over other measures. First, each separate inventory is quite brief, taking only 5 to 10 minutes to complete. It's suggested that children and adolescents may be more compliant in completing one or a combination of these shorter inventories over longer, more traditional self-report scales. Of particular note, the scores of the BANI-Y and BDBI-Y scales, of which few of these types of scales are available, are reliable and valid. The BYI-II covers a broad scope of potential difficulties experienced by youth and adolescents. Additionally, the measures were developed and co-normed with a sample of U.S. youth stratified in accordance with the U.S. Census data. The manual provides extensive validity information for the BYI-II scores. However, Henington (2007) noted that there is a lack of information on item development of the BYI-II. Overall, the BYI-II is a well-calibrated instrument that provides quality information in combination with other measures and methods for evaluations of children and adolescents as well as for research purposes.

Children's Depression Rating Scale-Revised

The Children's Depression Rating Scale—Revised (CDRS-R; Poznanski & Mokros, 1996) is a rating scale based on a 20- to 30-minute semi-structured interview designed to evaluate children, ages 6 to 12, for depression and dysthymia. The CDRS-R addresses 14 different areas of symptomatology (Impaired Schoolwork, Difficulty Having Fun, Social Withdrawal, Sleep Disturbance, Excessive Fatigue, Physical Complaints, Irritability, Excessive Guilt, Low Self-Esteem, Depressed Feelings, Morbid Ideation, Suicidal Ideation, Excessive Weeping, and Appetite Disturbance) and three areas of observable behavior (Depressed Facial Affect, Listless Speech, and Hypoactivity). A clinician provides a rating from 1 to 7 for each symptom and observable behavior. Higher scores indicate more severe symptoms or behaviors. For Sleep Disturbance, Appetite Disturbance, and Listless Speech, a rating from 1 to 5 is used, also based on severity. The raw scores for each symptom or behavior are then summed and converted to a T-score, the CDRS-R Summary score, to provide a standardized score for comparison to the norm group, as well as percentile rank. Besides the child, parents, significant other adults, and peers can also be interviewed regarding the presentation of symptoms by the targeted child (Poznanski & Mokros, 2005).

A nonclinical sample consisting of 223 children and their parents from an urban public school in Chicago, Illinois served as the norming sample. These students were selected using a stratified random sampling procedure, and they participated in a one-time evaluation. However, not all of the children who participated had parents who were interviewed. Only about 50% (n = 109) of the parents also participated in the interviews. Of the 223 children participating, approximately 33.3% were African-American, 27.3% were of other (primarily Hispanic) ethnicity, and 60.6% were White. Mean age of the respondents was approximately 10 years. In contrast, the clinical sample consisted of 78 children recruited from affective disorder clinics at two University medical centers in the Chicago area. Of these 78 children, 64% were male, 35% were Black, 7% were from other (primarily Hispanic) backgrounds, and 58% were White. Sixty of these children were identified as having depression, 90% (n = 54) with a Major Depressive Disorder. Of the remaining 18, 19% (n = 15) were identified as having another psychiatric diagnosis other than depression. Of the 60 children identified as having depression, 46.7% had another comorbid disorder. Mean age of the clinical sample respondents was 10 years (Poznanski & Mokros, 2005).

Three types of reliability (inter-rater, test-retest, and internal consistency) were examined for the clinical and nonclinical samples based on the CDRS-R ratings. Inter-rater reliability for the CDRS-R ratings was .92 for a sample of 25 children. A test score stability coefficient of .80 was reported for the CDRS-R Summary scores based on an intake and 2-week follow-up assessment. A coefficient alpha of .85 was found for the CDRS-R Summary scores in the nonclinical sample consisting of 223 children (Poznanski & Mokros, 2005). These reliability estimates are in the strong to very strong range.

Evidence supporting the validity of the CDRS-R Summary scores has been found. A moderate validity coefficient of .48 was reported between the CDRS-R Summary scores and the Hamilton Rating Scale for Depression (Warren, 1994) Total scores in the clinical sample. The validity of the CDRS-R Summary scores was also examined in relation to the Dexamethasone Suppression Test (DST; Carroll et al., 1981), a measure used to evaluate the biological markers of depression, in the clinical sample. Results of an analysis of variance (ANOVA) indicated significantly higher scores on the CDRS-R Summary scores for children displaying DST results indicative of depression. A contrasted group study was conducted to also evaluate the discriminant validity of the CDRS-R Summary scores using data from two groups of children from the clinical sample, one group of children with major depression or dysthymia (n = 60) and the other group of children diagnosed with other disorders other than depression (n = 18), and the group of children from the nonclinical sample (n = 223). Children in the major depression and dysthymia group scored significantly higher on the CDRS-R Summary scores than those in the other clinical and nonclinical groups, and the nonclinical sample had the lowest mean CDRS-R Summary scores of the three groups. Other evidence supporting the discriminant validity of the CDRS-R Summary scores for the clinical and nonclinical samples is provided in the manual (Poznanski & Mokros, 2005).

The CDRS-R has the advantage of being a revised version of the original Children's Depression Rating Scale (CDRS; Poznanski, Cook, & Carroll, 1979) that has been used in clinical and nonclinical settings for over 20 years. This most recent version of the CDRS has been updated in the following ways: the addition and renaming of symptom areas, revised rating scale anchors, additional interpretive and usage considerations, including development of suggested interview prompts and providing a means for integrating information from multiple informants, and revision of the calculation of the Summary score. It has a flexible method of administration, with emphasis on empathy with the child and fluidity in interviewing, appears to require more extensive training in administration than more traditional interviews or measures. Additionally, reviewers note that the manual is quite dense and could be organized in a more easily understood format (Dowd, 2001). One reviewer noted concerns about the diversity and representation of the sample, completely lacking of children from Asian-American and Native American backgrounds (Stovall, 2001).

Clinical Assessment of Depression

The Clinical Assessment of Depression (CAD; Bracken & Howell, 2004a) is a 50-item, multidimensional, self-report measure designed to assess depression in children, adolescents, and adults, ages 8 to 79. The CAD consists of eight scales — a Total scale, four Symptom scales (Depressed Mood, Anxiety/Worry, Diminished Interest, and Cognitive and Physical Fatigue), three validity scales (Inconsistency, Negative Impression, and Infrequency), and six critical item clusters (Hopelessness, Self-Devaluation, Sleep/Fatigue, Failure, Worry, and Nervousness). The purpose of the validity scales on the CAD is to assist clinicians in assessing the veracity of the rater's self-report, whereas the purpose of the six critical item clusters is to assist clinicians in addressing specific issues in therapy or in taking specific action to help their client (Bracken & Howell, 2004b).

The CAD is a comprehensive measure with application across a large portion of the child, adolescent, and adult life span. The authors of the CAD believe based on clinical practice and the literature in the area of depression that there are more symptoms of depression in common than not common across the life span and thus, they developed a measure (i.e. a single form) to assess depressive symptomatology found across the child, adolescent, and adult life span. However, the measure also assesses those unique features of depression found in specific age groups. The CAD's items were written to reflect the diagnostic criteria found in the DSM-IV-TR, as well as the current literature on depression in children, adolescents, and adults. The CAD's items were written at a third-grade reading level. The CAD is easy to administer and it can be administered on an individual basis or in a group setting. Little training is needed to administer and score the CAD. However, individuals with little training should receive professional supervision. During the administration of the measure, children, adolescents, and adults respond to the CAD items by indicating how they have felt lately. Respondents rate their responses on the CAD on a 4-point Likert scale, ranging from 1 (*strongly disagree*) to 4 (*strongly agree*). The CAD takes approximately 10 minutes to complete. Once completed, the CAD can be hand scored or computer scored and interpreted. Interpretation of the CAD scores and profiles involves a five-step process articulated in the manual and should be done by qualified professionals (Bracken & Howell, 2004b).

The standardization sample for the CAD consists of 1,900 individuals, 300 children (150 females and 150 males), ages 8 to 11, 400 adolescents (200 females and 200 males), ages 12 to 17, 400 older adolescents/young adults (200 females and 200 males), ages 18 to 25, and 800 young, middle, and older adults (400 females and 400 males), ages 26 to 79. These demographic characteristics of the standardization sample for the CAD matched closely the U.S. population demographics. Of those individuals, ages 18 to 79 in the standardization sample, 1.3% had eight or fewer years of education, 4.3% had 9 to 11 years of schooling, 18.9% had 12 years of education, 37.1% had 13 to 15 years of schooling, and 38.4% had more than 16 years of education. Based on these percentages, Bracken and Howell (2004b) noted that the standardization sample was slightly more highly educated than the U.S. population. The racial/ethnic composition of the sample was 70.2% Caucasian, 12.9% African American, 8.3% Hispanic, and 8.6% Other. The racial/ethnic composition of the standardization sample was comparable to the U.S. population. The standardization sample was recruited from 22 states in the U.S., 44% from the Midwest, 8.7% from the Northeast, 31.4% from the South, and 15.5% from the West. According to the authors of the CAD, the Midwest was oversampled and the Northeast was undersampled (Bracken & Howell, 2004b).

Overall, the reliability and validity of the CAD scores are solid. Internal consistency reliability estimates are reported for the standardization sample by age group, gender, and race/ethnicity. Coefficient alphas for the CAD Total scale scores and the four Symptom scale scores for the different groups ranged from .96 to .98 and from .78 to .96, respectively. Internal consistency reliability for the scores of the Total scale and the four Symptom scales for a clinical sample of 99 children were comparable to the coefficient alphas reported for the standardization sample and ranged from .85 to .98. The consistency of the CAD scores was also examined over a 7–36 day test-retest period for children and adolescents. Corrected test score stability coefficients for a sample of 40 children and adolescents, ages 8 to 18, ranged from .64 to .81 for the Total scale scores and the four Symptom scale scores, with only one test score stability coefficient falling below .70 (i.e. the Diminished Interest scale scores; Bracken & Howell, 2004b). Overall, the majority of these reliability estimates are in the strong to very strong range.

Evidence supporting the validity of the CAD scores was examined through content analysis, convergent validity studies, contrasted group studies, and factor analyses (Bracken & Howell, 2004b). Bracken and Howell note that the content validity of the CAD was ensured with the inclusion of items representing symptoms of depression supported in the literature and the DSM-IV-TR. Examination of the mean scores of a combined clinical sample of 30 children and adolescents, ages 8 to 18 and 37 adults, ages 19 to 79, and a non-clinical control sample of 66 children and adolescents, and 123 adults of comparable ages revealed that the clinical subsamples had mean CAD scores above the normative mean and the clinical control subsamples had mean CAD scores below the normative mean in all cases except two. These findings support the discriminant validity of the CAD scores. Convergent validity of the CAD scores was supported in studies conducted with scores of measures external to the test. Bowers (2004) administered the CAD and the BDI-II to 119 adolescents and reported moderate to strong validity coefficients (rs = .64 to .77) between the scores of the two measures. Likewise, Tinsley (2004) administered the CAD to 121 adolescents along with the Reynolds Adolescent Depression Scale (RADS; Reynolds, 1986) and found strong validity coefficients (rs = .71 to .88) between the scores of the two measures. Confirmatory factor analyses were also performed. The normative sample was divided into two age groups, ages 8 to 17 and 18 to 79, to form a child/adolescent and adult analysis groups. In addition, the entire normative sample served as a third analysis group. One-, two-, and four-factor models were compared and contrasted using the data. Results of the confirmatory factor analyses indicated that the four-factor model provided the best fit for the data for all groups. The four factors were Depressed Mood, Anxiety/Worry, Diminished Interest, and Cognitive and Physical Fatigue (Bracken & Howell, 2004b).

The CAD is a promising relatively brief, multidimensional measure used to assess depressive symptoms in children, adolescents, and adults. Several strengths of the CAD include the use of a single measure to assess depressive symptoms across the life span, the inclusion of validity scales for clinical interpretation, the ease of administration and scoring of the measure, a user-friendly manual, a large, fairly representative standardization sample, and good psychometric properties overall. In contrast, some weaknesses or limitations of the measure include limited description of the clinical normative sample, a low test score stability coefficient for the Diminished Interest scale scores in the child/adolescent sample, and possible breadth of coverage of depressive symptoms on the measure in comparison to some existing measures of depression. Furthermore, additional research is needed with the CAD to examine the reliability and validity of its scores and its clinical utility in treatment planning and progress monitoring (Kavan, 2007).

Fear Survey Schedule for Children—Revised

The Fear Survey Schedule for Children—Revised (FSSC-R; Ollendick, 1983) is a self-report measure designed to assess several types of fears and anxieties in children and adolescents. The FSSC-R was created as a revision of Scherer and Nakamura's (1968) Fear Survey Schedule for Children (FSS-FC), in an attempt to increase the scale's utility among younger children. The FSSC-R scale contains 80 items assessing children's fears and anxieties, to which raters respond using a 3-point Likert scale, ranging from 1 (*none*) to 3 (*a lot*). The normative sample consists of 126 children, ages 7 to 18 (Ollendick, Matson, & Helsel, 1985). In addition, data were gathered from 25 children, ages 7 to 12, who had received referrals for treatment of school phobia. These individuals make up the clinical sample of the FSSC-R (Ollendick, 1983).

Using a sample of 217 children, ages 8–11, Ollendick (1983) reported very strong internal consistency reliability for the FSCC-R scores, ranging from .92 to .95. In an independent study conducted by Muris, Merckelbach, Ollendick, King, and Bogie (2002), the FSSC-R scores demonstrated moderate to very strong internal consistency reliability across the Total scale ($\alpha = .96$) and five subscales – Fear of Failure and Criticism ($\alpha = .91$), Fear of the Unknown ($\alpha = .87$), Fear of Animals/Minor Injuries ($\alpha = .85$), Fear of Danger and Death ($\alpha = .89$), and Medical Fears ($\alpha = .65$). With regard to test score stability, Ollendick (1983) reported reliability estimates ranging from .81 to .89 over a 1-week test-retest interval and .55 to .62 over a 3-month test-retest interval.

A factor analysis of 217 children's responses on the FSSC-R supported a five-factor structure. The five factors are: Fear of Failure and Criticism, Fear of the Unknown, Fear of Injury and Small Animals, Fear of Danger and Death, and Medical Fears (Ollendick, 1983). These factors are similar to the factors found on Scherer and Nakamura's (1968) original FSS-FC scale and provide support for the construct validity of the FSCC-R scores. The factor structure of the FSSC-R has proven to be relatively stable across gender, age, and nationality among American and Australian youth (Ollendick, King, & Frary, 1989).

In addition, researchers have examined the convergent and discriminant validity of the FSSC-R scores. Ollendick (1983) reported moderate correlations ($rs = .32$ to $.56$) between the FSSC-R scores and the scores of the State-Trait Anxiety Inventory for Children (STAI-C; Spielberger, 1973)—Trait Scale, supporting the convergent validity of the FSSC-R scores. In contrast, Ollendick reported negative, moderate to strong validity coefficients between the FSCC-R scores and scores of a measure of self-esteem ($rs = -.62 - -.79$) and between the FSSC-R scores and the scores of a measure of internal locus of control ($rs = -.42 - -.74$) among female participants, providing support for the discriminant validity of the FSCC-R scores. Although the FSSC-R scores also demonstrated negative correlations with the scores of these two measures among male participants, they were not significant. Ollendick also reported the results of a contrasted group study in which children with school phobia had significantly higher scores on the FSSC-R than children without phobias. In contrast, Last, Francis, and Strauss (1989) reported mixed results in their contrasted group study with children with different types of anxiety disorders. Specifically, the FSSC-R scores appeared unable to detect differences in mean scale and subscale scores among children with different types of anxiety disorders. However, qualitative analysis of the data indicated that children with different types of anxiety disorders may be differentiated based on the number of intense fears reported.

The FSSC-R has been translated by researchers into several different languages to allow for clinical and research use with culturally and linguistically diverse populations, including Swedish (Svensson & Ost, 1999), Dutch (Bokhorst, Westernberg, Oosterlaan, & Heyne, 2008), Greek (Mellon, Koliadis, & Paraskevopoulos, 2004), Turkish (Erol, 1995), and Spanish-speaking children (Valiente, Sandin, Chorot, & Tabar, 2002). In addition, several new measures have been designed based on the FSSC-R, to allow its use in ethnically and culturally diverse populations. The Fear Survey Schedule for Children and Adolescents-II (FSSC-II; Gullone & King, 1992) is a 75-item self-report measure that includes updated item content, and it was normed on a sample of 918 Australian children and adolescents, ages 7 to 18. Gullone and King examined the technical adequacy of the measure, and the results suggest the measure has good psychometric properties. Gullone and King's FSSC-II was adapted for use with children in the U.S. (Burnham, 2005; Burnham & Gullone, 1997). The resulting American Fear Survey Schedule for Children (FSSC-AM; Burnham, 2005) contains 98 items and was normed on 720 U.S. children, ages 7 to 18. The psychometric properties reported for the FSSC-AM are similar to those of the FSSC-II (Burnham, 2005). Finally, Shore and Rapport (1998) developed a third revision of the FSSC-R, the 84-item Fear Survey Schedule for Children–Hawaii (FSSC-HI). The FSSC-HI's culturally diverse normative group includes 385 Hawaiian children, ages 7 to 16. Similar to the FSSC-R, the psychometric properties of the FSSC-HI are good. However, factor analysis of the FSSC-HI produced a seven-factor structure rather than the five-factor structure reported for the FSSC-R, FSSC-II (Gullone & King, 1992), and FSSC-AM (Burnham, 2005).

The FSSC-R is a useful instrument for both research and clinical purposes. Unlike other measures of general anxiety, the FSSC-R appears able to tap anxiety associated with fears and phobias found in children. In addition, qualitative data provided by the FSSC-R (i.e., numbers of intense fears) may be especially helpful in identifying children with or at risk for different types of anxiety disorders. An additional strength of the FSSC-R is its versatility, as it has been translated into other languages and normed on diverse populations. However, the multiple variations of the Fear Survey Schedule for Children may also represent a drawback. Specifically, the multiple variations of the scale may make it difficult for researchers and clinicians to identify the most appropriate instrument and normative data for use with various research and clinical populations. A review of the literature indicates that the FSSC-R, FSSC-II, FSSC-AM, and FSSC-HI each continue to be used in current research, and it is unclear what makes one scale more suitable for use than another (e.g. each instrument has updated norms, solid psychometric properties, and has been used successfully with diverse populations).

Internalizing Symptoms Scale for Children

The Internalizing Symptoms Scale for Children (ISSC, Merrell & Walters, 1998) is a 48-item, self-report measure for children in grades 3 through 6, ages 8 to 12. The instrument is used to assess children's perceptions of internalizing symptoms (i.e. depression, anxiety, social withdrawal, and somatic problems) and positive and negative affect. The ISSC was developed based on the behavioral dimension approach, an innovative, alternative approach, for classifying behavioral, social, and emotional problems. In this approach, externalizing and internalizing problems are viewed as representing large general behavioral clusters that account for many of the problems children experience. The ISSC assesses one of those general behavioral clusters (i.e. internalizing problems). The ISSC can be administered on an individual basis or in a group setting. Children may complete the ISSC independently or have the items read aloud to them by a test administrator. Children respond to the items on the ISSC using a 4-point Likert scale to indicate how "true" the items are for them: never true, hardly ever true, sometimes true, and often true. The ISSC takes approximately 10 to 15 minutes to complete. Scoring of the ISSC results in three scores: the Total score, the Negative Affect/General Distress score, and the Positive Affect score. The Positive Affect items are reverse scored, thus higher scores are associated with greater levels of distress. The Total, Negative Affect/General Distress, and Positive Affect raw scores are converted to percentile ranks, standard deviations, and standard scores (Merrell, 2008). Qualified professionals should only interpret the ISSC scores, using a four-step process articulated in the manual (Christopher, 2001).

The ISSC normative sample consisted of 2,149 students (1,109 boys and 1,040 girls), ages 8 to 13, in grades 3 through 6. The students were from several states, representing the four geographic regions of the U.S. The sample included a large percentage of children with learning disabilities. There are differing opinions as to whether or not the normative sample adequately represents the racial/ethnic composition of the general U.S. population as well as the distribution of students' special education status (Christopher, 2001a; & Merrell, 2008).

Extensive information is presented in the manual and literature on the reliability and validity of the ISCC scores. Internal consistency reliability for the ISCC Total scores (α = .91), Negative Affect/General Distress scores (α = .90), and Positive Affect scores (α = .86) were in the strong to very strong range (Merrell, 2008). Michael and Merrell (1998) reported on the test score stability of the ISSC scores over a 2-week, 4-week, and 12-week test-retest interval. For the ISCC Total scores, test score stability coefficients were .84, .76, and .74 over a 2-, 4-, and 12-week test-retest period. The test score stability coefficients for the Negative Affect/General Distress scores and the Positive Affect scores were .81, .73, and .70 and .79, .79, and .72 over a 2-, 4-, and 12-week test-retest interval, respectively. Michael and Merrell reported a general attenuation in symptom endorsement after the first administration of the ISSC.

Evidence supporting the construct validity of the ISSC scores has been found (Merrell, Crowley, & Walters, 1997). Merrell and colleagues used exploratory and confirmatory factor analytic procedures to examine the factor structure of the ISSC. Results of the factor analyses indicated that a two-factor structure provided the best fit for the data. The two factors were named Negative Affect/General Distress and Positive Affect.

Studies investigating the convergent and discriminant validity of the ISSC scores with scores of other measures have been conducted. Moderate to strong correlations with the RCMAS anxiety subscale scores (rs = .36 to .68) and the Reynolds Child Depression Scale (RCDS; W. M. Reynolds, 1989) scores (rs = .68 to .78; Crowley & Merrell, 2000), and strong correlations with the YSR Internalizing scale scores (rs = .71 to .86; Merrell, Anderson, & Michael, 1997) have been found, lending support to the convergent validity of the ISSC scores. In contrast, negligible correlations between the ISSC scores and the RCMAS Lie scale scores (rs = .08-.10), and negative, negligible to moderate correlations between the ISSC scores and the Social Skills Rating Scale Social subdomain scores (rs = -.51 to -.14; Crowley & Merrell, 2000) have been reported, supporting the discriminant validity of the ISSC scores. Sanders (1996) reported additional evidence of discriminant validity of the ISSC scores in differentiating students with emotional disturbance from students in regular education programs.

The ISSC has been shown to be a good measure for clinical and research purposes, with evidence supporting the reliability and validity of its scores (Merrell, 2008). The ease of administration and scoring of the ISSC make it a useful and attractive instrument to use in a variety of settings, including the schools. The ISSC is unique in that it was designed to assess a broad range of internalizing symptoms and positive and negative affect in the child population rather than assessing symptoms associated with specific disorders. However because the ISSC is a broad assessment tool, it should be used as a screening tool and used in conjunction with other measures for diagnostic purposes

(Christopher, 2001a). At the present time, the ISSC is being updated.

Multidimensional Anxiety Scale for Children

The Multidimensional Anxiety Scale for Children (MASC; March, Parker, Sullivan, Stallings, & Conners, 1997) is one of the most commonly used measures of childhood anxiety. The MASC is a 39 item, self-report measure designed for use with children and adolescents, ages 8 to 19. The MASC consists of four scales (Physical Harm, Harm Avoidance, Social Anxiety, and Panic/Separation Anxiety) and six subscales (Tense, Somatic, Perfectionism, Anxious Coping, Humiliation Fears, and Performance Fears). In addition, a Total Anxiety scale (consisting of all 39 items), an Anxiety Disorders Index (reflecting diagnostic criteria from the DSM-IV-TR), and a validity scale (assessing response inconsistency) are also available. Children and adolescents respond to the items on the MASC by indicating how "true" the items are for them using a 4-point Likert scale, ranging from 0 (never) to 3 (often). The MASC is written at a fourth grade reading level, and can be completed in approximately 15 minutes (Christopher, 2001b).

The MASC was normed on 2,698 children and adolescents. The norming sample included children of several racial/ethnic backgrounds: 53.5% Caucasian, 39.2% African American, .7% Hispanic/Latin American, 1.4% Asian American, 2.4% Native American, and 3% classified as Other. Hispanics and Asian Americans were underrepresented in the MASC norming sample and African Americans were overrepresented in the norming sample (Christopher, 2001b).

According to the test developers, moderate to very strong internal consistency reliability estimates (αs = .60 –.90) for the MASC scale scores were found. However, some MASC subscale scores, such as Perfectionism, Performance Fears, and Anxious Coping, had much lower internal consistency reliability estimates (αs = .62, .60, and .66, respectively; March et al., 1997), indicating that the items on certain subscales may not be homogenous in content. This may be due to the wide range of symptoms and characteristics inherent in some anxiety disorders, but it may also indicate a need for caution when interpreting the assessment results. March, Sullivan, and Parker (1999) examined the test score stability of the MASC scores among a community sample of 142 school children and reported strong to very strong test score stability coefficients over a 3-week test-retest interval (rs = .71 –.92).

During the development of the MASC, two confirmatory factor analyses were conducted. The results of the two confirmatory factor analyses indicated that a four-factor structure provided the best fit for the data for the norming sample of 2, 698 children and adolescents as well as a clinical sample of 390 individuals. The four factors are Physical Anxiety, Harm Avoidance, Social Anxiety, and Panic/Separation Anxiety (March et al., 1997). Further analyses identified six sub-factors, including Tense, Somatic, Perfectionism, Anxious Coping, Humiliation Fears, and Performance Fears. Independent studies have replicated the four-factor structure of the MASC among various clinical, racial, and ethnic groups (Baldwin & Dadds, 2007; Fincham et al., 2008; March, Conners, et al., 1999; Olason, Sighvatsson, & Smari, 2004; Rynn et al., 2006). In contrast, research involving African American adolescents did not support the four-factor structure, and instead supported a three-factor structure (Kingery, Ginsburg, & Burstein, 2009). These results suggest that the MASC factor structure may not be invariant across certain racial/ethnic groups.

Evidence supporting the convergent and discriminant validity of the MASC scores has been examined in relation to the scores of measures external to the test. March and colleagues (1997) reported that studies have compared the MASC scores with scores of other measures of anxiety, depression, and disruptive behaviors, with higher correlations found between the MASC scores and scores of other measures of anxiety overall and lower correlations reported between the MASC scores and the scores of measures of depression and disruptive behaviors. Furthermore, March and Sullivan (1999) conducted a contrasted group study with anxious children, non-anxious children, and children with other psychiatric disorders and found that the MASC scores were able to differentiate between children who were anxious and children who were non-anxious or who had other psychiatric disorders.

Limitations of the MASC include underrepresentation of Hispanic/Latino and Asian-American children and over-representation of African American children in the norming sample. The MASC scores demonstrate adequate reliability and validity in some areas, but exhibit low internal consistency reliability estimates for some of the MASC subscale scores, suggesting the need to interpret the MASC scores with caution. In addition, although the MASC scores demonstrate good discriminant validity, more data are needed to examine differences in the MASC scores among children

with different types of anxiety disorders (rather than simply differentiating between children with and without anxiety disorders). Furthermore, with the emergence of a three-factor structure in a sample of African American adolescents, the MASC scores may need to be interpreted with caution with certain racial/ethnic groups of children and adolescents.

Revised Children's Manifest Anxiety Scale-Second Edition

The Revised Children's Manifest Anxiety Scale-Second Edition (RCMAS-2; C. R. Reynolds & Richmond, 2008a) is a 49-item, self-report measure used to assess anxiety symptoms in children and adolescents, ages 6 to 19. Written for children and adolescents at a second-grade reading level, individuals respond to the items by simply circling "yes" or "no" to each statement. The RCMAS-2 is comprised of three anxiety subscales (Physiological Anxiety, Social Anxiety, and Worry), a Total Anxiety scale, and two validity indexes (Inconsistent Responding and Defensiveness). The Total Anxiety score is obtained by summing the raw scores from the three anxiety subscales and provides an overall measure of chronic, manifest anxiety. The RCMAS-2 can be administered on an individual basis or in groups, and the time to complete the measure is 10 to 15 minutes (C. R. Reynolds & Richmond, 2008b).

New additions to the RCMAS-2 from the original version of the RCMAS include the Inconsistency index and a Performance Anxiety scale. The Inconsistency index consists of nine pairs of items, eight of which are usually endorsed by the respondent in a similar manner and one pair of items endorsed in a dissimilar manner. The Inconsistency score indicates the number of incongruent response pairs. A high Inconsistency score may suggest careless responding, unfavorable testing conditions, or a reading barrier. The Performance Anxiety scale measures anxiety in performance situations. In contrast to the other scales and subscales, the Performance Anxiety scale does not provide a standard score. If the majority of the items are endorsed on this scale, follow-up assessment is encouraged. High scores on the Performance Anxiety scale may indicate anxiety that hinders academic or test performance. In the latest version of the RCMAS, the Social Anxiety subscale has replaced the Social Concerns/Concentration subscale and it assesses anxiety in social and performance situations. The new Social Anxiety subscale includes six items from the original RCMAS Social Concerns/Concentration subscale and six new items. Another new feature found on the RCMAS-2 is the Short Form Total Anxiety scale comprised of the first 10 items on the RCMAS-2. This scale provides a brief measure of chronic, manifest anxiety (C. R. Reynolds & Richmond, 2008b).

The RCMAS-2 standardization sample, which consists of 2,368 individuals, came from the full reference sample of over 3,000 children and adolescents. Demographic characteristics of the standardization sample are fairly representative of the U.S. population in 2000. The standardization sample includes roughly equal numbers of males and females (1,201 females and 1,185 males) and it consists of individuals from all major regions of the U.S. Ethnic/racial composition of the standardization sample includes 3.5% Asian, 14.8% Black, 17.1% Hispanic, 1.0% Native American, 61.5% White, and 1.9% Other. Parents' educational level is also reported and is fairly consistent with the educational level of the U.S. adult population in 2000. The RCMAS-2 also includes a clinical sample of 341 children and adolescents with Attention Deficit Disorders, Autism Spectrum Disorders, Anxiety disorders, Depression, Oppositional Defiant Disorders, and Conduct Disorders (C. R. Reynolds & Richmond, 2008b).

The strong correlations between the scores of the RCMAS and RCMAS-2 scales and subscales may portend to the psychometric properties of the RCMAS-2. Correlations between the scores of similar dimensions on the RCMAS and RCMAS-2 ranged from .88 to .96. The internal consistency reliability estimates for the RCMAS-2 scores ranged from .75 to .92 and test score stability coefficients over a one-week test-retest interval ranged from .64 to .76. Test score stability coefficient over the same one-week test-retest interval for the Short Form Total Anxiety scale scores was .54 (C. R. Reynolds & Richmond, 2008b). Overall, the test score stability coefficients are not strong, but the magnitude of these correlations may be due to the small sample size (n = 100) used to assess the consistency of the RCMAS-2 scores over time. Additional research with larger samples is needed in the future to explore the test score stability of the RCMAS-2 scores across different test-retest intervals.

Evidence supporting the validity of the RCMAS-2 scores is limited and additional research is needed. However, an exploratory factor analysis of the responses of the individuals in the full reference sample to the RCMAS-2 items produced a five-factor structure (C. R. Reynolds & Richmond, 2008b). The five factors include three anxiety factors (Physiological Anxiety, Social Anxiety, and Worry)

and two Defensiveness factors. The RCMAS-2 factor structure is similar to the RCMAS factor structure reported in the RCMAS manual in which the Lie factor split into two factors (C. R. Reynolds & Richmond, 1985). The three anxiety factors on the RCMAS-2 are comparable to the three anxiety factors found on the RCMAS (C. R. Reynolds & Richmond, 1979). A three-factor structure of anxiety has been consistently reported in the literature, not only for the RCMAS (e.g. Paget & C. R. Reynolds, 1984; C. R. Reynolds & Richmond, 1979; Scholwinski & C. R. Reynolds, 1985), but its predecessor the Children's Manifest Anxiety Scale (CMAS; Castaneda, McCandless, & Palermo, 1956; Finch, Kendall, & Montgomery, 1974).

The RCMAS-2 scores were further evaluated by convergent and discriminant validity comparisons with the scores of three separate measures: the Children's Measure of Obsessive-Compulsive Symptoms (CMOCS; C. R. Reynolds & Livingston, 2010, the Children's Depression Inventory-Short Form (CDI-Short Form; Kovacs & Multi-Health Systems, 2003), and the parent and teacher forms of the Conners' Rating Scales (CRS; Conners, 1989). The CMOCS scores correlated the highest with the RCMAS-2 Total Anxiety scale scores and the scores of conceptually similar subscales of the RCMAS-2 among 2,550 children and adolescents from the reference sample. The CDI-Short form scores were moderately correlated (rs = .45 to .68) with the RCMAS-2 anxiety scores in a sample of children with ADD (C. R. Reynolds & Richmond, 2008b). Moderate correlations were expected as the constructs of depression and anxiety overlap in the area of negative affectivity (Watson & Clark, 1984). In contrast, the correlations between the scores of the Conners' Parent and Teacher rating forms and the scores of the RCMAS-2 anxiety scale and subscales in the same sample of children with ADD ranged from -.37 to .32, supporting the discriminant validity of the RCMAS-2 scores (C. R. Reynolds & Richmond, 2008b). Finally, evidence supporting the discriminant validity of the scores of the RCMAS-2 comes from comparisons of children diagnosed with various clinical disorders and children in the standardization sample. Children with anxiety disorders had higher mean raw scores on the RCMAS-2 anxiety scale and subscales than the children in the standardization sample, and the children in the standardization sample had higher mean raw scores on the RCMAS-2 anxiety scale and subscales than children with externalizing disorders (C. R. Reynolds & Richmond, 2008b).

The RCMAS-2 provides encouraging evidence of improvement from the previous version of the measure. The standardization sample is exemplary and the manual provides excellent information regarding administration and interpretation. However, in some instances, the psychometric properties of the RCMAS-2 could be stronger, especially with regards to the test score stability coefficients. Additional research with larger samples of children and adolescents is needed to address the stability of the RCMAS-2 over time. Furthermore, replication of the factor structure of the RCMAS-2 is needed with large independent samples. Considering its brevity, the RCMAS-2 is a good measure, with the Total Anxiety scale scores providing the most sensitive and accurate indication of elevated levels of anxiety in children and adolescents.

Reynolds Adolescent Depression Scale-Second Edition

A self-report measure of depressive symptoms, the Reynolds Adolescent Depression Scale-Second Edition (RADS-2; W. M. Reynolds, 2002a), is the most recent iteration of the original 1986 Reynolds Adolescent Depression Scale (RADS; W. M. Reynolds, 1986). As a measure of adolescent depression, the RADS-2 is age inclusive, allowing administration among individuals, ages 11 to 20. The design of the 30 item RADS-2 is based upon converging depressive symptomatology across a number of formalized diagnostic paradigms (i.e. the DSM-IV, 1994; and the International Classification of Diseases-Tenth Edition, ICD-10; World Health Organization, 1992). Though based upon conceptual nosology of depressive symptoms, the RADS-2 is a measure that assesses the severity of depressive symptoms and should not be used as a diagnostic tool. Yet as a measure of symptom severity, the measure taps the following domains: Dysphoric Mood, Anhedonia/Negative Affect, Negative Self-Evaluation, and Somatic Complaints. In addition, the RADS-2 includes a Depression Total Scale. The RADS-2 is designed for use in individual or group settings. Respondents choose from one of the four available response options (*almost never, hardly ever, sometimes,* or *most of the time*) to describe the frequency of occurrence of depressive symptoms. Completing the RADS-2 requires approximately five minutes for most adolescents, though those who have difficulty reading may require additional time. However, most respondents will have little or no difficulty completing this measure, as the RADS-2 was written at a third grade reading level (W. M. Reynolds, 2002b).

The school-based restandardization sample of the RADS-2 was drawn from a sample of 9,052 adolescents from seven states and the Canadian province of British Columbia. The regional sampling method included states from the Eastern seaboard, the Midwest, and the Northwest. Test developers reduced this total sample to 3,300 participants (the school-based restandardization sample) using a stratified sampling procedure based on the 2000 U.S. Census to reflect the then current ethnic population rates. The three age groups described in the RADS-2 manual include 11 to 13, 14 to 16, and 17 to 20 year olds. Each of these three groups comprises 1,100 participants and contains an equal number of male and female adolescents (W. M. Reynolds, 2002b).

Reliability studies revealed strong to very strong reliability coefficients for the RADS-2 scores. Internal consistency reliability estimates for the RADS-2 Depression Total scores ranged from .91 to .96. Coefficient alphas for the RADS-2 four subscale scores ranged from .78 to .92. Test score stability coefficients for the RADS-2 Depression Total scale scores over a two-week test-retest interval ranged from .85 to .89. Temporal stability coefficients for the RADS-2 four subscale scores over the same test-retest period ranged from .77 to .85 (W. M. Reynolds, 2002b).

The RADS-2 manual provides extensive validity evidence for the scores of the RADS-2 and the original RADS. W. M. Reynolds (2002b) reported the results of a factor analysis of the responses of the total school sample to the RADS-2 items, producing a four-factor structure. The four factors were named Dysphoric Mood, Anhedonia/Negative Affect, Negative Self-Evaluation, and Somatic Complaints. The strong factor scores and organization of the items in the factor analysis provided additional nosological evidence supporting the use of the RADS-2 as a measure of depression. Strong evidence was also found for the convergent validity of the RADS-2 Depression Total scale scores. The RADS-2 Depression Total scale scores were compared to the scores of a number of other scales and interviews measuring psychological distress, including the Hamilton Depression Rating Scale (Hamilton, 1960) interview ($r = .82$), the MMPI Depression scale ($r = .78$), and the APS Major Depression ($r = .76$) and Dysthymic Disorder ($r = .74$) scales. In contrast, the RADS-2 scores were compared to scores of academic achievement and social desirability, and negligible to small validity coefficients of -.25 to .11 were reported (W. M. Reynolds, (2002b), lending support to the discriminant validity of the RADS-2 scores. Furthermore, the results of a study conducted by the author of the measure clearly demonstrated the clinical efficacy of the RADS-2 Depression Total scores in a group of 214 adolescents, 107 individuals with a primary diagnosis of a Major Depressive Disorder and a matched group of 107 non-referred individuals. The author considered several cutoff scores to differentiate the two groups. Ultimately, a RADS-2 Depression Total T score of 61 was selected and produced a hit rate of 88%, and a specificity and sensitivity level of 84% and 92%, respectively (Carlson, 2005).

The RADS-2 is an exemplary measure and serves as an excellent model for test developers to follow in designing future screening instruments to assess symptom severity in the adolescent population. The RADS-2 has many strengths including its brevity, efficient administration and scoring procedures, a clear and concise manual containing information and caveats about the scale's use and interpretation, a strong norming sample, and well-documented evidence in support of the RADS-2 psychometric properties and few, if any weaknesses or limitations. The RADS-2 is an excellent addition to the group of narrow-band instruments designed specifically to assess certain aspects of an adolescent's affect.

Reynolds Child Depression Scale-2nd Edition

The Reynolds Child Depression Scale-2nd Edition (RCDS-2; W. M. Reynolds, 2010a) is a brief paper-and-pencil measure used to assess depressive symptomatology in children. The RCDS-2 is suitable for children, ages 7 to 13, in grades 2 through 6 (W. M. Reynolds, 2010b). The items on the RCDS-2 consists of all 30 items found on the original RCDS and assesses the severity of a range of depressive symptoms, such as cognitive, vegetative, somatic and social-interpersonal symptoms. Children respond to 29 of the 30 items using a 4-point Likert scale, ranging from 1 (almost never) to 4 (all of the time). The other item consists of five smiley-type faces, with a very sad and a very happy smiley face serving as anchors. Children select the face that best represents how they have felt during the past two weeks. Seven of the 30 RCDS-2 items are reverse scored to provide a check for inconsistent responding. There are also

seven critical items on the RCDS-2 that discriminate between children who are depressed and not depressed. Items on the RCDS-2 were written at the second-grade level. However, for children in grades 2, 3 and 4, as well as children with learning difficulties, the RCDS-2 should be administered verbally. The RCDS-2 is suitable for individual and group administration and takes approximately 10 minutes to complete. Scoring of the RCDS-2 involves the use of built-in scoring keys and simply summing the raw scores of the items to obtain a Total raw score. A standard score and percentile rank can also be derived. Although the RCDS-2 does not provide for a formal diagnosis of depression, an empirically tested cutoff score (i.e. a T score of 65) is available to offer an indication of clinically relevant levels of depression (W. M Reynolds, 2010b).

The RCDS-2 also comes with a shortened version, the Reynolds Child Depression Scale—2nd Edition: Short Form (RCDS-2:SF; W. M. Reynolds, 2010c). Similar to the RCDS-2, the RCDS-2:SF assesses the severity of depressive symptomatology in children between the ages of 7 and 13 and in grades 2 through 6. The RCDS-2:SF, which takes approximately 2 to 3 minutes to complete, is billed as a quick screener for childhood depressive symptomatology. The RCDS-2:SF requires a second-grade reading level to complete. However, it is permissible for children with reading difficulties to be administered this measure verbally. The 11 items on the RCDS-2:SF were selected from the 30-item RCDS-2. The response format is similar to the RCDS-2, with children responding to 10 of the 11 items using a 4-point Likert scale, with 1 (almost never) and 4 (all the time) serving as anchors. Children respond to the last question by circling one of the five smiley-type faces, with a very sad face and a very happy face serving as anchors. Four items on the RCDS-2:SF were identified as critical items that discriminate between children who are depressed and not depressed. Two items on the RCDS-2:SF were reverse scored to reduce response pattern bias. A Total raw score (including a standard score and percentile rank) is derived by summing the raw scores for each item. This Total raw score is then compared with an associated cutoff score (i.e. a T score of 62) to identify children who might be exhibiting clinically significant levels of depressive symptomatology. Despite this metric, the RCDS-2:SF is emphasized as not being a diagnostic tool for depressive symptoms (W. M. Reynolds, 2010b).

The standardization sample for the RCDS-2 and RCDS-2:SF consists of 1,100 children (550 boys and 550 girls) between the ages of 6 and 13 (with 99% of the children between 7 and 12 years of age) and in grades 2 through 6. The sample approximates the 2007 U.S. Census in both gender and ethnic backgrounds. Approximately 43% of the standardization sample consists of children from different ethnic minority backgrounds (W. M. Reynolds, 2010b).

Studies on the reliability and validity of the RCDS-2 scores have been conducted. The internal consistency reliability estimates for the RCDS-2 Total scores for the standardization sample was .90. Coefficient alphas were also reported for the RCDS-2 Total scores in the standardization sample for children by gender (α = .89 for boys and α = .91 for girls), grade level (αs = .85 to .92 for grades 2 through 6) and ethnicity (αs = .87 to .93; W. M. Reynolds, 2010b). These internal consistency reliability estimates are in the strong to very strong range. To our knowledge, there is no study that has been conducted to examine the test score stability of the RCDS-2 scores.

For the RCDS-2:SF, the internal consistency reliability estimate for the Total scores was strong (α = .85). The internal consistency reliabilities were also reported for children by gender (α = .85 for boys and α = .86 for girls), grade level (αs = .74 to .89 for grades 2 through 6) and ethnicity (αs = .82 to .90; W. M. Reynolds, 2010b). These reliability estimates are in the strong to very strong range. Like the RCDS-2, temporal stability for the RCDS-2:SF scores has not been examined.

Evidence supporting the construct validity of the RCDS-2 and RCDS-2:SF scores has been found. Principal component analysis followed by the varimax rotation procedure of 1,100 children's responses on the RCDS-2 resulted in a four-factor solution—emotional or emotional self-directed cognitions factor, anhedonia factor, cognitive-behavioral factor, and somatic-vegetative factor (W. M. Reynolds, 2010b). Convergent and discriminant validity of the RCDS-2 scores have been examined in relation to scores external to the test. W. M. Reynolds reported moderate correlations of .44 to .60 between the scores of the RCDS-2 and RCDS-2:SF and the scores of the APS, the BVS Victimization scale and the Revised Body Esteem Scale for Children (Mendelson & White, 1993). These findings support the convergent validity of the RCDS-2 and RCDS-2:SF scores. In contrast, W. M. Reynolds (2010b) reported low validity coefficients between the RCDS-2 and RCDS-2:SF scores and the BVS

Bullying Scale scores (r = .29 and r = .24, respectively), and self-reported average school grades (r = -.30 and r = -.27, respectively). These findings lend support for the discriminant validity of the RCDS-2 and RCDS-2:SF scores.

Like its predecessor, the RCDS, strengths of the RCDS-2 and the RCDS-2:SF include the ease of administration and scoring, low reading level for younger children, and brevity of the measures. Limitations of the measures include the number of independent research studies conducted to date to address the psychometric properties of the measures. In addition, no studies are reported in the RCDS-2 manual on the test score stability of the RCDS-2 and RCDS-2:SF scores. Independent research studies need to be conducted in the future on these newly published, brief measures that assess the severity of depressive symptomatology in children.

Social Phobia and Anxiety Inventory for Children

The Social Phobia and Anxiety Inventory for Children (SPAI-C; Beidel, Turner, & Morris, 1998) was developed to screen for and measure the behavioral, cognitive and somatic aspects of social phobia in children and young adolescents in a variety of settings, including outpatient clinics, inpatient clinics, schools, juvenile detention facilities, and residential treatment settings. The SPAI-C is a 26 item self-report inventory for children and adolescents, ages 8 to 14. For those adolescents 14 and older who are socially anxious, the Social Phobia and Anxiety Inventory (SPAI; Turner, Beidel, Dancu, & Stanley, 1989) may be used. To complete the SPAI-C, children and young adolescents need to be able to read at least at a third-grade reading level. Individual test administration is recommended for the measure. However, the SPAI-C may be administered in a group setting. Test administrators can be clinical or non-clinical staff. In the administration of the measure, children read each statement on the SPAI-C and respond by circling how frequently each place or activity makes them feel nervous or scared. The SPAI-C uses a 3-point Likert scale, ranging from 0 (*never or hardly ever*) to 2 (*most of the time or always*). The SPAI-C takes approximately 20 to 30 minutes to complete. Scoring of the SPAI-C is relatively easy and involves the summing of the raw scores for each item. The SPAI-C Total score is obtained from the summing of these raw scores, and a SPAI-C Total score of 18 is recommended as the cut score for screening purposes. Qualified professionals should interpret the SPAI-C. While the SPAI-C Total score provides an overall assessment of symptom intensity across settings, clinicians may examine response patterns on the protocol to determine important aspects of children's fears in different social situations. Using this information qualitatively may assist in developing effective treatment plans (Beidel, Turner & Morris, 2000).

The normative sample for the SPAI-C included 154 children, ages 8 to 17 (M = 11.5). Fifty-three percent were female and 47% were male. Racial/ethnic composition of the sample included 83% Caucasian, 14% African American, 2% Asian American, and 1% Native American. A large portion of the normative sample included children and adolescents with psychiatric disorders, particularly children and adolescents with anxiety disorders (Beidel, Turner, & Morris, 1995).

Reliability and validity of the SPAI-C scores have been examined. Coefficient alphas for the SPAI-C Total scores in a sample of 148 children and adolescents and the normative sample of 154 children and youth were .92 (Beidel, Turner, & Fink, 1996) and .95 (Beidel, Turner, & Morris, 1995), respectively. Beidel and colleagues (1995) reported test score stability coefficients for the SPAI-C scores of .86 over a two-week test-retest interval among 62 individuals in the normative sample and .63 over a 10-month test-retest interval among 19 individuals in the normative sample who participated in the two-week test-retest session.

Beidel et al. (1995) conducted a number of studies to evaluate the validity of the SPAI-C scores. A principal-component factor analysis with varimax rotation of the responses of the 154 children and adolescents in the norming sample to the SPAI-C was performed. Results of the factor analysis indicated that a three-factor solution produced the best fit. The three factors (Assertiveness/General Conversation, Traditional Social Encounters, and Public Performance) together accounted for 60% of the variance. The Assertiveness/General Conversation factor consisted of items that measured negative assertion and general conversation skills, the Traditional Social Encounters factor included items that assessed fears of particular situations, and the Public Performance factor consisted of items that measured fears of performance situations. These findings provided support for the construct validity of the SPAI-C scores. Beidel and colleagues (1995) also found support for the convergent and discriminant validity of the SPAI-C scores. The authors reported a moderate validity

coefficient of .50 between the SPAI-C scores and the STAI-C Trait scale scores in a subsample of 38 children from the normative sample. In addition, the SPAI-C scores were compared to the scores of the five subscales (Fear of Failure and Criticism, Fear of the Unknown, Fear of Injury and Small Animals, Fear of Danger and Death, and Medical Fears) of the FSSC-R, and moderate correlations (rs = .41-.53) were noted in a subsample of 59 children from the normative sample. Also, children's scores on the SPAI-C were compared to parents' ratings on the CBCL in a subsample of 74 children from the normative sample. The SPAI-C scores correlated moderately with the CBCL Internalizing scale scores (r = .45), moderately and negatively with the CBCL Social Competence scale scores (r = -.33), and negligibly with the CBCL Externalizing scale scores (r = .18; Beidel et al., 1995). These findings provide support for the convergent and discriminant validity of the SPAI-C scores. Furthermore, a contrasted group study comparing children with social phobia to children with externalizing disorders and children without a diagnosis was conducted using the SPAI-C. Beidel and colleagues (1996) reported the mean score on the SPAI-C for children with social phobia (M = 24.6) was significantly higher than the mean score for children in the externalizing group (M = 12.8) and the no diagnosis group (M = 11.05), supporting the discriminant validity of the SPAI-C scores.

The strengths of the SPAI-C include a strong conceptual basis and theoretical rationale, assessment of a wide range of social fears across different settings, brevity of the measure, convenience and ease of use, quick administration and scoring (Allen, 2003), and availability of the measure in several different languages (English, French-Canadian, and Spanish; Spenciner, 2003). In contrast, limitations of the measure include a lack of detailed description of the test development sample (Spenciner, 2003), and few reliability and validity studies in comparison to comparable instruments presented in the manual (Allen, 2003), especially studies conducted by independent researchers. Overall, the SPAI-C has a number of strengths as a screener of children and young adolescents' social fears in a variety of settings and situations.

Clinical Interviews

Along with structured personality inventories, less formal (i.e. informal) methods such as clinical interviews are available to assess the personality and affect of children and adolescents. In this section, information on some of the most common semi-structured and structured interviews used with children and adolescents will be discussed.

Diagnostic Interview for Children and Adolescents—Fourth Edition

The Diagnostic Interview for Children and Adolescents-Fourth Edition (DICA-IV; Reich, Welner, & Herjanic, 1997) is a semi-structured instrument which assesses the psychiatric status of 6 to 18 year old children using the DSM-IV criteria. The purpose of the DICA-IV is to make psychiatric diagnoses; it can also be used in epidemiological and clinically-oriented research. Barbara Herjanic initially developed the DICA in the early 1970s. The original version of the DICA was highly structured and was designed to be administered by lay interviewers (Reich, 2000). The current computerized version was published in 1997 by Multi-Health Systems (Reich, Welner, & Herjanic, 1997). It can be administered by highly-trained lay persons or, if the respondent has adequate reading skills, can be self-administered.

There are two versions of the DICA-IV—one for the child/adolescent and one for the parent. The child/adolescent version assesses a wide variety of clinical diagnostic categories, including ADHD, substance use, depressive disorders, anxiety disorders, conduct disorders, eating disorders, gender identity, etc. There is also a critical items feature to aid in highlighting high-risk responses such as suicidal ideation, violent tendencies, and drug abuse. Scoring consists of linking the interviewee's responses to relevant diagnostic categories which, in turn, allows the clinician to determine the focus of a follow-up interview (M. Marocco, personal communication, June 30, 2009). In terms of response format, respondents can answer with a "firm yes" or "firm no." Less firm answers—or "evasive" answers—are probed (Reich, 2000). The DICA-IV format allows interviewers to probe responses with predefined probes; interviewee requests for information and clarification are answered with scripted material (Orvaschel, 2006). The child/adolescent version has 26 clinical diagnostic categories. A branching question structure is employed; the interview offers over 1,600 possible questions. Interviewers can choose to administer either some or all of the categories (M. Marocco, personal communication, June 30, 2009). The time required to administer the DICA-IV is between one and three hours, depending upon the number of categories of pathology that are probed.

For the self-administered computerized version, the child or adolescent must have at least a fourth-grade reading level. Interviewees with beginning reading skills and skill deficits need to have the material read aloud to them (Reich, Cottler, McCallum, Corwin, & VanEerdewegh, 1995). It is also recommended that a nearby assistant be available to answer questions for those interviewees who can read the material themselves.

Several limitations of the DICA-IV include no norming sample and no reliability and validity data for this version of the instrument (M. Marocco, personal communication, June 30, 2009). To its credit, the DICA-IV can be used to aid clinicians in their attempts to diagnose their clients. It is widely used in both research and clinical settings and can be used with both younger children and adolescents. The computerized version has been found to be acceptable to children and adolescents (Reich et al., 1995).

National Institute of Mental Health—Diagnostic Interview Schedule for Children Version IV

The National Institute of Mental Health Diagnostic Interview for Children Version IV (NIMH DISC-IV; National Institute of Mental Health, 1997) is a structured diagnostic interview instrument that addresses more than thirty psychiatric diagnoses possibly present in children and adolescents, ages 6 to 17 (Shaffer, Fisher, Lucas, Dulcan, & Schwab-Stone, 2000). It can be used in clinical studies for research purposes, in mental health settings to aid in diagnosis, and in schools as a prevention/screening instrument. It has six diagnostic sections based on the criteria of the DSM-IV and the ICD-10. These sections cover anxiety disorders, mood disorders, disruptive disorders, substance-abuse disorders, schizophrenia, and miscellaneous disorders such as eating and elimination disorders (National Institute of Mental Health, n.d.). The instrument includes parallel parent and child versions and is available in English and Spanish. It has been in development since 1979, was the product of an initiative by the NIMH Division of Biometry and Epidemiology, and was developed to be used for large-scale surveys whose purpose was to determine the prevalence of mental disorders and the need for related services for children (Shaffer et al., 2000).

The questions on this instrument are designed to be read exactly as written. Responses are typically limited to "yes," "no," and "sometimes" or "somewhat." The questions are organized in a branching-tree question structure. The categories of questions for the child version include: (1) 358 "stem" questions asked of everyone; (2) 1,341 contingent questions asked only if the previous stem question were answered positively; (3) 732 questions about age of onset, degree of impairment, and treatment; and (4) 499 "whole-life" questions—or questions that pertain to a past history of symptoms—which also employ a stem-contingent structure (National Institute of Mental Health, n.d.). The administration time for the NIMH DISC-IV is dependent upon the number of symptoms that are endorsed, and the interview averages approximately 70 to 120 minutes. Computers are utilized in the administration and scoring of the NIMH DISC-IV.

Depending on the disorder, informant, and sample tested, kappa test-retest reliability estimates range from. 05 to .93 (Shaffer et al., 2000). For combined (parent and child) informants in community samples, kappa statistics fall within the moderate range for some common disorders: ADHD (k = .48), Oppositional Defiant Disorder (k = .59), Conduct Disorder (k = .66), and social phobia (k = .44; Orvaschel, 2006). Orvaschel notes that there is a lack of validity studies for this instrument.

In listing advantages of the NIMH DISC-IV, Shaffer and colleagues (2000) indicate that it is relatively inexpensive to use in a research setting and it is standardized and thus minimizes the possibility of measurement error. The NIMH DISC-IV has a variety of parallel versions and translations and is widely used throughout the world, which allows international comparisons of prevalence and incidence data (Orvaschel, 2006). In terms of limitations, Shaffer and colleagues (2000) state that the instrument is unable to address invalid responses of an interviewee who misunderstands a question, and—since it is restricted to assessing the symptoms of the DSM and ICD systems—it is unable to allow atypical presentations to be revealed. Additionally, some researchers and clinicians consider it to be too structured, thus discouraging clinical judgment in a diagnostic instrument (Orvaschel, 2006).

Kiddie Schedule for Affective Disorders and Schizophrenia for School-Aged Children

The Kiddie Schedule for Affective Disorders and Schizophrenia for School-Aged Children (K-SADS; Orvaschel, 1995) is a semi-structured interview designed to aid in the identification and diagnosis of psychopathology in children and adolescents (Orvaschel, 2006). The interview format is designed to allow for the collection of information from children and adolescents, ages 7 to 18, and their parents in order to determine both present and lifetime versions of thirty-two DSM-IV Axis I psychiatric disorders (Reynolds, 2006). The initial version was designed in the late 1970s to provide a systematic method for identifying symptoms of depression in children who participated in a research program (Orvaschel, 2006). Various versions have been developed since that time.

The K-SADS is intended to be administered by trained clinicians rather than lay interviewers. It requires a brief (five minutes) unstructured time for the interviewer to develop rapport with the interviewee. The interviewer then moves on to sections on history of treatment and medication for emotional problems, then proceeds to specific topics of psychopathology, including mood disorders, psychoses, anxiety disorders, and so on (Orvaschel, 2006). The primary caregiver is interviewed before the child/adolescent. Responses of each are recorded and summary ratings for each symptom are made during the child's interview. Diagnoses are then based on the summary ratings of both respondents. The interviews of each informant may take from 30 to 60 minutes, depending upon the nature and extent of the symptoms of psychopathology endorsed.

Whereas reliability was initially established with patient populations in New York and Pittsburgh, there is no norming sample and the expectation is that reliability will be established at the research site (Orvaschel, personal communication, July 23, 2009). Orvaschel (2006) reported an interrater reliability mean kappa coefficient of .66 for version 5 of the K-SADS-Epidemiologic Version. Kappa coefficients for specific disorders range from .45 to .81. An important advantage of the K-SADS is that it has been widely used throughout the world in clinical and epidemiological research studies. The K-SADS is considered the "gold standard" among diagnostic interview instruments (Kessler et al., 2009). There are versions available in different languages throughout the world, not only in widely used languages such as Spanish (Ulloa et al., 2006) but also in less widely used languages such as Korean (Kim et al., 2004) and Icelandic (Lauth, Magnússon, Ferrari, & Pétursson, 2008). The various versions generate helpful data on "episode duration, age of onset, treatment characteristics, and syndrome-specific impairment" (Ambrosini, 2000, p. 56). Disadvantages include limited data on reliability and validity.

Anxiety Disorders Interview Schedule for DSM-IV

The Anxiety Disorders Interview Schedule for DSM-IV (ADIS; Silverman & Albano, 1996) is a semi-structured clinical interview derived from the DSM-IV. The purpose of the ADIS is to aid clinicians in diagnosing anxiety and related disorders in children, ages 6 to 18. The ADIS consists of two versions – a child version and parent version. The interview should be conducted by a trained clinician and it takes approximately one hour per respondent to administer.

The ADIS utilizes a yes/no response format for each diagnostic category, with follow-up probes used to obtain clarification. Endorsement of a "yes" response to an interview question directly corresponds to the DSM-IV diagnostic criteria. Scoring occurs by summing the number of "yes" responses. If a sufficient number of "yes" responses warrant a possible diagnosis, the clinician asks the respondent to rate the level of impairment or interference caused by the symptoms. Children rate the level of impairment of their symptoms on a 9-point "feelings thermometer", ranging from 0 (*no impairment*) to 8 (*severe impairment*). Parents respond on the same 9-point scale (0 to 8), as to the degree to which the child's symptoms interfere or "mess things up." Child and parent interviews are considered jointly when issuing a diagnosis as well as determining the level of impairment. When impairment ratings vary between the child and parent, the clinician defers to the higher rating.

The ADIS is an excellent and renowned tool for clinicians wanting corroborating evidence for diagnostic purposes, and researchers concerned with the psychometrics of instruments. Silverman, Saavedra, and Pina (2001) reported kappas of .61 to 1.00 and interclass correlations of .81 to .95 for the ADIS. Test-retest reliability coefficients over a 7 to 14 day test-retest interval for the child and parent impairment ratings ranged from .60 to .84, with one correlation coefficient falling below .60, and from .56 to .84, respectively (Silverman et al., 2001). Additionally, the ADIS has been shown to produce high agreement between the child and parent. However, research has shown that child-parent agreement and agreement consistency over time (child-child, parent-parent) varies across specific anxiety disorders diagnosed, research studies, and motivational level of the child (Reuterskiöld, Öst, & Ollendick, 2008; Silverman et al., 2001). Despite these differences, the ADIS is an important tool in the field for evaluating childhood anxiety (Orvaschel, 2006).

Behavioral Observations

Besides structured personality inventories and clinical interviews, there are other methods to assess children and adolescents' affect. Informal methods such as behavioral observations can be used to identify behavioral indicators of negative affect or emotion in children and adolescents. In this section, the use of informal methods to assess children and adolescents' affect will be reviewed. In addition, this chapter will close with a brief discussion of functional assessment and analysis and how this informal method of assessment can be used possibly in the future to gain a better understanding of the development and maintenance of negative affect and maladaptive thoughts in children and adolescents.

According to a recent survey by Shapiro and Heick (2004), behavioral observation is one of the most common assessment tools used by mental health professionals in the schools. Observations inform the assessment and treatment process through the gathering of baseline information, assisting in the determination of benchmarks for setting treatment goals, and validating of information from semi-structured and structured interviews and objective questionnaires. Martin and Pear (2003) outline two types of observation, direct and indirect. For issues of affect, direct observation can be problematic because of the covert nature of many symptoms, but some methods of observation for problems related to affect provide helpful information and will be discussed.

Direct Behavioral Observations

One way to gain a better understanding of a referral problem is to observe the behaviors of concern in the natural environment. Several observational techniques can be used depending on the problem behavior, the environment, or the time constraints involved. Direct informal observations involve writing down a description of behaviors and environmental events in sequence without any systematic measurement. While this technique is helpful in gathering descriptive information, it is not a reliable technique for gathering quantitative information (e.g. frequency or duration of behavior). However, direct informal observation can help the clinician better understand the behaviors of concern and the potential environmental factors that may trigger or maintain the behavior, and this may be an important step in designing a more systematic observation for future use.

A second way to record behavior in the natural environment is to create a systematic behavioral measurement system. This kind of direct observation requires an observable and measurable definition of the behavior in order to achieve consistent results over time. Guidelines outlining the development of reliable observation protocols are beyond the scope of this chapter, but these can be found in most books on behavior modification (e.g. Cooper, Heron, & Heward, 2007; Martin & Pear, 2003). Systematic behavioral observation is commonly used for externalizing disorders, but several researchers have indicated that there are observable behaviors related to problems of affect. For example, Kazdin (1988) identified several broad categories that may indicate symptoms of depression, including social activity, solitary behavior, and affect-related facial expression. Using these broad categories, it would be possible to create an observation form to record the amount of time a child spends interacting with others, the amount of time the child spends alone, and the frequency of different facial expressions. It is important for the clinician to also observe other same-sex peers who are in the vicinity. This allows the clinician to compare the behavior of the child to other peers in the same situation (Merrell, 2008).

Glennon and Weisz's (1978) work provides another example of using observable behaviors for affect related disorders. The authors designed a coding system for 30 anxiety-related behaviors in preschool children, including verbal expressions (e.g. physical complaints), affect-related expressions (e.g. facial expressions of fear), gratuitous bodily movements (e.g. moving of feet), and other behaviors such as nail-biting, chewing on other objects, and eye contact avoidance. Glennon and Weisz found that these behaviors could be reliably coded by independent observers, with interobserver agreement ranging form .66 to .99, with a .92 level of agreement across all categories.

Behavioral Avoidance Tasks

Observing behavior in the natural environment is not always an option, especially for affect-related problems. Another method to directly observe these behaviors is to create controlled analogue situations which will induce the behaviors of concern. One method that has been used frequently in research and practice is the Behavioral Avoidance Test (BAT; Schniering, Hudson, & Rapee, 2000). In a BAT, the clinician introduces the child to a stimulus or situation which brings about avoidance or anxious behaviors in the individual. It is then possible to record aspects of the child's behavior in the situation. For example, if a child is afraid of dogs, the clinician could have a small, tame dog in a room and have the child enter the room with the dog. Several types of measures can then be taken, such as length of time the child spends in the room, how close the child comes to the dog, how long it takes before the child begins to approach the dog, or percentage of steps completed in a standardized protocol that brings the child into more intimate interactions with the dog (Ollendick et al., 2009; Woodruff-Borden & Leyfer, 2006). In addition to the behavioral measures, BATs often include subjective scales, such as a fear thermometer, to assess the level of fear a person is experiencing (Walk, 1956). This allows the clinician to gather both observable measures and ratings of the child's subjective feelings in the feared situation. BATs can also be designed to include several different types of tasks which also have several graded steps to be performed (Steketee, Chambliss, Tran, Worden, & Gillis, 1996).

BATs have been used in research to assess behavioral symptoms of several disorders, including social anxiety (Compton, Grant, Chrisman, Gammon, Brown, & March, 2001), phobias (Ollendick et al. 2009), and obsessive compulsive disorders (Barrett, Healy, & March, 2003). Because BATs are not standardized, Schniering et al. (2000) suggests that BATs are most useful for assessing simple phobias because the nature of other anxiety disorders usually include a complex set of variables that would be difficult to recreate in a clinical setting. Also, because many of these tasks are often tailored to individual children, there has not been extensive research into the psychometric properties of BATs, but studies which have used them have reported acceptable levels of reliability and concurrent validity. For instance, Hamilton and King (1991) completed a test-retest reliability study using a BAT for children diagnosed with a phobia for dogs. In this study, the assessments were seven days apart and the reliability was .97 between the two administrations of the BAT, which indicates very strong temporal stability. Ollendick et al. (2009) also examined the reliability of the BAT over a one-hour test-retest interval and reported stability coefficients of .87 for the behavioral avoidance tasks and .92 for ratings of subjective levels of distress among a group of children with phobias. Although these coefficients are in the strong to very strong range, the test-retest period was relatively short and it is difficult to determine whether the BAT would have shown adequate temporal stability over extended periods of time. Steketee et al. (1996) found evidence to support the convergent validity of the BAT with individuals, adults not children, with obsessive-compulsive disorders. Moderate correlations were reported for the BAT and scores of the Maudsley Obsessional Compulsion Inventory (MOCI: Hodgson & Rachman, 1977) Composite scale (r = .46), and the Yale-Brown Obsessive Compulsive Scale (YBOCS; Goodman et al., 1989) Composite scale (r = .49), Avoidance subscale (r = .61) and Compulsions subscale (r = .63). These findings indicate that the BAT measures aspects of obsessions and compulsive behaviors that are similar but different from those assessed by standardized questionnaires.

One advantage of a BAT is that it allows the clinician to ask about subjective levels of fear or anxiety while the child is in the situation, which is not something that can happen easily with observations in the natural environment. Also, this helps the clinician view behaviors that may be difficult to observe in the natural environment because of their low frequency, such as a phobic reaction to animals. Each task should be tailored for the individual child based on his/her specific fears or anxieties, making this method most useful for pre/post-treatment assessment of behavior change. However, because BATs are analogue situations, the clinician must always keep in mind that it is possible that the child's behavior may differ if the individual was in the same situation, but in the natural environment. Because they are controlled situations, the child may feel more able to perform in the feared situation than he/she would outside of a clinical setting.

Family Anxiety Coding Schedule

The Family Anxiety Coding Schedule (FACS; Dadds, Ryan, Barrett, & Rappee, n.d) is an observational coding system that assesses child and parent reactions to ambiguous situations. It includes interviews for both the child and parents, and then it includes four discussions between family members about ambiguous situations and issues that may concern family members, also called "hot" issues (Dadds et al., n.d.). The purpose of the FACS is to analyze the way parents and children talk with each other when they are attempting to come up with solutions to problems they are presented with during a session. Initially, Barrett et al. (1996) found that children who are anxious tend to view ambiguous situations as threatening, and choose avoidant solutions to cope with those situations. They also found that parents contributed to their child's avoidance behavior when interacting with the child by rewarding or reciprocating avoidant verbal statements of the child, leading to avoidant solutions to

problems. Little research has been completed on the FACS psychometric properties, but Dadds et al. (1996) found adequate agreement between raters, with mean kappa indices for content and affect codes of .78 and .72, respectively.

The FACS can be helpful because it allows the clinician to observe how the child and parent interact when resolving problems. Previous research has shown that parents with anxiety disorders tend to have children with anxiety disorders (Beidel & Turner, 1997; Turner, Beidel, & Costello, 1987), and this procedure allows clinicians to investigate the possibility of familial contribution and maintenance of affect disorders, especially anxiety disorders.

Functional Assessment of Affective Symptoms

Similar to the research on direct observation, the use of functional assessment and functional analysis have been used mostly to analyze externalizing behaviors, but recent advances in behavioral theory (Hayes, Barnes-Holmes, & Roche, 2000) and therapy (Hayes, Strosahl, & Wilson, 1999) have provided a basis for gaining a better understanding of the development and maintenance of negative affect and maladaptive thoughts from a behavioral perspective. Merrell (2008) points out the possible importance of examining the antecedent events related to the development of affective issues such as depression and anxiety, as well as how the consequences of behaving in an anxious or depressed manner may maintain those behaviors. With further research, it may be possible to develop reliable methods to assess affective states from a functional perspective. Using a function-based assessment method for affective issues can help in the design of function-based interventions as well. For instance, an understanding of the antecedent conditions that predict anxious symptoms may help an individual recognize those situations and possibly implement a relaxation intervention on their own. Additionally, gaining an understanding of the consequences of the behaviors related to the internalizing symptoms may help with the design of interventions that help alter the maintaining consequences, such as removing aversive stimuli or providing social attention for appropriate behaviors. While there is still much work to do in this area, an effective and reliable function-based approach could provide promising outcomes for the treatment of affect-related disorders.

In summary, there are several helpful methods for observing the behavior of children who experience affective problems. There are specific overt behaviors that can be assessed through typical observation measures, and analogue sessions can be created to help determine how children may behave in natural environments. These methods are essential to the assessment process to help provide additional information beyond verbal reports, and they can help validate and extend upon the information gathered using other forms of assessment.

Conclusion

Over the years structured personality inventories designed for children and adolescents have increased in numbers and have become more sophisticated and more psychometrically sound. In this chapter, a wide array of established, newly developed, and updated objective personality inventories broad and narrow in scope were reviewed. Informal methods of assessing children and adolescents' affect were discussed, as well as methods not commonly used to assess affect but may have the potential in the future to contribute invaluable information in the assessment process. The use of and information gleaned from structured personality inventories, clinical interviews, and behavior observations assist professionals in their understanding of children and adolescents' behavior and in making sound decisions about the appropriate course of action to take to help children and adolescents lead healthy and productive lives. Future research directions include the development of more sophisticated and psychometrically sound instruments specifically designed to assess the personality and affect of children and adolescents and adapting structured personality inventories for use with children and adolescents from diverse cultural backgrounds.

References

Achenbach, T. M. (1991). *Youth Self-Report and 1991 Profile.* Burlington, VT: University of Vermont, Department of Psychiatry.

Achenbach, T. M., & Edelbrock, C. (1987). *Youth Self-Report and Profile.* Burlington, VT: University of Vermont, Department of Psychiatry.

Achenbach, T. M., & Mc Conaughy, S. H. (1992). Taxonomy of internalizing disorders of childhood and adolescence. In W. M. Reynolds (Ed.), *Internalizing disorders in children and adolescents* (pp. 19–60). New York: Wiley.

Achenbach, T. M., & Rescorla, L. A. (2001a). Child Behavior Checklist. Burlington, VT: University of Vermont, Research Center for Children, Youth, & Families.

Achenbach, T. M., & Rescorla, L. A. (2001b). *Manual for the ASEBA School-Age Forms & Profiles.* Burlington, VT: University of Vermont, Research Center for Children, Youth, & Families.

Achenbach, T. M., & Rescorla, L. A. (2001c). Teacher's Report Form. Burlington, VT: University of Vermont, Research Center for Children, Youth, & Families.

Achenbach, T. M., & Rescorla, L. A. (2001d). Youth Self-Report. Burlington, VT: University of Vermont, Research Center for Children, Youth, & Families.

Allen, S. J. (2003). Test Review: Social Phobia & Anxiety Inventory for Children. In B. S. Plake & J. C. Impara (Eds.), *The fifteenth mental measurements yearbook* [Electronic version]. Retrieved July 30, 2009 from the Buros Institute's Test Reviews Online website: http://www.unl.edu/buros.

American Psychiatric Association. (1987). *The diagnostic and statistical manual of mental disorders* (3rd ed. rev.). Washington, DC: Author.

American Psychiatric Association. (1994). *The diagnostic and statistical manual of mental disorders* (4th.ed.). Washington, DC: Author.

American Psychiatric Association. (2000). *The diagnostic and statistical manual of mental disorders* (4th ed., text rev.). Washington, DC: Author.

Ambrosini, P. (2000). Historical development and present status of the Schedule for Affective Disorders and Schizophrenia for School-Age Children (K-SADS). *Journal of the American Academy of Child and Adolescent Psychiatry, 39,* 49–58.

Anton, W. D., & Reed, J. R. (1990). *College Adjustment Scales.* Odessa, FL: Psychological Assessment Resources.

Archer, R. P., Belevich, J. K. S., & Elkins, D. E. (1994). Item-level and scale-level factor structures of the MMPI-A. *Journal of Personality Assessment, 62,* 332–345.

Archer, R. P., Bolinskey, K., Morton, T. L., & Farris, K. L. (2002). A factor structure for the MMPI-A: Replication with male delinquents. *Assessment, 9,* 319–326.

Arita, A. A., & Baer, R. A. (1998). Validity of selected MMPI-A content scales. *Psychological Assessment, 10,* 59–63.

Baldwin, J. S., & Dadds, M. R. (2007). Reliability and validity of parent and child versions of the Multidimensional Anxiety Scale for Children in community samples. *Journal of the American Academy of Child and Adolescent Psychiatry, 46,* 252–260.

Barrett, P. M., Rapee, R. M., Dadds, M. M., & Ryan, S. M. (1996). Family enhancement of cognitive style in anxious and aggressive children. *Journal of Abnormal Child Psychology, 24,* 187–203.

Barrett, P. M., Healy, L., & March, J. S. (2003). Behavioral avoidance test for childhood obsessive compulsive disorder: A home-based observation. *American Journal of Psychotherapy, 57,* 80–100.

Beck, A. T. (1988). *Beck Hopelessness Scale.* San Antonio, TX: The Psychological Corporation.

Beck, J. S., Beck, A. T., & Jolly, J. B. (2001). *Beck Youth Inventories for Children and Adolescents of Emotional and Social Impairment.* San Antonio, TX: The Psychological Corporation.

Beck, J. S., Beck, A. T., Jolly, J. B., & Steer, R. A. (2005a). *Beck Youth Inventories, Second Edition.* San Antonio, TX: Harcourt Assessments.

Beck, J. S., Beck, A. T., Jolly, J. B., & Steer, R. A. (2005b). *Beck Youth Inventories, Second Edition manual.* San Antonio, TX: Harcourt Assessments.

Beck, A. T., Kovacs, M., & Weissman, A. (1979). Assessment of suicidal intention: The Scale for Suicidal Ideation. *Journal of Consulting Clinical Psychology, 47,* 343–352.

Beck, A. T., Rush, A. J., Shaw, B. F., & Emery, G. (1979). *Cognitive therapy of depression.* New York: Guilford.

Beck, A. T., Steer, R. A., & Brown, G. K. (1996a). *Beck Depression Inventory-II.* San Antonio, TX: The Psychological Corporation.

Beck, A T., Steer, R. A., Brown, G. K. (1996b). *Manual for the Beck Depression Inventory II (BDI-II)*. San Antonio, TX: The Psychological Corporation.

Beck, A. T., Ward, C., Mendelson, M., Mock, J., & Erbaugh, J. (1961). An inventory for measuring depression. *Archives of General Psychiatry*, 4, 561–571.

Beidel, D. C., & Turner, S. M. (1997). At risk for anxiety: I. Psychopathology in the offspring of anxious parents. *Journal of the American Academy of Child and Adolescent Psychiatry*, 36, 918–924.

Beidel, D. C., Turner, S. M., & Fink, C. M. (1996). Assessment of childhood social phobia: Construct, convergent, and discriminant validity of the Social Phobia and Anxiety Inventory for Children (SPAI-C). *Psychological Assessment*, 8, 235–240.

Beidel, D. C., Turner, S. M., & Morris, T. L. (1995). A new inventory to assess social anxiety and phobia: The Social Phobia and Anxiety Inventory for Children. *Psychological Assessment*, 7, 73–79.

Beidel, D. C., Turner, S. M., & Morris, T. L. (1998). *Social Phobia & Anxiety Inventory for Children*. North Tonawanda, NY: Multi-Health Systems.

Beidel, D. C., Turner, S. M., & Morris, T. L. (2000). *SPAI-C: Social Phobia & Anxiety Inventory for Children manual*. North Towanda, New York: Multi-Health Systems.

Bokhorst, C. L., Westernberg, P. M., Oosterlaan, J., & Heyne, D. A. (2008). Changes in social fears across childhood and adolescence: Age-related differences in the factor structure of the Fear Survey Schedule for Children–Revised. *Journal of Anxiety Disorders*, 22, 135–142.

Bolinskey, P. K., Arnau, R. C., Archer, R. P., & Handel, R. W. (2004). A replication of the MMPI-A PSY-5 scales and development of facet subscales. *Assessment*, 11, 40–48.

Bowers, S. L. (2004). Concurrent validity of the Clinical Assessment of Depression with the Beck Depression Inventory-Second Edition. *Master's thesis*. Western Kentucky University, Bowling Green.

Bracken, B. A., & Howell, K. (2004a). *Clinical Assessment of Depression (CAD)*. Lutz, FL: Psychological Assessment Resources.

Bracken, B. A., & Howell, K. (2004b). *Clinical Assessment of Depression* (CAD): Professional manual. Lutz, FL: Psychological Assessment Resources.

Buckley, T. C., Parker, J. D., & Heggie, J. (2000). A psychometric evaluation of the BDI-II in treatment-seeking substance abusers. *Journal of Substance Abuse Treatment*, 20, 197–204.

Burney, D. M. (2001). *Adolescent Anger Rating Scale*. Odessa, FL: Psychological Assessment Resources.

Burnham, J. J. (2005). Fears of children in the United States: An examination of the American Fear Survey Schedule with 20 new contemporary fear items. *Measurement and Evaluation in Counseling and Development*, 38, 78–91.

Burnham, J. J., & Gullone, E. (1997). The Fear Survey Schedule for Children–II: A psychometric investigation with American data. *Behavior Research and Therapy*, 35, 165–173.

Butcher, J. N., Dahlstrom, W. G., Graham, J. R., Tellegen, A., & Kaemmer, B. (1989). *Minnesota Multiphasic Personality Inventory-2*. Minneapolis: University of Minnesota Press.

Butcher, J. N., Williams, C. L., Graham, J. R., Archer, R. P., Tellegen, A., Ben-Porath, Y. S., et al. (1992). *Minnesota Multiphasic Personality Inventory—Adolescent: Manual for administration, scoring, and interpretation*. Minneapolis: University of Minnesota Press.

Butcher, J. N., Williams, C. L., Graham, J. R., Kaemmer, B., Archer, R. P., Tellegen, A., et al. (1992). *Minnesota Multiphasic Personality Inventory—Adolescent*. Minneapolis: University of Minnesota Press.

Carroll, B. J., Feinberg, M., Greden, J. F., Tarika, J., Albala, A. A., Hakett, R. F. et al., (1981). A specific laboratory test for the diagnosis of melancholia: Standardization, validation, and clinical utility. *Archives of General Psychiatry*, 38, 15–22.

Carlson, J. F. (2005). Test review of the Reynolds Adolescent Depression Scale-Second Edition. In R. A. Spies & B. S. Plake (Eds.), *The sixteenth mental measurements yearbook*. [Electronic version]. Retrieved August 10, 2009 from the Buros Institute's Test Reviews Online website: http://www.unl.edu/buros.

Castaneda, A., McCandless, B., & Palermo, D. (1956). The children's form of the Manifest Anxiety Scale. *Child Development*, 27, 317–326.

Christopher, R. (2001a). Test review of the Internalizing Symptoms Scale for Children. In B. S. Plake & J. C. Impara (Eds.), *The fourteenth mental measurements yearbook*. [Electronic version]. Retrieved June 10, 2009 from the Buros Institute's Test Reviews Online website: http://www.unl.edu/buros.

Christopher, R. (2001b). Test review of the Multidimensional Anxiety Scale for Children. In B. S. Plake & J. C. Impara (Eds.), *The fourteenth mental measurements yearbook*. [Electronic version]. Retrieved July 15, 2009 from the Buros Institute's Test Reviews Online website: http://www.unl.edu/buros.

Claiborn, C. D. (1995). Test review of the Minnesota Multiphasic Personality Inventory-Adolescent. In J. C. Conoley & J. C. Impara (Eds.), *The twelfth mental measurements yearbook*. [Electronic version]. Retrieved July 20, 2009 from the Buros Institute's Test Reviews Online website: http://www.unl.edu/buros.

Compton, S. N., Grant, P. J., Chrisman, A. K., Gammon, P. J., Brown, V. L., & March, J. S. (2001). Sertraline in children and adolescents with social anxiety disorder: An open trial. *Journal of the American Academy of Child and Adolescent Psychiatry*, 40, 564–571.

Conners, C. K. (1989). *Conners' Rating Scales*. North Tonawanda, NY: Multi-Health Systems.

Conners, C. K. (1997). *Conners Rating Scales-Revised*. North Tonawanda, NY: Multi-Health Systems.

Conners, C. K., Erhardt, M. A., & Sparrow, M. A. (1999). *Conners' Adult ADHD Rating Scales* (CAARS). North Towanda, NY: Multi-Health Systems.

Conoley, J. C., & Impara, J. C. (1995). *The twelfth mental measurements yearbook*. [Electronic version]. Retrieved July 20, 2009 from the Buros Institute's Test Reviews Online website: http://www.unl.edu/buros.

Cooper, J. O., Heron, T. E., & Heward, W. L. (2007). *Applied behavior analysis* (2nd ed.). Upper Saddle River, NJ: Prentice Hall.

Costa, P. T., Jr., & McCrae, R. R. (1989). *The NEO Five Factor Inventory*. Odessa, FL: Psychological Assessment Resources.

Crowley, S. L., & Merrell, K. W. (2000). Convergent and discriminant validity of the Internalizing Symptoms Scale for Children. *Journal of Psychoeducational Assessment*, 18, 4–16.

Dadds, M. R., Barrett, P. M., Rapee, R. M., & Ryan, S. (1996) Family process and child anxiety and aggression: An observational analysis. *Journal of Abnormal Child Psychology*, 24, 715–734.

Dadds M. R., Ryan, S., Barrett, P. M., & Rapee, R. M. (n.d.). *Family anxiety coding schedule procedures manual*. Retrieved

July 21, 2009, from http://www2.psy.unsw.edu.au/Users/Mdadds/Resources/FACS.pdf

Davison, M. L., Bershadsky, B., Bieber, J., Silversmith, D., Maruish, M. E., & Kane, R. L. (1997). Development of a brief, multidimensional, self-report instrument for treatment outcomes assessment in psychiatric settings: Preliminary findings. *Assessment, 4*, 259–276.

Destefano, L. (2001). Test review of the Personality Inventory for Youth. In B. S. Plake & J. C. Impara (Eds.), *The fourteenth mental measurements yearbook*. [Electronic version]. Retrieved July 15, 2009 from the Buros Institute's Test Reviews Online website: http://www.unl.edu/buros.

Dowd, T. E. (2001). Review of the Children's Depression and Rating Scale-Revised. In B. S. Plake & J. C. Impara (Eds.), *The fourteenth mental measurements yearbook* [Electronic version]. Retrieved July 2, 2009 from the Buros Institute's Test Reviews Online website: http://www.unl.edu/buros.

Drummond, R. J., & Jones, K. D. (2010). *Assessment procedures for counselors and helping professionals* (7th ed.). Upper Saddle River, NJ: Pearson Education.

Dunn, L. M., & Dunn, L. M. (1981). *Peabody Picture Vocabulary Test-Revised Form*. Circle Pines, MN: American Guidance Service.

Erol, N. (1995). Fears of children and the cultural context: The Turkish norms. *European Child and Adolescent Psychiatry, 4*, 85–93.

Farmer, R. F. (2001). Test review of the Beck Depression Inventory II (BDI-II). In B. S. Plake & J. C. Impara (Eds.), *The fourteenth mental measurements yearbook* [Electronic version]. Retrieved July 9, 2009 from the Buros Institute's Test Reviews Online website: http://www.unl.edu/buros.

Finch, A. J., Kendall, P. C., & Montgomery, L. E. (1974). Multidimensionality of anxiety in children: Factor structure of the Children's Manifest Anxiety Scale. *Journal of Abnormal Child Psychology, 2*, 331–336.

Fincham, D., Schickerling, J., Temane, M., Nel, D., De Roover, W., & Seedat, S. (2008). Exploratory and confirmatory factor analysis of the Multidimensional Anxiety Scale for Children among adolescents in the Cape Town metropole of South Africa. *Depression and Anxiety, 25*, E147–E153.

Finger, M. S., & Ones, D. S. (1999). Psychometric equivalence of the computer and booklet forms of the MMPI: A meta-analysis. *Psychological Assessment, 11*, 58–66.

Flanagan, R. (2005). Test review of the Achenbach System of Empirically Based Assessment. In R. A. Spies & B. S. Plake (Eds.), *The sixteenth mental measurements yearbook* [Electronic version]. Retrieved August 4, 2009 from the Buros Institute's Test Reviews Online website: http://www.unl.edu/buros.

Fontaine, J. L., Archer, R. P., Elkins, D. E., & Johansen, J. (2001). The effects of MMPI-A T-score elevation on classification accuracy for normal and clinical adolescent samples. *Journal of Personality Assessment, 76*, 264–281.

Forbey, J. D., & Ben-Porath, Y. S. (2003). Incremental validity of the MMPI-A content scales in a residential treatment facility. *Assessment, 10*, 191–202.

Glennon, B., & Weisz, J. R. (1978). An observational approach to the assessment of anxiety in young children. *Journal of Consulting and Clinical Psychology, 46*, 1246–1257.

Goodman, W. K., Price, L. H., Rasmussen, S. A., Mazure, C., Fleischmann, R. L., Hill, C. L. et al. (1989). The Yale-Brown Obsessive Compulsive Scale I: Development, use and reliability. *Archives of General Psychiatry, 46*, 1006–1011.

Gullone, E., & King, N. J. (1992). Psychometric evaluation of a Revised Fear Survey Schedule for Children and Adolescents. *Journal of Child Psychology and Psychiatry and Allied Disciplines, 33*, 987–998.

Hamilton, D. I., & King, N. J. (1991). Reliability of a behavioral avoidance test for the assessment of dog phobic children. *Psychological Reports, 69*, 18.

Hamilton, M. (1959). The assessment of anxiety state by rating. *British Journal of Medicine Psychology, 32*, 50–55.

Hamilton, M. (1960). A rating scale for depression. *Journal of Neurology, Neurosurgery and Psychiatry, 23*, 56–62.

Hand, C. G., Archer, R. P., Handel, R. W., & Forbey, J. D. (2007). The classification accuracy of the Minnesota Multiphasic Personality Inventory-Adolescent: Effects of modifying the normative sample. *Assessment, 14*, 80–85.

Hathaway, S. R., & McKinley, J. C. (1943). *Minnesota Multiphasic Personality Inventory*. Minneapolis: University of Minnesota Press.

Hayes, S. C., Barnes-Holmes, D., & Roche, B. (Eds.) (2000). *Relational frame theory: A post-Skinnerian account of human language and cognition*. New York: Plenum Press.

Hayes, S. C., Strosahl, K. D., & Wilson, K. G. (1999). *Acceptance and commitment therapy: An experiential approach to behavior change*. New York: The Guilford Press.

Henington, C. (2007). Test review of the Beck Youth Inventories, Second Edition. In K. F. Geisinger, R. A. Spies, J. F. Carlson, & B. S. Plake ((Eds.), *The eighteenth mental measurements yearbook*. Retrieved July 2, 2009 from the Buros Institute's Test Review Online website: http://www.unl.edu/buros.

Hilts, D., & Moore, J. M. (2003). Normal range MMPI-A profiles among psychiatric inpatients. *Assessment, 10*, 266–272.

Hodgson, R. J., & Rachman, S. (1977). Obsessional-compulsive complaints. *Behaviour Research and Therapy, 15*, 389–395.

Kamphaus, R.W., & Frick, P. J. (2002). *Clinical assessment of child and adolescent personality and behavior, Second edition*. Boston: Allyn Bacon. 128–129.

Kavan, M. G. (2007). Test review of the Clinical Assessment of Depression. In K. F. Geisinger, R. A. Spies, J. F. Carlson, & B. S. Plake (Eds.), The seventeenth mental measurements yearbook [Electronic version]. Retrieved June 11, 2009 from the Buros Institute's Test Reviews Online website: http://www.unl.edu/buros.

Kazdin, A. E. (1988). Childhood depression. In E. J. Mash & L. G. Terdal (Eds.), Behavioral assessment of childhood disorders (2nd ed., pp. 157–195). New York: Guilford.

Kessler, R. C., Avenevoli, S., Green, J., Gruber, M. J., Guyer, M., He, Y., et al. (2009). National Comorbidity Survey Replication Adolescent Supplement (NCS-A): III. Concordance of DSM-IV/CIDI diagnoses with clinical reassessments. *Journal of the American Academy of Child & Adolescent Psychiatry, 48*, 386–399.

Kim, Y. S., Cheon, K. A., Kim, B. N., Chang, S. A., Yoo, H. J., Kim, J. W., et al. (2004). The reliability and validity of Kiddie-Schedule for Affective Disorders and Schizophrenia-Present and Lifetime Version-Korean version. *Yonsei Medical Journal, 45*, 81–89.

Kovacs, M. (1992). *Children's Depression Inventory*. Toronto, Canada: Multi-Health Systems.

Kovacs, M., & Multi-Health Systems. (2003). *Children's Depression Inventory—Short form*. North Towananda, NJ: Multi-Health Systems.

Kingery, J. N., Ginsburg, G. S., & Burstein, M. (2009). Factor structure and psychometric properties of the Multidimensional Anxiety Scale for Children in an African American adolescent sample. *Child Psychiatry and Human Development*, 40, 287–300.

Lachar, D. (1982). *Personality Inventory for Children (PIC): Revised*. Los Angeles: Western Psychological Services.

Lachar, D., & Gruber, C. P. (1995a). *Personality Inventory for Youth* (PIY). Los Angeles, CA: Western Psychological Services.

Lachar, D., & Gruber, C. P. (1995b). *Personality Inventory for Youth* (PIY): Administration and interpretation guide. Los Angeles, CA: Western Psychological Services.

Lachar, D., & Gruber, C. P. (1995c). *Personality Inventory for Youth* (PIY): Technical guide. Los Angeles, CA: Western Psychological Services.

Lachar, D., Harper, R. A., Green, B. A., Morgan, S. T., & Wheeler, A. C. (1996). *The Personality Inventory for Youth: Contributions to diagnosis.*. Paper presented at the annual meeting of the American Psychological Association, Toronto, Canada.

Lanyon, R. I. (1995). Test review of the Minnesota Multiphasic Personality Inventory-Adolescent. In J. C. Conoley & J. C. Impara (Eds.), *The twelfth mental measurements yearbook.* [Electronic version]. Retrieved July 20, 2009 from the Buros Institute's Test Reviews Online website: http://www.unl.edu/buros.

Last, C. G., Francis, G., & Strauss, C. C. (1989). Assessing fears in anxiety-disordered children with the Revised Fear Survey Schedule for Children (FSSC-R). *Journal of Clinical Child Psychology*, 18, 137–141.

Lauth, B., Magnússon, P., Ferrari, P., & Pétursson, H. (2008). An Icelandic version of the Kiddie-SADS-PL: Translation, cross-cultural adaptation and inter-rater reliability. *Nordic Journal of Psychiatry*, 62, 379–385.

March, J. S., Conners, C., Arnold, G., Epstein, J., Parker, J., Hinshaw, S., et al. (1999). The Multidimensional Anxiety Scale for Children (MASC): Confirmatory factor analysis in a pediatric ADHD sample. *Journal of Attention Disorders*, 3, 85–89.

March, J. S., Parker, J. D., Sullivan, K., Stallings, P., & Conners, C. K. (1997). The Multidimensional Anxiety Scale for Children (MASC): Factor structure, reliability, and validity. *Journal of the American Academy of Child and Adolescent Psychiatry*, 36, 554–565.

March, J. S., & Sullivan, K. (1999). Test-retest reliability of the Multidimensional Anxiety Scale for Children. *Journal of Anxiety Disorders, 13*, 349–358.

March, J. S., Sullivan, K., & Parker, J. (1999). Test-retest reliability of the Multidimensional Anxiety Scale for Children. *Journal of Anxiety Disorders*, 13, 349–358.

Marchant, G. J., & Ridenour, T. A. (2001). Test review of the Personality Inventory for Youth. In B. S. Plake & J. C. Impara (Eds.), *The fourteenth mental measurements yearbook.* [Electronic version]. Retrieved June 10, 2009 from the Buros Institute's Test Reviews Online website: http://www.unl.edu/buros.

Martin, G., & Pear, J. (2003). *Behavior modification: What it is and how to do it* (7th ed.). Upper Saddle River, NJ: Prentice Hall.

Mellon, R., Koliadis, E. A., & Paraskevopoulos, T. D. (2004). Normative development of fears in Greece: Self-reports on the Hellenic Fear Survey Schedule for Children. *Anxiety Disorders*, 18, 233–254.

McGrath, R. E., Pogge, D. L., & Stokes, J. M. (2002). Incremental validity of selected MMPI-A content scales in an inpatient setting. *Psychological Assessment*, 14, 401–409.

Mendelson, B. K., & White, D. R. (1993). *Manual for the Body-Esteem Scale for Children*. Montreal, Quebec, Canada: Concordia University.

Merrell, K. W. (2008). *Behavioral, social, and emotional assessment of children and adolescents* (3rd ed.). New York: Lawrence Erlbaum.

Merrell, K. W., Anderson, K. E., & Michael, K. D. (1997). Convergent validity of the Internalizing Symptoms Scale for Children with three self-report measures of internalizing problems. *Journal of Psychoeducational Assessment*, 15, 56–66.

Merrell, K. W., Crowley, S. L., & Walters, A. S. (1997). Development and factor structure of a self-report measure: For assessing internalizing symptoms of elementary-age children. *Psychology in the Schools*, 34, 197–210.

Merrell, K. W., & Walters, A. S. (1998). *Internalizing symptoms scale for children*. Austin, TX: PRO-ED.

Michael, K. D., & Merrell, K. W. (1998). Reliability of children's self-reported internalizing symptoms over short to medium-length time intervals. *Journal of the Academy of Child and Adolescent Psychiatry*, 37, 194–201.

Morey, L. C. (1991). *The Personality Assessment Inventory*. Odessa, FL: Psychological Assessment Resources.

Morey, L. C. (2007a). *The Personality Assessment Inventory-Adolescent*. Lutz, FL: Psychological Assessment Resources.

Morey, L. C. (2007b). *The Personality Assessment Inventory-Adolescent professional manual*. Lutz, FL: Psychological Assessment Resources.

Muris, P., Merckelbach, H., Ollendick, T., King, N., & Bogie, N. (2002). Three traditional and three new childhood anxiety questionnaires: Their reliability and validity in a normal adolescent sample. *Behaviour Research and Therapy*, 40, 753–772.

National Institute of Mental Health. (1997). *The National Institute of Mental Health Diagnostic Interview Schedule for Children-Fourth Edition*. New York: Author.

National Institute of Mental Health Diagnostic Interview Schedule for Children (n.d.). Retrieved July 13, 2009 from http://chipts.ucla.edu/assessment/pdf/assessments/discforth-eweb.pdf

Olason, D. T., Sighvatsson, M. B., & Smari, J. (2004). Psychometric properties of the Multidimensional Anxiety Scale for Children (MASC) among Icelandic schoolchildren. *Scandinavian Journal of Psychology*, 45, 429–436.

Ollendick, T. H. (1983). Reliability and validity of the revised Fear Survey Schedule for Children (FSSC-R). *Behavior Research and Therapy*, 21, 685–692.

Ollendick, T. H., King, N. J., & Frary, R. B. (1989). Fears in children and adolescents: Reliability and generalizability across gender, age, and nationality. *Behavior Research and Therapy*, 27, 19–26.

Ollendick, T. H., Matson, J. L., & Helsel, W. J. (1985). Fears in children and adolescents: Normative data. *Behavior Research and Therapy*, 23, 465–467.

Ollendick, T. H., Öst, L.G., Reuterskiöld, L., Costa, N., Cederlund, R., Sirbu, C., et al. (2009). One-session treatment of specific phobias in youth: A randomized clinical train in the United States and Sweden. *Journal of Consulting and Clinical Psychology*, 77, 504–516.

Orvaschel, H. (1995). *Schedule for Affective Disorders and Schizophrenia for School-Age Children—Epidemiologic Version 5* (K-SADA-E-5). Ft. Lauderdale, FL: Nova Southeastern University.

Orvaschel, H. (2006). Structured and semistructured interviews. In M. Hersen (Ed.) *Clinician's handbook of child behavioral assessment* (pp. 159–179). Burlington, MA: Elsevier Academic Press.

Paget, K. D., & Reynolds, C. R. (1984). Dimensions, levels and reliabilities on the Revised Children's Manifest Anxiety Scale with learning disabled children. *Journal of Learning Disabilities, 17*, 137–141.

Piers, E. V. (2002). *Piers-Harris Self-Concept Scale* (2nd ed.). Los Angeles, CA: Western Psychological Services.

Poznanski, E. O., Cook, S. C., & Carroll, B. J. (1979). A depression rating scale for children. *Pediatrics, 64*, 442–450.

Poznanski, E. O., & Mokros, H. B. (1996). *Children's Depression and Rating Scale-Revised.* Los Angeles, CA: Western Psychological Services.

Poznanski, E. O., & Mokros, H. B. (2005). *Children's Depression and Rating Scale-Revised manual.* Los Angeles, CA: Western Psychological Services.

Reich, W. (2000). Diagnostic Interview for Children and Adolescents (DICA). *Journal of the American Academy of Child and Adolescent Psychiatry, 39*, 59–66.

Reich, W., Cottler, L., McCallum, K., Corwin, D., & VanEerdewegh, M. (1995). Computerized interviews as a method of assessing psychopathology in children. *Comprehensive Psychiatry, 36*, 40–45.

Reich, W., Welner, Z., & Herjanic, B. (1997). *Diagnostic Interview for Children and Adolescents-IV Windows Version.* Toronto: Multi-Health Systems.

Reuterskiöld, L., Öst, L. G., & Ollendick, T. (2008). Exploring child and parent factors in the diagnostic agreement on the anxiety disorders interview schedule. *Journal of Psychopathology and Behavioral Assessment, 30*, 279–290.

Reynolds, C. R., & Kamphaus, R. W. (1992). *The Behavior Assessment System for Children.* Circle Pines, MN: AGS.

Reynolds, C. R., & Kamphaus, R. W. (2004a). *The Behavior Assessment System for Children* (2nd ed.). Circle Pines, MN: American Guidance Service.

Reynolds, C. R., & Kamphaus, R. W. (2004b). *The Behavior Assessment System for Children* (2nd ed.) *manual.* Circle Pines, MN: American Guidance Service.

Reynolds, C. R., & Kamphaus, R. W. (2005). *The Behavior Assessment System for Children* (2nd ed.): *Manual supplement for the Self-Report of Personality-Interviewl.* Circle Pines, MN: American Guidance Service.

Reynolds, C. R., & Livingston, R. B. (2010). *Children's Measure of Obsessive-Compulsive Symptoms.* Los Angeles: Western Psychological Services.

Reynolds, C. R., & Richmond, B. O. (1978). What I Think and Feel: A revised measure of children's manifest anxiety. *Journal of Abnormal Child Psychology, 6*, 271–280.

Reynolds, C. R., & Richmond, B. O. (1979). Factor structure and construct validity of What I Think and Feel: The Revised Children's Manifest Anxiety Scale. *Journal of Personality Assessment, 43*, 281–283.

Reynolds, C. R., & Richmond, B. O. (1985). *Revised Children's Manifest Anxiety Scale manual.* Los Angeles: Western Psychological Services.

Reynolds, C. R., & Richmond, B. O. (2008a). *Revised Children's Manifest Anxiety Scale, Second Edition.* Los Angeles: Western Psychological Services.

Reynolds, C. R., & Richmond, B. O. (2008b). *Revised Children's Manifest Anxiety Scale, Second Edition manual.* Los Angeles: Western Psychological Services.

Reynolds, W. M. (1986). *Reynolds Adolescent Depression Scale.* Odessa, FL: Psychological Assessment Resources.

Reynolds, W. M. (1989). *Reynolds Child Depression Scale: Professional manual.* Lutz, FL: Psychological Assessment Resources.

Reynolds, W. M. (1992). The study of internalizing disorders in children and adolescents. In W. M. Reynolds (Ed.), *Internalizing disorders in children and adolescents* (pp. 1–18). New York: Wiley.

Reynolds, W. M. (1998a). *Adolescent Psychopathology Scale.* Lutz, FL: Psychological Assessment Resources.

Reynolds, W. M. (1998b). *Adolescent Psychopathology Scale: Administration and interpretation manual.* Lutz, FL: Psychological Assessment Resources.

Reynolds, W. M. (1998c). *Adolescent Psychopathology Scale: Psychometric and technical manual.* Lutz, FL: Psychological Assessment Resources.

Reynolds, W. M. (2002a). *The Reynolds Adolescent Depression Scale-Second Edition.* Lutz, FL: Psychological Assessment Resources.

Reynolds, W. M. (2002b). *The Reynolds Adolescent Depression Scale-Second Edition manual.* Lutz, FL: Psychological Assessment Resources.

Reynolds, W. M. (2003). *Reynolds Bully Victimization Scales for Schools.* San Antonio, TX: Harcourt Assessments.

Reynolds, W. M. (2006). Depression. In M. Hersen (Eds.), *Clinician's handbook of child behavioral assessment* (pp. 291–311). Burlington, MA: Elsevier Academic Press.

Reynolds, W. M. (2010a). *Reynolds Child Depression Scale-2nd Edition.* Lutz, FL: Psychological Assessment Resources.

Reynolds, W. M. (2010b). *Reynolds Child Depression Scale-2nd Edition and Short Form Professional manual.* Lutz, FL: Psychological Assessment Resources.

Reynolds, W. M. (2010c). *Reynolds Child Depression Scale-2nd Edition: Short Form.* Lutz, FL: Psychological Assessment Resources.

Rinaldo, J. C. B., & Baer, R. A. (2003). Incremental validity of the MMPI-A content scales in the prediction of self-reported symptoms. *Journal of Personality Assessment, 80*, 309–318.

Riskind, J. H., Beck, A. T., Brown, G., & Steer, R. A. (1987). Taking the measure of anxiety and depression: Validity of reconstructed Hamilton scales. *Journal of Nervous and Mental Disease, 175*, 474–479.

Rowe, E. W. (2003). The Minnesota Multiphasic Personality Inventory-Adolescent. In C. R. Reynolds & R. W. Kamphaus (Eds.), *Handbook of psychological & educational assessment of children: Personality, behavior, and context* (2nd ed., pp. 368–386). New York: Guilford Press.

Rynn, M. A., Barber, J. P., Khalid-Khan, S., Siqueland, L., Dembiski, M., McCarthy, K. S., et al. (2006). The psychometric properties of the MASC in a pediatric psychiatric sample. *Journal of Anxiety Disorders, 20*, 139–157.

Sanders, D. E. (1996). *The Internalizing Symptoms Scale for Children: A validity study with urban, African-American, seriously emotionally disturbed and regular education students.* Unpublished doctoral dissertation, James Madison University, Harrisonburg, VA.

Scherer, M. W., & Nakamura, C. Y. (1968). A Fear Survey Schedule for Children (FSS-FC): A factor analytic comparison with manifest anxiety (CMAS). *Behavior Research and Therapy, 6*, 173–182.

Schniering, C. A., Hudson, J. L., & Rapee, R. M. (2000). Issues in the diagnosis and assessment of anxiety disorders in children and adolescents. *Clinical Psychology Review, 20,* 453–478.

Scholwinski, E., & Reynolds, C. R. (1985). Dimensions of anxiety among high IQ children. *Gifted Child Quarterly, 29,* 125–130.

Shaffer, D., Fisher, P., Lucas, C., Dulcan, M. K., & Schwab-Stone, M. E. (2000). NIMH Diagnostic Interview Schedule for Children Version IV (NIMH DISC-IV): Description, differences from previous versions, and reliability of some common diagnoses. *Journal of the American Academy of Child and Adolescent Psychiatry,39,* 28–38.

Shapiro, E. S., & Heick, P. F. (2004). School psychologist assessment practices in the evaluation of students referred for social/behavioral/emotional problems. *Psychology in the Schools, 41,* 551–561.

Shore, G. N., & Rapport, M. D. (1998). The Fear Survey Schedule for Children—Revised (FSSC-HI): Ethnocultural variations in children's fearfulness. *Journal of Anxiety Disorders, 12,* 437–461.

Silverman, W. K., & Albano, A. M. (1996). *Anxiety Disorders Interview Schedule for DSM IV.* Boulder, CO: Graywind Publications.

Silverman, W. K., Saavedra, L. M., & Pina, A. A. (2001). Test-retest reliability of anxiety symptoms and diagnoses with the Anxiety Disorders Interview Schedule for DSM-IV child and parent versions. *Journal of the American Academy of* Child *and* Adolescent Psychiatry, *40,* 937–944.

Spenciner, L. (2003). Test Review: Social Phobia & Anxiety Inventory for Children. In B. S. Plake & J. C. Impara (Eds.), *The fifteenth mental measurements yearbook* [Electronic version]. Retrieved July 30, 2009 from the Buros Institute's Test Reviews Online website: http://www.unl.edu/buros.

Spielberger, C. D. (1973). *The State-Trait Anxiety Inventory for Children.* Palo Alto, CA: Consulting Psychologists Press.

Spielberger, C. D. (1983). *The State-Trait Anxiety Inventory.* Palo Alto, CA: Consulting Psychologists Press.

Steketee, G., Chambliss, D. L., Tran, G. Q., Worden, H., & Gillis, M. M. (1996). Behavioral avoidance test for obsessive compulsive disorder. *Behaviour Research and Therapy, 34,* 73–83.

Stovall, D. L. (2001). Test Review of the Children's Depression and Rating Scale-Revised. In B.S. Plake & J. C. Impara (Eds.), *The fourteenth mental measurements yearbook* [Electronic version]. Retrieved July 2, 2009 from the Buros Institute's Test Reviews Online website: http://www.unl.edu/buros.

Svensson, L., & Ost, L. (1999). Fears in Swedish children: A normative study of the Fear Survey Schedule for Children-Revised. *Scandinavian Journal of Behaviour Therapy, 28,* 23–36.

Tinsley, B. W. (2004). Concurrent validity of the Clinical Assessment of Depression with the Reynolds Adolescent Depression Scale. Master's thesis, Western Kentucky University, Bowling Green.

Turner, S. M., Beidel, D. C., & Costello, A. (1987). Psychopathology in the offspring of anxiety disorders patients. *Journal of Consulting and Clinical Psychology, 55,* 229–235.

Turner, S. M., Beidel, D. C., Dancu, C. V., & Stanley, M. A. (1989). An empirically derived inventory to measure social fears and anxiety: The Social Phobia and Anxiety Inventory. *Psychological Assessment: A Journal of Consulting and Clinical Psychology, 1,* 35–40.

Ulloa, R. E., Ortiz, S., Higuera, F., Nogales, I., Fresán, A., Apiquian, R., et al. (2006). Estudio de fiabilidad interevaluador de la versión en español de la entrevista Schedule for Affective Disorders and Schizophrenia for School-Age Children—Present and Lifetime version (K-SADS-PL). *Actas Españolas De Psiquiatría, 34,* 36–40.

Valiente, R., Sandin, B., Chorot, P., & Tabar, A. (2002). Gender differences in prevalence and intensity of fears in a sample of children and adolescents: Data based on the FSSC-R. *Revista de Psicopatologia y Psicologia Clinica, 7,* 103–113.

Walk, R. D. (1956). Self ratings of fear in a fear-invoking situation. *Journal of Abnormal Psychology, 52,* 171–178.

Warren, W. L. (1994). *Revised Hamilton Rating Scale for Depression.* Los Angeles, CA: Western Psychological Services.

Watson, D., & Clark, L. A. (1984). Negative affectivity: The disposition to experience aversive emotional states. *Psychological Bulletin, 96,* 465–490.

Watson, T. S. (2005). Test review of the Achenbach System of Empirically Based Assessment. In R. A. Spies & B. S. Plake (Eds.), *The sixteenth mental measurements yearbook* [Electronic version]. Retrieved August 4, 2009 from the Buros Institute's Test Reviews Online website: http://www.unl.edu/buros.

Woodruff- Borden, J., & Leyfer, O. T. (2006). Anxiety and fear. In M. Hersen (Ed.), *Clinician's handbook of child behavioral assessment* (pp. 267–289). Burlington, MA: Elsevier Academic Press.

World Health Organization. (1992). *International classification of diseases and related health problems* (10th ed.). Geneva, Switzerland: Author.

Methods of Assessing Academic Achievement

Michelle A. Drefs, Tanya Beran, *and* Meghann Fior

Abstract

Academic assessment is a complex and intricate process owing to the various factors that need to be taken into consideration. Within this chapter, an overview is provided of the skills and knowledge areas that are typically viewed as essential to successful reading, writing, and mathematics achievement. Moreover, additional factors that are important to examine in explaining poor academic achievement are reviewed. Attention is given to more recent work linking various neuropsychological processes (e.g., executive functions, memory) to academic performance. The goal of this chapter is to provide a framework of the skills, knowledge, and cognitive processes that are essential to reading, writing, and mathematics achievement. It is the intent that this framework will assist the reader in making important decisions regarding methods of academic assessment and, relatedly, appropriate areas to target for Intervention.

Key Words: academic assessment, reading, writing, mathematics

The assessment of academic achievement has been of longstanding interest within the field of psychology. Along with cognitive and personality tests, academic assessments have long been considered a core component of psychological assessment (Halpern, 1960). At the same time, the attention and thoroughness given to the assessment of academic skills within the extant psychological assessment literature has lacked in comparison to that given to the assessment of such latent traits as cognition (Kamphaus, 2009). In particular, achievement testing has traditionally been addressed primarily within the field of education, serving as only a minor footnote within the psychology literature. Academic testing when completed by psychologists has tended to focus on large-scale standardized measures that provide an indication of one's status, progress, or accomplishments in relation to others, whereas detailed assessment of specific academic skills and knowledge has more commonly been viewed as

falling within the domain of classroom and special education teachers.

Interest in the measurement of academic achievement has heightened over the past number of years, however, owing to several factors. Among these are the increased emphasis placed on teacher and school accountability (Rury-Smith, 2001) and greater adoption of response-to-intervention (RTI) practices (e.g., universal screening and progress monitoring). Relatedly, considerable research has amassed to support the importance of the assessment and intervention for learning difficulties during the early grades. Young children with less developed skills in reading and mathematics, for example, are at-risk for continuing to underperform and struggle academically throughout their schooling without adequate assessment, intervention, and support (Duncan et al., 2007; Jordan, Kaplan, Ramineni, & Locuniak, 2009; Judge & Bell, 2011; Romano, Babchishin, Pagani, & Kohen, 2010; Vellutino, Scanlon, Small,

& Fanuele, 2006). Identifying early learning difficulties and providing appropriate remediation requires the assessment of specific academic skills and subskills. Also contributing to the increased attention on academic achievement are recent advances with respect to the tests and assessment procedures used. Academic assessments have long been used to identify *how* a child is performing, relative to other students or a set criterion. Contemporary methods and approaches to achievement testing are beginning to be developed that help to better understand *why* a child is performing at a particular level and, consequently, how best to intervene.

Within this chapter we provide an overview of what is currently known regarding the essential skills, knowledge, and cognitive processes important to consider in the assessment of academic achievement. At the outset, defining what is entailed in achievement testing appears to be a relatively simple task. Simply stated, achievement testing involves the assessment of an individual's understanding of information and proficiency with specific skills in accordance with established learning objectives within a specific academic domain (e.g., reading, writing, and mathematics) (Ebel & Frisbie, 1986) and/or in relation to other students. A distinction that is commonly made is between measures of academic achievement and measures of general abilities, such as intelligence, memory, and spatial skills. In fact, a significant discrepancy between an individual's performance on ability versus achievement tests has long served as an indicator of a specific learning disability (see Gridley & Roid, 1998). While the ability-achievement discrepancy model of diagnosis has been heavily criticized, the model is representative of the contrasts that have been and continue to be drawn between achievement and ability testing. Achievement testing is generally presumed to measure a domain of skills or knowledge that can be fully articulated and described (e.g., single-digit addition and subtraction) and that can be impacted by teaching and schooling. In contrast, ability measures are viewed as underlying traits that cannot be directly observed and, in general, are believed to be less amenable to intervention (Kamphaus, 2009).

In reality, such ability-achievement distinctions are overly simplistic. Ability and achievement are better viewed along a continuum (Hogan, 2007) or as interrelated skills and processes that are coordinated in optimal academic performance (Busse, Berninger, Smith, & Hildebrand, 2001). For example, the task of reading requires the execution of learned letter-sound correspondence skills (decoding), as well

as the recruitment of more general comprehension skills. Among the cognitive factors that have been identified as integral to an individual's ability to achieve academically are attention, memory, language skills, processing speed, and intelligence (see Alloway, Gathercole, Adams, Willis, Eaglen, & Lamont, 2005; Berg, 2008; Bull, Espy, & Wiebe, 2008; Monette, Bigras, & Guay, 2011; Park, 2011; von Aster & Shalev, 2007). Such capacities determine not only the rate and extent of learning, but also influence an individual's ability to successfully demonstrate the knowledge he or she possesses. As such, the assessment of academic achievement requires consideration of both domain-specific (e.g., decoding) and domain-general (e.g., attention, memory) capacities.

Aside from knowledge-based skills and neuropsychological factors, a comprehensive assessment of academic achievement must also give consideration to a number of individual (e.g., motivation, self-efficacy, behavior), educational (e.g., teacher-student relationship, instructional practices, teacher knowledge), and broader contextual (e.g., parent-child interactions, attitudes towards education) factors (Berninger & Hooper, 1993; Blevins-Knabe & Musun-Miller, 1996; Klibanoff, Levine, Huttenlocher, Vasilyeva, & Hedges, 2006; LeFevre et al. 2009; Ma, 1999). Of these, educational factors have garnered increased attention as of recent. In adopting response-to-intervention practices, practitioners are being encouraged to examine the quality of instruction, the breadth, pacing, and sequencing of the curriculum, and the school environment (e.g., classroom rules, school discipline policies) as possible factors impacting student academic performance (Upah, 2008). Mutlidirectional relationships exist between these various factors, resulting in both direct and indirect influences on student achievement. Using modeling methods, for example, Ellefsen and Beran (2007) found children's behaviours in terms of conscientiousness, homework completion, conduct, and attention to be directly related to academic achievement, whereas family factors were significant, albeit more distal factors. Related factors involved may also include a family history of particular academic problems, limited exposure to the language the child is learning in, and limited educational history. Consideration also needs to be given to the developmental aspects of academic achievement, with some academic problems resolving with time and others remaining more persistent (Geary, Hamson, & Hoard, 2000). Moreover, the hierarchical nature of academic learning, with later skills building upon and extending earlier skills, can result in the demonstration of varying skill levels across an individual's development. Comorbid conditions, such as attention deficit hyperactivity disorder (ADHD) and conduct disorder (CD), also factor into understanding a child's current level of academic performance (American Psychological Association, 2000; Klein & Mannuzza, 2000; Kooistra, Crawford, Dewey, Cantell, & Kaplan, 2005). Best practice entails an examination of these multiple processes and factors.

When determining what approach to take towards academic assessment, it is also imperative to identify the purpose for conducting the assessment. In general, academic achievement is used to evaluate: (a) overall achievement, (b) student growth, and/or (c) specific strengths and weaknesses in and across content domains. Once ascertained, such information is used for a variety of purposes, including screening, assisting with eligibility decisions and diagnoses, and informing the planning, design, and evaluation of educational interventions and individualized instructional plans (American Educational Research Association, American Psychological Association, & National Council on Measurement in Education, AERA, APA, NCME, 1999; Rury-Smith, 2001). The results can also be more broadly used to evaluate the quality and effectiveness of instruction and educational programming, as is often the case with system-wide testing programs. The amount and complexity of assessment data required are linked to the purpose for which they are being collected. Screening and program evaluation tend to require less comprehensive and involved procedures and fewer sources of information than is required for eligibility and intervention decisions (AERA, APA, & NCME). Clearly, academic assessment is a more complex and intricate process than it may at first appear.

The remainder of this chapter will focus on outlining specific areas that should be examined in the assessment of academic abilities, particularly as they relate to informing instructional practices. Certain delimitations exist with respect to the scope of this chapter that require discussion at the onset. First, this chapter is organized in accordance with the three most commonly assessed academic areas of reading, writing, and mathematics. Acknowledgement is given, however, to the importance of assessing content knowledge and skills in curricular areas, such as language arts, science, and history, as well as vocational areas particularly in the later elementary, middle, and high school grades (McLoughlin & Lewis, 2008).

Second, this chapter is not intended to be a comprehensive review of all relevant academic achievement instruments and methods. Given that there are more achievement tests than all other types of tests combined (Hogan, 2007), this should be a welcome relief to the reader. Rather, the intent is to provide a framework by which the reader can subsequently review and consider the adoption of various instruments and methods. Examples are also provided in the Appendix of assessment instruments that fit within the proposed framework. While these examples are primarily from standardized tests due to their prominent use within the field and familiarity amongst most readers, the skills and processes detailed within this chapter can readily be assessed through various formal and informal academic measures and approaches. As well, the reader should remain cognizant while reviewing this chapter that a comprehensive assessment of academic ability requires the additional consideration and attention to the full range of individual, educational, and broader contextual factors, as noted above.

Reading Assessment

Of the various academic skills, reading skills have undoubtedly received the majority of attention. This is perhaps owing to the significant contributions reading offers to learning and achievement across all subject areas as well as to successful functioning within society. It is generally acknowledged that reading is a complex cognitive activity, with successful reading involving the ability to identify words in text, know their meaning, connect represented ideas to prior knowledge, and retain this information long enough to comprehend the intention of the author. That is, requisite in the reading task is both the ability to successfully recognize the printed words on the page and the ability to make sense of those words. This section begins with a focus on core skills required in both decoding and reading comprehension. In particular, we discuss phonological awareness, which has received considerable attention in the research and is supported by many empirical findings. Three other important skills, orthographic awareness, morphological awareness, and linguistic comprehension, will also be discussed as will other skills that have received more recent attention. Finally, considerations and methods of assessing these various reading skills are discussed.

Core Processes: Decoding and Comprehension

Most researchers who have studied reading development agree that mastery of phonological awareness is critical (Adams, 1990; Bradley & Bryant, 1983). Phonological awareness entails "an understanding of the different ways that oral language can be divided into smaller components and manipulated" (Chard & Dickson, 1999, p. 261). Moving from larger to smaller speech units, this includes dividing sentences into words, (e.g., Billy / really / likes / to / sing), words into syllables (e.g., /real/, /ly/), onset-rime units (e.g., /s/ and /ing/), and individual phonemes (e.g., /s/, /i/, /ŋ/). It relies, in part, on an individual's ability to attend to the intonation, stress, and timing of speech. Individuals who have strong phonological awareness are readily able to rhyme words, segment words into syllables or individual sounds, omit sounds in the beginning, middle, and end of words, and substitute or blend sounds to form new words. This ability to distinguish and manipulate various parts of language is an important requisite skill in connecting oral sounds to written letters. Referred to as alphabetic knowledge, this awareness that certain names and sounds are associated with printed letters or combinations of letters allows an individual to begin to decode or "sound out" words (Reading & Deuren, 2007).

Successful readers also create and store visual representations of whole words, letters, or letter clusters (e.g., prefixes, suffixes; Apel, 2009; Berninger, 1990). Once formed, these visual mental representations permit the rapid recognition and decoding of words, in absence of sounding out. An example here is the preschool child who can readily recognize his or her own name and can visually distinguish it from similar looking words. Such representations are based on an orthographic awareness, "a specific understanding or knowledge of the rules and patterns that govern how individuals represent words in print" (Apel, Wilson-Fowler, Brimo, & Perrin, 2011, para. 5). For example, a pseudoword such as "blark" appears more plausible than a word "zjke" based on stored mental representations of commonly occurring letter combinations. Although it has been less examined, morphological awareness is another linguistic skill that has been linked to reading achievement (Apel et al., 2011; Berninger, Abbott, Nagy, & Carlisle, 2010). It refers to an understanding of the units of meaning within words (root words, compound words, prefixes, suffixes) and the relations between them (e.g., word derivations; Apel et al., 2011). Morphological awareness permits, for example, an individual to identify the difference between a "bicycle" and a "tricycle" due to knowledge of how the prefixes "bi" and "tri" contribute to the meaning of a word.

Together, these three metalinguistic factors (phonological awareness, orthographic awareness, morphological awareness) help foster reading development, although it is important to consider their relative influence. While prominence is often given to phonological awareness, all three kinds of linguistic awareness have been found to be important developments during the primary grades (Berninger et al., 2010) and to be associated with word-level reading at later grades (Roman, Kirby, Parrila, Wade-Woolley, & Deacon, 2009). Combined, it appears that the coordination of phonological, orthographic, and morphological awareness is required at both the initial stages of reading acquisition and throughout its development in order to optimize reading achievement.

Although necessary, word-level literacy skills are not sufficient for effective reading. As stated earlier, reading comprehension is also a key component of the reading process and is viewed by some as the "essence of reading" (Durkin, 1993, p. 4–1). Beyond deciphering the literal meaning of the passage, reading comprehension also refers to the higher-level processes in which an individual interprets, evaluates, synthesizes, infers, predicts, critically analyzes text, and considers alternative interpretations (Klinger, 2004; McLoughlin & Lewis, 2008).

According to the *simple view of reading* (Hoover & Gough, 1990), reading comprehension is the result of an interaction between decoding skills (i.e. word-level reading ability) and accurate linguistic comprehension. As such, reading comprehension relies heavily on the mastery of the word-level reading skills of phonological, orthographic, and morphological awareness, particularly at the younger ages when children are first learning to read (Betjemann et al., 2008). In terms of linguistic comprehension, successful reading relies on the ability to make meaning from and interpret language. It is viewed as a multidimensional construct involving awareness and interpretation of oral sounds, focused attention, and active participation (James, 1984). It is commonly assessed through listening comprehension tasks in which information is presented orally. This skill, in combination with decoding, has been found to be significantly related to reading comprehension (Hoover & Tunmer, 1993, see also Høien-Tengesdal, 2010).

Core Processes: Not So Simple View of Reading

More recent research has identified a number of additional skills and cognitive processes that account for variance in both reading comprehension and decoding. Among the most commonly identified are: vocabulary, fluency, naming speed, and working memory. An unresolved question is to whether these additional candidate skills are best subsumed within the simple view of reading model (e.g., vocabulary viewed as a subskill of language comprehension, see also Vellutino, Tunmer, Jaccard, & Chen's (2007) Convergent Skills Model of Reading Development) or whether they constitute distinctive components (see Pressley et al., 2009). Although this remains a debated area, there is accumulating evidence to support a *not-so-simple view of reading* in which these wider range of factors need to be considered as determinants of reading ability. In other words, although necessary, decoding and linguistic awareness may not be sufficient for effective reading (Blachman, 2000; National Reading Panel, 2000; Snow, Burns, & Griffin, 1998). In support of a less simple view of reading are, for example, longitudinal and factor analytic studies in which a number of factors have been found to account for variance in reading comprehension above that explained by either decoding or linguistic comprehension (e.g., Conners, 2009). Interventions targeting such candidate factors have also proven effective in improving reading comprehension (e.g., fluency interventions as reviewed by the National Reading Panel, 2000). It is also the case that individuals can have deficits in reading comprehension despite intact decoding and listening comprehension skills (e.g., Georgiou, Das, & Hayward, 2009). The importance of these additional factors may be greater in explaining individual differences in comprehension skills within the higher grades, as individuals become more proficient readers and text complexity increases, and within populations with more intransient reading problems (e.g., reading disabilities).

Of these additional skills, vocabulary has consistently been identified as an important factor in reading achievement. Vocabulary refers to knowledge of words and their corresponding meanings (Verhoeven & Perfetti, 2011). It has been found to be strongly associated with reading comprehension and also, albeit somewhat weaker, with decoding skills (Ouellette & Beers, 2010; Verhoeven, van Leeuw, Vermeer, 2011). With respect to the latter, a rich vocabulary is believed to aid in the successful identification of common words and helps facilitate the decoding processes of new or novel words when encountered in print (Simmons & Kame'enui, 1998). In turn, greater fluency and skill in the reading process assists in the acquisition of new

vocabulary (for further discussion of the relationship between lexical growth and reading skills, see Verhoeven et al., 2011). Both vocabulary breadth (number of words one knows) and vocabulary depth (how well one knows attributes, functions, and features of words) are important to examine (Ouellette & Beers, 2010; Tannenbaum, Torgesen, & Wagner, 2006).

It also appears that it is not just the ability to decode that is important for reading comprehension but also the rate at which decoding occurs. Reading fluency occurs when children can quickly and automatically identify words (Snow et al., 1998). Words are read with speed, accuracy, and proper expression (prosody) (National Reading Panel, 2000). While there is some debate regarding the direction of causality between fluency and comprehension, a generally supported view is that fluent or automatic reading frees up attentional resources required for the higher level comprehension of text. In other words, if a child can decode with relative ease he has more resources to divert towards understanding what he is reading. In addition to the rapid recognition of words, fluency at both the syntactic level (adeptness in processing phrases and sentences as syntactic units) and passage level (appropriate expressiveness and consistent mood and tone) have been linked to increased reading comprehension (Klauda & Guthrie, 2008).

In examining the underlying mechanisms of reading difficulties, considerable evidence has also amassed to support rapid automatized naming (RAN) tasks as predictive of reading ability (e.g., Barth, Catts, & Anthony, 2008; Compton, 2003; Joshi & Aaron, 2000). Poor performance on both naming speed and phonological tasks has been linked to more severe and intractable reading problems (e.g., Frijters et al., 2011), commonly referred to by the term "double deficit" (Wolf & Bowers, 1999). The proportion of variance in decoding and reading comprehension accounted for by RAN tasks has been found to vary depending upon the type of RAN tasks and reading outcomes utilized (Høien-Tengesdal, 2010), developmental factors (Wagner et al., 1997), and degree of reading impairment (e.g., Lervåg, Bråten, & Hulme, 2009 report RAN as an important predictor for the poorest readers). What is not clear at this juncture is the underlying processes that are shared between rapid naming tasks and the reading process. Among the hypotheses to account for the RAN-reading relationship is the importance of processing abilities in reading (Wolf, 1991). For example, speed of processing may underlie differences in letter naming speed. Researchers have argued that when naming is quick, automatic, and effortless it requires little cognitive load and concentration (Logan, 1988; Stanovich, 1990). This allows the reader to focus attention more on extracting meaning than on decoding. Indeed, difficulty fully automatizing skills may explain reading deficits (Nicolson & Fawcett, 1990; for alternative hypotheses regarding RAN and reading skills, see de Jong, 2011 and Georgiou, Parrilla, Kirby, & Stephenson, 2008).

In addition to the above processes, both short-term and working memories are cognitive processes that have been widely studied and are associated with poor reading ability (Dahlin, 2010; Ni, Crain, & Shankweiler, 1996; Swanson, Zheng, & Jerman, 2009). Deficits in these areas have been found to persist over time (Swanson et al., 2009) and to contribute to reading abilities independent of other reading skills and processes (Crews & D'Amato, 2009). It may be that difficulty retaining word information in memory while extracting meaning interferes with fluency and comprehension (Bayliss, Jarrold, Baddeley, & Leigh; 2005). Additional executive functions associated with the concurrent processing, monitoring, and storage of information have also been implicated in the reading process, such as attentional/inhibitory control processes (Conners, 2009), planning (Das, Georgiou, & Janzen, 2008), visual attention span/memory (Bosse, Tainturier, & Valdois, 2007; Vellutino et al., 2007), and (verbal) IQ (Frijters et al., 2011; Hulslander, Olson, Willcutt, & Wadsworth, 2010).

At present, consensus is lacking with respect to the neuropsychological factors of most importance to the reading process and the exact mechanisms by which they exert their influence. What is known, however, is that the reading process is multicomponential and relies on the integration of multiple linguistic and cognitive factors. Difficulty in any one can affect the understanding of text. Although all of these skills play a necessary role in comprehension, not one guarantees that comprehension will occur (Pressley, 2000). Clearly, reading is complex. There are a variety of skills and cognitive processes that comprise reading ability, and it is each one, along with their coordination that influences reading performance (Berninger, Abbott, & Stage, 1999).

Assessment Methods and Considerations

As reading is one of the most assessed academic skills (McLoughlin & Lewis, 2008), the large variety of tests and methods available to assess reading should not be surprising. They range from single-word decoding tasks to a wide-range of comprehension tasks on passages of varying length. Typically, word-level measures are used to assess accuracy and fluency and consist of words or pseudowords presented in list or text form. They can also include tasks that focus on certain components of a word, such as in the rhyming, sound blending, or sound deletion tasks commonly used in the assessment of phonological skills. Word reading measures tend to be highly correlated with each other. In contrast, lower correlations found between measures of reading comprehension suggest that they tap a broader range of cognitive skills (Johnston, Barnes, & Descrochers, 2008). Among the more diverse methods for assessing reading comprehension are the reading of a passage followed by short-answer, multiple-choice, cloze tasks (fill in blanks of omitted words), interviews and questionnaires, anecdotal records and observations, oral retelling, freewriting, and think-aloud procedures (for a review of advantages and limitations of these methods, see Klinger, 2004). In selecting such measures, it is important to ensure that the items assess both concrete (direct) ideas (e.g., word meaning, recognition of relevant information) and abstract (higher-level) thinking (e.g., inferences, critical analysis; Svetina, Gorin, & Tatsuoka, 2011). Also, the reading material must be within an individual's instructional reading level (Klingner, 2004).

While the focus of reading assessment is typically limited to decoding (accuracy and fluency) and reading comprehension, the following areas, as outlined in the foregoing review, are also important to examine in the assessment of children's reading ability: letter identification (orthography), listening comprehension, vocabulary, speed of processing, working memory, general knowledge, verbal ability, and intelligence. Provided in the Appendix is a listing of subtests from four commonly used standardized test instruments that assess these various skills and cognitive processes. As mentioned at the onset of this chapter, this listing is not intended to be exhaustive. It does not include all of the subtests from the four selected instruments nor does it reflect the wide range of available formal and informal measures. Rather, the chart is intended to serve as a guide in helping to select appropriate measures required for the comprehensive assessment of academic abilities. Specifically, it provides examples of the types of measures that can be used to examine the broader range of skills, knowledge, and cognitive processes detailed in this chapter. The reader is encouraged to add to this framework additional formal and informal measures and procedures. Since many of the skills and processes used in the reading process are also used in other academic areas, the example measures provided for reading, writing, and mathematics have been compiled into one chart for ease of reference and comparison.

In assessing these areas it is also important to stress that attention should not only be given to the various skills and cognitive processes listed in the Appendix, but also more broadly to the interaction between the reader and text (McLoughlin & Lewis, 2008). There are many factors about the text itself that may influence how children read. For example, clues in the text passage can be used meaningfully and systematically as aids to reading. Also, the context and meaning of the passage can assist in interpreting text (Baumann, Font, Edwards, & Boland, 2005). Successful reading also requires metacognitive awareness and control of strategic processes in planning, monitoring, and evaluating what is being read. Skilled readers effectively deploy a number of reading strategies, dependent on the goals of reading and the nature of the text being read, to make reading meaningful (e.g., establishing a purpose for reading, making predictions) and to deal effectively with difficult text (Mokhtari & Reichard, 2002). Such areas are most readily assessed through informal measures, such as interviews, questionnaires, and think-aloud procedures, but can also be observed during the administration of more standardized measures. For example, observations of a student reading aloud can provide immediate information on fluency and decoding skills, but can also provide invaluable information on self-monitoring and self-correction (Westwood, 2009). While a thorough review of the use of informal measures is beyond the scope of this chapter, more detailed discussion is given to this topic within the remaining writing and mathematics sections.

Written Expression

Similar to reading, writing is a complex process involving the integration of multiple requisite skills and mental processes. Among these, for instance, are oral language and visual-motor integration skills, background and discourse (e.g., story elements) knowledge, ability to generate and organize ideas and adhere to established writing conventions (e.g., spelling, punctuation, grammar), and self-monitoring strategies (Espin, Weissenburger, & Benson, 2004; Olinghouse & Graham, 2009).

Writing well involves a complex progression from ideation through to execution of an organized, planful, and compelling discourse. While a number of models exist by which to examine the manner in which these various skills and processes contribute to the writing process (for review of models, see Wagner et al., 2011), a useful division from an assessment perspective is between transcription (e.g., spelling, handwriting) and text generation skills (e.g., writing down one's ideas) (Berninger, 2009). In alignment with this approach is the considerable attention that has been given to the trifecta areas of handwriting, spelling (transcription), and written composition (text generation) in terms of the instruction and assessment of written expression (Berninger, Garcia, & Abbott, 2009; Berninger et al., 2002). This section outlines the core writing skills and processes within this simplified division of transcription and text generation skills before attending to methods for assessment.

Core Processes: Transcription Skills

Transcription skills, such as spelling, handwriting, and keyboarding, are considered lower-order text production skills that support a student's ability to successfully produce written work. The majority of research in this area supports handwriting and spelling as differentially impacting upon the quality and length (compositional fluency) of the written product (Graham, Berninger, Abbott, Abbott, & Whitaker, 1997). A commonly accepted position is that impairments in the mechanics of writing (e.g., handwriting, spelling) limit the attentional and cognitive resources available for other aspects of the writing process, such as idea generation, planning, and revising (Graham, Harris, & Chorzempa, 2002). There is some evidence to suggest that these constraints are particularly relevant for the beginning writer (Graham et al., 1997), although researchers have found both spelling and handwriting to continue to exert influence on the writing process well into the high school years (Dockrell, Lindsay, & Connelly, 2009).

In general, it appears that spelling skills are a common area that differentiates poor writers from more capable writers. While highly correlated with reading abilities (Ehri, 1989; 2000), spelling remains a separate and distinct process. For example, students with unimpaired reading abilities can struggle with spelling (Treiman, 1993), and although less common, the reverse also holds true (Bryant & Bradley, 1980). Moreover, "deficits in spelling tend to be more tenacious [and can] persist long after reading deficits have been ameliorated" (Joshi & Carreker, 2009, p. 113). This is likely owing to the fact that whereas reading is a recognition task in which context and word features may be of assistance, spelling constitutes a more complex recall task that requires the accurate production and sequencing of each letter (Joshi & Carreker, 2009).

Due to its close association with reading, it is not surprising that spelling shares with reading many of the cognitive and linguistic skills aforementioned in the reading section. Of these, phonological, morphological, and orthographic word-level skills are considered salient skills underlying competent spelling ability (Joshi & Carreker, 2009; Silliman, Bahr, & Peters, 2006). Phonemic awareness, in particular, has been identified as playing a strong role in spelling development (across the grades—early to high school, first and second languages) (Sparks, Patton, Ganschow, Humbach, & Javorsky, 2008), with arguments made for spelling as a phonologically guided process (Treiman, 2004).

While phonological awareness is an important contributor to spelling skills, it is not sufficient. Spellers must also be able to effectively use certain strategies and memory skills. Knowledge of the morphemic structure of words and how to manipulate that structure allows students to correctly spell words (Apel et al., 2011; Carlisle, 1995), particularly those that do not appear to adhere to a regular phoneme-grapheme correspondence pattern (Mather, Wendling, & Roberts, 2009). For instance, students are aided in the spelling process when they know that the suffix /ed/ denotes past tense in words that have a final end sound of /d/, /t/, or /id/ as in called, helped, and waited (Leong, 2009).

Likewise, an understanding of the basic orthographic properties of language, the way in which spoken language is visually represented, is also needed in spelling (Abbott & Berninger, 1993; Berninger et al., 2002). These visual representations of words or parts of words are of particular importance given the alternative spellings for the same phoneme, such as the /long e/ phoneme which can be spelt as *e* (be), *ee* (meet), *ea* (leaf), or *y* (baby). Once formed, they allow for the rapid recognition or retrieval of whole words, letters, and letter clusters (e.g., prefixes, suffixes) and can assist in the production of spellings that are consistent with commonly occurring letter patterns (Apel, 2009). In summary, although the order of acquisition and developmental processes are not well understood, learning to spell consists of the amalgamation of phonological, morphological,

and orthographic knowledge (Joshi & Carreker, 2009).

Turning to handwriting, both legibility (quality) and speed have been shown to be important components of handwriting (Berninger, Yates, Cartwright, Rutberg, Remy, & Abbott, 1992; Rosenblum, Weiss, & Parush, 2003). Quality measures include examination of such areas as letter size and proportion, line quality (pressure consistency), consistency of slant and style (manuscript, cursive), spacing between letters and words, and general merit (Mather et al., 2009; Rosenblum et al., 2003). Measures of speed are concerned with the number of letters or amount of text that can be generated within a set time period (Rosenblum et al., 2003). Reviews of comparative studies identify a number of spatial, pressure, and temporal characteristics that differentiate the handwritten output of typical children from those with writing difficulties (Engel-Yeger, Nagauker-Yanuv, & Rosenblum, 2009; Rosenblum et al., 2003). The general consensus is that writing tends to be a slower process and result in less legible product for the struggling writer.

Processes that contribute to handwriting competency include both intrinsic and extrinsic factors (Feder & Majnemer, 2007). The former of these appear to be largely related to fine motor coordination and visual motor integration (Van Hartingsveldt, De Grott, Aarts, & Nijhuis-Van Der Sanden, 2011), with some support also for visual perception/memory and kinesthesia[1] (Feder & Majnemer, 2007). There is also some initial evidence to suggest that handwriting is dependent upon an underlying mental representation of written words and letters to hand movements. These areas have been assessed through orthographic coding tasks, successive finger movements, and the automatic retrieval and production of legible letters (Berninger, 2009; Graham et al., 1997). Extrinsic considerations relate to the environment and biomechanics, such as sitting position, distance from copy source, lighting, and writing volume (Feder & Majnemer, 2007). It may be the case that early deficits in psychomotor skills persist over time (Smits-Engelsman & Van Galen, 1997) or, as suggested by the work of Overvelde and Hulstijn (2011), notable improvements occur over the primary grades with a general stabilization of handwriting quality towards the beginning of the third grade. What is clear, however, is that poor handwriting skills contribute to decrements in both compositional fluency and quality (Graham et al., 1997).

Core Processes: Text Composition

A second area for consideration in writing assessment is that of text composition, the process of selecting and organizing words "to convey and represent ideas for a particular purpose" (Mather et al., 2009, p. 23). To write well is an involved process in which higher–order attentional and cognitive skills are recruited in the recursive processes of planning, text generation (i.e., translating ideas into written words), and reviewing and editing (Scott, 2009). Also required is requisite verbal and background knowledge (e.g., established semantic and syntactical components of a particular text structure; Mather et al., 2009), an understanding of the writing goals (e.g., audience), and ability to evaluate and revise goals and strategies as required to meet one's writing objectives (Butler, Elaschuk, & Poole, 2000). "Because proficiency in written expression requires the integration of multiple skills, the assessment of writing is a complex endeavour. In fact, some view writing assessment as the most difficult domain in achievement testing" (Espin et al., 2004, p. 55). This fact is further compounded by a lack of concreteness in determining what constitutes successful text composition. While one can readily determine if a child has successfully summed "4 plus 6" or correctly read the word "circumference," a more challenging task is to determine the quality of an individual's written work.

Text composition is commonly assessed by evaluating the written product or *what* has been produced, most typically in response to a writing prompt or picture. In general, struggling writers tend to write less and have more poorly constructed composition than their typically developing peers (Amato & Watkins, 2011). When examining the writing product, measures can be qualitative, "requiring an assessor to rate a text as a whole (holistic assessment) or to rate several traits of at a text (organization, sentence fluency, etc.) according to a predetermined rubric" (Scott, 2009, p. 359). Measures can also be quantitative, with common indicators being compositional fluency (amount written under specific time conditions), lexical diversity (number of different words used), and accuracy measures (percentage of grammatically correct sentences produced) (Scott, 2009).

In assessing the written product, the primary concern is with the linguistic characteristic of the text (e.g., the extent to which the text includes rich vocabulary, varied sentences, a clear message, etc.). Recent work in this area points to the importance of the assessment of text composition at several linguistic levels, namely at the word, sentence, and text/discourse levels (Scott, 2009; Wagner et al., 2011). These levels appear to be somewhat dependent on separate processes (Whitaker, Berninger, Johnston, & Swanson, 1994), with performance in any one area not entirely predictive of performance in the others (Berninger, Mizokawa, Bragg, Cartwright, & Yates, 1994). Word-level measures tend to provide an assessment of an individual's vocabulary size and control, e.g., lexical diversity (number of different words used), word length, density (content words to total words), and word choice (maturity, interest, and variety). The emphasis in sentence-level measures is on the extent to which a thought can be effectively expressed in terms of the syntax, grammatical accuracy, and semantic relations (Scott, 2009). Simple fluency measures (total number of words written) have consistently been found to be valid indicators of writing proficiency at the elementary level; with more limited support for the use of complex fluency and accuracy measures (e.g., number of correct word sequences) at higher grade levels (for review, see Weissenburger & Espin, 2005, see also Amato & Watkins, 2011). At the discourse-level, attention is given to determining how effectively the author translates ideas into words to achieve the purpose and effectively communicate to the intended audience. In general, discourse-level measures tend to demonstrate effects of age and language ability more consistently than do word- and sentence-level measures (Scott, 2009).

Breaking text composition down further, what is receiving increased attention is the *process* by which the text is developed. Here, attention is given to the types of cognitive activities in which a writer is engaged (e.g., planning ideas, formulating sentences, revising the text) and the extent to which movement between these activities is done in a recursive and ongoing process throughout the writing process (Berninger, Mizokawa, & Bragg, 1991). Additional constraints include a writer's content knowledge (specific topic knowledge) and knowledge of the specific writing organizational structures (e.g., discourse/genre forms, such as narrative, descriptive, compare/contrast, and persuasive; Beers & Nagy, 2011; see also McCutchen, 1986). Studies examining differences between adept and struggling writers have identified a number of differences with respect to these processes. When compared with adept writers, struggling writings tend to spend less productive and uninterrupted time on these tasks (Garcia & Fidalgo, 2008; Troia, 2007). They also demonstrated a less sophisticated understanding of the purpose and goals of writing, defining quality writing in terms of lower order skills (handwriting, spelling, neatness) as opposed to its communicative importance (Lin, Monroe, Brandon, & Troia, 2007).

While there is general agreement that skilled and struggling writers differ in terms of both the writing product and processes, less is known regarding the factors that contribute to these differences. Certainly, as earlier detailed, there is evidence to support the important contributions of lower order transcription skills, such as spelling and handwriting, to the writing process (Graham et al., 1997; Wagner et al., 2011). Language and linguistic functions also impact text generation and are broadly recruited throughout the writing process. These include vocabulary, phonological processing, orthographic coding, word finding, sentence syntax, language pragmatics, and reading capabilities (see Hooper et al., 2011). This association begins early, with expressive vocabulary and other oral language skills already linked with fluency and productivity measures at the kindergarten years (Kim, Otaiba, Puranik, Folson, Greulich, & Wagner, 2011). This should not be surprising given that, pragmatically speaking, writing is language production (Kellogg, 2001).

More recent attention has been given to the importance of executive functions as an early and consistent neuropsychological contributor to written language expression (Berninger, 2009; Hooper et al., 2011, see also Berninger, Garcia, & Abbott's (2009) Not-So-Simple View of Writing). These include self-regulation of attention, inhibitory control, and planning (Berninger et al., 2009; Hooper et al., 2011). Subsumed within this category are also the various memory functions that are central to a functional writing system. Long-term memory processes influence the writing process by allowing access to the aforementioned content and discourse-specific knowledge. Working memory allows such information along with the writing goals to be held in an active state during the planning, reviewing, and revising processes (Alamargot, Caporossi, Chesnet, & Ros, 2011; Kellogg, 2001).

Assessment Methods and Considerations

There are considerably fewer assessments available for the assessment of writing skills than for reading and mathematics; with the majority of those available constituting more informal measures (McLoughlin & Lewis, 2008). Considerable diversity also exists with respect to the types of writing tasks utilized. Spelling and handwriting are commonly assessed as isolated skills (e.g., spelling lists, figure and letter formations) or examined within larger writing samples. Joshi (1995) suggests the inclusion of spelling tests that consist of familiar words, those words an individual can read, in order to allow for the examination of more than phonological skills within spelling production.

Text composition measures can vary from the production of a single sentence to the generation of longer text with opportunities for planning and revision (Scott, 2009). It is also the case that writing tasks can consist of "machine-scored multiple-choice judgment tasks that do not require writing per se" (p. 359). A common approach to word- and sentence-level measures is the use of curriculum-based measures (CBMs) of writing. The most common of these measures include counts of the total number of words written (TW), number of correct word sequences (CWS), and number of correct minus incorrect word sequences (CWS-ICWS) (Weissenburger & Espin, 2005). These areas are also indirectly measured on standardized assessments that examine, for example, word choice and varied sentence structure (Scott, 2009).

For discourse-level measures involving the generation of longer passages, effort should be given to ensuring that the writing task is authentic with a clear purpose and audience (Calfee & Miller, 2007). This transforms the writing task from a "test" to a substantive "real life" exercise with value to the student. Opportunities for support and feedback allows for greater insight into how an individual transitions between the planning, formulating, and revising stages. While discourse-level text can also be evaluated through such quantitative measures as fluency and productivity, it is more common for a composition to be assessed through the aforementioned holistic and analytic approaches. Of these, the analytic approach is viewed as having greater diagnostic utility as it provides a breakdown of the various writing features (trait) that are required for communicative competence. Commonly examined areas include; ideas, organization, voice, word choice, sentence fluency, conventions, and presentation (Calfee & Miller, 2007). It should be noted that some criticism has been levied against available writing rubrics as lacking a strong basis in a theory or model of language or writing development (see Knoch, 2011). Finally, it is important to mention that the assessment of writing skills should also be conducted across a number of diverse genres (e.g., narrative, expository, compare-and-contrast) given that the organization and components may vary, thus resulting in differing cognitive demands (Kellogg, 2001). The reader is again referred to the Appendix for a listing of the various skills and processes detailed above and corresponding measures.

Mathematics Assessment

Compared to reading and writing, limited consensus exists regarding the componential parts or processes of mathematics knowledge. This is likely owing, in large part, to the fact that mathematics is a broad discipline encompassing a wide range of concepts, skills, and procedures. At the broadest level, learning math requires an understanding of knowledge and skills across a number of content areas or strands, such as algebra or geometry. Students may demonstrate deficits within one or more of these strands, or with respect to a set of competencies within a given strand (Geary, 2004; see also Dowker, 2005). Even a seemingly simply task, such as determining the sum of two numbers, requires a number of diverse cognitive skills. These can include retrieving arithmetic facts from semantic memory, applying arithmetic procedures to solve multi-digit numbers, accessing a cognitive system of arithmetic signs, and possessing a conceptual understanding of what addition means (see Denes & Signorini, 2001).

Further contributing to the lack of consensus regarding what constitutes mathematical knowledge and how best to assess such abilities is the limited research attention that has traditionally been given to this area in comparison to that given to the development and assessment of reading skills (Donlan, 1998; Wilson & Dehaene, 2007). In general, research into mathematics abilities has almost exclusively focused on the development and assessment of basic numerical competencies (counting, number comparisons) and computational skills of children (Geary, 2004). While we know a great deal about the types and sophistication of children's strategies in solving single-digit addition problems (Siegler & Shrager, 1984), for example, considerably less is known about the processes and skill that contribute to poor performance in geometry or algebra.

Against this backdrop, the following section outlines two complementary orientations to assessing mathematics. The first, based primarily on psychological and educational perspectives, focuses on a general framework in which *types* of mathematical thinking and skills are detailed. The second, arising more from the cognitive neuropsychology field, focuses on the *processes* which underlie mathematical cognition. Methods of assessing these various math skills are also discussed.

Core Skills: Types of Mathematical Knowledge

As stated, the assessment of mathematics achievement at the broadest level is concerned with a student's current level of skills and abilities across content and domain areas. According to the National Council of Teachers of Mathematics (NCTM; 2000) these areas include: number and operations, algebra, geometry, measurement, and data analysis and probability. General consideration is given to ensuring that a child can demonstrate those skills and abilities that are in line with the curricular objectives for a particular grade level. An individual's level of mathematical development can be examined in terms of mastery of broad skills areas (e.g., arithmetic operations) or further examined in terms of more discrete skills and competencies (e.g., single-digit addition, double-digit addition). Given that math learning is generally considered a developmental process, in which higher-level mathematics skills and knowledge are predicated on the successful acquisition of rudimentary abilities (Duncan et al., 2007), central here is the determination and assessment of mathematical proficiency within a hierarchical sequence, as outlined within a curriculum resource or the research literature.

Another distinction that is commonly made for both assessment and intervention purposes is between an individual's procedural and conceptual knowledge (Burns, 2011). Procedural knowledge is defined as *knowing how* in terms of specific sequences, steps, or rules required for solving problems (e.g., the FOIL method to multiply polynomials). It is not only a student's ability to successfully execute a particular procedure, but the assessment of strategy selection and efficiency which can vary as a result of individual factors (e.g., age, cognitive processes, arithmetic skills) and problem features (e.g., format, problem type) (Imbo & Vandierendonck, 2007; Lemaire & Callies, 2009). While most students tend to employ a variety of strategies, children with math disabilities may be more limited in their range and flexible use of appropriate strategies (Ostad, 1997). Conceptual knowledge, in contrast, is an individual's *knowing why* in terms of implicitly or explicitly understanding the meaning of mathematical principles, facts, or procedures (e.g., understanding the FOIL method in terms of the distributive and commutative rules used to distribute the terms from one of the polynomials being multiplied to the other) (Rittle-Johnson & Siegler, 1998; Rittle-Johnson, Siegler, & Alibali, 2001).

While procedural and conceptual knowledge comprise the two most commonly identified types of mathematical knowledge, a number of additional types of mathematical knowledge have been proposed. A comprehensive psychological framework advanced by Byrnes (2007), for example, identifies three additional types of mathematical competencies: declarative knowledge, estimation skills, and ability to graphically depict and model mathematical relationships and outcomes. The former of these areas, declarative knowledge, is defined as an extensive storehouse of math knowledge, inclusive of basic number facts (e.g., 8 X 8 = 64) and more general mathematics information (e.g., number of sides in a triangle). A related skill, math fluency has also been linked to math achievement and refers to the "fast, accurate, and effortless computation with basic operations as well as appropriate and flexible application" (Jordan & Levine, 2009, p. 63).

When these various types of math knowledge are examined, areas of deficit may be identified in one or more of these areas. For those with math disabilities, the research supports impairments in fact retrieval and calculation fluency (Chong & Siegel, 1998; Jordan & Levine, 2009; Mabbot & Bisanz, 2008) and differences in retrieval strategy usage, rate, and accuracy (e.g., Geary, Hoard, Byrd-Craven, & DeSoto, 2004; Wu et al., 2008). Such weaknesses in basic arithmetic knowledge and computation skill may in turn impair the development of conceptual structures needed for advanced mathematics learning (Passolunghi, 2011), although conceptual deficits have not been found to be a constant feature of math disabilities (see Mabbott & Bisanz, 2008).

Core Processes: Not So Simple View of Mathematics

In contrast to the types of mathematical knowledge detailed above, a number of models have emerged primarily from the cognitive neuropsychology field that detail the brain structures and processes that underlie numerical and mathematical cognition (see Dehaene & Cohen, 1995; McCloskey, Caramazza, & Basili, 1985). One of the most influential of these, the triple-code theory, asserts mathematical knowledge as being influenced by linguistic, quantitative, and spatial processes

(Dehaene & Cohen, 1995; Dehaene, Piazza, Pinel, & Cohen, 2003). The application of this model to children has identified links between children's success on a range of mathematical outcomes with measures of linguistic (vocabulary and phonological processing), quantitative (rapid recognition of small number sets) and spatial attention processes (LeFevre et al., 2010). The research in this area remains tentative largely due to the relatively restrictive focus on arithmetic skills and impairments within adult populations. However, what is emerging is a cursory listing of core skills and processes in mathematics that is similar to those detailed earlier in the area of reading. Of these, number sense (supported by the core quantity system within Dehanene's model) has received heightened research interest and attention as of late.

Number sense refers to an awareness of what number means and the relationship between numbers (Malofeeva, Day, Saco, Young, & Ciancio, 2004). Children who have a well-developed number sense are able to count, compare quantities, estimate, do simple mental-computations, and use number flexibly (Politylo, White, & Marcotte, 2011). Children with less well-developed number sense than their same-aged peers by grade one are at risk of experiencing serious delays and performing below their peers through their schooling (Case & Griffin, 1990; Griffin, 2004; Griffin, Case, & Capodilupo, 1995; Griffin, Case, & Siegler, 1994; see also Jordan, 1995). Additional arguments have been made for the links between the obtainment of number sense and children's self-confidence and low anxiety in mathematics performance (Malofeeva et al., 2004). In general, it appears that number sense is one potential source of deficit for children who are experience difficulties in mathematics learning (Geary, 2010). In fact, Gersten and Chard (1999) draw an analogous comparison between phonemic awareness in reading and number sense in mathematics.

As with reading and writing, a number of additional cognitive processes have been identified as explanatory of differences in math achievement. Of these are measures of fluency (e.g., Methe, Hintze, & Floyd, 2008), rapid naming (e.g., Lago & DiPerna, 2010), processing speed (Bull & Johnston, 1997), visual spatial memory (e.g., Bull, Espy, & Wiebe, 2008), working memory (e.g., Fuchs, Geary, Compton, Fuchs, Hamlett, & Bryant, 2010; Wu et al., 2008), executive attention (e.g., LeFevre et al., 2013), and inhibitory processes (e.g., Passolunghi, 2011). It seems that "doing" mathematics, such as calculations and problem solving, requires involvement of the executive functions in the representation and manipulation of information and the inhibition of irrelevant associations. In alignment with this view, the retrieval errors commonly observed among children with math learning difficulties are not viewed as simply a storage-retrieval problem, but rather may be contributed to more general cognitive deficits, such as difficulties in inhibiting irrelevant number associations (Geary, Hoard, Byrd-Craven, Nugent, & Numtee, 2007). Geary et al. found that the number and extent of cognitive deficits is greatest for children with the most pervasive and severe math difficulties, although subtle differences in a more limited number of processes were also found for low achieving students. While our understandings of the contributions of cognitive functions to math achievement are still fairly modest, there is evidence to suggest that such domain-general processes may differentially impact the acquisition and growth of certain types of mathematical knowing (e.g., fluency versus procedural). For example, recent work by LeFevre and colleagues (2013) supports executive attention as playing a larger role in the initial acquisition of novel procedures as opposed to the execution of well-learned procedures. In sum, it appears that there are a number of underlying skills and cognitive processes that contribute in diverse ways to mathematical competence.

Methods of Math Assessment

As demonstrated in the foregoing review, there is less consensus and less presently known regarding key areas to examine in the assessment of children's mathematical abilities. It should not be surprising to the reader, therefore, to know that there is limited correspondence between the areas of mathematical knowledge detailed above and the types of tasks included within contemporary measures. The majority of assessment items have been designed to measure mastery of specific skills and mathematical abilities. Those that do so for a wide range of skills and across different mathematics strands (e.g., number and operations, algebra, geometry, measurement) are referred to as survey or diagnostic instruments (e.g., KeyMath-3; Connolly, 2007). While diagnostic instruments have not been included in the Appendix, selection of such tests should be done with attention given to the range of math content areas assessed and the number and type of items within each strand.

The correspondence between other types of mathematical knowledge and assessment subscales and headings may be somewhat obscure. That is, many of the available math instruments are not organized in terms of procedural, conceptual, and declarative knowledge (although fluency is a commonly assessed area). Rather, mathematical tasks are routinely organized within standardized measures in accordance with the broad headings of mathematical concepts, numerical operations/computation, application, and problem solving (Taylor, 2009). It is thus necessary to make determination as to how and the extent to which these knowledge types are assessed on various instruments. Dowker (1998), for example, extends the procedural-conceptual distinction as akin to the numerical facility and mathematical reasoning distinction commonly made on many standardized assessment instruments. In support of this comparison is the typical assessment of procedural knowledge through computational tasks (e.g., exact calculation, written problems, forced retrieval), with conceptual knowledge more often assessed through novel or applied tasks (e.g., approximate arithmetic, place value, calculations principles, story problems; see Jordan, Mulhern, & Wylie, 2009).

Finally, it should be noted that measures associated with some of the outlined neuropsychological processes (e.g., number sense) remain largely restricted to the research arena. Although additional instruments and methods are forthcoming (e.g., REMA, Clements et al., 2008) and items can be selected from larger batteries to assess particular competencies (e.g., quantity comparison and estimation tasks as indicators of early number sense), the instruments available to practitioners at this juncture remains limited. Again, the Appendix is provided to assist the reader in identifying measures that correspond to the skills and processes identified above as contributing to math achievement.

Echoing similar discussions in the preceding reading and writing sections, ascertaining a child's level of mathematical understanding and best informing instructional activities additionally requires attention to informal measures. Returning to the procedural and conceptual distinction, determining the extent of a student's mathematical understandings often requires extension beyond standardized measures to the use of informal techniques. That is, a response of "54 + 28 = 82" is not sufficient to conclude that a student has procedural proficiency in regrouping. Rather, observation of and discussion with the student with respect to the manner in which the problem was solved is required in identifying a student's level of conceptual and procedural knowledge. While of importance in the assessment of any academic area, informal techniques are essential in the assessment of mathematics given the wide range of steps, strategies, and thought processes that undergird both successful and unsuccessful responses.

Two informal assessment techniques that are widely used as part of a mathematics assessment are *error analysis* and *clinical interviewing*. With error analysis, the goal is to, first, identify if there is a pattern to an individual's incorrect responses and to, second, determine if such errors are due to systematic misunderstandings (McLoughlin & Lewis, 2008). Error analysis requires a sufficient number of items to permit the identification of an error pattern and subsequent classification of the type of errors being made. Within the math clinical interview, students are encouraged to "talk through" the processes they use while completing math tasks, either during or following task completion. When students are provided with manipulatives (i.e., coins, base-ten blocks, calculator, paper and pencil) greater insight can be gained regarding the individual's mathematical thinking, in addition to broader strategy approaches, attitudes about math, and perseverance. Both these techniques require substantive mathematics knowledge on behalf of the examiner to ensure a correct analysis and assessment of mathematical thinking (Fleischner & Manheimer, 1997).

Conclusion

Academic assessment is a complex and intricate process. Within this chapter we provided an overview of the skills, knowledge, and cognitive processes that are currently viewed as important contributors to academic achievement with the goal being to better inform academic assessment as well as intervention practices. A general direction that was taken in writing this chapter was to give less attention to the domain-general versus domain-specific distinctions that are often made within the literature. It is likely the case that many of the neuropsychological factors discussed may more broadly exert influence on learning and academic achievement (Fuchs et al., 2010). We share the view of Bull et al. (2008), however, that a "good estimate of a child's ability to learn and hence their future academic success" requires a combination of knowledge-based plus cognitive measures (p. 225). Awareness of cognitive limitations allows for modifications to be made to learning activities that reduce the cognitive demands and permits more targeted interventions to be delivered.

In review of the outlined skills, knowledge, and processes it is clear that significant advances have been made over the last 20 years with respect to our knowledge of and ability to assess those factors that contribute to both typical and atypical academic development. It is also the case, however, that research, particularly with respect to neuropsychological correlates, remains in its infancy. While a considerable amount is known about processes involved in the reading process, considerably less is known in the areas of writing and mathematics. Moreover, across all academic areas, continued work is needed to better explicate the specific neuropsychological processes of influence and the mechanisms by which they exert such influence. At present, moderate to strong correlations between assessment tasks and more global measures of academic achievement appear sufficient for their inclusion within academic models and theories, in absence of a clear understanding of what constructs are being measured by such tasks. An example of this is the rapid automatized naming (RAN) tasks in which debate continues as to whether the underlying processes involve phonological processing, general or more specific processing speed skills, response inhibition, or other as of yet indeterminate processes (Savage, Pillay, & Melidona, 2007). In other words, while evidence continues to accumulate regarding which neuropsychological factors influence performance on a variety of academic tasks, considerably less is known about the exact mechanisms or manner of the influence. It is likely that continued work in this area and refinement of assessment measures will reveal more nuanced relationships, with the various skills and processes contributing in both domain-general and domain-specific ways. Although continued research is needed to more fully understand and articulate such areas, this chapter serves as a roadmap based on the extant research in identifying essential areas to consider in the comprehensive and thorough examination of reading, writing, and math achievement.

Several cautionary notes are worth mentioning. It is generally acknowledged that insightful interpretation is dependent upon examination of interindividual differences in academic performance, as well as consideration for an individual's pattern of performance and processes used to arrive at a particular answer (Fiorello, Hale, & Snyder, 2006). Given that reading, writing, and mathematics are multicomponential, in terms of both the component parts (e.g., reading consists of word-level reading and comprehension) and diverse skills and processes required for successful performance, it is not uncommon to find asynchronous patterns of development within an academic domain. Jordan, Mulhern et al. (2009), for example, found typically achieving children to demonstrate marked variations in their learning trajectories across seven arithmetic tasks (e.g., exact calculation, story problems, and place value). As a greater number of factors are considered, it is possible that a greater number of discrepancies between such factors at the individual level will also be observed. In concert with examining the range and/or severity of discrepant performance within and across certain tasks, it is also important to examine whether such patterns of low achievement extend across successive academic years (Geary, 2004).

It is important to reiterate that the comprehensive assessment of academic achievement requires consideration of broader factors than were the focus of this chapter. In addition to both formal and informal tests, academic assessment should also include observing the student in and out of the classroom, interviewing the student, teacher, and parents, analyzing parent and teacher behavioural rating scales, reviewing work products and samples, as well as reviewing records for developmental, educational, and family history. These combined results, and their appropriate interpretation, provide a wealth of information about children's academic abilities. As mentioned at the onset of this chapter, a comprehensive and thorough academic assessment requires attention to a number of individual, educational, and broader contextual factors.

In writing this chapter, a decision was made to organize it along subject areas (in accordance with the three Rs), as is often the case in review and discussion of academic assessment. While helpful in highlighting skills and processes contributing to typical and atypical development within each academic area, such an approach attenuates the extent to which skills and processes common across subject areas are emphasized. For example, children with certain types of writing difficulties may also experience difficulties with such math specific writing skills as legible numeral writing and the visual-spatial placement of numerals during computation (Berninger, 2009). An alternative organizational approach that provides greater emphasis on common areas of deficits (e.g., orthographic coding) is to organize in terms of specific learning disabilities and hallmark phenotypes. For example, Berninger (2009) has categorized dyslexia as "a writing and reading disorder in which spelling is the persisting feature...and the gender differences are related to the writing problems rather than the reading problems" (p.75).

The reader interested in further examining specific phenotypes associated with such specific learning disabilities as Dysgraphia, Dyslexia, and Oral and Written Language Learning is referred to the works of Berninger and her colleagues (e.g., Berninger, 2009; Berninger & May, 2011).

Finally, it is important to return to the issue of the place of academic assessment within the broader context of psychology and psychological assessment. As mentioned in the introduction, academic assessment is often relegated to more minor status within psychological assessment. It should be evident in review of this chapter, however, that academic achievement is dependent on a complex interplay of domain-specific and domain-general skills and cognitive processes. As such, academic assessment requires more than a simple tally of the number of correct and incorrect responses to academic content questions. Rather, at the core of academic assessment is not only identification of areas of skill deficit, but also an exploration of the neuropsychological factors that are key to understanding an individual's performance and areas to target for intervention.

Note

1. "Proprioception/kinesthesia—'ability to discriminate position of body parts as well as amplitude and direction of their movements without visual or auditory cues" (Feder & Majnemer, 2007, p. 312)

References

Abbott, R., & Berninger, V. (1993). Structural equation modeling of relationships among developmental skills and writing skills in primary and intermediate grade writers. *Journal of Educational Psychology*, 85, 47–508. doi: 10.1037/0022–0663.85.3.478

Adams, M. (1990). *Beginning to read*. Cambridge, MA: MIT Press.

Alamargot, D., Caporossi, G., Chesnet, D., & Ros, C. (2011). What makes a skilled writer? Working memory and audience awareness during text composition. *Learning and Individual Differences*, 25(5), 505–516. doi:10.1016/j.lindif.2011.06.001

Alloway, T. P., Gathercole, S. E., Adams, A. M., Willis, C., Eaglen, R., & Lamont, E. (2005). Working memory and phonological awareness as predictors of progress towards early learning goals at school entry. *British Journal of Developmental psychology*, 23, 417–426. doi:10.1348/026151005X2680

Amato, J.M., & Watkins, M.W. (2011). The predictive validity of CBM writing indices for eight-grade students. *The Journal of Special Education*, 44, 195–204. doi: 10.1177/002246690 933351610.1177/0022466909333516

American Educational Research Association, American Psychological Association, & National Council on Measurement in Education. (1999). *Standards for educational and psychological testing*. Washington, DC: American Educational Research Association.

American Psychological Association. (2000). *Diagnostic and statistical manual of mental disorders* (4th ed., Text Revision). Washington, DC: Author.

Apel, K. (2009). The acquisition of mental orthographic representations for reading and spelling development. *Communication Disorders Quarterly, 31,* 42–52. doi: 10.1177/1525740108325553

Apel, K., Wilson-Fowler, B., Brimo, D., & Perrin, N. A. (2012). Metalinguistic contributions to reading and spelling in second and third grade students. *Reading and Writing: An Interdisciplinary Journal, 25,* 1283–1305.doi: 10.1007/s11145–011–9317–8

Barth, A. E., Catts, H. W., Anthony, J. C. (2008). The component skills underlying reading fluency in adolescent readers: a latent variable analysis. *Reading and Writing: An Interdisciplinary Journal, 22,* 567–590. doi: 10.1007/s11145–008–9125-y

Baumann, J. F., Font, G., Edwards, E. C., & Boland, E. (2005). Strategies for teaching middle-grade students to use word-part and context clues to expand reading vocabulary. In E. H. Hiebert & M. L. Kamil (Eds.), *Teaching and learning vocabulary: Bringing research to practice* (pp. 179–205). Mahwah, NJ, US: Lawrence Erlbaum.

Bayliss, D. M., Jarrold, C., Baddeley, A. D., & Leigh, E. (2005). Differential constraints on the working memory and reading abilities of individuals with learning difficulties and typically developing children. *Journal of Experimental Child Psychology, 92*(1), 76–99. doi:10.1016/j.jecp.2005.04.002

Beers, S. F., & Nagy, W. E. (2011). Writing development in four genres from grades three to seven: syntactic complexity and genre differentiation. *Reading and Writing: An Interdisciplinary Journal, 24,* 183–202. doi: 10.1007/s11145–010–9264–9

Berg, D. H. (2008). Working memory and arithmetic calculation in children: The contributory roles of processing speed, short-term memory, and reading. *Journal of Educational Psychology, 96,* 699–713. doi:10.1016/j.jecp.2007.12.002

Berninger, V. (1990). Multiple orthographic codes: key to alternative instructional methodologies for developing orthographic-phonological connections underlying word identification. *School Psychology Review, 19,* 518–533.

Berninger, V. W. (2007). *The Process Assessment of the Learner— Diagnostic Assessment for Reading and Writing (PAL-II).* San Antonio, TX: NCS Pearson.

Berninger, V. W. (2009). Highlights of programmatic, interdisciplinary research on writing. *Learning Disabilities Research & Practice, 24*(2), 69–80. doi: 10.1111/j.1540–5826.2009.00281.x

Berninger, V. W., Abbott, R. D., Nagy, W., & Carlisle, J. (2010). Growth in phonological, orthographic, and morphological awareness in grades 1 to 6. *Journal of Psycholinguistic Research, 39,* 141–163. doi: 10.1007/s10936–009–9130–6

Berninger, V. W., Abbott, R., & Stage, S. (1999). *Educational and biological factors in preventing and treating dyslexia.* Society for Research in Child development, Albuquerque, NM.

Berninger, V. W., Garcia, N. P., & Abbott, R. D. (2009). Multiple processes that matter in writing instruction and assessment. In G. A. Troia (Ed.), *Instruction and assessment for struggling writers: Evidence-based practices* (pp. 15–50). New York, Guilford Press.

Berninger, V. W., & Hooper, S. R. (1993). Preventing and remediating writing disabilities: Interdisciplinary frameworks for assessment, consultation, and intervention. *School Psychology Review, 22,* 590–595.

Berninger, V. M., & May, M. O. (2011). Evidence-based diagnosis and treatment for specific learning disabilities involving impairments in written and/or oral language. *Journal of Learning Disabilities, 44*(2), 167–183. doi:10.1177/00222/94/039/189

Berninger, V. W., Mizokawa, D., & Bragg, R. (1991). Theory-based diagnosis and remediation of writing, *Journal of School Psychology, 29,* 57–79. doi:10.1016/0022–4405(91)90016-K

Berninger, V., Mizokawa, D., Bragg, R., Cartwright, A., & Yates, C. (1994). Intraindividual differences in levels of written language. *Reading and Writing Quarterly, 10,* 259–275. doi: 10.1080/1057356940100307

Berninger, V. W., Vaughan K., Abbott, R. D., Begay, K., Coleman, K. B., Curtin, G., Hawkins, J. M., & Graham, S. (2002). Teaching spelling and composition alone and together: Implications for the simple view of writing. *Journal of Educational Psychology, 94,* 291–304. doi: 10.1037/0022–0663.94.2.291

Berninger, V., Yates, C., Cartwright, A., Rutberg, J., Remy, E., & Abbott, R. (1992). Lower-level developmental skills in beginning writing. *Reading and Writing: An Interdisciplinary Journal, 4,* 257–280. doi: 10.1007/BF01027151

Betjemann, R. S., Willcutt, E. G., Olson, R. K., Keenan, J. M., DeFries, J. C., & Wadsworth, S. J. (2008). Word reading and reading comprehension: stability, overlap and independence. *Reading and Writing: An Interdisciplinary Journal, 21,* 539–558. doi: 10.1007/s11145–007–9076–8

Blachman, B. A. (2000). Phonological awareness. In M. L. Kamil, P. B. Mosenthal, P. D. Pearson & R. Barr (Eds.), *Handbook of reading research, Vol. III* (pp. 483–502). Mahwah, New Jersey: Lawrence Erlbaum Associates.

Blevins-Knabe, B., & Musun-Miller, L. (1996). Number use at home by children and their parents and its relationship to early mathematical performance. *Early Development and Parenting, 5*(1), 35–45. doi: 10.1002/(SICI)1099–0917(19 9603)5:1<35::AID-EDP113>3.0.CO;2–0

Bosse, M-L., Tainturier, M. J., & Valdois, S. (2007). Developmental dyslexia: The visual attention span deficit hypothesis. *Cognition, 104,* 198–230. doi:10.1016/j.cognition.2006.05.009

Bradley, L., & Bryant, P. E. (1983). Categorizing sounds and learning to read—a causal connection. *Nature, 310,* 21–43. doi: 10.1038/301419a0

Bryant, P., & Bradley, L. (1980). Why children sometimes write words which they do not read. In U. Frith (Ed.), *Cognitive processes in spelling* (pp. 353–370). London: Academic Press.

Bull, R., Espy, L., Wiebe, S. A. (2008). Short-term memory, working memory, and executive functioning in preschoolers: Longitudinal predictors of mathematical achievement at age 7 years. *Developmental Neuropsychology, 33,* 205–228. doi: 10.1080/87565640801982312

Bull, R., & Johnston, R. S. (1997). Children's arithmetical difficulties: Contributions from processing speed, item identification, and short-term memory. *Journal of Experimental Child Psychology, 65,* 1–24. doi: 10.1.1006/jecp.1996.2358

Burns, M. K. (2011). Matching math interventions to students' skill deficits: A preliminary investigation of a conceptual and procedural heuristic. *Assessment for Effective Intervention, 36,* 201–218. doi: 10.1177/1534508411413255

Busse, J., Berninger, V. W., Smith, D. R., & Hildebrand, D. (2001). Assessment for math talent and disability: A developmental model. In J. J. W. Andrews, D. H. Saklofske, &

H. L. Janzen (Eds.), *Handbook of psychoeducational assessment: Ability, achievement, and behaviour in children* (pp. 225–253). New York: Academic Press. Butler, D. L., Elaschuk, C. L., Poole, S. (2000). Promoting strategic writing by postsecondary students with learning disabilities: A report of three case studies. *Learning Disability Quartery, 23,* 196–213. Retrieved from http://www.jstor.org/stable/1511164.

Byrnes, J. P. (2007). Some ways in which neuroscientific research can be relevant to education. In D. Coch, K. W. Fischer, & G. Dawson (Eds.), *Human behavior, learning, and the developing brain: Typical development* (pp. 30–49). New York: Guilford Press.

Calfee, R. C., & Miller. R.G. (2007). Best practices in writing assessment. In S. Graham, C. A. MacArthur, & J. Fitzgerald (Eds.), *Best practices in writing instruction* (pp. 265–286). New York: Guilford Press.

Carlisle, J. F. (1995). Morphological awareness and early reading achievement. In L. Feldman (Ed.), *Morphological aspects of language processing* (pp. 54–78). Hillsdale, NJ: Lawrence Erlbaum.

Case, R., & Griffin, S. (1990). Child cognitive development: The role of central conceptual structures in the development of scientific and social thought. In C. A. Haver (Ed.), *Advances in psychology: Developmental psychology* (pp. 193–220). North Holland: Elsevier.

Chard, D. J., & Dickson, S. V. (1999). Phonological awareness: Instructional and assessment guidelines. *Intervention in School and Clinic, 34,* 261–270. doi: 10.1177/105345129903400502

Chong, S. L., & Siegel, L. S. (1998). Stability of computational deficits in math learning disability from second through fifth grades. *Developmental Neuropsychology, 33*(3), 300–317. doi: 10.1080/87565640801982387

Clements, D. H. Sarama, J. H., & Liu, Z. H. (2008). Development of a measure of early mathematics achievement using the Rasch model: the Research-Based Early Maths Assessment. *Educational Psychology, 28,* 456–482. doi: 10.1080/01443410701777272

Compton, D. L. (2003). Modeling the relationship between growth in rapid naming speed and growth in decoding skill in first-grade children. *Journal of Educational Psychology, 95,* 225–239.

Conners, F. A. (2009). Attentional control and the simple view of reading. *Reading and Writing: An Interdisciplinary Journal, 22,* 591–613. doi: 10.1007/s11145-008-9126-x

Connolly, A. J. (2007). *KeyMath-3 diagnostic assessment: Manual forms A and B.* Minneapolis, MN: Pearson.

Crews, K. J., & D'Amato, R. C. (2009). Subtyping children's reading disabilities using a comprehensive neuropsychological measures. *International Journal of Neuroscience, 119,* 1615–1639. doi: 10.1080/00207450802319960

Dahlin, K. I. E. (2010). Effects of working memory training on reading in children with special needs. *Reading and writing: An Interdisciplinary Journal, 24,* 479–491. doi: 10.1007/s11145-010-9238-y

Das, J.P., Georgiou, G., & Janzen, T. (2008). Influence of distal and proximal cognitive processes on word reading. Reading Psychology, *29,* 366–393. doi: 10.1080/02702710802153412

de Jong, P.F. (2011). What discrete and serial rapid automatized naming can reveal about reading. *Scientific Studies of Reading, 15,* 314–337. doi: 10.1080/10888438.2010.485624

Dehaene, S., & Cohen, L. (1995). Towards an anatomical and functional model of number processing. *Mathematical Cognition, 1,* 83–120.

Dehaene, S., Piazza, M., Pinel, P., & Cohen, L. (2003). Three parietal circuits for number processing. *Cognitive Neuropsychology, 20,* 487–506. Retrieved from http://www.tandf.co.uk/journals/pp/02643294.html

Denes, G., & Signorini, M. (2001). Door but not four and 4: A category specific transcoding deficit in a pure acalculic patient. *Cortex, 37,* 267–277. doi:10.1016/S0010–9452(08)70572–0

Dockrell, J. E., Lindsay, G., Connelly, V. (2009). The impact of specific language impairment on adolescents' written text. *Exceptional Children, 75*(4), 427–446.

Donlan, C. (1998). *The development of mathematical skills: Studies in developmental psychology.* Hove, East Sussex, UK: Psychology Press Ltd.

Dowker, A. (1998). Individual differences in normal arithmetical development. In C. D. (Ed.), *The development of mathematical skills* (pp. 275–302). Hove, East Sussex, UK: Psychology Press.

Dowker, A. (2005). *Individual difference in arithmetic.* Hove, UK: Psychology Press.

Duncan, G. J., Dowsett, C. J., Claessenes, A., Magnuson, K., Huston, A. C. Klebanow, P., Pagnai, L. S., Feinstein, L., Engel, M., Brooks-Gunn, J., Sexton, Ho., Duckworth, K., & Japel, C. (2007). School readiness and later achievement. *Developmental Psychology, 43*(6),1428–1446. doi: 10.1037/0012–1649.43.6.1428

Durkin, D. (1993). *Teaching them to read* (6th ed.). Boston, MA: Allyn & Bacon.

Ebel, R. L., & Frisbie, D. A. (1986). *Essentials of educational measurement* (4th ed.). Englewood Cliffs, NJ: Prentice Hall.

Ehri, L. (1989). The development of spelling knowledge and its role in reading acquisition and reading disabilities. *Journal of Learning Disabilities, 22,* 356–365. doi: 10.1177/002221948902200606

Ehri, L. C. (2000). Learning to read and learning to spell: Two sides of a coin. *Topics in Learning Disorders, 20,* 19–49.

Ellefsen, G., & Beran, T. N. (2007) Individuals, families, and achievement: A comprehensive model in a Canadian context. *Canadian Journal of School Psychology, 22*(2), 167–181. doi: 10–1177/0829573507304875

Engel-Yeger, B., Nagauker-Yanuv, L., Rosenblum, S. (2009). Handwriting performance, self-reports, and perceived self-efficacy among children with dysgraphia. *American Journal of Occupational Therapy, 63,* 182–192. doi:10.5014/ajot.63.2.182

Espin, C. A., Weissenburger, J. W., & Benson, B. J. (2004). Assessing the writing performance of students in special education. *Exceptionality, 12,* 55–66. doi: 10.1207/s15327035ex1201_5

Feder, K. P., & Majnemer, A. (2007). Handwriting development, competency, and intervention. *Developmental Medicine & Child Neurology, 49*(4), 312–317. doi:10.1111/j.1469–8749.2007.00312.x

Fiorello, C. A., Hale, J. B., & Snyder, L. E. (2006). Cognitive hypothesis testing and response to intervention for children with reading problems. *Psychology in Schools, 43,* 835–853. doi:10.1002/pits.20192. doi: 10.1002/pits.20192

Fleischner, J. E., & Manheimer, M. A. (1997). Math interventions for students with learning disabilities: Myths and realities. *School Psychology Review, 26* (3), 397–413. Retrieved from http://www.nasponline.org/publications/spr/sprmain.aspx

Frijters, J. C., Lovett, M. W., Steinbach, K. A., Wolf, M., Sevcik, R. A., & Morris, R. D. (2011). Neurocognitive predictors of reading outcomes for children with reading disabilities. *Journal of Learning Disabilities, 44*, 150–166. doi: 10.1177/0022219410391185

Fuchs, L. S., Geary, D. C., Compton, D. L., Fuchs, D., Hamlett, C. L., & Bryant, J. D. (2010). The contributions of numerosity and domain-general abilities to school readiness. *Child Development, 81*, 1520–1533. doi: 10.1111/j.1467–8624.2010.01489.x

García, J-N., & Fidalgo, R. (2008). Orchestration of writing processes and writing products: A comparison of sixth-grade students with and without learning disabilities. *Learning Disabilities: A Contemporary Journal, 6*(2), 77–98. Retrieved from http://www.ldworldwide.org/research/learning-disabilities-a-contemporary-journal

Geary, D. C. (2004). Mathematics and learning disabilities. *Journal of Learning Disabilities, 37,* 4–15.

Geary, D. C. (2010). Mathematical disabilities: Reflections on cognitive, neuropsychological, and genetic components. *Learning and Individual Differences, 20*, 130–133. doi:10.1016/j.lindif.2009.10.008

Geary, D. C., Hamson, C. O., & Hoard, M. K. (2000). Numerical and arithmetic cognition: A longitudinal study of process and concept deficits in children with learning disabilities. *Journal of Experimental Child Psychology, 77*, 236–263. doi:10.1006/jecp.2000.2561

Geary, D. C., Hoard, M. K., Byrd-Craven, J., & DeSoto, M. C. (2004) Strategy choices in simple and complex addition: Contributions of working memory and counting knowledge for children with mathematical disability. *Journal of Experimental Child Psychology, 88*, 121–151. doi: 10.1016/j.jecp.2004.03.002

Geary, D. C., Hoard, M. K., Byrd- Craven, J., Nugent, L., & Numtee, C. (2007). Cognitive mechanisms underlying achievement deficits in children with mathematical learning disability. *Child Development, 78*, 1343–1359. doi: 10.1111/j.1467–8624.2007.01069.x

Georgiou, G. K., Das, J.P., & Hayward, D. (2009). Revisiting the "simple view of reading" with a group of children with poor reading comprehension. *Journal of Learning Disabilities, 42*, 76–84. doi: 10.1177/0022219408326210

Georgiou, G.K., Parrilla, R., Kirby, J.R., & Stephenson, K. (2008). Rapid naming components and their relationship with phonological awareness, orthographic knowledge, speed of processing, and different reading outcomes. *Scientific Study of Reading, 12*, 325–330. doi: 10.1080/10888430802378518

Gersten, R., & Chard, D. (1999). Numbers sense: Rethinking arithmetic instruction for students with mathematical disabilities. *The Journal of Special Education, 33*, 18–28. doi: 10.1177/002246699903300102

Graham, S., Berninger, V., Abbott, R. D., Abbott, S., & Whitaker, D. (1997). The role of mechanics in composing of elementary school students: A new methodological approach. *Journal of Educational Psychology, 89,* 170–182. doi: 10.1037/0022–0663.89.1.170

Graham, S., Harris, K. R., & Chorzempa, B. F. (2002). Contribution of spelling instruction to the spelling, writing, and reading of poor spellers. *Journal of Educational Psychology, 94*, 669–686. doi: 10.1037/0022–0663.94.4.669

Gridley, B. E., & Roid, G. H. (1998). The use of the WISC-III with achievement tests. In A. Prifitera & D. Saklofske (Eds.), *WISC-III: Clinical use and interpretation: Scientist-practitioner perspectives* (pp. 249–288). San Diego, CA: Academic Press.

Griffin, S. (2004). Teaching number sense. *Educational Leadership, 61*(5), 39–43. Retrieved from http://www.ascd.org/publications/educational-leadership.aspx

Griffin, S., Case, R., Capodilupo, A. (1995). Teaching for understanding: The importance of the central conceptual structures in the elementary mathematics curriculum. In A. McKeough, J. Lupart, & A. Marini (Eds.), *Teaching for transfer: Fostering generalization in learning.* New Jersey: Lawrence Erlbaum Associates.

Griffin, S., Case, R., & Siegler, R. S. (1994). Rightstart: Providing the central conceptual prerequisites for first formal learning of arithmetic to students at risk for school failure. In K. McGilly (Ed.), *classroom lessons: Integrating cognitive theory* (pp. 25–49). Cambridge, MA: Bradford Books, MIT Press.

Halpern, F. (1960). The individual psychological examination. In M.G. Gottsengen & G. B. Gottsengen (Eds.), *Professional school psychology.* New York: Grune & Stratton.

Hogan, T. P. (2007). *Psychological testing: A practical introduction.* Hoboken, NJ: Wiley.

Høien-Tengesdal, I. (2010). Is the simple view of reading too simple? *Scandinavian Journal of Educational Research, 54*, 451–469. doi: 10.1080/00313831.2010.508914

Hooper, S. R., Costa, L-J., McBee, M., Anderson, K. L., Yerby, D. C., Knuth, S. B., & Childress, A. (2011). Concurrent and longitudinal neuropsychological contributors to written language expression in first and second grade students. *Reading and Writing: An Interdisciplinary Journal, 24*(2), 221–252. doi: 10.1007/s11145–010–9263-x

Hoover, W. A., & Gough, P. B. (1990). The simple view of reading. *Reading and Writing: An Interdisciplinary Journal (2)*, 127–160.

Hoover, W. A., & Tunmer, W. E. (1993). The components of reading. In G. B. Thompson, W. E. Tunmer, & T. Nicholson (Eds.), *Reading acquisition processes* (pp. 1–19). Clevedon, England: Multilingual Matters.

Hulslander, J., Olson, R. K., Willcutt, E. G., Wadsworth, S. J. (2010). Longitudinal Stability of Reading-Related Skills and Their Prediction of Reading Development, *Scientific Studies of Reading, 14*, 111–136. doi: 10.1080/10888431003604058

Imbo, I., & Vandierendonck, A. (2007). The development of strategy use in elementary school children: Working memory and individual difference. *Journal of Experimental Child Psychology, 96*, 284–309. doi:10.1016/j.jecp.2006.09.001

James, C. J. (1984). Are you listening: The practical components of listening comprehension. *Foreign Language Annals, 17* (2), 129–133. doi: 10.1111/j.1944–9720.1984.tb01719.x

Johnston, A. M., Barnes, M. A., Descrochers, A. (2008). Reading comprehension: Developmental processes, individual differences, and interventions. *Canadian Psychology, 49*, 125–132. doi: 10.1037/0708–5591.49.2.125

Jordan, N. C. (1995). Clinical assessment of mathematical disabilities: Adding up the research findings. *Learning Disabilities Research & Practice, 10*(1), 59–69. Retrieved from http://www.wiley.com/bw/journal.asp?ref=0938–8982

Jordan, N. C., Kaplan, D., Ramineni, C., & Locuniak, M. N. (2009). Early math matters: Kindergarten number competence and later mathematics outcomes. *Developmental Psychology, 45*(3), 850–867. doi: 10.1037/a0014939

Jordan, N. C., & Levine, S. C. (2009). Socioeconomic variation, number competence, and mathematics learning difficulties in young children. *Developmental Disabilities Research Reviews, 15*, 60–68. doi: 10.1002/ddrr.46

Jordan, J-A., Mulhern, G., & Wylie, J. (2009). Individual differences in trajectories of arithmetical development in typically achieving 5- to 7-year-olds. *Journal of Experimental Child Psychology, 103*, 455–468. doi:10.1016/j.jecp.2009.01.011

Joshi, R. M. (1995). Assessing reading and spelling skills. *School Psychology Review, 24*, 361–375.

Joshi, R. M., & Aaron, P. G. (2000). The component model of reading: Simple view of reading made a little more complex. *Reading Psychology, 21*, 85–97. doi: 10.1080/02702710050084428

Joshi, R. M., & Carreker, S. (2009). Spelling: Development, assessment, and instruction. In G. Reid (Ed.). *The Routledge companion to dyslexia* (pp. 113–125). New York: Routledge.

Judge, S., & Bell, S. M. (2011). Reading achievement trajectories for student with learning disabilities during the elementary school years. *Reading & Writing Quarterly, 27*, 153–178. doi: 10.1080/10573569.2011.532722

Kamphaus, R. W. (2009). Assessment of intelligence and achievement. In T. B. Gutkin & C. R. Reyonds (Eds), *The handbook of school psychology* (4th ed., pp. 230–229). Hoboken, NJ: Wiley.

Kellogg, R. T. (2001). Psychology of writing process. In N. J. Smelser (Ed.), *International encyclopedia of the social & behavioural sciences* (pp. 16629–16633). doi:10.1016/B0–08–043076–7/01562-X

Kim, Y-S., Otaiba, S. A., Puranik, C., Folson, J. S., Greulich, L., & Wagner, R. K. (2011). Componential skills of beginning writing: An exploratory study at the end of kindergarten. *Learning and Individual Differences, 21,* 517–525. doi: 10.1016/j.lindif.2011.06.004

Klauda, S. L., & Guthrie, J.T. (2008). Relationships of three components of reading fluency to reading comprehension. *Journal of Educational Psychology, 100*, 31–321. doi: 10.1037/0022–0663.100.2.310

Klein, R. G., & Mannuzza, S. (2000). In L. L. Greenhill (Ed.), Children with uncomplicated reading disorders grown up: A prospective follow-up into adulthood. *Learning disabilities: Implications for psychiatric treatment* (pp. 1–32). American Psychiatric Association Review of Psychiatry Series. Volume 19, number 5; Washington, D.C.: American Psychiatric Press.

Klibanoff R. S., Levine S. C., Huttenlocher J., Vasilyeva M., Hedges L. V. (2006). Preschool children's mathematical knowledge: The effect of teacher "math talk." *Developmental Psychology, 42*, 59–69. doi: 10.1037/0012–1649.42.1.59

Klingner, J.K. (2004). Assessing reading comprehension. *Assessment for Effective Intervention, 29*, 59–70. doi: 10.1177/073724770402900408

Knoch, U. (2011). Rating scales for diagnostic assessment of writing: What should they look like and where should the criteria come from? *Assessing Writing, 16*, 81–96. doi: 10.1016/j.asw.2011.02.003

Kooistra, L. Crawford, S., Dewey, D., Cantell, M., & Kaplan, B. J. (2005). Motor Correlates of ADHD: Contribution of Reading Disability and Oppositional Defiant Disorder. *Journal of Learning Disabilities, 38*(3), 195–206. doi:10.1177/00222194050380030201

Korkman, M., Kirk, U., & Kemp, S. (2007). *NEPSY-II: A developmental neuropsychological assessment*. San Antonio, TX: The Psychological Corporation.

Lago, R. M. & DiPerna, J. C. (2010). Number sense in kindergarten: A factor analytic study of the construct. *School Psychology Review, 39*(2), 164–180.

LeFevre, J-A., Berrigan, L., Vendetti, C., Kamawar, D., Bisanz, J., Skwarchuk, S-L., & Smith-Chant, B. (2013). The role of executive attention in the acquisition of mathematical skills for children in Grades 2 and 4. *Journal of Experimental Child Psychology, 114*, 243–261.

LeFevre, J-A., Fast, L., Skwarchuk, S-L., Smith-Chant, B. L., Bisanz, J., Kamawar, D., & Penner-Wilger, M. (2010). Pathways to mathematics: Longitudinal predictors of performance. *Child Development, 81*(6), 1753–1767. doi: 10.1111/j.1467–8624.2010.01508.x

LeFevre, J-A., Skwarchuk, S-L., Smith-Chant, B. L., Fast, L., Kamawar, D., & Bisanz, J. (2009). Home numeracy experiences and children's math performance in the early school years. *Canadian Journal of Behavioural Science, 41*(2), 55–66. doi: 10.1037/a0014532

Lemaire, P., & Callies, S. (2009). Children's strategies in complex arithmetic. *Journal of Experimental Child Psychology, 103*, 49–65. doi: 10.1016/j.jecp.2008.09.007

Leong, C. K. (2009). The role of inflectional morphology in Canadian children's word reading and spelling. *Elementary School Journal, 109,* 343–358. doi: 10.1086/593937

Lervåg, A., Bråten, I., & Hulme, C. (2009). The cognitive and linguistic foundations of early reading development: A Norwegian latent variable longitudinal study. *Developmental Psychology, 45*, 764–781. doi: 10.1037/a0014132

Logan, G. (1988). Toward an instance theory of automatization. *Psychological Review, 95*, 492–527. doi: 10.1037/0033–295X.95.4.492

Ma, X. (1999). A meta-analysis of the relationship between anxiety toward mathematics and achievement in mathematics. *Journal for Research in Mathematics Education, 30*(5), 520–40. doi: 10.2307/749772

Mabbott, D. J., & Bisanz, J. (2008). Computational skills, working memory, and conceptual knowledge in older children with mathematics learning disabilities. *Journal of Learning Disabilities, 41*, 15–28. doi: 10.1177/0022219407311003

Malofeeva, E., Day, J., Saco, X., Young, L., & Ciancio, D. (2004). Construction and evaluation of a number sense test with head start children. *Journal of Educational Psychology, 96* 648–659. doi: 10.1037/0022–0663.96.4.648

Mather, N., Wendling, B. J., & Roberts, R. (2009). *Writing assessment and instruction for students with learning disabilities*. San Francisco, CA: John Wiley & Sons.

McCloskey M., Caramazza, A., & Basili, A. (1985). Cognitive mechanisms in number processing and calculation: Evidence from dyscalculia. *Brain and Cognition, 4*, 171–196. doi:10.1016/0278–2626(85)90069–7

McCutchen, D. (1986). Domain knowledge and linguistic knowledge in the development of writing ability. *Journal of Memory and Language, 25*, 431–444.

McLoughlin, J. A., & Lewis, R. B. (2008). *Assessing students with special needs* (7th ed.). Upper Saddle River, NJ: Pearson.

Methe, S. A., Hintze, J. A., & Floyd, R. G. (2008). Validation and decision accuracy of early numeracy skill indicators. *School Psychology Review, 37*(3), 359–373. Retrieved from http://www.nasponline.org/publications/spr/sprmain.aspx

Mokhtari, K., & Reichard, C.A. (2002). Assessing students' metacognitive awareness of reading strategies.

Journal of educational Psychology, 94, 249–259. doi: 10.1037/0022–0663.94.2.249

Monette, S., Bigras, M., & Guay, M. C. (2011). The role of the executive functions in school achievement at the end of grade 1. *Journal of Experimental Child Psychology, 109,* 18–173. doi:10.1016/j.jecp.2011.01.008

National Council of Teachers of Mathematics. (2000). *Principles and standards for school mathematics.* Reston, VA: Author.

National Early Literacy Panel (NELP) (2008). Developing early literacy: Report of the National Early Literacy Panel. Washington, DC. Retrieved from http://lincs.ed.gov/publications/pdf/NELPSummary.pdf

National Reading Panel (2000). *Teaching children to read: An evidence based assessment of the scientific research literature on reading and its implications for reading instruction.* Washington, DC: National Institute of Child Health and Human Development.

Ni, W., Crain, S., & Shankweiler, D. (1996). Sidestepping garden paths: Assessing the contributions of syntax, semantics and plausibility in resolving ambiguities. *Language and Cognitive Processes, 11*(3), 283–334. doi: 10.1080/016909696387196

Nicolson, R., & Fawcett, A. (1990). Automaticity: A new framework for dyslexia research? *Cognition, 35*(2), 159–182. doi:10.1016/0010–0277(90)90013-A

Olinghouse, N. G., & Graham, S. (2009). The relationship between the discourse knowledge and writing performance of elementary-grade students. *Journal of Educational Psychology, 101,* 37–50. doi:10.1037/a0013462

Ostad, S. (1997). Developmental differences in addition strategies: A comparison of mathematically disabled and mathematically normal children. *British Journal of Educational Psychology, 67,* 345–357. doi:10.1111/j.2044–8279.1997.tb01249.x

Ouellette, G., & Beers, A. (2010). A not-so-simple view of reading: How oral vocabulary and visual-word recognition complicate the story. *Reading and Writing: An Interdisciplinary Journal, 23,* 189–208. doi: 10.1007/s11145–008–9159–1

Overvelde, A., & Hulstijn, W. (2011). Handwriting development in grade 2 and grade 3 primary school children with normal, at risk, or dysgraphic characteristics. *Research in Developmental Disabilities, 32,* 540–548. doi:10.1016/j.ridd.2010.12.027

Park, Y. (2011). How motivational constructs interact to predict elementary student performance: Examples from attitudes and self-concept in reading. *Learning and Individual Differences, 21,* 347–358. doi: 10.1016/j.lindif.2011.02.009

Passolunghi, M. C., (2011). Cognitive and emotional factors in children with mathematical learning disabilities. *International Journal of Disability, Development, and Education, 58,* 61–73. doi: 10.1080/1034912X.2011.54351

Pearson. (2009). *Wechsler Individual Achievement Test–III.* San Antonio, TX: Author.

Polityło, B., White, K., & Marcotte, A. M. (2011, Feburary). An investigation of the construct of number sense. Poster submitted to the National Association of School Psychologists (NASP), San Francisco, CA.

Pressley, M. (2000). What should comprehension instruction be the instruction of? In M. L. Karnil, P. B. Mosenthal, P. D. Pearson, & R. Barr (Eds), *Handbook of reading research* (Vol.III, pp. 545–562). Mahwah, NJ: Lawrence Erlbaum Associates.

Pressley, M., Duke, N. K., Fingeret, L., Park, Y, Reffitt, K., Mohan, L., et al. (2009). Working with struggling readers: Why we must go beyond the simple view of reading and visions of how it might be done. In T. B. Gutkin & C. R. Reynolds (Eds.). *Handbook of school psychology* (4th ed., pp. 522–568). Hoboken, NJ: Wiley.

Reading, S., & Deuren, D. V. (2007). Phonemic awareness: When and how much to teach? *Reading Research and Instruction, 46*(3), 267–286. doi: 10.1080/19388070709558471

Rittle-Johnson, B., & Siegler, R. S. (1998) The relationship between conceptual and procedural knowledge in learning mathematics: A review. In C. Dolan (Ed.), *The development of mathematical skills: Studies in developmental psychology* (pp. 75–110). Hove, East Sussex, UK: Psychology Press Ltd.

Rittle-Johnson, B., Siegler, R., & Alibali, M. W. (2001). Developing conceptual understanding and procedural skill in mathematics: An iterative process. *Journal of Educational Psychology, 93*(2), 346–362. doi: 10.1037/0022–0663.93.2.346

Roman, A. A., Kirby, J. R., Parrila, R. K., Wade-Woolley, L. & Deacon, S. H. (2009). Toward a comprehensive view of the skills involved in word reading in grades 4, 6, and 8. *Journal of Experimental Child Psychology, 102,* 96–113.

Romano, E., Babchishin, L., Pagani, L. S., & Kohen, D. (2010). School readiness and later achievement: Replication and extension using a nationwide Canadian survey. *Developmental Psychology, 46*(4), 995–1007. doi: 10.1037/a0018880

Rosenblum, S., Weiss, P. L., & Parush, S. (2003). Product and process evaluation of handwriting difficulties. *Educational Psychology Review, 15,* 41–81. doi: 10.1023/A:1021371425220

Rury-Smith, D. (2001). Wechsler Individual Achievement Test. In J. J. W. Andrews, D. H. Saklofske, & H. L. Janzen (Eds), *Handbook of psychoeducational assessment: Ability, achievement and behavior in children* (pp. 169–197). New York: Academic Press.

Savage, R., Pillay, V., & Melidona, S. (2007). Deconstructing rapid automatized naming: Component processes and the prediction of reading difficulties. *Learning and Individual Differences, 17*(2), 129–146. doi: 10.1016/j.lindif.2007.04.001

Scott, C. M. (2009). Language-based assessment of written expression. In G. A. Troia (Ed.), *Instruction and assessment for struggling writers: Evidence-based practices* (pp. 358–385). New York, Guilford Press.

Siegler, R. S., & Shrager, J. (1984). Strategy choice in addition and subtraction: How do children know what to do? In C. Sophian (Ed.), *Origins of cognitive skills* (pp. 229–293). Mahway, NJ: Erlbaum.

Silliman, E. R., Bahr, R. H., Peters, M. L. (2006). Spelling patterns in preadolescents with atypical language skills: Phonological, morphological, and orthographic factors. *Developmental Neuropsychology, 29,* 93–123. doi: 10.1207/s15326942dn2901_6

Simmons, D. C., & Kame'enui, E. J. (1998). *What reading research tells us about children with diverse learning needs: Bases and basics.* Mahwah, NL: Erlbaum.

Smits-Engelsman, B.C.M., & Van Galen, G. P. (1997). Dysgraphia in children: Lasting psychomotor deficiency or transient developmental delay. *Journal of Experimental Child Psychology, 67*(2), 164–184. doi:10.1006/jecp.1997.2400

Snow, C. E., Burns, M. S., & Griffin, P. (Eds.). (1998). *Preventing reading difficulties in young children.* Washington, DC: National Academy Press.

Sparks, R. L., Patton, J., Ganschow, L., Humbach, N., & Javorsky, J. (2008). Early first-language reading and spelling skills predict later second-language reading and spelling skills. *Journal of Educational Psychology*, *100*, 162–174. doi: 10.1037/0022–0663.100.1.162

Stanovich, K. E. (1990). Concepts in developmental theories of reading skill: Cognitive resources, automaticity, and modularity. *Developmental Review*, *10*, 72–100. doi:10.1016/0273–2297(90)90005-O

Svetina, D., Gorin, J. S., & Tatsuoka, K. K. (2011). Defining and comparing the reading comprehension construct: A cognitive-psychometric modeling approach. *International Journal of Testing*, *11*, 1–23. doi: 10.1080/15305058.2010.518261

Swanson, H. L., Zheng, Z., & Jerman, O. (2009). Working memory, short-term memory, and reading disabilities. *Journal of Learning Disabilities*, *42*, 260–287. doi: 10.1177/0022219409331958

Tannenbaum, K. R., Torgesen, J. K., & Wagner, R. K. (2006). Relationships between word knowledge and reading comprehension in third-grade children. *Scientific Studies of Reading*, *10*, 381–398. doi: 10.1207/s1532799xssr1004_2

Taylor, R. L. (2009). *Assessment of exceptional students: Educational and psychological procedures* (8th ed.). Upper Saddle River, NJ: Pearson.

Treiman, R. (2004). Phonology and spelling. T. Nunes & P. Bryant (Eds.), *Handbook of children's literacy* (pp. 31–42). Dordrecht, Netherlands: Kluwer.

Treiman, R. (1993). *Beginning to spell*. New York: Oxford University Press.

Troia, G. A. (2007). Reading in writing instruction: What we know and what we need to know. In M. Pressley, A. K. Billman, K. H. Perry, K. E. Reffitt, & J. M. Reynolds (Eds.), *Shaping literacy achievement: Research we have, research we need* (pp. 129–156). New York: Guildford Press.

Upah, K. R. F. (2008). Best practices in designing, implementing, and evaluating quality interventions. In A. Thomas & J. Grimes (Eds.), *Best practices in school psychology V* (Vols. 2, pp. 209–224). Bethesda, MD: National Association of School Psychologists.

Van Hartingsveldt, M. J., De Groot, M. J. M., Aarts, P. B. M., & Nijhuis-Van Der Sanden, M. W. G. (2011). Standardized tests of handwriting readiness: A systematic review of the literature. *Developmental Medicine & Child Neurology*, *53*(6), 506–515. doi:10.1111/j.1469–8749.2010.03895.x

Vellutino, F. R., Scanlon, D. M., Small, S., & Fanuele, D. P. (2006). Response to intervention as a vehicle for distinguishing between children with and without reading disabilities: Evidence for the role of kindergarten and first-grade interventions. *Journal of Learning Disabilities*, *39*, 157–169. doi:1 0.1177/00222194060390020401

Vellutino, F.R., Tunmer, W.E., Jaccard, J.J., & Chen, R. (2007). Components of Reading Ability: Multivariate Evidence for a Convergent Skills Model of Reading Development, *Scientific Studies of Reading*, *11*, 3–32. doi: 10.1080/10888430709336632

Verhoeven, L. & Perfetti, C.A. (2011). Introduction to this special issue: Vocabulary growth and reading skill. *Scientific Studies of Reading*, *15*, 1–7. doi: 10.1080/10888438.2011.536124

Verhoeven, L, van Leeuwe J., & Vermeer, A. (2011). Vocabulary growth and reading development across the elementary school years. *Scientific Studies of Reading*, *15*, 8–25. doi: 10.1080/10888438.2011.536125

von Aster, M. G., & Shalev, R. S. (2007). Number development and developmental dyscalculia. *Developmental Medicine & Child Neurology*, *49*, 868–873. doi:10.1111/j.1469–8749.2007.00868.x

Wagner, R. K., Puranik, C. S., Foorman, B., Foster, E., Wilson, L. G., Tschinkel, E., & Kantor, P. T. (2011). Modeling the development of written language. *Reading and Writing: An Interdisciplinary Journal*, *24*(2), 203–220. doi: 10.1007/s11145–010–9266–7

Wagner, R.K., Torgesen, J.K., Rashotte, C.A., Hecht, S.A., Barker, T.A., Burgess, S.P., et al. (1997) Changing relations between phonological processing abilities and word-level reading as children develop from beginning to skilled readers: A 5-year longitudinal study. *Developmental Psychology*, *33*, 468–479.

Weissenburger, J. W., & Espin, C. A. (2005). Curriculum-based measures of writing across grade levels. *Journal of School Psychology*, *43*, 153–169. doi:10.1016/j.jsp.2005.03.002

Westwood, P. (2009). Arguing the case for a simple view of literacy assessment. *Australian Journal of Learning Difficulties*, *14*, 3–15. doi: 10.1080/19404150902783401

Whitaker, D., Berninger, V., Johnston, J., & Swanson, L. (1994). Intraindividual differences in levels of language in intermediate grade writers: Implications for translation process. *Learning and Individual Differences*, *6*, 107–130. doi:10.1016/1041–6080(94)90016–7

Wilson, A. J., & Dehaene, S. (2007). Number sense and developmental dyscalculia. In D. Coch, G. Dawson, K. W. Fischer (Eds.), *Human behavior, learning, and the developing brain: Atypical development* (pp. 212–238). New York: Guilford Press

Wolf, M. (1991). Naming speed and reading: The contribution of the cognitive neurosciences. *Reading Research Quarterly*, *26*(2), 123–141. doi:10.2307/747978

Wolf, M., & Bowers, P. G. (1999). The double-deficit hypothesis for the developmental dyslexias. *Journal of Educational Psychology*, *91*, 415–439.

Woodcock, R. W., McCrew, K. S., & Mather, N. (2001). *Woodcock-Johnson III tests of achievement*. Itasca, IL: Riverdale.

Wu, S. S., Meyer, M. L., Maeda, U., Salimpoor, V., Tomiyama, S., Geary, D. C., & M enon, V. (2008). Standardized assessment and strategy use and working memory in early mental arithmetic performance. *Developmental Neuropsychology*, *33*, 365–393. doi: 10.10 80/87565640801982445

Chapter 23: Appendix

Selected subtests from four assessment instruments, the *Weschler Individual Achievement Test-III* (WIAT-III; Pearson, 2009), *Woodcock-Johnson III Tests of Achievement* (WJ-III ACH; Woodcock, McCrew, & Mather, 2001), *The Process Assessment of the Learner—Diagnostic Assessment* (PAL-II; Berninger, 2007) and the *NEPSY-II* (Korkman, Kirk, & Kemp, 2007), and their correspondence with core skills/cognitive processes that should be considered in the assessment of reading (R), writing (W), and mathematics (M).

Core Skills / Cognitive Processes & Example Methods of Assessment		Academic Areas		
Phonological Awareness Decoding				
WIAT-III	Pseudoword Decoding—read nonsense words	R	W	
WJ-III	Sound Awareness (Rhyming)—produce rhyming words	R	W	
PAL-II	Syllables- pronounce polysyllabic word with targeted syllable deleted	R	W	
Orthographic Awareness				
WJ-III	Spelling Sounds—spell using frequently occurring spelling patterns	R	W	
PAL-II	Receptive Coding—recognize letters /words from prior presented words	R	W	
Morphological Awareness				
PAL-II	Are They Related—determine if one word is derived from another	R	W	
Reading Comprehension				
WIAT-III	Reading Comprehension—read passages and answer questions	R		
WJ-III	Passage Comprehension—identify a key missing word from a passage	R		
Listening Comprehension				
WIAT-III	Listening Comprehension—listen to sentences/passages and respond to comprehension questions	R	W	
WJ-III	Understanding Directions—listen to instructions and follow them	R	W	
PAL-II	Sentence Sense—identify sentences that make sense based on word choice/ context	R	W	
Vocabulary				
WIAT-III	Listening Comprehension Receptive Vocabulary—match pictures to orally presented words	R	W	M
WJ-III	Reading Vocabulary—provide synonyms, antonyms, analogies for words	R	W	M
Spelling (Transcription Skill)				
WIAT-III	Spelling—write out orally presented words		W	
WJ-III	Spelling—write out orally presented words		W	
PAL-II	Word Choice—identify correctly spelled word among distracters		W	

Core Skills / Cognitive Processes & Example Methods of Assessment		Academic Areas	
Handwriting (Transcription Skills)			
WIAT-III	Alphabet Writing Fluency—write the letters of the alphabet (timed)	W	
WJ-III	Handwriting Legibility Scale—evaluation of handwriting on the Writing Samples subtest based on legibility and general appearance.	W	
PAL-II	Finger Sense (Repetition)—imitate index finger to thumb finger movement	W	
Text Composition (Sentence Level)			
WIAT-III	Sentence Composition (Combining)—combine sentences to form one sentence that retains the meaning	W	
WJ-III	Punctuation/Capitalization—punctuate and capitalize items	W	
PAL-II	Sentence Structure—select plausible sentences based on word order/endings	W	
Text Generation (Text Level)			
WIAT-III	Essay Composition—write text in response to a prompt (analytic scoring)	W	
WJ-III	Writing Samples—write text in response to a prompt (holistic scoring)	W	
PAL-II	Expository Note Taking and Report Writing—write a report from notes	W	
Number Sense			
PAL-II	Oral Counting—count forwards/backwards by various increments		M
Math: Procedural			
WIAT-III	Numerical Operations—complete range of calculation tasks		M
WJ-III	Calculation—complete range of calculation tasks		M
PAL-II	Computation Operations—explain steps in solving written calculations		M
Math: Conceptual			
WIAT-III	Math Problem Solving—analyse and solve math problems		M
WJ-III	Applied Problems—analyse and solve math problems		M
PAL-II	Part-Whole (Fractions/Mixed Numbers)—report fraction/mixed number that represents the shaded portion of geometric shapes		M
Math: Declarative			
WJ-III	Quantitative Concepts—identify math terms, facts, and number sequences		M
PAL-II	Fact Retrieval—retrieve basic math facts		M
Fluency			
WIAT-III	Oral Reading Fluency—read passages aloud for comprehension (timed)	R	
WJ-III	Writing Fluency—formulate simple sentences quickly (timed)	W	
PAL-II	Oral Counting—count forwards/backwards by various increments (timed)		M

Core Skills / Cognitive Processes & Example Methods of Assessment			Academic Areas		
Speed of Processing					
	PAL-II	RAS—identify words or numbers	R	W	M
	NEPSY-II	Speeded Naming—produce names of colours/shapes/sizes/letters/ numbers	R	W	M
Working Memory					
	PAL-II	Spatial Working Memory—recall dot patterns/locations			M
	NEPSY-II	Word List Inference—repeat a series of unconnected words	R	W	M
Attention/Executive Functions					
	NEPSY-II	Inhibition—quickly read the names of shapes with changing rules	R	W	M

Methods of Assessing Learning and Study Strategies

Kathy C. Stroud

Abstract

This chapter seeks to provide an overview of theories of learning strategies and self-regulation. Learning strategies, academic motivation, and related constructs are defined, and their role in fostering academic achievement is discussed. For each construct, specific strategies are highlighted that have been shown empirically to academic performance. Incorporating learning strategies assessment in a battery of tests is crucial to the overall understanding of an individual, and the success achieved from using these strategies can be far-reaching. Only a few measures have been developed for the purpose of measuring learning strategies and/or self-regulated learning, and most have significant limitations in their utility. More commonly, measures are designed to measure one or two constructs, with little consideration given to the possible interactions of the factors measured. Others are developed primarily for research purposes and may change with a given hypothesis. The School Motivation and Learning Strategies Inventory (SMALSI; Stroud & Reynolds, 2006) was developed as means of providing a comprehensive assessment of learning strategies across a broad age range to be used both for assessment and clinical purposes.

Key Words: Learning strategies, Academic motivation, Study strategies, Test-taking strategies, School Motivation, and Learning Strategies Inventory

The purpose of psychological assessment in children is to, as accurately and completely as possible, describe the whole child in a way that is meaningful. For this reason, no assessment can be considered truly complete without giving consideration to school functioning. Academic achievement is an essential accomplishment of childhood, and success or failure is tied to numerous outcomes, including emotional adjustment, self-esteem, and self-efficacy. It is interesting that, given its importance, standard practice in measuring academic achievement has often reduced to the comparison between a standardized achievement test and an intellectual instrument. While the information obtained from these measurements can be invaluable, they fail to account for many of the other variables affecting student performance. Just as cognitive functioning is no longer considered

a one-dimensional entity, a more multifaceted approach is necessary in understanding the process of learning and ultimately academic achievement.

A universal definition of learning strategies has remained elusive, often being used interchangeably with similar but different terms (i.e., study skills, learning styles, cognitive skills). Understanding the qualitative differences in these terms is important when making inferences about a student. Learning strategies have been defined as "the purposeful behaviors of a learner that are intended to facilitate the acquisition and processing of information" (Stroud & Reynolds, 2006, p. 8). By contrast, learning styles are "characteristic cognitive, affective, and physiological behaviors that serve as relatively stable indicators of how learners perceive, interact with, and respond to the learning environment" (Keefe, 1979, p.4).

Learning style indicates a tendency to use a limited repertoire of strategies for learning (Schmeck, 1988). Learning styles may be more dependent on the preferences of the learner and may or may not be the most efficient means of learning, whereas learning strategies are more universal and necessary in their ability to improve learning. Learning styles imply more passive attributes of the learner whereas learning strategies require the student to actively manipulate and process the information being presented. Most notably for intervention, learning strategies are an empirically supported, objective set of skills that can be taught and engage the student in an active learning process.

Theories of Learning Strategies and Self-Regulation

Early theories (and measures) of study methods emerged in the mid-twentieth century (Entwistle & McCune, 2004). At that time, the source and responsibility for successful academic achievement was placed solely on the student. One of the first measures of learning strategies included scales measuring effective study procedures, completing work promptly, having positive attitudes about teachers, and adoption of educational objectives (Brown & Holtzman, 1966; Entwistle & McCune, 2004). Entwistle and McCune (2004) provide an interesting perspective on the evolution of "study habits" and differences in conceptualization for American and European researchers. Their discussion includes a comparison of recent inventories and a qualitative discussion of their common factors. A few of the more current conceptualizations of learning strategies and self-regulated learning are presented here.

Weinstein and Mayer (1986) presented a taxonomy of learning strategies with five distinct but related categories, including rehearsal, elaboration, and organization—specific techniques enabling the student to organize and learn information; comprehension monitoring, which is the learner's metacognitive awareness of learning and ability to control the use of strategies (Weinstein, Husman, & Dierking, 2000).; and affective strategies, which are used to "help focus the learner's attention and maintain the learner's motivation" (Weinstein et al., 2000, p. 732). Within this model, strategies are viewed in terms of their relationship with variables such as motivation and metacognition.

Weinstein's more recent "model of strategic learning has at its core the learner: a unique individual who brings to each learning situation a critical set of variables, including his or her personality,

prior knowledge, and school achievement history" (Weinstein et al., 2000, p. 733). This more comprehensive model includes three components: skills, will, and self-regulation. Skills include a learner's knowledge about himself/herself as a learner, understanding the characteristics of the academic task, learning strategies, prior knowledge, and learning content as well as skills in the use of learning strategies, discerning important information, reading and listening comprehension, listening and note-taking, study and test-taking skills, and reasoning (Weinstein, 1994). The second component, *will*, encompasses the development and use of goals, academic motivation, affect with respect to learning, beliefs, volition, and a positive attitude toward learning. *Self-regulation* incorporates metacognitive components such as concentration, time management, monitoring comprehension, a systematic approach to learning and accomplishing academic tasks, coping with academic stress, and managing motivation (Weinstein, 1994). Will and Self-regulation are particularly important factors in discriminating between high achievers and low achievers (Yip, 2009).

Although they have a different primary emphasis, theories of self-regulation include learning strategies. Self-regulated learning has the same origins in cognitive psychology as learning strategies. Self-regulated learners: monitor and adapt their learning according to the situation; are strategic and goal-oriented in their approach to learning tasks; and rely on intrinsic self-control of the situation rather than simply reacting to external controls (Purdie, Hattie, & Douglas, 1996). Zimmerman (1998) describes the learning process in three cycling consecutive phases: forethought, performance or volitional control, and self-reflection. Each phase is comprised of subprocesses that may be used to understand the differences between skilled and unskilled learners. Processes in the forethought phase include setting goals, strategic planning, self-efficacy beliefs, goal orientation, and intrinsic interest. For example, skilled self-regulators more often adopt a mastery orientation, or an intrinsic desire to improve their ability; non-skilled learners, on the other hand, demonstrate a performance orientation, or learning in response to the threat of evaluation (Pintrich & DeGroot, 1990). During the performance phase learners engage in the tasks of attention focusing, self-instruction, and self-monitoring. In this phase, differences in learning include unfocused or divided focus or a focus on performance, use of ineffective (handicapping) strategies or self-instruction as well as strategic learning, and monitoring of outcome or monitoring of success. The final phase, self-reflection, provides for self-evaluation regarding performance, including making attributions for success or failure, positive or negative self-reactions, and appropriate adaptation (Zimmerman, 1998). In this third phase, self-reflection for skilled learners involves self-evaluation and ultimately leads to appropriate attributions for the strategies used. The result is a positive self-reaction and an adaptive approach to subsequent tasks and differing situations (Zimmerman, 1998).

Winne and Hadwin (1998) also have proposed a theoretical model depicting self-regulated learning as an event with four phases: 1. defining the task (developing a perception of what factors relevant to the current task), 2. setting goals and devising a strategy for achieving them, 3. using tactics and strategies, and 4. monitoring, evaluating, and making changes as needed either during the task or in preparation for future learning (Winne, 2010). Students monitor themselves through the first three phases, making small or large scale changes to their learning as the task dictates. The fact that the primary measures of self-regulated learning are learning strategies inventories highlights the similarities of the theoretical constructs. Two measures used are the Learning and Study Strategies Inventory (LASSI: Weinstein, Schulte, & Palmer, 1987) and Motivated Strategies for Learning Questionnaire (MSLQ: Pintrich, Smith, Garcia, & McKeachie, 1991; Winne & Perry, 2000). Self-regulated learning as an aptitude has also been measured through structured interviews and teacher judgments or by using think aloud procedures, error detection tasks, and observations. Observations have been used to examine self-regulated learning in children as young as kindergarten (Whitebread, Coltman, Pasternak, Sangster, Grau, Bingham, Almeqdad, & Demetriou, 2009).

More recently, it has been argued that SRL must be considered in relation to context of internal environment and external environment. As such, self-regulated learning is an event that can be measured by traces, or "observable representations of cognitive, metacognitive and motivational events," during the task itself (Winne, 2010, 267).

Broekkamp and Van Hout-Wolters (2007). conceptualize learning as occurring through strategy adaptation. Strategy adaptability is defined as "the degree to which students are capable of selecting or revising strategies in ways that make these strategies match relevant external and internal characteristics

of study tasks" (Broekkamp & Van Hout-Wolters, 2007, p. 405). External characteristics are task demands or the goals of the task determined by others. Internal characteristics are the personal goals adopted by the student for a given task. For test preparation, the model identifies internal task processes including adaptation of study strategies, task perceptions, and implementation of study strategies. These internal task processes interact with the student's task dispositions (i.e., metacognitive skills, motivational beliefs, subject matter knowledge) as well as with external factors such as the student's task environment and contextual factors (i.e., test, teacher's task demands, test demands).

There has been some confusion regarding differences in the conceptualization of self-regulated learning (Roeser and Peck, 2009). Some view self-regulation in terms of content, including goals and self-efficacy; others describe volition or a self-regulatory process designed to "protect activated belief-goal systems (i.e., *intentions*) from competing demands and to bring them to fruition in action under favorable conditions" (Roeser & Peck, 2009, p. 121). The Basic Levels of Self model seeks to resolve this apparent inconsistency by referring to the I-Self (volitional) and Me-Self (automatic) systems. Roeser and Peck (2009) also introduce the concept of contemplative education which views self-regulated learning as a framework for cultivating "awareness and related volitional modes of attending, thinking, feeling, perceiving, acting, and interacting" in order to enhance functioning in society beyond the school setting.

Who Needs Learning Strategies?

The short answer—everyone. The assumption is often that students naturally develop learning strategies as they progress through school; this is not always the case however. Some typically achieving students make it through school without learning effective strategies for learning (Nicaise & Gettinger, 1995). Even students who have already developed study strategies demonstrate improved performance with explicit teaching of learning strategies. Students of all abilities benefit academically from learning to be strategic in their academic tasks (e.g., Gall et al., 1990; Weinstein & Hume, 1998; Faber, Morris, & Lieberman, 2000; Bail, Zhang, & Tachiyama, 2008). Children who struggle tend to adopt more passive and ineffective strategies; they fail to monitor their progress in studying and do not consider the purpose of studying (Gettinger & Seibert, 2002). For college students, explicit teaching in self-regulated learning strategies has been associated with higher cumulative grade point averages four semesters after taking the course, higher odds of graduation, and lower chances of receiving failing a course (Bail, Zhang, & Tachiyama, 2008)

While the routine teaching of learning strategies in regular education classrooms may well allow for incidental learning of some strategies for many children, special populations with particular needs or circumstances will likely require specific attention and intervention. The largest single group of students who have the capacity to benefit from explicit skill instruction would be those with learning disabilities. These students differ from their peers in their use of learning strategies. They lack confidence in their academic self-efficacy (Baird, Scott, Dearing, & Hamill, 2009; Lackaye, Margalit, Ziv, & Ziman, 2006) and their ability to monitor and regulate their learning, termed self-regulatory efficacy (Klassen 2010). Further, students with learning disabilities display significant difficulties with memory on academic tasks, highlighting the great need for instruction in test-taking and study skills, specifically mnemonic strategies (Scruggs & Mastropieri, 2000). Reading comprehension strategies instruction has also helped to improve understanding of science and social studies texts (Bakken, Mastropieri, & Scruggs, 1997). Other special populations for whom educational interventions related to learning strategies have been recommended include children who are survivors of childhood cancer (Jannoun & Chessells, 1987; Peckham, 1989), with traumatic brain injuries, (Powers, Vanetta, Noll, Cool, & Stehbens, 1995), with Attention-Deficit/ Hyperactivity Disorder (ADHD) (DuPaul & Stoner, 1994; Harrison, Thompson, & Vannest, 2009) and with other psychiatric disorders (Brackney & Karabenick, 1995; Vannest, Temple-Harvey, & Mason, 2009). Neuropsychological deficits can be wide-ranging, depending on the nature of the illness, disability, or injury for these children making accurate assessment of learning and study strategies is necessary for determining students' strengths as well as their weaknesses.

Learning Strategies and Related Constructs

Topics included in or related to learning strategies include academic motivation (Brophy, 2004; Pajares & Urdan, 2002), note-taking and listening skills (Kobayashi, 2006; Hughes & Suritsky, 1994; Bygrave, 1994; Hamilton, Seibert, Gardner, & Talbert-Johnson, 2000), time management (Boller, 2008; Britton & Tesser, 1991), test anxiety (Cassady & Johnson, 2002), research strategies (Quarton, 2003), concentration/attention (Reynolds & Voress, 2007; Reynolds & Shirey, 1988, Rabiner & Coie, 2000), organizational techniques (Bakunas and Holley, 2004; Ho & McMurtrie, 1991; Shapiro, DuPaul, & Bradley-Klug, 1998), test-taking strategies (Scruggs & Mastropieri, 1992), study strategies (Kirby, Silvestri, Allingham, Parrila, & La Fave, 2008; Sweidel, 1996), writing strategies (Graham and Perin, 2007) and reading and comprehension strategies (Scammacca, Roberts, Vaughn, Edmonds, Wexler, Reutebuch, & Torgesen, 2007; Gersten, Fuchs, Williams, & Baker, 2001). These constructs provide concrete, distinct areas that can be targeted for intervention. Success in these areas has broad academic implications for increasing academic achievement. The relationship of each of these topics to academic achievement and, in some instances to each other, has been empirically supported, requiring careful and integrated assessment in order to better understand the development and selective use of cognitive strategies.

Study Strategies

Perhaps the heart of learning, study is the process by which information is integrated with existing knowledge and committed to long-term memory. Studying is unique in several ways (Gettinger and Seibert, 2002). First, the act of study is skillful, requiring instruction to acquire and retain important information. Second, studying is a purposeful or intentional task requiring effort. Next, studying is an individual process that is highly dependent on the characteristics of the student. Finally, studying is dependent on a student's ability to self-regulate or monitor his learning. Studying in and of itself is not generally a requirement of high school. Therefore, it is up to the student to determine if it is needed, how much, and how best to accomplish it (Gettinger and Seibert, 2002).

Students receive a vast amount of academic information and must use study strategies that facilitate identifying important information when they study, making associations when learning, using a variety of resources when a concept is not understood, and using strategies for memory and encoding. Teaching students how to use a systematic, strategic approach to studying is important to learning clearly improves academic performance (e.g., Alexander & Murphy, 1999; Paris & Winegrad, 1990). Students need explicit instruction in how to organize information from different sources such as class notes, textbooks, and worksheets or homework, as well as how to use memory aids. Direct instruction maximizes strategy use and academic potential (Alexander & Murphy, 1999, Kirby et al., 2008). These rehearsal, elaboration, and organizational strategies are necessary to acquire and use information in a meaningful way (e.g., Weinstein & Hume, 1998). Students are then able to adapt and use the most appropriate strategies, given the demands of a particular situation or test (Ross, Green, Salisbury-Glennon, & Tollefson, 2006; Broekkamp & Van Hout-Wolters, 2007).

Evidenced-study strategies that lend themselves to direct teaching include: improving concentration, improving memorization, developing associations with prior learning, learning self-talk, using concept maps, and using multiple sources of information (Vannest, Stroud, & Reynolds, 2011). For example, memorization may be improved by using strategies that aid in storing and retrieving information. Mnemonics (e.g., acrostics, rhyme keys, keyword, image name, chaining) are helpful strategies for remembering information or necessary steps for other types of learning, particularly for special populations such as students with behavioral and emotional difficulties (Mastropieri & Scruggs, 1998, Kleinheksel & Summy, 2003). Mnemonics are valuable tools for transferring information from working memory to long term memory, the main goal of studying (Goll, 2004). Whereas other learning strategies may be learned spontaneously, mnemonic strategies should be taught explicitly (Levin, 1993), Younger children, in particular, are able to categorize information in some way but are much less likely to spontaneously use mnemonics.

Self-testing is also a powerful tool for learning information (Carpenter, Pashler, & Vul, 2006; Karpicke & Roediger, 2007; McDaniel, Roediger, & McDermott, 2007). It's superiority to more commonly used strategies such as rereading information has been documented, however, students are far more likely to use the latter strategy (Karpicke, Butler, and Roediger, 2009), again highlighting the need for explicit instruction, not only in how to use the strategy, but in its effectiveness relative to other strategies.

Reading Comprehension Strategies

The purpose of reading is to take of meaning from the printed word or text (Stroud & Reynolds, 2009). This simple but complete definition highlights comprehension as being the fundamental purpose of reading. The National Institute for Literacy (NIFL) identifies 5 areas of development critical for learning to read: phonemic awareness, phonics, fluency, vocabulary, and text comprehension (Armbruster, Lehr, & Osborn, 2003). Perhaps the most complex skill, reading comprehension is also ultimately the most important. After all, the goal of reading is to understand the content of what has been written. Therefore, it is surprising that, through classroom observations, Durkin (1979) asserted that less than 1% of instructional time in reading was used for actual instruction in comprehension. More recently, a study of the curriculum of schools in the United States (ACT, 2007) revealed that reading comprehension strategies are still not being taught in elementary and secondary classrooms and that the lack of these skills is a substantial stumbling block to success in post secondary education. A meta-analysis of intervention studies with students struggling in reading indicated that instruction in reading comprehension strategies had the greatest effect in improving comprehension (Scammacca et al., 2007).

In 2000, the National Reading Panel (NRP) released results from a review of more than 100,000 empirical studies of reading (Armbruster et al., 2003). Among their findings, good readers are identified as being purposeful or goal-directed and active thinkers who incorporate previous learning in their reading. Reading is an "active goal-directed problem-solving process in which the reader's task is to construct meaning from information contained in the text." (Samuels, 1989, p. 3). Six strategies critical to text comprehension include: monitoring comprehension, using graphic and semantic organizers, answering questions, generating questions, recognizing the structure of the material, and summarizing (Armbruster et al., 2003).

Monitor comprehension. Monitoring comprehension allows students to assess what they do and do not understand about what they are reading and to use strategies to adjust their approach to reading when necessary. Self-regulatory behaviors are components of metacognition during comprehension tasks (Baker and Brown, 1984). Students are asked to engage in a variety of self-regulatory behaviors, including comprehension monitoring, or self-checking during reading (to detect errors and monitor understanding) and comprehension regulation (the active use of strategies to help regulate the reader's comprehension).

Researchers have also studied the effects of working memory on reading comprehension. Students with comprehension difficulties do not demonstrate differences on short term memory measures, but they do have significantly lower performance on working memory measures (De Beni & Palladino, 2000). De Beni and Palladino (2000) demonstrated that students with poor comprehension made more intrusion errors than their peers. In fact, their recall of irrelevant information was better than their recall of relevant information. Intrusion errors were a predictor of reading comprehension performance one year later.

Using graphic and semantic organizers. Graphic organizers, including semantic organizers, are visual tools to help students focus on important concepts and their relationships with each other (Armbruster et al., 2003). The characteristics of text (i.e., representational illustrations, imagery, spatial organization, mnemonic illustrations) are helpful aids for improving comprehension and retention of material (Mastropieri & Scruggs, 1997). These tools may provide an additional mode of information to be encoded and a means of organizing the information for learning (Mastropieri & Scruggs, 1997). Mnemonic illustrations can also be an aid when students need to commit the material to memory (Scruggs & Mastropieri, 1992). Aside from the use of these illustrations, Mastropieri and Scruggs (1997) identified several adjunct aids that appear to improve comprehension. It is believed that these aids, such as study guides, audiotapes, underlining, and semantic feature relationship charts help students to discern more important facts, providing an additional chance for encoding.

Answering questions. Providing questions prior to or embedded within the text cues students to attend to the most important information in a text and improves retention (Duchastel & Nungester, 1984; Pressley, Tanenbaum, Mc Daniel, & Wood, 1990). The Question Answer Relationship (QAR; Ezell, Hunsicker, & Quinque, 1997) teaches students the need to use previously acquired knowledge together with information from the text. Students become proficient at (a) locating information, (b) recognizing text structures and how they present important information, and (c) deciding whether an inference is required or invited (Raphael, 1986). Students must be able to understand information that is both explicitly stated and implied. *Generating questions.* Questioning techniques have proven to be effective strategies for both students with learning disabilities and normally achieving students (Mastropieri and Scruggs, 1997; Rosenshine, Meister, and Chapman, 1996). Students are able to monitor their comprehension as well as improve their comprehension by generating questions for themselves before, during, and after reading. Rosenshine et al. (1996)

examined the effectiveness of five types of prompts: signal words, generic question stems/generic questions, main idea, question types, and story grammar categories. Signal words and generic stems/generic questions were the most effective prompts used followed by story grammar prompts, perhaps because these three prompts are easy to use and they provide students with a guide and a way to focus their attention without requiring strong cognitive skills. Rosenshine and his colleagues (1996) felt that more intensive instruction might have led to improved results of the other types of prompts that were less successful but could be more beneficial. Using generic questions would have more value than signal words "because they promote deeper processing, initiate recall of background knowledge, require integration of prior knowledge, and provide more direction for processing than might be obtained through the use of the more simplified signal words" (Rosenshine et al., 1996, p. 200).

Recognizing the structure of the material. Recognizing structure includes a learner's ability to identify the setting as well as to determine why he or she is reading the material and its purpose. Students should be taught how to recognize expository text, recognize the structure of text by looking for signal words or phrases, developing goals for understanding based on the purpose of the text, and selecting study strategies best suited for the structure (Bakken & Whedon, 2002). Recognizing structures and using them to comprehend text are more effective strategies than paragraph restatement and retelling the main idea and incidental information (Bakken & Whedon, 2002).

Summarizing. Summarization requires that students understand, process, and formulate their own interpretation of the material presented. Summarization and main idea strategies include a student asking questions (e.g., "Who?", "What's happening?") during reading, then summarizing the text in their own words (Gajria & Salvia, 1992; Jenkins, Heliotis, Stein, & Haynes, 1987). Summarization strategies have generally been effective as a singular technique as well as when combined with self-monitoring and attribution training (Mastropieri & Scruggs, 1997).

Writing/Research Skills

Writing is, perhaps, our best means of communicating an understanding of concepts. It is the most common way, from an academic perspective, of expressing one's own ideas or feelings. More than perhaps any other task in school, it is generative and original in nature. Writing requires coordination of numerous thought processes, including coordination and knowledge of material being presented, strategies of effective writing and revision, and the skills associated with the mechanics of writing (i.e., grammar, vocabulary use). Writing is also a common task carried over to many vocational pursuits. Given these important distinctions, it is frequently used for measuring academic achievement and is often included as part of most state tests required for grade advancement or graduation.

Prior to the 1990s, writing instruction was largely limited to the mechanics of writing (e.g., grammar, spelling) and little attention was given to the process of writing (e.g., planning, organization of ideas). In a meta-analysis, traditional school grammar was determined to have no effect in improving quality of writing (Hillocks, 1986). Writing activities that were more effective than traditional or free writing were building more complex sentences as well as using and internalizing scales, criteria, or specific questions to generate material. The most effective treatments, termed Inquiry treatments, included those of analyzing data, problem-solving, and generating arguments.

A rather dramatic shift to more process-centered approaches to writing was heralded with the widespread adoption of programs such as Writer's Workshop (Troia, 2002, Atwell, 1987, Graves, 1983). The results were impressive, with several differences noted. 1. The amount of time spent writing in school has increased. 2. Writing is seen as more purposeful by teachers. 3. Teachers respond more to content than error correction 4. Students engage in more writing for pleasure 5. Exemplary teachers are encouraging the use of more advanced writing practices such as planning prior to writing and editing during writing, writing journals, and portfolios of writing samples (Troia, 2002; Campbell, Voelkl, & Donahue, 1997; Pressley, Rankin, and Yokoi, 1996). The National Assessment of Educational Progress (NAEP) was conducted most recently in 2007 to assess writing proficiency for American students (Salahu-Din, Persky, and Miller, 2008). 88% of 8th graders obtained scores corresponding with at least basic achievement, defined as partial mastery of necessary skills to perform at grade level. Only 33% of students had proficient achievement, defined as solid academic performance and competency with challenging subject matter. In other words, 67% of 8th graders are not adequately equipped to competently navigate grade-level subject matter. Results for 12th graders are even more disheartening, with only 24%

of students having obtained proficiency in writing at grade level (Salahu-Din et al., 2008). These results represent a best-case-scenario, in that many students with learning and other disabilities (and likely lower writing achievement) are excluded from the results (Salahu-Din et al., 2008). Not all news is bad. These results represent clear trends of improvement from previous assessments. Improvements have also been demonstrated for some minority groups as well as low and middle achieving students. (Salahu-Din et al., 2008). Overall, the findings clearly underscore the need, not only for a widespread process-centered approach, but one that incorporates both writing strategies and self-regulated strategies.

Numerous descriptions of the writing process exist, and they range in levels of specificity (e.g., Harris, Graham, Mason, & Friedlander, 2008; Strichart & Mangrum, 2002; Tompkins, 1994). All include elements describing steps for planning and organizing information prior to writing, creating at least one draft, and revising drafts both for content and grammar prior to producing a final copy. While these models are presented in linear format, many steps may be revisited as needed during the process. During prewriting, students should make a plan for their composition. This may be accomplished by doing some initial reading or conducting interviews (Scott & Vitale, 2003). Then begins the process of collecting information through such means as brainstorming, answering appropriate questions, using software, or reading more information (Roberts, 2002; Scott & Vitale, 2003). Research skills are needed as part of composition during the planning process in order to obtain necessary information. Children are encouraged early in life to use libraries to increase general reading skills and interest in reading; equal attention should be given to learning basic skills to use other aspects of the library (Krapp, 1988). Wooden card catalogs have been replaced in libraries by various resources, including the internet, databases, reference books and materials, audio/video materials, archival documents, and others. College students will need to be able to independently use all of these resources effectively as soon as they start college. Not only must students learn how to find resources, it is important to teach students how to discern which sources are credible as well as how to effectively organize and narrow the information available (Quarton, 2003). These research skills are essential beginning skills in the initial process of writing. After the initial information gathering phase, students must be taught to efficiently organize the information to be used into a coherent plan or outline for writing (Scott & Vitale, 2003). Strategies utilized during the actual writing process are designed to narrow the topic, recognize the need for new information, or adapt a paper for a specific audience.

Research with students with learning disabilities yields alarming differences in their performance as compared to their normally achieving peers. Students with learning disabilities do not use writing strategies to the extent that nondisabled students do and they are not as purposeful in prewriting or revision activities; instead the majority of their focus is on grammar, spelling, and handwriting (Faigley, Cherry, Jolliffee, & Skinner, 1985; Graham, Schwartz, & MacArthur, 1993). Students with learning disabilities also spend much less time planning their writing prior to beginning a composition and have a tendency to write without pausing to rethink or read what they have written (MacArthur & Graham, 1987; Faigley et al., 1985). They are less likely than normally achieving peers to understand that the process of writing or the use of writing strategies is important (Graham et al., 1993). Students with learning disabilities are more prone to neglecting the more subtle nuances of writing, such as taking the perspective of their audience. When specifically directed to take their audience into account, they are more likely to examine surface level aspects of their writing; by contrast, normally achieving students typically suggest changes to the substance of the material.

Graham and Perin (2007) conducted a meta-analysis to delineate which elements of writing instruction improve student performance. Eleven elements emerged as being independently effective in improving student performance: writing strategies, summarization, collaborative writing, specific product goals, word processing, sentence combining, prewriting, inquiry activities, process writing approach, study of models, writing for content learning.

The effects of teaching writing strategies to normally achieving students and students with learning disabilities can be dramatic. Explicit teaching of skills such as considering their audience, developing a plan, evaluating the impact of content, and continuing to generate new content during the writing process increased their use from 10% of papers written prior to the intervention to 80% afterward (Graham and Harris, 1989). Measures of maintenance and generalization also yielded positive results. Self-regulated learning strategies including how to brainstorm, semantic webbing, setting writing goals, and revision have produced improvements in word production and quality of writing (Chalk, Hagan-Burke, & Burke, 2005). Combining writing strategies instruction with self-regulation strategies has also been effective (Glaser & Brunstein, 2007; De La Paz & Graham, 2002; Graham & Harris, 1993; Harris & Graham, 1996). Self-regulated strategies during the writing process include goal setting, self-monitoring, and self-instructions. The self-regulated strategy development model (SRSD; Harris & Graham, 1996, 1999) has been designed to offer explicit instruction of writing and self-regulatory strategies. The six stages of instruction include the following: 1. teach any background knowledge needed to learn the strategy, 2. discuss the benefits and purpose of the strategy, 3. model use of the strategy and introduce self-instruction, 4. memorize steps of the strategy, 5. teacher supports or scaffolds mastery of the strategy, and 6. where the students independently use the strategy (Graham, Harris, & MacArthur, 2006).

Test-taking Strategies

Given the increased use of high-stakes testing emerging across the United States to determine grade promotion and school funding, much more emphasis has been placed on individual student performance on tests. As states transition to requiring passing scores on state tests (e.g., Texas Assessment of Knowledge and Skills, TAKS; Florida Comprehensive Assessment Test, FCAT) to determine school funding and pupil progress, teachers and school personnel are faced with the increasing demands of promoting children and adolescents' academic knowledge, but also their test-taking abilities. Standardized testing remains a part of the requirements for acceptance at most colleges and universities as well, leading educators, parents, and students to place a premium on improving performance on tests.

Evaluating content knowledge is most often the purpose of giving a test; however, several factors may affect a person's score, including the students' level of confidence and motivation for success as well as knowledge and effective use of test-taking strategies. Test-taking strategies are a set of skills that allow a student to recognize differences in test format and the entire testing situation in order to improve his or her score (Millman, Bishop, & Ebell, 1965). Test-taking strategies and self-regulation strategies during tests are not a new concept and have been proven to be effective interventions (e.g., Beidel, Turner, & Taylor-Ferreira, 1999; Schraw, 1994).

The major types of test-taking skills include: time-using strategies, error avoidance strategies, guessing strategies, deductive reasoning strategies, intent consideration, and cue using (Millman et al., 1965). Intent consideration strategies and cue using strategies are skills specific to a particular testing situation or test author. Time-using strategies are the techniques designed to make monitor and make efficient use of time during a test. Students can be taught strategies such as monitoring their time during tests, answering questions they know first, and not spending too much time on one item or one section. Strategies used to minimize wrong answers due to mistakes are error avoidance strategies (i.e., reading and understanding directions, accurately selecting answers, and checking for mistakes). Guessing strategies increase a student's chance of answering a question correctly. Students can use deductive reasoning strategies to arrive at an answer by using the item content, eliminating unlikely answers, and recognizing similar responses. Intent consideration indicates a test-taker's awareness of the intent behind the test as a whole or the individual item. Finally, cue using strategies rely on the test-taker's awareness of the idiosyncrasies of the specific test author (Mastropieri & Scruggs, 1992).

Hong, Sas, and Sas (2006) delineated 3 types of test-taking strategies: structural organization, cognitive strategies, and motivational awareness. Structural organization includes tasks that assess and allocate time and that sequence tasks to be completed. High achievers were more likely to use these strategies than low achievers. Cognitive strategies include checking (for understanding, correctness, or mistakes), externalizing (writing down formulas, definitions), remembering material, repeating (redoing or checking items), eliminating wrong answers in multiple choice items, using memory aids such as mnemonics, and elaborating (relating material to something). High achievers used more cognitive strategies overall, with particular differences noted in checking for correctness. Motivational awareness is having the student make positive self-statements about putting forth effort and adopting a passive attitude with no method (hope). Low achievers tended to adopt a more passive approach to strategy use.

As with other learning strategies, test-taking strategies are essential in helping special populations such as students with learning disabilities, emotional or behavioral difficulties, and minorities (Hughes, 1993; Scruggs & Mastropieri, 1986; Scruggs & Tolfa, 1985). Teaching elementary students strategies that include "attending to directions, marking answers carefully, choosing the best answer carefully, using error avoidance strategies, and deciding appropriate situations for soliciting teacher attention" (Scruggs & Mastropieri, 1986, p. 65) resulted in significant increases from pretest to posttest on the Stanford Achievement Test Word Study subtest. Similar results were obtained in a much smaller study with middle school students identified as having an emotional behavioral disability; they were taught test-taking strategies using a mnemonic device (Hughes, 1993). Maintenance effects were seen at 11 weeks and generalization to class tests was noted. Research suggests that the effectiveness of an intervention is influenced by several factors, including length of time for instruction (Scruggs White, & Bennion, 1986). Also, when combining age and length of instruction, the performance of older children is much less dependent on length of instruction than younger children, with older elementary children appearing to benefit from even short instruction periods. The effectiveness of test-taking strategies is also likely dependent on the complexity or difficulty of the test design and material (Scruggs & Mastropieri, 1986).

Other variables, including socioeconomic and cultural factors also appear to influence learning and use of test-taking strategies. For example, children of low socioeconomic status appear to benefit from test-taking strategies instruction twice as much as much as their peers of higher socioeconomic status (Scruggs et al., 1986). One of few studies examining cultural factors examined differences in how students prepare for tests, use test-strategies, and self-efficacy and their effects on a cognitive ability test (Ellis & Ryan, 2003). Differences were most apparent between Caucasians and African Americans in their use of ineffective strategies with African Americans reporting much more frequent use of ineffective strategies. Both reported that they use effective test-taking skills. Strategy use can also be affected by motivation (Barnett, 2000) or a failure to understand when to use them (Winne & Jamieson-Noel, 2002). The variability in performance and lack of sufficient research underscore the need for additional study in this area.

Note-taking/Listening Strategies

"Notes may be defined as short condensations of a source material that are generated by writing them down while simultaneously listening, studying, or observing" (Piolat, Olive, & Kellogg, 2005, p. 292). Note-taking begins in elementary school and becomes a critical skill in secondary school and college as instruction shifts to primarily teacher lectures. Note-taking skills and text marking strategies are specific learning strategies associated with good listening skills and the ability to discern important versus non-important information (Stroud & Reynolds, 2006). Effective note-taking as a strategy is a higher level skill that requires manipulating information or reconstructing it in a way that is most meaningful for efficient learning (Porte, 2001). It incorporates both comprehension and written production similar in scope to an original composition (Piolat et al., 2005). Piolat et al. (2005) measured note-taking in terms of the cognitive effort it requires.

Early research on note-taking strategies took one of two perspectives: information processing and product perspective. Research adopting an information processing view focuses on the process or actual recording of information (Kiewra, 1985). This focus on the "process" of note-taking is assessed by comparing students who do take notes with students who do not take notes on a given measure (Kiewra, 1985). The "product" or "external storage" perspective evaluates the effectiveness of note-taking according to whether or not it improves achievement by aiding in review of the information recorded. It is typically evaluated by comparing students who review their notes prior to assessment with those who are not given the opportunity to review their notes (Kiewra, 1985).

Many strategies are designed specifically to decrease the amount of time needed to physically write notes. Piolat, Olive, and Kellogg discuss three levels of language that are available to be targeted: abbreviated procedures, syntax, and physical formatting. Examples of abbreviated procedures include end truncation, conservation of the frame of consonants, and suffix contractions (Piolat et al., 2005). These and other procedures serve the same purpose but are often tailored specifically to the individual. Syntax may be changed by leaving out unnecessary words (telegraphic style) or substitutive techniques using symbols. Finally, the physical format of notes involves altering the physical placement of notes on the page from a linear presentation to an organized layout of concepts (Piolat et al., 2005).

Meta-analyses evaluating the effectiveness of note-taking and note-taking interventions have indicated support for the efficacy of taking notes, and in particular taking and reviewing notes (Kobayashi, 2006; Kiewra, 1985; Hartley, 1983). Students appear to benefit more from interventions that include providing a graphic organizer or the instructor's notes (Robinson, Katayama, Beth, Odom, Ya-Ping, Vanderveen, 2006: Kobayashi, 2006). Also, students with low ability benefit much more from explicit teaching of strategies than high-achieving students do (Kobayashi, 2006; Shrager & Mayer, 1989; Kiewra & Benton, 1985; Wade & Trathen, 1989).

Note-takers differ in how well they are able to relate new information to that already learned, take effective notes, make note-taking an active process, and determine priorities of relevant information (Faber et al., 2000). Students shift their focus and the learning strategies they choose to employ with repetition of lecture material, suggesting that "students are active learners who have some metacognitive control over their learning strategies" (Kiewra, et al., 1991, p. 123). As might be expected, students with learning disabilities have significant difficulties taking notes, including their ability to record notes with sufficient speed, focus their attention on lectures, and use appropriate strategies such as a shorthand method (Suritsky, 1992; Hughes & Suritsky, 1993).

Acquisition of note-taking skills is a developmental process, particularly with regard to the way that students encode information as they hear and write it (Faber et al., 2000). Both encoding and external storage are important in learning as it relates to note-taking. In the encoding process, the learner processes the new information and assimilates it with previous related knowledge. Self-questioning is an important tool for monitoring comprehension and making associations with other information (Faber et al., 2000). Research suggests that students gradually transition from using notes in a primarily external storage function to a more efficient use of encoding, and younger students of both high and low ability can be taught to use skills such as how to apply prior knowledge to the current subject matter, (b) how to detect and write main ideas, and (c) how to monitor themselves for understanding. (Faber et al., 2000). Other methods used to help students develop complete and effective notes include the following: learning shorthand, writing faster, previewing the subject before class, using guided notes provided by the teacher, and strategic note-taking that cues the student what questions to ask himself about the lecture (Boyle, 2001).

Listening strategies are also important components of learning in the classroom. Perhaps more than any other strategies discussed here, listening is often viewed as a skill that develops naturally and does not require explicit instruction; alternatively it is viewed as an innate ability that cannot be taught (Opitz & Zbaracki, 2004). Research does not support either of these contentions. Listening strategies are often taught in the context of learning a second language (Field, 2008). Effective listening strategies that lend themselves well to explicit instruction include: preparing to listen, becoming an active listener, listening for teacher cues, and developing a comprehensive plan for listening (Vannest, Stroud, & Reynolds, 2011).

Attention/Concentration

Attention is a precursor to memory and learning (e. g., see Reynolds & Voress, 2007; Riccio, Reynolds, Lowe, & Moore, 2002). Most theories of learning include in their beginning phases the ability to attend adequately to the material or stimulus. Bandura's (1965) Social Learning Theory has four necessary components: attention, retention, reproduction, and motivation. Attention is dependent both on the characteristics of the learner and of the model. For learning to occur, the learner must be able to filter out extraneous information and focus on the salient elements to be learned. The Keller's ARCS Model (Attention, Relevance, Confidence, Satisfaction) integrates concepts, theories, strategies, and tactics related to the motivation to learn (Keller, 1997). According to Keller, learning is facilitated by capturing the learner's interest (perceptual arousal), stimulating inquiry (inquiry arousal), and maintaining attention (variability). Attention is composed of 4 factors: initiating focus or attention, sustaining attention, inhibiting responses to distractions, and shifting attention (Riccio, Reynolds, Low, & Moore, 2002). Concentration is the extended attention required for learning; this "paying attention" is a skill that can be taught to students (Vannest, Stroud, & Reynolds, 2011).

Attention problems relating to learning are often considered synonymous with Attention-Deficit/Hyperactivity Disorder (ADHD). Prevalence rates of ADHD range from 3–7% (American Psychiatric Association, 2000) to 10–20% of school-age children (Shaywitz & Shaywitz, 1992). ADHD is the most common clinical referral concern for children (Barkley & Murphy, 1998). Clearly, ADHD is a common problem in most classrooms; however, inattention is not limited to children with ADHD. In fact, attention problems impact many children suffering from other neurological and psychological disorders, including schizophrenia (Riccio et al., 2002), depression (American Psychological Association, 2000), anxiety (LaBerge, 2002), acute stress (Hancock & Warm, 1989) and brain injuries or dysfunction (Sohlberg, McLaughlin, Pavese, Heidrich, & Posner, 2000). Environmental or personal factors also impact attention (e.g., fatigue, medication) (Zentall, 2005). Indeed, the relationships between both internalizing and externalizing disorders and academic underachievement appear to be mediated by attention (Barriga, et al., 2002; Hinshaw, 1992). Given the role of attention in learning and the frequency of reported concerns, it is essential to include assessment of attention and intervention, if needed, with children who are struggling academically (Barriga et al., 2002).

Cognitive psychologists see the ability to self-monitor and adjust in a learning environment as an important skill in the development of effective learning strategies (e.g., Alexander & Murphy, 1999). The successful use of strategies is dependent on several processes, including identifying important information, allocating attention, and monitoring comprehension (Reynolds & Shirey, 1988). As a student learns skills in study, note-taking, and test-taking strategies their perception that attention and performance can be controlled is likely to increase.

Research and recommendations for strategies aimed at improving attention typically have been directed toward children with ADHD and are most often multimodal in nature. Numerous classroom strategies appear to be helpful in engaging children with attention problems. Such techniques target tasks including getting attention, focusing attention, sustaining attention, reducing distractions, teaching organizational skills, increasing time management skills, and increasing specific skills in content areas (Teeter, 1998).

Organizational Techniques

The ability to manage learning tasks is integral to academic success. Organization allows a student to be purposeful in the arrangement of his own environment and materials. It is much more than an academic skill; it is a work skill and a life skill. Organizational behaviors may be defined as the ability "to (a) plan and manage activities within a time framework, (b) systematically arrange objects and assignments within space for rapid retrieval, and (c) structure an approach to a task" (Zentall, Harper, and Stormont-Spurgin, 1993, p. 112). In this definition of organizational behavior 3 types of organization are introduced: time (time management which will be discussed shortly), object (a student's ability to maintain his possessions, including needed supplies), and idea (the management and structure of academic information to be learned). It is object organization that is the focus of this section.

Having weak organizational skills can result in problems with school, work, and personal life (Gureasko-Moore, DuPaul, & White, 2006). Organizational strategies are those techniques which are used to organize materials to be learned (Stroud & Reynolds, 2006). For example, students can be taught specific steps in order to be prepared for class; they may need help learning to keep their assignments in a designated place. Students who often come to class with one binder that has numerous assignments from every subject protruding from it, yet cannot find the one that is currently due will likely need specific instruction, modeling, and practice in order to learn better organization. Teaching students these basic organizational techniques provide students with a skill set for learning more complex organization tasks as adults (Slade, 1986). Students who are strategic in their organization of work in various environments are more apt to be efficient learners and to have more time to devote to academic tasks. They are also more likely to complete homework assignments and to turn in their work (Hughes, Ruhl, Schumaker, & Deshler, 2002). Object organizational strategies are also essential tools for learning other skills including time management (Richards, 1987).

Organizational techniques may be taught with other self-management strategies including filing and having materials accessible at school as well as defining a study space at home (Gall et al., 1990). Teachers can foster organization by requiring the use of a three-ring binder, providing lessons and games regarding organization of students' desks at school, teaching students ways to define and organize a place to study at home, providing incentives for using appropriate skills, and eliciting parent support. Bakunas and Holley (2004) identify specific organizational objectives to teach students. For example, teach students to bring needed supplies through methods such as making a list of supplies for the class and involving parents in making sure students are coming to school prepared. Teachers might also have students learn to organize their desks and lockers, cleaning them regularly. Suggestions include having students draw maps of their desks as they are and as they should be. Using class time allows different ideas to be compared and implementation to begin.

Time Management

Time management refers to the ability to identify tasks to be completed and to allocate sufficient time to each of those tasks. Most college students identify management of their time more effectively to be their greatest area of need (Weissberg, Berentsen, Cote, Cravey, and Heath, 1982). Having weak time management skills can result in problems with school, work, and personal life (Mauksch, Hillenburg, & Robins, 2001; Peeters & Rutte, 2005). To help address this need, numerous books and learning strategies classes for college students have included efficient time management skills as a focus. Most of these resources have offered very similar suggestions for improving the time management practices (Macan, Shahani, Dipboye, & Phillips, 1990).

While children are at home, their parents often monitor, at least to some degree, their allocation of time. Teachers provide oversight for larger projects in the classroom. As they progress through middle school and into high school, expectations for independent management of work and extracurricular activities gradually increase. That children naturally mature and develop effective time management practices tends to be assumed but not necessarily supported (Boller, 2008). Even children in elementary school benefit from learning time management techniques (Hoover, 1993). Instruction in effective time management, often included as a self-regulatory strategy, has been associated with higher course grades (Brackney & Karabenick, 1995; Zimmerman, Greenberg, & Weinstein, 1994), reduced anxiety (Macan, 1994), increased problem-solving abilities, effort, and self-efficacy (Jung, 2009) and better grades (Gureasko-Moore et al., 2006; Langberg et al., 2008).

Time management as a self-regulatory or self-management technique includes skills such as learning to organize a schedule, setting attainable goals and accurate timelines, deciding on priorities, arriving on time for class or other obligations, completing work on time, providing rewards or incentives for work completion, and breaking an assignment into manageable parts (Gall et al., 1990). To include these in the general classroom curriculum, teachers might teach students to: use an assignment sheet to keep track of tasks to be completed in their various classes, to schedule their time and encourage them to monitor their ability to stay on schedule, and break larger tasks into smaller more manageable ones. Whenever possible, it is important to draw the connection between students' goals and their academic effort, and incentives may be helpful in reinforcing the use of good skills. Finally, the need for parent involvement, by having them allocate and monitor study time, model good time management behavior, provide tools such as "to do" lists and assignment planners, and reinforce good time management practices at home, is critical, as it provides this reinforcement across settings (Gall et al., 1990).

Time management may also be viewed from an information processing perspective (Britton and Tesser, 1991). Given a limited amount of time and a set of tasks to be completed, it makes sense that a student who is able to efficiently allocate time to prioritized tasks would be able to accomplish more academically. Many different factors of tasks must be taken into account when prioritizing tasks, including task length, complexity, deadlines, and resources needed.

Measures of time management as a behavior have been used primarily for research purposes rather than a means of intervention. As such, they are not standardized measures. They are also almost exclusively designed for college-age students rather than younger students. The Time Management Behavior Scale (TMB; Macan and colleagues, 1990) includes items based on behaviors recommended by various sources on time management. Research with the TMB indicates that students' report of effective general time management behaviors are significantly correlated with factors including role ambiguity, somatic tension, job and life satisfaction, self-rated performance, and GPA. Greater perceived control over time was associated with less role ambiguity, job induced tension and somatic tension; it was also associated with higher scores on life and job satisfaction measures as well as self-reports of achievement and grade point average (Macan et al. 1990). The TMB also supported the effectiveness of a time management seminar while reading a book on time management was not helpful.

Academic Motivation

Among other things, motivation dictates a student's investment in the process of learning, which strategies are used, and the amount of effort put into carrying them out (Stroud & Reynolds, 2006). In addition, understanding motivation helps to explain the differential use of learning strategies, both between students and in one student across learning situations. The converse is also true. The effective use of learning strategies leads to academic success which leads to increased academic motivation.

Models of strategic learning include motivation as a key component (Weinstein et al., 2000). Weinstein et al.'s (2000) model has three components: skill, will, and self-regulation, with "Will" meaning the motivation to learn. Given the relationship between learning strategies and academic motivation, no assessment of one should be considered complete without including the other. An exhaustive review of academic motivation is beyond the scope of this chapter. The reader is referred to Brophy (2004) for a comprehensive discussion of theories of academic achievement motivation with a strong emphasis on how teachers can use aspects of each of these theories to adapt their teaching style and classroom environments to maximize student effort.

The definition of motivation differs according to one's theoretical orientation (Dembo & Eaton, 1996). Descriptions vary according to the frequency, duration, and/or intensity of behavior (behaviorist), as an unconscious drive (psychodynamic), or as a student's thoughts or feelings about a task (cognitive). Conceptualizations of motivation might also take into consideration the students' social or cultural experiences (Dembo & Eaton, 1996). In general, motivation can be considered the "process by which the individual's needs and desires are activated and, thus, directs their thoughts and their behaviors" (Alexander & Murphy, 1998, p. 33) or "an internal state that arouses, directs, and maintains behavior" (Dembo & Eaton, 1996, p. 68). Dembo and Eaton (1996) describe three components of motivation: (a) expectancy, or the student's attributions and self-efficacy for success/failure, (b) value, or the importance placed on the task, and (c) affective, or the emotional processes associated with the learning situation. Motivation is also a key component of models of self-regulation (Zimmerman, 2002). A student's beliefs are important in the forethought phase of learning and include self-efficacy, outcome expectations, intrinsic interest or value, and goal orientation.

Academic achievement motivation relates specifically to academic learning. Leading theories of achievement motivation include self-efficacy, attribution, and goal theories as well as self-determination and intrinsic motivation. While each of these has provided new insights into learning, they have similarities as well. Many have argued that much can be learned from integrating the practical points of these theories when the aim is for successful interventions in the classroom (Brophy, 2004; Roeser & Galloway, 2002). Others feel that there is merit in viewing academic motivation as a multidimensional construct (Bong, 2001). Brophy (2004) asserted that self-efficacy, attribution, and goal theories can all be conceptualized in the expectancy part of expectancy-value theory.

According to expectancy-value theory, an individual's expectations regarding success and the value he or she gives to succeeding are important factors affecting motivation to perform different achievement tasks (Wigfield & Tonks, 2002). Expectancy for success may depend largely on self-efficacy for the task. Self efficacy is defined as "people's judgments of their capabilities to organize and execute courses of action required to attain designated types of performances" (Bandura, 1986, p. 391). It is the culmination of both perceived performance in previous tasks and perceived control that a person feels he has had. Self-efficacy is independent of ability, and it affects numerous factors including students' choice of tasks, persistence, future performance, and their emotional reaction to the task or situation (Collins, 1982). Higher self-efficacy has been associated with both improved coping with stress and academic performance (Chemers, Hu, & Garcia, 2001). Given its independence from ability, it is an exciting consideration for intervention with students of all achievement levels.

Attribution theory refers to one's natural desire to understand why things happen and their beliefs about the causes of success or failure (Dembo & Eaton, 1996). As it applies to learning, attribution theory seeks to explain students' perceptions of the causes of academic success or failure. Weiner's (1979, 1986) achievement motivation theory is the most commonly accepted theory of attribution. Attributes are organized into three dimensions: internal/external, stable/unstable, and controllable/uncontrollable. Students base their beliefs and future actions on their judgment of events in these dimensions, and these attributions affect their expectancy of future performance, persistence in similar tasks, emotional responses, which tasks they choose, and students' self-efficacy (Dembo & Eaton, 1996; Weiner, 1976).

Goal theory has emerged as providing an important conceptualization of academic motivation (Anderman & Wolters, 2006; Elliot, 2005) Goal theory suggests that students adopt one of two distinct goals—performance or mastery (Brophy, 2004). Performance goals, otherwise known as ability or task goals, view learning as a means to an end. These goals focus on "one's ability and sense of self-worth" and pair evaluation of a student's ability with the process of learning (Ames, 1992, p. 262).

Mastery goals, or learning goals, are those adopted in which "individuals are oriented toward developing new skills, trying to understand their work, improving their level of competence, or achieving a sense of mastery based on self-referenced standards" (Ames, 1992, p. 262). Adoption of mastery goals has been associated with perceived lecture engagement and a lack of harsh or evaluative environment (which were associated with performance goals) (Church, Elliot, & Gable, 2001). Mastery goals are associated with a student's investment in tasks, seeking challenges, persisting longer, increased productivity, and increased positive feelings toward the task (Kaplan & Maehr, 2007). In fact, mastery goals are also associated with a more adaptive life orientation, including increased social behavior, positive feelings toward self, and a general sense of well-being (Kaplan & Maehr, 2007).

While Ames asserted that performance and mastery goals are contrasting goals that do not coexist (Ames, 1992), a 2 x 2 model refutes that notion, taking into account approach/avoidance goals as well as mastery/performance (Kaplan & Maehr, 2002). Learning or mastery approach goals appear to facilitate achievement, and performance avoidance goals hinder achievement (Brophy, 2004). The role of performance approach goals is not as clear; it may be that their usefulness or detrimental nature is related to situational factors including the age of the students (Pintrich, 2000). Research on mastery avoidance goals is needed (Kaplan & Maehr, 2002). Mastery avoidance goals may be associated with disorganized learning and test anxiety (Elliot & McGregor, 2001). Many studies suggest that students do not adopt goals in isolation; rather they often adopt multiple goals depending on the situation or context (Kaplan & Maehr, 2002). Obviously lacking in the 2 x 2 model of goal theory is that it does not take into account other goals that students have endorsed, including work completion and social goals. A more recent model takes personal and situational characteristics into account (Kaplan and Maehr, 2002). Three major components comprise what is referred to as a "personal achievement goal": 1. perceived purpose in the situation, 2. self-processes (i.e., self-efficacy, social identity), and 3. the available possibilities for action in the situation.

Developed by Deci and Ryan (1985, 2000), Self-Determination Theory (SDT) has also been a strong presence in academic motivation research. SDT is based on the proposition that humans have an innate desire to learn which is either encouraged or discouraged by an individual's environment. In order for intrinsic motivation to develop, fulfillment of three basic psychological needs is necessary—competency, relatedness, and autonomy (Deci & Ryan, 1985, 2000). SDT delineates intrinsic and extrinsic motivation but further suggests the existence of amotivation or the absence of any desire to pursue an activity. Rather than a simple dichotomy, these states exist on a continuum, with varying degrees of extrinsic motivation: external regulation, introjected regulation, identified regulation, and integrated regulation. There have been indications, however, that intrinsic motivation decreases as extrinsic motivation increases (Darner, 2009). Intrinsic motivation may be further divided into three categories: intrinsic motivation to know, intrinsic motivation to accomplish, and intrinsic motivation to experience stimulation (Vallerand, Pelletier, Blais, & Briere, 1992). It is intrinsic motivation, which elicits pleasure from the act of engaging in the behavior, that is the most self-determined (Vallerand & Ratelle, 2002). High levels of intrinsic motivation appear to be associated with greater academic motivation (Faye & Sharpe, 2008; Wang, 2008; Turner, Chandler, & Heffer, 2009).

A few measures have been designed specifically to assess academic motivation, primarily for research rather than clinical purposes and for use with college students. The Academic Motivation Scale (AMS; Vallerand et al., 1992) was developed to measure academic motivation for college students based on Self-Determination Theory. The AMS assesses 7 constructs which measure intrinsic motivation, extrinsic motivation, and amotivation. Research has indicated only partial support for the construct validity of the AMS (Cokley, Bernard, Cunningham, & Motoike, 2001, Cokley, 2000). In fact, some researchers have argued that validity studies of the AMS suggest that the constructs of SDT may not fit well along a continuum. A better alternative might be to conceptualize intrinsic and extrinsic motivation in a hierarchical manner (Fairchild, Horst, Finney, & Barron, 2005).

Interventions. Motivation is a behavior that can be learned. Which strategies one chooses to use for improving academic motivation largely depend to the theoretical orientation adopted. For example, learning strategies interventions appear to have a positive effect on self-efficacy (Corno & Mandinach, 1983; Pintrich & De Groot, 1990; Zimmerman & Martinez-Pons, 1990). Being able to use a strategy to accomplish a task provides a sense of control over performance outcomes. If the strategy is successful,

then the student's self-efficacy is improved and the learner is more likely to use the strategy again.

Attribution retraining with learning strategies instruction improved use of reading strategies in a group of children with learning disabilities (Borkowski, Weyhing, & Carr, 1988) and significantly increased the passing rate for final exams with a group of college freshmen (Van Overwalle & De Metsenaere, 1990). Attribution retraining has been less effective (Craske, 1985) or not supported by similar studies (Miranda, Villaescusa, & Vidal-Abarca, 1997; Short & Ryan, 1984) that incorporated self-regulation procedures as part of the intervention. It may be that the use of self-regulation strategies generated sufficient self-confidence, circumventing the need for additional training. Individual strategies such as self-talk, goal setting, and time management have been used effectively to increase academic motivation (Dembo & Eaton, 1996). In addition, classroom management strategies employed by teachers have a profound effect on students' academic achievement motivation (Brophy, 2004; Church et al., 2001).

Test Anxiety

Anxiety may be defined as "the tendency to be nervous, fearful, or worried about real or imagined problems" (Reynolds & Kamphaus, 2004). Anxiety may be described s general or specific. Test anxiety is a situation-specific form of anxiety. Simply put, test anxiety prevents a student from performing on a test at the level he or she is capable of. Assessment of test anxiety dates back to the mid-twentieth century and test anxiety as a construct was proposed much earlier (Sarason & Mandler, 1952; Mandler & Sarason, 1953). The increasing reliance on state-mandated testing in schools and the consequences for individual students as well as schools has transformed the issue of test anxiety from an individual concern to one that is shared by students, parents, and educators alike. As with so many other areas discussed in this chapter, test anxiety has been studied most in college-age students; however, test anxiety can be and a hindrance for students of all ages. Test anxiety has been associated with lower test scores as well as lower self-esteem (Marsh, 1990; Newbegin & Owens, 1996). Students who obtain high scores on measures of test anxiety are also more likely to report more pervasive psychological difficulties, including anxiety disorders and depressive symptoms (Beidel, Turner, & Trager, 1994; King, Mietz, Tinney, & Ollendick, 1995) and even suicidal thoughts (Keogh & French, 2001). Awareness of when students experience test anxiety has expanded as well to include the time before and after the test as well as during the test itself (Raffety, Smith, & Ptacek, 1997; Zeidner, 1998; Stöber, 2004). The incidence of test anxiety appears to be increasing, from estimates of 10 to 20 percent to more recent suggestions of 33 percent (e.g., Methia, 2004).

Models of test anxiety conceptualize the construct in one of three ways: a personality trait, an emotional state, a clinical disorder (Putwain, 2008). Four main theories have shaped the study of test anxiety (Jones & Petruzzi, 1995). The *cognitive-attentional model* includes the original worry-emotionality constructs, theorizing that excessive worries, self-coping statements, concern regarding physiological reactions, and other task-irrelevant thoughts interfere with optimal task performance (Naveh-Benjamin, 1991; Wine, 1971). The *learning deficit model* or *skill deficit model* suggests that test anxiety arises from a lack of adequate study and test-taking skills (Birenbaum, 2007; Hodapp & Henneberger, 1983). Although the relationship between poor study habits and test anxiety has been established, this model has not been able to adequately explain how high-achieving students who have good study skills can also experience test anxiety (Tobias, 1985). The *dual deficit* or *information processing model* seeks to bridge the gap between the first two models, proposing that both task-irrelevant thoughts and skills deficits may contribute to feelings of anxiety (Jones & Petruzzi, 1995). According to this view, test anxiety is caused by difficulties encoding and organizing material as well as retrieval during an evaluation (Naveh-Benjamin, 1991). Finally, the *social learning model* argues that the origins of test anxiety lie with a student's self-efficacy regarding a task and motivation to perform well.

Another integrative model of test anxiety is the Transactional Process Model, which describes the relationships among antecedents, student dispositions, cognitive processes, and the consequences associated with test anxiety (Spielberger & Vagg, 1995). Antecedents include the subject matter of the test, study skills, and test taking skills. During the evaluation, a student retrieves and processes information, continually assesses his situation, and may respond with an increase in worry and/or emotionality associated with test anxiety. The result of these processes will be behavior that is relevant or not relevant to the task.

The cause of test anxiety differs according to the characteristics of the student. For example, high achieving students and low achieving students may have test anxiety for very different reasons (Wigfield and Eccles, 1989). High achievers may experience heightened anxiety due to the unrealistic expectations placed on them by parents, peers, or self, while less able students may be anxious due to previous experiences of and future expectations of failure. Also, some anxious students may have good study habits but suffer from the pressure of being evaluated, whereas other students have poor study strategies which inhibit their learning (Naveh-Benjamin, McKeachie, & Lin, 1987).

Students with high anxiety divide their attention between task-relevant and task-irrelevant thoughts (Wine 1971). Children with high anxiety are similar to anxious adults in their increased reporting of negative self-evaluations (Galassi et al., 1981; Zatz & Chassin, 1983; Zatz & Chassin, 1985). Cognitive distortions, including catastrophizing, are particularly detrimental to performance on tests (Putwain, Connors, & Symes, 2010). Unfortunately, the coping statements that test anxious children so often make do not appear to improve their performance (Zatz & Chassin, 1985). Students with high test anxiety report significantly more self-coping statements than their peers, likely because they perceive the situation as stressful (Prins, Groot, & Hanewald, 1994). Research indicates that it is likely the absence of negative thoughts rather than the presence of positive thoughts that improves performance, a finding which highlights the need for intervention programs to decrease all off-task thoughts.

When assessing test anxiety, it should be considered that the relationship between anxiety and performance is likely not linear. Ball (1995) summarized the following points describing the relationship between the two factors: (a) "that test anxiety may be facilitating" (for some students), (b) that moderator variables including test difficulty and "the proficiency of the test taker" may be present, and (c) "the relation between test anxiety and performance may be curvilinear" (p. 109). Also of concern, students with test anxiety demonstrate poor study habits and organizational difficulties which inhibit information processing (Culler & Holahan, 1980; Naveh-Benjamin et al., 1987). Some distinguish between test anxiety, which they consider to always be debilitating and more mild fear of failure that facilitates better performance (Martin & Marsh, 2003).

Self-report methods remain the commonly used method of assessing test anxiety. Preferred for their efficiency and ease of administration, self-report methods are used more often for research than for diagnostic or intervention purposes. The most commonly used measures for children are the Test Anxiety Scale for Children (TASC; Sarason, Davidson, Lighthall, & Waite, 1958) and the Test Anxiety Inventory (TAI; Spielberger, 1980). The TAI was developed for use with college students but norms have been developed for high school students. The Children's Test Anxiety Scale (CTAS; Wren & Benson, 2004) is a newer measure of test anxiety. Developed for use with children in grades 3 to 6, the CTAS measures three dimensions of test anxiety: thoughts, autonomic reactions, and off-task behaviors.

Hembree's (1988) meta-analysis asserted that a variety of cognitive and behavioral interventions have had lasting effects in reducing anxiety and increasing academic performance. Unfortunately, as with studies regarding the antecedents and correlates of test anxiety, much of what we know about interventions with children and adolescents is inferred from studies with adults (Ergene, 2003).

Effective intervention most often utilizes a multi-component approach. Elements can include training in cognitive restructuring, relaxation, time management, attention control, test-taking, and study-skills (Dendato and Diener, 1986; Decker, 1987; Glanz, 1994; Wilson & Rotter, 1986). Results of teaching these combined skills appear to be decreased test anxiety and improved academic performance. Such multi-component approaches have effectively reduced test anxiety and increased self-esteem and academic performance (Wilson & Rotter, 1986). Teaching students as young as 3rd grade relaxation techniques can effectively reduce test anxiety (Larson, El Ramahi, Conn, Estes, & Ghibellini, 2010). Abbreviated Upright Behavioral Training, which offers explicit instruction in the use of 10 overt relaxed behaviors, has effectively reduced test anxiety for college students as well (2006).

Assessment Measures

The importance of learning strategies and their related constructs is hopefully evident at this point. The next logical consideration should be the accurate measurement of these constructs. Only a few measures currently exist for the purpose of measuring learning strategies and/or self-regulated learning, and most have significant limitations in their utility. More commonly, measures are designed to measure one or two constructs (Child Organization Scale, Zentall, 1993), with little consideration given to the possible interactions of these constructs. Others are developed primarily for research purposes and may

change with a given hypothesis (e.g., Approaches to Learning and Studying Inventory, Entwistle & McCune, 2004). The most widely used and more comprehensive assessment measures are the Learning and Study Strategies Inventory (LASSI, Weinstein, 1987), the Motivated Strategies for Learning Questionnaire (MSLQ; Pintrich, Smith, Garcia, & McKeachie, 1991), and the School Motivation and Learning Strategies Inventory (SMALSI; Stroud & Reynolds, 2006). As is the case with much work on learning strategies, the MSLQ was created to be used for college-age students. The LASSI, which is commercially available, was also originally designed for use with college students (Weinstein, 1987). The LASSI for high school students is a downward extension of a college level version of the instrument. The LASSI is an established method of measuring of learning strategies and a sound clinical tool, however, it and the other measures listed above leave much unanswered about children and the development of learning strategies and their related constructs.

A measure designed to assess learning strategies and study habits serves many purposes. Historic purposes for high school and college level inventories include: predicting academic performance, advising students about their use of strategies, and screening and progress measures for study skills courses (Weinstein, Zimmerman, and Palmer, 1988). Other reasons cited in the development of the LASSI include: assessment of a wide variety of topics related to and including learning strategies with sound psychometric properties, assessment of observable and modifiable behaviors that are reflective of current research in cognitive psychology, and use as a diagnostic instrument (Weinstein et al., 1988).

The Learning and Study Strategies Inventory—High School (LASSI-HS, Weinstein & Palmer, 1990) is a "diagnostic and prescriptive measure that assesses student thought processes and behaviors that impact studying and learning" (5). It is designed for adolescents entering the ninth grade to first year college students. The 76-item questionnaire has students rate themselves on a 5-point Likert scale. Reliability coefficients range from.68 to.82. Validity information was not available in the original manual. The LASSI has 10 scales: (1) Attitude, (2) Motivation, (3) Time Management principles for academic tasks, (4) Anxiety, (5) Concentration, (6) Information Processing, (7) Selecting Main Ideas, (8) Study Aids, (9) Self Testing, and (10) Test Strategies.

The LASSI and, by extension, the LASSI-HS have taught us much about the assessment of learning strategies and have provided invaluable clinical and empirical information; however, as useful as they are, they leave many questions about the nature of learning strategies and related constructs. The SMALSI (Stroud & Reynolds, 2006) was designed to enhance our understanding of the process of learning. For example, little is known about special populations such as children with ADHD, cancer, learning disabilities, or children with Traumatic Brain Injuries, and their individual needs. Perhaps the greatest potential for contribution of the SMALSI is that it covers a more broad range of child development. The ability to measure and compare these constructs across ages provides a greater understanding of the development of certain cognitive skills as well as an understanding of motivational factors and how they change from childhood to adolescence. Educators are able to assess and monitor learning strategies as they develop rather than only targeting them for remediation once difficulties have emerged.

Much of the practice of psychological assessment involves diagnosing the problem. A less tangible, but no less important aspect of the SMALSI is its focus on student strengths along with weaknesses. More than just allowing the clinician to "rule out" issues as being part of the problem, strengths on the SMALSI allow the clinician to tailor recommendations for intervention given the tools they already have for success.

Inventories prior to the SMALSI provided a reasonable understanding of learning strategies, but only from a remedial or reactive perspective. What remained missing was research to help understand the development of learning strategies in younger children (Weinstein et al., 2000). A psychometrically sound means of measuring such strategies and their associated features was necessary in order to accomplish this goal. The SMALSI was intended to help to identify which behaviors are consistent with academic success and how or if these behaviors vary according to age, gender, intelligence, motivation, attributions, and other relevant variables.

Finally, one might assume that learning strategies naturally increase as a student matures, regardless of instruction. This is certainly true for many learning strategies, but is not the case for all. In fact, self-regulated learning strategies appear to change as students progress through school, with some increasing while others increase then decrease over time (Zimmerman & Martinez-Pons, 1990). Research indicates that very effective reading comprehension strategies such as generating questions while reviewing texts or making visual representations of information do not improve over time (Thomas & Rowher, 1986). Also, how often students use some strategies are related to their use of other strategies (Zimmerman and Martinez-Pons, 1990). For example, during the transition from junior high to high school, students report declines in the practice of reviewing textbooks whereas their tendency to reviewing notes increases during this period. These two trends highlight the relationships among strategies how students base their strategic decisions on the nature of their changing learning activities. The SMALSI provides a means of further exploring such trends.

The Student Motivation and Learning Strategies Inventory

The SMALSI is comprised of two forms: one for children ages 8–12 (SMALSI-Form C) and one for adolescents ages 13–18 (SMALSI-Form T). The SMALSI-Child has 147 items and the SMALSI-Teen has 170 items. The SMALSI was designed to be a versatile and widely utilized measure. As such, it can be administered in a group or individual setting in a relatively short period of time. Typical administration time is 20–30 minutes.

The SMALSI includes seven strengths scales and three liabilities scales. Student Strengths scales include: Study Strategies, Reading/Comprehension Strategies, Note-taking/Listening Strategies, Writing/Research Strategies, Test-Taking Strategies, Organizational Techniques, and Time Management. Student Liabilities scales include Low Academic Motivation, Attention/Concentration, and Test Anxiety. On the Child Form, the Time Management and Organizational Techniques scales are combined to reflect developing but not yet distinct organizational behaviors. Scales are reported as T-scores, which allows for comparison of performance among constructs as well as for monitoring development or the effectiveness of an intervention. The SMALSI also has an Inconsistent Responding Index (INC) to indicate responses that are inconsistent, perhaps due to noncompliance, poor understanding, or carelessness. Definitions of these scales as used in the SMALSI are given in Table X.X.

Psychometric properties appear to be solid for both the SMALSI Form C and Form T (Stroud & Reynolds, 2006). Internal consistencies for the ten scales yielded estimates consistently above .7, indicating support for the structure of the SMALSI

Table 24.1 Definitions of the SMALSI Scales

Scale	Definition
Study Strategies	Selecting important information, relating new to previously learned information, and memory strategies for encoding.
Note-taking/Listening Skills	Discriminating important material when taking notes, organizing notes, efficiency in note-taking.
Reading and Comprehension Strategies	Previewing, monitoring, and reviewing texts, including self-testing to ensure understanding.
Writing-Research Skills	Researching topics in a variety of ways, organizing writing projects as well as monitoring and self-checking for errors.
Test-taking Strategies	Increasing efficiency in test-taking, including eliminating unlikely answers and strategic guessing.
Organizational Techniques	Organizing class and study materials, structuring assignments including homework and other projects.
Time Management	Effective use of time to complete assignments, understanding of time needed for academic tasks.
Academic Motivation	Level of intrinsic motivation to engage and succeed in academic tasks
Test Anxiety	Student's experience of debilitating symptoms of test anxiety, lower performance on tests due to excessive worry
Attention/Concentration	Attending to lectures and other academic tasks, monitoring and adjusting attention to performance, concentrating and the avoidance of distractions.

scales. These findings were consistent across ages and grades with the exception of one scale (SMALSI Form C Writing/Research Strategies). As might be expected, younger children had the most difficulty responding reliably regarding their use of writing strategies. This was the lowest scale in general; however, reliability on this scale tended to increase with age as would be expected from a developmental perspective. With this exception, younger children tended to respond in the same manner as older children to SMALSI constructs, further supporting the assertion that younger children are capable of reliably reporting their own attitudes and behaviors (Reynolds & Kamphaus, 1992, 2004; Reynolds & Richmond, 1985).

The reliability of the SMALSI scales was also generally robust across gender and across ethnicity (Stroud & Reynolds, 2006). The one exception to this was found in the American Indian sample. When ethnicity was taken into account, results were generally commensurate with the exception of the American Indian sample which produced higher reliability coefficients on several scales. This difference was observed to a small but consistent degree on both forms and was larger with the adolescent sample. Such a small difference alone did not indicate significant implications for individual interpretation; it does suggest that further study of differences in response patterns for different ethnic groups would be beneficial. Overall, the results of the initial standardization and validity studies suggested that the SMALSI has sufficient reliability and they indicate good confidence that the items comprising the SMALSI scales are accurate in estimating a student's current functioning on the constructs measured.

Validity is an equally important consideration when evaluating the utility of the SMALSI. The constructs measured by the SMALSI were determined by conducting a thorough review of literature in education, psychology, and related areas. Each construct was chosen due to empirical evidence establishing its role in fostering academic success. The content validity of the scales and items was also supported by expert review from multiple sources (Stroud & Reynolds, 2006).

Correlations between SMALSI scales supported the structure of the SMALSI as measuring individual constructs that fall within the two general areas of student strengths and student liabilities (Stroud & Reynolds, 2006). Similar results across forms indicated the presence of both common and distinctive constructs. As expected, student strengths scales were correlated with each other, while student liabilities scales were correlated with each other.

The validity of the SMALSI scales was further indicated by divergence of the SMALSI scales from measured clinical dimensions (i.e., depression) and convergence with academic measures. For example, School Liability (Low Academic Motivation, Attention/Concentration, and Test Anxiety) scales on the SMALSI were positively correlated with measures of clinical, personal, and school maladjustment, whereas the School Strength scales had negative associations with these scales. This pattern was consistent for younger and older students. In particular, academic motivation was highly correlated with students' attitudes toward school and teachers, further supporting previous literature asserting the critical roles that academic environment and characteristics of the teacher play in the level of students' academic motivation (e.g., Brophy, 2004; Pajares & Urdan, 2002). Also of note, children who reported increased depression also reported less frequent use of some strategies including test-taking strategies and note-taking strategies; these students also reported decreased concentration, attention skills, and academic motivation. This finding lends further support to the importance of direct teaching of learning strategies to students with psychiatric disorders (Brackney & Karabenick, 1995).

Of paramount importance was the relationship between SMALSI constructs and academic achievement. For example, student's use of study strategies, writing skills, and time management/organizational techniques were positively linked with reading abilities (Stroud & Reynolds, 2006). In addition, writing skills were associated positively with math abilities, whereas test anxiety impaired math performance. In the adolescent group, though, a shift was observed, with test anxiety playing a more prominent role; for these students, test anxiety negatively impacted reading, social studies, and science academic abilities. Academic motivation was a more prominent factor in the adolescent sample, particularly in the areas of reading and social studies.

The performance of different demographic groups on the SMALSI also produced interesting results. For example, girls consistently scored higher than boys on both the Child and Teen forms for several scales (Note-taking/Listening Strategies, Writing/Research Strategies, and Test-Taking Strategies. Differences for gender comparison of adolescents were more prevalent, with girls scoring higher on all student strengths scales. Adolescent girls also tended to report higher test anxiety. Effect sizes were all small but consistent and in line with previous research (Reynolds & Kamphaus, 1992, 2002, and 2004).

The SMALSI scores demonstrated reliability and validity across age and grades. In the child sample, scores on the SMALSI were stable, with little deviation aside from minor score fluctuations around the mean T-score of 50. In the adolescent group, a general trend toward increasing study strategies with age and grade was observed. This is to be expected, given that student's study strategies and abilities tend to improve with increased practice and refinement of skills with added exposure to the academic setting. It is worth noting, however, 8th grade students reported decreased study and learning strategies relative to other teen groups, a trend which invites future research and exploration in adolescent samples.

Interpreting the SMALSI

The SMALSI can be used in two main ways to determine which strategies may be most effective to focus on for an individual student. Individual items should be examined to determine if there appears to be a pattern to the strategies a student is already using. For example, does the student report using a variety of strategies but very infrequently? He or she may benefit from additional practice with these strategies to make their use more efficient and to increase the student's awareness of strategy effectiveness. Alternatively, does the student report relying heavily on just a few strategies, while not using other strategies at all? Some students may rely on the initial process of taking notes but lack essential skills for later review and organization.

After getting an idea of what strategies an individual is using, the results of each scale in relation to scores on other scales should be examined. These may also provide cues in deciding which specific strategies to focus on. For example, a child also demonstrating difficulties on the Organizational techniques scale may need additional help in developing organizational strategies as well as organizing information. On the other hand, a student who appears to have well-developed organizational skills may need less instruction in strategies used to organize information. Also, a student who endorses using note-taking/listening strategies, but relatively infrequently, and who has low academic motivation may already know the strategies necessary for success, but lack the motivation to use them regularly or effectively.

Implications of the SMALSI as a Measure of Learning Strategies

The SMALSI opens new doors for research in understanding learning strategies and their related construct. More importantly it is intended for clinical use in individuals and with groups. The SMALSI was intentionally designed to be used in a variety of settings and by different professions. In the school setting, for example, the SMALSI can be applied as a preventive measure at the classroom level. Teachers may use this measure in a group format to identify specific problem areas such as poor study or organizational habits for the class as a whole. Areas of weakness might then be incorporated into the teacher's class curriculum. Progress can then be monitored by re-administering the SMALSI following a specific intervention or later in the school year. Children struggling academically are often referred to school level teams designed to help implement interventions prior to referral for Special Education services. On this individual level, the SMALSI may be used to identify specific areas that may become the focus of pre-referral intervention. Such instruction may improve academic performance without the need for additional levels of academic support. In this venue in particular, the SMALSI is an excellent tool in response-to-intervention models. Further, given the emphasis on state-mandated testing to determine school funding and pupil progress, teachers and school personnel are faced with the increasing demands of facilitating both students' academic knowledge as well as their test-taking abilities. The SMALSI can be a valuable tool for helping teachers identify children's individual strengths and weaknesses in these areas to help tailor interventions to their specific needs. This measure provides teachers and administrators with a user-friendly method of assessing the skills of multiple children at one time, without the need for comprehensive one-on-one testing.

Psychologists and other professionals with formal training in assessment are able to use the SMALSI in a more diagnostic manner, depending upon their level of training. While the SMALSI is a helpful tool for teachers in the classroom, psychologists will likely use it as part of a complete diagnostic battery. The valuable relationships among constructs measured by the SMALSI and more global behavioral and emotional difficulties have been demonstrated. The child's use of learning strategies as well as the factors of academic motivation, test anxiety, and attention are useful adjuncts to academic achievement and intellectual measures. Results of the SMALSI can add unique insight into possible academic causes, consequences, or correlates of emotional and behavioral disorders.

Results of the SMALSI may be used by clinicians to make meaningful and measurable academic recommendations regarding interventions to use and classroom accommodations to make in the Individualized Education Plan (IEP). Struggling students who do not qualify for additional services under the Individuals with Disabilities Education Act (IDEA) or Section 504 equal access services are particularly susceptible to academic failure. School personnel will need specific and measurable recommendations about what areas to target given the constraints of available general education modifications (i.e., tutoring, reading programs, skill-building programs).

A significant strength of the SMALSI is its focus on strengths. It is easy to focus on "what is wrong" with a child in an assessment. Just as important is what is right, what is working. The importance of identifying a child's strengths cannot be understated. The aim of the SMALSI is to do both, to delineate both strengths and areas for improvement and to offer objective assessment in a comprehensive manner in areas that previously have been difficult to assess. Much can be done with this knowledge to increase students' skills in the classroom. Sound measurement affords us the opportunity to monitor progress in teaching and use of skills. The result is strategic learners who possess the flexibility and problem-solving skills that will lead to long term academic and vocational success.

Conclusions

The purpose of this chapter has been to present an overview of learning strategies and related constructs, emphasizing the need for and methods of assessment. Certainly with younger students, the focus to date has been on assessment of learning strategies for the broader purposes of research intended to understand the process of learning and effective methods of increasing student achievement. While these goals cannot be overstated, equally important is impact on the individual. Much can be discovered about the process of learning in an individual. Much can be done to intervene in specific areas of weakness for an individual. Assessment of children, in general, reveals many psychological processes that may not lend themselves to easy intervention. Learning strategies, on the other hand, can be quickly improved through direct group or individual instruction (Vannest, Stroud, & Reynolds, 2011). Incorporating learning strategies assessment in a battery of tests is crucial to the overall understanding of an individual, and the success achieved from learning these strategies can be far-reaching.

References

Alexander, P. A., & Murphy, P. K. (1998). The research base for APA's learner-centered psychological principles. In N. M. Lamberst & B. L. McCombs (Eds.), *How students learn: Reforming schools through learner-centered education* (pp. 25–60).Washington, DC: American Psychological Association.

Alexander, P. A., & Murphy, P. K. (1999).What cognitive psychology has to say to school psychology: Shifting perspectives and shared purposes. In C. R. Reynolds & T. B. Gutkin (Eds.), *The handbook of school psychology* (3rd ed., pp. 167–193). New York:Wiley.

American Psychiatric Association. (1994). *Diagnostic and statistical manual of mental disorders* (4th ed.). Washington, DC: Author.

Ames, C. (1992). Classrooms: Goals, structures, and student motivation. *Journal of Educational Psychology*, *84*(3), 261–271.

Anderman, E. M. & Wolters, C. A. (2006). Goals, values, and affect: Influences on student motivation. In P. Alexander & P. Winne (Eds.), Handbook of Educational Psychology (pp. 369–389). Mahwah, NJ: Erlbaum.

Armbruster, B. B., Lehr, F., & Osborn, J. (2003). Putting reading first: The research building blocks for teaching children to read (2nd ed.). Retrieved for http://www.nifl.gov/partnershipforreading/publications/PFRbookletBW.pdf

Atwell, N. (1987). In the middle: Reading, writing, and learning from adolescents. Portsmouth, NH: Heinemann.

Bail, F. T., Zhang, S., & Tachiyama, G. T. (2008). Effects of a self-regulated learning course on the academic performance and graduation rate of college students in an academic support program. *Journal of College Reading and Learning, 39*(1), 54–73.

Baird, G. L., Scott, W. D., Dearing, E., & Hamill, S. K. (2009). Cognitive self-regulation in youth with and without learning disabilities: Academic self-efficacy, theories of intelligence, learning vs. performance goal preferences, and effort attributions. *Journal of Social & Clinical Psychology, 28*(7), 881–908.

Baker, L., and Brown, A. (1984). Metacognitive skills in reading. In P. D. Pearson, R. Barr, M. L. Kamil, & P. Morenthal, P. (Eds.), *Handbook of reading research* (pp. 353–394). New York: Longman.

Bakken, J. P., Mastropieri, M. A., & Scruggs, T. E. (1997). Reading comprehension of expository science material and students with learning disabilities: A comparison of strategies. *Journal of Special Education, 31*(3), 300–324.

Bakken, J. P., & Whedon, C. K. (2002). Teaching text structure to improve reading comprehension. *Intervention in School and Clinic, 37*(4), 229–233.

Bakunas, B., & Holley, W. (2004). Teaching organizational skills. *Clearing House, 77*(3), 92–95.

Ball, S. (Ed.). (1995). *Anxiety and test performance*. Philadelphia, PA: Taylor & Francis.

Bandura, A. (1965). Behavioral modifications through modeling procedures. In L. Krasner & L. P. Ullman (Eds.) Research in behavior modification (pp. 310–340). New York: Holt, Rinehart, and Winston.

Bandura, (1986). *Social foundations of thought and action: A social cognitive theory*. Englewood Cliffs, NJ: Prentice-Hall.

Barkley, R. A., & Murphy, K. R. (1998). *Attention-Deficit Hyperactivity Disorder: A Handbook for Diagnosis and Treatment: A Clinical Workbook. Second Edition*. New York: The Guilford Press

Barnett, J. E., (2000). Self-regulated reading and test preparation among college students. *Journal of college reading and learning, 31*(1), 42–61.

Barriga, A. Q., Doran, J. W., Newell, S. R., Morrison, E. M., Barbetti, V., & Robbins, B. D. (2002). Relationships between problem behaviors and academic achievement in adolescents: The unique role of attention problems. *Journal of Emotional and Behavioral Disorders, 10*(4), 233–240.

Beidel, D. C., Turner, M.W., & Trager, K. N. (1994). Test anxiety and childhood anxiety in African American and white school children. *Journal of Anxiety Disorders, 8*(2), 169–179.

Birenbaum, M. (2007). Assessment and Instruction Preferences and Their Relationship with Test Anxiety and Learning Strategies, Higher Education: The International Journal of Higher Education and Educational Planning, v53 n6 p749–768

Boller, B. (2008). Teaching Organizational Skills in Middle School. *Education Digest: Essential Readings Condensed for Quick Review, 74*(2), 52–55.

Bong, M. (2001). Between- and within-domain relations of academic motivation among middle and high school students' self-efficacy, task-value, and achievement goals. *Journal of Educational Psychology, 93*(1), 23–34.

Borkowski, J. G., Weyhing, R. S., & Carr, M. (1988). Effects of attributional retraining on strategy-based reading comprehension in learning-disabled students. *Journal of Educational Psychology, 80*(1), 46–53.

Boyle, J. R. (2001). Enhancing the note-taking skills of students with mild disabilities. *Intervention of School and Clinic, 36*(4), 221–224.

Brackney, B. E., & Karabenick, S. A. (1995). Psychopathology and academic performance: The role of motivation and learning strategies. *Journal of Counseling Psychology, 42*(4), 456–465.

Britton, B. K., & Tesser, A. (1991). Effects of time-management practices on college grades. *Journal of Educational Psychology, 83*(3), 405–410.

Broekkamp, H., & Van Hout-Wolters, B. M. (2007). Students' adaptation of study strategies when preparing for classroom tests. *Educational Psychology Review, 19*(4), 401–428.

Brophy, J. (2004). *Motivating students to learn*, 2nd ed. Mahwah, NJ: Lawrence Erlbaum Associates.

Brown, W. F., & Holtzman, W. H. (1966). *Manual of the survey of study habits and attitudes*. New York: Psychological Corporation.

Bygrave, P. L. (1994). Development of listening skills in students in special education settings. *International Journal of Disability, Development and Education, 41*(1), 51–60.

Campbell, J. R., Voelkl, K. E., & Donahue, P. L. (1997). *NAEP 1996 trends in academic progress*. Washington, DC: National Center for Education Statistics.

Carpenter, S. K., Pashler, H., & Vul, E. (2006). What types of learning are enhanced by a cued recall test? *Psychonomic Bulletin & Review, 13*, 826–830.

Cassady, J. C., & Johnson, R. E. (2002). Cognitive test anxiety and academic performance. *Contemporary Educational Psychology, 27*(2), 270–295.

Chalk, J. C., Hagan-Burke, S., & Burke, M. D. (2005). The effects of self-regulated strategy development on the writing process for high school students with learning disabilities. *Learning Disability Quarterly, 28*(1), 75–87.

Chemers, M. M., Hu, L., & Garcia, B. F. (2001). Academic self-efficacy and first-year college student performance and adjustment. *Journal of Educational Psychology, 93*(1), 55–64.

Church, M. A., Elliot, A. J., & Gable, S. L. (2001). Perceptions of classroom environment, achievement goals, and achievement outcomes. *Journal of Educational Psychology, 93*(1), 43–54.

Cokley, K. O. (2000). Examining the validity of the academic motivation scale by comparing scale construction to . . . *Psychological Reports, 86*(2) 560.

Cokley, K. O., Bernard, N., Cunningham, D., & Motoike, J. (2001). A psychometric investigation of the academic motivation scale using a United States sample. *Measurement and Evaluation in Counseling and Development, 34*, 109–119.

Collins, W. (1982). Some correlates of achievement among students in a supplemental instruction program. *Journal of Learning Skills, 2*(1), 19–28.

Corno, L., & Mandinach, E. B. (1983). Using existing classroom data to explore relationships in a theoretical model of academic motivation. *Journal of Educational Research, 77*(1), 33–42.

Craske, M. L. (1985). Improving persistence through observational learning and attribution retraining. *British Journal of Educational Psychology, 55*, 138–147.

Culler, R. E., & Holahan, C. J. (1980). Test anxiety and academic performance: The effects of study-related behaviors. *Journal of Educational Psychology, 72*(1), 16–20.

Darner, R. (2009). Self-determination theory as a guide to fostering environmental motivation. *Journal of Environmental Education, 40*(2), 39–49.

De Beni, R., & Palladino, P. (2000). Intrusion errors in working memory tasks: Are they related to reading comprehension ability? *Learning and Individual Differences, 12*(2), 131–143.

De La Paz, S., & Graham, S. (2002). Explicitly teaching strategies, skills, and knowledge: Writing instruction in middle school classrooms. *Journal of Educational Psychology, 94*, 291–304.

Deci, E. L., & Ryan, R. M. (1985). The general causality orientations scale: Self-determination in personality. *Journal of Research in Personality, 19*(2), 109–134.

Decker, T.W. (1987). Multi-component treatment for academic underachievers. *Journal of College Student Psychotherapy, 1*(3), 29–37.

Dembo, M. H., & Eaton, M. J. (1996). School learning and motivation. In G. D. Phye (Ed.), *Handbook of academic learning: Construction of knowledge* (pp. 66–105). San Diego: Academic Press.

Dendato, K. M., & Diener, D. (1986). Effectiveness of cognitive/relaxation therapy and study-skills training in reducing self-reported anxiety and improving the academic performance of test-anxious students. *Journal of Counseling Psychology, 33*(2), 131–135.

Duchastel, P. C., & Nungester, R. J. (1984). Adjunct question effects with review. *Contemporary Educational Psychology, 9*(2), 97–103.

DuPaul, G. J., & Stoner, G. D. (1994). *ADHD in the schools: Assessment and intervention strategies*. New York: Guilford Press.

Durkin, D. (1979).What classroom observations reveal about reading comprehension instruction. *Reading Research Quarterly, 14*(4), 481–533.

Elliot, A. J. (2005). A conceptual history of the achievement goal construct. In A J. Elliot & C. S. Dweck (Eds.), Handbook of competence and motivation (pp. 52–72). New York: Guilford Press.

Elliot, A. J., & McGregor, H. A. (2001). A 2 × 2 achievement goal framework. *Journal of Personality and Social Psychology, 80*(3), 501–519.

Ellis, A. P., & Ryan, A. M. (2003). Race and cognitive-ability test performance: The mediating effects of test preparation, test-taking strategy use and self-efficacy. *Journal of Applied Social Psychology, 33*(12), 2607–2629.

Entwistle, N., & McCune, V. (2004). The conceptual bases of study strategy inventories. *Educational Psychology Review, 16*(4), 325–345.

Ergene, G. (2003). Effective interventions on test anxiety reduction: A meta-analysis. *School Psychology International, 24*(3), 313–328.

Ezell, H. K., Hunsicker, S. A., & Quinque, M. M. (1997). Comparison of two strategies for teaching reading comprehension skills. *Education and Treatment of Children, 20*(4), 365–82.

Faber, J. E., Morris, J. D., & Lieberman, M. G. (2000). The effect of note taking on ninth grade students' comprehension. *Reading Psychology, 21*, 257–270.

Faigley, L., Cherry, R. D., Jolliffee, D. A., & Skinner, A. M. (1985). *Assessing writers' knowledge and processes of composing*. Norwood, NJ: Ablex.

Fairchild, A. J., Horst, S. J., Finney, S. J., & Barron, K. E. (2005). Evaluating existing and new validity evidence for the academic motivation scale. *Contemporary Educational Psychology, 30*(3), 331–358.

Faye, C., & Sharpe, D. (2008). Academic motivation in university: The role of basic psychological needs and identity formation. *Canadian Journal of Behavioural Science, 40*(4), 189–199.

Field, J. (2008). *Listening in the language classroom*. Cambridge, UK: Cambridge University Press.

Gajria, M., & Salvia, J. (1992). The effects of summarization instruction on text comprehension of students with learning disabilities. *Exceptional Children, 58*(6), 508–516.

Galassi, J. P., Frierson, H. T., & Sharer, R. (1981). Behavior of high, moderate, and low test anxious students during an actual test situation. *Journal of Consulting and Clinical Psychology, 49*, 51–62.

Gall, M. D., Gall, J. P., Jacobsen, D. R., & Bullock, T. L. (1990). *Tools for learning: A guide to teaching study skills*. Alexandria, VA: Association for Supervision and Curriculum Development.

Gersten, R., Fuchs, L. S., Williams, J. P., & Baker, S. (2001). Teaching reading comprehension strategies to students with learning disabilities: A review of research. *Review of Educational Research, 71*(2), 279–320.

Gettinger, M., & Seibert, J. K. (2002). Contributions of study skills to academic competence. *School Psychology Review, 31*(3), 350–365.

Glanz, J. (1994). Effects of stress reduction strategies on reducing test-anxiety among learning-disabled students. *Journal of Instructional Psychology, 21*(4), 313–317.

Glaser, C., & Brunstein, J. C. (2007). Improving fourth-grade students' composition skills: Effects of strategy instruction and self-regulation procedures. *Journal of Educational Psychology, 99*(2), 297–310.

Goll, P. S. (2004). Mnemonic strategies: Creating schemata for learning enhancement. *Education, 125*(2), 306.

Graham, S., & Harris, K. R. (1989). Improving learning disabled students' skills at composing essays: Self-instructional strategy training. *Exceptional Children, 56*(3), 201–214.

Graham, S., & Harris, K. R. (1993). Self-regulated strategy development: Helping students with learning disabilities develop as writers. *Elementary School Journal, 94*, 169–181.

Graham, S., Harris, K. R., & MacArthur, C. (2006). Explicitly teaching struggling writers: Strategies for mastering the writing process. *Intervention in School & Clinic, 41*(5), 290–294.

Graham, S. & Perin, D. (2007). A meta-analysis of writing instruction for adolescent students, *Journal of Educational Psychology, 99*(3), 445–476.

Graham, S., Schwartz, S. S., & MacArthur, C. A. (1993). Knowledge of writing and the composing process, attitude toward writing, and self-efficacy for students with and without learning disabilities. *Journal of Learning Disabilities, 26*(4), 237–249.

Graves, D. H. (1983). *Writing: Teachers and children at work.* Exeter, NH: Heinemann.

Gureasko-Moore, S., DuPaul, G. J., & White, G. P. (2006). The effects of self-management in general education classrooms on the organizational skills of adolescents with ADHD. *Behavior Modification, 30*(2), 159–183.

Hancock, P. A. & Warm, J. S. (1989). A dynamic model of stress and sustained attention. *Human Factors, 31*, 519–537.

Harris, K. R., & Graham, S. (1996). Making the writing process work: Strategies for composition and self- regulation. Cambridge, MA: Brookline Books.

Harris, K. R., Graham, S., Mason, L., & Friedlander, B. (2008). *Powerful writing strategies for all students.* Baltimore, MD: Brookes.

Harrison, J., Thompson, B., & Vannest, K. J. (2009). Interpreting the Evidence for Effective Interventions to Increase the Academic Performance of Students with ADHD: Relevance of the Statistical Significance Controversy. *Review of Educational Research, 79*(2), 740–775.

Hartley, J. (1983). Note-taking research: Resetting the scoreboard. *Bulletin of the British Psychological Society, 36*, 13–14.

Hembree, R. (1988). Correlates, causes, effects, and treatment of test anxiety. *Review of Educational Research, 58*(1), 47–77.

Hinshaw, S. P. (1992). Externalizing behavior problems and academic underachievement in childhood and adolescence: Causal relationships and underlying mechanisms. *Psychological Bulletin, 111*(1), 127–155.

Hillocks, G. (1986). *Research on written composition: New directions for teaching.* Urbana, IL: ERIC Clearinghouse on Reading and Communication Skills and the National Conference on Research in English.

Ho, R., & McMurtrie, J. (1991). Attributional feedback and underachieving children: Differential effects on causal attributions, success expectancies, and learning processes. *Australian Journal of Psychology, 43*(2), 93–100.

Hodapp, V., & Henneberger, A. (1983). Test anxiety, study habits, and academic performance. In H. M. van der Ploeg, R. Schwarzer, & E. D. Spielberger (Eds.), *Advances in test anxiety research, Vol. 2* (pp. 119–127). Hillsdale, NJ: Erlbaum.

Hong, E., Sas, M., & Sas, J. C. (2006). Test-Taking Strategies of High and Low Mathematics Achievers. *Journal of Educational Research, 99*(3), 144–155.

Hoover, J. J. (1993). Helping Parents Develop a Home-Based Study Skills Program. *Intervention in School and Clinic, 28*(4), 238–245.

Hughes, C. A. (1993). Test-taking strategy instruction for adolescents with emotional and behavioral disorders. *Journal of Emotional & Behavioral Disorders, 1*(3), 189–198.

Hughes, C. A., & Suritsky, S. K. (1994). Note-taking skills of university students with and without learning disabilities. *Journal of Learning Disabilities, 27*(1), 20–24.

Hughes, C. A., & Suritsky, S. K. (1993). Note-taking skills and strategies for students with learning disabilities. *Preventing School Failure, 38*(1), 7–11.

Hughes, C. A., Ruhl, K. L., Schumaker, J. B., & Deshler, D. D. (2002). Effects of instruction in an assignment completion strategy on the homework performance of students with learning disabilities in general education classes. *Learning Disabilities Research & Practice, 17*(1), 1–18.

Hughes, C. A., & Suritsky, S. K. (1994). Note-taking skills of university students with and without learning disabilities. *Journal of Learning Disabilities, 27*(1), 20–24.

Jannoun, L., & Chessells, J. M. (1987). Long-term psychological effects of childhood leukemia and its treatment. *Pediatric Hematology and Oncology, 4*, 293–308.

Jenkins, J. R., Heliotis, J. D., Stein, M. L., & Haynes, M. C. (1987). Improving reading comprehension by using paragraph restatements. *Exceptional Children, 54*, 54–59.

Jones, L., & Petruzzi, D. C. (1995). Test anxiety: A review of theory and current treatment. *Journal of College Student Psychotherapy, 10*(1), 3–15.

Jung, M. (2009). The effects of integrating time management skills into a blended distance learning course. *Dissertation Abstracts International: Section A. Humanities and Social Sciences, 69*(9-A), 3454.

Kaplan, A., & Maehr, M. (2007). The Contributions and Prospects of Goal Orientation Theory. *Educational Psychology Review, 19*(2), 141–184.

Kaplan, A., & Maehr, M. L. (2002). *Adolescents' achievement goals: Situating motivation in sociocultural contexts.* Greenwich, CT: Information Age Publishing.

Karpicke, J. D., Butler, A. C., & Roediger III, H. L. (2009). Metacognitive strategies in student learning: Do students practice retrieval when they study on their own? *Memory, 17*(4), 471–479.

Karpicke, J. D., & Roediger, H. L. (2007). Repeated retrieval during learning is the key to long-term retention. *Journal of Memory and Language, 57*, 151–162.

Keefe, J. W. (1979). Learning style: An overview. In J. W. Keefe (Ed.), *Student learning styles: Diagnosing and prescribing programs* (pp. 1–17). Reston, VA: National Association of Secondary School Principals.

Keller, J. M. Motivational design and multimedia: Beyond the novelty effect. *Strategic Human Resource Development Review, 1997, 1* (1), 188–203.

Keogh, E., & French, C. C. (2001). Test anxiety, evaluative stress, and susceptibility to distraction from threat. *European Journal of Personality, 15*(2), 123–141.

Kiewra, K. A. (1985). Learning from a lecture: An investigation of note-taking, review and attendance at a lecture. *Human Learning: Journal of Practical Research & Applications, 4*(1), 73–77.

Kiewra, K. A., & Benton, S. L. (1985). The effects of higher-order review questions with feedback on achievement among learners who take notes or receive the instructor's notes. *Human Learning: Journal of Practical Research & Applications, 4*(3), 225–231.

Kiewra, K. A., Mayer, R. E., Christensen, M., Kim, S and Risch (1991). Effects of repetition on recall and note-taking: Strategies for learning from lectures. *Journal of Educational Psychology, 83*(1), 20–123.

King, N. J., Mietz, A., Tinney, L., & Ollendick, T. H. (1995). Psychopathology and cognition in adolescents experiencing severe test anxiety. *Journal of Clinical Child Psychology, 24*(1), 49–54.

Kirby, J. R., Silvestri, R., Allingham, B. H., Parrila, R., & La Fave, C. B. (2008). Learning Strategies and Study Approaches of Postsecondary Students With Dyslexia. *Journal of Learning Disabilities, 41*(1), 85–96.

Klassen, R. M. (2010). Confidence to Manage Learning: The Self-Efficacy for Self-Regulated Learning of Early Adolescents with Learning Disabilities. *Learning Disability Quarterly, 33*(1), 19–30.

Kleinheksel, K. A., & Summy, S. E. (2003). Enhancing student learning and social behavior through mnemonic strategies. *Teaching Exceptional Children, 36*(2), 30–35.

Kobayashi, K. (2006). Conditional effects of interventions in note-taking procedures on learning: A meta-analysis. *Japanese Psychological Research, 48*(2), 109–114.

Krapp, J. V. (1988). Teaching research skills: A critical-thinking approach. *School Library Journal, 34*(5), 32–35.

LaBerge, D. (2002). Attentional control: Brief and prolonged. *Psychological Research, 66*(4), 220–233.

Lackaye, T., Margalit, M., Ziv, O., & Ziman, T. (2006). Comparisons of Self-Efficacy, Mood, Effort, and Hope Between Students with Learning Disabilities and Their Non-LD-Matched Peers. *Learning Disabilities Research & Practice (Blackwell Publishing Limited), 21*(2), 111–121.

Langberg, J. M., Epstein, J. N., Urbanowicz, C. M., Simon, J. O., & Graham, A. J. (2008). Efficacy of an organization skills intervention to improve the academic functioning of students with attention-deficit/hyperactivity disorder. *School Psychology Quarterly, 23*(3), 407–417.

Larson, H. A., El Ramahi, M. K., Conn, S. R., Estes, L. A., & Ghibellini, A. B. (2010). Reducing Test Anxiety among Third Grade Students through the Implementation of Relaxation Techniques. *Journal of School Counseling, 8*(19), 1–19.

Levin, J. R. (1993). Mnemonic Strategies and Classroom Learning: A Twenty-Year Report Card. *Elementary School Journal, 94*(2), 235–44.

Macon, T. H. (1994). Time management: Test of a process model. *Journal of Applied Psychology, 79*(3), 381–391.

Macan, T. H., Shahani, C., Dipboye, R. L., & Phillips, A. P. (1990). College students' time management correlations with academic performance and stress. *Journal of Educational Psychology, 82*(4), 760–768.

MacArthur, C., & Graham, S. (1987). Learning disabled students' composing with three methods: Handwriting, dictation, and word processing. *Journal of Special Education, 21*, 22–42.

McDaniel, M. A., Roediger, H. L., & McDermott, K. B. (2007). Generalizing test-enhanced learning from the laboratory to the classroom. *Psychonomic Bulletin & Review, 14*, 200–206.

Mandler, G., & Sarason, S. B. (1953). The Effect of Prior Experience and Subjective Failure on the Evocation of Test Anxiety. *Journal of Personality, 21*(3), 336.

Marsh, H. W. (1990). Causal ordering of academic self-concept and academic achievement: A multiwave, longitudinal panel analysis. *Journal of Educational Psychology, 82*(4), 646–656.

Martin, A. J., & Marsh, H. W. (2003). Fear of Failure: Friend or Foe?. *Australian Psychologist, 38*(1), 31–38.

Mastropieri, M. A., & Scruggs, T. E. (1992). Science for students with disabilities. *Review of Educational Research, 62*(4), 377–411.

Mastropieri, M. A., & Scruggs, T. E. (1997). Best practices in promoting reading comprehension in students with learning disabilities: 1976 to 1996. *RASE: Remedial and Special Education, 18*(4), 197–214.

Mastropieri, M. A., & Scruggs, T. E. (1998). Enhancing school success with mnemonic strategies. *Intervention in School and Clinic, 33*(4), 201–208.

Mauksch, L. B., Hillenburg, L., & Robins, L. (2001). The establishing focus protocol: Training for collaborative agenda setting and time management in the medical interview. *Families, Systems, & Health, 19*(2), 147–157.

Methia, R. A. (2004). *Help your child overcome test anxiety and achieve higher test scores.* College Station, TX: VBW.

Millman, J., Bishop, C. H., & Ebel, R. (1965). An analysis of test-wiseness. *Educational and Psychological Measurement, 25*(3), 707–726.

Miranda, A., Villaescusa, M. I., & Vidal-Abarca, E. (1997). Is attribution retraining necessary? Use of self-regulation procedures for enhancing the reading comprehension strategies of children with learning disabilities. *Journal of Learning Disabilities, 30*(5), 503–512.

Naveh-Benjamin, M. (1991). A comparison of training programs intended for different types of test-anxious students: Further support for an information-processing model. *Journal of Educational Psychology, 83*(1), 134–139.

Naveh-Benjamin, M., McKeachie, W. J., & Lin, Y. (1987). Two types of test-anxious students: Support for an information processing model. *Journal of Educational Psychology, 79*(2), 131–136.

Newbegin, I., & Owens, A. (1996). Self-esteem and anxiety in secondary school achievement. *Journal of Social Behavior and Personality, 11*(3), 521–530.

Nicaise, M., & Gettinger, M. (1995). Fostering Reading Comprehension in College Students. *Reading Psychology, 16*(3), 283–337.

Opitz, M. F., & Zbaracki, M. D. (2004). *Listen hear! 25 effective listening comprehension strategies.* Portsmouth, NH: Heinemann.

Pajares, F., & Urdan, T., Eds. (2002). *Academic motivation of adolescents.* Greenwich, CT: Information Age Publishing.

Paris, S. G., & Winegrad, P. (1990). Dimensions of thinking and cognitive intervention. In B.F. Jones & L. Idol (Eds.), *How metacognition can promote academic learning and instruction* (pp. 15–51). Hillsdale, NJ: Erlbaum.

Peckham, V. C. (1989). Learning disabilities in long-term survivors of childhood cancer: Concerns for parents and teachers. *Journal of Reading, Writing, and Learning Disabilities International, 5*(4), 313–35.

Peeters, M. A. G., & Rutte, C. G. (2005). Time management behavior as a moderator for the job demand-control interaction. *Journal of Occupational Health Psychology, 10*(1), 64–75.

Pintrich, P. R. (2000). The role of goal orientation in self-regulated learning. In M. Boekaerts, P. R. Pintrich, & M. Zeidner (Eds.), *Handbook of self-regulation* (pp. 451–502), San Diego: Academic Press.

Pintrich, P. R., & De Groot, E. V. (1990). Motivational and self-regulated learning components of classroom academic performance. *Journal of Educational Psychology, 82*, 33–40.

Pintrich, P., Smith, D. E., Garcia, T., & McKeachie, W. (1991). *A manual for the use of the Motivated Strategies for Learning Questionnaire (MSLQ).* Ann Arbor, MI: The Regents of the University of Michigan.

Piolat, A., Olive, T., & Kellogg, R. T. (2005). Cognitive effort during note taking. *Applied Cognitive Psychology, 19*(3), 291–312.

Porte, L. K. (2001). Cut and paste 101: New strategies for note-taking and review. *Teaching Exceptional Children, 34*(2), 14–20.

Powers, S.W., Vanetta, K., Noll, R. B., Cool, V. A., & Stehbens, J. A. (1995). Leukemia and other childhood cancers. In M. C. Roberts (Ed.), *Handbook of pediatric psychology* (2nd ed., pp. 310–326). New York: The Guilford Press.

Pressley, M., Rankin, J., & Yokoi, L. (1996). A survey of instructional practices of primary teachers nominated as effective in promoting literacy. *Elementary School Journal, 96*(4), 363–384.

Pressley, M., Tanenbaum, R., McDaniel, M. A., & Wood, E. (1990).What happens when university students try to answer prequestions that accompany textbook material? *Contemporary Educational Psychology, 15*(1), 27–35.

Prins, P. J., Groot, M. J., & Hanewald, G. J. (1994). Cognition in test-anxious children: The role of on-task and coping cognition reconsidered. *Journal of Consulting and Clinical Psychology, 62*(2), 404–409.

Purdie, N., Hattie, J., & Douglas, G. (1996). Student conceptions of learning and their use of self-regulated learning strategies: A cross-cultural comparison. *Journal of Educational Psychology, 88*(1), 87–100.

Putwain, D. W. (2008). Deconstructing Test Anxiety. *Emotional & behavioural difficulties, 13*(2), 141–155.

Putwain, D., Connors, L., & Symes, W. (2010). Do cognitive distortions mediate the test anxiety-examination performance relationship?. *Educational Psychology, 30*(1), 11–26.

Quarton, B. (2003). Research skills and the new undergraduate. *Journal of Instructional Psychology, 30*(2), 120–124.

Rabiner, D., & Coie, J. D. (2000). Early attention problems and children's reading achievement: A longitudinal investigation. *Journal of the American Academy of Child & Adolescent Psychiatry, 39*(7), 859–867.

Raffety, B. D., Smith, R. E., & Ptacek, J. T. (1997). Facilitating and Debilitating Trait Anxiety, Situational Anxiety, and Coping With an Anticipated Stressor: A Process Analysis. *Journal of Personality & Social Psychology, 72*(4), 892–906.

Raphael, T. E., (1986). Teaching question answer relationships, revisited. *The Reading Teacher, 39*, 516–522.

Reynolds, C. R., & Kamphaus, R. W. (1992). *Behavior assessment system for children: BASC.* Circle Pines, MN: American Guidance Service.

Reynolds, C. R., & Kamphaus, R. W. (2002). *Reynolds intellectual assessment scales.* Lutz, FL: Par, Inc.

Reynolds, C. R., & Kamphaus, R. W. (2004). *Behavior Assessment System for Children–Second edition: BASC-2.* Circle Pines, MN: American Guidance Service.

Reynolds, C. R., & Richmond, B. O. (1985). *Revised Children's Manifest Anxiety Scale.* Los Angeles: Western Psychological Services.

Reynolds, C. R. & Voress, J. (2007). *Test of Memory and Learning—2.* Austin, TX: Pro-Ed.

Reynolds, R. E. & Shirey, L. L. (1988). The role of attention in studying and learning. In C. E. Weinstein, E. T. Goetz, & P. A. Alexander (Eds.), *Learning and study strategies: Issues in assessment, instruction, and evaluation* (pp. 77–100). San Diego: Academic Press.

Riccio, C. A., Reynolds, C. R., Lowe, P., & Moore, J. J. (2002). The continuous performance test: A window on the neural substrates for attention. *Archives of Clinical Neuropsychology, 17*(3), 235–272.

Richards, J. H. (1987). Time management: A review. *Work & Stress, 1*(1), 73–78.

Roberts, S. K. (2002). Taking a technological path to poetry pre-writing. *Reading Teacher, 55*(7), 678–688.

Robinson, D. H., Katayama, A. D., Beth, A., Odom, S., Ya-Ping, H., & Vanderveen, A. (2006). Increasing text comprehension and graphic note taking using a partial graphic organizer. *Journal of Educational Research, 100*(2), 103–111.

Roeser, R.W., & Galloway, M. K. (2002). *Studying motivation to learn during early adolescence: A holistic perspective.* Greenwich, CT: Information Age Publishing.

Roeser, R. W.; Peck, S. C. (2009). An education in awareness: Self, motivation, and self-regulated learning in contemplative perspective, *Educational Psychologist, 44*(2) 119–136.

Rosenshine, B., Meister, C., & Chapman, S. (1996). Teaching students to generate questions: A review of the intervention studies. *Journal of Educational Research, 66*(2), 181–221.

Ross, M., Green, S., Salisbury-Glennon, J., & Tollefson, N. (2006). College students' study strategies as a function of testing: An investigation into metacognitive self-regulation. *Innovative Higher Education, 30*(5), 361–375.

Salahu-Din, D., Persky, H. & Miller, J. (2008). The nation's report card: Writing 2007 (NCES 2008–468). Washington, DC: National Center for Education Statistics. Institute of Education Sciences. U. S. Department of Education.

Samuels, S. J. (1989). Training students how to understand what they read. *Reading Psychology, 10*(1), 1–17.

Sarason, S. B., Davidson, K., Lighthall, F., & Waite, R. (1958). A test anxiety scale for children. *Child Development, 29*, 105–113.

Sarason, S. B., & Mandler, G. (1952). Some correlates of test anxiety. *Journal of Abnormal & Social Psychology, 47*, 810–817.

Scammacca, N., Roberts, G., Vaughn, S., Edmonds, M., Wexler, J., Reutebuch, C. K., & Torgesen, J. K. (2007). Interventions for adolescent struggling readers: A meta-analysis with implications for practice, *Center on Instruction,* 49pp.

Schmeck, R. R. (1988). Individual differences and learning strategies. In C. E.Weinstein, E. T. Goetz, & P. A. Alexander (Eds.), *Learning and study strategies: Issues in assessment, instruction, and evaluation* (pp. 171–192). San Diego: Academic Press.

Schraw, G. (1994). The effect of metacognitive knowledge on local and global monitoring. *Contemporary Educational Psychology, 19*(2), 143–54.

Scott, B. J., & Vitale, M. R., (2003). Teaching the writing process to students with LD. *Intervention in School & Clinic*, *38*(4), 31–42.

Scruggs, T. E., & Mastropieri, M. A. (1986). Improving the test-taking skills of behaviorally disordered and learning disabled children. *Exceptional Children*, *53*(1), 63–68.

Scruggs, T. E., & Mastropieri, M. A. (1992). *Teaching test-taking skills: Helping children show what they know*. Brookline, MA: Brookline Books.

Scruggs, T. E., & Mastropieri, M. A. (2000). The effectiveness of mnemonic instruction for students with learning and behavior problems: An update and research synthesis. *Journal of Behavioral Education*, *10*(2–3), 163–173.

Scruggs, T. E., & Tolfa, D. (1985). Improving the test-taking skills of learning-disabled students. *Perceptual & Motor Skills*, *60*(3), 847–850.

Scruggs, T. E., White, K. R., & Bennion, K. (1986). Teaching test-taking skills to elementary-grade students: A meta-analysis. *Elementary School Journal*, *87*(1), 69–82.

Shapiro, E. S., DuPaul, G. J., & Bradley-Klug, K. L. (1998). Self-management as a strategy to improve the classroom behavior of adolescents with ADHD. *Journal of Learning Disabilities*, *31*(6), 545–555.

Shaywitz, S.E., & Shaywitz, B.A. (1992). *Attention-deficit disorder comes of age*. Austin, TX: Pro-Ed.

Short, E. J., & Ryan, E. B. (1984). Metacognitive differences between skilled and less skilled readers: Remediating deficits through story grammar and attribution training. *Journal of Educational Psychology*, *76*(2), 225–235.

Shrager, L., & Mayer, R. E. (1989). Note-taking fosters generative learning strategies in novices. *Journal of Educational Psychology*, *81*(2), 263–264.

Slade, D. L. (1986). Developing foundations for organizational skills. *Academic Therapy*, *21*(3), 261–66.

Sohlberg, M. M., McLaughlin, K., Pavese, A., Heidrich, A., & Posner, M. I. (2000). Rehabilitation of attention disorders with attention process therapy. *Journal of Clinical and Experimental Neuropsychology*, *22*(5), 656–676.

Spielberger, C. D. (1980). *Preliminary professional manual for the Test Anxiety Inventory*. Palo Alto, CA: Consulting Psychologists Press.

Spielberger, C. D., & Vagg, P. R., Eds. (1995). *Test anxiety: A transactional process model*. Philadelphia, PA: Taylor & Francis.

Stöber, J. (2004). Dimensions of Test Anxiety: Relations to Ways of Coping with Pre-Exam Anxiety and Uncertainty. *Anxiety, Stress & Coping*, *17*(3), 213–226.

Strichart, S. S., & Mangrum, C. T. (2002). Teaching learning strategies and study skills to students with learning disabilities, attention deficit disorder, or special needs (3rd ed.). Boston, MA: Allyn & Bacon.

Stroud, K. C., & Reynolds, C. R. (2006). *School motivation and learning strategies inventory*. Los Angeles: Western Psychological Services.

Stroud, K. C., & Reynolds, C. R. (2009). Assessment of learning strategies and related constructs in children and adolescents. In Gutkin, T. B. & C. R. Reynolds (Eds.), *The Handbook of school psychology* (4th ed., pp. 739–766). New York: Wiley.

Suritsky, S. K. (1992). Notetaking approaches and specific areas of difficulty reported by university students with learning disabilities. *Journal of Postsecondary Education and Disability*, *10*, 3–10.

Sweidel, G. B. (1996). Study strategy portfolio: A project to enhance study skills and time management. *Teaching of Psychology*, *23*(4), 246–248.

Teeter, P. A. (1998). *Interventions for ADHD: Treatment in developmental context*. New York: The Guilford Press.

Thomas, J.W., & Rowher, W. D. (1986). Academic studying: The role of learning strategies. *Educational Psychologist*, *21*, 19–41.

Tobias, S. (1985). Test anxiety: Interference, defective skills, and cognitive capacity. *Educational Psychologist*, *20*(3), 135–142.

Tompkins, G. E. (1994). *Teaching writing: Balancing process and product* (2nd ed.). New York: Macmillan.

Troia, G. A. (2002). Teaching writing strategies to children with disabilities: Setting generalization as the goal. *Exceptionality*, *10*(4), 249–269.

Turner, E. A., Chandler, M., & Heffer, R. W. (2009). Student perceptions and motivation in the classroom: Exploring relatedness and value. *Journal of College Student* Development, *50*(3), 337–346.

Vallerand, R. J., & Ratelle, C. F. (2002). Intrinsic and extrinsic motivation: A hierarchical model. In E. L. Deci & R. M. Ryan (Eds.), *The motivation and self-determination of behaviour: Theoretical and applied issues* (pp. 37–63). Rochester, NY: University of Rochester Press.

Vallerand, R. J., Pelletier, L. G., Blais, M. R., & Bri`ere, N. M. (1992). The academic motivation scale: A measure of intrinsic, extrinsic, and amotivation in education. *Educational and Psychological Measurement*, *52*(4), 1003–1017.

Van Overwalle, F. & De Metsenaere, M. (1990). The effects of attribution-based intervention and study strategy training on academic achievement in college freshmen. *British Journal of Educational Psychology*, *60*, 299–311.

Vannest, K.J., Stroud, K. C., & Reynolds, C.R. (2011). *Strategies for academic success: An instructional handbook for teaching k-12 students how to study, learn, and take tests*. Los Angeles: Western Psychological Services.

Vannest, K. J., Temple-Harvey, K. K., & Mason, B. A. (2009). Adequate yearly progress for students with emotional and behavioral disorders through research-based practices. *Preventing School Failure*, *53*(2), 73–84.

Wade, S. E. & Trathen, W. (1989). Effect of self-selected study methods on learning. *Journal of Educational Psychology*, *81*(1), 40–47.

Wang, F. (2008). Motivation and English achievement: An exploratory and confirmatory factor analysis of a new measurement for Chinese students of English learning. *North American Journal of Psychology*, *10*(3), 633–646.

Weiner, B. (1976). Attribution theory, achievement motivation, and the educational process. *Review of Educational Research*, *42*, 201–215.

Weiner, B. (1979). A theory of motivation for some classroom experiences. *Journal of Educational Psychology*, *71*, 3–25.

Weiner, B. (1986). *Attribution, emotion, and action*. New York: The Guilford Press.

Weinstein, C. E. (1987). *Learning and Study Strategies Inventory (LASSI)*. Clearwater, FL: H & H Publishing.

Weinstein, C. E. (1994). Strategic learning/strategic teaching: Flip sides of a coin. In P. R. Pintrich, D. R. Brown, & C. E.Weinstein (Eds.), *Student motivation, cognition, and learning: Essays in honor of Wilbert J. McKeachie* (pp. 257–273). Hillsdale, NJ: Erlbaum.

Weinstein, C. E., & Hume, L. M. (1998). *Study strategies for lifelong learning.* Washington, DC: American Psychological Association.

Weinstein, C. E., & Palmer, D. R. (1990). *Learning and Study Strategies Inventory-High School version: User's manual.* Clearwater, FL: H & H Publishing.

Weinstein, C. E., Husman, J., & Dierking, D. R. (Eds.). (2000). Self-regulation interventions with a focus on learning strategies. In M. Boekaerts, P. R. Pintrich, & M. Zeidner (Eds.), *Handbook of self-regulation.* (pp. 727–747). San Diego: Academic Press.

Weinstein, C. E., & Mayer, R. F. (1986). The teaching of learning strategies. In M. C. Wittrock (Ed.), *Handbook of research on teaching.* (pp. 315–327). New York: MacMillan.

Weinstein, C. E., Schulte, A. C., & Palmer, D. R. (1987). *LASSI: Learning and Study Strategies Inventory.* Clearwater, FL: H & H Publishing.

Weinstein, C. E. Zimmerman, S. A., and Palmer, D. R. (1988). Assessing learning strategies: The design and development of the LASSI. In C. E. Weinstein, E. T. Goetz, & P. A. Alexander (Eds.), *Learning and study strategies: issues in assessment, instruction, and evaluation* (pp. 25–40). San Diego: Academic Press.

Weissberg, M., Berentsen, M., Cote, A., Cravey, B. & Heath, K. (1982). An assessment of the personal, career, and academic needs of undergraduate students. *Journal of College Student Personnel, 23*, 115–122.

Whitebread, D., Coltman, P., Pasternak, D., Sangster, C., Grau, V., Bingham, S., & Demetriou, D. (2009). The development of two observational tools for assessing metacognition and self-regulated learning in young children. *Metacognition and Learning, 4*(1), 63–85.

Wigfield, A., & Eccles, J. S. (1989). Test anxiety in elementary and secondary school students. *Educational Psychologist, 24*(2), 159–183.

Wigfield, A., & Tonks, S. (2002). *Adolescents' expectancies for success and achievement task values during the middle and high school years.* Greenwich, CT: Information Age Publishing.

Wilson, N. H., & Rotter, J. C. (1986). Anxiety management training and study skills counseling for students on self-esteem and test anxiety and performance. *The School Counselor, 34*(1), 18–31.

Wine, J. (1971). Test anxiety and direction of attention. *Psychological Bulletin, 76*(2), 92–104.

Winne, P. H. (2010). Improving measurements of self-regulated learning. *Educational Psychologist, 45*(4), 267–276.

Winne, P. H., & Hadwin, A. F. (Eds.). (1998). *Studying as self-regulated learning.* Mahwah, NJ: Lawrence Erlbaum Associates.

Winne, P. H., & Jamieson-Noel, D. (2002). Exploring students' calibration of self reports about study tactics and achievement. *Contemporary Educational Psychology, 27*(4), 551. Retrieved from EBSCO*host*.

Winne, P. H., & Perry, N. E. (Eds.). (2000). *Measuring self-regulated learning.* San Diego: Academic Press.

Wren, D. G., & Benson, J. (2004). Measuring Test Anxiety in Children: Scale Development and Internal Construct Validation. *Anxiety, Stress & Coping, 17*(3), 227–240.

Yip, M. C. (2009). Differences between high and low academic achieving university students in learning and study strategies: A further investigation. *Educational Research and Evaluation, 15*(6), 561–570.

Zatz, S., & Chassin, S. (1983) Cognitions of test-anxious children. *Journal of Consulting and Clinical Psychology, 51*, 526–534.

Zatz, S., & Chassin, L. (1985). Cognitions of test-anxious children under naturalistic test-taking conditions. *Journal of Consulting and Clinical Psychology, 53*(3), 393–401.

Zeidner, M. (1998). *Test anxiety: The state of the art.* New York: Plenum Press

Zentall, S. S. (2005). Theory- and evidence-based strategies for children with attentional problems. *Psychology in the Schools, 42*(8), 821–836.

Zentall, S. S., Harper, G. W., and Stormont-Spurgin, M. (1993). Children with hyperactivity and their organizational abilities. *Journal of Educational Research, 87*(2), 112–117.

Zimmerman, B. J. (1998). Academic studying and the development of personal skill: A self-regulatory perspective. *Educational Psychologist, 33*(2–3), 73–86.

Zimmerman, B. J., Greenberg, D., & Weinstein, C. E. (Eds.). (1994). *Self-regulating academic study time: A strategy approach.* Hillsdale, NJ; England: Lawrence Erlbaum Associates, Inc.

Zimmerman, B. J. & Martinez-Pons, M. (1990). Student Differences in Self- Regulated Learning: Relating Grade, Sex, and Giftedness to Self-Efficacy and Strategy Use. *Journal of Educational Psychology, 82*(1), 51–59.

Models and Methods of Assessing Creativity

James C. Kaufman, Christina M. Russell, *and* Jonathan A. Plucker

Abstract

Creativity assessment has been studied for nearly as long as creativity itself. In this chapter, we review many different ways of measuring creativity. Most common are divergent thinking tests, including the Torrance Tests of Creative Thinking, although they are not without controversy. More recently, expert raters have been used to evaluate creative work, as outlined in the Consensual Assessment Technique. Peers, teachers, and parents have also been asked to assess a child's creativity, and self-ratings can be used as well. Finally, we provide a rationale for including creativity as part of a battery of assessments.

Key Words: creativity, assessment, creativity tests, divergent thinking, Consensual Assessment Technique, self assessments

Creativity is a key component of human cognition that is related to yet distinct from the construct of intelligence. Before discussing its measurement, however, we must define it. It is notable that so many studies on creativity do *not* define the construct. Plucker, Beghetto, and Dow (2004) selected 90 different articles that either appeared in the two top creativity journals or were articles in a different peer-reviewed journal with the word "creativity" in the title. Of these papers, only 38 percent explicitly defined what creativity was. For the purpose of this chapter, we will use the definition proposed by Plucker et al. (2004):

> Creativity is the interaction among aptitude, process, and environment by which an individual or group produces a perceptible product that is both novel and useful as defined within a social context. (p. 90)

Creativity assessment has been studied for nearly as long as creativity itself. Guilford (1950), one of the early pioneers of creativity research, placed creativity into a larger framework of intelligence in his Structure of the Intellect Model. He attempted to organize all of human cognition along three dimensions. The first dimension was called "operations," and simply meant the mental gymnastics needed for any kind of task. The second dimension, "content," referred to the general subject area. The third dimension, "product," represented the actual products that might result from different kinds of thinking in different kinds of subject matters. With five operations, four contents, and six products, Guilford's (1967) model had 120 different possible mental abilities. One of Guilford's operations (or thought processes) was "divergent thinking"—the ability to answer open-ended questions with both novel and useful responses. The assessment of divergent thinking remains the source of the most frequently used creativity tests (Hunsaker & Callahan, 1995).

Divergent Thinking (DT) Assessments

A lot of time, energy, and effort have been invested on developing and researching measures of divergent thinking (Plucker & Makel, 2010). Ironically, there is not much divergence in the history of creativity assessments. Divergent thinking is the backbone of creativity assessment and has held this position for many decades—many articles have been published on divergent thinking in the major creativity journals, most books on creativity include long discussions of divergent thinking; schools frequently use DT tests to identify the creative potential of students; and DT tests are used extensively around the world to assess creativity. The launching point for serious development efforts and large-scale application of divergent thinking into assessments were Guilford's Structure of the Intellect divergent production tests (1967), Wallach and Kogan's (1965) and Getzels and Jackson's divergent production tests, and Torrance's (1962, 1974) Tests of Creative Thinking (TTCT).

Guilford (1967) proposed the Structure of the Intellect model (SOI), in which he identified 24 distinct components of divergent thinking, one type for each combination of the four types of content (Figural, Symbolic, Semantic, Behavioral) and six types of product (Units, Classes, Relations, Systems, Transformations, Implications). The SOI Divergent Thinking battery consists of several dozen tests that correspond with the 24 distinct components. One example of a Guilford DT task is the Sketches subtest, which assesses the Figural Unit dimension by inviting the student to draw as many objects as possible using a basic figure, such as a circle. Many tests of DT were based on Guilford's SOI assessments, including the most widely studied of the DT assessments: the Torrance Tests of Creative Thinking.

During the 1960s, researchers published results of students that were "Guilford/SOI-like" assessments. For example, the Instances Test required students to list as many things that move on wheels (that make noise, etc.) as possible (Wallach & Kogan, 1965; Wallach & Wing, 1969). Another such example is the Uses Test, in which students provide answers to prompts such as "Tell me all the different ways you could use a chair" (Wallach & Kogan, 1965, p. 31) or bricks, pencils, and toothpicks (Getzels & Jackson, 1962). The greatest difference between the various batteries developed during this time was the conditions under which students take the tests. Wallach and Kogan (1965) preferred a more game-like, untimed administration of divergent thinking tasks, as they believed this allowed creativity to be measured distinctly from intelligence due to the creation of "a frame of reference which is relatively free from the coercion of time limits and relatively free from the stress of knowing that one's behavior is under close evaluation" (p. 24). This test-taking approach is in contrast to timed, test-like protocols used with most other DT measures, which addressed the concerns of scholars like Torrance (1970), who worried "children are so accustomed to the one correct of best answer that they may be reluctant to think of other possibilities or to build up a pool of ideas to be evaluated later" (p. 86).

The Torrance Tests of Creative Thinking (TTCT)

The Torrance Tests of Creative Thinking (Torrance, 1966, 1968, 1972, 1974, 1984, 1988, 1990, 2008) remain the most widely used assessment of creative talent (Sternberg, 2006). Torrance focused on divergent thinking as the basis for creativity, and constructed tests that emphasized the assessment of divergent thinking (Sternberg, 2006). Although based on the SOI assessments, Torrance (1968) wrote, these tests "represent a fairly sharp departure from the factor type tests developed by Guilford and his associates" (p. 167; Kaufman, Plucker, & Baer, 2008, p. 25).

The TTCT are the longest-running continually published assessments of DT, the most carefully studied, and the most widely used in educational settings of all tests of creativity (Kaufman et al., 2008). The Torrance Tests are commonly used in efficacy studies and meta-analyses of the impact of creativity training programs.

TEST ORGANIZATION

The TTCT includes a Form A and Form B that can be used alternatively. The test battery includes Verbal tests (thinking creatively with words) and Figural tests (thinking creatively with pictures). The Figural section includes three subtests:

- *Picture Construction*: participants use basic shape and expands on it to create a picture
- *Picture Completion*: the student is asked to finish and title incomplete drawings
- *Lines/Circles*: the participant is asked to modify many different series of lines (Form A) or circles (Form B)

The Verbal section of the TTCT has eight subtests:

- *Ask-and-Guess*: the examinee is asked to look at a picture (Ex.: Form A has a picture of an elf staring into a pool of water) at the beginning of the test booklet to complete three subtasks:

- Asking: participant asks as many questions as possible about the picture

- Guessing Causes: participant lists possible causes for the pictured action
- Guessing Consequences: participant lists possible consequences for the pictured action

- *Product Improvement;* participant is asked to make changes to improve a toy
- *Unusual Uses*: participant is asked to think of as many different uses for an ordinary item (ex. Cardboard box
- *Unusual Questions*: participant asks as many questions as possible about an ordinary item (this subtest does not appear in later editions)
- *Just Suppose*: participant is asked to "just suppose" an improbable situation has happened then list the possible ramifications.

The administration, scoring, and score reporting of the tests and forms are standardized and include detailed norms that were revised accordingly (Torrance, 1972, 1974; Torrance & Ball, 1984). While reading and understanding the manual allows novice raters to produce reliable scores, Torrance recommended that scorers be trained, as untrained raters tended to deviate from the scoring protocol when assessing originality. Novice scorers tended to unintentionally allow their personal judgments to affect scoring of individual responses.

SCORING

The original test produced scores in the traditional four DT areas. The current TTCT (2008) produces scores in five areas: Fluency, Elaboration, Originality, Resistance to Premature Closure, and Abstractedness of Titles. Revisions to the scoring protocol in 1984 streamlined the scoring process and flexibility was removed as a score, as these were undifferentiated from fluency scores.

Another change in the scoring protocol allowed for the Figural tests to be scored for Resistance to Premature Closure. Resistance to premature closure is determined by a participant's tendency to not immediately close the incomplete figures on the Figural Picture Completion Test. Torrance believed that this score reflected the examinee's ability to "keep open and delay closure long enough to make the mental leap that makes possible original ideas. Less creative people tend to leap to conclusions prematurely without considering the available information" (Torrance & Ball, 1984, p. 20). On the Picture Completion task, the responses are scored zero points for finishing the picture with the easiest, most direct route. One point is scored for indirectly finishing the figure. Two points are awarded for

never completing the picture or completing it with irregular lines that form part of the figure rather than with simple straight or curved lines.

Scoring for the abstractedness of the titles test takers give to the figures in the Picture Construction and Picture completion tasks ranges from zero points for common, obvious titles ("Shoe" or "River"), to one point for more descriptive titles ("The Dancing Cat"), two points for more descriptive or imaginative titles that reach beyond concrete labels ("The Giant's Finger Puppet") or three points for abstract but appropriate titles that go beyond the picture and tell a story ("The Time of Your Life").

There are thirteen other criterion-referenced scores that can be calculated, such as emotional expressiveness, humor, internal visualization, richness of imagery, and synthesis of incomplete figures. The Verbal tests can be scored for fluency, originality, and flexibility.

Remote Associates Test (RAT)

The Remote Associates Test (RAT) is different from traditional DT tests. It is based on the associative theory that "creative thinking…consists of forming mutually distant associative elements into new combinations which are useful and meet specified as well as unforeseen requirements" (Mednick, 1968, p. 213). Basically, more creative individuals tend to make meaningful, useful associations between disparate concepts and ideas to a greater extent than do less creative individuals.

The test consists of 30 items, each with three stimulus words. Examinees must identify a fourth word that links the groupings of words. For example, for one test item may include the three words wheel, electric, high. Potential answers could be "chair" or "wire," as these link together the three stimulus words. The RAT has been updated to modify out-of-date language. One revision is available for free on the internet: http://socrates.berkeley.edu/~kihlstrm/RATest.htm.

Other Divergent Thinking Assessments

The majority of DT assessments are borrowed from or are very similar to the TTCT and Guilford's SOI Assessments. One example is that the DT scores from the Profile of Creative Abilities (Ryser, 2007) are derived from Guilford's work and have tasks similar to those on the TTCT. One departure is real-world divergent thinking items, which are similar to those of Guilford and Wallach & Kogan verbal tasks, but are placed in a realistic, applied context. This format assumes that a more realistic assessment of DT skills should take place within a realistic context. Plucker, Runco, and Lim (2006) adapted a task from Chand and Runco (1993) and scored it for fluency and originality:

> Your friend Pat sits next to you in class. Pat really likes to talk to you and often bothers you while you are doing your work. Sometimes he distracts you and you miss an important part of a lecture, and many times you don't finish your work because he is bothering you. What should you do? How would you solve this problem? Remember to list as many ideas and solutions as you can.

Other DT assessments are more domain-specific, such as the Creative Engineering Design Assessment (CEDA; Charyton, Jagacinski, & Merrill, 2008).

Controversy Regarding Divergent Thinking Assessments

While DT tests are associated with evidence of reliability and concurrent validity, there is a perceived lack of predictive validity (Baer, 1993a, 1993b, 1994a, 1994b; Gardner, 1988, 1993; Kogan & Pankove, 1974; Weisberg, 1993). This has led researchers and educators to avoid using DT tests, and they continue to draw criticisms of the psychometric study of creativity (Plucker & Renzulli, 1999). Another controversial aspect of DT assessments is that people tend to over-generalize DT test performance to all other aspects of creativity. Potentially the historical focus on divergent thinking tests among academics and educators has had a negative effect on the influence of the field of creativity.

Consensual Assessment Technique (CAT)

Although divergent thinking is the most common way to assess creativity, it is far from the only way. The best assessment of creativity in a particular field is usually derived from the collective judgment of recognized experts in the field. This type of assessment emphasizes the creative product. One approach to evaluating the creative product is through rating scales (Besemer & O'Quin, 1993; Hargreaves, Galton & Robinson, 1996; Treffinger, 1989). Teacher rating scales, for example, ask teachers to rate the creativity of students' creative products (e.g., Creative Product Semantic Scale; Besemer & O'Quin, 1993). These instruments tend to be reliable; however, their validity remains to be addressed.

Another approach to evaluating the creative product is the Consensual Assessment Technique (CAT). The CAT is based on the idea that the best measure of the creativity of a work of art, theory, or any other artifact is the combined assessment of experts in that field to judge the work (Amabile, 1996). Subjects are asked to create something (a product) and experts independently evaluate the creativity of those products (Kaufman & Baer, 2012). Poems, collages, and stories are often evaluated in CAT studies. One example of how the CAT was used was in the field of children's writing. Students were given a simple drawing of a boy and a girl and were asked to write an original story involving both the girl and the boy. Experts in this field of children's writings were asked to evaluate the creativity of the stories written by students on a 1.0–5.0 scale. Judges were able to use fractions (e.g., 4.5) and were not asked to defend their ratings (Baer, 1994c).

The CAT does not have standardized scores, rather only comparative scoring among participants. This method is widely used in creativity research but less widely in schools. CAT ratings can be used in classrooms, however, to assess creativity for admission to special programs that look for people who excel in an area of creativity (e.g., poetry, art, inventing).

How to Use the CAT

1. *Choose an appropriate task*: This method is most appropriate if you are interested in assessing creativity in a specific domain. Consider more specific domains, such as collage-making instead of the more general artistic creativity. In some cases, you may use previously created artifacts.

2. *Collect the artifacts*: Subjects can work independently or in groups, as long as they do not observe competitors approaching the same task. It is important to ensure that the conditions for all participants are as identical as possible (i.e., time constraints, instructions, materials, any possible rewards).

3. *Assemble panel of experts*: This is one of the more challenging and time-consuming portions of the CAT. Judges should have a level of expertise clearly higher than the subjects' and have some familiarity with the populations from which the subjects are drawn. Judges of high school students, for example, should have some familiarity with production from that age range (Baer, Kaufman, & Riggs, 2009; Kaufman, Baer, & Cole, 2009; Kaufman, Baer, Cole, & Sexton, 2008). For most purposes, five to ten judges is adequate. Too few

judges may make inter-rater reliability difficult to produce.

4. *Organize the work of the expert judges*: All judges must receive identical directions and should not know the identity of the students; however, they should know the average age of the participants. Judges should approach the creative products in a different order.

Parent, Peer, and Teacher Measures: Assessments by Others

Whereas the CAT focused on products, Assessments by Others focus on the creative *person* (personality traits, creativity-relevant abilities, motivation, intelligence, thinking styles, emotional intelligence, or knowledge). This method of assessment can be as simple as having a teacher globally rank his or her students based on the teacher's knowledge of the students and implicit beliefs about the nature of creativity. This method emphasizes traits and abilities that are believed to be relevant to creativity and is domain-general (by its nature, CAT is always domain-specific). The assessors using this method are experts on the child (teachers, parents of the child), not experts in creativity.

One common way to assess creativity is via checklists. When using creativity checklists, there is reason to be wary of teacher, parent, and supervisor ratings of creativity based on global impressions of a student due to unintended bias. To limit this bias, raters are given checklists of traits to rate each child separately.

Creativity Checklist

There are many different creativity checklists, most of which were designed for use in schools. Many creativity checklists are sold commercially and copyright-protected. One freely available assessment is the Creativity Checklist by Proctor and Burnett (2004). The Creativity Checklist is composed of characteristics that are thought to be indicative of a creative person, both cognitive and dispositional traits. The items are defined in terms of classroom behaviors for teachers to use on elementary students. A 3-point Likert scale is used to rate whether each characteristic occurs *rarely* (score of 1), *sometimes* (score of 2), or *often* (score of 3). The total score is computed by summing the markings for the characteristics. For example, a *fluent thinker* item has a performance indicator such as, "The student is full of ideas"; and a *flexible thinker* performance indicator is "The student is versatile

and can cope with several ideas at once" (Proctor & Burnett, 2004). There were no norms established for this checklist and therefore it is only appropriate for making comparisons within groups of students. There also has been no criterion-related or predictive validity established.

Scales for Rating Behavioral Characteristics of Superior Students (SRBCSS)

The SRBCSS checklist is widely used in the selection of students for gifted and talented programs (Callahan et al., 1995; Hunsaker & Callahan, 1995). The first of these scales were designed to introduce teacher perspectives into the gifted and talented identification process (Bracken & Brown, 2006). The SRBCSS is based on a multiple-talent approach to identifying gifted students (Renzulli, 1986). The scales include following 14 scales to help identify student abilities: learning, motivation, creativity, leadership, art, music, drama, planning, communication (precision), communication (expression), math, reading, science, and technology. This creativity scale was based on a literature review as well as feedback from educators. Although the publisher reports no criterion-validity, the reliability has been found to be significant if those completing the assessment have been trained (Center for Creative Learning, 2002).

Williams Scale of Creativity Assessment Packet

The Williams Scale is a creativity checklist that is part of a larger assessment package widely used in selection of students for gifted and talented programs (Williams, 1980). It is composed of 48 items related to characteristics of creative students. It can be completed by a teacher, caregiver, or parent in 10 to 20 minutes. There are eight item types on this scale, including Fluency, Flexibility, Originality, Elaborativeness, Curiosity, Imagination, Complexity, and Courageousness/Risk Taking. The raters are instructed to place checkmarks depending on how often a characteristic is present: double checkmark when the characteristic is present most of the time, a single checkmark if it is present some of the time or a blank item if the characteristic is rarely or never present. The publisher of this scale provides neither reliability nor validity information.

Ideal Child Checklist

This checklist is not a measure of individual creativity; rather, it is a measure of attitudes toward creativity. The Ideal Child Checklist was developed to provide criteria of a productive, creative person and is most often used in research involving perceptions of parents, teachers, and children of what an ideal student is. A factor-analysis of the Ideal Child Checklist revealed four factors that are indicative of an "ideal child": confident/aggressive/well-adjusted, sociable, not stubborn/domineering/trouble-making, and creative/intuitive. Only the last of these factors relates to creativity, and it has the weakest reliability of the four (Paguio, 1983). While this checklist is appropriate to measure the values of students, teachers, or parents, caution should be exercised when using it as an indicator of creativity.

Several other rating scales outside of the previously mentioned measures exist; however, none has adequately been studied for validity or reliability, nor are they used in creativity literature. One such example is the Gifted Evaluation Scale–Second Edition (GES-2; Henage, McCarney & Anderson, 1998). This scale consists of 48 items. Raters assess areas of intellect, creativity, specific academic aptitude, leadership ability, and performing and visual arts.

Guidelines for Using Creativity Checklists

When using creativity checklists, it is crucial for the assessors to be familiar with the students whose creativity is being assessed. The raters should have had the opportunity to observe and work with the students in a variety of different contests and domains. The validity of creativity checklists depends on how well the assessors know the students, how well they understand the questions and the theory of creativity that underlies them, the objectivity of the assessors, and the appropriateness of the questions/theory of creativity that underlies them.

There currently is not a creativity checklist that has the criterion-related concurrent and predictive validity one would like in tests being used for decision-making purposes. It is helpful for several people to independently rate students. While checklists may not be the most psychometrically sound assessments, they can serve as a small piece of an assessment when combined with other measures like divergent thinking tests, self-assessments, and rating of creative artifacts to help paint a picture of the student's creative abilities.

Self-Assessment

Self-assessment is one of the simplest ways to assess creativity—all that one needs to do is ask people how creative they are. This method, however, seems too easy and good to be true, and depending the purpose of the assessment, it may be exactly that.

Creative Personality Assessment

Personality inventories are some of the most prevalent forms of self-assessment. The Five-Factor Theory is the leading theory in personality (Costa & McCrae, 1992). It organizes *personality* into five components: neuroticism (emotional stability), extraversion, openness to experience, conscientiousness, and agreeableness. Openness to experience is the personality component most associated with creativity. There is a near-universal finding that openness to experience is associated with creativity, including self-reports of creative acts (Griffin & McDermott, 1998), verbal creativity (King, McKee-Walker, & Broyles, 1996), being in a creative profession (Domino, 1974), analysis of participants' daydreams (Zhiyan & Singer, 1996), creativity ratings on stories (Wolfradt & Pretz, 2001), creative activities and behaviors throughout life (Soldz & Vaillant, 1999), self-estimates of creativity (Furnham, 1999), and psychometric tests (McCrae, 1987). The NEO Personality Inventory and the briefer NEO Five-Factor Inventory are the most popular measures of the five-factor personality theory (Costa & McCrae, 1992).

Another type of creativity personality assessment is to assess one's *creativity style*, which refers to the ways in which people choose their creativity (Hourtz et al., 2003; Isaksen & Dorval, 1993; Selby, Treffinger, Isaksen, & Powers, 1993). One assessment of this nature is the Creativity Styles Questionnaire–Revised (Kumar, Kemmler, & Holman, 1997; Kumar & Holman, 1989). This is a 76-item self-assessed questionnaire with seven subscales: Belief in the Unconscious Process, Use of Techniques, Use of Other People, Final Product Orientation, Superstition, Environmental Control, and Uses of Senses. For example, on the Belief in the Unconscious Process subscale, a sample item is, "I have had insights, the sources of which I am unable to explain or understand" (Kumar, Kemmler, & Holman, 1997). One study examined the Creative Styles Questionnaire (the original survey) and found more creative students used more techniques and were less guided by the goal of the final project (Kumar, Holman, & Rudegeair, 1991).

The Kirton Adaption-Innovation Inventory (KAI; Kirton, 1999) was developed to measure a personality dimension ranging from adaption (ability to do things better) to innovation (ability to do things differently (Kirton, 1994b). This assessment is often used in organizations, as it is relevant to organizational change (Kirton, 1994b). This inventory is constructed of 32 items that produce a score ranging from 32 to 160, although the observed range has been 45 to 146, with an average of 96 and a distribution approaching normality (Kirton, 1994a).

Creative Behavior Checklists

Rather than asking people questions regarding personality, another method for self-assessment of creativity is through creative behavior checklists, which ask people to rate their past or current creative accomplishments. The author of the Creative Behavior Inventory argued that self-reports of activities and attainments are among the best techniques for measuring creativity (Hocevar, 1979a, 1979b; Hocevar, 1981; Hocevar & Bachelor, 1989). This inventory is constructed of 90 items that assess creative behavior in literature, music, crafts, art, performing arts, and math/science. The Creativity Achievement Questionnaire is a second creative behavior checklist (CAQ; Carson, Peterson, & Higgins, 2005). This instrument assesses creativity through 96 items across nine domains that load on two factors: the arts (drama, writing, humor, dance, visual arts) and science (invention, science, and culinary). The tenth domain (architecture) did not load on a factor. This test has a test-retest reliability of .81 and internal consistency of .96. CAQ items ask people to mark their highest level of achievement on a scale that ranges from "I do not have recognized talent in this area" to "My XXX has been recognized as a national publication."

The Runco Ideational Behavioral Scale (RIBS; Runco, 2008) was developed in response to Runco's (2007) perceived need for a more appropriate criterion in studies of predictive validity for divergent thinking tests. Runco hypothesized that researchers were using divergent thinking tests to predict inappropriate criteria, such as those traditionally used in studies of the predictive validity of intelligence tests. Runco reasoned that a more appropriate criterion would be one that emphasizes ideation: the use of, appreciation of, and skill of generating ideas. Runco reduced a pool of 100 items to 23 after initial pilot testing. All of the items describe actual overt behavior related to ideation, such as, "I have many wild ideas," or "I come up with a lot of ideas or solutions to problems."

The Kaufman Domains of Creativity Scale (K-DOCS; Kaufman, 2012), is a recent self-report scale that asks people to rate their creativity across multiple behaviors and domains. The K-DOCS is 50 items and covers the broad domains of Self/Everyday, Scholarly, Performance (encompassing Writing and Music), Mechanical/Scientific, and Artistic.

Conclusion

All of the assessments we have covered have several limitations that prevent them from being a perfect test. Some have poor reliability or validity; others are impractical. Given these restrictions, why would anyone want to include a measure of creativity in their battery of assessments?

We believe, however, that there are many compelling reasons and situations where using a measure of creativity could greatly benefit an overall evaluation. For example, we advise the use of a creativity measure when:

• There is reason to think that traditional IQ or achievement tests may not tap all of a person's potential. Divergent-thinking tests may help give a more comprehensive understanding of a person's overall abilities. The same can be said of creativity checklists completed by teachers.

• A test-taker is at risk for a stereotype threat reaction to traditional tests. Almost all measures of creativity show fewer ethnicity and gender biases than standard IQ and achievement tests.

• Parents, teachers, or peers describe an individual as being especially creative.

• A test-taker has a learning disability that may impact their scores on a traditional ability or achievement measure.

• You are trying to assess creative abilities in a particular area, such as creative writing, artistic creativity, or musical creativity. Giving people a chance to show what they can do (using a real-world task such as writing a short story or making a collage, then judging their creations using the Consensual Assessment Technique) can help you spotlight creative talent that might be overlooked in a traditional battery of assessments.

• You need to judge the creativity of a group of artifacts (poems, musical compositions, science fair projects, etc.) as part of a competition, and you want to include (or focus on) creativity in your assessment. This is a perfect opportunity to use the Consensual Assessment Technique.

• You are selecting students for a gifted/talented program and want to follow national guidelines to use multiple selection criteria (rather than relying solely on IQ and achievement data). Most creativity measures, although not necessarily the only solution for such selections, may serve as part of a broader evaluation that can add to the overall picture of each candidate.

It is important to reiterate that we do not support administering a creativity test instead of a traditional IQ, achievement, or behavior test. We believe that all of these measures can work together to create the fullest possible picture of an individual. Creativity assessment is a work in progress—we know far less about creativity and its measurement than we would like to know—yet there is still a multitude of tools available for a dedicated test administrator.

References

Amabile, T. M. (1996). *Creativity in context: Update to the social psychology of creativity.* Boulder, CO: Westview.

Baer, J. (1993a). *Creativity and divergent thinking: A task-specific approach.* Hillsdale, NJ: Lawrence Erlbaum Associates.

Baer, J. (1993b). Why you shouldn't trust creativity tests. *Educational Leadership, 51,* 80–83.

Baer, J. (1994a). Performance assessments of creativity: Do they have long-term stability? *Roeper Review, 7,* 7–11.

Baer, J. (1994b). Why you *still* shouldn't trust creativity tests. *Educational Leadership, 52,* 72–73.

Baer, J. (1994c). Divergent thinking is not a general trait: A multi-domain training experiment. *Creativity Research Journal, 7,* 35–46.

Baer, J., Kaufman, J. C., & Riggs, M. (2009). Rater-domain interactions in the Consensual Assessment Technique. *International Journal of Creativity & Problem Solving, 19,* 87–92.

Besemer, S. P., & O'Quin, K. (1993). Assessing creative products: Progress and potentials. In S. G. Isaksen, M. C. Murdock, R. L. Firestien, & D. J. Treffinger (Eds.), *Nurturing and developing creativity: The emergence of a discipline* (pp. 331–349). Norwood, NJ: Ablex Publishing Company.

Bracken, B. A., & Brown, E. F. (2006). Behavioral identification and assessment of gifted and talented students. *Journal of Psychoeducational Assessment, 24,* 112–122.

Callahan, C. M., Hunsaker, S. L., Adams, C. M., Moore, S. D., & Bland, L. C. (1995). *Instruments used in the identification of gifted and talented students* (Report No. RM-95130). Charlottesville, VA: National Research Center on the Gifted and Talented.

Carson, S. H., Peterson, J. B., & Higgins, D. M. (2005). Reliability, validity, and factor structure of the creative achievement questionnaire. *Creativity Research Journal, 17,* 37–50.

Center for Creative Learning. (2002). *Review of the Scales for Rating Behavioral Characteristics of Superior Students.* Retrieved November 10, 2007, from the Center for Creative Learning website: http://www.creativelearning.com/Assess/test55.htm.

Chand, I., & Runco, M. A. (1993). Problem finding skills as components in the creative process. *Personality & Individual Differences, 14,* 155–162.

Charyton, C., Jagacinski, R. J., & Merrill, J. A. (2008). CEDA: A research instrument for creative engineering design assessment. *Psychology of Aesthetics, Creativity, & the Arts, 2,* 147–154.

Costa, P. T., & Mc Crae, R. R. (1992). Normal personality assessment in clinical practice: The NEO personality inventory. *Psychological Assessment, 4,* 5–13.

Domino, G. (1974). Assessment of cinematographic creativity. *Journal of Personality & Social Psychology, 30,* 150–154.

Furnham, A. (1999). Personality and creativity. *Perceptual & Motor Skills, 88,* 407–408.

Gardner, H. (1988). Creativity: An interdisciplinary perspective. *Creativity Research Journal, 1,* 8–26.

Gardner, H. (1993). *Creating minds.* New York: Basic Books.

Getzels, J. W., & Jackson, P. W. (1962). *Creativity and intelligence: Explorations with gifted students.* New York: Wiley.

Griffin, M., & McDermott, M. R. (1998). Exploring a tripartite relationship between rebelliousness, openness to experience and creativity. *Social Behavior & Personality, 26,* 347–356.

Guilford, J. P. (1950). Creativity. *American Psychologist, 5,* 444–544.

Guilford, J. P. (1967). *The nature of human intelligence.* New York: McGraw-Hill.

Hargreaves, D. J., Galton, M. J., & Robinson, S. (1996). Teachers' assessments of primary children's classroom work in the creative arts. *Educational Research, 38,* 199–211.

Henage, D., McCarney, S. B., & Anderson, P. D. (1998). *Gifted Evaluation Scale* (2nd ed.). Columbia, MO: Hawthorne Educational Services.

Hocevar, D. (1979a, April). *The development of the Creative Behavior Inventory.* Paper presented at the annual meeting of the Rocky Mountain Psychological Association. (ERIC Document Reproduction Service No. ED 170 350)

Hocevar, D. (1979b). The unidimensional nature of creative thinking in fifth grade children. *Child Study Journal, 9,* 273–277.

Hocevar, D. (1981). Measurement of creativity: Review and critique. *Journal of Personality Assessment, 45,* 450–464.

Hocevar, D., & Bachelor, P. (1989). A taxonomy and critique of measurements used in the study of creativity. In J. A. Glover, R. R. Ronning, & C. R. Reynolds (Eds.), *Handbook of creativity* (pp. 53–75). New York: Plenum Press.

Hunsaker, S. L., & Callahan, C. M. (1995). Creativity and giftedness: Published instrument uses and abuses. *Gifted Child Quarterly, 39,* 110–114.

Hourtz, J. C. Shelby, E., Esquivel, G. B., Okoye, R. A., Peters, K. M., & Treffinger, D. J. (2003). Creativity styles, personal type. *Creativity Research Journal, 15,* 321–330.

Isaksen, S. G., & Dorval, K. B. (1993). Toward an improved understanding of creativity within people: The level–style distinction. In S. G. Isaksen, M. C. Murdock, S. L. Firestien, & D. J. Treffinger (Eds.), *Understanding and recognizing creativity: The emergence of a discipline* (pp. 299–230). Norwood, NJ: Ablex.

Kaufman, J. C. (2012). Counting the muses: Development of the Kaufman-Domains of Creativity Scale (K-DOCS). *Psychology of Aesthetics, Creativity, and the Arts, 6,* 298–308.

Kaufman, J. C., & Baer, J. (2012). Beyond new and appropriate: Who decides what is creative? *Creativity Research Journal, 24,* 83–91.

Kaufman, J. C., Baer, J., & Cole, J. C. (2009). Expertise, domains, and the Consensual Assessment Technique. *Journal of Creative Behavior, 43,* 223–233.

Kaufman, J. C., Baer, J., Cole, J. C., & Sexton, J. D. (2008). A comparison of expert and non-expert raters using the

Consensual Assessment Technique. *Creativity Research Journal, 20,* 171–178.

Kaufman, J. C., Plucker, J. A., & Baer, J. (2008). *Essentials of creativity assessment.* New York: Wiley.

King, L. A., McKee Walker, L., & Broyles, S. J. (1996). Creativity and the five-factor model. *Journal of Research in Personality, 30,* 189–203.

Kirton, M. J. (Ed.). (1994a). *Adaptors and innovators: Styles of creativity and problem solving.* New York: Routledge.

Kirton, M. J. (1994b). A theory of cognitive style. In Kirton, M. J. (Ed.) (1994a), *Adaptors and innovators: Styles of creativity and problem solving* (pp. 1–33). New York: Routledge.

Kirton, M. J. (1999). *Kirton Adaption-Innovation Inventory (KAI)* (3rd ed.). Hertfordshire, UK: KAI Distribution Centre.

Kogan, N., & Pankove, E. (1974). Long-term predictive validity of divergent-thinking tests: Some negative evidence. *Journal of Educational Psychology, 66,* 802–810.

Kumar, V. K., & Holman, E. R. (1989). *Creativity Styles Questionnaire.* Unpublished instrument.

Kumar, V. K., Holman, E. R., & Rudegeair, P. (1991). Creativity styles of freshmen students. *Journal of Creative Behavior, 25,* 320–323.

Kumar, V. K., Kemmler, D., & Holman, E. R. (1997). The Creativity Styles Questionnaire–Revised. *Creativity Research Journal, 10,* 51–58.

Mednick, S. A. (1968). The Remote Associates Test. *Journal of Creative Behavior, 2,* 213–214.

McCrae, R. R. (1987). Creativity, divergent thinking, and openness to experience. *Journal of Personality & Social Psychology, 52,* 509–516.

Paguio, L. P. (1983). The influence of gender of child and parent on perceptions of the ideal child. *Child Study Journal, 13,* 187–194.

Plucker, J. A., & Makel, M. C. (2010). Assessment of creativity. In J. C. Kaufman & R. J. Sternberg (Eds.), *Cambridge handbook of creativity* (pp. 48–73). New York: Cambridge University Press.

Plucker, J. A., Beghetto, R. A., & Dow, G. (2004). Why isn't creativity more important to educational psychologists? Potential, pitfalls, and future directions in creativity research. *Educational Psychologist, 39,* 83–96.

Plucker, J. A., & Renzulli, J. S. (1999). Psychometric approaches to the study of human creativity. In R. J. Sternberg (Ed.), *Handbook of creativity* (pp. 35–60). New York: Cambridge University Press.

Plucker, J. A., Runco, M. A., & Lim, W. (2006). Predicting ideational behavior from divergent thinking and discretionary time on task. *Creativity Research Journal, 18,* 55–63.

Proctor, R. M. J., & Burnett, P. C. (2004). Measuring cognitive and dispositional characteristics of creativity in elementary students. *Creativity Research Journal, 16,* 421–429.

Renzulli, J. S. (1986). The three-ring conception of giftedness: A developmental model for creative productivity. In R. J. Sternberg & J. Davidson (Eds.), *Conceptions of giftedness* (pp. 53–92). New York: Cambridge University Press.

Runco, M. A. (2007). *Creativity: Theories and themes: Research, development, and practice.* San Diego, CA: Elsevier Academic Press.

Runco, M. A. (2008). Divergent thinking is not synonymous with creativity [Commentary]. *Psychology of Aesthetics, Creativity, & the Arts, 2,* 93–96.

Ryser, G. R. (2007). *Profiles of Creative Abilities: Examiner's Manual.* Austin, TX: Pro-Ed.

Selby, E. C., Treffinger, D. J., Isaksen, S. G. & Powers, S. V. (1993). Use of the Kirton Adaption-Innovation Inventory with middle school students. *Journal of Creative Behavior, 27,* 223–235.

Soldz, S., & Vaillant, G. E. (1999). The big five personality traits and the life course: A 45-year longitudinal study. *Journal of Research in Personality, 33,* 208–232.

Sternberg, R. J. (2006). The nature of creativity. *Creativity Research Journal, 18,* 87–98.

Torrance, E. P. (1962). *Guiding creative talent.* Englewood Cliffs, NJ: Prentice-Hall.

Torrance, E. P. (1966). *The Torrance Tests of Creative Thinking—Norms—Technical Manual Research Edition—Verbal Tests, Forms A and B—Figural Tests, Forms A and B.* Princeton, NJ: Personnel Press.

Torrance, E. P. (1968). A longitudinal examination of the fourth grade slump in creativity. *Gifted Child Quarterly, 12,* 195–199.

Torrance, E. P. (1970). *Encouraging creativity in the classroom.* Dubuque, IA: William C. Brown Company Publishers.

Torrance, E. P. (1972). *Torrance Tests of Creative Thinking: Directions manual and scoring guide. Figural test booklet A* (Rev ed.). Bensenville, IL: Scholastic Testing Service.

Torrance, E. P. (1974). *Torrance Tests of Creative Thinking: Norms-technical manual.* Bensenville, IL: Scholastic Testing Service.

Torrance, E. P. (1984). Sounds and images productions of elementary school pupils as predictors of the creative achievements of young adults. *Creative Child & Adult Quarterly, 7,* 8–14.

Torrance, E. P. (1990). *The Torrance Tests of Creative Thinking–Norms–Technical Manual–Figural (Streamlined) Forms A and B.* Bensenville, IL: Scholastic Testing Service.

Torrance, E. P. (2008). *The Torrance Tests of Creative Thinking–Norms–Technical Manual–Figural (Streamlined) Forms A and B.* Bensenville, IL: Scholastic Testing Service.

Torrance, E. P., & Ball, O. E. (1984). *Torrance Tests of Creative Thinking: Streamlined administration and scoring manual* (rev. ed.). Bensonville, IL: Scholastic Testing Service.

Treffinger, D. J. (1989). *Student invention evaluation kit: Field test edition.* Sarasota, FL: Center for Creative Learning.

Wallach, M. A., & Kogan, N. (1965). *Modes of thinking in young children: A study of the creativity–intelligence distinction.* New York: Holt, Rinehart & Winston.

Wallach, M. A., & Wing, C. W., Jr. (1969). *The talented student: A validation of the creativity–intelligence distinction.* New York: Holt, Rinehart and Winston.

Weisberg, R. W. (1993). *Creativity: Beyond the myth of genius.* New York: W. H. Freeman and Company.

Williams, F. E. (1980). *Creativity assessment packet.* Buffalo, NY: DOK Publishers.

Wolfradt, U., & Pretz, J. E. (2001). Individual differences in creativity: Personality, story writing, and hobbies. *European Journal of Personality, 15,* 297–310.

Zhiyan, T., & Singer, J. L. (1996). Daydreaming styles, emotionality, and the big five personality dimensions. *Imagination, Cognition, & Personality, 16,* 399–414.

Methods of Assessing Behavior: Observations and Rating Scales

Erin Dowdy, Jennifer Twyford, *and* Jill D. Sharkey

Abstract

This chapter discusses two primary methods of behavioral assessment: observations and rating scales. The popularity of these behavioral assessment techniques is on the rise, and information is provided to clinicians and clinicians-in-training on the basic tenets of behavioral observations and rating scales. Specifically, the advantages and limitations of behavioral observations and rating scales, key considerations when preparing for and conducting an observation or collecting behavioral rating scales, measurement issues, information on frequently utilized tools, and recommendations for practice are provided. The chapter concludes with possible future directions for the use of behavioral observations and rating scales.

Key Words: assessment, behavior, observations, rating scales, measurement

Introduction

This chapter provides an overview of two primary methods that are frequently used to assess behavior: behavioral observations and rating scales. The necessity of this chapter is reflective of current trends among psychologists toward an increased use of both behavioral observations and rating scales when conducting assessments in the behavioral, social, and emotional domains of functioning (Shapiro & Heick, 2004). In fact, a wide variety of studies surveying psychologists about their assessment practices have demonstrated an increase in the use of both direct observation and behavior rating scales over time (Hutton, Dubes, & Muir, 1992; Shapiro & Heick, 2004; Stinnett, Havey, & Oehler-Stinnett, 1994; Wilson & Reschly, 1996). For example, in a recent survey focused on their last eight social/emotional/behavioral cases, school psychologists reported they administered parent and/or teacher behavior rating scales or checklists 76% of the time, direct observations 69% of the time, and student rating scales 67% of the time (Shapiro & Heick, 2004). As observations and rating scales are gaining popularity, their methods are also becoming more advanced, structured, and refined. Given the widespread use and growing sophistication of observations and behavior rating scales in the psychological assessment of children and adolescents, it is increasingly critical for practitioners to understand methods and issues concerning their use.

Although conducting an observation or interpreting the results of a rating scale might be treated as simplistic, significant training and practice is needed to become fluent in their use (Hintze, Volpe, & Shapiro, 2008). Clinicians need to be aware of the various types of behavioral information that can be gathered through the use of observations and rating scales, as well as their limitations and when specific techniques are most appropriately used. From defining target behaviors to understanding the psychometric properties of instruments available for use, there are considerable skills that must be learned. This chapter aims to provide clinicians and clinicians-in-training with a solid foundation on the central tenets of both behavioral observations and rating scales so that clinicians can begin to understand and employ these critical components of a behavioral assessment. Towards this end, we highlight the advantages and limitations of behavioral observations and rating scales, key considerations when preparing for and conducting an observation or collecting behavioral rating scales, measurement issues, frequently utilized tools, and recommendations for practice. To aid clinicians and clinicians-in-training, specific considerations for practice and information on commonly utilized observation systems and rating scales are provided in Tables 26.1–26.5.

Preliminary Considerations
An Ecologically Valid Approach

The field of psychology has long operated under the medical model, in which the "problem" is viewed as existing within the child and clinicians have been individually focused in case conceptualization as well as intervention. Accordingly, behavioral observations and rating scales have been primarily implemented to determine what are assumed to be client-based behavioral problem(s). However, it is necessary to move beyond simply viewing the problem as existing within the child to taking a more comprehensive, ecological approach (Sheridan & Gutkin, 2000). An ecological approach allows for the examination of the contextual variables that might also be affecting the child's behavior (Bronfenbrenner, 1992). The transaction between the child and others is considered, as well as an assumption that problems can occur when a child is placed in an environment where unable to meet the expectations of the environment. The problem is therefore not viewed as the client's, but rather as a problem of "environmental mismatch." Ecological approaches are also advocated for within the nondiscriminatory-assessment literature that touts the benefits of first assuming that the problem behavior is not due to a child's characteristic, but is rather due to the environment or an environmental mismatch (Ortiz, 2008). An assessment of the problem behavior within the ecological approach does not conclude with the assessment of the client's behaviors. Rather, such an approach considers the various contexts in which the client functions.

Although the majority of behavioral assessment tools currently available were designed under the medical model and primarily provide information on the individual's maladaptive or adaptive functioning, the central techniques of behavioral observations and rating scales can be applied in an ecological approach. Take, for example, the case of a client who demonstrates significant hyperactivity and inattentiveness within the reading classroom but is calm, attentive, and responsive in a variety of other environments including at home, in church, and at the community center that the family frequently visits. Conducting behavioral observations in a variety of these settings with attention to environmental characteristics, as opposed to solely focusing on the client in the reading classroom, would reveal that the "problem" is not, in fact, the client's activity level. Perhaps the child is unable to read and is assigned tasks are too challenging. Or perhaps there is an ongoing conflict between the client and the teacher. The approach to treatment is dramatically different depending on the identified problem(s). Within the medical model, perhaps psycho-stimulant medication and behavioral modification would be advocated; while within an ecological approach, the intervention team decides to move the client to a different reading classroom. By adopting an ecological approach to observation, the astute clinician observes the variety of environments in which a client functions, in addition to observing the unique characteristics and behaviors of the client.

Behavioral rating scales also can be utilized within an ecological approach. In fact, collecting information from a variety of sources can provide insight into the likelihood of the problem's truly existing within the child, or within the environment. Achenbach and colleagues (1987) argued that each informant within a multi-informant system offers a unique and important perspective. Thus, an ecological perspective elucidates those behaviors with higher inconsistency across raters as being more contextually relevant. Taking the aforementioned example, if the teacher, parent, and community center worker each completed a behavior rating scale examining characteristics of inattention, hyperactivity, and impulsivity, the client may have only received scores in the clinical or at-risk range when rated by the reading teacher. This would lend further credibility to the hypothesis that the client does not, in fact, have sufficient symptoms of Attention Deficit Hyperactivity Disorder, Combined Type to warrant a diagnosis, but that the problem appears to be more related to an environmental mismatch. Furthermore, rating scales examining characteristics of classroom climate and/or home environments, when used in combination with behavioral rating scales, can provide a more comprehensive assessment of functioning. When examining rating scales and behavioral observation techniques throughout this chapter, a focus on applying these techniques within an ecological approach will be provided.

A Strength-Based Approach

In part due to the influence of the medical model, observations and behavior rating scales have typically focused on risk, problems, and pathology and neglected human adaptation and development (Masten, 2001). However, longitudinal studies have found that strengths are as important as risks to understanding developmental pathways (Garmezy, 1993), encouraging research into resilience and positive psychology. Thus, comprehensive assessment of child behavior should take into consideration both positive and negative aspects of functioning for a complete understanding of child well-being (Huebner & Gilman, 2003). Moreover, understanding strengths may allow for more accurate and effective intervention plans (Jimerson, Sharkey, Nyborg, & Furlong, 2004); help participants feel more empowered and motivated (Epstein, Hertzog, & Reid, 2001); result in a more positive parent-student-professional relationship (LeBuffe & Shapiro, 2004); communicate respect for families and their children (Weick & Chamberlain, 2002); and lead to developing interventions that are more acceptable to children, families, and external service providers (Walrath, Mandell, Holden, & Santiago, 2004). Observations of desired behavior have been increasingly popular, particularly as a way for students to monitor their own success, as they focus attention on the desired goal rather than an undesired behavior. In terms of behavior rating scales, there are far more psychometrically validated problem-based behavior rating scales than strength-based measures. However, as the importance of understanding strengths has become clear, researchers have begun to invest considerable time and resources to develop and psychometrically test strength-based measures in order to balance efforts to understand and treat mental health problems. Clinicians should consider integrating strengths into behavioral observations and identifying psychometrically solid rating scales that include adaptive skills or other strengths.

A Legally Defensible Approach

Collecting functional information on students' performance and behaviors using techniques and instruments with established validity and reliability is a routine and necessary part of many behavioral assessments. At times, the inclusion of behavioral observational data is a legal requirement. For example, behavioral observations are a requisite part of psychoeducational assessments as specified in the Individuals with Disabilities Education Act (IDEA). Specifically, IDEA mandates that assessment professionals "review existing evaluation data on the child, including … classroom-based observations; and observations by teachers and related services providers" (IDEA, 2004, S. 614, c1A). For students with suspected learning disabilities, a trained professional must observe the student and the learning environment to document their academic and behavioral performance in the areas of difficulty. For students with problematic behaviors, school personnel must conduct functional behavioral assessments under specific circumstances, including when determining if a student's conduct is a manifestation of his or her disability. Additionally, no single procedure or assessment tool may be used to make eligibility determinations for special education. While behavior rating scales are frequently utilized as one component of a comprehensive behavioral assessment, the use of rating scales alone is not sufficient. The necessity and utility of understanding how to conduct and interpret behavioral observations and rating scales is clear, not only to obtain valid behavioral data but also to ensure a legally defensible assessment approach.

Features of Observations and Rating Scales

Observations and rating scales both provide behavioral assessment information, but the information is gathered through different methods. Observations can be conducted in a variety of settings, with the goal of providing a snapshot of what certain behaviors look like, with what frequency they are taking place, and whether they are appropriate under the observed circumstances. With an underlying assumption that behavior is specific to a certain situation, multiple observations over time in diverse contexts are necessary to accurately define the problem (Hintze et al., 2008). On the other hand, behavior rating scales are administered to parents, teachers, or youth to gain information on the youth's current or past functioning from a particular person's perspective. Thus, behavior rating scales allow for a summary of past observations across contexts familiar to the rater. Information on the frequency, duration, or appropriateness of the behaviors is provided in an indirect manner by asking the informant to reflect on past observations. Observations and behavior rating scales are fundamentally different in that observations collect direct information, while behavior rating scales gather information from indirect sources. There are clear advantages and disadvantages to both observations and rating scales, depending on the situation and information to be obtained. When administered together, behavioral rating scales and observations allow for a more comprehensive view of behavioral functioning. The following sections will provide more detailed information on the specific features of behavioral observations and rating scales. For practice considerations that align with the content in the following sections, refer to Table 26.1.

Table 26.1 Considerations for Practice

Step	Considerations for Practice
1. Collect information on referred behavior	• Interview others in the setting where the behavior does and does not occur • Conduct a narrative recording to gather global data about the environment • Define target behavior
2. Select and disseminate broad rating scales to collect information for differential diagnosis	• Select rating scales with items which represent behavior, not consequences of behavior, inferences of behavior, or assumptions, or guesses (McConaughy & Ritter, 2008) • Use scales that have been psychometrically tested and validated for the purpose intended • Ensure normative sample adequately represents the client and is up-to-date • Use behavior rating scales, not checklists • Consider options for multiple raters
3. Empirically record behavioral observations	*Considerations to have before selecting an observation system:* • Is the behavior continuous? Or is it discrete? • Is the behavior frequent? Overt? • When does the behavior occur? • Review time and training requirements of the system • How many subjects are to be observed at once? • Select observer

4. Systematically collect direct observation data about the behavior, the child, and the environment in settings with and without the targeted behavior	• Select time and setting for observations
	• Collect information on severity, intensity, frequency, duration, antecedents, consequences, interpersonal interactions, ecological observations, positive behaviors, other problematic behaviors
	• Interpret information in light of potential:
	  • Observer bias
	  • Inter-observer reliability
	  • Reactivity

5. Analyze behavioral data from observations and rating scales	• Use patterns from behavioral data and broad rating scales to determine if more assessment is necessary *Consider if:* • Narrow rating scales are necessary to provide more specific information about an identified problematic behavior or for differential diagnosis • More observation or a different system of data collection is needed • Collect baseline data about specific targeted behavior(s)
6. Analyze information from additional observations or rating scales if applicable	• Establish level of severity for the behavior • Establish antecedents triggering behavior • Establish consequences maintaining the behavior • Determine if there is enough information available to diagnose and create an intervention plan
7. Create and implement an intervention or treatment plan	• Use data collected on antecedents, consequences, severity, frequency, intensity, and diagnostics
8. Collect data during treatment	• Analyze data to inform treatment planning • Adjust intervention as indicated by data collected

Behavioral Observations
Advantages and Limitations of Behavioral Observations

The most direct way to assess behavior is through the use of observations in the setting where the behavior naturally occurs (Skinner, Rhymer, & McDaniel, 2000). However, the most direct way may not always be the most desirable or feasible way, and choosing an observation approach as part of a behavioral assessment depends on the reason for referral, the time and resources available, and the behavior that has been targeted for change. A brief review of the advantages and limitations of behavioral observations is provided.

Direct observations have distinct advantages, which probably contribute to, and maintain, their popularity among both clinicians and researchers. Advantages of direct observations include the amount of information that can be collected during an observation, including information on the frequency and duration of behaviors as well as information on the environmental factors that are maintaining or exacerbating the behaviors (Bloomquist & Schnell, 2002). Observations can focus on the psychological and physical characteristics of the setting where the behavior occurs, and provide a particularly thorough ecological assessment (Sattler & Hoge, 2006). The ability to determine the function of the behavior while also allowing an assessment of the environmental contingencies is among the most attractive features of behavioral observations. Additionally, clinicians often view observations as pure measures of behavior and are thus not subjected to bias through someone else's (parent, teacher, youth) ratings and perceptions (Winsor, 2003).

Behavioral observations are also advantageous in that they can have direct implications for treatment planning and they allow for a more authentic or outcome-based assessment (Stein & Karno, 1994). Gathering information that children in one classroom are, on average, out of their seats 10 times over a 40-minute observation period provides specific baseline information that can be utilized in treatment planning. For example, after obtaining this baseline data, a positive reinforcement system could be implemented in which the children are offered reinforcement for every ten minutes that passes without their getting out their seat. Furthermore, direct observation can allow a clinician to evaluate the effectiveness of an intervention and/or monitor progress towards a specified goal. If, following an intervention, the children are observed to get out of their seats only one time over a 40-minute observation, the effectiveness of the intervention is documented.

Along with distinct advantages, direct observations are replete with disadvantages. Most notably, direct observations are costly both in terms of professional time and labor. Observers must be trained, inter-rater reliability checks often need to be established, and travel to and from multiple settings to conduct observations can be time-consuming. Due to time constraints, it is not possible to sample a comprehensive variety of behaviors or settings, thus the information obtained is limited. In general, direct observation procedures are not useful to gather information about behaviors that occur infrequently or internally (e.g., depressive mood). Furthermore, if the incorrect method of sampling is employed, the information obtained may not be accurate or representative of the behavior being targeted. For example, if an observer chose to implement a time-sampling procedure to observe a child's hitting, and the hitting did not occur during the specified time period, then it might seem as if the target behavior (hitting) was not problematic. Direct observations might also provide inaccurate information if the person or family under observation is aware that an observation is taking place. The act of being observed can cause a reaction or a change in behavior due to an awareness of being observed (Kazdin, 1981). The presence alone of an observer can change the behavior being observed (Reid, Baldwin, Patterson, & Dishion, 1988). Thus, observations are only a "pure" measure of behavior in a particular setting in the presence of the observer. Overall, the results and interpretations of observations must be considered in light of the advantages and disadvantages of behavioral observations.

Preparing for an Observation: Things to Consider

While the novice clinician might consider starting an observation by simply walking into a classroom with a notepad and watching a child referred for an assessment, there are many things that should be considered prior to conducting an observation. Information on the reason for referral, the target behaviors to be observed, the setting and timing of observations, and who will be conducting the observation must be considered.

REASON FOR REFERRAL

First, the reason for referral and the referral source are likely to shape decisions regarding types of observational data collected. The referral question, for example, could lead to a short observation to determine if behaviors are indicative of motor or vocal tics or if a behavior is developmentally inappropriate. Alternatively, the referral question could lead to a more intensive observation in which the intention and the function of the behavior are analyzed and determined. The reason for referral might be related to a problem of frequency (e.g., how often a hand is raised), timing (e.g., when requests for drinks of water are made), or environmental mismatch (e.g., failure to complete tasks in one class) and observations need to be tailored accordingly. The referral source (person) also shapes the observation by labeling the behavior as problematic.

TARGET BEHAVIORS

One of the first key tasks the observer encounters is to identify what to observe. For example, it might be necessary to observe an individual, an interaction between individuals (teacher/student, parent/child), the characteristics of an environment, or the events surrounding the target behaviors or situational context. The target behavior of interest can range from a single, isolated behavior to an interaction between individuals, and it should not be unnecessarily limited. An observation can be structured to collect information about multiple things, including the environment, interactions, and behaviors.

When a behavior is the target of observation, it should be operationally defined with a clear, concise description that is observable, measurable, and specific, to minimize the likelihood of misunderstanding and bias (Winsor, 2003). However, providing too much specificity can also be detrimental to observations. Using too much specificity to define a behavior (e.g., 10 subcategories for "on task" behaviors) can make data recording difficult, and the ultimate goal should be to find a balance between being too global or too specific (Chafouleas, Riley-Tillman, & Sugai, 2007). In general, the ability to provide a clear and operational definition of the behavior will allow for reliable and valid data collection. For example, stating that "aggression" is the target behavior could result in widely varying results during an observation session. One observer might solely indicate that the target behavior occurred only when the child hit another student, while another observer might take "aggression" to encompass a wide range of behaviors, including making fun of another child or refusing to share toys. To provide further clarification, examples of the target behavior, along with inclusionary and exclusionary criteria, can be considered.

SETTING AND TIMING OF OBSERVATIONS

The setting in which the observation is going to occur and the timing of the observation should also be well thought-out. Observations can be conducted in both naturalistic and controlled settings. Observations conducted in naturalistic settings, such as within a classroom or home environment, can provide contextually relevant information and are generally preferred. The observer can see the behavior in its naturally occurring environment, and information on the environment and interactions between individuals in the environment, in addition to the target behaviors, can be recorded. Controlled observations involve observing a child in a staged environment where conditions can be created to elicit the target behavior. Advantages of this approach include not having to wait for the behavior to occur naturally, and the ability to examine how multiple individuals will respond to the same conditions; disadvantages include participants' not behaving spontaneously, and not allowing for additional, potentially informative events to take place (Sattler & Hoge, 2006).

When considering the timing of the observation, it is beneficial to observe at a time when the behavior is likely to occur. For example, if a child were referred for off-task behavior that occurs during math class, observing during math class would make logical sense. However, comparison data gathered during a different class period can provide more information from which to draw conclusions. It might be meaningful to indicate that off-task behavior is not problematic throughout the day and in a variety of settings, but rather solely during math class. Another timing consideration involves the length of the observation. Observers should not schedule overly short observational periods, to ensure that there is adequate time to observe the target behaviors (Winsor, 2003). To obtain a more representative sample of the child's behavior, observations should be conducted within multiple settings and at various times throughout the day. However, it is prudent to remember the resources required to carry out multiple observations at multiple time points and an effort at balance should be sought.

THE OBSERVER

Who is going to conduct the observation is another preliminary question to be answered. Both internal and external observers are frequently utilized to collect observational data. The person-nel resources required to collect observational data might lead to having an internal observer, such as a teacher or a peer, collect data. Alternatively, obser-vations are collected by external observers, such as a psychologist or other trained observer, in which an outside person enters the situation that they are not normally a part of.

External observers, such as a school psycholo-gist, are often chosen due to their objectivity and training in conducting behavioral observations. However, their presence in the new environment can cause reactivity, disruptions in the environ-ment, and further affect the validity of the observa-tional information obtained. Additionally, external observers can be costly in terms of time to conduct the observation, travel to and from the natural set-ting, and training needed.

The advantages of an internal observer include their knowledge of the context and the degree to which they can unobtrusively observe in their own natural environment (Winsor, 2003). Internal observers can remain in an environment for an extended period of time to collect frequency data on low-frequency behaviors, and they can plan to conduct a more structured observation at a suit-able time. However, internal observers, such as teachers, often have limited time to conduct inten-sive observations without disrupting their other responsibilities; thus, teacher recordings are best accomplished when data can be recorded infre-quently and through simple methods (Skinner et al., 2000).

Observational Recording Procedures

Following the specification of the target behavior, setting, and timing, observers must decide which data collection method is optimal. Towards this end, pro-fessionals should (a) ensure targeted behaviors align with the purpose of the instrument, (b) examine the reliability and validity of the system for adequacy, and (c) review the amount of time and training required to learn the system (Volpe, DiPerna, Hintze, & Shapiro, 2005). A variety of different methods of behavioral observation are available, including nar-rative and empirical recording techniques. Examples of recording procedures, along with a summary of general properties of these selected observation sys-tems, are provided in Table 26.2.

Narrative Recording Procedures

Also called *anecdotal recordings*, narrative record-ings simply describe what happens (Bloomquist & Schnell, 2002). This is generally accomplished by observing in a natural setting and recording a detailed narrative of the observed sequence of events. Following a referral, the school psycholo-gist might observe in the classroom to record the sequence of events preceding and following behav-ioral outbursts. The school psychologist might note precipitating factors and resulting consequences, list classroom characteristics, and delineate what other students were doing at the time of the outburst.

Skinner and colleagues (2000) indicated five main purposes for recording behaviors through narrative means: to (a) confirm the presence of problems, (b) define target behaviors, (c) develop

Table 26.2 General Properties of Selected Observation Systems

Title	Author	Age	Behaviors Observed	Length of Observation	Recording Methods
Behavior Assessment System for Children–Student Observation System (BASC-2–SOS)	Reynolds & Kamphaus (2004)	Preschool to High School	• Classroom environment • 65 behaviors within 9 categories of problem behaviors • 4 categories of positive/adaptive behaviors	15 minutes	Momentary time sample at 30-sec. intervals
Child Behavior Checklist–Direct Observation Form (DOF)	Achenbach (1986)	Ages 5 thru 14	• 97 Problematic and on-task behaviors	10 minutes	Likert scale
Behavior Observation of Students in Schools (BOSS)	Shapiro (2004)	Grades Pre-K thru 12	• Problematic Behaviors • Positive behaviors • On-task behaviors and engaged academic time	15 minutes	Momentary time sample at 15-sec. intervals

empirical recording procedures, (d) develop procedures for future observations, and (e) identify the antecedents and consequences of behaviors. Describing what the behavioral outburst looks like (e.g., flailing one's arms and throwing oneself on the floor, versus screaming in a high-pitched voice) informs a more systematic and precise strategy for future observations. The psychologist might notice that the behavioral outbursts occur more frequently during physical education class or the psychologist might have been able to determine where to sit in the classroom to be able to observe the behaviors most easily (Skinner et al., 2000). Hypotheses regarding the function of the behavior and what might maintain the behavior can begin to take shape by analyzing the antecedents and consequences and recording what is taking place in the classroom. An "ABC" chart with three columns of notes describes in depth what happened immediately preceding the behavior (antecedents), a description of the target behavior (behavior), and what happened immediately following the behavior (consequences). Observing and recording the ABCs can help determine the function of a behavior or generate hypotheses about what might contribute to the frequency of the behavior. For example, a school psychologist might receive a referral to observe a child who tells inappropriate jokes during instructional time. During the observation, when the teacher turns around to write on the board (antecedent), the child tells an inappropriate joke (behavior), at which time the entire class may laugh (consequence). The ABC analysis leads to the conclusion that peer attention in the form of laughter is reinforcing the problem behavior. In an alternative scenario, classmates ignore the joke but the teacher punishes the offending student by taking away recess. Through repeated observations in multiple settings, the observer finds that the student wants to skip recess to avoid confrontations with a bully. The ABC analysis leads to the conclusion that taking away recess is reinforcing rather than deterring the student's inappropriate behavior. By recognizing the antecedents and consequences contributing to problematic behavior, an intervention that considers the function of problem behavior (teaches a replacement behavior or manipulates antecedents and/or consequences) is much more likely to succeed than if the problem behavior is simply punished.

Narrative recording procedures are advantageous, particularly with regard to the minimal amount of training required and the ease with which descriptions of observations can be recorded. Conducting a general, global observation is often recommended prior to honing in on specific behaviors to observe, particularly when provided with a non-specific referral question (Sattler & Hoge, 2006); this type of general observation could be accomplished with a narrative recording. Specifically, Sattler & Hoge recommend that when a child is first referred for a behavior problem, the initial observation should be broad enough to allow for an observation of the child's overall behavior and the behavior of other children and adults in the setting. This allows for the observer to note specific behaviors that might need to be observed more closely, as well as make an assessment of the context in which the child's behaviors exist.

Disadvantages of narrative recordings include an end result of imprecise data subject to observers' biases. The descriptive record of behaviors and events and the sequence in which they occurred provides a limited amount of information leading to limited interpretations, particularly if quantitative data are desirable. Furthermore, anecdotal and descriptive accounts can be subject to over-interpretation (making inferences from an unstandardized and limited sample of behavior) and should not be used in high-stakes decisions (Hintze et al., 2008). Therefore, when narrative recording procedures are used it, is important to consider limitations of the information gained and to build upon this information to collect additional empirical data when appropriate.

Empirical Recording Procedures

Although narrative recording procedures are often implemented and can provide meaningful descriptions, empirical recording procedures provide more precise data instead of simply recording the presence or absence of exceptional behavior (Skinner et al., 2000). Empirical procedures allow professionals to monitor goals that must be objective and measurable. The frequency (how often a hand is raised), latency (following a teacher request, how long it takes to initiate the desired behavior), and duration (how long a tantrum lasts) of behaviors can be recorded in a systematic fashion.

EVENT OR FREQUENCY RECORDING

Event or frequency recording provides information on the number of times a behavior occurs during a specified time period. The flexibility of the time period makes an event or frequency recording optimal for a variety of observers and is especially conducive for behaviors that occur at a low frequency. The observer (e.g., parent, teacher, daycare worker, psychologist) can simply tally the number of times that the event occurs in the specified time period. The number of occurrences can be summed, and frequency data can be provided. If the frequency data are divided by the total time observed, an indicator of behavioral rate is provided. For example, frequency data might show that a child hit his sibling six times during a two-hour period, a behavioral rate of three times per hour. Intervention monitoring could include regular observations to check the frequency of behavior with the goal to reduce the frequency to a more desirable level.

Three criteria should be met to select an event or frequency recording: (1) the target behavior should have a clear and specified beginning and end; (2) the behavior should be relatively similar in length and intensity at each instance, and (3) the target behavior should occur in distinct instances (Merrell, 2003). The first criterion provides further reason for having a pre-specified operational definition of the target behavior. A behavior with a discrete beginning and end, such as raising one's hand, could easily be tallied in terms of the number of times that it occurs. However, a behavior such as tapping one's pencil might be ongoing and frequently varies in the length of occurrence and even perhaps its intensity. This inconsistency (criterion 2) leads to challenges such as whether the observer places a tally every time the pencil hits the desk or waits until the student stops tapping. If the behavior occurs too frequently, such as every second, recording the frequency of occurrence would be too burdensome (criterion 3). A different strategy, such as interval recording, would be more appropriate in this instance.

INTERVAL RECORDING AND TIME SAMPLING

Interval recording procedures measure whether a behavior occurs during a specified time period, and they have also been referred to as *time sampling procedures* since they only record a sample of the behavior (Sattler & Hoge, 2006). An observational period is divided into equal intervals, and the observer records if the predetermined behavior occurs at any time during the interval. For example, an observation period totaling fifteen minutes may be divided into 30-second intervals, providing for a total of 30 intervals. The observer would observe and note, during each interval, if the student displayed the target behavior.

Interval recording techniques are most useful with behaviors that occur at moderate to high or steady rates, and/or if the observer is interested in observing multiple behaviors simultaneously. The observer can record the presence or absence of several behaviors (e.g., raising hand, out of seat, talking to neighbor, inappropriate movements) during each interval. The observer can also observe multiple students during a specified interval. Direct observation data can be collected on the target student, as well as on peers to facilitate comparisons. Data on one or several comparison students can be collected simultaneously (observe if the target student is on task while also observing if a peer is on task) or discontinuously (alternative intervals observing the target student and the peer) (Skinner et al., 2000). Simultaneous recording is easier if students are proximal, whereas discontinuous recording can allow for the rotation of comparison students across intervals, thereby including a wider sample of students.

Interval recording techniques require intensive attention by the observer and are facilitated by the use of a stopwatch or time-recording device. Earphones connected to a looped tape in which a beep denotes the beginning of the interval can be helpful to signal the observer that a new interval is starting. Alternatively, personal digital assistants (PDAs) or other hand-held computers can be programmed to provide a checklist of behaviors under observation and to alert the observer when to observe and when to record. Increasingly advanced technologies allow for user-friendly observations in which the observer is not responsible for juggling multiple forms, timepieces, and recording devices. Software is available for some observations systems (e.g., the Behavior Assessment System for Children–2 Student Observation System and Portable Observation Program; Reynolds & Kamphaus, 2004) that enables downloading to hand-held computers and charting and reporting of results from completed observations.

There are three main types of interval recording: partial-interval recording, whole-interval recording, and momentary time sampling. During a *partial-interval* recording, the observer records a behavior as occurring only once during that interval, whether or not it occurred multiple times, or lasted the entire duration of the interval. During a *whole-interval* recording, in order for the observer to record the behavior as occurring, the behavior must last throughout the interval. If the behavior was occurring at the beginning of the interval, but stopped in the middle of the interval, the behavior would be recorded as "not occurring." Similarly, if the behavior occurred for 25 seconds out of the 30-second interval, it would be coded as a non-occurrence. A *momentary time sampling* involves paying particular attention to the exact moment in which the timed interval begins or ends and recording whether or not the behavior occurred during that brief instant. For example, given a 30-second interval, the only momentary time of interest is that first second. If the behavior is occurring at the beginning of the interval, it is recorded. However, if the behavior was not occurring during the first few seconds of the interval, but started during the fifth second of the interval and lasted the remainder of the interval, it would be recorded as a non-occurrence.

Each interval-recording technique yields an approximation rather than an entirely accurate estimate of the behavior. Whole-interval procedures may underestimate the true occurrence of the behavior, partial-interval procedures may overestimate the true occurrence of the behavior, and momentary time sampling techniques may miss behaviors that occur infrequently (Chafouleas et al., 2007). The choice of interval recording strategy depends on the characteristics of the behavior being observed and how frequently the behavior occurs. Whole-interval procedures are most useful if the behavior occurs continuously and the intervals are fairly short, while partial-interval procedures are best utilized with lower-frequency behaviors when the intervals are over a long period of time (Shapiro & Skinner, 1990).

DURATION AND LATENCY RECORDING

In comparison to event recording and time sampling procedures, duration and latency recording procedures are focused on the temporal aspects of the behaviors, rather than the frequency with which the behaviors occur (Merrell, 2003). Specifically, with duration recording, the observer measures the amount of time a behavior lasts, and with latency recording, the observer notes the amount of time between the onset of a stimulus and the behavior initiation. Behaviors that have discrete beginnings and endings are conducive to these types of recording procedures.

Duration recordings are helpful when the behavior is a problem, primarily due to its duration. For example, it might not be disruptive for a student to walk around the classroom on occasion; however, if the student is walking around for twenty minutes during a sixty-minute instructional period, it may disrupt classroom learning. Other examples of behaviors in which duration might be of interest include temper tantrums (how long they last), time actively engaged in a subject, and arguing following being assigned a task or chore. Both total duration in which the behavior occurs and the average duration of the occurrence can be computed (Hintze et al., 2008) to inform intervention planning.

Latency recordings are helpful when the primary problem is the amount of time it takes to begin a behavior after a stimulus, such as a request. This type of recording can be employed to track a student's ability to comply with directions (Allessi, 1988) or to measure the amount of time between a response and an antagonistic stimulus in an aggression scenario (Stein & Karno, 1994). For example, consider a mother who asks her child to take out the trash. The latency recording records the amount of time following the directive ("Please take out the trash now") to the time in which the behavior is performed. The observer records how long it takes for the behavior to begin after the prompt, and this can be averaged across multiple events. The mother starts recording as soon as she gives the directive and stops recording as soon as the behavior is initiated. Over the course of five observations, it takes her child an average of thirty minutes to initiate the behavior of taking out the trash. A specific reinforcement system could be put into place to encourage her child to initiate the behavior within ten minutes. Ongoing observations will inform intervention success. For example, when the child is able to take out the trash within an average of 10 minutes of a request over three observations, the child can earn a reward.

Reliability and Validity of Observation Procedures

The importance of reliable and valid data cannot be overstated, particularly when the data inform a diagnostic or placement evaluation. The reliability and validity of an observation can be affected by a variety of things, including the type of recording system and observation method selected, the setting, the observer, the target person or persons being observed, and the interaction between these sources (Sattler & Hoge, 2006). We provide a brief discussion of psychometric issues affecting observations as an introduction to some of the common issues when empirically evaluating the reliability and validity of observational data. See Table 26.3 for a summary of psychometric information for select published observational systems.

Reliability involves the extent to which the observations collected are consistent and replicable.

Table 26.3 Psychometric Properties of Observation Coding Systems

Observation Coding System	Setting	Norming Information	Reliability	Validity	
			Inter-observer agreement	Convergent	Discriminate
BASC-2–SOS	• School	Authors recommend use of 2–3 randomly selected peers	• No published data	• No published data	• Discriminated ADHD from non-disabled children
CBCL-DOF	• School • Home	Authors recommend observing comparison peers 10 minutes before and 10 minutes after target child	• Average correlations across 4 studies inter-observer agreement r = .90 for total behavior problems and r = .84 for on-task scores	• TRF total behavior problems score (r = −.26 to −.53) • TRF school performance (r = .14 to .66) • TRF adaptive functioning composite (r = .48 to .72)	• Discriminated boys referred for problem behaviors from typically developing boys matched for age, grade, and race
BOSS	• School	Authors recommend use of classroom comparison child at every 5th interval	• Kappas between .93 and .98	• No published data	• Discriminated children with ADHD from their non-disabled peers

Information can be obtained to measure the degree to which behaviors are consistent across times and situations (test-retest reliability), although it is likely that the behaviors being observed might not be consistent across time points or settings. Regardless of behaviors changing across testing situations, the observers should be consistent in their recordings of observations (Skinner et al., 2000). The degree to which independent observers who are observing the same student at the same time are consistent with one another is referred to as "inter-observer reliability" or "agreement."

Inter-observer agreement is important to establish the reliability of a behavioral observation technique. It is generally reported as the mean percentage of agreement amongst observers along with the range of agreement across sessions. Inter-observer agreement is calculated by dividing the number of agreements by the number of agreements plus the number of disagreements and then multiplying by 100 to yield a percentage (House, House, & Campbell, 1981). High inter-observer agreement confirms that data are due to actual behavior rather than biases or inaccuracies of the observer (Stein & Karno, 1994). Potential biases include expectancy effects, in which the observer's expectations influence recordings, or observer drift, in which the observer changes the criteria for judging the behavior due to fatigue or other variables (Sattler & Hoge, 2006). Additional threats include problems of omission or commission when the observer fails to record a behavior or miscodes a behavior (Sattler & Hoge).

Inter-observer agreement data are relatively easy to collect, although the procedure does require having at least two observers trained in a single method of observation collect data simultaneously. An inter-observer accordance of 80 percent is generally acceptable, and inter-observer agreement data are generally collected during a minimum of 20 percent of observation sessions (Skinner et al., 2000). Techniques to improve inter-observer agreement include: altering the recording system, providing improved operational definitions, reducing the number of behaviors recorded, increasing the amount of time training observers, and providing corrective feedback to observers during trainings (Skinner et al., 2000). Inter-observer agreement is not sufficient to demonstrate the validity of an observation system. There could be a high level of agreement between observers, but the observational system might still be flawed or the observations recorded might not be useful (Sattler & Hoge, 2006).

Whereas *reliability* generally refers to consistency, *validity* demonstrates if the test (or observation) measures what it is supposed to theoretically measure. When considering behavioral observations, validity can be affected by whether observations are representative of behavior in a particular situation and across situations (Sattler & Hoge, 2006). Clinicians conducting or overseeing behavioral observations should be aware of some of the potential threats to the validity of behavioral observations. For example, *reactivity* occurs when behaviors change as a result of being observed. In observer reactivity, the observer changes recording style when aware of being observed. For example, when observers are aware that their ratings will be compared to other observers or if their observation is being observed by a supervisor, they tend to be more attentive, careful, and accurate (Sattler & Hoge, 2006). In subject reactivity, the subject changes their behavior as a result of the presence of the observer. For example, consider the teacher who frequently yells at students but, when observed, maintains an even tone because yelling would be inappropriate. Similarly, children who frequently get out of their seat at inappropriate times might be more inclined to stay seated if they are aware of being observed. These changes in behavior affect the validity of the findings; thus, reactivity should be minimized to the degree possible by conducting observations in an unobtrusive and discreet manner (Merrell, 2003) or by allowing the client to get accustomed to the presence of the observer (Keller, 1986). Specifically, observers can practice techniques such as shifting attention away from the target child periodically, entering the setting in a non-disruptive way (during breaks or class changes), observing from a distance or through one-way mirrors, avoiding interactions with others during the observation, and finding an inconspicuous location from which to observe (Sattler & Hoge, 2006).

In addition to minimizing the effects of reactivity during an observation, clinicians should consider how to increase the likelihood that the behaviors sampled are representative of the child's behavior as a whole. This can be accomplished by conducting observations in multiple settings and at multiple time points and by not making broad generalizations from limited data (Merrell, 2003). It might also be useful to collect social comparison data, in which information on the behavior of peers is also collected. These comparison data can allow for more meaningful descriptions of the behaviors observed (e.g., how this student behaves in comparison to

his or her classmates) and can place the behaviors within a meaningful context (Sattler & Hoge, 2006). Comparison data should ideally be collected in the same setting and during the same time period as the observation. The variety of potential threats to validity and reliability is extensive; thus it is critical to consider the variety of ways to minimize these threats and to report data in light of these limitations to behavioral observations.

Behavioral Rating Scales

Unlike behavioral observations, which provide data regarding behavior in a specific context during a limited time frame, behavior rating scales provide a summary of behavioral characteristics of a student that may occur in one or more settings as observed by a particular informant over a longer period of time (Merrell, 2000). Rating scales are different from personality tests in that they focus on patterns of overt behavior rather than underlying personality traits (Sattler & Hoge, 2006). Rating scales provide an efficient summary of a person's behavior by a specific rater. Possible raters include the person who is being assessed (self-report), teachers, parents, and other key informants who have specialized knowledge about an individual. A brief explanation of scale development is necessary to explain the complexity of behavior rating scales and highlight the importance of limiting their use to well-trained professionals.

Development and Types of Behavioral Rating Scales

Behavioral rating scales consist of statistically grouped behavioral and emotional problems or strengths that represent patterns of functioning. Scores indicate how different a person's behavioral and emotional functioning is compared to large normative samples that are most often separated by gender and age. The utility of a scale's published/stated purpose must be tested thoroughly with a normative sample prior to its use with true clients. Before implementing a rating scale, it is crucial that practitioners review its development and select one with empirically validated scales and large normative samples that are representative of the client being tested in terms of demographic characteristics such as gender, age, race, language status, and region of the country.

In the beginning stages of scale development, researchers generate a broad list of behavioral and emotional problems or skills related to the purpose of assessment. For example, to develop a depression inventory, a scientist generates a list of behavioral and emotional symptoms or characteristics of depression such as being sad or tired. In order to generate items, the scientist might look at case files of clinically depressed clients, review the literature, include diagnostic criteria, or survey experts in the field. Once a comprehensive list is identified, the scale developer may or may not want to shorten the list of potential items prior to expensive norming procedures and statistical analyses. Thus, scale developers often use experts to rate the relevance of items to the construct under investigation. For example, the developer might send a list of potential depression items to 100 clinical psychologists with expertise in depression to rate each item for its relevance to the disorder. The highest-rated items are assigned response options so raters can identify the frequency with which a particular symptom or characteristic is present. Multiple responses such as "never, sometimes, often" or "never, rarely, sometimes, often, always" allow the rater to weigh the presence of a symptom more precisely than a yes or no option. Having multiple responses is one of the key characteristics of a behavior rating scale that differentiate it from a checklist, and this allows for more precise measurement of symptom frequency or intensity (Merrell, 1999).

Once a list of potential items has been identified, the developer must conduct a study to isolate and group a final list of items through statistical analyses. The developer recruits a large, diverse sample of participants who each provide responses to every item. Once data are collected, a statistician conducts various analyses, which may include item response theory, differential item functioning, or factor analysis, to evaluate the psychometric properties of the scale. For example, factor analysis is guided by decisions such as how many scales are desirable and which items fit together based on theory and expert knowledge. In creating a depression scale, if a single depression scale is predicted, any item that does not fit within a single factor might get eliminated. However, if statistics reveal unexpected results, such as two distinct factors, the scale developers would need to consider how the two scales fit within the existing knowledge and research regarding depression. Ultimately, psychometric analysis yields a final abbreviated scale that is ready to be tested. Scale developers assign labels to the *factors*, or *subscales*, that describe their contents. For example, all items that describe symptoms of inattention might be labeled "inattention," and all aggressive behaviors might be named "delinquency," "aggression," or

"conduct problems." Note that scales with different names might measure similar behaviors and scales with similar names might measure quite different behaviors. It is up to the test user to review items and scales to understand what is being measured and how it compares to other tests and measures.

In the final stage, the scale developer must recruit a large sample of participants whose demographic characteristics (e.g., gender, age, race, geographical location) are representative of the types of clients who will complete the final version of the scale, yet who are drawn from the general population, so the developer can determine the full range of responses, including what are typical ratings for the average person. This sample is termed the *normative sample* and sets the standard for identifying average, at-risk, and clinical levels of symptoms. The data collected from the normative sample are examined to determine the distribution of scores. A number of reliability and validity analyses are crucial at this step; see Chapter 3 for a thorough discussion of related measurement issues. Behavior-rating scales all have somewhat different development procedures and psychometric properties. It is the responsibility of an assessment professional to carefully review the procedures and psychometric properties to ensure an assessment is valid for the purpose intended.

BROADBAND VERSUS NARROWBAND SCALES

In general, broadband scales assess multiple syndromes that may have overlapping symptoms and characteristics and allow for an assessment of multiple behaviors simultaneously. Using a broadband scale, an assessor can develop a better understanding of the pattern of behaviors displayed by a student. For example, a teacher might refer a student for having difficulty paying attention. Giving a broadband behavior rating scale with multiple informants, the assessor might determine that the student has inattentive behaviors from the teacher's viewpoint; inattentive, emotional, and depressed behaviors from the parent perspective; and emotional ups and downs from the self-report. If a unidimensional attention rating scale had been administered, the practitioner might have concluded that the student has symptoms of attention-deficit hyperactivity disorder (ADHD). Using the broadband scale allowed the user to identify internalizing problems as the source of inattention, which requires a different course of treatment than ADHD.

In contrast to the omnibus measurement of a broadband rating scale, narrowband behavior rating scales are disorder- or category-specific, assessing for subtypes or precise traits within a focused problem area. The implementation of more specific narrowband scales as a second step might help focus the assessment on the internalizing problems and further detail eligibility or treatment needs. As comorbidity (co-occurring disorders) tends to be the rule rather than the exception in these cases (Sroufe, 1997), it is important to assess broadly at first, and only narrow in once preliminary results are examined. See Table 26.4 for examples of broadband and narrowband rating

scales, including information on their general properties.

CHECKLISTS VERSUS RATING SCALES

Checklists are not rating scales; rather, they allow for simple ratings of the presence or absence of emotional or behavioral characteristics that represent a particular syndrome, diagnosis, or area of strength. The DSM-IV-TR and IDEA represent categorical classification systems that require a specific diagnosis for access to funding streams such as mental health or special education services. A categorical approach

Table 26.4 General Properties of Selected Rating Scales

Scale	Authors	Type	Behaviors Assessed	Age	Informants	# of items
ASEBA (CBCL, TRF, and YSR)	Achenbach & Rescorla (2001)	Broad	• Multi-disorder syndrome scales • Adaptive scales • Competency scales	1½ to 18 1½ to 90+ 11 to 90+	Teacher & parent Self	Ages 6–18: 112 Ages 11–18: 110
BASC-2 (TRS, PRS, and SRP)	Reynolds & Kamphaus (2004)	Broad	• Multi-disorder syndrome scales • Adaptive scales • Competency scales	2 to 21:11 8 to college	Teacher & parent Self	100 or 139 (teacher) 134, 160, or 150 (parent) 139, 176, or 185 (self-report)
Conners Third Edition (Conners 3)	Conners (2008)	Narrow	• ADHD • Externalizing	6 to 18 8 to 18	Teacher, Parent Self	Short Form: 39–43 Long Form: 59–115
ADHD Rating Scale-IV (ADHD RS IV)	DuPaul, Power, & Anastopoulos (1998)	Narrow	• ADHD	5 to 17 5 to 17	Parent Teacher	18
Reynolds Adolescent Depression Scale, Second Edition (RADS-2)	Reynolds (2002)	Narrow	• Depression	11 to 20	Self	30
Children's Depression Inventory (CDI)	Kovacs (2001)	Narrow	• Depression	6 to 17	Self	27
Social Skills Improvement System, Social Skills Rating System (SSIS)	Gresham & Elliot (1990)	Narrow	• Social skills • Problem behaviors • Academic competence	3 to 18 3 to 18 8 to 18	Parent Teacher Self	34–57
Piers-Harris Self Concept Scale, Second Edition (Piers-Harris 2)	Piers, Harris, & Herzberg (2002)	Narrow	• Self-concept	7 to 18	Self	60

assumes disorders are either present or not, and does not acknowledge subsyndromal levels of pathology (Kamphaus, VanDeventer, Brueggemann, & Barry, 2007). Although behavior rating scales can be used to complete a behavior checklist such as one used to make a diagnosis according to the DSM-IV-TR, behavior rating scales are much more complex and have many more uses than a behavior checklist. (See Chapter 9 for a more thorough description of classification systems and diagnosis.) Depending on the purpose of assessment, behavioral rating scales may be used in combination with observations, interviews, records reviews, and other types of direct and indirect measures of functioning. It is critical that behavior rating scales be validated for each specific purpose they are used for.

Purpose of Assessment

Behavior-rating scales play an important role in the psychological assessment of children and adolescents. As previously mentioned, psychological assessment has historically focused on deficit-based, or "medical," models for understanding behavioral functioning. The most accurate and legally defensible assessment takes into account ecological variables and includes a breadth of strengths and deficits. The main uses of behavior rating scales are screening, diagnosis, treatment planning, and progress monitoring.

SCREENING

The purpose of screening is to efficiently identify those who are likely to be at-risk for problems and therefore need intervention. Schools are ideal settings for universal screening of children and adolescents, as they serve the entire youth population. Although few schools systematically screen for mental health problems (Romer & McIntosh, 2005), screening is a highly beneficial and cost-effective strategy that all schools should consider. This is particularly important as early identification and intervention of mental health problems attenuates the long-term consequences associated with mental illnesses, such as academic failure and healthcare costs (Campaign for Mental Health Reform, 2005). Schools routinely screen for other health challenges that may impede learning, such as vision, hearing, fitness, and language development; screening for mental health is the next step in allocating early intervention services to promote academic excellence.

For screening, a brief behavior rating scale is administered to a whole group. For instance, a school may wish to determine which students could most benefit from school-based counseling services.

A behavior rating scale is administered to the entire student population, and students whose scores fall a standard deviation above a preset cutoff point (e.g., one standard deviation above the mean) are selected for more intensive assessment. Through a multi-gating approach, students pass through increasingly more intensive assessments and interventions as needed to address problems. By assessing the entire population, screeners can identify challenges for students who may have been missed by less structured methods such as parent or teacher referral. For accuracy, the behavior rating scale needs to be validated for the purpose of screening.

One example of a systematic behavioral screening system is the Behavior Assessment System for Children, Second Edition–Behavior and Emotional Screening System (BESS; Kamphaus & Reynolds, 2007). The BESS consists of brief rating scales for students, parents, and teachers with 25 to 30 items. Elevated results provided by T scores and interpreted through cut-scores indicate which children demonstrate precursors for emotional and behavioral problems and can be used in the systematic identification of children in need for intervention. (For more information on screening, see Chapter 9.)

DIAGNOSIS

Behavior-rating scales are important to help professionals categorize and diagnose behavior according to classification schemes such as the *Diagnostic and Statistical Manual of Mental Disorders–Fourth Edition, Text Revision* (DSM-IV-TR; American Psychiatric Association, 2000) or Individuals with Disabilities Education Act (IDEA; PL 101–476). The DSM-IV-TR is a comprehensive list of all recognized mental health disorders with their diagnostic criteria. If a certain number of behavioral criteria are met to a marked degree and over a sufficiently long period of time and causing significant disruptions to functioning, a person is assigned a mental health disorder. If criteria are not met, the individual is thought not to have a mental health disorder. The IDEA provides diagnostic criteria for children from birth to 21 years of age to access special-education services in the public schools setting. To receive services, children must meet criteria for one of 13 disabilities and be unable to access regular education without special-education supports and services. Although the DSM-IV-TR and IDEA overlap in terms of disabilities covered, the criteria are different, and it is possible, for example, to meet DSM-IV-TR criteria but not IDEA criteria.

Diagnoses are often tied to access to services and funding streams.

A sequence of steps is necessary to use behavioral rating scales as part of a diagnostic decision (Kamphaus et al., 2007). First, a broadband scale, which assesses several syndromes in one scale, can be used to assess multiple groupings of behavior (e.g., depression, anxiety, social skills; examples are provided in Tables 26.4 and 26.5). Level of functioning on the various scales/syndromes allows the assessor to determine the breadth and depth of difficulties. Score profiles indicate if a single disorder emerges as problematic or is accompanied by co-occurring problems, or if behavior that looks like one disorder is actually caused by an alternative disorder (e.g., aggression masking depression). If scores on one or more syndromes falls in the at-risk or clinical range, the assessor must determine if the score is consistent with other sources of information including other informants and/or other assessment strategies (e.g., observations, interviews, records review). Narrowband scales, which assess a particular disorder, can be used as a second step in the assessment process to obtain more in-depth data regarding a particular problem, such as inattention, depression, or aggression (examples are provided in Tables 26.4 and 26.5). Prior to making a diagnosis based on rating scale results, alternative reasons for elevated scores should be considered and ruled out,

Table 26.5 Psychometric Properties of Selected Rating Scales

Scale	Results	Reliability	Validity	Normative Properties	Additional Considerations
Broadband Rating Scales					
ASEBA	T scores and percentile ranks for subscales and composites Syndrome scales DSM scales	• Internal consistency on school-age forms CBCL, YSR, TRS: α = .55–.97 • Test-retest CBCL, YSR, TRF: mean r = .60–.96 • Inter-rater CBCL and TRF mean r Pre-school: r = .40–.65 School age: r = .19–.59	• Convergent validity: Across subscales compared to DSM-IV-TR checklist r = .43–.80	• Nationally representative non-referred sample from 1999 survey of stratified random sampling • Non-referred/referred sample matched for age, gender, and ethnicity • Borderline clinical rage developed to lessen false positives (Achenbach & McConaughy, 2003)	69 different languages Syndrome scales DSM categories Multicultural module, supplements, and manual
BASC-2	Cutoff scores for clinically significant and at-risk behaviors T scores and percentile ranks for subscales and composites	• Internal consistency (mean across SRP, TRS, PRS) α = .84 • Test-retest (all 3 form types) r = .79 • Inter-rater (teacher forms) r = .56 • Inter-rater (parent forms) r = .76 (Reynolds & Kamphaus, 2004; Sattler & Hoge, 2006)	• Content, Construct, and Criterion-related validities = satisfactory • Composite scale contain indices to detect threats to internal validity (Sattler & Hoge, 2006)	• Normed on population comparative to 2001 census data for age, ethnicity, and gender. • Clinical norm sample to compare T-scores to general, gender, age, and clinical combined or separated for ADHD and LD	• Spanish form versions

(continued)

Table 26.5 (Continued)

Scale	Results	Reliability	Validity	Normative Properties	Additional Considerations
Narrowband Rating Scales: Externalizing					
Conners 3	Cut-scores for clinically significant and at-risk behaviors Impairment items DSM-IV TR subscales T scores and percentile ranks for subscales and composites	Across content & DSM-IV TR scales all • Internal consistency: α = .85–.91 • Test-retest r = .76–.89 • Inter-rater r = .70–.81	Convergent validity with other measures: • BASC-2 Attention Problems scale: r = .52 to .89 • ASEBA Attention Problems scale: r = .73–.96 • BASC-2 Hyperactivity/ Impulsivity: r = .46–.91 • ASEBA Aggression scale: r = .69 to .93 • BASC-2 Aggression: r = .77–.95	• Normed on sample representative of U.S. population (n = 3,400)	• Short forms • Index forms (10 item ADHD screener) • Spanish versions of parent and self-report • Linked to IDEIA • Linked to DSM-IV-TR symptom scales
ADHD RS IV	Compatible with DSM IV ADHD criteria Yields 1 broad score and 2 subscale scores of hyperactivity/ impulsivity and attention	• Internal consistency α = .86–.96 • Test-retest across teacher and parent over 4 weeks r = .78–.90 (Lindskog, 2003)	• Concurrent/predictive across other ADHD scale r = .25–.88 • Convergent across other ADHD scale r = .81 parent r = .76–.85	• Normed on over 2000 children, mirrored 1990 census for ethnicity and region of residence • English and Spanish forms available; may be used for progress monitoring and screening (DuPaul et al., 1998)	• English and Spanish forms available • Progress monitoring and screening • Home and school versions
Narrowband Rating Scales: Internalizing					
RADS-2	Current severity of symptoms: dysphoric mood, anhedonia/ negative affect, negative self-evaluation, somatic complaints	• Internal consistency α = .87–.96 • Test-retest over 12 weeks r = .79 • Inter-rater is not reported	• Predictive validity: r = .40–.75 on self-esteem, loneliness, suicidal ideation, hopelessness • Convergent validity: r = .70–.89 with other measures of depression (Holmbeck et al., 2008)	• Re-standardized in U.S. and Canada on 3,300 adolescents ages 11–20	

(continued)

Table 26.5 (Continued)

Scale	Results	Reliability	Validity	Normative Properties	Additional Considerations
CDI	5 clinical subscales; composite scores can determine severity	• Internal consistency $\alpha = .71–.89$ • Test-retest r = .38–.87 • Inter-rater r = .40 across parent and child	• Predictive: Differentiated clinical and normal cases and depressed versus non-depressed patients • Convergent validity: r = .20–.60 across anxiety, anger, and depression measures	• Limited normative sample (Eckert, Dunn, Codding, & Guiney, 2000)	• Short 10-item form available
Narrowband Rating Scales: Social Skills					
SSIS	Social Skills subdomains: social skills, problem behaviors, academic competence	Across all forms, all 3 subdomains: • Internal consistency $\alpha = .73–.95$ • Test-retest r = .65–.93 • Inter-rater is not reported	• Specific psychometric properties for validity not reported	• Standardization sample based on U.S. 1988 census data • Sample included over-sample of special needs populations	• Spanish version of parent and student forms • National preschool norms
Narrowband Rating Scales: Self-concept					
Piers-Harris 2	T-scores reported for domain scales: behavioral adjustment, intellectual and school status, physical appearance and attributes, freedom from anxiety, popularity, happiness and satisfaction, and total score	• Internal consistency for Total Scale $\alpha = .91$ • Test-retest additional reliability studies needed with this version • Previous version has supporting reliability (Spies & Plake, 2005)	• Convergent validity as inverse measure to other studies • Additional validity studies needed with this version (previous version has supporting reliability)	• Standardized representative national sample of 1,400 students based on 2001 U.S. census • Hispanic students from Western U.S. are under-represented	• Spanish version • Used as a screener • Group or individual administration

such as rater bias, environmental mismatch, or temporary stress.

TREATMENT PLANNING AND PROGRESS MONITORING

Behavior-rating scales may be useful for treatment planning and progress monitoring. Ideally, scales that provide data useful for diagnosis could also inform the next step: deciding what evidence-based strategies can be implemented to help the individual being assessed. Unfortunately, not much empirical research has examined behavior-rating scales for this purpose (Merrell, 2000). A challenge with treatment identification is that there may be several treatment options for a youth with a particular disorder depending on additional factors such as age, intelligence, and comorbidity. Thus, an expert may need to make a judgment based on a comprehensive set of data. A challenge with treatment monitoring is that ratings might not be sensitive to change, as behavior rating scales rely on rater memory of past behavior over a broad period of time (Chafouleas et al., 2007). With the recent focus on response-to-intervention strategies, however, some behavior rating scales are being developed for use with treatment planning and progress monitoring. Others have been revised and re-normed with more frequent assessment in mind.

When data gathered from behavior rating scales can be used to design interventions that improve behavior, the scale has *intervention validity* (Elliott, Gresham, Frank, & Beddow, 2008). When they are designed and validated for use in planning and monitoring intervention, behavior rating scales can add value and efficiency to the assessment-treatment process. For example, item wording can impact how valid a measure is for treatment planning. "Molar" items represent a series of behaviors ("Make friends easily"; Gresham & Elliott, 1990), whereas "molecular" items represent a specific skill set ("Raises hand to request a turn"). Although molar items are useful for classification and diagnosis, molecular items are more useful for treatment planning (Elliott et al., 2008). Strategies that encourage intervention validity are (a) basing scale development on theory for problem solution, (b) targeting behavior that is socially important, and (c) organizing results to facilitate treatment planning (Elliott et al., 2008). Further research is needed to validate the use of behavior rating scales for treatment planning and progress monitoring, but it is a promising approach to streamline the assessment to intervention process, which historically has been quite disconnected.

In response to the multitude of ways to identify children and the need for intervention, the authors of the Behavior Assessment System for Children, Second Edition (BASC-2; Reynolds & Kamphaus, 2004) have also recently published the BASC-2 Progress Monitor (BASC-2 PM; Kamphaus & Reynolds, 2009) and the BASC-2 Intervention Guide (BASC-2 IG; Vannest, Reynolds, & Kamphaus, 2009). The BASC-2 PM has been developed as a means to collect additional behavioral information for a variety of purposes. It contains different form versions containing 15 to 20 items, gathering brief ratings completed by students, parents, and parents and teachers. These ratings provide scores in the following domains: externalizing behaviors and ADHD problems, internalizing problems, social withdrawal, and adaptive skills. Information is reported through raw scores, T scores, and percentile ranks. Results render mental health professionals with the information necessary to monitor the changes in an individual's behavior over time. The BASC-2 IG provides recommendations on methods of intervention, prevention, and management of behavioral problems corresponding to BASC-2 TRS and PRS subcategories (see "Observation Systems and Rating Scales" section below for additional information on the BASC-2) and is grounded in empirically validated research.

Merrell (2003) proposes specific strategies for using behavior rating scales to inform treatment decisions. First, data gathered through behavior rating scales identify a set of problem behaviors that are interrelated. Subsequently, professionals could use a Keystone Behavior Strategy (Nelson & Hayes, 1986) to select interventions that target a subset of behaviors effective at reducing the entire set of problem behaviors. A Keystone Behavior Strategy includes reducing risk through identifying a behavior deficit and enhancing the missing skills to translate into improved outcomes broadly. For example, a psychologist could teach a child with aggressive tendencies anger-management and relaxation strategies. The increase in skills will reduce the problematic instances where aggression was once displayed, in exchange for more pro-social behaviors.

Alternatively, clinicians could use data from behavior rating scales to inform a Template-Matching Strategy (Hoier & Cone, 1987), which involves targeting skills to the level of those consistently displayed by behaviorally high-functioning children. A Template Matching procedure may include collecting baseline information on molecular behavior such as disruptively speaking out in class. After an assessment of how frequently a typical peer in the class engages in the same speaking out behavior, the goal for intervention could be to decrease the behavior and enhance skills of the targeted child to an acceptable level as established by matching the template of an average peer. Both strategies require monitoring to determine if interventions selected by using the rating scale lead to treatment improvement. Although treatments are often assessed for their "face value," or apparent worthiness based on common sense, careful research is needed to validate the selection and implementation of a treatment and avoid potential iatrogenic effects.

Measurement Issues with Behavioral Rating Scales

Behavioral rating scales can provide rich information from multiple sources regarding a variety of student behaviors. However, the quality of rating scale development varies greatly from scale to scale. Numerous scales are marketed to clinicians, and it is tempting to purchase and implement measures based on the advertised benefits. However, not all published scales have psychometric properties adequate for making decisions about individual clients. Alternatively, there exist many unpublished scales that are thoroughly developed for multiple purposes. Thus, it is critical for any professional who uses behavioral rating scales to understand how scales are developed and validated in general, and the psychometric properties of any particular scale selected for use. Assessment professionals must be able to discern whether an assessment tool has the reliability and validity adequate for the purpose intended. This section will review some of the measurement issues that need to be considered by test developers and understood by test consumers. (See Table 26.5 for a summary of the psychometric properties of selected published rating scales.)

Although the target of the measure is the subject being rated, behavioral rating scales may also provide information about the person providing the information on the rating scale. Results reflect a rater's perspective of another person's behavior, as the rating can be biased by inaccurate memory. Behavior-rating scales are susceptible to several types of effects that lead to bias and reduce the accuracy of results (Merrell, 1999). "Halo effects" occur when a rater's overall opinion of a student who is being rated as good or bad influences all the ratings. For example, if a teacher feels a student is particularly out of control, the teacher might rate the student poorly on all indices, due to his or her knowledge of the student's poor behavior. The same could be true of a teacher rating a popular or well-liked student; the teacher might rate all indices positively due to his or her overall good feeling about a student. Leniency or severity effects occur when a rater is consistently lenient or severe across ratings of various students. Central-tendency biases occur as well, because raters tend to avoid judgments at the far ends of the scale. Schwartz (1999) hypothesized that survey respondents also are most likely to choose response options near the middle of Likert scales because they may interpret them to convey "normative" behavior. Finally, a self-serving bias may occur if the rater responds in a manner designed to gain or avoid services (Furlong & Smith, 1994).

Behavior-rating scales are also susceptible to various types of error variance. *Source error* reflects the subjectivity of the rater, *setting variance* reflects the phenomenon that the environment has a unique interaction with behavior, and *temporal variance* notes that behaviors vary and are inconsistent over time and across settings. Instrument variance acknowledges that different scales measure related but slightly different constructs and represent distinct normative samples, and thus, should not be expected to completely align with each other (Merrell, 1999). Although threats to validity are a fact of behavior rating scales, serious errors can be avoided by constructing scales that encourage accurate responding.

Format of Rating Scales

Survey design and implementation has a critical impact on how accurately people respond to behavior rating scales. Long- and short-term memory limitations, emotional reactions to items, item wording, response wording, and time frames all might affect responses (Furlong & Smith, 1994). Instructions on the rating scale itself can influence accuracy (Merrell, 2003). Directions should be succinct yet clear, and provide decision rules when deciding between multiple response options. By understanding the research related to various development and administration procedures, clinicians can select the most accurate behavior rating scales possible for their purpose.

ADMINISTRATION

When administered individually by a trained professional, behavior rating scales are most likely completed carefully and relatively accurately. Unfortunately, when administered in large group settings by untrained professionals, research has demonstrated that the accuracy of ratings may suffer. Cross and Newman-Gonchar (2004) compared rates of invalid responses to surveys administered by trained versus untrained teachers. Results indicated that the trained administrators obtained far lower rates of highly suspect responses (3%) than did the untrained administrators (28%). Thus, it is important to train survey administrators regarding the importance of accurate ratings and procedures for how to obtain accurate results.

PRESENTATION FORMAT

The presentations of information to be rated can significantly affect the ratings. In a study by Hilton, Harris, and Rice (1998), the authors examined the consistency of youth self-reports of violence victimization and perpetration and compared prevalence rates derived from traditional paper-and-pencil reports to those provoked by the same experience modeled in an audio vignette. They found that the same youths reported two to three times more violence perpetration and victimization using the self-report format. Perhaps hearing the information made it more salient than reading about the perpetration. Turner et al. (1998) provided one of few investigations regarding how traditional paper-and-pencil formats and computer-assisted presentation influence response rates. Turner and colleagues found that the computer format produced statistically significantly higher prevalence rates than did the paper-and-pencil format for weapon-carrying, acts of violence, and threatened violence. It is possible that the computer format promotes more accurate and less socially desirable responses, as responses may seem more confidential to respondents; more research is needed to draw firm conclusions.

RATING SCALE TIME FRAME

Behavior scales sometimes include items that refer to past behavior using a particular time frame (e.g., 30 days, six months, one year). Presumably, respondents would report higher incidents of behaviors over a much longer period of time. However, research on the issue has found some counter-intuitive results. Hilton, Harris, and Rice (1998) examined differences in self-reports across one-month, six-month, and one-year time periods and found that rates of interpersonal violence were insensitive to time frame. Their participants reported the same number of violent acts over the past year as in the past month. Multiple factors affect student recollection of school experiences, and respondents may find it difficult to accurately remember past events (Cornell & Loper, 1998; Fowler, 1993). Raters tend to place priority on more recent events than on more distant events and remember unusual rather than ordinary behavior (Worthen, Borg, & White, 1993). It is also possible that respondents interpret response time frames as providing subtle cues about the types of events the researchers are interested in. Asking about the past month may convey to respondents that researchers want to know about less serious but common events. In contrast, students may interpret asking about the past year as seeking information about less frequent but more serious incidents (Schwartz, 1999).

RESPONSE OPTIONS

Response options on behavior rating scales are formatted so raters can provide their level of agreement on a scale with multiple options. With only two options, the scale acts more as a checklist than a rating scale. With too many options, it is difficult to establish inter-rater reliability. Thus, a three-point scale tends to be common (Elliott et al., 2008). More accurate ratings are obtained when each rating is well operationalized so it is easy for raters to distinguish between options and select the one that best fits the ratee (Merrell, 2003).

WORDING OF QUESTIONS

How the question is asked influences the response. For example, ratings of specific behaviors (e.g., the student says "please" when making a request) may be more accurate than ratings of global judgments (e.g., "the student is polite"; Sattler & Hoge, 2006). When test developers create items, they should have a rationale for the wording of items and carefully consider whether molecular or molar items are required for the purpose intended. Test consumers should review test manuals to determine the quality of item development and if the wording of questions was adequately considered for the intended goal of assessment.

DATA SCREENING

Data screening methods can be used to help professionals detect response inconsistencies or implausibly extreme patterns of responding. Some surveys ask raters directly if they are responding honestly. Survey methods should include strategies to detect if youths respond in a socially desirable way (under-reporting negative behavior) and recognize that youths involved with antisocial and aggressive peers may *exaggerate* their involvement in delinquent activities as an alternative form of social desirability (Furlong & Sharkey, 2006). Procedures can be built into scale analyses that detect patterns of responding or significant inconsistencies among similar items.

Informants

Behavior-rating scales are indirect measures of behavior, as they rely on a rater's memory of behavior over time rather than recording behavior as it occurs. Thus, ratings are only as accurate as the person or "informant" who does the rating. Research indicates that there is low agreement between parent, teacher, and self-respondents to the same rating system. For example, weak correlations of .27 between teacher and parent, .25 between parent and self-report, and .20 between teacher and self-report ratings have been found, while more modest correlations of .59 were found between two parents and .64 between two teachers (Achenbach et al., 1987). This phenomenon is based on several factors: (a) behaviors occur within specific environments, (b) the restricted number of response options might not fit the behavior of a particular child, and (c) there is error associated with measurement. Merrell (2000) identified six findings related to behavior ratings across informants: correlations are modest, agreement in ratings across raters in similar roles (e.g., two parents) is more likely than across raters in different roles (e.g., parent and teacher), agreement is stronger for externalizing than internalizing problems, agreement between child self-report and adult raters is low, gender of rater or student does not impact ratings, and age of student may be important but the influence of age is not yet understood. All of these factors should be taken into consideration when selecting measures and informants for the purpose of assessment.

Given that consistent ratings across informants is the exception rather than the rule, when this does happen, results indicate areas of consistency across environments and expectations (McConaughy & Ritter, 2008). Differences should be examined for factors affecting a respondent's perceptions. Perhaps there are different behavioral expectations in different settings. A teacher sees dozens of children in the school context. When teacher ratings are in the normal range and parent scores are elevated, this result may be because teachers may have a more realistic sense of what a typical child feels and does. Parents may be comparing their child to a well-behaved or high-functioning sibling. On the other hand, teachers may have higher expectations for behavioral conformity given the structured setting, and rate students as more extreme than parents who provide their children lots of unstructured time to play freely where focus on required tasks is not necessary. Clinicians should look for explanations for different results across informants using observational data and interviews to corroborate hypotheses.

When considering who should complete ratings for a particular client, practitioners should consider who knows the person well enough to respond accurately to the questions. Some informants may not know the child well enough or for long enough to accurately report on the behaviors in question. Informants may not have the opportunity to know about the child's behavior outside the setting, so a rating scale developed for any adult to complete may be difficult for a teacher to complete if there are questions about free-time activities, or for a parent to complete if there are questions about classroom behaviors. Superior rating scales are developed and validated specifically for a particular user to a user class, such as teachers, parents, or self.

Self-reports are the most direct assessment of a person's behavioral and emotional functioning. Self-reports are particularly useful when trying to understand an individual's internal state of functioning, including thoughts and feelings that might otherwise not be visible. However, for information gathered from self-report to be accurate, the developmental and cognitive ability of the respondent must be taken into consideration. In general, self-reports are not accurate for children under eight years of age (McConaughy & Ritter, 2008). Older children are more able to self-reflect, yet reading ability, self-awareness, meta-cognitive skills, interest and motivation may all impact the accuracy of their responses. Moreover, children often do not initiate the assessment process, but are referred by parents, teachers, or others close to them. Thus, children may be fearful or anxious about the testing situation, particularly since testing is generally a high-stakes process. That is, results may be used to make significant and life-altering placement and treatment decisions. Placed in a one-on-one testing situation, children may respond to please or get the "right" response rather than responding freely (Smith & Handler, 2007). Building rapport and establishing a relationship with the child can help offset some of these challenges. Additionally, children's report of their feelings may represent only the moment (Smith & Handler). For example, if a child recently was reprimanded by the teacher, the child might report that school is not fun. However, this could be a temporary response, and the child might normally enjoy school.

Overall, practitioners should take care to observe respondents for any signs that reports may not be accurate, and provide observational data regarding testing behavior as part of any comprehensive evaluation. Any data that may be compromised by lack of understanding or inattentive behavior should be interpreted with caution. In general, a multi-informant approach provides the most balanced view of an individual's behavior in multiple contexts with raters who have different priorities.

Strengths of Behavioral Rating Scales

In general, behavior rating scales posses a number of strengths that make them a popular and defensible choice for a variety of purposes. Behavioral rating scales provide quantifiable data regarding the frequency or intensity of a behavior or emotion. Thus, psychometric analyses can examine the reliability and validity of measurements to promote consistent findings (McConaughy & Ritter, 2008). The structured format increases objectivity and reliability (Furlong & Smith, 1994), and results are more reliable than unstructured types of data (Merrell, 1999). For practitioners, once the time-consuming rigorous development process is complete, rating scales can take just minutes to complete and can oftentimes be scored by computer (McConaughy & Ritter). Saving additional time and resources, rating scales can be administered by paraprofessionals or in group settings.

By identifying syndromes, behavior rating scales represent what occurs in normative samples rather than clinician-derived or diagnostic code–derived checklists, which may be more realistic (McConaughy & Ritter, 2008). Results yield information about comorbidity, as scales acknowledge overlapping symptoms for various syndromes (McConaughy & Ritter). Using rating scales, professionals can judge the severity of a problem compared to a large normative group rather than a particular classroom or school where clusters of problems or a lack of problems might bias observations (McConaughy & Ritter). Moreover, rating scales can measure low-frequency behaviors that might not be seen in a series of observations in a particular setting, such as delinquent behavior in the school setting (Merrell, 1999). This ensures that potentially important behaviors are not missed or overlooked (Furlong & Smith, 1994). It is also possible for raters to provide data regarding the frequency or intensity of behaviors over a period of time in a natural environment that may not be accessible to a clinician (Merrell, 1999).

Behavior-rating scale systems may include related scales developed for multi-informants, allowing for a cross-informant approach with data that are comparable when scales are developed together (McConaughy & Ritter, 2008). This cross-informant approach allows for the input and perspective of important others in a person's life, such as parents or teachers (Merrell, 1999), leading to a more ecologically valid approach (Furlong & Smith, 1994). When differences are found, data can help provide an understanding of setting-specific behavior; these benefits are particularly important when the subject of assessment will not participate in self-report or does not exhibit typical behavior when under observation (Furlong & Smith).

Limitations of Behavioral Rating Scales

Despite numerous strengths to using behavior rating scales for a variety of purposes, professionals must be trained in their use and proceed with caution when interpreting results. Although the implementation of behavior rating scales seems simple, they are in fact quite complex and may be used inaccurately. Published scales do not always have the best reliability and validity, despite their potentially high costs, yet they are easy to access and use by anyone without the training truly needed for accurate interpretation

of results (McConaughy & Ritter, 2008). One considerable limitation of behavior rating scales is that scales are only valid for use with the population included in the norming sample. Unless extensive testing has been conducted with numerous individuals across demographic groups, a scale's use should be limited to the population represented by the norming sample. Otherwise, a threat to validity termed *measurement inequivalence* may occur. Measurement inequivalence occurs when a specific group, such as English-language-learners, responds differently to the latent constructs measured by an instrument than did the original norm group. This differential item functioning is expected when cultural values related to behavioral functioning are quite different across ethnic groups. Thus, it is important for test users to check the norms to make sure they are representative of any particular child being assessed.

Accurate interpretation of behavior rating scales rests on the reliability and validity of the measure and the objectivity of the rater. Behavior-rating scales measure the perception, not reality of a behavior (McConaughy & Ritter, 2008; Merrell, 1999) and are not very sensitive to change since responses are based on perception of behavior over time (Chafouleas et al., 2007). Measurement issues of response bias and error variance also impair accuracy, and clinicians must carefully review validation procedures to determine if scales have been developed for the purpose intended. For example, behavior rating scales do not identify the causes of behaviors (McConaughy & Ritter). Professionals must gather additional information about the antecedent and consequences for specific problems as well as environmental causes. Moreover, additional data are most often needed to determine and design effective intervention (McConaughy & Ritter).

Observation Systems and Rating Scales

Following a determination of the type of behavioral information of interest, a mental health professional might choose to use published observation systems and/or rating scales to facilitate data collection. In clinical and school practice, particular scales have become frequently selected for various reasons including superior psychometric properties; standardized norm samples on special populations of concern; low cost; easy administration; and the ability to obtain specific information that can aid in diagnosis, intervention, and treatment planning. Although using commercially available observation systems and rating scales may increase ease of use, mental health professionals are cautioned to remember threats to reliability and validity remain, and each system warrants independent evaluation.

To provide the clinician and clinician-in-training with some information on available behavioral assessment systems, this chapter highlights two frequently utilized systems: the Behavior Assessment System for Children, Second Edition (BASC-2; Reynolds & Kamphaus, 2004), and the Achenbach System of Empirically Based Assessment (ASEBA; Achenbach & Rescorla, 2001). The BASC-2 and the ASEBA have emerged as two of the more popular scales, in part due to their extensive research base (Hosp, Howell, & Hosp, 2003), psychometric properties, and ability to provide behavioral information from multiple informants across multiple environments. Tables 26.2–26.5 provide information regarding additional published behavioral observations systems and rating scales.

Achenbach System of Empirically Based Assessment

The Achenbach System of Empirically Based Assessment (ASEBA) is a multi-informant assessment that offers comprehensive, evidence-based assessment of adaptive and maladaptive functioning in children and adolescents. It is considered a comprehensive assessment system due to the multi-modal approach of information collected through rating scales, self-report forms, interview schedules, and observation forms (Achenbach & McConaughy, 2003). Multiple raters can provide information on a child's (ages 1½ to 18 years) functioning in a variety of applicable settings including the home (Child Behavior Checklist; CBCL), school (Teacher's Report Form; TRF), community, and any other setting where the child spends time (Achenbach & McConaughy). The ASEBA also includes self-report information on the Youth Self-Report (YSR) for youth ages 11 to 18. The ASEBA includes features such as computer scoring and a fifth-grade readability level on the rating forms, which increase ease of use and administration. The normative sample is nationally representative in terms of demographics including age, ethnicity, regional location, and gender. Extensive psychometric information is available in the manual (Achenbach & Rescorla, 2001).

Three overarching scores are provided for the CBCL, TRF, and YSR: an Internalizing behavior score, an Externalizing behavior score, and a composite Total Problems behavior score. These broader scores break down into eight subscales: the Externalizing scales include Aggressive Behavior, Attention Problems, and Delinquent Behavior and the Internalizing Scales contain the Social Problems, Anxious/Depressed, Somatic Complaints, Thought Problems, and Withdrawn narrow subscales. The ASEBA also contains three scales for identifying adaptive and competency behaviors: Activities, Social, and School, which yield an overarching composite Total Competence score. Alternative methods of scoring allow for forms to be scored in terms of DSM-oriented scales targeted for diagnostic purposes. The following six DSM-oriented scales are based on the CBCL, YSR, and TRF for ages 6 to 18: Affective Problems, Anxiety Problems, Somatic Problems, Attention Deficit Hyperactivity Problems, Oppositional Defiant Problems, and Conduct Problems (Achenbach, 2007; Achenbach & Rescorla, 2001).

In addition to behavioral rating scales, the ASEBA includes the Direct Observation Form (DOF; Achenbach, 1986) to aid in the collection of behavioral observation data. The DOF employs narrative and time sampling recording procedures to observe on-task and 96 problem behaviors across 10-minute periods. The user conducts time sample recordings of on- and off-task behavior at the end of each minute for the duration of the observation and records narrative observations throughout the observation. Observers provide ratings on a 4-point Likert scale where 0 signifies the behavior is not observed, and 3 signifies a definite behavioral occurrence with severe intensity or for a behavior with greater than a 3-minute duration. The authors recommend conducting three to six 10-minute observations yielding an average score calculated across occasions. Also recommended is the use of comparison peers as "controls" for 10-minute observations before and after observing the targeted child. The sum of observation ratings provides raw scores corresponding with cutoff points for clinical levels of behavior across the problem behavior syndrome scales. These cutoff points were derived from both a referred and a non-referred control sample, and the DOF differentiates between referred and non-referred children (McConaughy, Achenbach, & Gent, 1988). Tables 26.2–26.5 summarize properties of the ASEBA.

Behavior Assessment System for Children, Second Edition

The Behavior Assessment System for Children, Second Edition (BASC-2; Reynolds & Kamphaus, 2004) consists of multi-rater forms, a structured developmental history, and a systematic observation system that results in a multi-perspective report of problem and adaptive behaviors for youth ages

2 to 21 years spanning preschool through college. BASC-2 rating scales are available for multiple informants including teachers (Teacher Rating Scale; TRS), parents (Parent Rating Scales; PRS), and self-report (Self-Report of Personality; SRP) with different age-based forms for ages 8 to 25 years. Additional components of the BASC-2 include the Structured Developmental History (SDH), the Systematic Observation System (SOS), the Progress Monitor (PM), and the Intervention Guide (IG). See previous section on treatment planning and progress monitoring for information on the PM and IG.

The items of the BASC-2 TRS, PRS, and SRP are rated on a four-point response scale of frequency, ranging from "Never" to "Almost Always." The results from the parent and teacher rating scales yield T-scores across five composite scales: Externalizing Problems Composite, Internalizing Problems Composite, School Problems Composite, Behavioral Symptoms Index, and an Adaptive Skills Composite. The SRP provides the following composite scores: School Problems, Internalizing Problems, Inattention/Hyperactivity, Emotional Symptoms Index, and Personal Adjustment. In addition to problematic behavior identification, the BASC-2 assesses for positive characteristics and functional behaviors using the Adaptive Skills Composite score. Results from the BASC-2 ratings provide cut-scores utilized as thresholds to label levels of behavior as within the following ranges: Low (T scores 10 to 60 for problem behaviors; > 40 for adaptive behaviors), At-Risk (T scores 61 to 69 for problem behavior; 30–39 for adaptive behaviors), or Clinically Significant (T scores > 69; < 30 for adaptive behaviors). By identifying severity of problematic behaviors in this way, the BASC-2 provides information regarding subsyndromal levels of behaviors not severe enough to meet DSM-IV-TR diagnostic criteria levels. Subscales and composites align with symptomology and characteristics of IDEA categorization for special education regulations and DSM-IV-TR diagnosis, aiding clinicians with categorization and diagnosis in both educational and clinical settings.

The BASC-2 forms are written at a fourth grade readability level and computer scoring is available. Internal validity indices, which detect internal threats such as "faking bad" (F-index), "faking good" (L-index), or responses that are nonsensical (V-index), are available. The BASC-2 manual provides extensive data on standardization, norms, reliability, and validity (Reynolds & Kamphaus, 2004).

The BASC-2-Systematic Observation System (BASC-SOS; Reynolds & Kamphaus, 2004) is a momentary time sample observation occurring at 30-second intervals requiring a 15-minute observation. BASC-SOS users can choose between the paper protocol and a computerized version called the BASC-Portable Observation Program (BASC-POP). At the end of a 15-minute observation, in addition to the time sampling data recorded, observers rate 65 adaptive and problem behaviors observed utilizing a 3-point scale from "never observed" (NO) to "sometimes observed" (SO), or "frequently observed" (FO). In addition to the behaviors delineated on the form for rating, users can also choose to observe and record information on additional behaviors that they specify. During the observation, observers can note directly onto the protocol specifics about teacher–student interactions and the classroom environment in addition to prioritizing which behavior is the most bothersome or is the focus of the observation. The BASC-SOS may also be utilized to measure changes in a child's behavior following an intervention. Normative data are not provided, but the manual recommends including two to three comparison peers for normative data. Although a paucity of reliability and validity data are available, the authors recommend repeated observations to increase reliability. Additionally, users should ensure threats to validity are minimized through inter-rater checks and checking for reactivity threats during an observation. Tables 26.2–26.5 provide information on the properties of the BASC-2. Information on additional observation systems and rating scales are also provided in Tables 26.2–26.5.

Conclusions and Future Directions

It is likely that continual progress will be made in the development and use of behavioral observation systems and rating scales. More sophisticated tools will be developed to integrate future technologies that will make observation of behavior more efficient to collect and accurate to interpret. Behavioral rating scales of the future might be gathered solely through the use of PDAs, which would allow for immediate feedback, graphing, and progress monitoring. Or perhaps brief questionnaires will be sent via cell phone to gather information that is specific to the situation that the adolescent is currently in. Similarly, behavioral observation systems might implement software where video from the classroom is streaming live and advanced technology systematically codes how often students are out of their seats. Tracking devices might be attached to shoes or desks to see how frequently hyperactive students move in comparison to their peers. Although advances seem limitless, the use of rating scales and observation systems will ultimately be decided by unsophisticated practicalities such as ease of use, ability to provide meaningful information, and cost in terms of time, materials, and personnel.

Realizing that new tools are frequently developed, it is imperative that clinicians and clinicians-in-training have the requisite tools and knowledge to be able to thoroughly evaluate new assessments. Throughout this chapter, a variety of issues were presented to highlight some of the critical concerns that should be attended to, such as the psychometric properties and limitations of assessments. Clinicians must guard against the adoption of a new tool prior to an extensive review of its psychometric properties, regardless of its popularity or face validity. Users will have to consider how to combine information gained from multiple sources and methods throughout the assessment process in a way that can be meaningfully digested and understood. Additionally, users will have to weigh actuarial data obtained with clinical judgments, recognizing that both can be biased and subjective. Above all else, great caution should be exercised when making diagnostic decisions that could potentially impact the delivery of future services.

Regardless of the assessment tool chosen, the actual behavioral assessment process should begin long before the observation period or the delivery of a rating scale and end long after the results are obtained. Prior to collecting information, a thorough evaluation of the selected tool, in light of the purpose for the assessment, is needed. Clinicians should engage in an iterative, problem-solving process until sufficient behavioral information is gained and results should be combined with other sources of information to provide a comprehensive assessment. Feedback from team members including parents should be solicited and incorporated into treatment planning and progress should be evaluated systematically. A psychologist is not simply a psychometrician gathering and reporting behavioral data. On the contrary, skilled clinicians utilize their full breadth of training and knowledge to conduct behavioral assessments as one part of a multifaceted assessment. We hope the concepts and recommendations discussed in this chapter will stimulate psychologists to critically evaluate and reflect upon how to improve current practices for behavioral assessment.

Author Note

Address correspondence to University of California Santa Barbara, Gevirtz Graduate School of Education, Department of Counseling, Clinical, and School Psychology, Santa Barbara, CA 93106 Phone/Fax: 805–893–2703; e-mail: edowdy@education.ucsb.edu.

Further Reading

Chafouleas, S., Riley-Tillman, T. C., & Sugai, G. (2007). *School-based behavioral assessment: Informing intervention and instruction.* New York: Guilford Press.

McConaughy, S. H., & Ritter, D. R. (2008). Best practices in multimethod assessment of emotional and behavioral disorders. In A. Thomas & J. Grimes (Eds.), *Best practices in school psychology V* (Vol. 2). Bethesda, MD: National Association of School Psychologists.

Merrell, K. W. (2003). *Behavioral, social, and emotional assessment of children and adolescents* (2nd ed.). Mahwah, NJ: Lawrence Erlbaum Associates.

Sattler, J. M., & Hoge, R. D. (2006). *Assessment of children: Behavioral, social, and clinical foundations* (5th ed.). San Diego, CA: Jerome M. Sattler, Publisher.

References

Achenbach, T. M. (1986). *Child Behavior Checklist—Direct Observation Form* (Rev. ed.). Burlington: University of Vermont Press.

Achenbach, T. M. (2007). Applications of the Achenbach System of Empirically Based Assessment to children, adolescents, and their parents. In S. R. Smith & L. Handler (Eds.), *The clinical assessment of children and adolescents: A practitioner's handbook* (Vol. XV; pp. 327–344). Mahwah, NJ: Lawrence Erlbaum Associates, Publishers.

Achenbach, T. M., & McConaughy, S. H. (2003). The Achenbach System of Empirically Based Assessment. In C. R. Reynolds & R. W. Kamphaus (Eds.), *Handbook of psychological and educational assessment of children: Personality, behavior, and context* (2nd ed.; pp. 406–430). New York, NY: Guilford Press.

Achenbach, T. M., McConaughy, S. H., & Howell, C. T. (1987). Child/adolescent behavioral and emotional problems: Implications of cross-informant correlations for situational specificity. *Psychological Bulletin, 101,* 213–232.

Achenbach, T. M., & Rescorla, L. A. (2001). *Manual for the ASEBA school-age forms and profiles.* Burlington, VT: University of Vermont, Research Center for Children, Youth, & Families.

Allessi, G. (1988). Direct observation methods for emotional/behavior problems. In E. S. Shapiro & T. R. Kratochwill (Eds.), *Behavioral assessment in schools* (pp. 14–75). New York, NY: Guilford.

American Psychiatric Association. (2000). *Diagnostic and statistical manual of mental disorders* (4th ed., text rev.). Washington, DC: APA.

Bloomquist, M. L., & Schnell, S. V. (2002). *Helping children with aggression and conduct problems: Best practices for intervention.* New York, NY: The Guilford Press.

Bronfenbrenner, U. (1992). Ecological systems theory. In R. Vasta (Ed.), *Six theories of child development: Revised formulations and current issues* (pp. 187–249). Philadelphia, PA: Jessica Kingsley.

Campaign for Mental Health Reform. (2005). A public health crisis: Children and adolescents with mental disorders. Congressional briefing. Retrieved September 1, 2005, from http://www.mhreform.org/kids.

Chafouleas, S., Riley-Tillman, T. C., & Sugai, G. (2007). *School-based behavioral assessment: Informing intervention and instruction.* New York: Guilford Press.

Conners, C. K. (2008). *Conners third edition manual.* Los Angeles: Western Psychological Services.

Cornell, D. G., & Loper, A. B. (1998). Assessment of violence and other high-risk behaviors with a school survey. *The School Psychology Review, 27,* 317–330.

Cross, J. E., & Newman-Gonchar, R. (2004). Data quality in student risk behavior surveys and administrator training. *Journal of School Violence, 3,* 89–108.

DuPaul, G. J., Power, T. J., Anastopoulos, A. D., & Reid, R. (1998). *ADHD Rating Scale IV: Checklists, norms, and clinical interpretation.* New York, NY: Guilford Press.

Eckert, T. L., Dunn, E. K., Codding, R. S., & Guiney, K. M. (2000). Self-report: Rating scale measures. In E. S. Shapiro & T. R. Kratochwill (Eds.), *Conducting school-based assessments of children and adolescent behavior.* New York, NY: Guilford Press.

Elliott, S. N., Gresham, F. M., Frank, J. L., & Beddow, P. A. (2008). Intervention validity of social behavior rating scales: Features of assessments that link results to treatment plans. *Assessment for Effective Intervention, 34*(1), 15–24.

Epstein, M., Hertzog, M., & Reid, R. (2001). The Behavioral and Emotional Rating Scale: Long term test-retest reliability. *Behavioral Disorders, 26*(4), 314–320.

Fisher, D. L., & Fraser, B. J. (1983). Validity and use of the Classroom Environment Scale. *Educational Evaluation and Policy Analysis, 5,* 261–271.

Fowler, F. J., Jr. (1993). *Survey research methods* (2nd ed.). Newbury Park, CA: Sage Publishers.

Furlong, M. J., & Sharkey, J. D. (2006). A review of methods to assess student self-report of weapons on school campuses. In S. R. Jimerson & M. J. Furlong (Eds.), *Handbook of school violence and school safety: From research to practice* (pp. 235–256). Mahwah, NJ: Lawrence Erlbaum Associates.

Furlong, M. J., & Smith, D. C. (Eds.). (1994). *Anger, hostility and aggression: Assessment, prevention, and intervention strategies for youth.* Brandon, VT: Clinical Psychology Publishing Company.

Garmezy, N. (1993). Children in poverty: Resilience despite risk. *Psychiatry, 56,* 127–136.

Gresham, F. M., & Elliott, S. N. (1990). *The Social Skills Rating System.* Bloomington, MN: Pearson Assessments.

Hilton, N. Z., Harris, G. T., & Rice, M. E. (1998). On the validity of self-reported rates of interpersonal violence. *Journal of Interpersonal Violence, 13,* 58–72.

Hintze, J. M., Volpe, R. J., & Shapiro, E. S. (2008). Best practices in the systematic direct observation of student behavior. In A. Thomas & J. Grimes (Eds.), *Best practices in school psychology V.* Bethesda, MD: National Association of School Psychologists.

Hoier, T. S., & Cone, J. D. (1987). Target selection of social skills for children: The template-matching procedure. *Behavior Modification, 11,* 137–154.

Holmbeck, G. N., Thill, A. W., Bachanas, P., Garber, J., Miller, K. B., Abad, M., et al. (2008). Evidence-based assessment in pediatric psychology: Measures of psychosocial adjustment and psychopathology. *Journal of Pediatric Psychology, 33,* 958–980.

Hosp, J. L., Howell, K. W., & Hosp, M. K. (2003). Characteristics of behavior rating scales: Implications for practice in assessment and behavioral support. *Journal of Positive Behavioral Interventions, 5,* 201–208.

House, A. E., House, B. J., & Campbell, M. B. (1981). Measures of inter-observer agreement: Calculation formulas and distribution effects. *Journal of Behavioral Assessment, 3,* 37–58.

Huebner, E., S., & Gilman, R. (2003). Toward a focus on positive psychology in school psychology. *School Psychology Quarterly, 18*(2), 99–102.

Hutton, J. B., Dubes, R., & Muir, S. (1992). Assessment practices of school psychologists: Ten years later. *School Psychology Review, 21,* 271–284.

Individuals with Disabilities Education Improvement Act. (2004). 20 U.S.C. 1400 *et seq.*

Jimerson, S., Sharkey, J., Nyborg, V., & Furlong, M. (2004). Strength-based assessment and school psychology: A summary and synthesis. *California School Psychologist, 9,* 9–19.

Kamphaus, R. W., & Reynolds, C. R. (2007). *Behavior Assessment System for Children, Second Edition: Behavioral and Emotional Screening System* (BASC-2 BESS). Bloomington, MN: Pearson.

Kamphaus, R. W., & Reynolds, C. R. (2009). *Behavior Assessment System for Children, Second Edition: Progress Monitor* (BASC-2 PM). Bloomington, MN: Pearson.

Kamphaus, R. W., VanDeventer, M. C., Brueggemann, A., & Barry, M. (2007). Behavior Assessment System for Children–Second Edition. In S. R. Smith & L. Handler (Eds.), *The clinical assessment of children and adolescents: A practitioner's handbook* (pp. 311–326). Mahwah, NJ: Lawrence Erlbaum Associates.

Kazdin, A. E. (1981). Behavioral observation. In M. Hersen & A. S. Bellack (Eds.), *Behavioral assessment: A practical handbook* (pp. 59–100). New York, NY: Pergamon Press.

Keller, H. R. (1986). Behavioral observation approaches to personality assessment. In H. M. Knoff (Ed.), *The assessment of child and adolescent personality* (pp. 353–390). New York, NY: The Guilford Press.

Kovacs, M. (2001). *Children's Depression Inventory (CDI).* Tonawanda, NY: Multi-Health Systems.

LeBuffe, P., & Shapiro, V. (2004). Lending "strength" to the assessment of preschool social-emotional health. *California School Psychologist, 9,* 51–61.

Lindskog, C. (2003). A review of ADHD Rating Scale-IV. In B. S. Plake, J. C. Impara & R. A. Spies (Eds.), *The fifteenth mental measurements yearbook* (pp. 23–25). Lincoln, NE: University of Nebraska Press.

Masten, A. S. (2001). Ordinary magic: Resilience processes in development. *American Psychologist, 56*(3), 227–238.

McConaughy, S. H., Achenbach, T. M., & Gent, C. L. (1988). Multiaxial empirically based assessment: Parent, teacher, observational, cognitive, and personality correlates of child profile types for 6- to 11-year-old boys. *Journal of Abnormal Child Psychology, 16,* 485–509.

McConaughy, S. H., & Ritter, D. R. (2008). Best practices in multimethod assessment of emotional and behavioral disorders. In A. Thomas & J. Grimes (Eds.), *Best Practices in School Psychology V* (Vol. 2). Bethesda, MD: National Association of School Psychologists.

Merrell, K. W. (1999). *Behavioral, social, and emotional assessment of children and adolescents.* Mahwah, NJ: Lawrence Erlbaum Associates, Publishers.

Merrell, K. W. (2000). Informant report: Rating scale measures. In E. S. Shapiro & T. R. Kratochwill (Eds.), *Conducting school-based assessment of child and adolescent behaviors* (pp. 203–234). New York, NY: The Guilford Press.

Merrell, K. W. (2003). *Behavioral, social, and emotional assessment of children and adolescents* (2nd ed.). Mahwah, NJ: Lawrence Erlbaum Associates.

Nelson, R. O., & Hayes, S. C. (Eds.). (1986). *Conceptual foundations of behavioral assessment*. New York, NY: The Guilford Press.

Ortiz, S. O. (2008). Best practices in nondiscriminatory assessment. In A. Thomas & J. Grimes (Eds.), *Best practices in school psychology V* (pp. 1321–1336). Bethesda, MD: National Association of School Psychologists.

Piers, E. V., Harris, D. B., & Herzberg, D. S. (2002). *Piers-Harris Children's Self-Concept Scale, Second Edition: Manual*. Los Angeles, CA: Western Psychological Services.

Reid, J. B., Baldwin, D. V., Patterson, G. R., & Dishion, T. J. (1988). Observations in the assessment of childhood disorders. In M. Rutter, A. H. Tuma & I. A. Lann (Eds.), *Assessment and diagnosis in child psychopathology* (pp. 156–195). New York, NY: Guilford Press.

Reynolds, C. R., & Kamphaus, R. W. (2004). *The Behavior Assessment System for Children—Second Edition* (BASC-2). Circle Pines, MN: AGS.

Reynolds, W. M. (2002). *Reynolds Adolescent Depression Scale—Second Edition*. Lutz, FL: Psychological Assessment Resources.

Romer, D., & McIntosh, M. (2005). The roles and perspectives of school mental health professionals in promoting adolescent mental health. In D. L. Evans, E. B. Foa, R. E. Gur, H. Hendin, C. P. O'Brien, M. E. P. Seligman & B. T. Walsh (Eds.), *Treating and preventing adolescent mental health disorders: What we know and what we don't know* (pp. 598–615). New York, NY: Oxford University Press.

Sattler, J. M., & Hoge, R. D. (2006). *Assessment of children: Behavioral, social, and clinical foundations* (5th ed.). San Diego, CA: Jerome M. Sattler, Publisher.

Schwartz, N. (1999). Self reports: How the questions shape the answers. *American Psychologist, 54*, 93–105.

Shapiro, E. S. (2004). *Academic skills problem workbook* (Rev. ed.). New York, NY: The Guilford Press.

Shapiro, E. S., & Heick, P. F. (2004). School psychologist assessment practices in the evaluation of students referred for social/behavioral/emotional problems. *Psychology in the Schools, 41*, 551–561.

Shapiro, E. S., & Skinner, C. H. (1990). Best practices in observation and ecological assessment. In A. Thomas & J. Grimes (Eds.), *Best practices in school psychology II* (pp. 507–518). Washington, DC: National Association of School Psychologists.

Sheridan, S. M., & Gutkin, T. B. (2000). The ecology of school psychology: Examining and changing our

paradigm for the 21st century. *School Psychology Review, 29*, 485–501.

Skinner, C. H., Rhymer, K. N., & Mc Daniel, E. C. (2000). Naturalistic direct observation in educational settings. In E. S. Shapiro & T. R. Kratochwill (Eds.), *Behavioral assessment in schools: Theory, research, and clinical foundations* (2nd ed.; pp. 21–54). New York, NY: The Guilford Press.

Smith, S. R., & Handler, L. (Eds.). (2007). *The clinical assessment of children and adolescents: A practitioner's handbook*. Mahwah, NJ: Lawrence Erlbaum Associates.

Spies, R. A., & Plake, B. S. (Eds.). (2005). *Review of the Piers-Harris Self Concept Scale—2nd Edition (The way I feel about myself)*. Lincoln, NE: University of Nebraska Press.

Sroufe, L. A. (1997). Psychopathology as an outcome of development. *Developmental Psychopathology, 9*, 251–268.

Stein, S., & Karno, M. (1994). Behavioral observation of anger and aggression. In M. Furlong & D. Smith (Eds.), *Anger, hostility, and aggression: Assessment, prevention, and intervention strategies for youth* (pp. 245–283). Brandon, VT: Clinical Psychology Publishing Co., Inc.

Stinnett, T. A., Havey, J. M., & Oehler-Stinnett, J. (1994). Current test usage by practicing school psychologist: A national survey. *Journal of Psychoeducational Assessment, 12*, 331–350.

Turner, C. F., Ku, L., Rogers, S. M., Lindberg, L. D., & Pleck, J. H. (1998). Adolescent sexual behavior, drug use, and violence: Increased reporting with computer survey technology. *Science, 280*, 867–873.

Vannest, K., Reynolds, C. R., & Kamphaus, R. W. (2009). *Behavior Assessment System for Children—Second Edition: Intervention guide*. Bloomington, MN: Pearson.

Volpe, R. J., DiPerna, J. C., Hintze, J. M., & Shapiro, E. S. (2005). Observing students in classroom settings: A review of seven coding schemes. *School Psychology Review, 34*, 454–474.

Walrath, C. M., Mandell, D., Holden, E. W., & Santiago, R. L. (2004). Assessing the strengths of children referred for community-based mental health services. *Mental Health Services Research, 6*(1), 1–8.

Weick, A., & Chamberlain, R. (2002). Putting problems in their place: Further explorations in the strengths perspective. In D. Saleebey (Ed.), *The strength perspective in social work practice* (pp. 95–105). New York, NY: Longman Publishing Group.

Wilson, M. S., & Reschly, D. J. (1996). Assessment in school psychology. *School Psychology Review, 25*, 9–23.

Winsor, A. P. (2003). Direct behavioral observation for classrooms. In C. R. Reynolds & R. W. Kamphaus (Eds.), *Handbook of psychological & educational assessment of children* (pp. 248–255). New York, NY: The Guilford Press.

Worthen, B. R., Borg, W. R., & White, K. (1993). *Measurement and evaluation in the schools: A practical guide*. White Plains, NY: Longman.

Models and Methods of Assessing Adaptive Behavior

Jason Hangauer, Jonathan Worcester, *and* Kathleen Hague Armstrong

Abstract

This chapter will summarize contemporary models and methods used for the assessment of adaptive behavior functioning in children and adolescents. This chapter will also emphasize how to best use such assessment information for diagnostic and eligibility purposes and in developing interventions and support plans. We will review the use of traditional, norm-referenced adaptive behavior assessment tools as well as what will be referred to as "supplemental methods," including the direct observation of adaptive skill functioning. The assessment of adaptive behavior with respect to developmental expectations, cultural expectations, systems of care, and legislation will also be discussed. Lastly, case studies will be presented to illustrate the usefulness of these methods in assessing individuals and planning effective interventions and services.

Key Words: adaptive behavior, assessment, children, models, methods

Definition of Adaptive Behavior

One of the most widely accepted definitions of adaptive behavior was first developed by the American Association on Mental Retardation (AAMR; 1992, 2002). As defined by the AAMR (2002), *adaptive behavior* is " the collection of conceptual, social, and practical skills that have been learned by people in order to function in their everyday lives" (p. 73). As such, adaptive behavior reflects one's competence in dealing with social expectations and across environments. Limitations in adaptive behavior affect one's daily life, one's ability to respond to life changes and environmental demands, and the degree to which an individual can be independent. The AAMR defines *conceptual skills* as the ability to understand and communicate via spoken and non-verbal language, the ability to plan out one's day-to-day activities, and performance of academic skills such as reading or writing. *Social skills* are defined as one's ability to relate to others, hold a conversation, and initiate dialogue for the purpose of communicating one's ideas or needs and wants. Additionally, social skills

include the ability to obey rules of an organization, such as family or school, as well as obey the laws of society. *Practical skills* include independence in performance of daily functions such as planning and preparing meals, putting on clothing, toileting, managing one's own finances, using the telephone, and ability to take needed medications. Adaptive behavior emphasizes the developmental nature of skills, which become more complex as individuals mature and are faced with new demands from their environment. Ultimately, adaptive behavior assessment must take into account the culture and social standards of the community in which the individual lives and functions.

Adaptive Behavior and Its Relationship with Intelligence

Adaptive behavior assessment evolved out of a concern voiced over 50 years ago, speaking to the need for nonbiased assessment beyond the IQ test for diagnosis, and linking to effective interventions for individuals with intellectual and developmental disabilities (IDD). The first accepted definition of adaptive behavior from the AAMR was developed in 1961) (Heber, 1961), born out of the recognized bias of diagnosing individuals with IDD based upon the results of IQ tests alone, without examining their day-to-day functioning in society. With the advent of the Education for All Handicapped Children Act in 1975 (Public Law 94–142), concern for the over-identification and labeling of some minorities by the sole use of IQ testing lead to several court cases, and subsequently to the inclusion of adaptive behavior in assessing children for IDD (Reschley, Kicklighter & McKee, 1988). Over the years, adaptive behavior has become a required element in determining eligibility for other special education programs besides IDD, as well as in qualifying for federal assistance programs, such as Social Security benefits. Therefore, legislation and litigation came to establish the critical importance of assessment of adaptive behavior in diagnosis, program eligibility, and intervention for individuals with IDD, in that it not only identified limitations, but provided a basis for developing interventions and services towards developing competencies and strengths.

For the past 30 years, several researchers have examined the relationship between adaptive behavior assessment and IQ tests, particularly with respect to individuals with IDD. Across multiple studies, comparing several instruments, the correlations between IQ and adaptive behavior scores were found to be in the low to moderate range (Coulter, 1980; Harrison, 1990; Lambert, Nihira, & Leland, 1993). Some reasons for these findings may be a function of the differences between the construct for intelligence (innate abilities, maximal performance potential, and stability of scores) and the construct for adaptive behavior (daily living skills, typical performance, and developmental/modifiable). Individuals with similar IQ scores will often demonstrate very different skills related to their adaptive behavior functioning, as a result of their opportunities, expectations, or motivation (Harrison & Oakland, 2003). With proper intervention, individuals can be taught and will learn adaptive behavior skills aimed to help them to function more successfully in new environments and situations. (Bruininks, Thurlow, & Gilman, 1987; Kamphaus, 1987).

While the assessment of adaptive behavior has been primarily used in individuals with IDD, it has also been found useful in assessing the strengths and needs of other clinical groups, including autism spectrum disorders (ASD; Harrison & Boney, 2002; Holman & Bruininks, 1985), Attention-Deficit/

Hyperactivity Disorder (ADHD; Harrison & Oakland, 2003), as well as emotional and behavioral disorders (EBD; Armstrong, Dedrick & Greenbaum, 2003). For example, deficits in adaptive behavior functioning are apparent in the early childhood years, and as such have become an integral part of early childhood assessment, diagnosis, and intervention (Harrison & Raineri, 2007). Young children who do not receive intervention to assist in increasing their adaptive skills are at greater risk for later behavior problems (Grossman, 1983). Adolescents with poor adaptive skills are less successful in completing school and assuming adult roles, including independent living, employment, and achieving satisfactory relationships (Armstrong, Dedrick, & Greenbaum, 2003). Furthermore, Armstrong and colleagues found that improvement in adaptive skill functioning was a better predictor of successful adult outcomes than either reduction of behavior problems or IQ scores.

Thus, meeting the demands and expectations for one's environment is important at all ages, and is critical to consider in providing supports and services that promote adaptation. Everyone, regardless of their age or disability, must learn to take care of themselves and get along with others to the extent that is possible. Interventions specifically designed to address limitations in adaptive skills and build strengths become key to successful and independent functioning, and so become a critical function of special education supports and services (Eldevik et al., 2010; Gresham & Elliott, 1987).

Purpose of Adaptive Behavior Assessment

The overarching purpose of adaptive behavior assessment is to develop supports and services to meet the needs of the individual. To accomplish this, it becomes essential to identify the individual's functional strengths and needs in relation to their family, culture, and community expectations. Often, adaptive behavior assessment is needed to help establish a diagnosis that may assist in explaining the reasons for the differences. Standard classification systems, including the American Psychiatric Association's Diagnostic and Statistical Manual of Mental Disorders, Fourth Edition, Text Revision (DSM-IV-TR; 2000), and the International Classification of Diseases, Ninth Revision (ICD-9; 1998) include the assessment of adaptive behavior for the diagnosis of IDD. Establishing a diagnosis can help link the individual and family to specific support groups, determine eligibility for supports and services, and supply a deeper understanding of the nature of the individual's differences. The latest revision of the DSM has kept its current definition of mental retardation (now known as IDD) and requires documentation of deficits in adaptive functioning along with deficits in IQ for diagnosis. The DSM-5, which is expected to be released in 2013, is proposing only minor changes in the definition of IDD, and will likely increase its emphasis on adaptive functioning. The DSM-IV-TR stresses that effectiveness in adaptive functioning should be considered within the context of one's age and cultural expectations, in areas of communication, self-care, home living, social skills, use of community resources, self-direction, functional academic skills, work, leisure, health, and safety.

A second emphasis of adaptive behavior assessment is to establish the level of an individual's functioning in order to determine their eligibility for special-education programs and to set goals and objectives. The Individuals with Disabilities Education Act (IDEA, 2004) is a federal law that mandates that all children aged birth to 21 receive free and appropriate services in the least restrictive environment. Part B of IDEA refers to regulations pertaining to children from three to 21 years of age, while Part C addresses regulations for infants and toddlers, from birth to age three. Lastly, there has been an increased focus on educational accountability extending from preschool to high school years, which requires assessment information that documents what children know and can do as part of the No Child Left Behind (NCLB) act of 2004 (NCLB, 2004). Given the developmental nature of adaptive behavior and presumed malleability, the emphasis on early identification and intervention with evidence-based strategies, adaptive behavior assessment becomes crucial. What children can and do perform in their everyday routines must be examined for the purposes of diagnosis and eligibility, as well as to establish interventions and supports needed to address specific functioning, and their response to the intervention (Harman, Smith-Bonahue, & Oakland, 2010).

Both the DSM-IV-TR, as well as the upcoming fifth revision, DSM-5, along with IDEA (2004) strongly emphasize the assessment of adaptive behavior for diagnostic purposes or when assessing an individual for special education services. This emphasis is not accidental. Adaptive behavior assessment initially was developed as a way to prevent misdiagnosing individuals, placing them in more restrictive settings, or giving them inappropriate services. Adaptive behavior assessment provides information both about an individual's weaknesses and strengths, is useful in planning and evaluating interventions, and helps document progress towards goals.

Standardized and Supplemental Adaptive Behavior Assessment Tools and Techniques

There are many well-standardized instruments that have been developed over the past two decades that are very useful in assessing adaptive behavior in individuals ranging in age from infants to senior citizens. As with other standardized assessment tools, adaptive behavior measures gather information about an individual's functioning to compare with those from national standardization samples and from certain clinical groups. Additionally, newer assessment techniques have been developed that allow for more in-depth assessment of key adaptive skills, which may be more useful for intervention planning and progress monitoring. Given the rapid changes in technology, and what is needed to interact with the environment and society, the construct of adaptive behavior is constantly changing and being modified (Oakland & Daley, 2010).

Standardized, Norm-based Assessment Methods

Among the most contemporary, well-standardized, and widely used norm-based adaptive behavior assessment instruments are the Adaptive Behavior Assessment System–Second Edition (ABAS-II; Harrison & Oakland, 2003), and the Vineland Adaptive Behavior Scales–Second Edition (VABS-II; Sparrow, Cicchetti & Balla, 2005). In addition, the Battelle Developmental Inventory–Second Edition (BDI-2; Newborg, 2004), and the Behavior Assessment System for Children–Second Edition (BASC-2; Reynolds & Kamphaus, 2004), include measures of adaptive behavior as one of the domains within those assessments. These tools are similar in that they rely on gaining information from caregivers familiar with the individual, such as parents or teachers, obtained through survey and semi-structured interview methods. The strengths and weaknesses of each of these tools will be discussed in the following section, and are outlined in Tables 27.1 and 27.2.

The VABS-II measures adaptive behavior in four domains and eleven subdomains. Scores from the four domains (Communication, Daily Living Skills, Socialization Skills, and Motor Skills) are combined to from the Adaptive Behavior Composite,

Table 27.1 Standardized Assessment Tools for Adaptive Behavior

Instrument Name	Age Range, Areas Assessed, and Materials	Strengths	Weaknesses
Adaptive Behavior Assessment System (ABAS-II), 2nd Edition (Harrison & Oakland, 2003)	Age range: Birth–72 Years Areas Assessed: Domains: General Adaptive Composite: Adaptive Domains—Conceptual (Communication, Functional Academics, Self-Direction, Social (Leisure, Social,); Practical (Community Use, Home Living, Health & Safety, Self-care, Work,) Motor domain for children birth–5 Used in Bayley-3	Strong standardization sample Internal consistency and factor score coefficients were high across all subdomains Inter-scorer reliability is above .90 Number of clinical samples included Four-point Likert-type scale (is not able, never or almost never when needed, sometimes when needed, and always or almost always when needed) to assess each skill area rather than simply "yes/no"	Additional data are required to assess utility of using the ABAS-II for progress monitoring Technical adequacy may be improved by norming the instrument on a larger sample size
Vineland Adaptive Behavior Scales–Second Edition (VABS-II; Sparrow, Cicchetti, & Balla, 2005)	Age range: Birth–90 years of age Areas Assessed: Four main domains: communication, daily living skills, socialization, and motor skills (only used for individuals birth- 6 years 11 months) Optional maladaptive behavior domain available	Number of clinical samples included Both clinical interview and parent/caregiver rating forms available Comprehensive, life span	Manual scoring is cumbersome and can lead to error Inter-rater reliability is relatively weak May be more accurate at measuring adaptive skill deficits versus high levels of performance

or overall measure of adaptive behavior. There are three forms: the Survey Form, the Expanded Form, and the Classroom Edition, which are selected by the evaluator based on the age of the individual. The Survey Form gathers information about adaptive functioning from caregivers, is normed for children birth through 18 years of age, and may be used for lower-functioning adults. The Expanded Form offers much more detailed information about adaptive behavior, and is normed for infants through adults up to age 77 years. The Classroom Edition is useful for children ages three to 12, and uses teacher report to assess adaptive functioning within the classroom. Both the Survey and the Expanded Forms include a maladaptive behavior domain for children age five and older, titled the Social-Emotional Early Childhood Scale (SEEC; Sparrow, Balla, Cicchetti, 1998).

The VABS-II used a representative, national sample of 3,000 individuals, selected by sex, race, socioeconomic status, geographic region, and community size. Standard scores are used to express adaptive behavior functioning, with a mean of 100, and standard deviation of 15, percentile ranks, stanines, and age equivalents. Internal consistency, test-retest reliability and inter-rater reliability, and validity data are adequate, and provided in more detail in Table 27.1. The SEEC is available for children birth through age five, and provides standard scores, percentile ranks, stanines, and age equivalents similar to those of the VABS-II.

The ABAS-II measures adaptive behavior in three domains: Conceptual, Social, and Practical, consistent with the American Association of Intellectual and Developmental Disabilities (AAID; 2007)definition of adaptive behavior. Each of the domains is factored into 11 subdomains, including Communication, Functional Academics, Self-Direction, Leisure, Social, Community Use, Home Living, Health and Safety, Self-care, Motor,

Instrument Name	Age Range, Areas Assessed,Strengths and Materials		Weaknesses
Battelle Developmental Inventory–Second Edition (BDI-2; Newborg, 2004) Behavior Assessment System for Children, Second Edition (BASC-2; Reynolds & Kamphaus, 2004)	Age Range: Birth–7 years 11 months Areas Assessed: Adaptive, Social-Emotional, Language, Motor, and Cognitive Age Range: 2–25 years Areas Assessed: Adaptive skills and overall behavioral assessment of maladaptive behaviors.	Representative norm sample of 2,500 children in the U.S. 19% of children were identified as of Hispanic origin Adaptive domain assessed via multiple methods: Structured (child performs the behavior in front of you), Observation (observe the child performing the behavior as part of their daily activities), or Interview (caregiver provides the information) Internal consistency, test-retest reliability, high validity comparisons with other instruments and inter-rater reliability is medium–high Representative norm sample including a clinical sample of children and adolescents with a variety of behavioral, emotional, and physical disorders and/or disabilities Internal consistency, test-retest reliability, high validity comparisons with other instruments and inter-rater reliability is high Allows for direct observation of a child's behavior in addition to caregiver/ teacher report	Norm sample did not include children at risk for developmental delays No test-retest reliability data provided for children under the age of 2. Item gradients for children 23 months old vs. 24 months can change substantially (e.g., earning significantly different scores between 23 and 24 months of age) Standard scores do not go below 55 thus limiting use with children who are very low-functioning Interpretation of results from multiple respondents can be difficult for professionals not experienced with the instrument Smaller sample size reported by authors for ages 2–5. However, authors note this had an insignificant effect on the norm sample overall

and Work (adults only). Scores from the three major domains are combined into a General Adaptive Composite score to represent overall adaptive behavior functioning.

There are five available forms, which are selected based upon the individual's age and the respondent. The Parent/Primary Caregiver Form is administered to parents or caregivers of children to age five. This form is used to assess adaptive behavior by the Bayley Scales of Infant and Toddler Development–Third Edition (Bayley-III; Bayley, 2006). The Parent

Form is given to parents of children ages five to 21, so there is some overlap with the younger ages. The Teacher/Daycare Provider is used by teachers of children ages two to 5. The Teacher Form is completed by teachers of children ages five to 21. Lastly, the Adult Form may be used for adults ages 16 to 89 years, and may be completed by the individual when able, or by someone familiar with them.

The ABAS-II was standardized with data gathered from national samples of parents and teachers, which were stratified based upon sex, race, education level, and geographic region. Internal consistency, inter-rater and test-rest reliability, and validity studies are reported in the manual and are acceptable. Table 27.1 summarizes these estimates. In addition, several studies have compared differences between scores of individuals in clinical groups, including ADHD, autism and developmental delay.

In addition to broad-adaptive behavior measures that can be used with individuals from birth onward through geriatric populations, several behavioral and developmental assessment tools also include adaptive behavior as a component within the evaluation. Two of these tools, the BDI-2, and the BASC-2, may be used to provide supplemental information about children's adaptive behavior.

The BDI-2 measures adaptive behavior as a component of a comprehensive assessment of five domains of development (adaptive, personal-social, communication, motor, and cognitive skills). The adaptive component of the BDI-II assesses adaptive behavior in two sub-domains: Adaptive and Personal Responsibility. Scores derived from each subdomain creates a composite score that is expressed as a developmental quotient with a mean of 100 and standard deviation of 15. The BDI-II may be used with children ages birth through age 7 years 11 months. A single form is utilized with the BDI-II. However, with respect to adaptive behavior, the BDI-II assesses only adaptive behavior related to activities of daily living in children under two (e.g., feeding and helping with dressing) while children over two are assessed with the sub-domain Personal Responsibility (e.g., understanding common dangers). The BDI-2 uses caregiver interview, direct observation, or a structured format face-to-face with the child to determine whether or not children have attained a developmental skill. The BDI-II was standardized with a representative sample of the U.S. population of 2,500 children. Internal consistency, test-retest reliability and inter-rater reliability, and validity data are adequate and provided in more detail in Table 27.2.

The BASC-2 measures adaptive behavior as a component of an overall behavioral assessment in five domains: activities of daily living, adaptability, functional communication, leadership, social skills, and study skills. Scores derived from these subdomains create a composite of Adaptive Behavior. There are five available forms that the user selects based on the age of the respondent. The Teacher Rating Scale (TRS) is separated into three forms: Preschool (ages 2–5), Child (ages 6–11), and Adolescent (ages 12–21). All items are rated

on a four-point scale of behavioral frequency from "Never" to "Almost Always." The Parent Rating Scale (PRS) follows the same format as the TRS as well as using the same four-point scale. The Self-Report of Personality (SRP) consists of three separate forms: Child (ages 8–11), Adolescent (ages 12–21) and College (ages 18–25). An interview format (SRP-I) is used for the Child form in which a child is asked to answer simply "yes" or "no" to each item. A Parent Relationship Questionnaire (PRQ) is also available and is designed to gather information about the relationship between a child or adolescent and his or her parents.

The BASC-2 was standardized with two populations: (1) A representative general population of children, adolescents, and young adults in the U.S. from a variety of public/private schools, mental health clinics, and preschools; and (2) A additional clinical norm sample was also used in the standardization process consisting of children and adolescents diagnosed with a variety of behavioral, emotional, and physical disorders or disabilities. T-scores are used to express adaptive behavior functioning. Internal consistency, test-retest reliability and inter-rater reliability, and validity data are adequate and provided in more detail in Table 27.2.

Supplemental Methods Assessing Adaptive Behavior

In addition to traditional norm-referenced methods that typically rely on caregiver reports to obtain information about an individual's functioning, it is possible to obtain meaningful and practical estimates of an individual's acquisition of adaptive skills through more objective methods. Specifically, two methods deserve consideration: (a) criterion-referenced assessments, as illustrated by The Assessment of Basic Language and Learning Skills–Revised (ABLLS-R; Partington, 2006); and (b) direct-observation data collected during probes teaching specific adaptive skills. Although these nontraditional methods have their own strengths and weaknesses, they offer clinicians a valid supplement to more traditional assessment methodologies of adaptive behavior assessment.

The ABLLS-R is a combined assessment, curriculum, and progress-monitoring system that was designed for children with language delays. Twenty-five different skill areas are grouped into four different assessments that are used to benchmark a child's acquisition of developmental skills. These include (1) the Basic Learner Skills Assessment; (2) the Academic Skills Assessment;

(3) the Self-Help Skills Assessment; and (4) the Motor Skills Assessment. The Basic Learner Skills Assessment comprises the following skill areas: cooperation and reinforcer effectiveness, visual performance, receptive language, motor imitation, vocal imitation, labeling, intraverbals, spontaneous vocalizations, syntax and grammar, play and leisure, social interaction, group interaction, following classroom routines, and generalized responding. The Academic Skills Assessment includes sections dedicated to reading, math, writing, and spelling, while the Self-Help Skills Assessment measures dressing, eating, grooming, and toileting skills. Finally, both gross motor and fine motor skills are assessed via the Motor Skills Assessment.

Skill areas on the ABLLS-R are composed of a series of discrete tasks. Each skill is defined operationally, has an interview question, an illustrative example, and a set of scoring criteria. Clinicians, educators, and parents are able to use three different sources of information to address scoring criteria, including interview, direct observation, and presentation of the task itself (i.e., an intervention probe). Data are then transferred into a skill-tracking grid for subsequent analysis.

The ABLLS-R has several distinct advantages. First, the ABLLS-R is versatile, serving several important functions, including as an assessment, instructional curriculum, and progress monitoring system. In this regard, the design of the ABLLS-R allows one to link assessment to intervention with relative ease (e.g., individualized educational plans, behavior intervention plans). Second, the ABLLS-R enhances its validity and utility through multi-method assessment, using a combination of interview, direct observation, and intervention probes. Third, its scoring criteria are highly observable and measurable, a feature that can be traced back to the behavior-analytic origins of the ABLLS-R's design. Fourth, the ABLLS-R allows for comprehensive analysis of a child's skill acquisition/ progress. Data can be analyzed within the task itself, as well as both within and across skill areas across a maximum of four separate administrations using the same protocol. Not only does the ABLLS-R allow for fine-grained analysis of skill acquisition within a specific skill area, but its criterion-referenced design is also sensitive to changes in growth over time.

However, the ABLLS-R cannot be used to compare a child's performance to a normative sample, and consequently, it cannot be used to document a delay or an intellectual disability, as is the case with norm-referenced assessments of adaptive behavior. In addition, the ABLLS-R only purports to offer approximations of the actual developmental sequence of a child's skill acquisition with a specific skill area (i.e., it is not necessarily an exhaustive list of tasks associated with the developmental progression of skill acquisition relative to a specific skill area). Another limitation pertains to the scope of the Self-Help Skills Assessment. The ABLLS-R addresses dressing, eating, grooming, and toileting skill areas, but does not include assessments of domestic and community-based skills. Finally, the ABLLS-R does not discriminate between performance and skill deficits. For example, if a child demonstrated challenging behavior when presented with demands to perform a specific task, it is not possible to use the ABLLS-R to determine whether or not a child's behavior may be predicted by the difficulty of the task, gaps in prerequisite skill acquisition, or other features of the child's environment. In such situations, a functional behavior assessment would be indicated either as an alternative or in conjunction with an ABLLS-R assessment.

Behavioral observations in the individual's natural environment offer another strategy to assess adaptive behavior functioning. In addition, one can administer specific probes across several periods of time, to assess skill mastery and response to intervention. Several steps are required in order to conduct adaptive skill probes, and are described by Table 27.3.

Using intervention probes of specific adaptive skills as a nontraditional method of assessing adaptive behavior presents both advantages and disadvantages. Given that the intervention itself is intended to take place within the person's natural environment, the most significant advantage involves generalization. Specifically, skills taught using this method are more likely to successfully generalize because they are trained within the natural environment during naturally occurring routines (e.g., mealtime, personal hygiene,

Table 27.3 Steps to Generate Adaptive Skill Probes

Step 1. Identify and observe the specific skill to be targeted for acquisition.

Step 2. Create operational definition.

Step 3. Set criterion for mastery.

Step 4. Select or generate training materials.

Step 5. Teach the skill (modeling, role play, performance feedback).

Step 6. Collect observation data.

Step 7. Evaluate relative to mastery criterion.

shopping, completing chores); they can incorporate multiple caregivers and/or examples; and they can be trained via variations in stimuli, responses, and reinforcers. In addition, this method allows for efficient error analysis. Through direct observation during intervention probes, it is possible to pinpoint which specific steps or prerequisite skills that have yet to be mastered may be inhibiting a child from acquiring a more complex skill. These skills can then be taught directly within the context of naturally occurring routines (with increased levels of prompting) or in isolation through discrete trials.

The first step involves identifying the specific skill to be targeted for acquisition. Skills can be selected in several ways, including from norm-referenced assessments of adaptive behavior, direct observations of prerequisite and targeted skills, or interviews (e.g., with parents, teachers, or therapists). Selection of skills targeted for acquisition should consider patterns of prerequisite skill acquisition, the child's needs and preferences, linkage into more complex skills, and the overall utility of the skill for the child and family (i.e., whether or not the skill will contribute toward incremental improvements in the individual child or family's quality of life). The skill should be observed with baseline data collected (e.g., percent accuracy) in order to both document the need for skill acquisition and establish a baseline. Once the target skill is identified and baseline data are obtained, the next step is to create an operational definition and set a criterion for mastery. The operational definition should be observable and measurable in order to lend itself to direct observation and measurement. The criterion for mastery should be defined prior to instruction and reflect a minimum degree of accuracy that would indicate the child is able to independently demonstrate the skill.

The next step entails selecting or generating materials for use in training. Depending on the skill targeted for acquisition, materials may either be readily available (e.g., Mannix, 1992; Mannix, 1995; Stages Learning Materials, 2004) or require custom development. With regard to the latter, some materials may only require modification to meet the needs of the child (e.g., enlarged size, using digital pictures instead of drawings, adding text to a stimulus). In other situations, materials may need to be developed, such as creating a pictorial/text task analysis of steps to demonstrate a complex skill (e.g., steps to brush teeth, steps to tie shoes, steps to load/unload the dishwasher),

or arranging and modifying materials for instructional purposes (e.g., using color-coded laundry baskets to teach sorting dirty laundry). The goal of materials selection/generation is to use materials that are both cost-effective and typically used by the child/family during naturally occurring routines. Once materials are available, teaching should proceed, using a combination of modeling the skill and subsequently delivering prompts and performance feedback. Given that the new skill has not been mastered, most-to-least prompts should be used and systematically faded over time in order to promote both mastery and independence. Data collection resumes (using the same metric as collected during baseline), and data are compared to the baseline in order to document the evaluee's response to intervention/skill acquisition.

Finally, treatment plans generated based on nontraditional assessments possess a greater degree of contextual fit than those developed using more traditional methods. Referring to the degree to which a treatment plan is congruent or compatible with variables related to an individual or environment (Albin et al., 1996), contextual fit takes three sets of variables into account: (1) characteristics related to the child and his or her patterns of behavior; (2) variables related to the people involved in the development and implementation of the intervention plan; and (3) features of the environments where the plan will be implemented and the systems in place within those environments. Treatment plans taking such variables into account may be more consistently implemented over time since they address potential barriers to treatment integrity on an *a priori* basis (e.g., considering the intervention strengths and weaknesses of natural intervention agents, considering how well the intervention could fit within the child's routines).

With regard to disadvantages of nontraditional assessments of adaptive behavior, the greatest barrier to their use is their greatest strength—they require that clinicians have access to a home- and community-based service delivery model. Clinicians who work in clinics, schools, and analogous settings would therefore have greater difficulties using a nontraditional method. Conversely, some community-based settings present with unique features that may limit or reduce the degree to which they are accessible or amenable to intervention (e.g., airports, hospitals). Aside from these disadvantages, concerns can be raised with potential risks of prompt dependence, dependence on resources (both time and material), and the need to have a fluent knowledge of prerequisite skills (in order to effectively identify and account for gaps in individual skills encapsulated within complex skills.

In an effort to illustrate the differences between both traditional and nontraditional methods of assessing adaptive behavior, two cases studies are presented below. For the sake of illustration, both cases describe assessment of community-based adaptive skills.

Case Study of a 12 Year-Old Boy with Autism and Seizure Disorder

"GT," a 12-year-old boy, presented with autism and seizure disorder, and challenging behaviors. These behaviors included a combination of aggression, self-injury, property destruction, tantrums, and non-compliance. Compounding the occurrences of these behaviors was the fact that GT did not have expressive language and relied on a combination of nonverbal functional communication training (e.g., picture exchange) and use of an augmentative communication device. These behaviors were exhibited across individuals, times of day, tasks/activities, and settings. In response to a parental request, a functional behavior assessment (FBA) and behavior intervention plan were developed in effort to both reduce occurrences of challenging behavior and to increase acquisition of age- and socially appropriate replacement behaviors.

With respect to medical and educational history, GT received medical care provided by a primary care pediatrician and pediatric neurologist. Relative to seizure history, the pediatric neurologist noted that seizures had not been reported in over two years and were considered well controlled with anticonvulsant medication. GT did not have any history of accidents, injuries, or surgical procedures. Hearing and vision were considered functional. In addition, a psychological evaluation conducted at age 14 revealed a non-verbal IQ score of 115 (which was indicative of average to above-average intellectual ability).

GT received a combination of speech language, occupational, and physical therapies, all of which were provided in a clinic. Inconsistent progress had been reported in all three therapies, particularly speech and occupational therapies. Therapists reported that GT's receptive language was far better developed than his expressive language and fine-motor skills.

In addition, GT received special education services and supports. He was served in a full-day program, with additional support including speech language therapy, occupational therapy, daily living skills training, and social skills training.

Given reports from parents and caregivers that GT's development appeared to have hit a plateau, a norm-referenced assessment of adaptive behavior was conducted and incorporated into his FBA (Vineland Adaptive Behavior Scales, 2nd ed.; Sparrow, Cicchetti, & Balla, 2005). Results of GT's adaptive behavior assessment are reported below, in Figure 27.1.

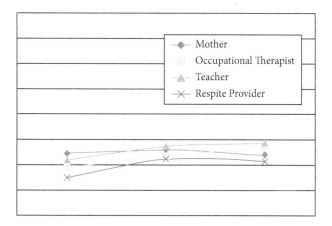

Figure 27.1 Results of the Vineland Adaptive Behavior Scales, 2nd Edition (VABS-II)

On the VABS-II, data were obtained from multiple caregivers, including GT's mother, occupational therapist, teacher, and respite provider. Specifically, GT's communication skills ranged between 30 and 49, with strengths noted relative to receptive language and written language skills (in contrast to his expressive language skills). Daily living skill standard scores ranged between 45 and 55 across caregivers, with higher ratings obtained within the personal and school community domains (as compared to academic, domestic, and community skills). On the socialization domain, GT's skills ranged between 43 and 57, with strengths noted relative to coping skills (in comparison to interpersonal relations and play/leisure skills). Estimates of motor skill functioning (range = 48–64) revealed scores indicating that GT's gross motor skills are currently better developed than his fine motor skills. Finally, Adaptive Behavior Composite scores ranged between 37 and 50, which confirmed that GT's present level of adaptive functioning fell well below age-level expectations, not to mention his measured learning potential. These data supported the clinician's hypothesis that the presenting challenging behaviors were potentially triggered by demands that were difficult for GT due to his skill deficits with adaptive behavior.

Based on these results, four skills measured by the VABS-II were selected and targeted for intervention by the clinician and GT's parents: (1) understanding the function of money; (2) understanding that some items cost more than others; (3) ordering meals; and (4) evaluating prices while making purchases. A treatment plan was developed articulating interventions and goals specifically designed to teach each skill.

In effort to provide the parents with tools to use for intervention, the clinician chose reproducible lessons from published resources teaching life skills (Mannix, 1992; Mannix, 1995). Specific lessons and worksheets included recognizing the value of items, eating in restaurants, shopping for food, buying stamps, and using the public library. Lessons and worksheets were reviewed and practiced with role play and performance feedback at the clinic with the clinician over the course of five intervention sessions, and then at home with GT and his parents. Intervention data are presented below, in Figure 27.2.

The data in Figure 27.2 indicated that GT had acquired two of the skills (i.e., demonstrating an understanding of the function of money; ordering meals), while demonstrating progress toward the pre-established mastery criterion (i.e., demonstrating his understanding that some items cost more than others; evaluating and comparing prices while making purchases). Together, these data are suggestive of a positive response to intervention. Instruction continued at home with GT's parents until mastery of each worksheet was achieved (i.e., 80% accuracy or greater). Once GT reached mastery demonstrating these skills, intervention sessions were faded, and additional lessons and worksheets were provided for practice at home with his parents.

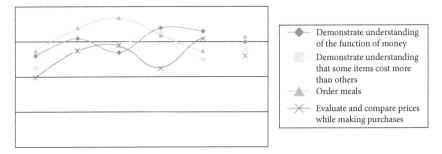

Figure 27.2 Intervention Data Collected At Clinic

Case Study of a 16-Year-Old Boy with Autism

"RV" is a happy, intelligent, and increasingly independent 16-year-old bilingual adolescent, with a diagnosis of autism and disruptive behavior problems. Behavior problems included a combination of noncompliance, inappropriate socializations, property destruction, and tantrums, which were reported by caregivers, across times of day, tasks/activities, and settings. RV's parents requested help in both preventing challenging behavior and teaching him social, communicative, and adaptive replacement behaviors.

A review of medical and educational records indicated that RV was in good health overall, with no history of medication, accidents, injuries, surgeries, or seizures. Hearing and vision were both considered functional. RV had received both clinic-based speech language and occupational therapies in the past, and currently was provided care through applied behavior analysis services in his home and community. RV also received services and supports through the school district, and was placed in a full-time, self-contained program for students with autism. RV's parents were interested in learning how to teach adaptive skills to their son. At the same time, they did not feel that previous standardized assessments were helpful in developing interventions. In response to this request, the clinician conducted direct observations during daily living skill routines in both the home and community. With these data, the RV's parents and the clinician targeted the following skills for intervention: (1) discriminating function of community helpers; (2) discriminating function of community locations; (3) ordering and purchasing goods and services; and (4) determining whether items cost more or less than a given sum of money. A treatment plan was developed articulating interventions and goals specifically designed to teach each skill. Included within RV's treatment plan were two operational definitions for community-based skills, which are presented in Table 27.4.

After setting a criterion for mastery (80% mean accuracy), the clinician selected published materials to teach identification and discrimination of community helpers (Freeman & Dake 1997; Stages Learning Materials, 2004). Training was then provided to RV at home using a combination of modeling, prompting, and performance feedback (e.g., praise, verbal prompts, nonverbal prompts, modeling, redirection). The clinician obtained accuracy data regarding community helpers and locations, which is shown in Figure 27.3.

As seen in Figure 27.3, RV was proficient in labeling common community helpers. Data for eight of 19 community helpers met the stated mastery criteria, while his identification of 11 of 19 community helpers fell below the target level. In general, RV had demonstrated a familiarity with community helpers whom he was most likely to come into direct contact with or to see regularly in his natural environment (e.g., police officers, firemen, doctor, mail carrier, librarian, teacher, school bus driver). It was also suspected that his skill acquisition was enhanced by the degree to which a specific community

Table 27.4 Operational Definitions

Community-Based Skill	Operational Definition
Community Helpers/Locations	Defined as any occurrence in which RV completes multi-step directions associated with functional community-based tasks using receptive, expressive, and written response formats (with fading prompts). Examples include: Identifying and/or discriminating basic community helpers by matching, sorting, and labeling; discriminating functions of community helpers and locations by matching, sorting, and labeling.
Purchasing/Ordering	Defined as any occurrence in which RV completes multi-step directions associated with functional community-based using both receptive and expressive response formats (with fading prompts). Examples include: Ordering goods/services, using setting-specific media to obtain information (e.g., ads, menus, coupons, catalogs, labels, and packages), and exchanging money in order to purchase and acquire products/services.

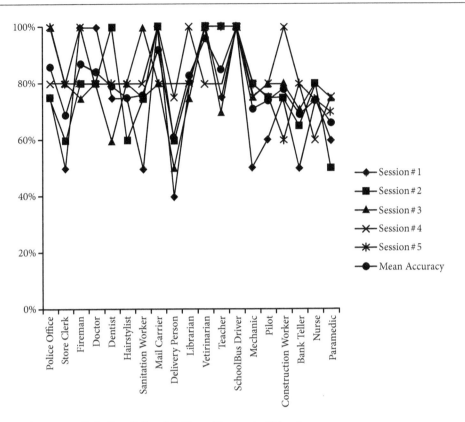

Figure 27.3 Intervention Probe Data Collected At Home (Community Helpers)

provider was associated with uniforms or any other visually identifiable characteristics that were easier for the child to identify (e.g., a police officer's uniform/badge/police car, a fireman's uniform/hat/fire engine, a mail carrier's uniform/mail truck, a doctor's white coat/stethoscope). If these types of concrete stimuli were not present, RV was less successful discriminating the type of community helper (e.g., bank teller, store clerk, delivery person).

In conjunction with the administration of intervention probes assessing mastery of community helpers, instruction was provided using written materials generated for the purpose of teaching RV to compare differences between community helpers relative to their role, location, tools associated with their role, and other relevant features (e.g., clothing, specific tasks). The clinician administered each of these probes, obtaining data are reported below in Figure 27.4.

Using these stimuli, probe data indicated that RV continued the same general trend as observed with community helper discrimination training, and appeared to have a better understanding of the general role/function that a specific community helper serves rather than the specific locations where they worked, the tools that they used, the uniforms/professional dress that they wore, or the more specific activities in which they are engaged.

Building on these results, intervention probes were custom-developed for RV for use within his natural environment. Probes consisted of multiple choice and open-ended questions that addressed a specific location (e.g., doctor's office; see Appendix of this chapter). In addition, specific activities were embedded within the probes so as to require RV to interact with and become more familiar with the setting itself. Data obtained through these individual probes are reported below in Figure 27.5.

Data obtained from these probes indicated that RV was most successful at the retail store, a library, at a restaurant, at the mall, at a hair salon, and at the doctor's office. While these probe data are limited

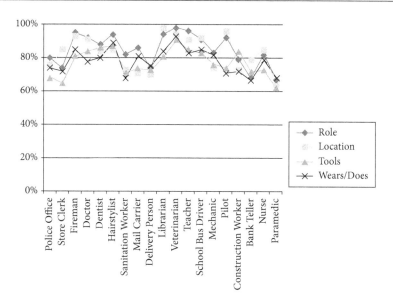

Figure 27.4 Intervention Probe Data Collected At Home (Community Locations/Community Helpers)

in that they represent performance during a single visit to each location, they provide an initial estimate of RV's familiarity and comfort with a specific community location, as well as the child's ability to navigate complex community environments in the presence of structured routines/activities (i.e., activities specified on the intervention probes).

Overall, data obtained through intervention probes administered in home and community environments indicated that RV was generally more proficient identifying or discriminating community helpers than he was at comparing community helpers, or engaging specific community helpers within complex community environments. These data also identified specific skill gaps; namely, mastery of the specific locations where a community helper works, the tools that are used, the uniforms/professional dress that are worn, or the more specific activities associated with their role. As a result of these

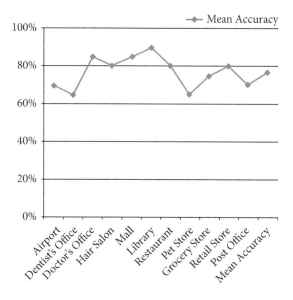

Figure 27.5 Accuracy of Intervention Probe Data Collected In Community (Community Locations/Community Helpers)

data, the clinician was able to recommend both additional activities and continued opportunities for practice with the aforementioned stimuli in order to sufficiently train RV to acquire a greater understanding of each skill gap. It is equally important to note that the clinician was able to transfer training to RV's parents, since they were present for each intervention session and became familiar with the clinician's instructional methods. Most importantly, RV's parents were confident that they could replicate the instruction alone with their son, since they were coached by the clinician and were encouraged to participate in treatment sessions.

Conclusion

In response to changes in social, legal, and educational conditions over the past 50 years, the significance of the assessment of adaptive behavior has intensified. No longer is adaptive behavior assessment limited to diagnosis and program eligibility, but it is increasingly recognized as critical to understanding development and needs of the individual. Furthermore, adaptive behavior assessment has gained notice outside the world of IDD, and is now recognized for its key role in identifying strengths and needs of all persons, with or without disabilities. As a result of this attention, adaptive behavior assessment approaches have become more sophisticated, comprehensive, and useful, and they may combine standardized and alternative assessment approaches. Whereas, in the past, psychometric concerns relative to the instruments were of primary concern for researchers, current and future interests are likely to focus on the utility of using adaptive behavior assessment information in understanding the needs of the individual, and in planning, monitoring, and evaluating interventions.

A central purpose of this chapter was to describe models and methods for assessing adaptive behavior. As compared to other domains of assessment, such as cognitive or personality, adaptive behavior assessments offer a natural link to intervention by targeting skills that are underdeveloped, and preventing further problems by addressing those needs within intervention plans. The links between assessment, intervention, and supports should be addressed within an ongoing, problem-solving process that improves outcomes.

Traditionally, clinicians have relied on information gathered from traditional, norm-referenced methods for diagnostic, intervention planning, and progress monitoring purposes. A second purpose of this chapter was to describe and illustrate nontraditional methods and tools that can also used to pinpoint specific skills or skill deficits within the context of naturally occurring routines and environments. Both traditional and nontraditional techniques have their tradeoffs as well; namely, limitations due to restrictions in scope of practice (traditional), and both available time and resources (nontraditional). However, a third option may be most efficacious—using a combination of both approaches. Using a combined approach enhances the traditional method's scope of assessment and access to feedback from multiple respondents, while also incorporating essential nontraditional elements that allow one to directly assess skills within the child's natural environment and facilitate generalization/transfer of training. Armed with these tools and techniques, clinicians will be able to customize assessment methods in order to obtain a more comprehensive understanding of the individual's strengths and needs, and ensure that interventions that are being provided are effective at improving outcomes.

References

Albin, R. W., Luchysyn, J. M., Horner, R. H., & Flannery, K. B. (1996). Contextual fit for behavioral support plans. In L. K. Koegel, R. L. Koegel, & G. Dunlap (Eds.), *Positive behavioral support: Including people with difficult behavior in the community* (pp. 81–98), Baltimore, MD: Paul H. Brookes Publishing Co.

American Psychiatric Association. (2000). *Diagnostic and statistical manual of mental disorders* (4th ed., text revision). Washington, DC: APA.

American Psychiatric Association. (2010). DSM-5 development. Retrieved March 2, 2011, from http://www.dsm5.org/ ProposedRevisions/Pages/proposed revision.

American Association on Mental Retardation. (1992). *Mental retardation: Definition, classification, and systems of support.* Washington, DC: AAMR.

American Association on Mental Retardation. (2002). *Mental retardation: Definition, classification, and systems of support* (10th ed.). Washington, DC: AAMR.

Armstrong, K., Dedrick, R., & Greenbaum, P. (2003). Factors associated with community adjustment of young adults with serious emotional disturbance: A longitudinal analysis. *Journal of Emotional & Behavioral Disorders, 11,* 66–76.

Bayley, N. (2006). *Bayley Scales of infant and toddler development* (3rd ed.). San Antonio, TX: Harcourt Assessment, Inc.

Bruininks, R., Thurlow, M., & Gilman, C. (1987). Adaptive behavior and mental retardation. *Journal of Special Education, 21*, 69–88.

Coulter, W. (1980). Adaptive behavior and professional disfavor: Controversies and trends for school psychologists. *School Psychology Review, 9*, 67–74.

Eldevik S., Hastings, R., Hughes, J., Jahr E., Eikeseth, S., & Cross, S. (2010). Using participant data to extend the evidence base for intwnsive behavioral intervention for children with autism. *American Journal on Intellectual and Developmental Disabilities, 115*, 381–405.

Freeman, S. & Dake, L. (1997). *Teach me language* (2nd ed). Langley, BC, Canada: SKF Books, Inc.

Gresham, F., & Elliott, S. (1987). The relationship between adaptive behavior and social skills: Issues in definition and assessment. *Journal of Special Education, 21*, 167–181.

Grossman, H. J. (Ed.). (1983). *Classification in mental retardation* (rev. ed.). Washington, DC: American Association on Mental Deficiency.

Harman, J.L.,Smith-Bonahue, T.M., & Oakland, T. (2010). Adaptive behavior assessment in young children. In E. Mpofu & T. Oakland (Eds.), *Rehabilitation and Health Assessment: Applying ICF guidelines*. New York: Springer Publishing.

Harrison, P. L. & Raineri, G. (2007). Adaptive behavior assessment for preschool children. In B. A. Bracken & R. J. Nagle (Eds.), *Psychoeducational assessment of preschool children* (4th ed.). Mahwah, NJ: Lawrence Erlbaum Associates.

Harrison, P. L. & Oakland, T. (2003). *Adaptive Behavior Assessment System* (2nd ed.). San Antonio, TX: The Psychological Corporation.

Harrison, P. L. & Boney, T. (2002). Best practices in the assessment of adaptive behavior. In A. Thomas & J. Grimes (Eds.), *Best practices in school psychology (4th ed.)*. Bethesda, MD: NASP.

Harrison, P. L. (1990). Mental retardation, adaptive behavior assessment, and giftedness. In A.S. Kaufman (Ed.), *Assessing adolescent and adult intelligence* (pp. 533–585). Boston, MA: Allyn & Bacon.

Heber, R. (1961). A manual on terminology and classification in mental retardation [Monograph Supplement]. American Association of Mental Deficiency.

Holman, J., & Bruininks, R. (1985). Assessing and training adaptive behaviors. In K. C. Lakin & R. H. Bruininks (Eds.), *Strategies for achieving community integration for developmentally disabled citizens* (pp. 73–104). Baltimore, MD: Paul H. Brookes.

Individuals with Disabilities Education Improvement Act (IDEIA) (2004). Retrieved February 16, 2011, from http://edworkforce.hourse.gove/issues/108th/education/idea/conference report/confrep.htm.

Kamphaus, R. (1987). Conceptual and psychometric issues in the assessment of adaptive behavior. *Journal of Special Education, 21*, 27–35.

Lambert, N., Nihira, K., & Leland, H. (1993). *AAMR Adaptive Behavior Scale, School* (2nd ed.). Austin, TX: PRO-ED.

Mannix, D. (1995). *Life skills activities for secondary students with special needs*. San Francisco, CA: Jossey-Bass, Inc.

Mannix, D. (1992). *Life skills activities for special children*. San Francisco, CA: Jossey-Bass, Inc.

Newborg, J. (2004). *Battelle Developmental Inventory, Second Edition*. Itasca, IL: Riverside Publishing.

Oakland, T., & Daley, M. (2010). Adaptive Behavior: Its history, concepts, assessment, and applications. In K. F. Geisinger (Ed.), *APA hand book of testing and assessment in psychology*. Washington DC: American Psychological Association.

Partington, J. W., (2006). *The Assessment of Basic Language and Learning Skills–Revised*. Pleasant Hill, CA: Behavior Analysts, Inc.

Reynolds, C. R., & Kamphaus, R. W. (2004). *BASC-2: Behavioral Assessment System for Children manual* (2nd ed.). Circle Pines, MN: AGS.

Reschly, D. J, Kicklighter, R. H., & Mckee, P. (1988). Recent placement litigation, Part III: Analysis of differences in Larry P, Marshall, and S-I. Implications for future practices. *School Psychology Review 17*, 37–48.

Sparrow, S., Cicchetti, D., & Balla, D. (2005). *Vineland Adaptive Behavior Scales* (2nd ed.). Minneapolis, MN: Pearson Assessment.

Sparrow, S., Balla, D., & Cicchetti, D. (1998). *Vineland Social-Emotional Early Childhood Scales*. Circle Pines, MN: American Guidance Service.

Stages Learning Materials. (2004). *Language builder: Occupation cards*. Chico, CA: Stages Learning Materials, Inc.

Westling, D. L., & Fox, L. (1995). *Teaching students with severe disabilities*. Englewood Cliffs, NJ: Prentice-Hall.

Chapter 27: Appendix

Name: _____

Which community helper works at this location?

A. Dentists
B. Postal Workers
C. Veterinarians
D. Doctors
E. Librarians

Which other type of community helper works at this location?

A. Dental Hygienists
B. Postal Workers
C. Veterinarians
D. Construction workers
E. Nurses

What are the Doctor Office's hours Monday through Friday?

_____

What are the Doctor Office's hours Saturday and Sunday?

_____

What is the first thing you should do when you walk into the office?

a. Watch TV
b. Sign in at the counter and tell the receptionist your name
c. Read a book
d. Sit down quietly

Look around the waiting room, what can you do while you are waiting for your turn to see the doctor? ____

_____

Does this doctor's office accept insurance? _____ If so, what kinds of insurance do they take?

_____
_____

Look at your insurance card. Do they accept your insurance?_____

Give your insurance card to the receptionist.

How do you know when it's your turn to see the doctor?

a. You wait for your mom to tell you it's your turn.
b. Someone comes on the TV and tells you it's your turn.
c. The nurse comes out to the waiting room and tells you it's your turn.
d. You just walk back whenever you feel like it.

What is your doctor's name?_____

Are there other doctors who work in this office? _____

If so, what are their names?

_____

_____

What is your nurse's name? _____
What can you do if you need to take a break during your visit?

_____

If you are not sick and are at the doctor's office for a simple check-up, which of the following can you expect the doctor to do?(HINT: There can be more than one correct answer)

  a. Check your weight
  b. Check your blood pressure
  c. Give you medicine
  d. Clean your teeth

Are you able to get your teeth cleaned at the Doctor's Office?

  a. Yes
  b. No

Are you able to get vaccines at the Doctor's Office?

  a. Yes
  b. No

Are you able to get X-rays at the Doctor's Office?

  a. Yes
  b. No

If you feel sick and have a fever but you do not have another doctor's appointment for 2 months, what should you do?

  a. Hope it gets better on its own.
  b. Call your dentist and schedule an appointment.
  c. Call your pediatrician (doctor) and schedule an appointment.
  d. Don't do anything.

How often should you go to the doctor's office for a check-up?

  a. Every 6 months
  b. Once a year
  c. Only when you need vaccinations
  d. I don't need to go to the doctor's office

Great work! You are all done!

PART 4

Special and Emergent Topics in Child and Adolescent Assessment

The Authentic Alternative for Assessment in Early Childhood Intervention

Marisa Macy *and* Stephen J. Bagnato

Abstract

Conventional tests and testing practices are at odds with professional "best practice" standards in early childhood intervention. Moreover, conventional tests have been neither developed for nor field-validated on young children with disabilities for early intervention purposes.

Dramatic changes are emerging in the assessment of young children, particularly those with developmental delays/disabilities. Interdisciplinary professionals must know and adhere to the professional practice standards for assessment in early childhood intervention. The National Association for the Education of Young Children (NAEYC) and the Division for Early Childhood (DEC) standards promote *authentic assessment* as the evidence-based alternative for young children to prevent the misrepresentation of young children with disabilities—the mismeasure of young children (Bagnato, Neisworth & Pretti-Frontczak, 2010).

Key Words: authentic assessment, alternative assessment, early childhood intervention, curriculum-based assessment

Conventional Tests and Testing

Aziano, a 36-month-old boy born with cerebral palsy, was enrolled in his neighborhood early childhood program. His parents soon realized his special needs were not being adequately addressed. Staff recommended that he be referred to the lead agency for testing to determine his eligibility for special IDEA services. Soon Aziano was tested by professionals unfamiliar to him. A standardized, norm-referenced test was used. Aziano struggled to respond to the prompts, but his communicative attempts could not be interpreted by the assessors. He cried when asked to perform specific tasks from the test. The tabletop testing format restricted his movements, and the assessor eliminated items he could not perform. Since so few items were appropriate for Aziano, the psychologist prorated the test, and Aziano's functioning was determined to be at about 11 months in most areas. His parents felt the test failed to reflect all of their son's capabilities they had seen at home, school, and in community settings. Aziano and his parents were frustrated by the testing experience. Eventually, he was deemed eligible for services, and results from the conventional test were used by his teachers and related specialists to design an individualized education plan (IEP). When his team implemented interventions to address IEP goals and objectives, they discovered he had already mastered many of the skills. It was also discovered that there were other areas of learning and development that were not addressed in Aziano's

IEP. The teachers and service delivery providers used some curriculum-based assessments, conducted another IEP meeting with Aziano's team, rewrote goals and objectives, and refocused their intervention efforts to address Aziano's "actual" capabilities and needs. The IEP team was mystified by results from the test, and disappointed that the test had failed to provide the information needed to develop program goals and inform intervention.

The scenario above illustrates a common practice wherein young children are assessed using rigid testing procedures and measures. Aziano was found eligible for services; however, the information collected during the eligibility assessment was not the functional information needed to develop a quality program for him and his family. Perhaps more important, the conventional test *misrepresented* Aziano's actual strong hidden capabilities, so that the teachers were expecting a child with severe disabilities. He was subsequently tested to determine: (a) specific supports needed in his inclusive classroom, (b) educational and developmental goals, (c) services for him and his family, and (d) where to enter the curriculum being used in his early childhood program.

Eligibility assessments should be linked to programmatic content in order to optimally serve children and their families. Early childhood is a unique and critical period when assessment efforts have the potential to make a positive difference for a child. We propose an alternative to the eligibility assessment process experienced by Aziano and his parents. In this chapter, we will describe salient features of early childhood assessment, research on conventional and authentic assessments, and conclude with recommendations for designing meaningful and authentic assessment practices.

Early Childhood Assessment Features

Young children are assessed to examine their learning and development levels. The purpose of conducting early childhood assessment may be to determine: (a) if further assessment is warranted—*developmental screening*, (b) if a child is eligible for special services—*eligibility assessment*, and (c) program goals, intervention/treatment content, and evaluation of program performance—*programmatic assessment*. Although there are some points of similarity between assessment practices used for school-age students and young children, there are at least two salient features of early childhood assessment practices that are non-diagnostic and non-categorical approaches.

Non-Diagnostic Feature

A distinguishing feature of assessing infants, toddlers, and preschooler is the non-diagnostic approach used to determine a child's eligibility for services. The Individuals with Disabilities Education Improvement Act (IDEA) first introduced infants and toddlers in the 1986 amendment (P.L. 99–457), which was about ten years after the initial legislation was passed for individuals age three to 21. School-age individuals with disabilities, or at risk, are typically educated in school settings, making it easier to find eligible candidates for IDEA services, since students are educated in one location—schools. Conversely, children who are too young to attend formal school are more difficult to locate in order to serve the eligible population of IDEA candidates. Therefore, IDEA indicates that states serving children and families under Part C (early intervention; birth to age three) must implement a *child find* system. Developmental screenings are used to identify children in need of comprehensive eligibility assessment.

Finding young children who are eligible for special services is a priority for Part C and Part B, Section 619 (early childhood special education; ages 3–6) programs. Children are identified as eligible for services based on their performance on eligibility assessments. A specific diagnosis is not necessary in order for the child and family to receive early intervention. A child who meets their state criteria (e.g., 2 standard deviations below the mean in one or more developmental domains) could become eligible for IDEA special services. Early intervention is available to children who meet state criteria for identification of a disabling condition/delay, or are at risk for developing a disability (Losardo & Notari-Syverson, 2001; McLean, Wolery, & Bailey, 2004).

The three types of risk conditions are *biological, established,* and *environmental*. A child is at an increased likelihood for developmental delay if they have experienced problems during prenatal, perinatal, or postnatal development (e.g., prematurity, "small for gestational age" status). In contrast, established risk is related to a known etiology with documented expectations for development. For example, a child born with Down syndrome may be at increased risk for developing atypical patterns of growth and learning. Environmental risk occurs when a healthy child has unhealthy living conditions (e.g., teratogens—radiation, pollution, illegal drug activity in household, etc.) and/or experiences (e.g., poverty). If left unaddressed, risk conditions could result in developmental delay. Part B of IDEA does not serve children with risk conditions, only those with identified disabilities. Part C of IDEA allows states to serve children at risk for developing a delay/disability. The majority of states/territories do not serve infants and toddlers with risk conditions; however, there are approximately eight that do serve children at risk, shown in Figure 28.1.

States and territories providing IDEA services have adopted guidelines and criteria for the eligible population of infants, toddlers, and preschoolers (Danaher, 2005; Danaher, Shakelford, & Harbin, 2004; Shakelford, 2006). The law allows three ways of deciding if a child qualifies for IDEA services: (1)

informed clinical opinion, (2) standard deviations, and (3) percent delay.

Informed clinical opinion involves an experienced practitioner making a judgment about a child's need for special services (Bagnato, Smith-Jones, Matesa, & McKeating-Esterle, 2006; Bagnato, McKeating-Esterle, Fevola, Bartalomasi, & Neisworth, 2008; Dunst & Hamby, 2004; Shakelford, 2002). It does not require direct testing of the child in order to render a decision. About 38 states and territories use informed clinical opinion for Part C eligibility determination process (Shakelford, 2006); and about 10 for Part B (Danaher, 2005).

Determining standard deviation and percent delay require a process where a practitioner administers a comprehensive assessment to the child in order to gather information needed for making decisions about eligibility. States and territories commonly use percent delay for Part C (i.e., $n = 43$), and fewer use standard deviation (i.e., $n = 28$) (Danaher, 2005; Shakelford, 2006). A different trend is found with Part B, where both percent delay (i.e., $n = 27$) and standard deviation (i.e., $n = 38$) are used by

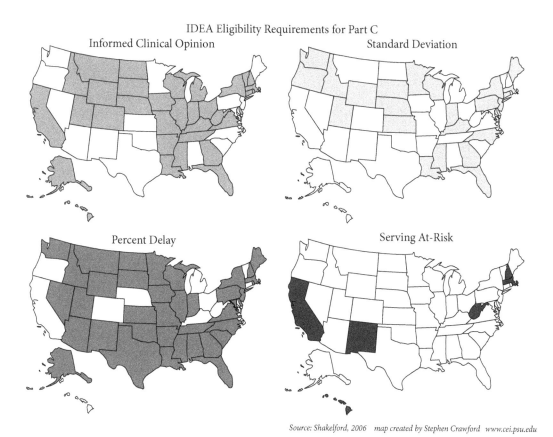

IDEA Eligibility Requirements for Part C

Informed Clinical Opinion

Standard Deviation

Percent Delay

Serving At-Risk

Source: Shakelford, 2006   map created by Stephen Crawford   www.cei.psu.edu

Figure 28.1 IDEA Eligibility Requirements for Part C

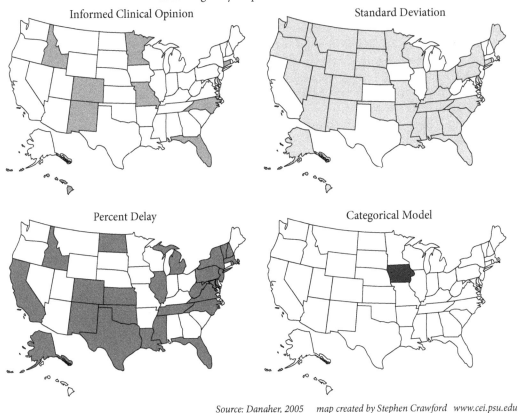

IDEA Eligibility Requirements for Part B

Informed Clinical Opinion

Standard Deviation

Percent Delay

Categorical Model

Source: Danaher, 2005   map created by Stephen Crawford   www.cei.psu.edu

Figure 28.2 IDEA Eligibility Requirements for Part B

states and territories to establish the eligible population of children (Danaher, 2005; Shakelford, 2006). Some states and territories use all three options as part of their eligibility determination process. For example, Idaho uses all options for both parts of IDEA. Figures 28.1 and 28.2 show use of the three formats used for Parts C and B.

Non-Categorical Feature

The second distinctive early childhood assessment feature is the absence of categorical labeling. Unlike the IDEA Part B requirement for school-age students to provide a disability category from a menu of 14 categories, it is unnecessary to provide a specific category of disability. States and territories have discretion in how they define the "developmental delay" (DD) category under Section 619 of Part B IDEA, and can choose to use the non-categorical option up to age nine.

There are several advantages of a non-categorical approach. First, the absence of defining a category at such a young age allows the child's team to focus on functional aspects of development by building on the child's strengths, rather than exerting efforts on

deficit-oriented labels that could tend to drive services. Categorical labels for defining an eligible population are potentially detrimental to young children (Haring, Lovett, Haney, Algozzine, Smith, & Clarke, 1992). Labels can create a stigma for families and have a lasting impact on a young child. It might be helpful to label hurricanes (e.g., Katrina) and earthquakes (e.g., 5.2 on the Richter scale), but not young children.

Second, early intervention programs can continue to serve children who may not meet specific categorical criteria. Therefore, children can be served earlier who would later be found eligible for special education. Children, like weather, are dynamic and constantly changing. They learn and develop at their own rate. It is important to give children time before rushing to categorize them with arbitrary social constructs that are meaningless to their overall development and learning.

Third, a non-categorical approach allows for smoother horizontal and vertical transitions. Parents who have a child in a Part C infant/toddler program who move to another location will probably experience a seamless, non-categorical transition in service delivery. Vertical transitions from infant/toddler program to preschool, or preschool to kindergarten, or kindergarten to first grade are easier to navigate without categorical distinctions.

Finally, developmentally appropriate assessments are possible because instruments for determining some specific disability categories are limited or nonexistent for young children. The use of authentic assessment for determining eligibility for special services is preferred over using standardized, norm-referenced assessment, in part because authentic measures have an eye toward programmatic components (Bagnato et al., 2007; Neisworth & Bagnato, 2004; Macy & Hoyt-Gonzales, 2007; Pretti-Frontczak, 2002). Using standardized/norm-referenced (hereafter referred to as *conventional*) tests simply answers a yes/no question—"Is the child eligible for services?" Conventional tests do not necessarily lend themselves to creating learning or developmental goals for a young child, nor do they have accompanying curricula or interventions to facilitate learning and development. An alternative to conventional testing is authentic assessment.

Authentic Assessment

Authentic assessment refers to the "systematic recording of developmental observations over time about the naturally occurring behaviors of young children in daily routines by familiar and knowledgeable caregivers in the child's life" (Bagnato & Yeh-Ho, 2006, p. 16). Authentic assessment is commonly used for goal development, intervention, curriculum, and/or program evaluation (Bagnato, 2007; Grisham-Brown, Hallam, & Pretti-Frontczak, 2008). Authentic assessment links to a curriculum framework to promote positive developmental outcomes in young children (Bredekamp & Copple, 2009; DEC, 2008; Grisham-Brown, Hallam, & Brookshire, 2006; NAEYC & NASDE, 2003). Treatment validity is improved when authentic methods are used.

Authentic assessment can identify children eligible for early childhood services (Bricker, Clifford, Yovanoff, Pretti-Frontczak, Waddell, Allen, & Hoselton, 2008; Macy, Bricker, & Squires, 2005). Using authentic assessment at the time of eligibility determination obviates the need to assess the child again once s/he starts the early childhood program. This saves time, resources, and unnecessary stress on the child and family. The next section of this chapter will expand on the comparisons between conventional and authentic assessment by presenting research related to eligibility assessment practices for young children.

Research in Early Childhood Assessment: Growing Evidence for Authentic Practices

Since the 1970s, a paradigm shift has occurred in relation to education and services for individuals with disabilities. People with disabilities did not consistently have access to appropriate and inclusive services prior to IDEA and other important legislation. Over time, special services have become more accessible. Now there is a trend toward ensuring that education and services for individuals with disabilities are of high quality. The early childhood field now has quality standards as well as accountability procedures in place (Greenwood, Walker, Hornbeck, Hebbeler, & Spiker, 2007; Harbin, Rous, & McLean, 2005; Head Start Bureau, 1992; Hebbeler, Barton, & Mallik, 2008; Meisels, 2007; National Early Childhood Accountability Task Force, 2007; Rous, Lobianco, Moffett, & Lund, 2005; Rous, McCormick, Gooden, & Townley, 2007). In addition, funding agencies, federal and state policy guidelines, and professional organizations (e.g., National Association for the Education of Young Children and Division for Early Childhood) advocate the use of research-based practices in early childhood programs.

There is a lack of research available on early childhood assessment practices used to determine if a young child is eligible for IDEA services. It has been a prevailing belief that the use of standardized, norm-referenced (hereafter referred to as *conventional*) measures is superior to other types of assessments designed to determine eligibility for services. Research does not substantiate the myth that conventional assessment has a more robust experimental base.

Bagnato and his colleagues conducted research syntheses on conventional (2007a) and authentic (2007b) assessments used to determine eligibility for IDEA early childhood services. The work was part of the Tracking, Referral, and Assessment Center for Excellence (Dunst, Trivette, & Cutspe, 2002). Research studies on conventional and authentic assessments were identified from the fields of child development, early intervention, psychology, special education, physical therapy, pediatrics, and behavioral development. A variety of widely used measures were chosen for each synthesis, displayed in Table 28.1. What follows are some highlights from both research syntheses.

Table 28.1 Conventional and Authentic Measures

Conventional Measures	Authentic Measures
1. Battelle Developmental Inventory (BDI) 2. Bayley Scales of Infant and Toddler Development (BSID) 3. Mullen Scales of Early Learning, AGS Edition (MSEL) 4. Stanford-Binet Intelligence Scales (SB) 5. Wechsler Preschool & Primary Scales of Intelligence (WPPSI)	1. Adaptive Behavior Assessment System (ABAS) 2. Assessment Evaluation and Programming System (AEPS) 3. Carolina Curriculum for Preschoolers with Special Needs (Carolina) 4. Child Observation Record (COR) 5. Developmental Observation Checklist System (DOCS) 6. Hawaii Early Learning Profile (HELP) 7. Pediatric Evaluation of Disability Inventory (PEDI) 8. Transdisciplinary Play-Based Assessment (TPBA) 9. Work Sampling System (WSS)/Ounce

Research on Conventional Testing

A total of 29 studies met search criteria for conventional assessment (Bagnato, Macy, Salaway, & Lehman, 2007a). Overall, there were 3,150 young children who participated in the conventional assessment research. Children's ages ranged from birth to 132 months. Twenty studies (69%) included children with identified disabilities or delays, and 12 studies (41%) included children at risk[1]. Table 28.2 shows the studies by each of the conventional tests examined in the research synthesis.

Each study reported in this synthesis examined some aspect of accuracy and/or effectiveness related to one or more of the conventional tests that were identified. Bagnato et al. (2007a) found ten studies (34.48%) that examined the *accuracy* of conventional measures; and 26 studies (89.65%) that looked at the *effectiveness* of conventional measures. The number of studies exceeds 29 because some studies examined both the accuracy and effectiveness

of conventional tests. The types of studies included five inter-item/inter-rater reliability, two test-retest reliability, two sensitivity/specificity, 14 concurrent validity, seven predictive validity, three construct and one criterion validity, and two utility studies.

Research on Authentic Assessment

A total of 27 studies met search criteria for authentic assessment (Bagnato, Macy, Salaway, & Lehman, 2007b; Macy & Bagnato, 2010). There were 10,272 young children who participated in the authentic assessment research. Children's ages ranged from birth to 224 months. Children were identified with various disabilities, and there were several studies that included children without disabilities and children who were at risk for developing a disability. Table 28.3 shows the studies by each of the authentic measures examined in the research synthesis.

There were 17 studies (59.26%) that examined the *accuracy* of authentic measures. Twenty

Table 28.2 Conventional Testing Studies

Measure	# of Studies	Publication Years	Children's Age Range (in months)	Sample Size (children)
BDI	16	1984–2000	birth to 95	1,637
BSID	11	1985–2004	2 weeks to 77	1,043
MSEL	2	1995–1999	0 to 48	237
SB	6	1992–2003	18 to 132	734
WPPSI	3	1992–2000	36 to 72	450

Note: BDI = Battelle Developmental Inventory; BSID = Bayley Scales of Infant Development; MSEL = Mullen Scales of Early Learning, AGS Edition; SB = Stanford-Binet–Fourth Edition; WPPSI = Wechsler Preschool and Primary Scale of Intelligence.

Table 28.3 Authentic Assessment Studies

Measure	# of Studies	Publication Years	Children's Age Range (in months)	Sample Size (children)
ABAS	2	2006–2007	33 to 216	151
AEPS	9	1986–2008	0 to 72	2,897
Carolina	1	2006	4.5	47
COR	3	1993–2005	48 to 68	4,902
DOCS	5	1997–2005	1 to 72	2,000+
HELP	2	1995–1996	22 to 34	29
PEDI	2	1993–1998	36 to 224	50
TPBA	4	1994–2003	6 to 46	74
WSS/Ounce	1	In progress	45 to 60	112

Note: ABAS = Adaptive Behavior Assessment System; AEPS = Assessment Evaluation & Programming System; Carolina Curriculum for Infants/Toddlers/Preschoolers with Special Needs; COR = Child Observation Record; DOCS = Developmental Observation Checklist System; HELP = Hawaii Early Learning Profile; PEDI = Pediatric Evaluation of Disability Inventory; TPBA = Transdisciplinary Play-Based Assessment; WSS = Work Sampling System/Ounce.

studies (74.07%) looked at the *effectiveness* of authentic measures. The number of studies exceeds 27 because some studies examined both accuracy and effectiveness. Researchers found the following types of studies: 13 inter-item/inter-rater reliability, five test-retest reliability, four sensitivity/specificity, 15 concurrent validity, three predictive validity, and six construct/criterion validity.

In general, the lack of research on assessments used for eligibility determination is troubling. More research is needed to examine the (1) extent to which assessments are used for Part B and Part C eligibility decisions; (2) ways in which assessments are used; and (3) degree to which assessments facilitate eligibility, placement, and early programming decisions. Conventional intellectual measures are less reliable with infants and preschoolers and no more functional in providing data for interventions and progress monitoring than with older students. It is important to note there is building evidence in support of an authentic assessment approach.

Early Childhood Authentic Assessment in Action

Evaluating a child to determine her or his eligibility using conventional testing practices presents

Authentic Assessment Approach

Eligibility

Aziano's familiar caregivers and professionals used an authentic assessment approach for eligibility determination. The current edition of the AEPS has cutoff scores used to decide if Aziano is eligible for IDEA services. The team selected the AEPS and used it over a two-week period to collect data across six developmental areas (i.e., adaptive, cognitive, social, social-communication, fine and gross moto r). They found the authentic assessment more accurately represented Aziano's actual functioning and lead to a more useful program plan.

Five-Step Programmatic Process

Step 1—Develop IEP goals and objectives. Data obtained from the AEPS were directly used to create an IEP for Aziano to include: present levels of performance, goals, and objectives. Information from the authic assessment helped the team decide specific supports, modifications, accommodations, and intervention strategies to use. They also linked their state standards for learning to his IEP.

Step 2—Create an intervention plan. His team created an intervention plan that included routines during the day for intervention efforts. The AEPS curriculum was used for instruction whereby the team planned out a developmental scope and sequence based on Aziano's assessment information. Activity-based intervention strategies were identified for use across settings (e.g., school, home, community), people, materials, and events. A combination of routines and child-initiated, adult-directed, and planned activities were planned. There were also interventions planned to occur during individual, small group, and large group activities. The team discussed specific strategies and supports to address Aziano's mobility and communication needs, like physical prompts, a picture-exchange communication system, and voice-output devices. Target behaviors/skills were a priority for all members of Aziano's team, not likely to develop without intervention, addressed numerous areas, and matched his developmental level.

Step 3—Collect ongoing data. His parents and professionals decided on procedures for data collection. They identified who would be responsible for collecting data, where data collection would take place, which activities to target for data collection, how often to collect data (e.g., which days/times, daily/weekly/monthly/etc.), and methods for collecting data.

Step 4—Monitor the child's learning. The team decided to monitor Aziano's progress every three months using the AEPS. His parents also decided they would use the AEPS Family Report on the same schedule to capture his performance from their perspective and his behavior repertoire at home. The diverse and multiple data points would allow the team to see change over time.

Step 5—Make data-based decisions and recommendations. Decision rules would be considered if adequate progress did not occur within a specified timeframe. The team may make changes to the following when they review his program: (a) target goals/behaviors, (b) intervention strategies, (c) modifications/accommodations, (d) how frequently intervention opportunities occur, and (e) where intervention takes place. Table 28.4 shows a sample of how the authentic assessment approach could be used for Aziano across typical routines in his day.

the following problems not usually found with an authentic assessment approach:

• It takes the child away from meaningful learning activities and experiences,
• does not engage the child by building on their interests and motivations, and
• requires the child to attend to tasks that are adult-directed.

Authentic assessment is becoming a favored alternative to conventional testing. When authentic assessments are used, professionals can focus their efforts on program (i.e., IEP or IFSP) development and implementation without having to administer additional, unnecessary tests. Children will enter their program with relevant initial eligibility assessment information that will lead to the creation of tailored learning and developmental goals, objectives, and interventions. The scenario described at the beginning of the chapter under-represented Aziano's abilities in many areas of his learning and development. His team discovered the inaccuracies

of the conventional test based on Aziano's response to intervention. The assessment process described earlier in the chapter has been revamped to show how an authentic assessment approach can be used instead of the conventional eligibility assessment.

There are several advantages to authentic assessment. For instance, the assessment takes place during familiar activities, with familiar people and caregivers, and uses familiar materials with children. Naturalistic observations become the core method for gathering information. Monitoring the efficacy of the program should be frequent and ongoing. By using authentic assessment practices, assessment teams can gather meaningful information about children like Aziano. Here are five recommendations for creating authentic assessment practices.

1. Early Learning Standards

Become familiar with federal, state, and local early learning standards for children. Knowing what expectations are for learning and development can help take eligibility assessment results and create individualized goals for children. It is often necessary to refer to such standards when creating IEPs and IFSPs.

2. Become a "Programmer"

Get to know the early childhood program. Become an expert on the program's philosophy, mission, goals, and all things related to the organization. This will help when translating assessment results into relevant content. Some of the best assessment reports are developed by those who know the program inside-out.

3. Partner with Families and Team Members

Involve parents and families in meaningful ways. Communicate with families and other professionals using common terms. Written and verbal communication related to authentic assessment should avoid the use of technical language or acronyms so that information is accessible to a wide audience. Jargon-free materials make it easier to communicate content as well as build positive relationships by facilitating clear communication.

4. Collaborate Effectively with Other Professionals and Team

Interdisciplinary teams typically use curriculum-based assessments to guide the authentic assessment process (Keilty, LaRocco, & Casell, 2009). Curriculum-based instruments link assessment to programming and intervention planning. Curriculum-based assessments are also designed to gather information from various sources, including parents and teachers, and can be used for progress monitoring.

5. Use Sensitive and Universal Measures

Gather information from several different situations (Bagnato & Macy, 2010). Before his team used authentic assessment, Aziano was observed only once. That event was only a snapshot of what he can do and the current skills he possessed at that point in time. Children need to be assessed across multiple events and time points to get a good understanding of what they can do and what they need to learn. It is also important to gain multiple perspectives from different people who know the child. A variety of views on the child's development can help the team gather useful data that make sense to those using the information.

Selecting a measure is part of the authentic assessment process (Bagnato, Neisworth, & Pretti-Frontczak, 2010). When deciding on which tool to use it is important to consider six questions.

First, does the measure include individuals with disabilities in the sample? It is important that persons with disabilities were part of the standardization sample. Read the assessment manual to determine if young children with delays/disabilities were included in the normative group and any field-validation samples. Research indicates that it is critical that children with functional characteristics similar to those of the child being tested be included in the standardization/field-validation sample. The sample should have at least 100 people per each age interval.

Does the measure have procedural flexibility? Young children with special needs require flexible procedures. "Procedural flexibility" refers to the extent to which the administration procedures allow professionals to modify the method of assessment (i.e., tabletop vs. play), the stimulus attributes of items, and the response modes of the young child to accommodate their functional impairments leading to a more realistic and representative estimate of capabilities.

Does the measure have comprehensive coverage? The results of eligibility assessment must reflect the "whole child." Choose an authentic assessment that contains assessment items from multiple domains of developmental functioning. Such broad coverage generates results that profile the young child's capabilities across multiple and interrelated functional competencies (i.e., cognitive, motor, adaptive, communication, self-regulatory).

Does the measure have functional content? One way to find out if the content is functional is to try to write IEP and IFSP goals and objectives. Functional content from the measure allows meaningful goal development that can be incorporated into a child's daily routines and family life. Avoid measures that focus on discrete and isolated tasks, like placing a peg in a pegboard. This is not a behavior that the intervention team would spend a lot of time teaching a child, since it does not help the child increase his/her independence. Rather, functional content might examine the child's use of pincer grasp, which could be observed during snack time when raisins are presented on the high-chair tray and the child picks up to eat. The measurement item is functional and could be turned into a goal, as well as intervention/curricular content.

Does the measure have item density? It is necessary that assessments have enough items of varying complexity in each developmental domain. A dense bank of items allows even low functional levels to be profiled. The lowest range of standard scores can be obtained when a child does not pass

Table 28.4 Authentic Assessment Approach During Selected Routine Activities for Aziano

Typical Routines	Developmental Domain(s)	Early Learning Foundations	Goals & Objectives	Intervention Plan	Progress Monitoring
Indoor play	Social Communication	Initiate communicative exchange with peers	IEP	Daily	AEPS
Bathing	Cognitive	Anticipate familiar routines	IEP	Daily	AEPS Family Report
Mealtime	Motor	Begin to feed finger foods to self	IEP	3x daily	AEPS
Nap	Social Emotional/ Attachment	Learn to comfort self	IEP	1x daily	AEPS & AEPS Family Report

assessment items, or only a few items were scored correctly on a measure or sub-domains. The assessment items should be low enough to discriminate age (i.e., very young children) and level of functioning. There should also be a comprehensive set of items in each age interval to describe a child's performance.

Does the measure have a graduated scoring system? A graduated scoring system provides more information about the child's skills. For example, a three-point scoring rubric (e.g., *yes, emerging,* and *not yet*) provides more information about a child's development when compared to a simple two-point scale (e.g., *yes/no*). It may also indicate

the conditions under which a young child can or cannot perform (i.e., with physical prompts, with verbal prompts, with general assistance, independently). These six practice characteristics are necessary to ensure accurate identification of eligible children. Table 28.5 shows these characteristics mapped onto various authentic early childhood measures.

Early childhood eligibility assessment is an essential component to creating quality programs for young children and their families. Non-diagnostic and non-categorical factors make assessment in early childhood distinctive from a school-age context. The use of an authentic approach to eligibility

Table 28.5 Practice Characteristics of Authentic Measures

Measures (N = 9)	Standardization Includes Children with Disabilities	Procedural Flexibility	Comprehensive Coverage	Functional Content	Item Density	Graduated Scoring
ABAS	Yes	Yes	Yes	Yes	Yes	Yes
AEPS	Yes	Yes	Yes	Yes	Yes	Yes
Carolina	Yes	Yes	Yes	Yes	Yes	Yes
COR	No	Yes	Yes	Yes	No	Yes
DOCS	Yes	Yes	Yes	Yes	No	No
HELP	Yes	Yes	Yes	Yes	Yes	Yes
PEDI	Yes	Yes	Yes	Yes	Yes	No
TPBA	No	Yes	Yes	Yes	Yes	Yes
WSS/Ounce	No	Yes	Yes	Yes	No	Yes

Note: Adaptive Behavior Assessment System (ABAS); Assessment Evaluation & Programming System (AEPS); Carolina Curriculum for Infants/Toddlers/Preschoolers with Special Needs (Carolina); Child Observation Record (COR); Developmental Observation Checklist System (DOCS); Hawaii Early Learning Profile (HELP); Pediatric Evaluation of Disability Inventory (PEDI); Transdisciplinary Play-Based Assessment (TPBA); Work Sampling System (WSS)/Ounce.

and programmatic assessments is supported in the research literature. Practice characteristics are useful to practitioners who are implementing authentic assessment. Young children and families will have a better eligibility assessment experience given the authentic assessment framework.

Note

1. Some studies included both children with *disabilities* and those *at risk* for developing a disability due to medical (e.g., low birthweight) or environmental (e.g., exposure to illegal drug use, teen parent) conditions. Therefore, the overall percentage of children included in sample exceeds 100%.

References

Bagnato, S. J. (2007). *Authentic assessment for early childhood intervention: Best practices.* New York: Guilford Press.

Bagnato, S., & Macy, M. (2010). Authentic assessment in action: A "R-E-A-L" solution. *National Head Start Association Dialogue, 13*(1), 1–4.

Bagnato, S. J., Macy, M., Salaway, J., & Lehman, C. (2007a). *Research foundations for conventional tests and testing to ensure accurate and representative early intervention eligibility.* Pittsburgh, PA: Children's Hospital of Pittsburgh of UPMC; Early Childhood Partnerships—TRACE Center for Excellence, and US Department of Education, Office of Special Education Programs.

Bagnato, S. J., Macy, M., Salaway, J., & Lehman, C. (2007b). *Research foundations for authentic assessments to ensure accurate and representative early intervention eligibility.* Pittsburgh, PA: Children's Hospital of Pittsburgh of UPMC; Early Childhood Partnerships—TRACE Center for Excellence, and US Department of Education, Office of Special Education Programs.

Bagnato, S. J., Neisworth, J. T., & Pretti-Frontczak, K. (2010). *Linking authentic assessment and early childhood intervention: Best measures for best practices.* Baltimore, MD: Paul Brookes Publishing.

Bagnato, S. J., Smith-Jones, J., Matesa, M., & McKeating-Esterle, E. (2006). Research foundations for using clinical judgment (informed opinion) for early intervention eligibility determination. *Cornerstones, 2*(3), 1–14.

Bagnato, S. J., McKeating-Esterle, E., Fevola, A. F., Bartalomasi, M., & Neisworth, J. T. (2008). Valid use of clinical judgment (informed opinion) for early intervention eligibility: Evidence-base and practice characteristics. *Infants & Young Children, 21*(4), 334–348.

Bagnato, S. J., & Yeh-Ho, H. (2006). High-stakes testing with preschool children: Violation of professional standards for evidence-based practice in early childhood intervention. *KEDI International Journal of Educational Policy, 3*(1), 23–43.

Bredekamp, S., & Copple, C. (2009). *Developmentally appropriate practice in early childhood programs* (3rd ed.). Washington, DC: National Association for the Education of Young Children.

Bricker, D., Clifford, J., Yovanoff, P., Pretti-Frontczak, K., Waddell, M., Allen, D., et al. (2008). Eligibility determination using a curriculum-based assessment: A further examination. *Journal of Early Intervention, 31*(1), 3–21.

DEC (2008). *Promoting positive progress outcomes for children with disabilities: Recommendations for curriculum, assessment, and program evaluation.* Missoula, MT: Division for Early Childhood.

Danaher, J. (2005). *Eligibility policies and practices for young children under Part B of IDEA* (NECTAC Note No. 15). Chapel Hill: The University of North Carolina, Frank Porter Graham Child Development Institute, National Early Childhood Technical Assistance Center.

Danaher, J., Shakelford, J., & Harbin, G. (2004). Revisiting a comparison of eligibility policies for infant/toddler programs and preschool special education programs. *Topics in Early Childhood Special Education, 24*(2), 59–67.

Dunst, C. J., & Hamby, D. W. (2004). States' Part C eligibility definitions account for differences in the percentage of children participating in early intervention programs. *TRACE Snapshots, 1*(4), 1–5.

Dunst, C. J., Trivette, C. M., & Cutspe, P. A. (2002). An evidence-based approach to documenting the characteristics and consequences of early intervention practices. *Centerscope, 1*(2), 1–6. Available at http://www.evidencebasepractices.org/centerscope/centerscopevol1no2.pdf.

Grisham-Brown, J., Hallam, R., & Pretti-Frontczak, K. (2008). Preparing Head Start personnel to use a curriculum-based assessment: An innovative practice in the "age of accountability." *Journal of Early Intervention, 30*(4), 271–281.

Grisham-Brown, J., Hallam, R., & Brookshire, R. (2006). Using authentic assessment to evidence children's progress toward early learning standards. *Early Childhood Education Journal, 34*(1), 45–51.

Greenwood, C. R., Walker, D., Hornbeck, M., Hebbeler, K., & Spiker, D. (2007). Progress developing the Kansas early childhood special education accountability system: Initial findings using ECO and COSF. *Topics in Early Childhood Special Education, 27*(1), 2–18.

Harbin, G., Rous, B., & Mc Lean, M. (2005). Issues in designing state accountability systems. *Journal of Early Intervention, 27*(3), 137–164.

Haring, K. A., Lovett, D. L., Haney, K. F., Algozzine, B., Smith, D. D. & Clarke, J. (1992). Labeling preschoolers as learning disabled: A cautionary position. *Topics in Early Childhood Special Education, 12*, 151–173.

Head Start Bureau (1992). *Head Start program performance standards* (DHHS Publication No. ACF92–31131). Washington, DC: Department of Health and Human Services.

Hebbeler, K., Barton, L. R., & Mallik, S. (2008). Assessment and accountability for programs serving young children with disabilities. *Exceptionality, 16*(1), 48–63.

Keilty, B., LaRocco, D. J., & Casell, F. B. (2009). Early interventionists reports of authentic assessment methods through focus group research. *Topics in Early Childhood Special Education, 28*(4), 244–256.

Losardo, A., & Notari-Syverson, A. (2001). *Alternative approaches to assessing young children.* Baltimore, MD: Brookes.

Macy, M., & Bagnato, S. (2010). Keeping it "R-E-A-L" with authentic assessment. *National Head Start Association Dialogue, 13*(1), 1–21.

Macy, M., Bricker, D., & Squires, J. (2005). Validity and reliability of a curriculum-based assessment approach to determine eligibility for Part C services. *Journal of Early Intervention, 28*(1), 1–16.

Macy, M., & Hoyt-Gonzales, K. (2007). A linked system approach to early childhood special education eligibility assessment. *TEACHING Exceptional Children, 39*(3), 40–44.

McLean, M., Wolery, M., & Bailey, D. B. (Eds.). (2004). *Assessing infants and preschoolers with special needs.* Upper Saddle River, NJ: Pearson Merrill Prentice Hall.

Meisels, S. J. (2007). Accountability in early childhood: No easy answers. In R. C. Pianta, M. J. Cox, and K. L. Snow (Eds.), *School readiness and the transition to kindergarten in the era of accountability* (pp. 31–47). Baltimore, MD: Brookes.

NAEYC & NASDE (2003). Early childhood curriculum, assessment and program evaluation: Building and effective and accountable system in programs for children birth to 8 years of age. Washington, DC: National Association for the Education of Young Children.

National Early Childhood Accountability Task Force. (2007). Taking stock: Assessing and improving early childhood learning and program quality. *The PEW Charitable Trusts.* Retrieved February 8, 2009, from http://www.pewtrusts.org/uploadedFiles/wwwpewtrustsorg/Reports/Pre-k_education/task_force_report1.pdf.

Neisworth, J. T., & Bagnato, S. J. (2004). The mismeasure of young children: The authentic assessment alternative. *Infants & Young Children, 17*(3), 198–212.

Pretti-Frontczak, K. L. (2002). Using curriculum-based measures to promote a linked system approach. *Assessment for Effective Intervention, 27*(4), 15–21.

Rous, B., Lobianco, T., Moffett, C. L., & Lund, I. (2005). Building preschool accountability systems: Guidelines resulting from a national study. *Journal of Early Intervention, 28*(1), 50–64.

Rous, B., McCormick, K., Gooden, C., & Townley, K. F. (2007). Kentucky's early childhood continuous assessment and accountability system: Local decisions and state supports. *Topics in Early Childhood Special Education, 27*(1), 19–33.

Shakelford, J. (2002). *Informed clinical opinion* (NECTAC Note No. 10). Chapel Hill: The University of North Carolina, Frank Porter Graham Child Development Institute, National Early Childhood Technical Assistance Center.

Shakelford, J. (2006). *State and jurisdictional eligibility definitions for infants and toddlers with disabilities under IDEA* (NECTAC Note No. 21). Chapel Hill: The University of North Carolina, Frank Porter Graham Child Development Institute, National Early Childhood Technical Assistance Center.

Assessing Mild Intellectual Disability: Issues and Best Practices

Daniel J. Reschly

Abstract

Broad consensus exists today regarding the conceptual definition of the diagnostic construct of intellectual disability (ID) as a disability with three prongs: intellectual functioning, adaptive behavior, and developmental origin (Luckasson et al., 2002; Reschly, Myers, & Hartel, 2002; Schalock et al., 2010). Less consensus and frequent controversy exist over the classification criteria used to operationalize the three prongs and how the prongs should be assessed in different contexts (education, law, social services). This chapter focuses on the ID diagnostic construct and classification criteria, with primary emphasis on the mild level of ID where the most controversy exists regarding classification criteria and assessment. Different approaches to the definition and assessment of the classification criteria are discussed, along with an evaluation of the implications of different options. Finally, persistent issues in ID are discussed as contributors to the decline in the identification of mild ID over the last 40 years.

Key Words: intellectual disability, mental retardation, death penalty, intellectual functioning, adaptive behavior

Intellectual Disability Diagnostic Construct: Conceptual Definition

Kanner's (1964) history of the treatment of the mentally retarded describes the occasional reference to persons with significant mental disabilities prior to the eighteenth century, but few or no systematic attempts were made to understand the nature and characteristics of persons now understood as ID, and even less effort to treat the symptoms. The late eighteenth and most of the nineteenth century were marked by initial efforts at description and treatment, but these efforts were isolated events with little or no actual impact on most persons with ID. In the latter part of the nineteenth century in the United States and Europe, some persons with ID were put in institutions that were designed to provide protective care and humane living conditions, but the majority lived with their families in communities without formal recognition of ID, often

as subjects of derision, fear, and condemnation. Prior to the early twentieth century, nearly all of the concern was with what would later be described as more severe levels of ID.

The conceptual definition of a diagnostic construct specifies what it is, its key dimensions, and its boundaries. For example, the modern conceptions of ID specify that it must have a developmental origin, thereby excluding persons who function as ID due to, for example, a brain injury during the adult years. Moreover, a proper diagnosis of ID involves deficits in *both* intellectual functioning and adaptive behavior, not either one or the other. The modern ID conceptual definition was reasonably well established as early as the 1940s in Doll's (1941) famous six criteria for mental deficiency: (1) social incompetence due to (2) mental subnormality that is (3) developmentally arrested, (4) obtains at maturity, is of (5) constitutional origin, and is (6) essentially incurable. Two of Doll's criteria were eliminated in subsequent formulations of ID; that is, constitutional origin and permanence were dropped beginning in the early 1960s (Heber, 1959, 1961). Both were inconsistent with the expanding literature that some persons with mild ID, properly diagnosed at one point in life (usually childhood), performed within broadly defined "normal" limits as adults. For some time in the 1940s and 1950s, these persons were designated as *pseudo-feebleminded*, a concept that was thoroughly discredited by Benton (1956). Since the 1959–1961 definitions of ID, all subsequent revisions have recognized that ID has diverse etiologies, refers to the current behavior of the individual, and is not necessarily permanent.

American Association on Intellectual and Developmental Disabilities (AAIDD) Classification Manuals

The primary organization in the United States that formulates the ID conceptual definition and classification criteria is the [1]American Association on Intellectual and Developmental Disabilities (AAIDD). The latest version is the eleventh edition of the classification manual (Schalock et al., 2010). The AAIDD classification manuals influence the Diagnostic and Statistical Manual of Mental Disorders (DSM; American Psychiatric Association [APA], 2000). Changes in the DSM ID criteria always follow rather than lead the AAIDD classification manual. For example, the current DSM mental retardation formulation is nearly identical to that in the Luckasson et al. (1992) classification manual, and it is expected that the DSM V, (anticipated publication in 2013) will closely reflect the eleventh edition of the AAIDD. Other formulations of ID criteria also are markedly influenced by the AAIDD, including state legal definitions (Duvall & Morris, 2006), Social Security disability criteria (Reschly et al., 2002), and education (Denning, Chamberlain, & Polloway, 2000).

THREE DIMENSIONS

The current conceptual definition of ID reflects the influences of the earlier definition by Doll (1941) in its emphasis on social competence (adaptive behavior), intellectual functioning, and developmental origin. Significant limitations in both intellectual functioning and adaptive behavior are required and both appear to receive equal weight. "Intellectual disability is characterized by significant limitations both in intellectual functioning and in adaptive behavior as expressed in conceptual, social, and practical adaptive skills. This disability originates before age 18" (Schalock et al., 2010, p. 3).

QUALIFICATIONS ON THE DEFINITION

Although the definition appears to be straightforward, further significant qualifications appeared in Schalock et al. (2010) regarding the conceptual definition. At p. 1, these qualifications are stated (paraphrased here). First, contextual influences from the community, peers, and culture are to be considered. Second, assessment of the intellectual and adaptive behavior prongs must consider cultural and linguistic diversity as well as communication, sensory, motor, and behavioral factors. Third, it is recognized that significant limitations can appear with strengths. Fourth, the purpose of describing limitations is to develop a profile of needed supports; and fifth, provision of needed supports generally improves the functioning of persons with ID.

CURRENT BEHAVIOR

The diagnosis of ID since the 1959–1961 formulation (Heber, 1959, 1961) and continuing today (Schalock et al., 2010) clearly refers to *current* behavior. The AAIDD clearly acknowledges that a person may be validly classified ID at one point and not at another across the life span. This provision overcomes the concern with the pseudo-feebleminded that puzzled the field in the 1940–1960 era.

LEVELS OF ID

Levels are based on the degree of need for supports to attain improved functioning and to achieve mastery of the daily activities of living to as normal a degree as possible. Levels of ID have been part of research and practice in this area since the late nineteenth and early twentieth century when the levels of *idiot, imbecile,* and *moron* (from most to least severe) were used (Kanner, 1964). Later levels were defined by the degree of deviation from normal using intellectual functioning standard deviation criteria (Grossman, 1973, 1983; Heber, 1959, 1961). Since 1992, levels of ID are described by degrees of needed support (Luckasson et al., 1992, 2002; Schalock et al., 2010). The similarity in levels specified by intellectual functioning deviations and needed levels of support is unmistakable (see Table 29.1). The mild level with a traditional IQ range of about 55 to 70 (+/−5) is analogous to the intermittent level of needed supports, and so on.

Table 29.1 Comparison of Pre- and Post-1992 AAIDD Levels of ID

Pre-1992 AAIDD Levels	Description: Levels of Intellectual Functioning	Post-1992 AAIDD Levels	Description: Levels of Support
Mild	IQ of approximately 55 to 70–75	Intermittent	Episodic, short-term
Moderate	IQ of approximately 40–54	Limited	Consistent over time; daily
Severe	IQ approximately 25–39	Extensive	Consistent, daily, most social roles
Profound	IQ approximately <25	Pervasive	Intense, consistent, daily, all social roles

MILD VS. MORE SEVERE ID

The current and 1992 and 2002 AAIDD classification manuals (Schalock et al., 2010) imply that all ID is on a continuum, differing only in degree. In fact the mild level of ID is significantly different from the more severe levels in more than quantity—qualitatively as well. From the lay perspective, the adjective "mild" is misleading, perhaps suggesting an insignificant degree of impairment. In fact, persons with mild ID have substantial and chronic problems with everyday coping due to limited thinking, conceptual understanding, and poor literacy skills, leading to adaptive behavior deficiencies. Most important, mild ID limits the person's ability to reason abstractly and make sound judgments about everyday activities and responsibilities and, thereby, limits their capacity to consider the likely consequences of their behaviors and increases the vulnerability of the person to exploitation by others (Greenspan, 2006).

In addition, individuals with mild ID often have developed a keen ability to mask their significant limitations, making the proper recognition and diagnosis all the more challenging. The masking phenomenon is well known in the research on mild ID and was described extensively in a monograph by Robert Edgerton, "The Cloak of Competence: Stigma in the Lives of the Mentally Retarded" (Edgerton, 1967, 1993). Persons with mild ID and their parents typically would prefer a diagnosis of some other mental disorder, such as emotional disturbance, autism, or physical disability (Reschly et al., 2002).

Mild ID is different from *normal development* in the level and quality of intellectual functioning and adaptive behavior performance. Persons with significant limitations in intellectual functioning have a significantly reduced capacity to learn,

recall, and reason (Campione, Brown, & Ferrara, 1982; Campione, Brown, Ferrara, & Bryant, 1985; Reschly, 1987). Such persons are particularly limited in applying abstract reasoning (e.g., moral or ethical principles) to practical situations and in spontaneously recalling thinking strategies to solve problems. These fundamental intellectual deficits affect everyday activities and responsibilities. Other learning deficits reported frequently with persons with low intellectual ability include difficulty in applying basic learning to new situations, and chronic, severe limitations in literacy skills.

Mild ID is different from *severe levels of ID* both qualitatively and quantitatively. Severe levels of ID are more easily identified and, hence, more familiar to the general public. Persons with more severe levels of ID nearly always show:

(a)   Significant physical stigmata (i.e., their appearance usually shows anomalies associated with ID),

(b)   Identifiable underlying biological disorders that can be said to "cause" the ID,

(c)   Comprehensive deficits in all adaptive behavior domains, including very basic self-help skills,

(d)   Early identification, usually by age two, nearly always by health care professionals, and

(e)   Need for permanent, daily guidance and protection.

In contrast to the characteristics of persons at severe levels of ID, persons with mild ID typically:

(a)   Do not show physical stigmata (they look normal) and cannot be identified as likely cases of ID from physical appearance,

(b)   Do not have identifiable biological disorders that can be regarded as "causes" of the ID,

(c) Often have areas of strength as well as weaknesses in adaptive behaviors; e.g., adequate self-care (grooming, eating, toileting),

(d) Significant deficits in more complex reasoning and judgment that interfere significantly with personal independence and social responsibility,

(e) Typically are identified by school psychologists (if at all) after age five, following entrance to public school, through referrals by teachers due to poor academic and social performance in the classroom,

(f) Often are misplaced in school programs for specific learning disability (SLD) and receive the "SLD" diagnosis, and

(g) Typically need short-term, usually *intermittent*, guidance and protection in the community in order to avoid exploitation and to cope adequately. The person(s) providing this guidance were identified as "benefactors" in the literature over the last 50 years (Baller, Charles, & Miller, 1967; Charles, 1953; Edgerton 1967, 1984; Edgerton, Ballinger, & Herr, 1984; Koegel & Edgerton, 1984).

Diagnosis of ID at the severe levels is rarely difficult. Significant limitations that reflect functioning in adaptive behavior and intelligence of that severity typically are recognizable by lay persons and readily diagnosed by medical personnel when these children are preschool age. In contrast, diagnosis of mild ID is much more challenging, for the reasons that will be discussed shortly.

Mild ID was first formally recognized in the early 1900s and soon thereafter added to the classification scheme that existed at that time (Kanner, 1964; Reschly, 1992). Mild ID was controversial then and is now, particularly the presumed etiology and recommended diagnoses and treatments. During the first 80 years of the twentieth century, mild ID, or as it was known previously, mild or educable mental retardation, was the most prominent reason for the identification of disabilities in educational settings, leading to placement of most of these children in special education. This pattern began to change dramatically in the last 30 years, such that mild ID is identified in school today far less often. The evolution of the mild ID construct and the controversies associated with it are relevant to the large decline in educational settings and to contemporary assessment practices that will be discussed later.

Assessment and Conceptual Criteria

Significant issues exist in the classification criteria and assessment of each of the three prongs of the conceptual definition of ID. Issues with each and recommended best practices are discussed in the next section.

Intellectual Functioning Assessment and Criteria

The current AAIDD classification manual requires a significant limitation in intellectual functioning to meet the intelligence prong of ID. Significant limitation is described as, "an IQ score that is approximately two standard deviations below the mean, considering the standard error of measurement for the specific instruments used and the instruments' strengths and limitations" (Schalock et al., 2010, p. 27). This criterion is further described as not specifying a hard, immutable cutoff point for ID, but rather as an *approximate* score that needs to considered in light of the inherent error in psychological tests and interpreted in relation to other factors such as cultural background, social environment, and overall health. The current classification manual further describes 10 factors that must be considered in interpreting IQ test results: measurement error, test fairness, the Flynn effect, comparability of scores from different tests, practice effect, extreme scores, determining a cutoff score, evaluating the role of tests in the diagnosis, assessor credentials, and test selection. Thorough discussion of all 10 challenges is beyond the scope of this chapter, but several of the most important are analyzed below.

INTELLECTUAL CUTOFF SCORE

Clearly, there is considerable controversy around the interpretation of the −2 SD criterion and the cutoff score. AAIDD unequivocally endorses clinical interpretation of the intellectual performance, not automatic application of a precise cutoff score. The question remains, how much flexibility should exist around the score of −2 SD, or with modern tests, IQ = 70? The current DSM-IV-TR (APA, 2000) suggests a score of approximately 70 to 75, implying that scores above 75 should not be the basis for an ID diagnosis.

Consideration of context further complicates the problem. Precise, rigid cutoff scores are established in some contexts, including the educational criteria in some states for special-education eligibility under ID (Denning et al., 2000) and legal specifications of ID for the consideration of death penalty appeals (Duvall & Morris, 2006). These rigid specifications can lead to what most would consider as irrational decisions, such as determining one person as

ID-eligible with an IQ of 69 and another person ineligible with a score of 71. Virtually no psychologist would argue that the two-point IQ difference is meaningful in any practical sense, yet this trivial difference can have large consequences, even life or death in capital crime appeals.

Psychologists must explain the nature of ID to interested parties and decision makers, noting that human intellectual performance exists on a broad continuum with fine gradations in performance from very low to very high. Moreover, choosing any precise point on this continuum to define a disability or giftedness is arbitrary, meaning that large distinctions are being made at the margins of the cutoff score that have little meaning in terms of human performance.

Closely related to issues with the cutoff score is the interpretation of the results of different scales on the same test. For example, most modern tests are organized around two broad factors of intelligence: *crystallized* and *fluid general ability*, although the names given on specific tests may differ. The recent revisions of the Wechsler Scales use the names Perceptual Reasoning Index and Verbal Comprehension Index for what are essentially fluid and crystallized general abilities (Wechsler, 2003, 2008). First, scales in addition to crystallized and fluid are provided on several recent tests, typically Processing Speed/Accuracy and Working Memory. Both are important, but the processing speed measure on the Wechsler scales has a lower loading than the other scales with general intellectual ability. The AAIDD classification manual stresses reliance on a general factor of ability rather than more specific abilities like processing speed (Schalock et al., 2010, p 34). One option on the Wechsler adult scale is to use the General Ability Index, which is a composite of the Verbal and Perceptual Reasoning Scales. Procedures and norms for deriving this score appear in the *WAIS Technical and Interpretative Manual* (Wechsler, 2008).

Now consider this dilemma. What should be done regarding ID identification for a 35-year-old with, for example, a Verbal Reasoning Index of 61, the Perceptual Reasoning Index of 92, and a composite or General Ability Index of 76? Can the Verbal Reasoning scale be used to determine ID, or do the higher scores on Perceptual Reasoning and the composite score rule out ID? The answer depends on the examiner's clinical judgment and the context. In some contexts, the pattern of performance would not justify an ID diagnosis; while in others, especially those that allow scale scores from broad-band measures of intellectual functioning, the person might be diagnosed legitimately as ID. There is no easy answer to this dilemma other than to emphasize using informed judgment involving the consideration of the consequences of different decisions and the context of the decision.

The National Research Council report *Mental Retardation: Determining Social Security Benefits* (Reschly et al., 2002) suggested a set of guidelines for making decisions when differing scores on broad ability scales from the same test were obtained. These guidelines may provide some useful information for psychologists making an ID diagnostic decision.

- *Composite score is 70 or below*: If the composite or total test score meets this criterion, then the individual has met the intellectual eligibility component of ID.
- *Composite score is between 71 and 75*: If the composite score is suspected to be an invalid indicator of the person's intellectual disability and falls in the range of 71–75, a part score of 70 or below can be used to satisfy the intellectual eligibility component.
- *Composite score is 76 or above*: No individual can be eligible on the intellectual criterion if the composite score is 76 or above, regardless of part scores.
- The committee recommends continuation of the presumptive eligibility for persons with IQs below 60.

IMPLICATIONS OF VARYING CUTOFF SCORES

The recommended AAIDD classification manual cutoff scores for ID have varied significantly over the last 50 years. The most liberal cutoff was set as only one standard deviation below the mean (IQ ≤ 85) in the 1959–1961 classification manual (Heber 1959, 1961). This cutoff markedly influenced ID criteria in schools (Patrick & Reschly, 1982) and was the subject of much criticism in the courts (*Diana*, 1970; *Guadalupe*, 1972; *Larry P.*, 1972, 1979*)* and by researchers (e. g., Mercer, 1973) as being too inclusive and stigmatizing excessive numbers of persons. In the 1973 and 1983 AAIDD classification manuals, the more traditional –2SD criterion was reestablished, with relatively little discussion of using flexibility and clinical judgment in applying that criterion (Grossman, 1973, 1983). In more recent versions, the intellectual criterion has been stated as *approximately* –2 SDs, with discussion of flexibility and clinical judgment. The differences between an IQ cutoff score of 70, 75, 80,

Table 29.2 Proportions of Population Eligible for ID at Different IQ Cutoff Scores

Cutoff Score	Percent at or Below:
< 60	0.38% (38 per 10,000)
≤ 60	0.47%
60–69	1.90%
< 70	2.28%
≤ 70	2.68%
< 75	4.75%
≤ 75	5.48%

or 85 may seem trivial until the implications are specified. In Table 29.2, the proportions of persons eligible on the intellectual prong of the ID diagnostic construct at and below different cutoff scores are given. Surprising to most is the fact that a five-point change in the cutoff score doubles the number of persons potentially eligible on the intellectual prong of ID. The actual prevalence, of course, has always been far below the theoretical prevalence based on the IQ score distribution (Larson et al., 2001).

FLYNN EFFECT

The Flynn Effect was named after the New Zealand social scientist who described the phenomenon of norms for intellectual functioning tests' becoming less stringent over time at the rate of approximately 0.3 points per year (Flynn, 1984, 1985, 1987, 1999, 2009a, 2009b). Although most psychologists through their clinical experience knew that new norms for a test typically yielded lower scores for individual clients, no one prior to Flynn established systematically the breadth and historical persistence of this effect as well as its impact on decisions about ID eligibility.

It must be noted that the Flynn Effect is a group phenomenon, much like regression to the mean, which may or may not apply to a specific score for an individual. The Flynn Effect can be understood from two perspectives: the inflation of the mean score over time or the likely impact on individual scores. For example, the most widely used adult test, the Wechsler Adult Intelligence Test (WAIS) third and fourth editions were published in 1991 and 2008, respectively (Wechsler, 1991, 2008). The norms for the third edition (1991) were actually established in 1989. When the WAIS (1991) was administered to a client in 2007, the norms were

then 18 years old, and the population mean in 2007 on the test with norms from 1989 was not 100, but rather 105.4 (0.3 x 18 years = 5.4). The point in the distribution that was −2 standard deviations (SD) was no longer 70, but had changed to 75.4. The likely impact on an individual score can also be estimated by taking the original score, e. g., IQ = 74, subtracting 5.4 points for the Flynn Effect, yielding a score of 68.6.

The Flynn Effect can have dramatic effects on the interpretation of individual scores in contexts with serious consequences for using a rigid cutoff score. [2]In the Virginia death penalty appeal of Kevin Green, the court heard competing arguments about whether Mr. Green met the criterion for ID during the developmental period. Although ample evidence existed of significant adaptive behavior limitations during the developmental period—e. g., he was 14 years old in the fourth grade where a teacher described him as fitting in well socially with children four to five years younger than he—there was a dispute over the interpretation of a Wechsler Intelligence Scale for Children–Revised IQ score of 71. The prosecution argued that the score of 71 did not meet the Virginia death penalty appeal statutory definition of IQ ≤ 70. Undisputed facts were that Mr. Green obtained an IQ of 71 in 1991 on the WISC-R, which was normed in 1972 (Wechsler, 1974). A sharp dispute ensued over whether the Flynn Effect should be considered in interpreting the score from a test whose norms were 19 years out of date. Adjusting the obtained WISC-R score for the Flynn Effect would have yielded a score of 65.3, clearly meeting the Virginia statutory standard. Recognition of an IQ score of 65 rather than 71 probably would have increased the likelihood of a successful appeal of Mr. Green's death sentence. In fact, the Flynn-adjusted score was rejected by the court, and Mr. Green was executed on May 27, 2008.

Although the Flynn Effect is a fact (Gresham, 2009) acknowledged by critics of test score corrections (Weiss, 2010), sharp disputes exist over whether it should be applied to individual cases in legal, social welfare, and educational settings (Hagan, Drogin, & Guilmette, 2008, 2010). One of the harshest critics of applying the Flynn Effect (Hagan), an expert witness in *Green* for the prosecution, argued that the Flynn Effect cannot be applied to any individual with certainty and that adjustments for the Flynn Effect do not meet the psychology standard-of-practice criterion. The standard-of-practice argument is advanced by

Hagan et al. based on a survey of the use of the Flynn correction method in psychological assessment textbooks (e. g., Sattler, 2001), journal articles, graduate courses for professional psychologists, and clinical practice. When the survey was completed in 2006 or 2007, the Flynn Effect was not mentioned in most of those sources, and none recommended correcting IQ scores. Standard of practice cannot, however, be based solely on what is done currently (Gresham & Reschly, 2011). Research findings also must inform psychological practice, including the fact of the Flynn Effect.

Consensus among psychologists exists. The Flynn Effect is a scientific fact (Gresham & Reschly, 2011). Test norms become obsolete with the passage of time. Although some disagreement exists about its origins and causes (Kaufman, 2010a; Zhou, Zhu, & Weiss, 2010), the guest editors of this special issue both endorsed Flynn corrections to scores on intellectual functioning measures in death penalty situations (Kaufman, 2010b; Weiss, 2010). It is important to note that Kaufman is an author of children and adult intelligence tests and Weiss has been intimately involved with the last two restandardizations of the Wechsler Adult Intelligence Scale. Psychological practice needs to reflect psychological science.

Other research documents the effects of outdated norms on the identification of ID in educational settings (Kanaya, Scullin, & Ceci, 2003; Scullin, 2006). In school settings, the WISC is used far more often than any other instrument as part of ID diagnosis for special education eligibility. These researchers documented the increase in ID with new norms on the WISC and gradual decline in ID identification as norms aged over time. Clearly, the Flynn Effect has significant influences on ID identification at both the individual and system levels.

Arguments about the application of the Flynn Effect therefore have real consequences in practical situations such as death penalty appeals, Social Security benefits, and special education eligibility. The AAIDD endorses consideration of the Flynn Effect, particularly as norms on current tests age (Schalock et al., 2007, 2010). "In cases where a test with aging norms is used, a correction for the age of the norms is warranted" (Schalock et al., 2007, p. 20). Schalock et al. concluded, "Thus the clinician needs to use the most current version of an individually administered test of intelligence and take into consideration the Flynn Effect as well as the standard error of measurement when estimating an individual's true IQ score" (p. 21). This appears to be sound advice to persons making diagnostic decisions about persons with ID, particularly when the consequences are substantial and the application of a rigid cutoff score is required. Unanswered questions remain about the kinds of ability to which the Flynn Effect is most applicable (perhaps it has more impact on fluid than crystallized abilities) and the age of the norms when the Flynn Correction should be applied (3, 5, or 10 years out of date). Best practice certainly requires the use of recently normed tests and, I contend, applying the Flynn correction as soon as the norms are three or more years out of date, particularly when a rigid cutoff score is specified.

This discussion of assessing intellectual functioning for ID determination could be expanded significantly. Here, only the most controversial issues were addressed. Other important considerations described in Reschly et al. (2002) include:

(a) Selection of reliable and valid *individually administered* intellectual assessment instruments that yield a composite IQ score composed of two or more group factors of intelligence, including crystallized and fluid general ability;

(b) Administration and interpretation of tests in high-stakes ID determination by properly credentialed psychologists who have background and experience with ID;

(c) Administration and interpretation of tests using standardized procedures;

(d) Interpretation of results considering the client's motivation, effort, cultural background, health, and sensory status;

(e) Consideration of test results in the context of other evidence of intellectual functioning;

(f) Consideration of context factors that may or may not bias results; and

(g) Application of the convergent validity principle in formulating conclusions about significant limitations in intellectual functioning; that is, determining the consistency or inconsistency of data from a variety of sources and methods of collecting information.

Adaptive Behavior Assessment and Criteria

Although the concept of *social competence* was well established as early as the 1940s, the term *adaptive behavior* was first used in the AAIDD classification in Heber (1961). Over the last 50 years, the conception and prominence of adaptive behavior in the conceptual definition and classification criteria for ID have evolved and strengthened. Today adaptive behavior is equal in importance to intellectual functioning in both conception of and classification criteria for ID.

EVOLUTION OF CONCEPTIONS AND CRITERIA

Some prior conceptions of adaptive behavior and classification criteria inform this discussion of the current assessment of adaptive behavior in ID diagnoses. In the AAIDD classification manuals in 1973 and 1983 (Grossman, 1973, 1983), adaptive behavior was defined as "the effectiveness or degree with which individuals meet the standards of personal independence and social responsibility expected for age and cultural group" (Grossman, 1983, p. 1). Guidance was then provided in defining the major domains of adaptive behavior developmentally; that is:

Infancy and Childhood: Sensorimotor skills, communication skills, self-help skills, and socialization

Childhood and Early Adolescence: Application of basic academic skills, application of appropriate reasoning and judgment, and social skills.

Late Adolescence and Adult Life: Vocational and social responsibilities and performance.

The criteria were cumulative. At each developmental level, the criteria from prior levels were included, as well as more advanced expectations. The language connecting adaptive behavior to intelligence in the 1973 and 1983 classification manuals was the phrase "existing concurrently"; that is, "Mental retardation refers to significantly sub-average general intellectual functioning *existing concurrently* with deficits in adaptive behavior...." (emphasis added; Grossman, 1983, p. 1). Significantly sub-average intellectual functioning was defined as approximately −2SD, but no *quantitative* guidance was provided regarding what constituted an adaptive behavior deficit.

The role of adaptive behavior subtly changed in the classification manuals published over the last 20 years (Luckasson et al., 1992, 2002; Schalock et al., 2010). In 1992, adaptive behavior was defined by 10 skill areas (communication, self-care, home living, social skills, community use, self-direction, health and safety, functional academics, leisure, and work). Limitations in two or more of the 10 areas were required for the diagnosis of ID, but no numerical guidance was provided regarding the degree of limitation. The Luckasson et al. (1992) definition of ID was criticized by several authors who pointed to the absence of a theoretical or psychometric rationale

for the 10 adaptive skills areas, varying importance of each to child and adult functioning, psychometric flaws in specifying so many skills areas, and the likely misapplication of the skills areas in decision-making about ID (Macmillan, Gresham, & Siperstein, 1993, 1995).

CURRENT ADAPTIVE BEHAVIOR DOMAINS

The conception of adaptive behavior changed again in the 2002 and 2010 classification manuals in at least two important ways (Luckasson et al., 2002; Schalock et al., 2010). The 1992 conception of 10 adaptive skills areas was abandoned, replaced by specification of three broad domains of adaptive behavior, applying in part a conceptual scheme by Greenspan (1981a, 1981b) that had been validated in a factor analysis of adaptive behavior measures (McGrew, Bruininks, & Johnson, 1996). The second change, subtle but potentially highly impactful, was to specify significant limitations in both intellectual functioning and adaptive behavior and to add for the first time a numerical cutoff for adaptive behavior at approximately −2SD, making it consistent with the traditional criterion for intellectual functioning and encouraging the use of the results from current adaptive behavior inventories in determining limitations in adaptive behavior. As will be explained later, the second change has vast potential implications for the existence of mild ID.

The three domains of adaptive behavior were described in Schalock et al. (2010, p. 44) as follows:

Conceptual skills: language; reading and writing; and money, time, and number concepts.

Social skills: interpersonal skills, social responsibility, self-esteem, gullibility, naiveté (i.e., wariness), follows rules/obeys laws, avoids being victimized, and social problem solving.

Practical: activities of daily living (personal care), occupational skills, use of money, safety, health care, travel/transportation, schedules/routines, and use of the telephone.

The same caveats regarding intellectual function tion were stated for adaptive behavior, including interpretation of specific scores as a range bounded by a confidence interval, consideration of culture and diversity in selection and interpretation of an instrument, flexibility around a cutoff score of 70, and so on.

MAXIMUM AND TYPICAL PERFORMANCE

Although the recent AAIDD classification manuals imply that assessments of intellectual functioning and adaptive behavior are analogous, the two areas are markedly different in several important respects. First, and perhaps most important, intellectual assessment along with assessment of achievement and aptitude are part of a genre of *maximum performance* tests (Cronbach, 1990). Maximum performance tests are given directly to the client, who is encouraged to give her or his best effort to do well. Individually administered tests given by appropriately credentialed psychologists, as recommended by AAIDD, provide a context to observe the individual's effort and persistence in attempting to perform well. "Faking bad" or malingering is not completely prevented by the close observation, but it is much less likely, particularly when judicious use is made of effort measures and full developmental information is considered (Salekin & Doane, 2009). Although faking a bad performance on a maximum performance measure is possible, it is generally unlikely when tests are given according to standardized procedures with the further safeguards recommended by AAIDD.

In contrast, adaptive behavior inventories as they have been developed over the last 30 years are *typical performance* measures, meaning that there is an attempt to assess the individual's day-to-day, usual display of competencies. An example may clarify the distinction. A contemporary adaptive behavior item might be skill in using a cell phone. Persons without this skill are at a disadvantage in many situations. We could provide a cell phone and ask to the client to demonstrate its use. Alternatively, we could ask someone else about whether the client uses a cell phone. In the former version we are using a "can do" question similar to those on maximum performance measures. In the latter, the question is "does s/he do it?" The first could be observed, while the second requires a knowledgeable third-party respondent. Adaptive behavior measures nearly always ask the "does do" rather than the "can do" question, typically using third-party respondents such as a parent, teacher, relative, caretaker, neighbor, etc. Some instruments have an option of self-reporting, which is problematic with persons with mild ID due to reading level limitations and their tendency to deny adaptive behavior limitations (Edgerton, 1993; Tasse, 2009). Although current adaptive behavior measures represent significant advances in terms of reliability, validity, and norms (Bruininks, Woodcock, Weatherman, & Hill, 1996; Harrison & Oakland, 2003; Sparrow, Cicchetti, & Balla, 2005), none are adequate as the sole assessment of adaptive behavior as conceptualized by AAIDD (Schalock et al., 2010).

Assessment in the conceptual domain is particularly difficult with third-party respondents. Determining the client's skills in "language, reading and writing, money, time, and number concepts" (Schalock et al., 2010, p. 44) is much more accurate and enlightening through *direct* administration of tasks and use of maximum performance tests than asking a third-party respondent to report his or her perceptions of these literacy skills that may or may not be based on direct observation. Moreover, with many clients there are inconsistencies between third-party respondents and actual tests of competencies in the conceptual skills domains. It seems obvious that the actual behavior rather than a third party's perception of the behavior is more useful in making a decision about performance in the conceptual skills domain and for some aspects of skills in the social and practical domains, such as knowledge of and use of money.

LIMITATIONS OF ADAPTIVE BEHAVIOR MEASURES

Existing adaptive measures have significant limitations that were discussed thoroughly by Reschly et al. (2002). A brief description of these limitations follows. First, the item format frequently mixes "can do" and "does do" responses. For example, the following response format is used in the highly structured Scales of Independent Behavior–Revised (SIB-R) (Bruininks et al., 1996). How should this item be scored: "fills car with gas when needed," which the client does very well, but only about 50 percent of the time, given the following SIB-R response format? Similar formats are used on other structured adaptive behavior inventories.

Score = 1: does the task, but not well, or about 25 percent of the time (may need to be asked)
Score = 2: does the task fairly well, or about 75 percent of the time (may need to be asked)
Score = 3: does the task very well always or almost always (without being asked).

The appropriate response to this item is not clear. Moreover, a response to this kind of item requires deep and broad knowledge of the individual's everyday functioning in a variety of settings that frequently is not available in any third-party respondent. Often, the adaptive behavior inventory has to be administered to the most knowledgeable person available, who may have relevant knowledge about adaptive skills in one context, but not in others.

Third, some instruments urge respondents to make estimations or even guess about the client's capabilities regarding specific items if they do not have direct knowledge of them. Such estimates or guesses undermine the validity of the inventory results. Fourth, response sets can subtly bias the results. For items and instruments with a three- or five-choice response format, there is a tendency to select the middle response when uncertain of the client's actual capabilities. Other well-known response sets include social desirability when items have negative or positive connotations, and halo effects that arise when the reporter has more positive or negative feelings about the client. Some response sets may be conscious. In assessment of adaptive behavior with relatives of individuals advancing death penalty appeals or claims for Social Security disability assistance, answering the questions in a particular direction has obvious advantages for the client and, frequently, for the family.

In addition to problems with third-party respondents, current adaptive behavior measures frequently have relative low ceilings, so that persons with mild ID pass easily, or a few items at the ceiling levels leading to superficial assessment and large changes in scores, depending on the success or failure on very few items (Reschly et al., 2002).

Although Schalock et al. (2010) recommend the use of currently available adaptive behavior measures, considerable caution is needed due to the limitations just discussed. No single score on an adaptive behavior measure should be the sole deciding factor in making a decision about limitations. All adaptive behavior measures must be supplemented with additional information from existing records, interviews with significant others, interviews with the client, and objective, maximum performance tests. It bears emphasizing that standardized achievement test results are highly relevant to assessing performance in the conceptual skills domain (literacy skills, language use). Determination of adaptive behavior limitations must be based on collecting a wide variety of relevant data, which are analyzed using the convergent validity principle.

ADAPTIVE BEHAVIOR CUTOFF AND CLASSIFICATION EFFECTS

The 2002 and 2010 AAIDD classification manuals require a significant limitation in only *one* of the three adaptive behavior domains: conceptual, social, and practical (Luckasson et al., 2002; Schalock et al., 2010). Using a standardized inventory and other information, an individual can be determined as displaying a significant adaptive behavior limitation if the result is a limitation in any of the three

domains or in the overall composite score. It is crucial to note that the AAIDD does *not* require significant limitations in all domains or in a composite score; significant limitation in one domain meets the AAIDD criterion.

These criteria seemed transparent and easily applied until the practical consequences of the –2SD standards on both the intellectual and adaptive behavior prongs were analyzed (Reschly et al., 2002). The 2002 and 2010 AIDD classification manual adaptive behavior requirement of the approximately –2SD (Luckasson et al., 2002; Schalock et al., 2010) on both intellectual functioning and adaptive behavior was not accompanied by any compelling justification or consideration of possible effects on the identification of mild ID. Persons with more severe ID, e.g., IQs below 55, nearly always show pervasive and significant adaptive behavior limitations, meaning that the –2SD criterion will have little or no influence on identifying persons at the severe levels of ID.

The largely unexplored issue is the likelihood of any client meeting simultaneously *both* the intellectual and adaptive functioning prongs required in AAIDD's recent ID classification criteria. An analysis in Reschly et al. (2002), led by panel member Keith Wildman, established that simultaneous application of both quantitative cutoffs would render ineligible most persons currently eligible for ID with IQs at 75, 70, 65, and even 60. It is highly unlikely that this result was intended by the AAIDD committees. Further consideration is needed to determine an appropriate cutoff with adaptive behavior, along with caution for the present in applying the current AAIDD criteria.

The appropriate assessment of adaptive behavior including the application of cutoff scores must go beyond the recommendations of the AAIDD (Schalock et al., 2010). Standardized adaptive behavior inventories are relevant when there are measures that match the age and functioning level of the client and knowledgeable third-party respondents are available. In most cases there are important limitations in the available inventories and third-party respondents, rendering highly tentative the interpretations of client's adaptive behavior status based on the results of an adaptive behavior inventory. Additional information about adaptive behavior must be gathered through other means, including standardized tests of conceptual skills, client interviews, client work products (e. g., letters actually written by the client), and observations in natural settings. The diverse information that results must be interpreted through clinical judgment; that is, consideration of all the data in relation to whether significant limitations exist. Direct application of cutoff scores is not appropriate.

Determination of Developmental Origin of Mild ID

The existence of a developmental origin has been an essential prong in the conceptual definition and classification criteria of ID for the last 50 years (Doll, 1941; Schalock et al., 2010). For some clients, particularly those at the more severe levels of ID, developmental origin is easily documented through a formal diagnosis of ID throughout the preschool and school-age years that appears in medical, school, and social service records. For many adult clients, however, determining developmental origin of *mild* ID is much more complicated, due to a variety of factors discussed below (Reschly, 2009a).

SCHOOL RECORDS

Schools are more likely to diagnose mild ID than any other agency or service (Denning et al., 2000; Mercer, 1973; Reschly & Ward, 1991). Some public schools in the United States provided special classes for students we now would recognize as having mild ID in the late nineteenth and early twentieth century, even before intelligence tests were used as part of ID identification (Kode, 2002). Since enactment in the 1970s of mandatory special-education legislation in the states and by the federal government (Education of the Handicapped Act; 1975, 1977), reauthorized as the Individuals with Disabilities Education Act (IDEA; 1990, 1997, 2004), all schools have to identify students with disabilities and provide special education services. ID is included in every state plan for providing special education services, although the terminology may vary from state to state. School records reflecting education performance, special-education referral, psychological evaluation, and special education programming are, therefore, a potential treasure trove of information relevant to the developmental origin of mild ID. In many situations this is the case, but in many others there are significant problems in using school records.

The first limitation is that relevant school records for adults may no longer exist. The 2006 IDEA regulations at 34 C.F.R. 300.624, guided by the earlier Family Education Rights and Privacy Act (FERPA) (1994), permits the destruction of most school records pertaining to an individual in accordance with state law. A permanent record *may* be retained by the school. Most states allow and some require destruction of individual records after three to five years have elapsed since the individual was enrolled. Most schools do retain a permanent record that contains only "the student's name, address, and phone number, his or her grades, attendance record, classes attended, grade level completed, and year completed." (34 C.F.R. 300.624). Important information such as referral, psychological and educational evaluations, test scores, and special-education participation frequently are not in the permanent school record. Some permanent school records (in the author's experience) may contain indications of special-education placement, special-education categorical diagnosis, grades in classes, grade retention information, and scores on standardized achievement tests. Although more information such as psychological and educational evaluations would be extremely helpful in determining the developmental origins of ID with adults, this information typically has been destroyed by the school. In some cases the school records may be preserved by another agency such as social services, private school, or state residential facility.

Interpretation of school records often is an art that draws on extensive prior experience in that setting. For example, teachers, administrators, and other school officials can interpret cryptic entries in the record that might not be understood by psychologists and others with little school experience. For example, some records may have a second letter by a grade indicating the student's placement, such as an S to indicate special-education placement or a B to denote that a course was at the basic level. Moreover, further information may exist about whether the student could pass the state high-stakes tests in designated areas, again through what may be ambiguous, cryptic designations. Assistance in interpreting school records clearly is useful in gathering information to establish the developmental origin of ID.

USE OF SCHOOL DIAGNOSES

For a variety of reasons, schools over the past 40 years have been increasingly reluctant to identify students as mild ID (Donovan & Cross, 2002; Reschly, 2009b). Several influences are responsible, including litigation regarding overrepresentation of minority students in ID and, to a lesser extent, to emotional disturbance. Since special-education prevalence data were first collected nationally in 1977, the number of students identified in all levels of ID has declined 50%, from about 950,000 to 425,000, while the prevalence of SLD has grown by 400%, from approximately 450,000 to 2.5 million. The prevalence trends are connected. Many students formerly diagnosed as ID now are determined to be SLD, even when the psychological and educational evaluation data are consistent with a mild ID diagnosis (MacMillan, Gresham, Siperstein, & Bocian, 1996). The discrepancy between school diagnoses of disabilities and AAIDD criteria for ID was the basis for the NRC Panel to recommend that objective school data be considered carefully in ID determination, but that school diagnoses should be treated more skeptically (Reschly et al., 2002).

EDUCATIONAL TERMINOLOGY AND CLASSIFICATION CRITERIA

Terminology for ID differs in the state special education statutes and rules. In some states, older terminology such as *mental retardation, mental handicap*, and *mental disability* are used to refer to ID (Denning et al., 2000). Moreover, many states have more lenient criteria for the intellectual functioning prong such as IQ ≤ 80 or IQ 1.5 SD below the mean. States also differ significantly in how adaptive behavior is conceptualized, assessed, and determined to reflect significant limitations. Knowledge of state rules and guidelines for each of the special education disability categories, including ID, is essential to understanding school records.

RETROSPECTIVE ADAPTIVE BEHAVIOR ASSESSMENT AND INTERVIEWS

Because adults who are functioning at the mild ID level may be misdiagnosed or not diagnosed prior to the age of 18, some kind of retrospective account of behavior from significant others is often sought. Retrospective accounts of behavior, whether using a formal standardized inventory or a more informal interview outline, are subject to several limitations and potential distortions (Olley, 2009; Tasse, 2009). Interviewing parents who often have had several children, sometimes in conditions of extreme poverty and social instability, will probably contain many guesses and unreliable information. Other retrospective reporters often are available such as general and special-education teachers who may recall the client vividly, but in a specific setting (school). These accounts may have greater credibility because they come from college-educated persons who have an informed perspective and ample experience with both normal and abnormal development. The general problems of retrospective accounts still exist, including biases, faulty memory, and insufficient opportunity to observe relevant behaviors.

SOCIAL SERVICES AND RECORDS

Most persons with mild ID come from low socioeconomic circumstances, regardless of race or ethnicity (Donovan & Cross, 2002; Edgerton, 1984, 1993; Reschly et al., 2002; Richardson, 1981). Many of the families have other children performing at or close to the mild ID level, and some will have been involved with social services agencies. Records at these agencies, with proper consent of the client, may be available. Other adults with mild ID have been placed in juvenile correction facilities or other state facilities prior to age 18. Records from these sources may include psychological evaluations and educational records pertaining to the existence of mild ID in the developmental period.

SUMMARY

Determination of the existence of mild ID during the developmental period from birth to age 18 is complicated by a number of factors, including the destruction of much of the school record, inadequate retrospective reporters, and the use of other diagnoses when mild ID would be more appropriate. The challenge to psychologists again is complex, requiring deep knowledge of ID and intimate knowledge of educational, social service, and legal agencies. In some cases, the records from these agencies provide unequivocal evidence; however, in many others, the evidence of ID will be incomplete and ambiguous. Consideration of a broad variety of information using the previously described convergent validity principle is essential to making sound judgments about the existence of ID during the developmental period.

Conclusion

The mild ID diagnostic construct has been recognized for slightly over 100 years. The essential features of the conceptual definition are well established by authoritative sources, particularly the AAIDD. ID is a status marked by significant limitations in intellectual functioning and adaptive behavior that appears during the developmental period. The classification criteria are broadly in line with the conceptual definition; however, significant disagreement and controversy exist over specific classification criteria. These disagreements have vast implications for individual clients who may or may not be diagnosed as having mild ID by psychologists, with accompanying high-stakes consequences for the client. High-stakes consequences include application of the death penalty, income assistance and health system support, and placement in appropriate educational services.

No easy answers exist to complex determinations of mild ID eligibility in diverse settings with inconsistent classification criteria. Direct application of test results, even with well-developed intelligence tests, using rigid cutoff scores is undesirable and inappropriate for many reasons. Rigid application of scores from less accurate and less well-developed adaptive behavior inventories is even less justified by the existing research.

Use of a wide range of information gathered through the methods of testing, observing, interviewing, and reviewing records, drawing on diverse sources, including the client and significant others, is required for sound diagnosis of mild ID. Appropriate interpretation of this diverse information requires clinical judgment informed by research on and experience with ID. Application of the convergent validity principle in weighing the information is the best approach to making sound ID diagnostic decisions that are justifiable to the general public and acceptable in educational, legal, and social service settings.

Notes

1. The organization that now is AAIDD had at least two prior titles in the twentieth century—American Association on Mental Retardation until 2008, and American Association on Mental Deficiency, previously.

2. The author was an expert witness for the defense in the *Green v. Johnson* 2006 death penalty appeal.

References

American Psychiatric Association. (2000). *Diagnostic and statistical manual of mental disorders* (4th ed.–Text Revision). Washington, DC: APA.

Baller, W., Charles, D., & Miller, E. (1967). Mid-life attainment of the mentally retarded. *Genetic Psychology Monographs, 75*, 235–329.

Benton, A. (1956). The concept of pseudo feeblemindedness. *Archives of Neurology & Psychiatry, 75*, 379–388.

Bruininks, R. K., Woodcock, R. W., Weatherman, R. F., & Hill, B. K. (1996). *Scales of Independent Behavior–Revised*. Itasca, IL: Riverside Publishing.

Campione, J. C., Brown, A. L., & Ferrara, R. A. (1982). Mental retardation and intelligence. In R. J. Sternberg (Ed.), *Handbook of human intelligence* (pp. 392–490). Cambridge, England: Cambridge University Press.

Campione, J. C., Brown, A. L., Ferrara, R. A., & Bryant, N. R. (1985). Breakdowns in flexible use of information: Intelligence-related differences in transfer following equivalent learning performances. *Intelligence, 9*, 297–315.

Charles, D. C. (1953). Ability and accomplishment of persons earlier judged mentally deficient. *Genetic Psychology Monographs, 47*, 3–71.

Cronbach, L. J. (1990). *Essentials of psychological testing* (5th ed.). New York: Harper & Row.

Diana vs. State Board of Education, No. C-70-37 RFP U.S. District Court, Northern District of California, Consent Decree, February 3, 1970.

Doll, E. A. (1941). The essentials of an inclusive concept of mental deficiency. *American Journal of Mental Deficiency, 46*, 214–219.

Denning, C. B., Chamberlain, J. A., & Polloway, E. A. (2000). An evaluation of state guidelines for mental retardation: Focus on definition and classification practices. *Education & Training in Mental Retardation & Developmental Disabilities, 35*, 226–232.

Donovan, M. S., & Cross, C. T. (Eds.). (2002). *Minority students in special and gifted education*. Washington, DC: National Academy Press.

Duvall, J. C., & Morris, R. J. (2006). Assessing mental retardation in death penalty cases: Critical issues for psychology and psychological practice. *Professional Psychology: Research & Practice, 37*, 658–665.

Edgerton, R. B. (1967). *The cloak of competence: Stigma in the lives of the mentally retarded*. Berkeley, CA: University of California Press.

Edgerton, R. B. (Ed.). (1984). *Lives in process: Mentally retarded adults in a large city*. Washington, DC: American Association on Mental Deficiency.

Edgerton, R. B. (1993). *The cloak of competence: Stigma in the lives of the mentally retarded* (revised and updated). Berkeley, CA: University of California Press.

Edgerton, R. B., Ballinger, M., & Herr, B. (1984). The cloak of competence: After two decades. *American Journal of Mental Deficiency, 88*, 345–351.

Education of the Handicapped Act. (1975, 1977). PL 94–142, 20 U.S.C. 1400–1485, 34 CFR-300.

Family Educational Rights and Privacy Act, 20 USC $1232g. (1994).

Flynn, J. R. (1984). The mean IQ of Americans: Massive gains 1932 to 1978. *Psychological Bulletin, 95*, 29–51.

Flynn, J. R. (1985). Wechsler intelligence tests: Do we really have a criterion of mental retardation? *American Journal on Mental Deficiency, 90*, 236–244.

Flynn, J. R. (1987). Massive IQ gains in 14 nations: What IQ tests really measure. *Psychological Bulletin, 95*, 29–51.

Flynn, J. R. (1999). Searching for justice: The discovery of IQ gains over time. *American Psychologist, 51*, 5–20.

Flynn, J. R. (2009a). The WAIS-III and WAIS-IV *Daubert* motions favor the certainly false over the approximately true. *Applied Neuropsychology, 19*, 98–104.

Flynn, J. R. (2009b). *What is intelligence? Beyond the Flynn Effect* (expanded paperback ed.). Cambridge, England: Cambridge University Press.

Green v. Johnson, 2006 U.S. Dist. LEXIS 90644 (E.D. Va.), adopted by, 2007 U.S. Dist. LEXIS 21711 (E.D. Va.), aff'd., 2008 U.S. App. LEXIS 2967 (4th Cir.), cert. denied, 128 S. Ct. 2527 (2008).

Greenspan, S. (1981a). Defining childhood social competence: A proposed working model. In B. K. Keogh (Ed.), *Advances in special education* (Vol. 3; pp. 1–39). Greenwich, CT: JAI Press.

Greenspan, S. (1981b). Social competence and handicapped individuals: Practical implications of a proposed model.

B. K. Keogh (Ed.), *Advances in special education* (Vol. 3; pp. 41–82). Greenwich, CT: JAI Press.

Greenspan, S. (2006). Mental retardation in the real world: Why the AAMR definition is not there yet. In H. N. Switzky and S. Greenspan (Eds.), *What is MR: Ideas for an evolving disability* (pp. 165–183). Washington, DC: American Association on Mental Retardation.

Gresham, F. M. (2009). Interpretation of intelligence test scores in *Atkins* cases: Conceptual and psychometric issues. *Applied Neuropsychology, 16*, 91–97.

Gresham, F. M., & Reschly, D. J. (2011). Standard of practice and Flynn Effect testimony in death penalty cases. *Intellectual & Developmental Disabilities, 49(3),* 131–140.

Grossman, H. (Ed.). (1973). *Manual on terminology and classification in mental retardation.* Washington, DE: American Association on Mental Deficiency. (Also see 1977 revision.)

Grossman, H. J. (Ed.). (1983). *Classification in mental retardation.* Washington, DC: American Association on Mental Deficiency.

Guadalupe Organization v. Tempe Elementary School District No. 3, No. 71–435 (D. Ariz., January 24, 1972) (consent decree).

Hagan, L. D., Drogin, E. Y., & Guilmette, T. J. (2008). Adjusting scores for the Flynn Effect: Consistent with the standard of practice? *Professional Psychology: Research & Practice, 39*, 619–625.

Hagan, L. D., & Drogin, E. Y., & Guilmette, T. J. (2010). Science rather that advocacy when reporting IQ scores. *Professional Psychology: Research and Practice, 41,* 420–423.

Harrison, P. L., & Oakland, T. (2003). *Adaptive Behavior Assessment System II manual* (2nd ed.). San Antonio, TX: Harcourt Assessments, Psychological Corporation.

Heber, R. (1959). A manual on terminology and classification in mental retardation. *American Journal of Mental Deficiency Monograph Supplement, 64*(2).

Heber, R. (1961). Modification of the "Manual on terminology and classification in mental retardation." *American Journal of Mental Deficiency, 65*, 499–500.

Individuals with Disabilities Education Act (1990, 1997, 2004). 20 U.S.C. 1400 et. Seq. (Statute). 34 C.F.R. 300 (Regulations).

Kanaya, T., Scullin, M. H., & Ceci, S. J. (2003). The Flynn effect and U.S. policies: The impact of rising IQs on American society via mental retardation diagnoses. *American Psychologist, 58*, 778–790.

Kanner, L. (1964). *A history of the care and study of the mentally retarded.* Springfield, IL: Charles C. Thomas.

Kaufman, A. S. (2010a). "In what way are apples and oranges alike?" A critique of Flynn's interpretation of the Flynn Effect. *Journal of Psychoeducational Assessment, 28*, 382–398.

Kaufman, A. S. (2010b). Looking through Flynn's rose-colored scientific spectacles. *Journal of Psychoeducational Assessment, 28,* 494–505.

Koegel, P., & Edgerton, R. B. (1984). Black "six hour retarded children" as young adults. In R. B. Edgerton (Ed.), *Lives in process: Mildly retarded adults in a large city* (pp. 145–171). Washington, DC: American Association on Mental Deficiency.

Kode, K. (2002). *Elizabeth Farrell and the history of special education.* Arlington, VA: Council for Exceptional Children

Larson, S. A., Lakin, K. C., Anderson, L., Kwak, N., Lee, J. H., & Anderson, D. (2001). Prevalence of mental retardation and developmental disabilities: Estimates from the 1994/1995 national health interview survey disability supplements. *American Journal on Mental Retardation, 106*, 231–252.

Larry P. v. Riles, 343 F. Supp. 1306 (N. D. Cal. 1972) (preliminary injunction). aff'd 502 F. 2d 963 (9th cir. 1974); 495 F. Supp. 926 (N. D. Cal. 1979) (decision on merits) aff'd (9th cir. no. 80–427 Jan. 23, 1984).

Luckasson, R., Coulter, D. L., Polloway, E. A., Reiss, S., Schalock, R. L., Snell, M. E., Spitalnik, D. M., & Stark, J. A. (1992). *Mental retardation: Definition, classification, and systems of support* (9th ed.). Washington, DC: American Association on Mental Retardation.

Luckasson, R., Brothwick-Duffy, S., Buntinx, W. H. E., Coulter, D. L., Craig, E. M., Reeve, A., et al. (2002). *Mental retardation: Definition, classification, and systems of support* (10th ed.). Washington, DC: American Association on Mental Retardation.

MacMillan, D. L., Gresham, F. M., Siperstein, G. N., & Bocian, K. M. (1996). The labyrinth of IDEA: School decisions on referred students with subaverage general intelligence. *American Journal on Mental Retardation, 101*, 161–174.

MacMillan, D. L., Gresham, F. L., & Siperstein, G. N. (1993). Conceptual and psychometric concerns about the 1992 AAMR definition of mental retardation. *American Journal on Mental Retardation, 98*, 325–335.

MacMillan, D. L., Gresham, F. M., & Siperstein, G. N. (1995). Heightened concerns over the 1992 AAMR definition: Advocacy versus precision. *American Journal of Mental Retardation, 100*, 87–97.

McGrew, K. S., Bruininks, R. H., & Johnson, D. R. (1996). Confirmatory factor analytic investigation of Greenspan's model of personal competence. *American Journal of Mental Retardation, 100*, 533–545.

Mercer, J. (1973). *Labeling the mentally retarded.* Berkeley, CA: University of California Press.

Olley, J. G. (2009). Challenges in implementing the *Atkins* decision. *American Journal of Forensic Psychology, 29*, 63–73.

Patrick, J., & Reschly, D. (1982). Relationship of state educational criteria and demographic variables to school-system prevalence of mental retardation. *American Journal of Mental Deficiency, 86*, 351–360.

Reschly, D. J. (1987). Learning characteristics of mildly handicapped students: Implications for classification, placement, and programming. In M. C. Wang, M. C. Reynolds, & H. J. Walberg (Eds.), *The handbook of special education: Research and practice* (Vol. I; pp. 35–58). Oxford, England: Pergamon Press.

Reschly, D. J. (1992). Mental retardation: Conceptual foundations, definitional criteria, and diagnostic operations. In S. R. Hooper, G. W. Hynd, & R. E. Mattison (Eds.), *Developmental disorders: Diagnostic criteria and clinical assessment* (pp. 23–67). Hillsdale, NJ: Lawrence Erlbaum Associates.

Reschly, D. J. (2009a). Documenting the developmental origins of mild mental retardation. *Applied Neuropsychology, 16*, 124–134.

Reschly, D. J. (2009b). *Prevention of disproportionate special education representation using response to intervention.* Washington, DC: Learning Point Associates. Available at http://www.tqsource.org/forum/documents/TQ_Issue_Paper_RTI_Disproportionality.pdf.

Reschly, D. J., Myers, T. G., & Hartel, C. R. (Eds.). (2002). *Mental retardation: Determining eligibility for Social Security benefits.* Washington, DC: National Academy Press.

Reschly, D. J., & Ward, S. M. (1991). Use of adaptive measures and overrepresentation of black students in programs for students with mild mental retardation. *American Journal of Mental Retardation, 96*, 257–268.

Richardson, S. (1981). Family characteristics associated with mild mental retardation. In M. Begab, H. C. Haywood, & H. Graber (Eds.), *Psychosocial influences in retarded performance* (Vol. II; pp. 29–43). Baltimore, MD: University Park Press.

Salekin, K. L., & Doane, B. M. (2009). Malingering intellectual disability: The value of available measures and methods. *Applied Neuropsychology, 16*, 105–113.

Sattler, J. M. (2001). *Assessment of children: Cognitive applications* (4th ed.). San Diego, CA: Jerome M. Sattler Publisher.

Schalock, R. L., Buntinx, W. H. E., Borthwick-Duffy, S. L., Luckasson, R., Snell, M. E., Tasse, M. J., et al., (2007). *User's guide: Mental retardation definition, classification, and systems of support.* Washington, DC: American Association on Intellectual and Developmental Disabilities. Schalock, R. L., Borthwick-Duffy, S. L., Bradley, V. J., Buntinx, W. H. E., Coulter, D. L., et al., (2010). *Intellectual disability: Definition, classification, and system of supports* (11th ed.). Washington D. C.: American Association on Intellectual and Developmental Disability.

Scullin, M. H. (2006). Large state-level fluctuations in mental retardation classifications related to introduction of renormed intelligence test. *American Journal on Mental Retardation, 111*, 322–335.

Sparrow, S. A., Balla, D. A., & Cicchetti, D. V. (2005). *Vineland-II Adaptive Behavior Scales* (2nd ed.). Minneapolis, MN: Pearson.

Tasse, M. J. (2009). Adaptive behavior assessment and the diagnosis of mental retardation in capital cases. *Applied Neuropsychology, 16*, 114–123.

Wechsler, D. (1974). *Manual for the Wechsler Intelligence Scale for Children–Revised.* San Antonio, TX: Psychological Corporation.

Wechsler, D. (1991). *Wechsler Intelligence Scale for Children–Third Edition.* San Antonio, TX: Psychological Corporation.

Wechsler, D. (2003). *Wechsler Intelligence Scale for Children–Fourth Edition.* San Antonio, TX: The Psychological Corporation.

Wechsler, D. (2008). *Wechsler Adult Intelligence Scale–Fourth Edition Technical and Interpretative Manual.* San Antonio, TX: Pearson, Psychological Corporation.

Weiss, L. G. (2010). Considerations on the Flynn Effect. *Journal of Psychoeducational Assessment, 28*, 482–493.

CHAPTER 2

Toward a Synthesis of Cognitive-Psychological, Medical/ Neurobiological, and Educational Models for the Diagnosis and Management of Dyslexia

Nancy Mather, Bennett A. Shaywitz, *and* Sally E. Shaywitz

Abstract

The most common and best understood specific learning disability is dyslexia, or specific reading disability, a disorder that affects the development of word-level reading, reading rate, spelling, and certain aspects of oral language, particularly phonological awareness and word retrieval, but with verbal reasoning and listening comprehension intact. Both the assessment and the treatment of dyslexia have interested researchers for over a century, not only in education, but also in the fields of psychology and neurology. This chapter reviews this disorder from three varying theoretical, scientific, and practical perspectives or models: cognitive-psychological, which emphasizes exploration of a learner's strengths and weaknesses in an attempt to understand the reasons for the reading failure; medical/neurobiological, which addresses the etiology, basis and mechanisms, explaining and predicting the symptoms; and educational, which is driven by legal mandates, as well as services provided by school systems. Each model offers insights into and contributes to the fullest understanding of the nature of this disability, as well as the conceptual and methodological frameworks that can contribute to the formulation of a diagnosis.

Key Words: dyslexia, specific reading disability, response-to-intervention, ability–achievement discrepancies, intra-individual variations, neural organization in reading and dyslexia, learning disability

Specific learning disability (SLD) is a diagnostic category that encompasses a group of heterogeneous cognitive and linguistic disorders that typically affect some aspect of academic performance (e.g., reading, written language, mathematics). Although different types of SLD exist, the most common and well researched is a word-level reading problem often referred to as *dyslexia* (developmental dyslexia) or *specific reading disability* (SRD). The word "specific" is critical, as it indicates that individuals with dyslexia have specific cognitive assets but also specific deficits that lead to poor reading; this differentiates individuals with SLD from those

who have lower global intelligence (Hale, Kaufman, Naglieri, & Kavale, 2006). Because it is the most common learning disability (Lerner, 1989) and considerable evidence has accumulated regarding how children learn to read and why some experience difficulties (Bradley & Bryant, 1983; Hooper, 1996; Torgesen et al., 1999), the focus of this chapter is on dyslexia.

The definition of dyslexia as an *unexpected* difficulty in reading (Critchley 1970; Lyon 1995; Lyon, Shaywitz, & Shaywitz, 2003; Monroe, 1932; Peterson & Pennington, 2012) has remained invariant over the century since its first description

(Morgan, 1896). Dyslexia is found in readers of all languages, including both alphabetic and logographic scripts. Dyslexia is defined as a specific reading disability that is neurobiological in origin and characterized by difficulties with accurate and/or fluent word-recognition and spelling. The addition of the adjective *specific* implies that the poor reading performance emanates from a limited number of underlying deficits (Kavale & Forness, 2000), most typically from a deficit in the phonological component of language that is "unexpected" in relation to the person's other cognitive abilities.

Historical Perspective

One of the first descriptions of dyslexia is credited to an English general practitioner, W. Pringle Morgan (Morgan, 1896). Shortly thereafter, James Hinshelwood, a Scottish ophthalmologist at the Glasgow Eye Infirmary, presented additional cases of children and adults with dyslexia (termed *congenital word blindness* in that era). Hinshelwood not only described the cases but made recommendations regarding treatment. For example, in a monograph describing two cases of children with "word blindness," Hinshelwood (1902) concluded that:

(a) particular areas of the brain appear to be involved;

(b) the children often have average or above-average intelligence and good memory in other respects;

(c) the problem with reading is localized, not generalized to all areas of academic performance;

(d) the children do not learn to read with the same rapidity as other children;

(e) the earlier the problem is identified, the better, so as not to waste valuable instructional time;

(f) the children must be taught by special methods adapted to help them overcome their difficulties;

(g) the sense of touch can help children retain visual impressions; and

(h) persistent and persevering attempts will often help children improve their reading.

By 1917, Hinshelwood concluded that, "With the possession of a knowledge of the symptoms, there is little difficulty in the diagnosis of congenital word-blindness when the cases are met with, since the general picture of the condition stands out as clear-cut and distinct as that of any pathological condition in the whole range of medicine" (p. 88). This same sentiment was expressed over 85 years later:

"The diagnosis of dyslexia is as precise and scientifically informed as almost any diagnosis in medicine" (Shaywitz, 2003, p. 165).

These early case studies described individuals who often had normal intelligence and even excelled in other areas, but their poor reading and spelling performance were in sharp contrast to their other abilities. Through the analyses of case studies of individuals over several decades, two basic concepts emerged: (1) the concept of unexpected under-achievement (that reading performance was unexpected or unpredicted based upon the person's higher cognitive abilities); and (2) the notion of variations among learning abilities (intra-individual variations).

Prevalence and Course of Dyslexia

As with other disabilities, the specific prevalence rate for dyslexia will reflect the particular definition and cut-points established as criteria for identification. Data emanating from multiple sources indicate that, for large segments of the population, reading remains effortful, and skilled reading elusive. For example, results of the 2005 National Assessment of Educational Progress (NAEP) indicated that 27% of high school seniors are reading below the most basic levels (i.e., the minimum level at which a student can demonstrate an understanding of what has been read (Grigg, Donahue, & Dion, 2007), and 36% of fourth-grade children are reading below basic levels (Perie, Grigg, & Donahue, 2005). In the Connecticut Longitudinal Study sample survey in which each participant was individually assessed, 17.5% of students were reading below age or ability levels (S. Shaywitz, Fletcher, & Shaywitz, 1994). This population has been followed continuously since 1983 with yearly individual assessments of their cognitive, academic, behavioral, social, and more recently, neurobiological characteristics. Accordingly, these longitudinal data permit examination of issues relating to the developmental course of reading difficulties and indicate the persistence and chronicity of reading problems, refuting the notion, long and tightly held, that reading difficulties can be "outgrown" or merely reflect a developmental lag (Francis, Shaywitz, Stuebing, Shaywitz, & Fletcher, 1996; B. Shaywitz, Fletcher, & Shaywitz, 1995). While the problems are persistent, it is important to keep in mind that the expression of the reading difficulty may change with time, so that difficulties with reading accuracy, especially in very bright children, often evolve into relatively accurate, but dysfluent, reading (S. Shaywitz,

Morris, & Shaywitz, 2008). Spelling difficulties also persist. In fact, poor spelling is often described as a hallmark of dyslexia (Gregg, 2009). Difficulties with word retrieval, fluent reading, and spelling persist throughout adulthood.

These explanatory and causative factors of dyslexia have interested researchers in the fields of psychology, neurology, and education for over a century (Hinshelwood, 1917; Monroe, 1935; Morgan, 1896; Orton, 1925). Thus, the assessment and diagnosis of dyslexia can be viewed from varying perspectives. Each perspective offers insights into the multifaceted perceptions and nature of this disability, as well as the conceptual, philosophical, and methodological frameworks that may be incorporated into the diagnostic process.

Cognitive-Psychological Models

Cognitive-psychological models of dyslexia attempt to explain human variability in terms of both the consistencies and inconsistencies within performance. From this perspective, researchers and practitioners have attempted to answer the central question of *why* some people struggle to learn to read. Typically, the basic information for psychological study is gathered through a comprehensive evaluation that addresses both the intrinsic and extrinsic factors related to reading, considering areas of strength as well as areas of weakness. In fact, from a cognitive-psychological perspective, the primary goal of a cognitive assessment is to acquire data specific to understanding the core cognitive constructs and traits that underlie reading development and achievement (Feifer, 2008; Semrud-Clikeman, 2005; Witsken, Stoeckel, & D'Amato, 2008). The results from a comprehensive evaluation can help determine the nature of the individual's difficulties, whether or not special education is necessary, and the type of individualized instruction that will be most beneficial.

The basic defining component of nearly all cognitive-psychological definitions of SLD in general and dyslexia specifically has been that one or more specific disorders exist in the basic psychological processes involved in learning. Because development is uneven, with some abilities being far more advanced than others, a *discrepancy*, then, often exists between a set of intact cognitive processes and one or more disordered processes (Hale, Kaufman, Naglieri, & Kavale, 2006; Hale, Naglieri, Kaufman, & Kavale, 2004). These weaknesses in basic psychological processes, compared to strengths in other processes, often referred to as intra-cognitive or intra-individual discrepancies or variations (unexpected differences), are considered to be the hallmark of SLD (A. S. Kaufman & Kaufman, 2001; Kavale, Kaufman, Naglieri, & Hale, 2005). Thus, in the case of dyslexia, the central purpose of a comprehensive cognitive-psychological assessment is to document cognitive integrities and unexpected deficits within the basic cognitive-psychological processes that are linked to the reading difficulties (Hale et al., 2004; Kaufman, 2004). This type of evaluation documents the learning abilities, as well as the learning disabilities (Kaufman, 2008).

Figure 30.1 represents the major goal of a cognitive-psychological dyslexia assessment, the basis for a pattern of strengths and weaknesses (PSW) approach. The purpose is to examine patterns of cognitive strengths and weaknesses and determine how these patterns relate to and affect

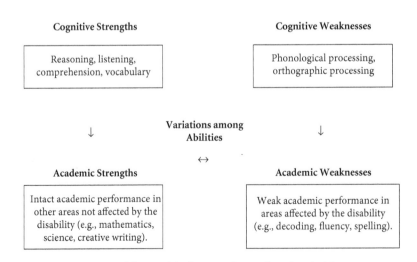

Figure 30.1 Relationships among cognitive abilities and the diagnosis of a specific reading disability.

reading development. A PSW approach involves several steps: (a) identifying an academic need; (b) determining if areas of cognitive weakness exist that have a research-based link to academic performance; (c) establishing cognitive and linguistic strengths; and (d) analyzing the results to see if the pattern is consistent with a profile of SLD (Schultz, Simpson, & Lynch, 2012). Essentially, the evaluator is attempting to explain the interrelationships among and between the individual's stronger and weaker cognitive and academic abilities.

In fact, the regulations of the Individuals with Disabilities Education Act (IDEA) §300.309(a)(2)(ii) also permit identification of a specific learning disability from consideration of whether or not the child exhibits a pattern of strengths and weaknesses in performance, achievement, or both, relative to her or his intellectual development. This provision is in line with the concept of intra-individual variations. This type of approach aligns the definition of SLD, as a deficit in basic psychological processing, with a possible way to operationalize identification. Kavale, Kauffman, Bachmeier, and Lefever (2008) noted: "Cognitive processing assessment aligns diagnostic procedures with a clearly articulated SLD definitional component: a disorder in one or more of the basic psychological processes" (p. 144). Children with SLD and dyslexia have *specific* cognitive deficits that lead to poorer academic performance than would be expected given their *specific* cognitive assets. This differentiates children with SLD from those with intellectual impairments (Hale et al., 2006, 2008).

In some aspects, the diagnosis of dyslexia falls within the framework of a PSW approach; however, the evaluator must have knowledge of the specific strengths and weaknesses that typify dyslexia. In the evaluation of children for dyslexia, the goal is to determine whether or not the particular PSW is symptomatic of dyslexia, such as a child with weaknesses in phonological processing, but strengths in listening comprehension and reasoning, a pattern consistent with an unexpected difficulty in reading. Proper use and interpretation of a PSW approach, incorporating the unexpected difficulty that characterizes dyslexia, could result in a true synthesis of the cognitive-psychological, the medical, and the educational models.

In the case of dyslexia, the central academic problems are difficulties with accurate and/or fluent word recognition and poor decoding and spelling abilities, as well as difficulties in word retrieval (Hanly & Vandenberg, 2010). This weakness in word reading is often surrounded by a "sea of strengths," wherein the individual's reasoning, general knowledge, and critical thinking abilities are intact, or even advanced (Shaywitz, 2003). For example, in many cases, often what distinguishes individuals with dyslexia from other poor readers is that their listening comprehension ability is significantly higher than their ability to decode nonsense words (Rack, Snowling, & Olson, 1992).

Though difficulties in phonological processing are most common in dyslexia, other factors may be associated with the poor reading. For example, one student may have poor phonological awareness, but strengths in listening comprehension and vocabulary, which may serve as partial compensation for the weakness in phonological processing. In another case, a student may have advanced reasoning and linguistic abilities, but poor orthographic awareness that may be exacerbated by overall slow processing speed (Konold, Juel, McKinnon, & Deffes, 2003). Variations, then, often exist between and among the person's intact and deficient cognitive and academic abilities. Konold et al. explained that learning to read is a multivariate phenomenon that is best understood by joint consideration of these processes and their influences on reading outcomes. Although much is known, questions still remain about the exact nature of the interrelationships among these variables (Bell, McCallum, & Cox, 2003).

Intra-Individual Variations

Intra-individual variations are determined through an analysis of a profile of cognitive-psychological abilities. In order to identify the unique abilities of an individual, the first line of analysis is the individual case study (Fawcett & Nicolson, 2007). An essential element of this diagnostic study is an exploration of the individual's cognitive and linguistic abilities to determine not only the unexpected nature of the reading difficulties but also how these other cognitive-psychological abilities may be related to the reading difficulties. Within the cognitive-psychological model, Ferrer, Shaywitz, Holahan, Marchione, and Shaywitz (2010) used dynamic modeling within a longitudinal framework to examine the relationship between cognitive and academic (reading) ability in different groups of readers. The findings confirmed the uncoupling of cognitive ability and reading ability in subjects with dyslexia. Specifically, using data from the Connecticut Longitudinal Study, Ferrer and associates provided empirical evidence demonstrating differences in the dynamics of reading and cognition between typical readers and those with dyslexia. Typical readers manifest mutual dynamics between reading and intelligence (IQ) with positive interrelations between both over time. For readers with dyslexia, however, such interrelationships are not perceptible, suggesting that reading and cognition develop more independently. These new data, based on dynamic models, provide an explanation for the "unexpected" nature of developmental dyslexia and provide the long-sought empirical evidence for the seeming paradox involving cognition and reading in individuals with developmental dyslexia.

Thus, valid dyslexia diagnosis uses data including both cognitive and achievement information. The assessment often reveals discrepancies among intact processes and those that are disordered (Hale et al., 2004); for example, the evaluator may find difficulties in phonological processing and reading fluency in comparison to strengths in other cognitive abilities. Some factors, such as working memory (Baddeley, 2007; Baddeley, 2012; Baddeley, Eysenck, & Anderon, 2009), have been associated with poor reading. Poor working memory may be particularly characteristic of students who have both dyslexia and attention deficit/hyperactivity disorder (ADHD) (Bental & Tirosh, 2007). Cognitive factors, such as phonological awareness, verbal short-term memory, orthographic awareness, rapid naming, and processing speed, have been shown to be correlates of reading failure, or in essence, factors contributing to specific reading impairments. In addition, problems with attention can also play a critical role. We briefly review each of these examples of cognitive correlates below.

PHONOLOGICAL PROCESSING

As noted above, difficulties with phonological processing represent the most commonly reported problem in dyslexia (Morris et al., 1998). "Phonological processing" includes phonological awareness, a component of oral language ability that encompasses the abilities to attend to, discriminate, and manipulate individual speech sounds. This metacognitive understanding involves the realization that spoken language is composed of a series of discrete speech sounds (phonemes) that are arranged in a particular sequence (Clark & Uhry, 1995). *Phonemic awareness* refers to the ability to discern and identify the smallest individual speech sounds or phonemes, whereas *phonological awareness* is a broader term that includes phonemes, as well as all types of larger elements of speech that can be assessed by asking the child to rhyme words or

count the number of syllables in a word. Both types of awareness involve the understanding that speech can be divided into sounds and these sounds can then be sequenced into a series to form syllables and words. In addition, working-memory abilities may influence some phonemic awareness tasks, such as phoneme-deletion tasks in which the person says a word while omitting a sound (e.g., say the word "nice," without the /n/ sound) or phoneme-reversal tasks in which the person reorders the sounds in a word to make a new word (e.g., Say the word "tip." Now say the sounds in the word "tip" backwards), since these tasks involve both storing and manipulating phonemes (Gathercole & Alloway, 2008; Savage, Lavers, & Pillay, 2007; Tunmer & Hoover, 1992).

Weaknesses in phonological processing play a critical role in dyslexia (Shaywitz, 2003; Willcutt, Pennington, Olson, Chhabildas, & Hulslander, 2005). While spoken language is natural and instinctive, print or written language is artificial and must be learned (Shaywitz, 2003). Brain mechanisms are in place to process the sounds of language automatically, but not the letters and words that make up print. Accordingly, these printed elements must link to something that is accepted by the neural machinery and has inherent meaning—the sounds of spoken language. To read, a child first must pull apart the spoken words into their individual sounds, link the letters to their appropriate sound (phonics), and then blend the sounds together. Thus, the awareness that spoken words come apart and the ability to notice and identify phonemes, these smallest elements of sound, allow the child to link letters to sound. In order to read, a child first must master what is referred to as "the alphabetic principle"; i.e., develop the awareness that the printed word has the same number and sequence of sounds as the spoken word. Phonemic awareness abilities have their primary impact on the development of phonics skills, or knowledge of the ways that letters represent the sounds in printed words (Torgesen & Mathes, 2000), as well as on encoding or spelling development (Bailet, 2001).

Reflecting the core phonological deficit, a range of downstream effects is observed in spoken as well as in written language (S. Shaywitz et al., 2008). Phonological processing is critical to both spoken and written language. While most attention has centered on print difficulties, the ability to notice, manipulate, and retrieve phonological elements also has an important function in speaking. For example, uttering a spoken word requires a two-step mechanism involving, first, semantic and then, phonological components (Levelt, Roelofs, & Meyer, 1999).

In dyslexia, it is the second step involving phonology that is affected (Hanly & Vandenberg, 2010). First, one must generate the concept of what one wants to communicate; this in turn triggers activation of the semantic or meaning-based representation of the word in the speaker's lexicon. However, in order to speak the word, once the concept and associated semantic form are activated, the lexical representations must be transformed into their phonological codes. To accomplish this, in the second step, the speaker accesses and retrieves the phonological representations (phonological codes) that link to the semantic structures, a necessary step in order to generate the articulatory (motor) patterns that are ultimately put into action by the articulatory muscles, resulting in the production of the spoken word.

In dyslexia, activation of the concept and its semantic representation proceeds smoothly; however, it is the second step, the transformation of the semantic (meaning) into the phonological (sound) code that is disrupted. A feedback mechanism enables the speaker to monitor his or her own speech and exercise some output control to correct errors. However, if the individual is anxious, as often is the case in dyslexia, word retrieval is further negatively affected. In fact, a considerable body of research indicates that anxiety disorders are frequently observed in individuals with dyslexia. Thus, higher levels of anxiety have been found in college students with dyslexia as compared to control college students, particularly in social situations and during interviews (Carroll & Iles, 2006). In adolescents, anxiety disorders were three times more prevalent in readers with dyslexia; in particular, social phobia and generalized anxiety disorder were both five times more prevalent among readers with dyslexia than among typical readers. In this study, many of the students with social phobia indicated that rather than have to talk in front of the class or make presentations, they would often skip classes or even accept lower grades (Goldston et al., 2007). More recently, the association between SLD and anxiety was further buttressed using meta-analysis, concluding that students with SLD had statistically significant increased scores on measures of anxiety (Nelson & Harwood, 2011).

As a consequence of this sound-based difficulty in accessing and retrieving the phonological codes, an individual with dyslexia, no matter how intelligent or well educated, may exhibit difficulties in word retrieval, so that his/her verbal output does not represent his/her abilities and knowledge. Thus,

it should not be surprising that problems with spoken language are often observed. These include late speaking, mispronunciations, difficulties with word retrieval, needing time to summon an oral response, and confusing words that sound alike, such as saying "recession" when the individual means to say "reception" (Faust, Dimitrovsky, & Shacht, 2003; Faust & Sharfstein-Friedman, 2003). Dyslexia is conceptualized as a "sea of strengths" in higher cognitive functions surrounding weaknesses in phonological awareness and fluent reading (Shaywitz, 2003). Thus, the same individual who struggles to retrieve words and reads slowly with effort may have great strengths in conceptual abilities, problem solving, verbal reasoning, the ability to grasp the big picture, and what has been referred to as creative or out-of-the-box thinking. Indeed, it is just these higher-level strengths that make it imperative for individuals who have dyslexia to receive the accommodations (e.g., extra time) they require in order to demonstrate their abilities (S. Shaywitz et al., 2008). When individuals have weaknesses in phonological awareness, interventions often focus on improving phonological awareness, accompanied by specific instruction in phoneme-grapheme relationships (phonics).

VERBAL SHORT-TERM MEMORY

In addition to phonologically related processes, memory-related processes also appear to contribute to dyslexia (Crews & D'Amato, 2009; Swanson, Zheng, & Jerman, 2009). Children with dyslexia have weaknesses in verbal short-term memory or the immediate serial recall of unrelated words (Kibby & Cohen, 2008; Steinbrink & Klatte, 2008). In a meta-analysis that included 43 studies between 1963 and 2006, Swanson et al. (2009) found that children with reading disabilities performed poorly on tasks that required non-word repetition as well as the immediate recall of letter, number, and word strings. A weakness in repeating nonsense words may indicate a problem in the overall quality of the phonological storage system, which would then relate to both phonological processing and word learning (Gathercole, 2006).

ORTHOGRAPHIC AWARENESS

Although difficulties in phonological processing are often described as the most common cause of reading disability, other cognitive and linguistic domains can also be involved (Friedmann & Lukov, 2008). For example, word recognition skill begins with phonological awareness, but then in skilled reading, orthographic representations take on an increasingly important role (Perfetti, 2011). Some have suggested that, in addition to phonological awareness, orthographic awareness should be viewed as a unique factor in the assessment and diagnosis of developmental dyslexia (Badian, 2005: Mano & Osmon, 2008; Roberts & Mather, 1997). High-functioning college students with dyslexia make some use of phonological skills to spell familiar words, but they still have difficulty memorizing orthographic patterns and recalling spelling rules, which results in inconsistent spellings of irregular and less familiar words (Kemp, Parrila, & Kirby, 2009).

Whereas phonological processing addresses acquisition of the sound system, orthographic processing reflects one's knowledge of the spelling system and the relationships between the speech sounds and print. Orthographic processing permits a reader to access from memory a whole word unit, a letter cluster unit, or a component letter (Berninger, 1996). Because orthographic knowledge enables instant recognition of letter chunks or whole words, it is more related to measures of reading speed than to measures of reading accuracy (Georgiou, Parrila, Kirby, & Stephenson, 2008). Students with weaknesses in orthography have particular difficulties remembering letter sequences and reading and spelling words that contain irregular spelling patterns (e.g., "once"), some believe because they do not have mental images of words stored in memory or word-specific memory (Ehri, 2000). This ability to store the orthographic forms of words in memory may play a role in attaining fluency in reading (Reitsma, 1989), as it helps readers establish detailed visual or mental representations of words that then allow rapid access to these representations. Individuals who fail to develop appropriate representations in the phonological and semantic regions of the brain may struggle to read because the brain lacks the hierarchial connections required to make predictions based on visual stimuli and contextual cues (Price & Devlin, 2011). Later in the chapter, we discuss the neurobiological correlate of this process in a specific neural system—the word-form area.

Successful spelling involves the abilities to remember the position of each letter in the word and to recall the letters in the correct sequence. Knowledge of orthographic structure (the constraints of permissible letter sequences) is evidenced by the ability to place common letter strings in the correct order (e.g., the letters "ck" would be used to end a word, but not to begin a word). Although unexpected letters and irregular spelling patterns may be stored in these representations, securing these images is more difficult than securing words that conform to common spelling patterns (Ehri, 2000). Even when accuracy improves for students with dyslexia, their reading remains effortful and slow even into late adolescence, and difficulties persist throughout adulthood (S. Shaywitz & Shaywitz, 2008).

In addition, students with weaknesses in orthography tend to regularize the element of the word that does not conform to a language's spelling rules. Their attempted spellings often violate the underlying rules of English spelling. Thus, they spell words the way they sound, rather than the way they look (e.g., spelling "houses" as "howssis"). Common methods for assessing orthographic awareness involve reading and spelling exception words and homophone choice tasks (e.g., Which is a flower?—*rows* or *rose*?) (Barker, Torgesen, & Wagner, 1992; Stanovich, West, & Cunningham, 1991). Because the pronunciation leads to the same sounds, phonological mediation does not help one identify the correct spelling; the reader must consult the orthographic input lexicon to know which spelling is correct (Friedmann & Lukov, 2008). In addition, the speed of perception of letter, word, and word-like stimuli is an important component of visual word recognition (Mano & Osmon, 2008). In individuals with poor orthographic awareness, interventions often focus on mastering common spelling patterns, as well as increasing the rate of word perception.

RAPID AUTOMATIZED NAMING (RAN)

Naming speed, also known as rapid automatized naming (RAN), is another cognitive variable that appears to be related to reading difficulties (Denckla & Cutting, 1999). RAN is often measured by asking an individual to name a series of repeating randomly ordered colors, objects, letters, or digits, as quickly as possible. As with poor orthographic awareness, slow RAN performance seems to be more related to reading speed than reading accuracy (Georgiou et al., 2008). RAN is a good predictor of orthographic skills, but not untimed non-word reading (Abu-Hamour, 2009; Abu-Hamour, Urso, & Mather, 2012). Early on in reading development, RAN reflects both phonological and orthographic processing, but later on RAN primarily relates to orthographic processing and reading speed (Georgiou et al., 2008).

Bowers and Wolf (1993) hypothesized that slow RAN signifies disruption of the automatic processes that result in quick word recognition. Morris et al. (1998) described these individuals as having a "rate deficit" because they were impaired on tasks requiring rapid serial naming but not on measures of phonological awareness. Bowers, Sunseth, and Golden (1999) concluded that their results give some support to the notion that (a) students with RAN impairments have less knowledge of orthographic patterns and are slower readers than students with poor phonemic awareness, and (b) orthographic pattern knowledge may depend, in part, on the processes tapped by naming speed. Further research has suggested that the significance of the relationship between RAN and word reading may be attributable to the fact that both require fast cross-modal matching of visual symbols and phonological codes, a process that is not measured by phonological awareness tasks (Vaessen, Gerretsen, & Blomert, 2009).

PROCESSING SPEED

Processing speed is another important cognitive mediator and a correlate of reading failure in children and adults (Evans, Floyd, McGrew, & LeForgee, 2002; Gregg, Coleman, Davis, Lindstrom, & Hartwig, 2006; Kail, 1991; Kail, Hall, & Caskey, 1999; Konold et al., 2003; Shanahan et al, 2006; Trainin & Swanson, 2005; Urso, 2008; Willcutt et al., 2005). In analyzing processing speed performance in a group of poor readers, Urso (2008) found that processing speed was a significant weakness in over one-third of the sample. Although less research has addressed processing speed, the impact of slow processing speed on reading performance appears to be most related to reading speed. Based on a cross-sectional study using structural equation modeling, processing speed has been suggested to have a direct effect on reading fluency that increases with each grade (Benson, 2007). However, given that this was a cross-sectional study, this finding needs to be replicated using longitudinal data.

Children with dyslexia have problems making reading-related skills automatic through practice. Their difficulty lies not just in decoding the words, but also in the rate and ease of decoding; their basic reading skills do not become effortless and automatic over time (Semrud-Clikeman, 2005; S. Shaywitz & Shaywitz, 2008). Processing speed may be related to the reading of words with irregular spelling patterns (e.g., "once"), but not to the reading of nonsense words that conform to English spelling patterns (e.g., "flib") (Abu-Hamour, 2009; Abu-Hamour et al., 2012). Poor performance on processing speed tasks could be attributable to several different factors, including slow motor speed, inefficiency of visual scanning, or weaknesses in attention.

Slow processing speed has also been described as a common characteristic of students with ADHD (Shanahan et al., 2006; Willcutt et al., 2005). In a large sample of 395 children with dyslexia and/ or ADHD, Shanahan et al. found that slow processing speed was a shared cognitive risk factor for both disorders, but that children with dyslexia had greater impairments than did children with ADHD. Good evidence relates automaticity of reading to the development of the word-form area in the left occipito-temporal brain region; however, while processing speed may relate to automaticity of reading, the neurobiological evidence for this relationship is yet to be demonstrated. As described later in the chapter, readers with dyslexia exhibit an inefficiency of functioning in this region, suggesting that the inefficient functioning of the left occipito-temporal word-form area is the neural correlate of the lack of automaticity of reading in dyslexia.

ATTENTION

Disruption of attentional mechanisms may also play an important role in reading and dyslexia (S. Shaywitz & Shaywitz, 2008). Although ADHD and dyslexia are distinct disorders, 15% to 40% of students with dyslexia also meet the criteria for ADHD (Bental & Tirosh, 2007; B. A. Shaywitz, Fletcher, & Shaywitz, 1995; Willcutt & Pennington, 2000). Although progress has been made, the neuropsychological profile for ADHD is not as well understood as the correlates of dyslexia (Willcutt et al., 2005). Results from preliminary studies suggest that pharmacotherapeutic agents used for the treatment of ADHD may also prove to be valuable for potentially new adjunct treatment options for dyslexia (S. Shaywitz & Shaywitz, 2008).

Academic and Classroom Functioning

Within the classroom, a teacher will note a range of difficulties in reading (e.g., misreading especially small function words and unfamiliar words, slow reading); spelling; the ability to master a foreign language; oral language (retrieving spoken words, lack of glibness); handwriting; and attention (Shaywitz 2003). The lack of reading fluency brings with it a need to read "manually" (a process consuming great effort), rather than automatically; the cost of such reading is a tremendous drain on the student's attentional resources. This is often observed in the classroom when struggling readers are asked to read quietly; they deplete their attentional resources as they struggle to decipher the print, and, as a consequence, appear to be daydreaming or not attending to the assigned reading.

In contrast to these difficulties, and consistent with the unexpected nature of dyslexia, other cognitive abilities, including thinking, reasoning, vocabulary, and listening comprehension are intact, and in fact may even be superior. Intact higher-level abilities offer an explanation of why reading comprehension is often appreciably better than single-word reading accuracy and fluency in individuals with dyslexia (reviewed in Shaywitz, 2003). As children mature, compensation often occurs, resulting in relatively accurate, but not fluent, reading. Awareness of this developmental pattern is critically important for the diagnosis of dyslexia in older children, young adults, and beyond. The consequence is that older children with dyslexia may appear to perform reasonably well on an untimed test of word reading or decoding because these tests give credit for a response regardless of how long it takes the individual to pronounce the word or whether the person corrects his or her initial word reading errors. Accordingly, tests of reading fluency that measure how quickly and accurately individual words and passages are read and tests assessing reading rate are essential assessment components

for an accurate diagnosis of dyslexia (Mather & Wendling, 2012; S. Shaywitz et al., 2008).

In summary, the essence of the cognitive-psychological perspective is the development of a thorough case study that explores an individual's unique learning profile. The elements of the cognitive and psychological strengths and weaknesses forming the individual's learning profile coalesce to explain that individual's reading difficulties, as well as his or her academic functioning in classroom settings. Together, the results of the cognitive-psychological assessment and the clinical history provide the elements for the diagnosis of dyslexia. Dyslexia is a clinical diagnosis, best made by an experienced clinician who has taken a careful history, observed the individual speaking and reading, and administered a battery of tests that assess cognitive abilities; academic skills including reading accuracy, fluency, and comprehension, spelling, mathematics (which is often average or high); and language skills, particularly phonological processing (Marzola & Shepherd, 2005; Shaywitz, 2003). The uneven peaks and valleys of cognitive and academic functioning contribute to the clinical picture of dyslexia: a weakness in phonologically based or orthographically based skills in the

Table 30.1 Assessment for Dyslexia*

The School-Age Child: Grade 2 and beyond
1. History: *** Ask about weaknesses in:*
Spoken language:
History of delayed speech
Mispronunciations of words
Lack of verbal fluency, hesitations before responding, lack of glibness
Word retrieval difficulties
Needing time to summon an oral response when questioned
Reading:
Difficulty learning letters and learning to associate letters with their sounds
Slow progress in acquiring reading skills
Trouble reading (pronouncing) new or unfamiliar words that must be sounded out
Omitting parts of words when reading
Confusing words of similar appearance (e.g. *who* and *how*)
Needing substantial repetition and review to develop a sight-reading vocabulary
Relying on use of context to discern the meaning of what is read

(continued)

Table 30.1 (Continued)

Disproportionately poor performance on multiple-choice tests
Reading slowly with much effort—even with improvement in reading accuracy
Having good knowledge of the material but nevertheless unable to finish tests on time
Fear of reading out loud
Avoiding reading
Messy and illegible handwriting
Spelling difficulties
Difficulty learning foreign languages
Increasing anxiety related to testing situations and to speaking on demand, reading and spelling
History: Ask about strengths in higher-level conceptualization and abstract, out-of-the box thinking
Strong ability to conceptualize, excellent reasoning skills
Strong ability to grasp the "big picture"
Listening comprehension that is much higher than reading comprehension
Excellence in areas not dependent on reading—visual arts, conceptual (versus fact-driven) subjects such as biology, philosophy, social studies, neuroscience, and creative writing (ignoring spelling errors and focusing on content)
2. Observation of individual speaking and reading aloud
Spoken language not fluent, hesitations, mispronunciations, not glib
Reading aloud—mispronunciations, omission and insertion of words, pauses, labored and choppy, poor prosody (phrasing and expression)
3. Cognitive and academic testing
Intelligence and linguistic abilities—pattern of peaks and valleys: strengths in abstract thinking; reasoning, vocabulary; information. Indications of ability to think and reason above ability to read accurately or fluently, reflecting the unexpected nature of dyslexia.
Weaknesses in oral language (e.g., phonological processing) and written language (orthographic processing, e.g., spelling)
Weaknesses in:
Basic reading skills: word identification; word attack (nonsense words)
Reading fluency: real and nonsense words
Reading passages out loud
Reading rate in connected text
Reading comprehension with and without time constraints
Spelling: real and nonsense words
Assessment for potential strengths (e.g., math problem-solving; reasoning; listening comprehension).

*The testing and interpretation will vary according to the age and education of the person. The approach above is relevant to school-age children in Grade 2 and higher. (Symptoms of spoken-language difficulties may be present in preschool children, and reading accuracy may significantly improve in young adults and adults while substantial problems in reading fluency persist.)

**Adapted with permission from © S. Shaywitz, "Overcoming Dyslexia" (Knopt, 2003) context of stronger cognitive and academic skills in non-reading-related areas. Dyslexia is more than simply a score on a reading test. Accordingly, the focus of a cognitive-psychological approach is not solely on test scores, but rather on understanding the unique learning profile, history, characteristics, and circumstances of an individual so that instruction can be tailored to meet his or her individual needs. Table 30.1 provides an overview of questions and characteristics to consider in the assessment of dyslexia.

Exceptionally bright and capable students with dyslexia, who are sometimes referred to as being "twice exceptional," may fail to meet current school-based criteria if a rigid psychometric approach is taken that ignores that individual's functioning in a full range of psychometric and clinical areas. In order to make an accurate diagnosis, an evaluator must, when comparing higher-level cognitive functions to reading related difficulties such as phonological processing and reading fluency, keep in mind that dyslexia reflects an *unexpected* difficulty within the individual. As such, the evaluator must consider the person's special circumstances, unique abilities, educational history, and outstanding areas of competence (Mather & Gerner, 2009; S. Shaywitz & Shaywitz, 2012). Psychological and cognitive tests are diagnostic tools that help people understand and explain the reasons for an individual's reading difficulties, the types of reading difficulties present, as well as the severity of the disability. These measures can help us understand the reasons why a student is struggling (Mather & Kaufman, 2006). At the same time, such measures are only proxies, attempts to reflect cognitive processes; they take second place to the reality of life experiences.

A variety of cognitive skills can be implicated in the acquisition of reading skills (Bell et al., 2003). An analysis of the assessment results of an individual often leads to an increased understanding of the cause or causes of the reading disability, as well as providing pertinent information related to treatment and the need for accommodations. Over seventy years ago, Stanger and Donohue (1937) made the following observation: "If these tests will give us a basis from which we can start to understand a child's difficulties, they will have justified the time spent on them. Anything which helps educators or parents to *understand* any phase of development or lack of development is of immeasurable value" (p. 189).

Additionally, after careful consideration of all factors, the evaluator attempts to select the most appropriate accommodations and interventions for the individual. (See Mather & Wendling, 2012; and Shaywitz, 2003, for descriptions of effective interventions for the treatment of dyslexia.) Clearly, the primary goal of an assessment is to enhance intervention (Shaywitz, 2003). Over seven decades ago, Monroe (1935) observed: "After proper diagnosis of the child's difficulty, remedial work, if carried out consistently, is usually highly successful. The foundation of remedial success is careful observation of the pupil, with thorough diagnostic analysis, careful tabulation and study of his errors, and ingenuity in applying specific treatment" (p. 228). Identifying cognitive integrities, as well as specific needs, is a prerequisite of intervention efficacy, as is having a deep understanding of the condition, such as dyslexia, that is impacting reading development (Hale et al., 2004). In the case of adults who have a long-standing diagnosis of dyslexia and who have a good understanding of their learning profile, as well as their need for accommodations, a new or re-evaluation should not be necessary or required. Dyslexia is established as a persistent chronic condition characterized by a lack of fluency and slow reading, poor spelling, and word retrieval difficulties that persist throughout the lifespan.

Medical/Neurobiological Models

The term *medical model* is often mentioned in reference to education. Unfortunately, the term is sometimes used pejoratively, suggesting that somehow use of this model is trying to "medicalize" what is primarily an educational concern. In our view, "medical model" refers to an approach that considers the many facets of an entity in a systematic, organized manner, including its definition, prevalence, course, etiology, symptoms, signs, diagnosis, intervention, and management. Importantly, the medical model is a diagnostic one that synthesizes all available information—neurobiological, clinical, and assessment—to arrive at a cohesive, integrated, big-picture understanding of an individual's symptoms. A diagnosis provides much more than a listing of psychological processes; a diagnosis provides critical information about "the whole." Awareness of the diagnosis provides both the individual and treaters, including educators, a link to the large body of knowledge relating to that diagnosis, including its underlying neurobiological mechanisms, prevalence, developmental course, outcome, and effective treatments. Some of these issues were examined above within the cognitive-psychological model. Here we will focus on one very vital and specific component of the medical model, the rapidly accumulating and converging evidence demonstrating the neural systems implicated in dyslexia. Perhaps most importantly, the information emerging from functional brain imaging has the unique power to provide the critical glue allowing synthesis of the cognitive-psychological and the medical model into a unified whole.

Neural Systems for Reading

Neural systems for reading were demonstrated more than a century ago, with descriptions of adults who (usually due to a stroke) suddenly lost their ability to read, a condition termed *acquired alexia* (Dejerine, 1891, 1892). Within the last two decades, the development of functional brain imaging, particularly functional magnetic resonance imaging (fMRI), has provided the most consistent and replicable data on the localization of the neural systems for reading and how they differ in readers with dyslexia. FMRI is non-invasive and safe and can be used repeatedly, properties that make it ideal for studying people, especially children. The signal used to construct MRI images derives from the determination of the blood-oxygen-level-dependent (BOLD) response; the increase in BOLD signal in brain regions that are activated by a stimulus or task results from the combined effects of increases in the tissue blood flow, volume, and oxygenation. On cognitive tasks, BOLD changes are typically in the order of 1%–5%. Details of fMRI are reviewed in several sources (e.g., Anderson & Gore, 1997; Frackowiak et al., 2004; Jezzard, Matthews, & Smith, 2001).

Reflecting the language basis for reading and dyslexia, three critical neural systems are localized in the left hemisphere: two left-hemisphere posterior systems, one around the parieto-temporal region and another in the left occipito-temporal region; and an anterior system around the inferior frontal gyrus (Broca's area) (Brambati et al., 2006; Kronbichler et al., 2006; Nakamura, Dehaene, Jobert, Le Bihan, & Kouider, 2007; Nakamura et al., 2006; Paulesu et al., 2001; Rumsey et al., 1992; Seki et al., 2001; B. Shaywitz et al., 2002; S. Shaywitz et al., 1998; S. Shaywitz et al., 2003). (See Figure 30.2.)

Many brain imaging studies in patients with developmental dyslexia (see below) have documented the importance of the parieto-temporal system in reading, properties involving word analysis, operating on individual units of words (e.g., phonemes). The parieto-temporal system encompasses portions of the supramarginal gyrus in the inferior parietal lobule, portions of the posterior aspect of the superior temporal gyrus, and the angular gyrus in the parietal lobe. The second posterior reading system is localized in the occipito-temporal area, which Cohen and Dehaene have termed the *visual word-form area* (VWFA; Cohen et al., 2000; Dehaene, Cohen, Sigman, & Vinckier, 2005; Dehaene et al., 2001; Gaillard et al., 2006; Vinckier et al., 2007) and their colleagues refer to as the *ventral occipito-temporal cortex* [(reviewed in Price & Devlin, 2011)]. Still another reading-related neural circuit involves an anterior

Neural Systems for Reading

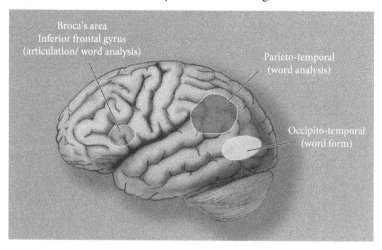

Figure 30.2 Neural systems for reading. This figure illustrates three neural systems for reading on the surface of the left hemisphere: an anterior system in the region of the inferior frontal gyrus (Broca's area) believed to serve articulation and word analysis; and two posterior systems, one in the parieto-temporal region believed to serve word analysis, and a second in the occipito-temporal region (termed the "word-form area") believed to serve for the rapid, automatic, fluent identification of words. (Reprinted from S. Shaywitz, 2003, with permission.)

system in the inferior frontal gyrus (Broca's area), a system that has long been associated with articulation and also serves an important function in word analysis (Fiez & Peterson, 1998; Frackowiak et al., 2004). In recent studies inspired by Levelt's two-step model of language (Levelt et al., 1999), Heim and his colleagues (Heim et al., 2008) have further examined the function of two architectonic regions of the inferior frontal gyrus, BA 44 and BA 45.

The Reading Systems in Dyslexia

Converging evidence from many laboratories around the world has demonstrated what has been termed "a neural signature for dyslexia"; that is, a disruption of posterior reading systems during reading real words and pseudowords, and often what has been considered a compensatory over-activation in other parts of the reading system (see Figure 30.3). This evidence from fMRI has for the first time made visible what previously was a hidden disability. In a study from our own research group, we (B. Shaywitz et al., 2002) used fMRI to study 144 children, approximately half of whom had dyslexia and half of whom were typical readers. The children were asked to read pseudowords and real words. Our results indicated significantly greater activation in typical readers than in readers with dyslexia during phonological analysis in the posterior reading systems.

Other studies report similar findings in German and Italian readers with dyslexia. For example, Kronbichler et al. (2006) used sentences to study dysfluent compared to fluent German readers. Individuals with dyslexia demonstrated reduced activation in the left supramarginal gyrus (parieto-temporal system) and left occipito-temporal system with compensatory activation in left inferior frontal area. Brambati et al. (2006), studying Italian adults with dyslexia as well as a family history of dyslexia, found reduced activation in posterior reading systems, paralleling results in English-speaking and German-speaking readers with dyslexia. Studies in Chinese readers with dyslexia show some differences, though the systems are generally the same. For example, in both typical Chinese readers and Chinese readers with dyslexia, there is more involvement of the left-middle frontal, superior parietal, and bilateral posterior visual regions and less for the inferior frontal and superior parietal regions (Perfetti, 2011). Thus, these data from fMRI studies in children with dyslexia reported by our group converge with reports from many investigators using fMRI that show a failure of left-hemisphere posterior brain systems to function properly during reading, particularly the systems in the left-hemisphere occipito-temporal region. (See Peterson & Pennington, 2012; Price & Mechelli, 2005; Richlan, Kronbichler, & Wimmer, 2009; 2011; S. Shaywitz & Shaywitz, 2005, for reviews.)

Recent findings indicate differences between readers with dyslexia and typical readers in connectivity of the visual word-form area (VWFA) and other components of the reading system. In typical readers, the VWFA was connected to distant and as well as adjacent reading systems in the left and right hemispheres. In contrast, functional connectivity in readers with dyslexia was significantly reduced to primarily adjacent areas in the left VWFA (van der Mark et al., 2011).

Neural Signature for Dyslexia: Disruption of Posterior Reading Systems

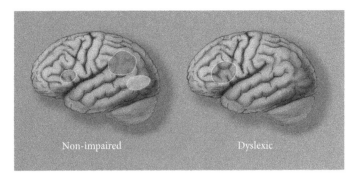

Figure 30.3 Neural signature for dyslexia. This schematic view depicts the left-hemisphere brain systems in both non-impaired readers (left) and readers with dyslexia (right). In non-impaired readers, the three systems are shown in Figure 30.2 In readers with dyslexia, the anterior system is slightly over-activated compared with systems of non-impaired readers; in contrast, the two posterior systems are under-activated. This pattern of under-activation in left-posterior reading systems is referred to as the "neural signature for dyslexia." (Reprinted from S. Shaywitz, 2003, with permission.)

Although readers with dyslexia exhibit an inefficiency of functioning in the left occipito-temporal word-form area, they appear to develop ancillary systems in other brain regions (B. Shaywitz et al., 2002). While these ancillary systems allow the reader to read accurately, readers with dyslexia continue to read dysfluently. Inefficient functioning in this essential system for skilled reading has very important practical implications for individuals with dyslexia—it provides the neurobiological evidence for the biological necessity for the accommodation of additional time on high-stakes tests (see Figure 30.4).

DEVELOPMENT OF READING SYSTEMS AND THE OCCIPITO-TEMPORAL READING SYSTEM

We examined just how the neural systems for reading develop in typical readers compared to those with dyslexia. We used fMRI to study age-related changes in reading in a cross-sectional study of 232 children (B. Shaywitz et al., 2007), comprising a group with dyslexia and a group of typical readers as they read pseudowords. Findings indicated that the neural systems for reading that develop with age in non-impaired readers differ from those that develop in readers with dyslexia. These findings noted below now permit a more fine-grained analysis of the word-form area by identifying two systems within the greater word-form area. Specifically, a system for reading that develops with age in readers with dyslexia differs from that in non-impaired readers,

primarily to being a more *posterior and medial system*, rather than a more *anterior and lateral system* within the left occipito-temporal area.

Interestingly, this difference in activation patterns between the two groups of readers has parallels to reported brain activation differences observed during reading of two Japanese writing systems: *Kana* and *Kanji*. Consideration of the mechanisms used for reading *Kanji* compared to *Kana* provides insights into potentially different mechanisms that develop with age in children with dyslexia as contrasted to non-impaired readers. Left anterior lateral occipito-temporal activation, similar to that seen in non-impaired readers, occurred during reading *Kana* (Nakamura, Dehaene, Jobert, Le Bihan, & Kouider, 2005). *Kana* script employs symbols that are linked to the sound or phonological element (comparable to English and other alphabetic scripts). In *Kana* and in alphabetic scripts, children initially learn to read words by learning how letters or symbols and sounds are linked, and then, over time, these linkages are integrated and permanently instantiated as a word form. In contrast, posterior medial occipito-temporal activation, comparable to that observed in readers with dyslexia, was noted during reading of *Kanji* script (Nakamura et al., 2005). *Kanji* script uses ideographs where each character must be memorized, suggesting that the posterior medial occipito-temporal system functions as a memory-based system.

Neural Basis for Extended Time

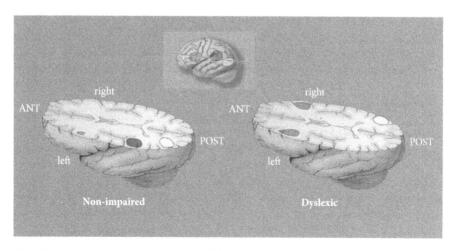

Figure 30.4 Neural basis for the requirement for extended time for students with dyslexia on high-stakes testing. This image shows a cutaway view of the brain so that both left and right hemispheres are visible. Non-impaired readers (*left panel*) activate three left-hemisphere neural systems for reading, an anterior system and two posterior systems. Readers with dyslexia (*right panel*) have inefficient functioning in the left-hemisphere posterior neural systems for reading but compensate by developing anterior systems in left and right hemispheres and the posterior homologue of the visual word-form area in the right hemisphere. This compensates for accuracy, but fluent reading remains impaired. (Reprinted from S. Shaywitz, 2003, with permission.)

Perhaps as children with dyslexia mature, this posterior medial system supports memorization rather than the progressive sound-symbol linkages observed in non-impaired readers. These findings are consonant with other evidence that readers with dyslexia are unable to make good use of sound-symbol linkages as they mature and instead come to rely on memorized words as they enter adolescence and adult life (Bruck, 1992; S. Shaywitz et al., 1999). Thus, persistently poor adult readers read words by memorization so that they are able to read familiar words but have difficulty reading unfamiliar words (S. Shaywitz et al., 2003). Furthermore, these data may help explain and confirm what many clinicians have observed; that is, the reliance by readers with dyslexia on memorization rather than phonological analysis in reading. This represents an example of neurobiological, cognitive-psychological, and educational findings and observations coalescing.

These results support and now extend previous findings to indicate that the system responsible for the fluent, automatic integration of letters and sounds, the word-form area in the anterior lateral occipito-temporal system, is the neural circuit that develops with age in typical readers. Just how the VWFA functions is the subject of intense investigation. Price and Devlin (2011), in what they term "the Interactive Account," suggest that this region acts to integrate phonological, orthographic, and semantic information, though some have suggested that visual familiarity, phonological processing, and semantic processing all make significant but different contributions to activation of the word-form region (Cohen et al., 2003; Cohen & Dehaene, 2004; Henry et al., 2005; Johnson & Rayner, 2007; Xue, Chen, Jin, & Dong, 2006). Readers with dyslexia who struggle to read new or unfamiliar words come to rely on an alternate system, the posterior medial occipito-temporal system that functions via memory networks.

IMPLICATIONS OF BRAIN IMAGING STUDIES

The brain imaging studies reviewed above provide neurobiological evidence that illuminates and clarifies our current understanding of the nature of dyslexia and its treatment. For example, brain imaging has taken dyslexia from what had previously been considered a hidden disability to one that is visible—as noted, these findings of a disruption in left-hemisphere posterior reading systems are often referred to as a "neural signature for dyslexia." These results should eliminate any speculation of whether or not dyslexia is a real or a "valid" diagnosis; even more so, these cutting-edge

converging data from imaging laboratories worldwide should encourage the use of the word *dyslexia*, as it has meaning and relevance at all levels, including the basic neural architecture essential for fluent reading and its disruption in struggling readers. As noted above, these findings, too, are universal, having been demonstrated in not only readers of English, but in readers of Italian, French, and German (Brambati et al., 2006; Kronbichler et al., 2006; Paulesu et al., 2001) and with similar findings in readers of logographic languages as well. In addition, the disruption of the neural systems for reading is found in younger and older readers; providing strong evidence for the persistence of reading difficulties, particularly the lack of fluency and with it, slow reading, throughout life. Here, an added implication is that past high school or the early years of post-secondary schooling, further assessment should not be needed to confirm the diagnosis or the need for accommodations.

Educational Models

Since the early descriptions of dyslexia (Morgan, 1896), a large body of research has shed much light on the nature, expression, and ontogeny of dyslexia, as well as on evidence-based approaches to treatment. The challenge is to reconcile this scientific knowledge with the constraints of educational settings. The goal is to honor the science and to translate it into a framework that will be practical and applicable in an educational setting with the primary objective of ensuring that struggling readers who require and would benefit from intervention are not overlooked. How can this be accomplished? Consistent with research and based on the fundamental concept of an unexpected difficulty in reading characterizing dyslexia, the discrepancy model—a discrepancy between cognitive ability and reading achievement—was applied to help determine if students had dyslexia and required educational intervention. Under IDEA 2004, in addition to an ability–achievement discrepancy, two alternative approaches have been proposed as potential methodologies for dyslexia identification: response to intervention (RTI) and alternative research-based methodologies (typically defined as a pattern of strengths and weaknesses [PSW] approach, described earlier).

Unexpected Nature of Dyslexia: Ability–Achievement Discrepancy

The purpose of the ability–achievement discrepancy in dyslexia diagnosis is to demonstrate whether a person's poor reading performance is unexpected in relationship to an estimate of cognitive ability. Although the concept is fundamental to SLD, the challenge becomes how to operationalize this discrepancy (S. Shaywitz et al., 2008). Ever since its incorporation in 1975 in PL 94–142, concern and dissatisfaction have been expressed regarding the use of a mathematical formula as the sole diagnostic criterion for SLD (e.g., Aaron, 1997; Bateman, 1992; Lyon, 1995; Mather & Healey, 1990; Stanovich, 1991). For the last three decades, the field seemingly has been focused more on developing specific mathematical formulae for SLD identification, by comparing intelligence and achievement test scores, rather than on the underlying concept of an unexpected difficulty in reading which was what the discrepancy was intended to represent. This rigid emphasis on global test scores and formulae often resulted in decreased attention to a careful analysis of both qualitative and quantitative information. Some have argued that focusing assessment on this type of discrepancy alone is too narrow, does not necessarily lead to instructional recommendations, and ignores the cognitive and linguistic abilities underlying academic achievement (Mather & Gregg, 2006; Semrud-Clikeman, 2005). In addition, the size of the required discrepancy has varied among states, as well as among school districts within states. Thus, a child might be identified as having an SRD in one school district, but not in another, depending upon the state or local guidelines or the personal philosophy of an independent evaluator (Berninger, 1996). These criticisms, however, are directed to *how* the discrepancy has been operationalized but *not* to the construct of unexpected underachievement or the use of an ability–achievement discrepancy as one component of an overall assessment that considers a person's history, observes the person speaking and reading aloud, and reviews his or her unique cognitive-psychological profile. This, once again, reinforces the diagnosis of dyslexia as a clinical diagnosis. While tests are helpful, they are only proxies for the real-life experiences and abilities and weaknesses of the person. Because this point is so often overlooked and lost sight of, we emphasize that we are talking about individuals and not isolated numbers. Thus, we reiterate, dyslexia is a clinical diagnosis, based on clinical judgement, made by an experienced clinician who considers both the individual's history and symptoms and his/her learning profile, including cognitive and achievement abilities that may point to an unexpected difficulty in reading, as well as the reasons for this difficulty.

Thus, a major criticism associated with use of the ability–achievement discrepancy has been the focus on various formulae as the key to eligibility for special services, and not the construct itself. As noted by Willis and Dumont (2002), the determination of a disability should be far more than "…an exercise in arithmetic" (p. 173), nor should students who truly have SRD be denied services "…simply because of the results of a statistical exercise" (Dumont, Willis, & McBride, 2001, p. 13).

In addition, the use of an ability–achievement discrepancy may reduce the chances of early reading intervention because the child had to fall behind his or her expected reading achievement before he or she would be eligible for services.. As a result, identification was often delayed and services were denied until the requisite discrepancy had developed, resulting in what has been described as a "wait-to-fail" approach. By the time a child was identified, he or she was often far behind peers in reading skill. So, for the most part, concerns focused on the mechanics—that is, how the discrepancy or unexpected condition was to be operationalized—as well as on the delay of identification of children in the first years of school. On the other hand, accumulating empirical evidence supports the fundamental concept of dyslexia as an unexpected difficulty in reading, and the use of a discrepancy as one key diagnostic element to demonstrate unexpected reading difficulty.

As noted above, for the first time, strong empirical evidence demonstrates that differential relationships exist between IQ and reading in groups of typical readers versus readers with dyslexia. Moreover, these differences go directly to the definition of dyslexia as an unexpected difficulty in reading as typically operationalized as an ability–achievement discrepancy. Whereas cognition and reading are dynamically linked in good readers, they are uncoupled in readers with dyslexia, so that individuals with high intelligence, for example, may demonstrate poor reading, which in turn, in assessment, is operationalized as an ability–achievement discrepancy (Ferrer et al., 2010). These new data provide a strong scientific basis and validation for use of an ability–achievement discrepancy to help identify children who have dyslexia and argue strongly for its importance and maintenance as a component of the assessment of a child for the presence of a dyslexia. Particularly for bright or gifted children, the ability–achievement discrepancy signals the unexpected underachievement of children who appear to be reading on par with their classmates but are underachieving in relation to their academic potential and intellect. For younger children, in kindergarten through the second grade, a discrepancy may not be present, because many children have not fallen behind sufficiently to reveal a disparity between their ability and achievement (S. Shaywitz et al., 2008). Here, as elsewhere, it is important to note that, for the initial identification of such children, it is critical to consider the whole child, which requires a synthesis of the child's history, observation of the child speaking and reading out loud, and the results of a cognitive-psychological assessment administered by an individual who has a contemporary understanding of dyslexia. Given that an ability–achievement discrepancy may not be present in some young children who have dyslexia, it should not be used as the sole diagnostic criterion. In addition, cases exist where the lack of reading lowers performance on measures of knowledge and vocabulary, and/or where the processing or attentional problems (e.g., slow processing speed) lower the overall ability score, so that a discrepancy does not exist. In contrast, longitudinal data indicate that those students who have dyslexia and have higher ability may actually maintain and even increase their ability scores, including their scores on subtests measuring, for example, vocabulary. Such students may catch up in their reading comprehension scores, but they continue to be slow, dysfluent readers (Shaywitz, 2003; S. Shaywitz et al., 2003).

Thus, if present, an ability–achievement discrepancy is helpful in demonstrating an unexpected difficulty in reading and should continue to be used as one component of the assessment for the determination and diagnosis of dyslexia. These new results of an uncoupling of IQ and reading in children with dyslexia are in addition to other empirical evidence demonstrating that IQ is important in the consideration of the existence of a SLD. For example, after reviewing major syntheses of the literature, Swanson (2008) noted: "My point in reviewing these major syntheses of the literature is to suggest that removing IQ as an aptitude measure in classifying children as LD, especially, Verbal IQ, from assessment procedures is not uniformly supported by the literature" (p. 36). This statement counters the critics who argue for the removal of IQ from such diagnostic procedures and to indicate that "…intelligence mediates responsiveness to intervention in reading instruction" (Reynolds & Shaywitz, 2009). Continuing, Swanson (2008) notes: "The obvious implication is that IQ does have relevance to any policy definitions of LD" (p. 37).

With the reauthorization of IDEA 2004, the mandate of an ability–achievement discrepancy was removed (while still permitting it as an option), potentially providing more flexibility in identification procedures, but at the same time creating a new set of issues and concerns regarding SLD identification procedures. Although the use of a discrepancy procedure is still permitted under federal law, some states have passed guidelines that do not allow a discrepancy model to be used at all (Berkeley, Bender, Peaster, & Saunders, 2009). This is unfortunate because it ignores the science and, even more important, ignores the bright student with dyslexia. As discussed, the concept of ability–achievement discrepancy is related to a major criterion that is a marker for SLD identification—that is, the concept of "unexpected" underachievement. In many cases, measures of cognitive ability can help evaluators determine students' "potential" for academic success and identify those with unexpectedly low achievement levels relative to their abilities. Such discrepancies strongly suggest the existence of SLD, particularly, as children progress in school (Kavale & Spaulding, 2008).

A suggested potential replacement is what has been referred to as response-to-intervention, an approach many consider to be a premature adoption of a large-scale change without the requisite scientific data and evidence of effectiveness. We note especially the lack of large-scale studies supporting its procedures or efficacy, and its inherent structural flaws that may only result in significant groups of struggling readers' failing to be identified.

Response-to-Intervention

As one possible alternative to the ability–achievement discrepancy, IDEA 2004 allows states to permit a process that theoretically examines whether or not a student responds to scientific, research-based interventions as *part* of the SLD evaluation procedure. This process is most often referred to as response-to-intervention (RTI). In principle, RTI involves the systematic use of data-based decision-making to identify struggling readers within a school and then provide a series of more intensive interventions for those in need (Burns & Van Der Heyden, 2007). Many questions, issues, and concerns, however, have been raised regarding the use and implementation of RTI (Barth et al., 2008; Berninger, O'Donnell, & Holdnack, 2008; Feifer, 2008; Franzen, 2008; Johns & Kauffmann, 2009; Kavale, 2005; Kavale, Holdnack, & Mostert, 2005; Kavale, Kauffman, Bachmeier, & Lefever, 2008;

McKenzie, 2009; Pass & Dean, 2008; Reynolds, 2008; Reynolds & Shaywitz, 2009; Schatschneider, Wagner, & Crawford, 2008; Speece & Walker, 2007; Suhr, 2008; Vaughn & Fuchs, 2003).

When viewed in the context of dyslexia evaluations, RTI has serious shortcomings as a means of diagnosis or determination of a disability. If followed to its ultimate conclusion, the approach and definition embedded in RTI have the strong probability of eliminating the basic concept of SLD as it was intended, as it is empirically supported, and as it is currently understood. This would be extraordinarily unfortunate, particularly since so much progress has been made in neuroscience in understanding and validating dyslexia.

The RTI approach fosters the dangerous concept of relativity of a disability in the context of the individual classroom as opposed to the long-accepted concept of a disability as a neuro-psychological condition residing *within* the individual. This fundamentally alters the concept of disability at its very roots. The RTI model focuses on the failure of a child–school interaction that is complex and modified by the overall achievement level of an individual classroom that will vary within schools and across schools. Consequently, a child may be identified by RTI in one classroom but not be found to require intervention in the classroom next door, depending on the make-up of each class. This approach represents a fundamental alteration and cuts out the very roots basic to the concept of dyslexia as an unexpected difficulty in learning to read that is intrinsic to the child. As an approach to diagnosis, RTI does not have proven value as either a rule-out or a rule-in process for a disability. Simply stated, a student who is not identified as having dyslexia through the RTI procedure, especially if he or she is above the classmates in ability or achievement, may have a reading disability. Conversely, one who fails in RTI may or may not have a reading disability, and the nature of the disability, when one is present, is unknown, following a failed RTI. A failed RTI is neither a necessary nor a sufficient condition for determination of the presence or absence of dyslexia. Whereas it is intuitively appealing to argue that RTI is a strong process for ruling out a disability, RTI, in its relativistic form for comparisons, cannot be applied accurately even in this manner. More unfortunately, it is becoming the sole or major criterion for the identification of an SLD. In fact, the regulations appear more concerned with the provision of adequate instruction, rather than accurate SLD diagnosis leading to effective instruction (Kavale & Spaulding, 2008). IDEA

2004 does not provide diagnostic criteria for SLD, but instead focuses on the issue of special education eligibility (Berninger & Wolf, 2009). RTI should not be viewed as a method for diagnosing dyslexia, but rather as a potential school-wide prevention model designed to provide early intervention and potentially reduce the number of children who are struggling to learn to read—a notion that awaits empirical support. An added concern is that RTI is a very large non-empirically supported experiment to apply on a national scale to tens of thousands of students.

One more serious concern is that RTI ignores bright struggling readers in the identification process. In the RTI process itself, consider the impact of so-called peer comparison to classmates if a specific child is highly intelligent or even gifted. What if such a child is in a class of "peers" who are functioning at lower cognitive levels? Such a bright student might be struggling and functioning well below his or her own capabilities, but at an absolute level that is comparable to the class average of his or her less-able peers. That struggling reader would be entirely invisible and overlooked in an RTI process. Within the RTI process, such students would never be detected, much less referred for a full evaluation of their cognitive and psychological processing abilities. Most critically, such struggling readers would not receive helpful interventions or accommodations, "despite the fact that their relative deficit in a particular domain could cause severe psychological distress as well as unexpected underachievement" (Boada, Riddle, & Pennington, 2008, p. 185) which could be ameliorated through interventions and accommodations. In fact, often the only way such struggling readers are identified is through a complete, comprehensive assessment in which their history, cognitive abilities, and psychological processes are evaluated. The data clearly show these bright students, although reading at higher levels, still are performing below their ability and share many qualities (e.g., phonological deficits) with lower-functioning struggling readers (Hoskyn & Swanson, 2000; Stuebing et al., 2002). It would be no fairer to leave out these bright struggling readers than it would be to leave out their lower-functioning classmates.

Conclusion

Time is of the essence. It is critical to identify dyslexia early and accurately. This means getting a careful synthesis of the individual's history, observing the individual's speaking and reading, and analyzing the results of an assessment of cognitive and academic abilities. To accurately diagnose dyslexia requires first and foremost the awareness that dyslexia represents an unexpected difficulty within the individual, together with the knowledge of the basic underlying difficulties of getting to the sounds of spoken words, and the resultant symptoms. Identification of that individual's cognitive abilities along with his or her strengths and weaknesses, together with associated difficulties such as anxiety, will help ensure accurate diagnosis followed by effective interventions and accommodations. To accomplish this goal, the assessment of a dyslexia requires an individualized approach, not just the use of group-based assessments. If we forego individualization in assessment, the essence of special education is lost and " the SLD category becomes the convenient home for those who otherwise might be left behind, something that perverts the category and is consistent only with the fantasy world of NCLB" (Kavale et al., 2008, p. 141). Students with disabilities will not disappear, but if they are not identified, their rights certainly will (Johns & Kauffman, 2009).

The ultimate goal of an assessment is to provide better services to children in need (Hooper, 1996). To accomplish this goal, we need competent evaluators who understand and can identify individuals who have dyslexia. An accurate diagnosis requires a deep understanding of the cognitive-psychological, neurobiological-medical, and educational factors underlying dyslexia. We want to emphasize that dyslexia is real—it exists, and thus, it not only makes sense but is imperative for evaluators to diagnose this disability. Without specific diagnoses, we have no way of talking about problems or solutions (Johns & Kauffman, 2009). Dyslexia needs to be accurately diagnosed. To not do so would be an injustice to the affected individuals. In discussing his own realization that he had dyslexia, Schultz (2011), a Pulitzer prize–winning poet, reflected: "My ignorance of my dyslexia only intensified my sense of isolation and hopelessness. Ignorance is perhaps the most painful aspect of a learning disability" (p. 64). Most scientists and educators would agree that the first step in solving a problem is to define it and understand its nature (Boada et al., 2008).

The concept of dyslexia is valid and supported by strong converging evidence. Dyslexia conveys specific meaning emerging from its definition, cognitive-psychological profile, and now neurobiological imprint. We now have knowledge of its epidemiology, including its prevalence and developmental course, the educational impact, and the importance of providing early evidence-based treatments, as well as the provision of accommodations. Dyslexia provides a common language with which a range of relevant individuals—educators, parents, psychologists, physicians, affected children, and others—can converse and collaborate. Many of these students with dyslexia will lose their identity as individuals with an SLD if they are not accurately identified; moreover, they will continue to struggle needlessly. By combining knowledge from the cognitive-psychological and neurobiological-medical models and recognizing that interventions will be applied within school settings, practitioners will be better prepared to make accurate diagnoses that identify the problem and propose the most efficacious solutions based upon a careful examination of all of the influences and variables.

Acknowledgements

We would like to acknowledge the support of the National Institutes of Health (RO1 HD 057655), Eli Lilly Ltd., and the Yale Center for Dyslexia and Creativity to Sally E. Shaywitz and Bennett A. Shaywitz. In addition, Michael E. Gerner and Deborah Schneider provided valuable editorial suggestions on the penultimate draft of this chapter.

References

Aaron, P. G. (1997). The impending demise of the discrepancy formula. *Review of Educational Research, 67*, 461–502.

Abu-Hamour, B. (2009). The relationships among cognitive ability measures and irregular word, non-word, and word reading. Unpublished doctoral dissertation, University of Arizona, Tucson.

Abu-Hamour, B., Urso, A., & Mather, N. (2012). The relationships among cognitive correlates and irregular word, non-word, and word reading. *International Journal of Special Education, 27*(1), 144–159.

Anderson, A., & Gore, J. (1997). The physical basis of neuroimaging techniques. In M. Lewis & B. Peterson (Eds.), *Child and adolescent psychiatric clinics of North America* (Vol. 6; pp. 213–264). Philadelphia; PA: W. B. Saunders Co.

Baddeley, A. (2007). *Working memory, thought, and action.* Oxford, UK: Oxford University Press.

Baddeley, A. (2012). Working memory: Theories, models, and controversies. *Annual Review of Psychology, 63*, 1–29.

Baddeley, A., Eysenck, M., & Anderon, M. (2009). *Memory.* New York: Psychology Press.

Badian, N. (2005). Does a visual-orthographic deficit contribute to reading disability? *Annals of Dyslexia, 55*, 28–52.

Bailet, L. L. (2001). Development and disorders of spelling in the beginning school years. In A. M. Bain, L. L. Bailet, & L. C. Moats (Eds.), *Written language disorders: Theory into practice* (2nd ed.; pp. 1–41). Austin, TX: PRO-ED.

Barker, T. A., Torgesen, J. K., & Wagner, R. K. (1992). The role of orthographic processing skills on five different reading tasks. *Reading Research Quarterly, 27*, 335–345.

Barth, A. E., Stuebing, K. K., Anthony, J. L., Denton, C. A., Mathes, P. G., Fletcher, J. M., et al. (2008). Agreement among response to intervention criteria for identifying responder status. *Learning & Individual Differences, 18,* 296–307.

Bateman, B. (1992). Learning disabilities: The changing landscape. *Journal of Learning Disabilities, 25,* 29–36.

Bell, S. M., McCallum, R. S., & Cox, E. A. (2003). Toward a research-based assessment of dyslexia: Using cognitive measures to identify reading disabilities. *Journal of Learning Disabilities, 36,* 505–516.

Benson, N. (2007). Cattell-Horn-Carroll cognitive abilities and reading achievement. *Journal of Psychoeducational Assessment, 26,* 27–41.

Bental, B., & Tirosh, E. (2007). The relationship between attention, executive functions and reading domain abilities in attention deficit hyperactivity disorder and reading disorder: A comparative study. *Journal of Child Psychology & Psychiatry, 48,* 455–463.

Berkeley, S., Bender, W. N., Peaster, L. G., & Saunders, L. (2009). Implementation of responsive to intervention: A snapshot of progress. *Journal of Learning Disabilities, 42,* 85–95.

Berninger, V. W. (1996). *Reading and writing acquisition: A developmental neuropsychological perspective.* Oxford: Westview Press.

Berninger, V. W., O'Donnell, L., & Holdnack, J. (2008). Research-supported differential diagnosis of specific learning disabilities and implications for instruction and response to instruction. In A. Prifitera, D. H. Saklofske, & L. G. Weiss (Eds.), *WISC-IV clinical assessment and intervention* (2nd ed., pp. 69–108). San Antonio, TX: Pearson Assessment.

Berninger, V. W., & Wolf, B. J. (2009). *Teaching students with dyslexia and dysgraphia: Lessons from teaching and science.* Baltimore, MD: Paul H. Brookes Publishing Company.

Boada, R., Riddle, M., & Pennington, B. F. (2008). Integrating science and practice in education. In E. Fletcher-Janzen & C. R. Reynolds (Eds.), *Neuropsychological perspectives on learning disabilities in the era of RTI: Recommendations for diagnosis and intervention* (pp. 179–191). Hoboken, NJ: John Wiley & Sons.

Bowers, P. G., Sunseth, K., & Golden, J. (1999). The route between rapid naming and reading progress. *Scientific Studies of Reading, 3,* 31–53.

Bowers, P. G., & Wolf, M. (1993). Theoretical links between naming speed, precise timing mechanisms, and orthographic skill in dyslexia. *Reading & Writing: An Interdisciplinary Journal, 5,* 69–85.

Bradley, L., & Bryant, P. E. (1983). Categorizing sounds and learning to read—a causal connection. *Nature, 301,* 419–421.

Brambati, S., Termine, C., Ruffino, M., Danna, M., Lanzi, G., Stella, G., et al. (2006). Neuropsychological deficits and neural dysfunction in familial dyslexia. *Brain Research, 1113*(1), 174–185.

Bruck, M. (1992). Persistence of dyslexics' phonological awareness deficits. *Developmental Psychology, 28,* 874–886.

Burns, M. K., & VanDerHeyden, A. M. (2007). Using response to intervention to assess learning disabilities. *Assessment for Effective Intervention, 32,* 3–5.

Carroll, J. M., & Iles, J. E. (2006). An assessment of anxiety levels in dyslexic students in higher education. *British Journal of Educational Psychology, 76,* 651–662.

Clark, D. B., & Uhry, J. K. (1995). *Dyslexia: Theory and practice of remedial instruction* (2nd ed.). Timonium, MD: York Press.

Cohen, L., & Dehaene, S. (2004). Specialization within the ventral stream: The case for the visual word-form area. *Neuroimage, 22*(1), 466–476.

Cohen, L., Dehaene, S., Naccache, L., Lehericy, S., Dehaene-Lambertz, G., Henaff, M. A., et al. (2000). The visual word-form area: Spatial and temporal characterization of an initial stage of reading in normal subjects and posterior split-brain patients. *Brain, 123,* 291–307.

Cohen, L., Martinaud, O., Lemer, C., Lehericy, S., Samson, Y., Obadia, M., et al. (2003). Visual word recognition in the left and right hemispheres: Anatomical and functional correlates of peripheral alexias. *Cerebral Cortex, 13,* 1313–1333.

Crews, K., & D'Amato, R. C. (2009). Subtyping children's reading disabilities using a comprehensive neuropsychological measure. *International Journal of Neuroscience, 119,* 1615–1639.

Critchley, M. (1970). *The dyslexic child.* Springfield, IL: Charles C. Thomas.

Dehaene, S., Cohen, L., Sigman, M., & Vinckier, F. (2005). The neural code for written words: A proposal. *Trends in Cognitive Sciences, 9,* 335–341.

Dehaene, S., Naccache, L., Cohen, L., Bihan, D. L., Mangin, J. F., Poline, J. B., et al. (2001). Cerebral mechanisms of word masking and unconscious repetition priming. *Nature Neuroscience, 4,* 752–758.

Dejerine, J. (1891). Sur un cas de cécité verbale avec agraphie, suivi d'autopsie. *C. R. Société du Biologie, 43,* 197–201.

Dejerine, J. (1892). Contribution a l'étude anatomo-pathologique et clinique des differentes variétés de cécité verbale. *Memoires de la Société de Biologie, 4,* 61–90.

Denckla, M. B., & Cutting, L. E. (1999). History and significance of rapid automatized naming. *Annals of Dyslexia, 49,* 29–42.

Dumont, R., Willis, J., & McBride, G. (2001). Yes, Virginia, there is a severe discrepancy clause, but is it too much ado about something? *The School Psychologist, APA Division of School Psychology, 55*(1), 1, 4–13, 15.

Ehri, L. C. (2000). Learning to read and learning to spell: Two sides of a coin. *Topics in Language Disorders, 20*(3), 19–36.

Evans, J. J., Floyd, R. G., McGrew, K. S., & Leforgee, M. H. (2002). The relations between measures of Cattell-Horn-Carroll (CHC) cognitive abilities and reading achievement during childhood and adolescence. *School Psychology Review, 31,* 246–262.

Faust, M., Dimitrovsky, L., & Shacht, T. (2003). Naming difficulties in children with dyslexia: Application of the tip-of-the-tongue paradigm. *Journal of Learning Disabilities, 36,* 203–215.

Faust, M., & Scharfstein-Friedman, S. (2003). Naming difficulties in adolescents with dyslexia: Application of the tip-of-the tongue paradigm. *Brain & Cognition, 53,* 211–217.

Fawcett, A. J., & Nicolson, R. I. (2007). Dyslexia, learning, and pedagogical neuroscience. *Developmental Medicine & Child Neurology, 49,* 306–311.

Feifer, S. G. (2008). Integrating response to intervention (RTI) with neuropsychology: A scientific approach to reading. *Psychology in the Schools, 45,* 812–825.

Ferrer, E., Shaywitz, B., Holahan, J., Marchione, K., & Shaywitz, S. (2010). Uncoupling of reading and IQ over time: Empirical evidence for a definition of dyslexia. *Psychological Science, 21,* 93–101.

Fiez, J. A., & Peterson, S. E. (1998). Neuroimaging studies of word reading. *Proceedings of the National Academy of Sciences, 95,* 914–921.

Frackowiak, R. S. J., Friston, K. J., Frith, C., Dolan, R., Friston, K. J., Price, C. J., et al. (2004). *Human brain function* (2nd ed.). San Diego: Academic Press, Elsevier Science.

Francis, D., Shaywitz, S., Stuebing, K., Shaywitz, B., & Fletcher, J. (1996). Developmental lag versus deficit models of reading disability: A longitudinal, individual growth curves analysis. *Journal of Educational Psychology, 88*(1), 3–17.

Franzen, M. D. (2008). Neuroscience, neuropsychology, and education: Learning to work and play well with each other. In E. Fletcher-Janzen & C. R. Reynolds (Eds.), *Neuropsychological perspectives on learning disabilities in the era of RTI: Recommendations for diagnosis and intervention* (pp. 247–254). Hoboken, NJ: John Wiley & Sons.

Friedmann, N., & Lukov, L. (2008). Developmental surface dyslexias. *Cortex, 44*, 1146–1160.

Gaillard, R., Naccache, L., Pinel, P., Clemenceau, S., Volle, E., Hasboun, D., et al. (2006). Direct intracranial, FMRI, and lesion evidence for the causal role of left inferotemporal cortex in reading. *Neuron, 50*, 191–204.

Gathercole, S. E. (2006). Nonword repetition and word learning: The nature of the relationship. *Applied Psycholinguistics, 27*, 513–543.

Gathercole, S., & Alloway, T. (2008). *Working memory & learning.* London: Sage Publications.

Georgiou, G. K., Parrila, R., Kirby, K. R., & Stephenson, K. (2008). Rapid naming components and their relationship with phonological awareness, orthographic knowledge, speed of processing, and different reading outcomes. *Scientific Studies of Reading, 12*, 325–350.

Goldston, D. B., Walsh, A., Arnold, E. M. Reboussin, B., Daniel, S. S., Erkanli, A., Nutter, D., et al. (2007). Reading problems, psychiatric disorders, and functional impairment from mid- to late adolescence. *Journal of the American Academy of Child & Adolescent. Psychiatry, 46*(1), 25–32.

Gregg, N. (2009). *Adolescents and adults with learning disabilities and ADHD: Assessment and accommodation.* New York: Guilford Press.

Gregg, N., Coleman, C., Davis, M., Lindstrom, W., & Hartwig, J. (2006). Critical issues for the diagnosis of learning disabilities in the adult population. *Psychology in the Schools, 43*, 889–899.

Grigg, W., Donahue, P., & Dion, G. (2007). *The nation's report card: 12th-grade reading and mathematics, 2005.* Washington, DC: National Center for Education Statistics. U.S. Department of Education.

Hale, J. B., Fiorello, C., Miller, J. A., Wenrich, K., Teodori, A., & Henzel, J. (2008). WISC-IV interpretation for specific learning disabilities; Identification and intervention: A cognitive hypothesis testing approach. In A. Prifitera, D. H. Saklofske, & L. G. Weiss (Eds.), *WISC-IV clinical assessment and intervention* (2nd ed.; pp. 109–171). San Antonio, TX: Pearson Assessment.

Hale, J. B., Kaufman, A. S., Naglieri, J. A., & Kavale, K. A. (2006). Implementation of IDEA: Response to intervention and cognitive assessment methods. *Psychology in the Schools, 43*, 753–770.

Hale, J. B., Naglieri, J. A., Kaufman, A. S., & Kavale, K. A. (2004). Specific learning disability classifications in the new Individuals with Disabilities Education Act: The danger of good ideas. *The School Psychologist, 58*(1), 6–13, 29.

Hanly. S. & Vandenberg, B. (2010). Tip of the tongue and word retrieval deficits in dyslexia. *Journal of Learning Disability, 43*, 15–23.

Heim, S., Eickhoff, S. B., & Amunts, K. (2008). Specialisation in Broca's region for semantic, phonological, and syntactic fluency? *NeuroImage, 40*, 1362–1368.

Henry, C., Gaillard, R., Volle, E., Chiras, J., Ferrieux, S., Dehaene, S., et al. (2005). Brain activations during letter-by-letter reading: A follow-up study. *Neuropsychologia, 43*, 1983–1989.

Hinshelwood, J. (1902). *Congenital word-blindness with reports of two cases.* London: John Bale, Sons & Danielsson.

Hinshelwood, J. (1917). *Congenital word-blindness.* London: H. K. Lewis.

Hooper, S. R. (1996). Subtyping specific reading disabilities: Classification approaches, recent advances, and current status. *Mental Retardation & Developmental Disabilities, 2*, 14–20.

Hoskyn, M., & Swanson, H. (2000). Cognitive processing of low achievers and children with reading disabilities: A selective meta-analytic review of the published literature. *School Psychology Review, 29*, 102–119.

Jezzard, P., Matthews, P., & Smith, S. (2001). *Functional MRI: An introduction to methods.* Oxford: Oxford University Press.

Johns, B. H., & Kauffman, J. M. (2009). Caution: Response to intervention (RtI). *Learning Disabilities: A Multidisciplinary Journal, 15*, 157–160.

Johnson, R., & Rayner, K. (2007). Top-down and bottom-up effects in pure alexia: Evidence from eye movements. *Neuropsychologia, 45*, 2246–2257.

Kail, R. (1991). Developmental change in speed of processing during childhood and adolescence. *Psychological Bulletin, 109*, 490–501.

Kail, R., Hall, L. K., & Caskey, B. J. (1999). Processing speed, exposure to print, and naming speed. *Applied Psycholinguistics, 20*, 303–314.

Kaufman, A. S. (2004). Standardized cognitive assessment and the new IDEA guidelines—Fit or misfit? Presentation at the National Association of School Psychologists Annual Convention, April 1, Dallas, TX.

Kaufman, A. S. (2008). Neuropsychology and specific learning disabilities: Lessons from the past as a guide to present controversies and future clinical practice. In E. Fletcher-Janzen & C. R. Reynolds (Eds.), *Neuropsychological perspectives on learning disabilities in the era of RTI: Recommendations for diagnosis and intervention* (pp. 1–13). Hoboken, NJ: John Wiley & Sons.

Kaufman, A. S., & Kaufman, N. L. (2001). Assessment of specific learning disabilities in the new millennium: Issues, conflicts, and controversies. In A. S. Kaufman & N. L. Kaufman (Eds.), *Specific learning disabilities: Psychological assessment and evaluation* (pp. 433–461). Cambridge Monographs in Child and Adolescent Psychiatry. Cambridge, England: Cambridge University Press.

Kavale, K. A. (2005). Identifying specific learning disability: Is responsiveness to intervention the answer? *Journal of Learning Disabilities, 38*, 553–562.

Kavale, K. A., & Forness, S. R. (2000). What definitions of learning disability say and don't say. *Journal of Learning Disabilities, 33*, 239–256.

Kavale, K. A., Holdnack, J. A., & Mostert, M. P. (2005). Responsiveness to intervention and the identification of specific learning disability: A critique and alternative proposal. *Learning Disability Quarterly, 28*, 2–16.

Kavale, K. A., Kauffman, J. M., Bachmeier, R. J., & Lefever, G. B. (2008). Response-to-intervention: Separating the rhetoric of self-congratulation from the reality of specific learning disability identification. *Learning Disability Quarterly, 31*, 135–150.

Kavale, K. A., Kaufman, A. S., Naglieri, J. A., & Hale, J. (2005). Changing procedures for identifying learning disabilities: The danger of poorly supported ideas. *The School Psychologist, 59*, 16–25.

Kavale, K. A., & Spaulding, L. S. (2008). Is response to intervention good policy for specific learning disability? *Learning Disabilities Research & Practice, 23*, 169–179.

Kemp N., Parrila, R. K., & Kirby J. R. (2009). Phonological and orthographic spelling in high-functioning adult dyslexics. *Dyslexia: The Journal of the British Dyslexia Association, 15*, 105–128.

Kibby, M. Y., & Cohen, M. J. (2008). Memory functioning in children with reading disabilities and/or Attention Deficit/Hyperactivity Disorder: A clinical investigation of their working memory and long-term memory functioning. *Child Neuropsychology, 14*, 525–546.

Konold, T. R., Juel, C., McKinnon, M., & Deffes, R. (2003). A multivariate model of early reading acquisition. *Applied Psycholinguistics, 24*, 89–112.

Kronbichler, M., Hutzler, F., Staffen, W., Mair, A., Ladurner, G., & Wimmer, H. (2006). Evidence for a dysfunction of left posterior reading areas in German dyslexic readers. *Neuropsychologia, 44*, 1822–1832.

Lerner, J. (1989). Educational interventions in learning disabilities. *Journal of the American Academy of Child & Adolescent Psychiatry, 28*, 326–331.

Levelt, W. J., Roelofs, A., & Meyer, A. S. (1999). A theory of lexical access in speech production. *Behavioral & Brain Sciences, 22*, 1–75.

Lyon, G. R. (1995). Toward a definition of dyslexia. *Annals of Dyslexia, 45*, 3–27.

Lyon, G. R., Shaywitz, S. E., & Shaywitz, B. A. (2003). A definition of dyslexia. *Annals of Dyslexia, 53*, 1–14.

Mano, Q. R., & Osmon, D. C. (2008). Visuoperceptual-orthographic reading abilities: A confirmatory factor analysis study. *Journal of Clinical & Experimental Neuropsychology, 30*, 421–434.

Marzola, E., & Shepherd, M. (2005). *Assessment of reading difficulties.* Baltimore, MD: Paul H. Brookes Publishing Company.

Mather, N., & Gerner, M. E. (2009). Postsecondary students with high abilities and reading disabilities: Case analyses and commentary. *Learning Disabilities: A Multidisciplinary Journal, 15*, 121–129.

Mather, N., & Gregg, N. (2006). Specific learning disabilities: Clarifying, not eliminating, a construct. *Professional Psychology, 37*, 99–106.

Mather, N., & Healey, W. C. (1990). Deposing aptitude-achievement discrepancy as the imperial criterion for learning disabilities. *Learning Disabilities: A Multidisciplinary Journal, 1*(2), 40–48.

Mather, N., & Kaufman, N. (2006). It's about the what, the how well, and the why. *Psychology in the Schools, 43*, 747–752.

Mather, N., & Wendling, B. (2012). *Essentials of dyslexia: Assessment and intervention.* New York, NY: John Wiley & Sons.

McKenzie, R. G. (2009). Obscuring vital distinctions: The oversimplification of learning disabilities within RTI. *Learning Disability Quarterly, 32*, 203–215.

Monroe, M. (1932). *Children who cannot read.* Chicago, IL: University of Chicago Press.

Monroe, M. (1935). Diagnosis and treatment of reading disabilities. In G. M. Whipple (Ed.), *The Thirty-fourth yearbook of the National Society for the Study of Education: Educational diagnosis* (pp. 201–228). Bloomington, IL: Public School Publishing Company.

Morgan, W. P. (1896). A case of congenital word blindness. *British Medical Journal*, November 7, 1378.

Morris, R. D., Stuebing, K. K., Fletcher, J. M., Shaywitz, S. E., Lyon, G. R., Shankweiler, D. P., et al. (1998). Subtypes of reading disability: Variability around a phonological core. *Journal of Educational Psychology, 90*, 347–373.

Nakamura, K., Dehaene, S., Jobert, A., Le Bihan, D., & Kouider, S. (2005). Subliminal convergence of Kanji and Kana words: Further evidence for functional parcellation of the posterior temporal cortex in visual word perception. *Journal of Cognitive Neuroscience, 17*, 954–968.

Nakamura, K., Dehaene, S., Jobert, A., Le Bihan, D., & Kouider, S. (2007). Task-specific change of unconscious neural priming in the cerebral language network. *Proceedings of the National Academy of Sciences, USA, 104*, 19643–19648.

Nakamura, K., Hara, N., Kouider, S., Takayama, Y., Hanajima, R., Sakai, K., & Ugawa, Y. (2006). Task-guided selection of the dual neural pathways for reading. *Neuron, 52*, 557–564.

Nelson, J. M., & Harwood, H. (2011). Learning disabilities and anxiety: A meta-analysis. *Journal of Learning Disabilities, 44*, 3–17.

Orton, S. T. (1925). "Word-blindness" in school children. *Archives of Neurology & Psychiatry, 14*, 581–615.

Pass, L. A., & Dean, R. S. (2008). Neuropsychology and RTI: LD policy, diagnosis, and interventions. In E. Fletcher-Janzen & C. R. Reynolds (Eds.), *Neuropsychological perspectives on learning disabilities in the era of RTI: Recommendations for diagnosis and intervention* (pp. 238–246). Hoboken, NJ: John Wiley & Sons.

Paulesu, E., Demonet, J. F., Fazio, F., McCrory, E., Chanoine, V., Brunswick, N., et al. (2001). Dyslexia-cultural diversity and biological unity. *Science, 291*, 2165–2167.

Perfetti, C. (2011). Phonology is critical in reading: But a phonological deficit is not the only source of low reading skill. In S. A. Brady, D. Braze, & C. A. Fowler (Eds.). *Explaining individual differences in reading: Theory and evidence* (pp. 153–171). New York: Psychology Press.

Perie, M., Grigg, W., & Donahue, P. (2005). *National assessment of educational progress: The nation's report card, Reading 2005.* U.S Government Printing Office.

Peterson, R. L., & Pennington, B. F. (2012). Developmental dyslexia. *Lancet, published online,* April 17, 2012. doi:10.1016/S0140-6736(12)60198-6

Price, C. J., & Devlin, J. T. (2011), The Interactive Account of ventral occipito-temporal contributions to reading. *Trends in Cognitive Sciences, 15*, 246–253.

Price, C., & Mechelli, A. (2005). Reading and reading disturbance. *Current Opinion in Neurobiology, 15*, 231–238.

Rack, J. P., Snowling, M. J., & Olson, R. K. (1992). The nonword reading deficit in developmental dyslexia: A review. *Reading Research Quarterly, 27*, 28–53.

Reitsma, P. (1989). Orthographic memory and learning to read. In P. G. Aaron & R. M. Joshi (Eds.), *Reading and writing disorders in different orthographic systems* (pp. 51–73). New York, NY: Kluwer Academic/Plenum Publishers.

Reynolds, C. R. (2008). RTI, neuroscience, and sense: Chaos in the diagnosis and treatment of learning disabilities. In E. Fletcher-Janzen & C. R. Reynolds (Eds.), *Neuropsychological perspectives on learning disabilities in the era of RTI:*

Recommendations for diagnosis and intervention (pp. 14–27). Hoboken, NJ: John Wiley & Sons.

Reynolds, C. R., & Shaywitz, S. (2009). Response to intervention: Ready or not? Or, from wait-to-fail to watch-them-fail. *School Psychology Quarterly, 24*, 130–145.

Richlan, F., Kronbichler, M., & Wimmer, H, (2009). Functional abnormalities in the dyslexic brain: A quantitative meta-analysis of neuroimaging studies. *Human Brain Mapping, 30*, 3299–3308.

Richlan, F., Kronbichler, M., & Wimmer, H, (2011). Meta-analyzing brain dysfunctions in dyslexic children and adults. *NeuroImage, 56*, 1735–1742.

Roberts, R., & Mather, N. (1997). Orthographic dyslexia: The neglected subtype. *Learning Disabilities Research & Practice, 12*, 236–250.

Rumsey, J. M., Andreason, P., Zametkin, A. J., Aquino, T., King, A. C., Hamburger, S. D., et al. (1992). Failure to activate the left temporo-parietal cortex in dyslexia. *Archives of Neurology, 49*, 527–534.

Savage, R., Lavers, N., & Pillay, V. (2007). Working memory and reading difficulties: What we know and what we don't know about the relationship. *Educational Psychology Review, 19*, 185–221.

Schatschneider, C., Wagner, R., & Crawford, E. (2008). The importance of measuring growth in response to intervention models: Testing a core assumption. *Learning & Individual Differences, 18*, 308–315.

Schultz, K. S., Simpson, C., & Lynch, S. (2012). Specific learning disability identification: What constitutes a pattern of strengths and weaknesses? *Learning Disabilities: A Multidisciplinary Journal, 18,* 87–97.

Schultz, P. (2011). *My dyslexia.* New York, NY: W. W. Norton & Company.

Seki, A., Koeda, T., Sugihara, S., Kamba, M., Hirata, Y., Ogawa, T., & Takeshita, K. (2001). A functional magnetic resonance imaging study during sentence reading in Japanese dyslexic children. *Brain & Development, 23*, 312–316.

Semrud-Clikeman, M. (2005). Neuropsychological aspects for evaluating learning disabilities. *Journal of Learning Disabilities, 38*, 563–568.

Shanahan, M. A., Pennington, B. F., Yerys, B. E., Scott, A., Boada, R., Willcutt, E. G., et al. (2006). Processing speed deficits in Attention Deficit/Hyperactivity Disorder and reading disability. *Journal of Abnormal Child Psychology, 34*, 585–602.

Shaywitz, B. A., Fletcher, J. M., & Shaywitz, S. E. (1995). Defining and classifying learning disabilities and attention-deficit/hyperactivity disorder. *Journal of Child Neurology, 10*, S50–S57.

Shaywitz, B. A., Shaywitz, S. E., Pugh, K. R., Mencl, W. E., Fulbright, R. K., Skudlarski, P., et al. (2002). Disruption of posterior brain systems for reading in children with developmental dyslexia. *Biological Psychiatry, 52*(2), 101–110.

Shaywitz, B. A., Skudlarski, P., Holahan, J. M., Marchione, K. E., Constable, R. T., Fulbright, R. K, et al. (2007). Age-related changes in reading systems of dyslexic children. *Annals of Neurology, 61*, 363–370.

Shaywitz, S. (2003). *Overcoming dyslexia: A new and complete science-based program for overcoming reading problems at any level.* New York: Alfred Knopf.

Shaywitz, S. E., Fletcher, J. M., Holahan, J. M., Shneider, A. E., Marchione, K. E., Stuebing, K. K., et al. (1999). Persistence of dyslexia: the Connecticut Longitudinal Study at adolescence. *Pediatrics, 104*, 1351–1359.

Shaywitz, S., Fletcher, J., & Shaywitz, B. (1994). Issues in the definition and classification of attention deficit disorder. *Topics in Language Disorders, 14*(4), 1–25.

Shaywitz, S., Morris, R., & Shaywitz, B. (2008). The education of dyslexic children from childhood to young adulthood. *Annual Review of Psychology, 59*, 451–475.

Shaywitz, S., & Shaywitz, B. (2005). Dyslexia (specific reading disability). *Biological Psychiatry, 57*, 1301–1309.

Shaywitz, S. E., & Shaywitz, B. A. (2008). Paying attention to reading: The neurobiology of reading and dyslexia. *Development & Psychopathology, 20*, 1329–1349.

Shaywitz, S. E., & Shaywitz, B. A. (2012). Dyslexia. In K. F. Swaiman, S. Ashwal, D. M. Ferriero, & N. F. Schor (Eds.), *Pediatric neurology: Principles and practice* (5th ed.). (pp. 613–621). Philadelphia, PA: Elsevier.

Shaywitz, S. E., Shaywitz, B. A., Fulbright, R. K., Skudlarski, P., Mencl, W. E., Constable, R. T., et al. (2003). Neural systems for compensation and persistence: young adult outcome of childhood reading disability. *Biological Psychiatry, 54*(1), 25–33.

Shaywitz, S. E., Shaywitz, B. A., Pugh, K. R., Fulbright, R. K., Constable, R. T., Mencl, W. E., et al. (1998). Functional disruption in the organization of the brain for reading in dyslexia. *Proceedings of the National Academy of Science, USA, 95*, 2636–2641.

Speece, D. L., & Walker, C. Y. (2007). What are the issues in response to intervention research? In D. Haager, J. Klingner, & S. Vaughn (Eds.), *Evidence-based reading practices for response to intervention* (pp. 287–301). Baltimore, MD: Paul H. Brookes Publishing Company.

Stanger, M. A., & Donohue, E. K. (1937). *Prediction and prevention of reading difficulties.* New York: Oxford University Press.

Stanovich, K. E. (1991). Conceptual and empirical problems with discrepancy definitions of reading disability. *Learning Disability Quarterly, 14*, 269–280.

Stanovich, K. E., West, R. F., & Cunningham, A. E. (1991). *Beyond phonological processes: Print exposure and orthographic processing.* Hillsdale, NJ: Erlbaum.

Steinbrink, C., & Klatte, M. (2008). Phonological working memory in German children with poor reading and spelling abilities. *Dyslexia, 14*, 271–290.

Stuebing, K. K., Fletcher, J. M., LeDoux, J. M., Lyon, G. R., Shaywitz, S. E., & Shaywitz, B. A. (2002). Validity of IQ-discrepancy classifications of reading disabilities: A meta-analysis. *American Educational Research Journal, 39*, 469–518.

Suhr, J. A. (2008). Assessment versus testing and its importance in learning disability diagnosis. In E. Fletcher-Janzen & C. R. Reynolds (Eds.), *Neuropsychological perspectives on learning disabilities in the era of RTI: Recommendations for diagnosis and intervention* (pp. 99–114). Hoboken, NJ: John Wiley & Sons.

Swanson, H. (2008). Neuroscience and response to instruction (RTI): A complementary role. In E. Fletcher-Janzen & C. Reynolds (Eds.), *Neuropsychological perspectives on learning disabilities in the era of RTI: Recommendations for diagnosis and intervention* (pp. 28–53). New York: John Wiley & Sons.

Swanson, H. L., Zheng, X., & Jerman, O. (2009). Working memory, short-term memory, and reading disabilities: A selective meta-analysis of the literature. *Journal of Learning Disabilities, 42*, 260–287.

Torgesen, J. K., & Mathes, P. G. (2000). *A basic guide to understanding, assessing, and teaching phonological awareness.* Austin, TX: PRO-ED.

Torgesen, J. K., Wagner, R. K., Rashotte, C. A., Rose, E., Lindamood, P., Conway, T., & Garvan, C. (1999). Preventing reading failure in young children with phonological processing disabilities. *Journal of Educational Psychology, 91*, 579–593.

Trainin, G., & Swanson, H. L. (2005). Cognition, metacognition, and achievement of college students with learning disabilities. *Learning Disability Quarterly, 28*, 261–272.

Tunmer, W. E., & Hoover, W. (1992). Cognitive and linguistic factors in learning to read. In P. B. Gough, L. C. Ehri, & R. Treiman (Eds.). *Reading acquisition* (pp. 175–224). Hillsdale, NJ: Erlbaum.

Urso, A. (2008). Processing speed as a predictor of poor reading. Unpublished doctoral dissertation, University of Arizona, Tucson.

Vaessen, A., Gerretsen, P., & Blomert, L. (2009). Naming problems do not reflect a second independent core deficit in dyslexia: Double deficits explored. *Journal of Experimental Child Psychology, 103*, 202–221.

van der Mark, S., Klaver, P., Bucher, K., Maurer, U., Schulz, E., Brem, S., et al. (2011). The left occipito-temporal system in reading: Disruption of focal fMRI connectivity to left inferior frontal and inferior parietal language areas in children with dyslexia. *NeuroImage, 54*, 2426–2436.

Vaughn, S., & Fuchs, L. S. (2003). Redefining learning disabilities as inadequate response to instruction: The promise and potential problems. *Learning Disabilities Research & Practice, 18*, 137–146.

Vinckier, F., Dehaene, S., Jobert, A., Dubus, J., Sigman, M., & Cohen, L. (2007). Hierarchical coding of letter strings in the ventral stream: Dissecting the inner organization of the visual word-form system. *Neuron, 55*(1), 143–156.

Willcutt, E. G., & Pennington, B. F. (2000). Comorbidity of reading disability and attention deficit/hyperactivity disorder: Differences by gender and subtype. *Journal of Learning Disabilities, 33*, 179–191.

Willcutt. E. G., Pennington, B. F., Olson, R. K., Chhabildas, N., & Hulslander, J. (2005). Neuropsychological analyses of comorbidity between reading disability and attention deficit hyperactivity disorder: In search of the common deficit. *Developmental Neuropsychology, 27*, 35–78.

Willis, J. O., & Dumont, R. P. (2002). *Guide to identification of learning disabilities* (3rd ed.). Peterborough, NH: Authors. Available from authors: print copy from johnzerowillis@yahoo.com or CD from dumont@fdu.edu.

Witsken, D., Stoeckel, A., & D'Amato, R. C. (2008). Leading educational change using a neuropsychological response-to-intervention approach: Linking our past, present, and future. *Psychology in the Schools, 45*, 781–798.

Xue, G., Chen, C., Jin, Z., & Dong, Q. (2006). Language experience shapes fusiform activation when processing a logographic artificial language: An fMRI training study. *Neuroimage, 31*, 1315–1326.

Testing Accommodations for Children with Disabilities

Brian C. McKevitt, Stephen N. Elliott, *and* Ryan J. Kettler

Abstract

Educators have a responsibility for including all students, including those in special education, in assessment programs designed to hold states, school districts, and schools accountable for student learning. Testing accommodations often are used to facilitate the participation of students with disabilities in these testing programs. Testing accommodations are changes to the conditions under which a test is administered or responded to by a student. This chapter discusses the use of testing accommodations with students with disabilities, including information about types of accommodations, research about accommodations, and psychometric issues associated with using accommodations on standardized tests. The chapter demonstrates how the use of testing accommodations can be a valid and fair method for including students with disabilities in testing.

Key Words: accommodations, accountability, assessment, disabilities, special education, standardized, students, testing

Introduction

Now more than ever, educators are required to document student learning outcomes. Recent federal education legislation in the United States, including the No Child Left Behind Act of 2002 (NCLB) and the Individuals with Disabilities Education Improvement Act (IDEA 2004), emphasizes the importance of regular testing of all students. Such large-scale standardized testing is intended to demonstrate students' educational progress so that schools and school districts may be held accountable for the academic performance of their students. If schools and school districts fail to meet annual goals for student achievement and participation in the testing, then corrective procedures must be undertaken.

One hallmark of NCLB and IDEA 2004 is that, in order for a school or district to meet annual achievement and participation goals, *all* students, including those with disabilities, must take the

required tests. Before these laws, it was common practice to exclude children with disabilities from large-scale testing, perhaps because of parents' not wanting their children to experience failure or because a school did not want its test scores to be negatively impacted by lower-achieving students (Kettler & Elliott, 2010; Pitoniak & Royer, 2001). However, excluding students with disabilities violated the spirit of inclusion and participation in the general education curriculum that IDEA espoused for these students. In addition, if students with disabilities did not participate in the testing, little was known about their academic outcomes, making it virtually impossible to hold schools accountable for academic achievement and to compare performance of students with disabilities across schools and school districts. As a result, educators must now enable students with disabilities to participate meaningfully in large-scale standardized testing programs.

Unfortunately, students with disabilities may have characteristics that interfere with their ability to successfully show what they know on a test. For example, a student with a learning disability in reading may have difficulty reading items that test math knowledge, thus potentially affecting his performance. A student with a behavior disability might not be able to sit quietly for a full hour to complete a long standardized test. Thus, testing accommodations may be used to facilitate the participation of students with disabilities in a school's testing program. Testing accommodations are changes in the way a test is administered, or the way that a student responds to the test, with the intent of offsetting any distortions in performance caused by the student's disability (Elliott, Kratochwill, & Schulte, 1999). The changes are *not* intended to change what the test is measuring or invalidate resulting scores, but rather to "level the playing field" for students with disabilities so they may show their true abilities on a test without the characteristics of their disabilities interfering with their performance (Elliott, Braden, & White, 2001).

Inherent in the use of testing accommodations are questions about their validity and fairness (Elliott, McKevitt, & Kettler, 2002). Obviously, standardized tests are supposed to be given in a uniform way to all students to allow for comparability of students' scores across classrooms, schools, districts, and states. If some students take the tests with accommodations and others do not, are those resulting scores truly compatible? In other words, does a score from an accommodated test have the same meaning as a score from a non-accommodated test? Can the same inferences be made about the scores? Is it fair for some students to receive accommodations while others do not?

The purpose of this chapter is to explore the use of testing accommodations on large-scale standardized tests and address the aforementioned questions. First, types of accommodations used and how educators select those accommodations will be discussed. Next, research concerning the effect that accommodations have on students' test performance and on students' and teachers' perceptions of testing will be reviewed. Finally, psychometric issues associated with testing accommodations will be presented, and in particular, issues surrounding their reliability, validity, and fairness of use. Suggestions for future directions in research and practice in the use of testing accommodations will be offered.

The Use of Testing Accommodations
Types of Accommodations

As stated earlier, a testing accommodation is a change to a test or testing situation that is intended to allow the test taker to demonstrate her or his knowledge and skills pertaining to the construct being measured. Testing accommodations can include alterations to the presentation and response format, timing and scheduling, setting, and assistive technology, but such alterations are not intended to change the construct reflected by the test score.

An important distinction between *accommodations* and *modifications* must be made. A test *modification* commonly refers to alteration of the test *content*. Because the content is changed, a modification usually changes to a certain degree the construct that is measured, thereby potentially impacting the validity of the resulting score and inferences that can be made about a student relative to that construct (Elliott et al., 1999). Appropriate accommodations, on the other hand, are not intended to alter item content. For example, reading a test of decoding skills aloud to students with reading disabilities is a *modification* to the test that changes the skill measured by the items; the test items become listening-comprehension items rather than reading-decoding items, thereby changing the construct of the test (McKevitt & Elliott, 2003). Reading aloud a math test to students with reading disabilities, however, is an appropriate *accommodation* because the test is intended to measure math skills, not reading skills. The read-aloud accommodation simply removes the barrier created by a student's reading disability when demonstrating math skills.

Testing accommodations are commonly grouped into four categories: (a) time accommodations; (b) environmental accommodations; (c) presentation format accommodations; and (d) response format accommodations (Elliott, 2007; Kettler & Elliott, 2010). Accommodations that address time typically extend the time allowed to complete a test, eliminate the time requirement altogether, or allow for more frequent breaks during testing. Environmental accommodations change aspects of the test-taking environment, such as providing a quiet, distraction-free space to complete a test, or having students take the test in a small-group setting. Accommodations that change the presentation format address how the test is administered or presented, such as reading directions aloud to a student or enlarging the text for those with a visual impairment. Finally, accommodations that address how students respond to a test include using an adult to record answers on a bubble sheet or dictating responses orally.

The Assessment Accommodations Checklist (AAC; Elliott et al., 1999) is a tool that lists 67 common testing accommodations to help educators and parents make decisions about choosing accommodations for individual students. Accommodations are selected based on student need, the accommodations that are used during regular classroom instruction, and the nature of the test that is being considered for accommodations. The AAC groups accommodations into the following categories: (a) assistance prior to test administration; (b) motivation; (c) scheduling; (d) setting; (e) assessment directions; (f) assistance during assessment; (g) equipment or assistive technology; and (h) changes in test format. Examples of accommodations listed on the AAC are provided in Table 31.1.

While not intended to affect the validity of resulting test score interpretations, accommodations may still impact the comparability of scores (and thus the validity), depending on their nature and how they are used. Testing experts at CTB/McGraw-Hill

(2000) developed a useful taxonomy for categorizing accommodations relative to the likelihood that they would change the interpretation of the resulting test score if they were used. A Category 1 accommodation under this taxonomy should not impact the score's validity and interpretation. An example of a Category 1 accommodation is moving a student to a distraction-free space to complete a test; it is unlikely a distraction-free space will change the nature of the resulting score. A Category 2 accommodation *may* influence score interpretation, depending on how it is used. Providing extra time on a test is an example of a Category 2 accommodation; it may influence score interpretation depending on how much of a departure from standardized administration the extra time was. A Category 3 accommodation almost always affects score interpretation and probably alters the construct itself. Paraphrasing directions for a student is an example of a Category 3 accommodation; by restating the directions in a way other than stated in the test manual, the test-giver may provide unintended clues or significantly change standardization, thus making the resulting score incomparable to other scores from the same test.

Table 31.1 Examples of Testing Accommodations Listed on the Assessment Accommodations Checklist

Accommodation Category	Example of Accommodations
Assistance Prior to Administering the Test	Teach test-taking skills
Motivational Accommodations	Provide verbal encouragement of effort
	Provide treats, snacks, or prizes
Scheduling Accommodations	Provide extra time
	Schedule testing over several days
Setting Accommodations	Provide a distraction-free space
	Provide special lighting
Assistance with Test Directions	Read directions to the student
	Circle or highlight the task in the directions
Assistance During the Assessment	Read questions and content to the student
	Turn pages for the student
Equipment or Assistive Technology	Tape recorder
	Calculator
Test Format Accommodations	Use large-print answer document
	Mark responses in test book rather than on a separate answer sheet

Frequency of the Use of Accommodations

Testing accommodations typically are provided as packages to students (Elliott, Kratochwill, & McKevitt, 2001). Rarely does a student receive just one accommodation (e.g., extra time); it is a more common practice for a student to receive multiple accommodations for a single test (e.g., extra time, distraction-free space, reading directions aloud to the student). In a 2005 study, Gibson, Haeberli, Glover, and Witter examined the frequency with which various accommodations were selected by students' individualized education program (IEP) teams. The IEP team has the primary responsibility for determining the participation of a student with disability in large-scale standardized testing and the accommodations required for that participation. The researchers used the AAC to track accommodations selected and categorized them according to the CTB/McGraw-Hill model described above.

Gibson et al. (2005) found that the five most-recommended accommodations were (a) providing extra testing time; (b) reading directions to students; (c) providing a distraction-free space or alternative location for the student; (d) reading questions and content to student; and (e) simplifying language in directions (paraphrasing). Each of these accommodations, except providing a distraction-free space, is considered a Category 2 or 3 accommodation, thus potentially affecting the validity of the resulting score and its interpretation. The authors caution that educators must consider the validity of accommodations when selecting them and question whether a particular accommodation is truly necessary for a given student.

Decision-Making about Using Accommodations

As stated above, IEP team members are charged with choosing testing accommodations for students. Keeping in mind that accommodations are intended to *enhance* the validity of score interpretations, educators must be careful to avoid accommodations that *decrease* the validity of score interpretations. As indicated by Gibson et al. (2005), the latter choices can be quite common. To assist with decision making, Elliott (2007) suggested six areas of knowledge that educators should have when choosing accommodations:

(a) knowledge about the student and the characteristics of the student's disability;

(b) knowledge about accommodations the student typically uses during classroom instruction;

(c) knowledge about state or district regulations;

(d) knowledge about the test items and format;

(e) an understanding about the concept of validity in score interpretation; and

(f) knowledge about previously used accommodations and their effectiveness for the student.

State and district regulations are important considerations for IEP teams when choosing accommodations. All 50 U.S. states have policies or guidelines in place about the use of testing accommodations for large-scale standardized tests (Crawford, 2007). However, state policies are quite variable. Christensen, Lazarus, Crone, and Thurlow (2008) summarized the most recent state policies on testing accommodations. They found that state policies are paying closer attention to validity issues than in the past. However, certain controversial accommodations (i.e., those that are Category 2 or 3 and may impact score interpretation) are still allowed by several states with or without restrictions. For example, reading aloud questions and content is allowed with no restrictions in three states, while 24 states allow it under certain circumstances (e.g., on math tests). Simplifying or paraphrasing directions is allowed without restrictions in 13 states, yet prohibited in one state. Using a calculator is allowed by 10 states without restrictions and 19 states with restrictions. Finally, the use of a spell checker on a test is allowed without restrictions by seven states and prohibited completely by one state.

Also according to Christensen et al. (2008), state policies are increasingly providing recommendations for scribes, readers, and sign-language interpreters to enhance the validity of scores when these accommodations are used. These changes are indicators that state policies are evolving to carefully consider issues of validity when deciding which accommodations are allowable and which are not. Such variability among states, however, may have consequences (Crawford, 2007). Scores from tests given with allowable accommodations may be reported for a school or school district's NCLB accountability requirements. Variability among states in allowable accommodations may degrade the comparability of scores between states and may inflate scores in states where certain controversial accommodations are allowed. Next, if a student moves from one state to another, he or she may not be allowed an accommodation that was once allowable, causing potential frustration and disappointment. Finally, teachers may avoid using non-allowed testing accommodations during classroom instruction, a time during which such accommodations could be beneficial for a student, thus affecting the quality of his or her education.

IEP teams must select accommodations within the parameters of state guidelines and policies, as well as their own knowledge about the student and the test. Empirical research on the effect of testing accommodations should also play a role in the selection of accommodations for individual students. Over the past 15 years, research has been conducted using a variety of designs to test the effect that various accommodations, used in isolation or in packages, have on the scores of students with and without disabilities. Research has also informed educators about students' and teachers' perceptions of testing accommodations and their validity and fairness of use.

The Effects of Testing Accommodations

In 2000, Thurlow, McGrew, Tindal, Thompson, Ysseldyke, and J. Elliott wrote a monograph for the National Center on Educational Outcomes (NCEO) to address the state of assessment accommodations research. The researchers indicated that future research should (a) focus on accommodations of most interest, (b) focus on students who compose a large part of the population needing accommodations, (c) use students without disabilities as a group in any comparison designs, and (d) collect other measures to help clarify findings. Thurlow et al. (2000) identified four group-research designs, all including participants taking tests under both accommodated and non-accommodated conditions, to address the matter of whether assessment accommodations work. Since the Thurlow et al. report, research on the effects of such accommodations has become more abundant. A review of the relevant literature reveals numerous studies examining the use of testing accommodations and the validity of score interpretations on tests given with accommodations (e.g., Elliott, McKevitt, & Kettler, 2002; Fletcher et al., 2006; Kosciolek & Ysseldyke, 2000; Lang, Elliott, Bolt, & Kratochwill, 2007; McKevitt & Elliott, 2003; Mehrens, 2002; Pitoniak & Royer, 2001). Another suggestion by Thurlow et al. was that work on assessment accommodations needs to be done as part of a program: "Even with the best research designs, we will not get nice answers unless we have a program of research to follow up with additional questions" (p. 28). Two of the most active and systematic programs of research have been conducted by Fuchs, Fuchs,

and colleagues and S. Elliott and colleagues. These investigators' research is featured next, along with a few other key studies.

Fuchs, Fuchs, and colleagues have done a number of research studies on assessment accommodations, in addition to their development of *Dynamic Assessment Tool for Accommodations* (DATA; a decision-making framework about using accommodations). In a meta-analytic study, Tindal and Fuchs (2000) found that the most effective accommodations included providing large-print or Braille tests for the visually impaired, as well as reading problems aloud for students with disabilities in math. Rather than examining accommodations in packages, Fuchs, Fuchs, and Capizzi (2006) indicated that research should be done on one accommodation at a time, with work on packages only commencing after individual accommodations have been validated. Findings from their studies include that:

(a) extended time does not provide a differential boost (i.e., it does not improve the scores of students with disabilities more than students without disabilities),

(b) reading a test orally helps students with disabilities more than it does students without disabilities,

(c) heterogeneity among students with disabilities reduces the likelihood of one set of accommodations' being appropriate for the entire group,

(d) student demographic characteristics may influence teachers' accommodation recommendations, and

(e) students with severe disabilities and severe reading deficits may benefit from reading a test aloud.

Based on a review of assessment accommodations literature, Fuchs, Fuchs, and Capizzi (2006) concluded that decisions about testing accommodations must be individualized, that the meaningfulness of test scores must be of primary importance when selecting accommodations; also that the mandated inclusion of students with disabilities in educational outcomes testing makes this area of research critical.

Elliott and colleagues have examined the effects of testing accommodations on the performance of students with and without disabilities in more than eight studies. In an early study, Elliott, Kratochwill, and McKevitt (2001) showed that the majority of students both with and without disabilities performed better on an achievement test when they were provided accommodations. Notably however, the average effect size of accommodations provided to students with disabilities (SWDs) was 0.88, while the effect size for students without disabilities (SWODs) was only 0.45.

In a second study, Schulte, Elliott, and Kratochwill (2001) had students with and without disabilities complete two equivalent forms of math achievement tests, one with accommodations and one without accommodations. The results of this study showed that on the constructed response tasks, most students performed better under the accommodated condition than under the non-accommodated condition. The largest interaction effect was found when responses to multiple-choice questions were compared across the two disability groups. For this type of question, accommodations produced an effect size of 0.41 for SWDs and an effect size of 0.00 for SWODs.

In a related study, McKevitt and Elliott (2003) examined the effect of testing accommodations on students' performance on the reading portion of the same achievement test. In this study, students with and without disabilities were administered the reading test either with or without accommodations. The group that received the test with accommodations was further divided into two groups—one that received a teacher-recommended accommodations package, and one that received a teacher-recommended accommodations package plus a read-aloud accommodation. Findings from this study revealed that (a) the teacher-recommended accommodations did not significantly improve scores for either disability status group, (b) the read-aloud accommodation significantly improved scores for both disability status groups, and (c) there was no significant interaction effect between disability status and the accommodation package with the read-aloud accommodation.

Expanding on the McKevitt and Elliott study, Elliott and Marquart (2004) examined the effects of a specific accommodation—extended time—on students' test performance and also on their perceptions of testing and testing accommodations. Results from this study showed that when students were grouped according to disability status, there was no significant effect of the accommodations on test performance for either group. When SWODs were grouped as at-risk and at-grade-level groups, however, the effect size of testing accommodations for the at-risk group was 0.48, whereas the effect size for the grade-level group was 0.20. Overall,

students in this study reported they felt more motivated and less frustrated, thought they performed better, thought the test was easier, and preferred taking the test when accommodations were provided.

Fletcher and colleagues (2006) examined the effects of accommodations on the high-stakes test results of Texas students with reading disabilities. Specifically, they examined the effects of accommodations on the reading performance of third-grade students, half of whom had word-decoding difficulties with dyslexia and half of whom were considered average decoders. Only students with decoding problems were found to benefit from the accommodation package, showing a significant increase in average performance and a sevenfold increase in the odds of passing the test. The authors suggested that these results demonstrated that "accommodations designed for a clearly defined academic disability can enhance performance on a high-stakes assessment" (p. 136).

A study conducted by Kosciolek and Ysseldyke (2000) added an important variable to testing accommodation research. These investigators examined students' attitudes towards the provision of testing accommodations and the alignment between the students' perceptions of accommodations and their test performance. Results based on a small sample of students indicated that most students preferred taking an accommodated test, but that SWDs showed a stronger preference for the accommodated condition. There was also a difference between the two student groups in the reason they gave for their preferences. While SWDs claimed that the accommodations made the test easier, SWODs said that the accommodations enabled them to take the test at their own pace. Overall, previous research on testing accommodations has produced mixed outcomes, and a great deal is yet to be determined about their effects and the means by which those effects are produced.

One hypothesis regarding the means by which accommodations may affect students' test performance is that accommodations affect specific thoughts and attitudes that students have about the tests and about their own test-taking abilities. Specifically, this hypothesis draws on social cognitive theory, in which self-efficacy plays a key role in task performance (Bandura, 1997). With achievement testing, a student who has low test-related self-efficacy may be less motivated to work hard on the tests, may lack persistence to work steadily on the more challenging problems, may have insufficient perseverance to continue working when the test gets hard, may have little interest in the test, may be likely to put forth only minimal effort, and may be extremely anxious about the test. As a result, this student's score on the test might not accurately reflect the student's true ability in the targeted skill area, but would be influenced by many other extraneous factors that can affect the construct being measured, particularly in comparison with the score obtained by a student with high test-related self-efficacy who was not hindered in a similar manner. Recently, Elliott and several colleagues have focused on the potential consequences of large-scale achievement testing on the self-efficacy of students who take the tests.

Lang et al. (2008) provided one of the first experimental examinations of the effects of testing accommodations on a number of student characteristics, as well as on performance outcomes. Most notably, Lang and her colleagues examined responses to questionnaire items completed by both fourth- and eighth-grade students following a test administration. Results demonstrated that testing accommodations improved most students' performance on the tests and showed that the effects of testing accommodations on student performance were larger for SWDs than for SWODs (i.e., a differential boost). Lang and colleagues also found that students both with and without disabilities preferred the accommodated testing condition, but that this preference was stronger among SWDs. Lang et al. also reported no significant correlation between disability status and the effect of testing accommodations on students' self-reported motivation.

In a follow-up experimental study to Lang et al. and using similar tests, Feldman, Kim, and Elliott (2008) examined the effects of testing accommodations on eighth-grade students' performance on large-scale achievement tests and also on the students' attitudes and reactions related to taking such tests. Their findings revealed significant differences in the ways in which students with and without disabilities experienced the testing, and in the ways that testing accommodations affected students' attitudes toward and beliefs about the tests. Specifically, results suggested that (a) students with disabilities had significantly lower test-related self-efficacy than students without disabilities; (b) self-efficacy was positively correlated with test performance for all students; and (c) the provision of accommodations improved the test performance of all students and exerted a differential boost for students with disabilities on constructs such as test-related self-efficacy and motivation. Collectively, these findings suggested

that testing accommodations may have a positive effect on students' test performance by improving their attitudinal constructs such as test-related self-efficacy and motivation, especially for students with learning disabilities.

Psychometric Issues Associated with Testing Accommodations

Testing accommodations are used to improve the measurement of abilities for students for whom tests administered without accommodations may not yield scores from which inferences are as reliable, valid, or fair. Testing accommodations are not intended to provide an advantage for SWDs, but are intended to make inferences yielded by test scores for SWDs comparable to those yielded by scores that SWODs obtain without accommodations. This section of the chapter addresses the issues of reliability and validity, as well as fairness, which must be considered with testing accommodations. To illustrate these issues, we revisit the example of students with reading disabilities taking a math test with a read-aloud accommodation.

The Impact of Testing Accommodations on Reliability and Validity

The variance in a set of scores can be subdivided into variance based on the construct being measured, or *true-score* variance, and variance based on other factors, or *error-score* variance. In our example, true-score variance corresponds to variance in students' abilities in mathematics. Error-score variance can be further subdivided into that which is from systematic sources (e.g., reading ability), and that which is from random sources (e.g., inconsistency in accommodation administration). One danger in using testing accommodations is that if they are applied inconsistently, the accommodations may increase the amount of error from random sources, therefore decreasing the reliability or consistency of test scores. Suppose that the administrators of the read-aloud accommodation in the example were not explicitly trained, but were only told that the students are allowed to have the test read aloud. To one person, this might mean that the directions, item stems, and answer choices can be read aloud, but not text in the item stimulus. A second person might think that everything can be read aloud, including the item stimulus, unless it contains key mathematics vocabulary words that are grade-appropriate for the students. A third person might interpret the accommodation to mean that absolutely everything can be read aloud. Other sources of confusion might be distinctions between whether the item must be read aloud or should only be read aloud upon student request, whether the item can be reread upon request, and whether the meaning of the text can be clarified by the administrator. Without explicit rules and training, the application of this accommodation would probably vary from person to person, as well as when administered by the same person at different points in time. The impact of this inconsistency of administration on the students taking the test is unpredictable, and the reliability of the resulting scores would almost certainly be reduced.

The most direct, intended psychometric impact of testing accommodations is to reduce error-score variance that is from systematic sources. Appropriate accommodations should be designed to match these sources, in order to help the student get around these barriers to good measurement, so that a higher proportion of the variance in scores is true-score variance. In our example of students with reading disabilities, a math test with a moderate to high reading load would be likely to yield scores that are indicative partially of mathematics ability and partially of reading ability (along with error from random sources). Some form of read-aloud accommodation could reduce the amount of variance that is connected to variance in reading ability, so that a larger proportion of the variance in the scores would be due to variance in mathematics ability, the target construct.

A few notes are important to consider when interpreting this example. The first is that this read-aloud accommodation would only be effective when applied to students who have reading problems. While the read-aloud accommodation may be appropriate for this group, it would probably not lead to more valid inferences if used with students who have a different disability. For example, students who are good readers but who have fine-motor deficits that cause difficulty holding a pencil are not likely to be helped. Another group who would probably not be helped are students with mathematics disabilities who are good readers. The variance in these students' scores would be largely composed of variance in mathematics abilities, as is appropriate for good measurement. Accommodations are not intended to distort students' abilities on the construct the test score is intended to reflect. Finally, it is important to note that although SWODs would not be helped by the read-aloud accommodation, they are not likely to be hurt by it, either. These students' scores on the non-accommodated test would be highly dependent on their mathematics abilities,

because reading would not be a barrier to them. The effect of the read-aloud accommodation for students with reading problems would be to make their scores more dependent on their mathematics ability, and thus more comparable to the scores of SWODs.

Once a model has been established for how testing accommodations should affect the reliability and validity of inferences drawn from test scores, the next logical question is how to evaluate whether testing accommodations are actually working in this fashion. The Standards for Educational and Psychological Testing (the Standards; American Educational Research Association [AERA], American Psychological Association [APA], & National Council on Measurement in Education [NCME], 1999) prescribe an evidence evaluation orientation toward establishing validity, including the collection of evidence based on relationships with other variables. "Evidence based on relationships with other variables" is the degree to which scores from the newly developed or accommodated test converge with scores for measures of similar constructs (e.g., other tests, known groups), but diverge with scores from dissimilar constructs. A special case of validity evidence based on relationships with other variables, the *interaction paradigm* (i.e., differential boost), has been used as a framework for evaluating improved access based on accommodations or modifications (Kettler & Elliott, 2010; Phillips, 1994), and is the focus of the next section.

The Interaction Paradigm

The interaction paradigm indicates that the gap between scores from SWDs and scores from SWODs should be reduced through the use of appropriate accommodations, because these accommodations would directly address sources of systematic error-score variance. An example from an authentic research study can illustrate the interaction paradigm: Kettler et al. (2005) administered research versions of standardized reading and mathematics tests to SWDs and SWODs, in a condition that included a package of accommodations identified by Individualized Education Programs and the students' teachers, as well as in a non-accommodated condition. In the non-accommodated condition of the fourth-grade reading test, SWDs ($n = 49$) had a mean score of 600 ($SD = 45$) and SWODs ($n = 69$) had a mean score of 662 ($SD = 37$). An ideal result from an interaction paradigm perspective, indicating that the packages of accommodations worked perfectly, would be for both groups of students to

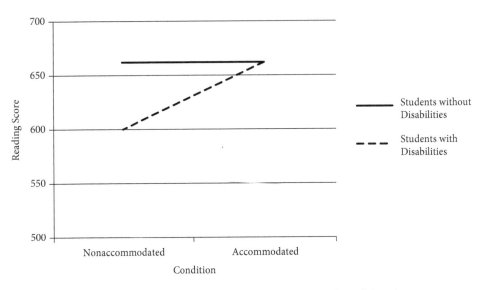

Figure 31.1 Ideal interaction between accommodation condition and group status in Kettler et al. (2005).

have a mean score of 662 in the accommodated condition. The effect size in that case would have been 1.38 for SWDs and 0.00 for SWODs. Figure 31.1 depicts this hypothetical, ideal finding.

While the aforementioned results would have been ideal evidence that the package of accommodations in Kettler et al. (2005) was appropriate, there are many reasons why consistently finding large effects for SWDs and no effects for SWODs is unlikely. The first of these reasons is the assumption that the SWDs and SWODs compose two completely non-overlapping groups, such that the accommodations used are helpful for SWDs, but do not make any difference to SWODs. In reality, it is very likely that the SWOD group will be composed of students with a continuum of abilities on skills that are related to the target construct, and that lower-performing or at-risk SWODs may very well benefit from some of the accommodations designed for SWDs. A second reason that finding the ideal interaction paradigm is unlikely is that it assumes that SWDs as a group have equal ability to that of the SWODs on the construct being measured. Such a scenario is unlikely, because SWDs often face more barriers in accessing classroom material, and to the degree that access to learning the material is limited, SWDs are likely to have lower achievement than SWODs, even if measurement is nearly perfect. A final complication is that many content areas (e.g., reading, mathematics) and sub-areas (e.g. fluency, comprehension) are closely related, so that students with one type of learning problem often struggle in other areas. All three of these complications make it

unlikely that SWODs and SWDs would have the same scores, even in the accommodated condition.

In Kettler et al. (2005), a significant interaction was found between accommodation condition and disability group on the fourth-grade reading test (significant interactions were not found on the other tests), indicating that the accommodations helped SWDs more than they helped SWODs. In the accommodated condition, SWDs had a mean score of 619 ($SD = 25$), and SWODs had a mean score of 666 ($SD = 34$). Cohen's d for SWDs (.42) was larger than Cohen's d for SWODs (0.13). Figure 31.2 depicts the observed interaction between accommodation and disability group, with the slope of the line for the SWD group being greater than the slope of the line for the SWOD group. The SWOD group probably improved on average because some students were relatively low performing and at-risk for academic problems. The SWD group likely did not reach mean score of SWODs in the non-accommodated condition (662) because the same barriers that make testing difficult have affected their access to instruction over the years, and because accommodations cannot change the reality that students who have difficulty with vocabulary are at a disadvantage for showing how well they comprehend, and vice versa. It is difficult to imagine accommodations that could overcome this discrepancy and have SWDs performing at the same level as SWODs, while improving the validity of inferences that can be drawn from the test scores. How to select fair accommodations, given these limitations, is the subject of the next section.

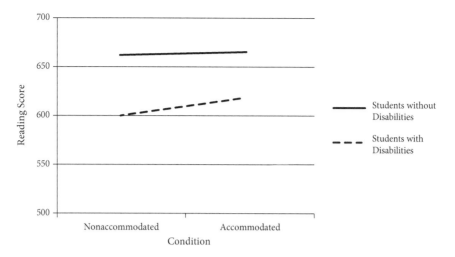

Figure 31.2 Actual interaction between accommodation condition and group status in Kettler et al. (2005).

Fairness of Testing Accommodation Use

The issue of which testing accommodations are fair is more subjective than are issues of reliability and validity, but determination of fairness should begin with the intention of measuring each construct as accurately as possible. For all tests, this means minimizing sources of error-score variance, both random and systematic. Maximizing measurement accuracy also means that, for some groups of students, testing accommodations need to be used for a test score to reflect the same construct that it reflects for most students in the non-accommodated condition. While SWODs reading and responding to a hypothetical math test may provide interpretable scores, SWDs may need to take the test under different conditions in order to obtain comparable scores. This is fair in the sense that the conditions under which a test is taken are not as important as the interpretability of the resulting scores. It is by this logic that using the interaction paradigm is a sensible method for evaluating testing accommodation fairness.

Researchers have used a couple of techniques to address the issue of fairness and testing accommodations. Lang et al. (2007) surveyed students ($n = 170$) who had taken a test with and without accommodations about whether testing accommodations are fair. On a five-point scale from 1 (*strongly disagree*) to 5 (*strongly agree*), the mean rating for the statement that "accommodations are fair for students who need them" ranged from 3.69 to 3.98 across grades and disability groups. Ratings were slightly higher for the statement that "accommodations are fair for students with disabilities," ranging from 4.19 to 4.41. These findings indicate that students believe accommodations are fair, and perhaps even fairer for SWDs.

Lang et al. (2007) did not address the fairness of any isolated accommodations used outside of a package. One almost universally accepted, if not empirically proven, method for considering the fairness of isolated accommodations is to only use testing accommodations that have been used as instructional accommodations prior to testing. A National Center on Educational Outcomes (NCEO) report on the peer review of progress in meeting NCLB requirements indicated that 39 states had acceptable language in their policies, indicating that testing accommodations should match instructional accommodations (Thurlow, Christensen, & Lail, 2008). For example, the State of Florida included a table linking student behavior with possible instructional and testing accommodations. The theory is that error-score variance could emerge if students see an accommodation for the first time in a testing situation. While the vast majority of states have language in their policies addressing this issue, it is debatable whether the match between instructional and assessment accommodations is very close. Based on an analysis of the Special Education Elementary Longitudinal Study (SEELS), Bottsford-Miller, Thurlow, Stout, and Quenemoen (2006) reported that the percentage of students with accommodations on IEPs was very close to the percentage of students who received instructional accommodations, but in most cases exceeded the percentage of students who received assessment accommodations. These data imply that many students are receiving instructional accommodations that they do not receive on assessments. It is less likely, based on these data, that students are often seeing accommodations for the first time in a testing situation. However, no direct analysis of which students were receiving which accommodations was done.

Conclusion

Research on the use and effects of testing accommodations has come a long way since the educational accountability movement began. As long as there is a requirement to include all students in large-scale assessment, educators will rely on testing accommodations to facilitate the participation of students with disabilities in those assessments. Research on testing accommodations has demonstrated that they can have a measurable impact on test scores for students with disabilities, and in some cases, for students without disabilities. Examining the impact of testing accommodations on the performance of students without disabilities is a useful way to assess the validity of accommodations, given that accommodations generally should not impact the scores of these students. When they do, questions about validity and fairness of accommodations may be raised. As educators continue to grapple with using accommodations appropriately, researchers and policy makers will continue to add new knowledge to our understanding of this complex assessment tool. Ultimately, however, knowledge about the student being tested, the test being used, local policies, and validity and fairness in measurement must be used in the provision of testing accommodations.

Future Directions

Research on the use and effects of testing accommodations still needs to be conducted. Such research should focus on students with and without disabilities, using single-subject and large-group designs. Ultimately, the research needs to help educators decide which accommodations to use for which students, and when to use them. State policies also may inform educators about using accommodations based on continuing research. As Christensen et al. (2008) reported, state policies are improving in the attention they pay to issues of validity and fairness with the use of accommodations. Still, more states need to develop specific accommodation policies that account for validity issues identified in the research.

There is also a need to examine the use of accommodations with other student groups, such as English language learners or students with more severe disabilities. Like students with disabilities, English language learners must be included in state and district accountability assessments.

Accommodations may be used in some cases to facilitate their participation as well. Research is needed to test the impact of accommodations with this group of students. Furthermore, the law allows a small percentage of students with disabilities to participate in an alternate assessment because of the severity of their disabilities. Research and policy are needed to help inform educators about how to design these alternate assessments and what role, if any, testing accommodations may play in their use.

The use of testing accommodations may seem, at first, a simple and effective way to help students with disabilities demonstrate their true knowledge on a test. However, the use of accommodations is anything but simple. Educators have a legal responsibility to include all students in testing and an ethical responsibility to attend to the validity and fairness of testing. Research on the use and effects of testing accommodations has shown that these two responsibilities may be difficult to reconcile in harmony with one another. Only with the continued efforts of researchers, policy makers, and educators will our understanding of the use and effects of testing accommodations continue to evolve in a positive direction.

Glossary and Abbreviations

Accommodation. A change in the way a test is administered or a student responds to it with the intent of offsetting any construct-irrelevant distortion on test performance caused by a student's disability.

Alternate assessment. A method of assessment for students with severe disabilities that is an alternative to a traditional large-scale standardized test. Alternate assessments can take many forms and vary between and within states.

Assistive technology. Any device that can be used to help students respond to test items (e.g., a pointer).

Construct. The characteristic that is being measured by a test.

Differential boost. See *interaction paradigm*.

Fairness. A judgement about whether the use of accommodations is equal for all those using them.

IDEA. The Individuals with Disabilities Education Act.

IEP. Individualized Education Program.

Interaction paradigm. An expected phenomenon in the use of testing accommodations wherein students with disabilities should experience greater gain in test scores when using accommodations than do students without disabilities who receive the same accommodations.

Modification. An alteration to the content of a test, thus changing the construct being measured.

NCLB. No Child Left Behind Act.

Standardized test. A test given and scored with uniform directions and procedures to all those taking it.

Student with a disability. A student who has undergone a school-based evaluation and has been determined to have one or more of 13 possible disabilities identified by IDEA.

Validity. The degree to which a test score reflects the construct that it is intended to measure, and allows accurate inferences to be made.

Author Note

Please direct all correspondence concerning this chapter to Brian C. McKevitt, Department of Psychology, University of Nebraska at Omaha, 6001 Dodge St., Omaha, NE 68137, (402) 554-2498, bmckevitt@unomaha.edu.

References

American Educational Research Association, American Psychological Association, & National Council on Measurement in Education (1999). *Standards for educational and psychological testing.* Washington, DC: AERA, APA & NCME.

Bandura, A. (1997). *Self-efficacy: The exercise of control.* New York: W.H. Freeman.

Bottsford-Miller, N. Thurlow, M. L., Stout, K. E., & Quenemoen, R. F. (2006). *A comparison of IEP/504 accommodations under classroom and standardized testing conditions: A preliminary report on SEELS data* (Synthesis Report 63). Minneapolis, MN: University of Minnesota, National Center on Educational Outcomes.

Christensen, L. L., Lazarus, S. S., Crone, M., & Thurlow, M. L. (2008). *2007 state policies on assessment participation and accommodations for students with disabilities* (Synthesis Report 69). Minneapolis, MN: University of Minnesota, National Center on Educational Outcomes.

Crawford, L. (2007). *State testing accommodations: A look at their value and validity.* New York: National Center for Learning Disabilities. Available online at www.ld.org.

CTB/McGraw-Hill (2000). *Guidelines for using the results of standardized tests administered under nonstandard conditions.* Monterey, CA: CTB/McGraw-Hill.

Elliott, S. N. (2007). Selecting and using testing accommodations to facilitate meaningful participation of all students in state and district assessments. In L. Cook & C. Cahalan (Eds.), *Large scale assessment and accommodations: What works?* (pp. 1–9). Princeton, NJ: Educational Testing Service.

Elliott, S. N., Braden, J. P., & White, J. L. (2001). *Assessing one and all: Educational accountability for students with disabilities.* Alexandria, VA: Council for Exceptional Children.

Elliott, S. N., Kratochwill, T. R., & McKevitt, B. C. (2001). Experimental analysis of the effects of testing accommodations

on the scores of students with and without disabilities. *Journal of School Psychology, 39,* 3–24.

Elliott, S. N., Kratochwill, T. R., & Schulte, A. G. (1999). *Assessment accommodations checklist.* Monterey, CA: CTB/McGraw-Hill.

Elliott, S. N., & Marquart, A. M. (2004). Extended time as an accommodation on a standardized mathematics test: An investigation of its effects on scores and perceived consequences for students with varying mathematical skills. *Exceptional Children, 70,* 349–367.

Elliott, S. N., McKevitt, B. C., & Kettler, R. (2002). Testing accommodations research and decision-making: The case of "good" scores being highly valued but difficult to achieve for all students. *Measurement & Evaluation in Counseling & Development, 35,* 156–166.

Feldman, E., Kim, J. S., & Elliott, S. N. (2008). Attitudes and reactions to large-scale assessments: An experimental investigation of the effects of accommodations on adolescents' self-efficacy and test performance. Unpublished manuscript, University of Wisconsin-Madison.

Fletcher, J. M., Francis, D. J., Boudousquie, A., Copeland, K., Young, V., Kalinowski, S., & Vaughn, S. (2006). Effects of accommodations on high-stakes testing for students with reading disabilities. *Exceptional Children, 72,* 136–150.

Fuchs, L. S., Fuchs, D., & Capizzi, A. M. (2006). Identifying appropriate test accommodations for students with learning disabilities. *Focus on Exceptional Children, 37,* 1–8.

Gibson, D., Haeberli, F. B., Glover, T. A., & Witter, E. A. (2005). Use of recommended and provided testing accommodations. *Assessment for Effective Instruction, 31,* 19–36.

Kettler, R., J., & Elliott, S. N. (2010). Assessment accommodations for children with special needs. In E. Baker, P. Peterson, & B. McGaw (Eds.), *International encyclopedia of education: 3rd Edition* (pp. 530–536). Oxford, UK: Elsevier Limited.

Kettler, R. J., Niebling, B. C., Mroch, A. A., Feldman, E. S., Newell, M. L., Elliott, S. N., et al. (2005). Effects of testing accommodations on math and reading scores: An experimental analysis of the performance of fourth- and eighth-grade students with and without disabilities. *Assessment for Effective Intervention, 31,*37–48.

Kosciolek, S. & Ysseldyke, J. E. (2000). *Effects of a reading accommodation on the validity of a reading test* (Technical Report 28). Minneapolis, MN: University of Minnesota, National Center on Educational Outcomes.

Lang, S. C., Elliott, S. N., Bolt, D. M., & Kratochwill, T. R. (2007). The effects of testing accommodations on students' performances and reactions to testing. *School Psychology Quarterly, 14,* 1–28.

McKevitt, B. C., & Elliott, S. N. (2003). Effects and perceived consequences of using read-aloud and teacher-recommended testing accommodations on a reading achievement test. *School Psychology Review, 32,* 583–600.

Mehrens, W. A. (2002). Consequences of assessment: What is the evidence? In G. Tindal & T. M. Haladyna (Eds.), *Large-scale assessment programs for all students: Validity, technical adequacy, and implementation* (pp. 149–177). Mahwah, NJ: Lawrence Erlbaum Associates.

Phillips, S. E. (1994). High-stakes testing accommodations: Validity versus disabled rights. *Applied Measurement in Education, 7,* 93–120.

Pitoniak, M. J., & Royer, J. M. (2001). Testing accommodations for examinees with disabilities: A review of psychometric, legal, and social policy issues. *Review of Educational Research, 71,* 53–104.

Schulte, A. G., Elliott, S. N., & Kratochwill, T. R. (2001). Experimental analysis of the effects of testing accommodations on students; standardized achievement test scores. *School Psychology Review, 30,* 527–547.

Thurlow, M. L., Christensen, L. L., & Lail, K. E. (2008). *An analysis of accommodations issues from the standards and assessments peer review* (Technical Report 51). Minneapolis, MN: University of Minnesota, National Center on Educational Outcomes.

Thurlow, M. L., McGrew, K. S., Tindal, G., Thompson, S.J., Ysseldyke, J. E., and Elliott, J. L. (2000). *Assessment accommodations research: Considerations for data analysis* (Tech. Rep. No. 26). Minneapolis, MN: University of Minnesota, National Center on Educational Outcomes.

Tindal, G., & Fuchs, L. S. (2000). *A summary of research on test changes: An empirical basis for defining accommodations.* Lexington, KY: Mid-South Regional resource Center Interdisciplinary Human Development Institute.

Special Issues in the Forensic Assessment of Children and Adolescents

Kathryn Kuehnle, Steven N. Sparta, H. D. Kirkpatrick, *and* Monica Epstein

Abstract

This chapter describes the forensic mental health assessment of children and adolescents related to psycholegal questions in three areas of civil law and one area of criminal judicial proceedings. The authors describe general principles of forensic assessment, including considerations of tests and methods, as well as special assessment issues applied to each of four common areas of assessment. In the forensic assessment for child custody, evaluation procedures are described for how best to assess the relationship between a child and each parent, where a broad consideration exists for the child's best interests. Child abuse and neglect cases, a second type of case calling for a forensic assessment, are usually heard in child dependency departments of the legal system. This chapter describes the assessment of the child's and/or the parents' psychological functioning, with particular reference to the child's safety and well-being. Forensic assessment also is described regarding certain types of civil matters, usually involving personal injury cases and how the psychological functioning of individuals may be affected by legally relevant events in the person's life. Finally, the authors describe the forensic assessment for determining the competency to stand trial of children or adolescents in criminal proceedings, including the individual's capacity to understand and meaningfully participate in the legal proceedings.

Key Words: forensic assessment of children and adolescents, civil judicial proceedings involving children, criminal judicial proceedings involving children, child abuse

The purpose of forensic evaluations conducted by mental health professionals is to be helpful to the legal decision-maker (i.e., judge, jury, or other hearing officer) or helpful to the retaining authority (e.g., attorney). In contrast, the purpose of the clinical evaluation is to be helpful to the patient. It has sometimes been said that the forensic evaluator "advocates for the data," striving for an objective and informed opinion, utilizing, when available, empirical data to form opinions. Forensic mental health evaluators may perform evaluations in many different psycholegal contexts.

To avoid confusing the reader with terms that may be inconsistent across various jurisdictions, we offer a brief description of the terminology we have used in this chapter to identify various judicial proceedings. In the adjudicative process, there are four major types of judicial proceedings: *criminal, civil, administrative,* and *quasi-criminal* (e.g., therapeutic courts) (Melton, Petrila, Poythress, & Slobogin, 2007). States vary in how they organize court divisions of civil judicial proceedings. Various states may hold cases for child custody (i.e., parent responsibility and timesharing), adoption, and potentially other family matters in "Family Courts," child protection matters in "Dependency Courts," juvenile delinquency cases in "Juvenile Courts," and personal injury or tort proceedings in "General Civil Courts." Other states may combine child custody and child protection cases in "Unified Family

Courts" and handle juvenile delinquency cases in a different court. In this article, we will refer to child custody cases (parenting plan and child-access cases) as *family law matters*, child protection cases as *dependency law matters*, and personal injury cases as *tort law matters*.

The following areas of forensic assessment are the focus of this chapter:

- Family law—Family dissolution and parenting plans
- Dependency law—Child abuse and neglect
- Tort law—Psychological injury: intentional and negligent
- Criminal law—Juvenile competency

General Principles of Forensic Assessment

In all forensic contexts when the legal proceedings involve children, there are two essential and necessary components: (1) skilled and developmentally appropriate interviewing of children and (2) the acquisition of sufficient information from the evaluation—including collateral sources—combined with an appropriate analysis adequate to support the opinions proffered regarding the child. Generally speaking, the following methods and procedures are applied in the forensic assessment of children and adolescents in a forensic context:

1. A competent forensic assessment usually involves the utilization of multiple methods to consider diverse sources of independent data. The utilization of collateral sources is often the *sine qua non* of forensic methodology—i.e., without collateral data, the forensic assessment fails the test of adequacy (Heilbrun, Warren, & Picarello, 2003).

2. To guard against confirmatory bias, a forensic evaluator considers multiple hypotheses when collecting and analyzing the data, including consideration of the limitations of existing data.

3. Collateral data are obtained from two general sources—*collateral persons* who may have relevant information pertaining to the child/adolescent, and *collateral information* that may provide useful data about the child. Relevant collateral persons may include parents, step-parents, extended-family members, babysitters, day-care providers, teachers, neighbors, other families who have had contact with the child or the child's family, or law enforcement personnel having contact with one or more family members. Relevant collateral information could include information from school, mental health treatment, medical, legal, child protection or other sources.

4. A forensic mental health evaluator of children and adolescents must always consider the evaluation context of the psycholegal question, and therefore guard against accepting at face value any information from a single source, e.g., one parent involved in a parenting dispute.

5. A forensic expert who engages in the assessment of children and adolescents in a psycholegal context recognizes that an adequate informed consent requires greater consideration that the relevant parties understand and agree upon matters such as the scope of the evaluation, the methods, fees and costs and how they are to be paid, the limits of confidentiality for all involved, and other relevant information. Because of the serious issues and associated emotional tension which accompany such matters, a careful execution of informed consent will help protect the forensic expert from risk derived from misunderstandings, distortion or unfounded accusations.

6. Forensic evaluators should adequately document the evaluation methods and results, and in cases involving investigations of child maltreatment, electronic recording of child interviews is essential. Empirical evidence is robust in showing that note-taking is not a reliable means of capturing the important data from children's interviews regarding alleged maltreatment (Berliner & Lieb, 2001; Lamb, Orbach, Sternberg, Hershkowitz, & Horowitz, 2000).

7. Psychological testing can contribute valuable norm-referenced data regarding a child's or parent's functioning. When considering such testing, forensic evaluators recognize many potential instruments may not have been developed for a specific forensic purpose, or that tests that do have some relevance may not answer ultimate psychological or psycholegal questions, but only limited elements of the questions.

8. Quasi-assessment tools, such as children's doll play, drawings, and sand play, should not be misrepresented as "tests," implying measurement validity beyond their value. To the extent such methods are ever used in a forensic assessment, the evaluator must recognize the reliability and validity limitations of quasi-assessment methods, and not communicate an unfounded or misleading justification for an opinion based on their limited use. Sometimes a forensic evaluator uses such techniques for rapport building, especially with young or psychologically defended children. Quasi-assessment tools should not be used to

answer ultimate psycholegal issues, e.g., the child was or was not abused.

9. The forensic evaluator recognizes that psychological testing should not be interpreted in isolation of other data, especially in a forensic context. In a forensic evaluation, the same test results can have different relevance or meaning, depending upon the case context and the nature and extent of other information associated with the forensic questions.

Assessment Instruments

Tests and measures should strive to meet *Daubert* (1993)[1] and *Kumho* (1999)[2] criteria of relevance and reliability for the context in which they are used—they should add valid and reliable information to the psycholegal question under consideration—even if the local jurisdiction does not adopt the federal rules. Appropriate, valid test data may add *incremental* validity to other data obtained in the evaluation, e.g., observations and interviewing of the child, collateral interviews, collateral records review, and application of relevant social sciences research. First and foremost, the forensic assessment of children and adolescents requires valid methods and procedures that demand consideration in case specific contexts. Consideration of the instruments' validity for the particular psycholegal question must be considered (Grisso, 2005, cited in Sparta & Koocher, 2006).

Melton, Petrila, Poythress, and Slobogin (2007, p. 48) identified 12 factors evaluators should consider before selecting a psychological test or assessment technique as part of a forensic evaluation:

1. What is the construct to be assessed?
2. How directly does the instrument assess the construct of interest?
3. Are there alternative methods that assess the construct of interest in more direct ways?
4. Does the use of this instrument require an unacceptable degree of inference between the construct it assesses and the relevant psycholegal issue(s)?
5. Is the instrument commercially published?
6. Is a comprehensive user's manual available?
7. Have adequate levels of reliability been established?
8. Have adequate levels of validity been demonstrated?
9. Is the instrument valid for the purpose for which it will be used?
10. What are the qualifications necessary to use the instrument?
11. Has the instrument been subject to peer review?
12. Does the instrument include measures of response style?

Examples of techniques sometimes relied upon by mental health providers in clinical settings that would fail in meeting the above criteria include play therapy and its derivatives. Play therapy (e.g., sand play/sand tray therapy, doll play), when employed as a projective assessment technique, meets few, if any, of these guidelines for forensic assessment tools (see Kuehnle, 1996, 2002). These techniques are not objective and reliable measures of concepts that are of relevance to the court, nor are they reliable indicators of external events. There are no established psychometric properties, manuals for use, or measures of response style for these techniques (Murray, Martindale, & Epstein, 2009). Children's drawings also meet few, if any, of the criteria set forth by Melton and his colleagues (2007). Despite this absence of empirical support, it is not uncommon for quasi-assessment projective techniques to play a role in forensic evaluations in the context of child maltreatment and parenting plan evaluations. Bow and colleagues found that, among experienced doctoral-level forensic specialists, approximately one in five reported they used projective drawings such as the House-Tree-Person Drawing or Human Figure Drawing (21%) or the Family Drawing (19%) (Bow, Quinnell, Zaroff, & Assemany, 2002; see also Murray, et al, 2009, and Weiner & Kuehnle, 1998, for psychometric information on these instruments).

There is an absence of standardized instruments to assess toddlers or preschool-age children other than checklists typically completed by respondent caretakers. With elementary school–age children, standardized testing appropriate for use in forensic cases also is limited to checklists with parents and teachers as the respondents and self-report checklists with the child as the respondent. Although the authors of several projective instruments for children have attempted to develop a quantifiable scoring system with sound psychometric properties, none of the currently published projective instruments (e.g., Roberts Apperception Test for Children, 2nd Edition; Children's Apperception Test; Thematic Apperception Test) show acceptable psychometric properties (e.g., norms, reliability, and validity) for evaluating children in forensic settings and in answering psycholegal questions. (for reviews, see Buros Institute of Mental Measurements, http://buros.unl.edu/buros/ jsp/search.jsp). The use of these projective instruments should be avoided.

Similarly, there are insufficient standardized assessment instruments for use with adolescents in forensic matters. Although there are some widely used personality tests that, depending on the adolescent's response style, may provide the evaluator with some useful data about the teen's emotional status, normative data on adolescents involved in legal proceedings are limited. The evaluator who contemplates using standardized personality measures for adolescents in legal contexts is encouraged to be knowledgeable about considerations and controversies in the professional community; for example, it might be useful to consider reviews included in Sparta and Koocher's volume on forensic assessment of children wherein two specific adolescent measures—the Minnesota Muliphasic Personality Inventory–Adolescent (MMPI-A) and the Millon Adolescent Clinical Inventory (MACI)—are discussed (2006; see Chapters 24 and 26) or review the evolving literature contained in forensic psychological journals and reviews in Buros Institute of Mental Measurements. (http://buros.unl.edu/buros/jsp/search.jsp).

Interviewing Children and Adolescents

The child's interviews may produce some of the most crucial data in the forensic evaluation. Forensic mental health evaluators must approach the task of interviewing children with a solid knowledge of forensic child interview techniques in order to avoid contamination of a valuable source of information. (For further information, refer to Kuehnle and Connell, (2009; see Chapters 12, 13, and 14). Furthermore, knowledge of empirically based interview techniques is important when reviewing the quality of other interviewers' methods. The ability of adults to elicit accurate information from children depends, in large part, on the degree to which children's limitations and abilities are understood. The quality of children's reports is a co-mingled product of their cognitive and social maturity, their experiences outside formal interviews, and the interview context (Lamb, Sternberg, & Esplin, 1998). When the interview goal is to gather precise information, young children may not possess the cognitive and language skills to answer accurately many specific content-type questions (e.g., "when" or "how often"). When interviewing does not match the developmental capabilities of the child, inaccurate responses are more likely to be given by the child (Friedman & Lyon, 2005; Quas & Schaaf, 2002; also refer to Malloy and Quas, 2009, for a discussion of children's suggestibility). This is an extremely important consideration, because a child not only might fail to report important information, but also inadequate interviewing may produce misleading or inaccurate information.

Parent Responsibility and Time Sharing— Best Interests of the Child

In assessing the best interests of children and adolescents, forensically, in a family law context, there are numerous variables that should be considered, including but not limited to the following:

1. The child's *best interests* (a legal construct);
2. The child's *psychological best interests* (CPBI) (a psychological construct);
3. The child's *expressed* interests (both a legal and subjective construct);
4. The context of the assessment (an environmental construct);
5. What methods of assessment to utilize?

Two obvious elements that should be considered in a best interests analysis are the functional capabilities of each parent and how his/her abilities do or do not match with the child's best interests (sometimes referred to as "goodness of fit"). An examination of these two elements is beyond the scope of this chapter. The APA Guidelines for Child Custody in Family Law Proceedings (2010) recommend that the evaluation focus on parenting qualities, the child's psychological needs, and the resulting fit between them.

Definitions of Legal and Psychological Constructs

The reader is referred to primary professional documents that address mental health professions' approaches to the assessment of the CPBI in custody and visitation matters, including the American Psychological Association's child custody "guidelines" (APA, 2010), the American Academy of Child and Adolescent Psychiatry's "parameters" (AACAP, 1997); and the American Association of Family and Conciliation Courts "standards" (AFCC, 2006). Forensic mental health practitioners would do well to be mindful of what standards do exist in constructing an assessment within a family law context. Some states—for example, California—have adopted Superior Court Rules that specify the minimum criteria that must be addressed in all child custody evaluation reports to the court. There are other models available to courts for obtaining a child custody and visitation evaluation. For a discussion of these alternatives, see Kirkpatrick, 2004; see also Rohrbaugh (2008).

The Child's Best Interests (CBI)

Despite the fact the CBI is the basis for deciding child custody or parenting schedules in disputed proceedings, the best interests of the child (BIC) is a well known and well established legal construct that ironically remains without a consensus definition within the practice of family law in the United States and other countries. In an initial definition of the BIC, the Uniform Marriage and Divorce Act (1973; 1979) stated that the court shall consider:

- The wishes of the child's parent or parents as to the child's custody
- The wishes of the child as to his custodian
- The interaction and interrelationship of the child with his parent, his siblings, and any other person who may significantly affect the child's best interest
- The child's adjustment to his home, school, and community
- The mental and physical health of all individuals involved

The American Law Institute (ALI) referred to the BIC standard as "elastic" and "too subjective to produce predictable results," advocating for its refinement (ALI, 2002). Nevertheless, the BIC standard is the "polar star" by which family courts are guided to make decisions about the custody, well-being, and welfare of children whose parents are divorcing, or who are engaging in post-divorce litigation. There are circumstances, too, wherein the child's parents are not married and the BIC may not involve a "divorce," but may pertain to custody and child access. The BIC might be viewed as a large umbrella held by the court under which all other constructs and factors pertaining to the child's welfare are contained. Courts are encouraged "to consider 'all relevant factors' that they view as important in any given case, and to weight those factors in any manner they choose" (Rohrbaugh, 2008, p. 44).

Its definition notwithstanding, the clear consensus about the BIC is the presiding judge may exercise considerable discretion about what it means. The forensic evaluator should be aware of his/her local and state jurisdictional definitions and relevant case law pertaining to the BIC standard.

The Child's Psychological Best Interests (CPBI)

The American Psychological Association Guidelines for Child Custody Evaluations in Family Law Proceedings (2010) encourages psychologists to weigh and incorporate a variety of factors, including the following: family dynamics and interactions; cultural and environmental variables; relevant aptitudes for all examined parties; and the child's educational, physical and psychological needs. Psychologists focus on an array of conditions and capacities related to the child's psychological best interests, recognizing that the court will ultimately decide which factors will be considered and to what degree.

The Child's Expressed Interests (CEI)

A court may consider and give considerable weight to the interests and wishes of a child of sufficient age in choosing a custodian. However, in the totality of the case, the child's wishes are rarely, if ever, controlling. While the expressed preferences of older children in many states must be given greater weight, there is no absolute recognition for such preference, nor are there uniform ages when such preferences should be given priority (Sparta, 1998).

The forensic mental health evaluator may be asked to aid the court in addressing the child's wishes. The court may ask for help in determining whether or not the child should be allowed to make a statement to the court as to his or her wishes or thoughts about custody and visitation. There is no consensus about an age at which a child is of sufficient age to exercise discretion in giving an opinion about custody. The "test" on this matter is not the child's chronological age. In considering a child's expressed interest, the evaluator considers the child's mental capacity and comprehension to make a reasoned opinion, and whether the wishes are a product of the child's independent considerations or parent/caretaker manipulation.

The above factors are a subset of competency, and a court may require proof of a child's competency. While some states provide a presumption of lack of competency below a specific age, a child of any age may demonstrate competence if he or she understands the difference between truth and lies, understands the requirement of the oath to tell the truth, and is able to testify reasonably accurately (Haralambie, 1999, 2005; for a more general discussion of children's competency, see Myers, 1997).

In considering the child's expressed wishes, courts may want to know what is the level of conflict between the parents in relation to the child's wishes, what factors may be influencing the child's wishes, and what is the child's vulnerability to suggestibility?

The Context of the Assessment

There are many potential contextual factors that define a thorough assessment of a child's best interests in family law matters. As used here, the *context* is defined as the cultural, legal, and environmental factors within which and about which the child is being assessed forensically. The following is a partial list of some of the more salient contextual factors that may be relevant to a particular case:

1. The history, duration, and tone of the litigation;
2. The level, degree and history of the parental conflict;
3. The nature of the child's psychological attachment with each parent at different times in the child's life;
4. Domestic violence allegations and issues;
5. Abuse and neglect allegations and issues;
6. Estrangement, alienation, or resistance issues;
7. Normal developmental stages and dynamics of the child;
8. Relocation, interstate, and international custody disputes;
9. Effects of parents' personalities on child;
10. Remarriage and blended family relationships;
11. Child abduction/kidnapping;
12. Alcohol/substance abuse history or allegations;
13. The child's stability within different schools and neighborhoods, as well as community bonds.

Assessment Procedures

Almost without exception, the forensic evaluator in a family law case should seek to be agreed upon by the parties through a consent order, or be appointed by court order. Some jurisdictions require advanced court appointment either by stipulated agreement of the parties, which is subsequently made into the court's order, or the order is made directly by motion of the court. While there are instances where an evaluator may be retained by one party—e.g., as a consulting expert whose role and identity is under the aegis of the attorney work product privilege—most forensic assessments of children and adolescents in family law will involve an expert who is court-appointed, impartial, and whose "client" is the court, the child's guardian, the child's attorney, or a child protection agency.

Generally speaking, the following methods and procedures are typically applied in the forensic assessment of children and adolescents in a family law context:

1. A forensic expert who engages in the assessment of children and adolescents in a family law context has established a comprehensive and clearly written policy statement that delineates the scope, methods, associated fees and costs, limits of confidentiality, and other relevant information that, in effect, become the "contract" between the evaluator and the parties in the specific case. Many evaluators have found it prudent to have their protocol attached to or referenced within the court order appointing the evaluator.

2. Collateral data are obtained from two general sources—*collateral persons* and *collateral information* (refer to definitions above).

3. Absent a compelling reason, the evaluator must conduct interviews with each parent and or caretaker and conduct/administer similar interviews, observations, and testing. To this end, the evaluator should obtain and be familiar with the relevant pleadings—especially the controlling custody and visitation order.

4. In a post-divorce, high-conflict case in which there are allegations of alienation, abuse, domestic violence, and/or estrangement, as in other forensic evaluations, the forensic evaluator must guard against accepting at face value information provided by the child or adolescent, because the child or adolescent's account may be influenced by one parent over or against the other, or the child or adolescent may have her/his own agenda.

5. Absent a compelling reason, the forensic evaluator, when asked to evaluate a parent–child relationship, should conduct an interview/observation of each parent–child dyad, even in instances where the evaluator has been asked to address child sexual abuse allegations. To be sure, this situation is extremely complex. On one hand, the professional should not participate in a harmful action against the child, such as, for example, coercing a child beyond their current coping capacity to engage in an experience that the child is incapable of dealing with. On the other hand, the evaluation is ordered by a court when there are not yet adjudicated findings of abuse, and it is the allegation that is pending before the court, not the conclusion. When a parent in family law litigation is the object of abuse allegations that have not been substantiated or adjudicated, forensic mental health evaluators should not prematurely avoid conducting a

standardized evaluation, which includes individual and joint sessions with both parents, including the accused. To avoid or omit a parent–child observation under such circumstances runs the risk of omitting essential data. 6. The forensic evaluator recognizes that psychological testing should not be used in isolation, should be considered as but one source of data, and should not solely be used to make custody, access, or visitation recommendations. Evaluators use assessment techniques or tests within the appropriate boundaries of what each method can contribute, neither over-interpreting data nor ignoring information contrary to conclusions.

Child Maltreatment—the Best Interests of the Child

In assessing the best interests of children and adolescents in a dependency case, there are numerous variables, similar to variables that should be considered in family law cases, including (but not limited to) the following:

1. The child's *best interests* (a legal construct);
2. The child's *physical safety* and *welfare* (a legal construct);
3. The child's *physical, psychological* and *emotional functions* (legal and psychological constructs);
4. The child's *expressed* interests (both a legal and subjective construct);
5. The context of the assessment (an environmental construct);
6. What methods of assessment to utilize?

Families found in the Dependency Court system are more often at the lower end of the socio-economic spectrum and receiving services from other community agencies (Sedlak & Broadhurst, 1996). This may make these impoverished families more visible to outside authorities, compared to families at the middle and upper end of the socioeconomic spectrum. The reader is referred to primary professional associations which have addressed mental health professions' approaches to the assessment of the CPBI in child protection and dependency matters, including: (a) the American Psychological Association (APA, 1998), (b) the American Academy of Child and Adolescent Psychiatry (AACAP, 1997), (c) the American Professional Society on the Abuse of Children (APSAC, 1995, 1997, 2002, 2008) and (d) the National Association of Counsel for Children (Duquette & Haralambie, 2010). Forensic examiners would do well to be mindful of what standards do exist in constructing an assessment within a child protection context.

In child custody cases, the primary goal of the mental health evaluator is to assess the best fit between the child's needs and each parent's abilities to meet the child's needs toward developing the child to his or her fullest potential. In child dependency cases, the goal is to assess the child's needs and the parents' abilities, and to make recommendations that assist the court and participants in determining the child's "best interest" specifically related to the child's psychological functioning, attachment relationships, and "safety" from future harm (Kuehnle, Coulter, & Firestone, 2000). As identified by Budd, Connell, and Clarke (2011), generally the concept of "best interest" in child dependency proceedings is invoked in consideration of disposition, visitation, and permanency planning, and the termination of parental rights. Elements in state statutes typically include the child's:

(a) age and developmental needs;
(b) physical safety and welfare;
(c) emotional, physical, and mental status or condition;
(d) background and ties, including family, culture, and religion;
(e) sense of attachments;
(f) wishes and long-term goals;
(g) need for permanence, stability, and continuity of relationships, including with siblings.

For "definitions of legal and psychological concepts, refer to this subsection within the above section, "Parent Responsibility and Time Sharing—Best Interests of the Child."

Assessment Procedures

In assessing the best interests of children and adolescents forensically in a child dependency context, there are several variables that should be considered:

1. Focus on minimally adequate parenting.
2. Identify clinical and forensic issues of short- and long-term planning.
3. Assess the child's psychological functioning, interpersonal attachments, and safety.

Focus on Minimally Adequate Parenting

Although the standard for deciding cases of child maltreatment is to determine what is in the "best interest of the child," the focus of the forensic evaluation in these matters is often on the parents and whether they are likely to be able to remedy deficits in their parenting capacity in order to achieve a minimally adequate level of parenting (Budd, Connell, & Clark, 2011). Within child maltreatment cases, the assessment of children and adolescents is typically conducted for purposes of initial treatment, annual evaluations of children in out-of-home placements, and, when parental deficits are not remedied, long-term placement.

Clinical and Forensic Issues of Short- and Long-Term Planning

The forensic evaluator may address treatment needs, placement needs, and the potential impact of visitation with parents or the absence of visitation, when the child has been temporarily removed from the parents. The forensic assessment of the child may shift to a focus on long-term planning. If the parental deficits that led to intervention cannot be remedied, long-term foster care, residential placement, or adoption may be under consideration, and the determination of a successful placement may be assisted by the forensic evaluation. The evaluator may be asked to focus on the potential impact on the child of permanent severance of the child's relationship with a parent, for example, or the child's long-term placement needs.

Assessment of the Child's Psychological Functioning, Interpersonal Attachments, and Safety

Forensic evaluations of children during out-of-home placement may occur annually or at other intervals in order to comply with statutorily defined reviews or because of facility licensing requirements. Evaluations are required in order to insure that the child's needs are being addressed, including educational, psychosocial, and behavioral needs. The evaluator may need to gather records of earlier evaluations from other providers. In contrast to a parenting plan evaluation conducted during divorce litigation, evaluations conducted for dependency proceedings may focus on whether the child's intellectual and academic development are delayed due to neglect or whether the history of the child's parenting has created psychopathology interfering in the child's adequate adjustment to living in a normal family environment, or co-existing well with society in general.

Evaluators conducting dependency evaluations also may be asked to address, specifically, the child's attachment to the parent whose parenting is considered to be deficient, to the foster parent, or to a relative with whom the child has lived or may be placed. Specialized understanding of manifestations of healthy attachment and of techniques for assessment of parent–child relationships should be sought by evaluators undertaking such evaluations. There is a rich literature on attachment, and evaluators bear an obligation to undertake these evaluations, like all other psychological services, only when they have the necessary knowledge, training, and experience to competently provide the service. Courts often order individual evaluations of only the child or parent, and, whenever there is not an opportunity to observe the parent–child interaction, the evaluator should recognize and identify the potential limitations in a dependency evaluation. Similar to family court parenting-plan evaluations, evaluators use collateral information, assessment techniques, or tests within the appropriate boundaries of what each method can contribute.

Psychological Injury—Tort Law

In assessing psychological injury of children and adolescents in a civil law context, there are certain variables that should be considered:

1. Psychological or emotional injury (a legal and psychological construct)
2. Negligence (a legal construct—a part of the law of torts)
3. Intentional tort (a legal construct)

Personal injury law is also known as *tort* law. Forensic evaluators may be involved in personal injury lawsuits related to psychological injury. Psychological injuries consist of stress-related emotional conditions, damaged self-esteem, or self-damaging behaviors as a result of imagined or real threats or injuries having the potential to become the subjects of legal attention, such as personal injury litigation. In the legal system, it is not required to prove an event is the sole cause of psychological injury. In personal injury litigation, the concept of *proximate cause* is important, reflecting an understanding that a contested event in the litigation was the cause for the claimed psychological injury, as opposed to alternative explanations, such as preexisting or coexisting causes (Sparta, 2003). These concepts are further explained in the next section (and for a further review, see Greenberg, 2003).

Definitions of Legal and Psychological Constructs

The legal claim or complaint, in the form of a lawsuit, is technically known as a *tort* (a "wrong"). A tort is an area of law in which the victims seek compensation for civil "wrongs" allegedly imposed on them. The viability of the claim usually requires a showing that the defendant has breached a legal duty that was owed to the plaintiff by the defendant (Greenberg & Brodsky, 2001). Personal injury claims fall into two stages—liability and compensation (Sawaya, 2010–2011).

TORT LAW

"Personal injury" is a legal term for an injury to the body, mind, or emotions, as distinct from an injury to property. A tort is an area of law in which the victim seeks compensation for civil "wrongs" imposed on him or her. There is a distinction between wrongs and wrongdoings—a difference between committing a wrong and acting wrongfully. To "act wrongfully" is to act without justification or excuse. To commit a *legal* wrong is to breach a duty, to invade another's right. One can breach a duty for good reason, with adequate justification, or under excusing conditions. Rights, in other words, can be invaded innocently (or justifiably) on one hand, or wrongfully (or unjustifiably) on the other (Sawaya, 2010–2011).

The person who sustains injury as the result of tortious conduct is known as the *plaintiff*, and the person who is responsible for inflicting the injury and incurs liability for the damage is known as the *defendant* or *tortfeasor* (Black et al., 1979; Trawick, 2010; Sawaya, 2010–2011). Torts or legal wrongs are legally defined. There are two kinds of torts: intentional and negligence.

Tort—Intentional

An intentional tort is a wrong perpetrated by a person who intends to do an act that the law has declared wrong, as contrasted with negligence, in which the person fails to exercise that degree of care in doing what is otherwise permissible (Black et al., 1979). Intentional "wrongs" may include physical or sexual abuse of a child or adolescent; intentional neglect such as confinement of a child from social interactions—e.g., confining a child 24 hours a day to a cage, room or house—or keeping a child from receiving an education or adequate food, which may result in mental handicaps.

Tort—Negligence

In tort law, *negligence* may be defined as the failure to act reasonably (Black et al., 1979; Sawaya, 2010–2011; Florida Standard Jury Instructions in Civil Cases, 2007). Depending on the individual facts of a case, failure by a mental health professional to intervene on a patient's threat during therapy to commit suicide may be an act of negligence, if the patient acted on his or her threat.

Negligence has three requirements, and a person claiming negligence must prove all three to hold the alleged wrongdoer (i.e., the defendant or tortfeasor) accountable (Sawaya, 2010–2011; Trawick, 2010). The elements of negligence are (a) duty, (b) breach of duty, and (c) causation (Myers, 1998; Trawick, 2010; Sawaya, 2010–2011). Negligence is a type of tort in which most children seek compensation in personal injury claims.

Context of the Assessment

The majority of torts have five legal requirements in order to prove liability (Trawick, 2010). These requirements differ greatly from other forensic cases. For example, in child custody cases, the sole legal criterion is typically based upon "the best interest of the child(ren)." The five requirements for torts are listed below (Goldberg, 2006):

1. Legal duty
2. Breach or dereliction of that duty
3. Proximate cause
4. Actual damage
5. Compensability

LEGAL DUTY

This criterion refers to an obligation that requires one individual to conform to a standard with respect to another person.

BREACH OR DERELICTION OF DUTY

After determining that the defendant owed a legal duty to the plaintiff, the plaintiff is required to prove that the defendant failed to complete his duty or acted in omission.

Proximate Cause

Forensic psychological evaluators are often asked for their expert opinion when it comes to the issue of causation. Under tort law, "proximate cause" requires a determination of cause and linking that cause as "proximate" to the psychological injury. To determine causation, experts often use the "but for" test. This test requires determination that the injury/damage would not have happened "but for" the defendant's actions (Black et al., 1979; Sawaya, 2010–2011).

ACTUAL DAMAGE

The law does not compensate for negligent behavior unless the plaintiff has truly suffered an injury. According to the law, no liability for damage exists if no harm occurred (Black et al.,1979; Trawick, 2010; Sawaya, 2010–2011).

COMPENSABILITY

In order to prove liability, one must determine that the complaint constitutes a type that the legal system sees as compensable. Once it is determined that the defendant did, in fact, have liability, the compensation process begins. Compensatory losses focus on the actual losses suffered by the plaintiff. There are two types of general compensatory damages in the context of psychological injury (Florida Standard Jury Instructions in Civil Cases, 2007). These include:

1. Loss of consortium: compensation for losing the companionship and love of a close relative.

2. Hedonic damage: how the injury will impact the individual's ability to enjoy life.

Assessment Methods

A systematic approach to the forensic assessment of emotional injuries includes viewing the claimant's life through three windows of time:

1. Who the child was and how he/she was functioning prior to the alleged tort;

2. Reconstruction of the events that surrounded and possibly created the alleged "tort";

3. The likely impact of experiencing such an event and the child's current level of functioning post-event.

Psychological evaluations in personal injury litigation primarily focus on whether or not an injury has occurred, the defendant's role in the injury, and the prognosis for rehabilitation and functioning in the future. Three primary types of data used in assessment of personal injury include: interviews and observations (discussed above), collateral data, and psychological testing.

COLLATERAL DATA

The collateral data collected for personal injury evaluations will, at times, have a different focus than the collateral data collected for child custody and dependency cases. In personal injury cases, the forensic evaluator will need to obtain information related to the developmental and clinical background of the child in order to contrast the child's assessed emotional, behavioral, cognitive, learning, social, or psychosomatic functioning against the child's normal expected functioning. Information from a variety of sources would document the child's actual functioning at different times, including any information related to the child's family environment, educational history, diagnosis of mental disorder

and/or substance abuse, history of prior involvement with the legal system, and medical/health issues. This information can be obtained from collateral interviews with current or past caregivers, teachers, mental health providers, or other parties familiar with the child or adolescent plaintiff. Past and current academic records, previous psychological reports, medical records, videotaped interviews or depositions of the plaintiff or other persons related to the case, and legal documents relevant to the case are essential to review. It is important to ask for such records, as sometimes an attorney would not necessarily identify the relevance of such data. Greenberg (2003, p. 241) provides the following data-organizational system related to five conceptual parts of the examination:

Pre-Allegation History
- Strengths and competencies
- Preexisting vulnerabilities
- Preexisting impairments in functioning

Trauma and Distress
- What the child (plaintiff) was exposed to

Sequelae
- Substantial impairments in functioning that the child (plaintiff) suffered
- Ways in which the child (plaintiff) was resilient

Proximate Cause
- Impairments that would not have occurred but for the alleged events
- Impairments that would have occurred otherwise

Prognosis
- Degree of future impairments (partial or complete, temporary or permanent)
- Interventions or accommodations indicated

TESTING

There is no universally accepted set of assessment tools to be used in personal injury examinations. Furthermore, there are no tests that directly answer the legally relevant questions regarding preexisting conditions, proximately caused damage, or the severity or the distress caused by the defendant's behavior (Greenberg, 2003). Personal injury forensic examiners tend to use the same core battery of tests for adults that are used in adult clinical assessments. The most commonly used instruments for adult assessments are the MMPI-2, the WAIS-R or III, MCMI-II or III, Rorschach, Beck Depression Inventory, Trauma Stress Inventory, and the Symptom Checklist 90–Revised (Boccaccini & Brodsky, 1999). The Minnesota Multiphasic Personality Inventory–2nd Edition-Restructured Form (MMPI-2-RF) (Ben-Porath & Tellegen, 2008) is emerging as a useful measure in adult personal injury assessments. Similar surveys have not been conducted on identifying the test battery most commonly used with children and adolescents in personal injury cases.

Several instruments have been developed in an attempt to measure traumatic experiences in children and identify the presence of post-traumatic stress disorder (PTSD). These include: Trauma Symptom Checklist for Children, with both child respondent and parent respondent forms (there is also a preschool-age version); the Clinician-Administered PTSD Scale for Children; the Child Dissociative Checklist; the Child Post-Traumatic Stress Reaction Scale; Child Rating Scales of Exposure to Interpersonal Abuse; and the Child's Reaction to Traumatic Events Scale. Shuman (2003) identifies a heightened criticism of PTSD claims in personal injury lawsuits, given the perception of the increased frequency of PTSD claims, as well as increased challenges to the expert testimony presented in support of PTSD claims.

As identified in reviews published by Buros Institute of Mental Measurements (http://buros.unl.edu/buros/jsp/search.jsp), the above-listed checklists and scales all have psychometric weaknesses, about which the forensic evaluator should be knowledgeable. Furthermore, any test result should be used to formulate hypotheses and not be used as a diagnostic tool in isolation from the myriad other data collected.

Juvenile Competency—Criminal Law

In *Dusky v. United States* (1960), the Supreme Court of the United States ruled that a defendant must have "sufficient present ability to consult with his attorney with a reasonable degree of rational understanding," and have a "rational as well as factual understanding of the proceedings against him" (p. 402). The Supreme Court further decided in *In re Gault* (1967) that juveniles are afforded the same rights as adults, which enabled the courts to consider competency to proceed for juveniles. In the forensic assessment of the competency of children and adolescents in a criminal law context, there are certain variables that should be considered:

1. Defendant's capacity to meet the *Dusky* standard (a legal construct)

2. Developmental and functional capacities: i.e., mental illness, mental retardation, or cognitive immaturity (legal and psychological constructs)

3. Interpersonal: i.e., to what degree can a juvenile interact and communicate with his/her counsel (legal and psychological construct)

DEFINITIONS OF LEGAL AND PSYCHOLOGICAL CONCEPTS

Grisso (2005) identified the following characteristics of competency:

- Functional—specific knowledge or understanding
- Causal—cause(s) of functional inabilities
- Contextual—the specific environment in which functional abilities are necessary
- Conclusive—based on information provided by a forensic evaluator, the court will determine the competency issue

Functional Capacities

Significant to issues of immaturity, Grisso and colleagues (2003) reported that juveniles between the ages of 16 and 17 typically had an understanding of the legal process comparable to that of adults; however, juveniles under the age of 15 demonstrated significant difficulty with understanding and participating in the legal process (Melton et al, 2007).

Causal capacities: Causes of Functional Inabilities

While statutes governing the legal construct of competency vary from state to state, whether a defendant has the capacity to meet the *Dusky* standard is typically associated with cognitive ability; i.e., the impact of mental illness or mental retardation (McGaha, Otto, McClaren, & Petrila, 2001), as well as developmental limitations and physical disabilities (Geraghty, Kraus, & Fink, 2007). Some courts are beginning to recognize cognitive or developmental immaturity as factors in juvenile incompetency, with relevant factors varying from case to case (Grisso, et al., 2003; Poythress, Lexcen, Grisso, & Steinberg, 2006).

Contextual

Given the adversarial nature of criminal courts, the ability of younger juveniles and juveniles with cognitive or developmental disabilities to recall information and testify relevantly may be significantly challenging. Juveniles also show greater brain activity in the limbic system compared to adults, which can have a significant influence on courtroom behavior, including emotionally charged behavior, emotional rather than logical thinking, and difficulty weighing decisions (Mayzer, Bradley, Rusinko, & Ertelt, 2009).

THE CONTEXT OF THE ASSESSMENT

All fifty U.S. states have a statute that delineates the procedures to be followed when the question of competency is raised in criminal court (Geraghty et al., 2007). The objective of the competency evaluation is to determine the defendant's *current* level of functioning, not to evaluate retrospective capacity (e.g., when the alleged crime was committed) or to predict future behavior. Forensic examiners are called upon to determine whether the juvenile defendant has a mental illness or is mentally handicapped and to determine whether the defendant lacks developmental maturity to the degree that this would interfere with the juvenile defendant's ability to meet criteria for "competence to proceed" in his or her criminal trial. The forensic evaluator must be familiar with the relevant state statutes and definitions of legal terms as they relate to the evaluation.

Conclusive

It is up to the judge or jury, not the evaluator, to answer the ultimate question: is the defendant competent?

ASSESSMENT METHODS

When addressing issues of competency, the forensic examiner considers and reports upon the defendant's capacity to:

1. Appreciate the charges or allegations
2. Appreciate the range and nature of possible penalties
3. Understand the adversarial nature of the legal process and the roles of the various participants
4. Disclose to counsel facts pertinent to the proceedings at issue
5. Manifest appropriate courtroom behavior
6. Testify relevantly if necessary

The following methods and procedures are typically used to address the competency criteria listed above when conducting a juvenile competency evaluation:

Interviews

Structured and semi-structured interviews have been developed for assessing competency. A semi-structured interview developed by Grisso (2005), the Juvenile Adjudicative Competency Interview (JACI), is structured to obtain information about the juvenile's abilities in twelve (12) areas relevant to competence to stand trial, and includes the assessment of developmental immaturity (e.g., perceived autonomy, perceptions of risk, time perspective, and abstract/concrete thinking), mental disorder, and intelligence.

Forensic evaluators who interview juveniles facing legal charges should be aware of the difficulties they might encounter when trying to communicate with the defendant—e.g., inaccurate understanding of the legal system, which might cause suspicion of the evaluation process; refusal to talk; threats to self-esteem for being suspected of having a mental disorder; or a lack of motivation to cooperate with the evaluator (Melton et al, 2007). Furthermore, it is essential to assess a juvenile's response style, i.e., how the juvenile approaches being evaluated in a criminal context and to determine if the defendant is responding in an honest and forthright manner (Melton, et al, 2007). Reasonably accurate hypotheses about an individual's response style can be developed by a confluence of data from validity scales from standardized assessment measures, collateral information, and clinical observation.

Observation

The forensic evaluator may reasonably infer that a juvenile can or cannot be cooperative when interacting with legal counsel or during court proceedings, or that the juvenile can or cannot understand and retain information based on demonstrated behavior during the evaluation (Otto, 2006). Observation of physical or developmental disabilities that may interfere with the defendant's capacity should be duly noted, as well as the juvenile's ability to accurately recall and communicate information. Behaviors suggestive of responses to stress, depression, delusions, or unusual behaviors should also be specifically noted as they relate to the defendant's ability to interact during the criminal process.

Testing

A greater proportion of juveniles of below-average intelligence are found in the juvenile justice system, and they are more likely to demonstrate impaired abilities relevant to competency, compared to juveniles of average intelligence (Grisso, et al. 2003; Melton et al., 2007). Therefore, tests of intelligence (e.g., Wechsler Intelligence Scale for Children) are useful in establishing intellectual and cognitive functioning. Tests of achievement and cognition may also be useful in identifying specific deficits significant to the juvenile's capacity; e.g., verbal abilities, comprehension, reasoning. Personality testing or neuropsychological testing may be warranted. When using psychological tests, the findings must be integrated with other assessment data (Gudas & Sattler, 2006).

Historical Information

Information regarding the family environment, educational history, psychosocial, cognitive, and emotional functioning, history of delinquency, mental disorders, and/or substance abuse, and physical health are factors that may contribute to the present capacity of the defendant. This information can be obtained from collateral interviews with past and/or current caregivers, teachers, healthcare providers, or other parties familiar with the defendant. Additionally, information can be gleaned from a review of records, e.g., police records, academic (including discipline) records, previous psychological reports or medical records, after obtaining the necessary consent from the parent or legal guardian.

Summary

The purpose of forensic evaluations conducted by mental health professionals is to be helpful to the legal decision-maker (i.e., judge, jury, other hearing officer) or retaining authority. In contrast, the purpose of the clinical evaluation is to be helpful to the patient. Forensic mental health evaluators may perform evaluations of children and adolescents in many different psycholegal contexts. This chapter described the forensic assessment of children and adolescents related to psycholegal questions in three areas of civil judicial proceedings and one area of criminal judicial proceedings. Forensic mental health evaluators of children and adolescents attempting to answer psycholegal questions must be familiar with the relevant state statutes and definitions of legal terms as they relate to the evaluation. They must also utilize multiple methods to consider diverse sources of independent data, multiple hypotheses when collecting and analyzing the data, and an awareness of the evaluation context of the psycholegal question—guarding against accepting at face value any information from a single source. A competent forensic evaluator utilizes a healthy dollop of skepticism as part of the assessment. Assessment of children in forensic contexts requires clarity of focus and adherence to general forensic guidelines and standards for objectivity. Instruments should be chosen with consideration for their relevance to the psycholegal construct and reliability for the purpose for which they are used. Whether the assessment procedures and instruments are also used in clinical assessments or are designed specifically for use in forensic contexts, their use in the forensic context must be undertaken thoughtfully and with good foundation. Ultimately, the evaluator should be able to draw a clear connection between the data collected and the resulting findings and opinions.

Notes

1. In 1993, in *Daubert v. Merrell Dow Pharmaceuticals*, the U.S. Supreme Court determined that the Federal Rules of Evidence (FRE) focus on *reliability* was the proper standard for determining admissibility of expert testimony (Flens, 2005).

2. In 1999, in *Kumho Tire Co. v. Carmichael*, the U.S. Supreme Court clarified that the court's "gatekeeping" role should encompass all expert testimony, not just "scientific" testimony (Flens, 2005).

References

American Academy of Child and Adolescent Psychiatry (AACAP). (1997). Practice parameters for child custody evaluation. *Journal of American Academy of Child & Adolescent Psychiatry, 36,* 10 S.

American Academy of Child and Adolescent Psychiatry. (1997). Practice parameters for the forensic evaluation of children and adolescents who may have been physically or sexually abused. *Journal of American Academy of Child & Adolescent Psychiatry, 36,* 423–444.

American Law Institute (2002). *Principles of the law of family dissolution: Analysis and recommendations.* Newark, NJ: Matthew Bender/Lexis Nexis.

American Professional Society on the Abuse of Children. (1997). *Guidelines for psychosocial evaluation of suspected sexual abuse in young children* (2nd ed.). Chicago, IL: APSAC.

American Psychological Association. (1998). *Guidelines for psychological evaluations in child protection matters.* Washington, DC: APA.

American Psychological Association (APA). (1994). Committee on Professional Practice and Standards Guidelines for child custody evaluations in divorce proceedings. *American Psychologist, 49,* 677–680. Washington, DC: American Psychological Association.

American Psychological Association (APA). (2010). Guidelines for child custody evaluations in family law proceedings. *American Psychologist, 65*(9), 863–867. Washington, DC: American Psychological Association.

American Professional Society on the Abuse of Children. (1995) *Psychosocial evaluation of suspected psychological maltreatment in children and adolescents.* Chicago, IL: APSAC.

American Professional Society on the Abuse of Children. (1997) *Psychosocial evaluation of suspected sexual abuse in children,* (2nd ed.). Chicago, IL: APSAC.

American Professional Society on the Abuse of Children. (2002) *Investigative interviewing in cases of alleged child abuse.* Chicago, IL: APSAC.

American Professional Society on the Abuse of Children. (2008) *Challenges in the evaluation of child neglect.* Chicago, IL: APSAC.

Association of Family and Conciliation Courts (AFCC), Task Force for Model Standards of Practice for Child Custody Evaluation. (2007). Model standards of practice for child custody evaluation. *Family Court Review, 45*(1), 70–91.

Ben-Porath, Y. S., & Tellegen, A. (2008). *MMPI-2-RF: Manual for administration, scoring, and interpretation*. Minneapolis, MN: University of Minnesota Press.

Berliner, L., & Lieb, R. (2001). *Child sexual abuse investigations: Testing documentation methods* (Document No. 01–0104102). Olympia, WA: Washington State Institute for Public Policy (www.wsipp.wa.gov). Retrieved March 8, 2011, from www. wsipp.wa.gov/rptfiles/PilotProjects.pdf

Black, H. C., Nolan, J. R., & Nolan-Haley, J. M. (Eds.). (1979). *Black's law dictionary*. St. Paul, MN: West Publishing Co.

Boccaccini, M. T., & Brodsky, S. L. (1999). Diagnostic test usage by forensic psychologists in emotional injury cases. *Professional Psychology: Research & Practice, 30*(3), 253–259.

Bow, J. N., Quinnell, F. A., Zaroff, M., & Assemany, A. (2002). Assessment of sexual abuse allegations in child custody cases. *Professional Psychology: Research & Practice, 33*, 566–575.

Budd, K., Connell, M., & Clark, J. (2011). *Evaluation of parenting capacity in child protection*. New York: Oxford University Press

Buros Institute of Mental Measurements (http://buros.unl.edu/buros/jsp/search.jsp) *Daubert v. Merrell Dow Pharmaceuticals*, 509 U.S. 579 (1993).

Duquette, D. N., & Haralambie, A. M. (Eds.) (2010). Child welfare law and practice: Representing children, parents, and state agencies in abuse, neglect, and dependency cases. Denver, CO: Bradford Publishing Company.

Dusky v. United States, 362 U.S. 402 (1960).

Friedman, W. J., & Lyon, T. D. (2005). Development of temporal-reconstructive abilities. *Child Development, 76*, 1202–1216.

Geraghty, T. F., Kraus, L. J., & Fink, P. (2007). Assessing children's competence to stand trial and to waive Miranda rights: new directions for legal and medical decision-making in juvenile courts. In Kessler, C. I. & Kraus, L. J. (Eds), *The mental health needs of young offenders: Forging paths toward reintegration and rehabilitation* (pp. 79–121). New York: Cambridge University Press.

Goldberg, M. (2006). Examining children in personal injury claims. In S. Sparta and G. Koocher (Eds.), *Forensic mental health assessment of children and adolescents* (pp. 245–259). New York: Oxford University Press.

Grisso, T., Steinberg, L., Woolard, J., Cauffman, E., Scott, E., Graham, S., Lexcen, F., Reppucci, N. D., & Schwartz, R. (2003). Juveniles' competence to stand trial: A comparison of adolescents' and adults' capacities as trial defendents. *Law and Human Behavior, 27*, 333–341.

Grisso, T. (2005). *Evaluating juveniles' adjudicative competence: A guide for clinical practice*. Sarasota, FL: Professional Resources Press.

Greenberg, S. (2003). Personal injury examination in torts for emotional distress. In A. M. Goldstein & I. B. Weiner (Eds.), *Handbook of psychology, Vol. 11: Forensic psychology* (pp. 233–257). New York: Wiley & Sons.

Greenberg, S. A., & Brodsky, S. (2001). *The practice of civil forensic psychology*. Washington, DC: American Psychological Association.

Gudas, L. S. & Sattler, J. M. (2006). Forensic interviewing of children and adolescents. In S. N. Sparta & G. P. Koocher (Eds.), *Forensic mental health assessment of children and adolescents* (pp. 115–128). New York: Oxford University Press.

Haralambie, A. M. (1999). *Child sexual abuses in civil cases: A guide to custody and tort cases*. Chicago, IL: American Bar Association.

Haralambie, A. M. (2005). Dependency court jurisdiction and interstate and international proceedings. In M. Ventrell & D. N. Duquette (Eds.), *Child welfare law and practice: Representing children, parents, and state agencies in abuse, neglect, and dependency cases* (pp. 235–246). Denver, CO: Bradford Publishing.

Heilbrun, K., Warren, J., & Picarello, K. (2003). The use of third party information in forensic assessment. In I. B. Weiner & A. M. Goldstein (Eds.), *Handbook of psychology, Vol. 11, Forensic Psychology* (pp. 69–86). New York: John Wiley & Sons Ltd.

In re Gault, 387 U.S. 1, 28 (1967).

Kirkpatrick, H. D. (2004). A floor, not a ceiling: Beyond guidelines—An argument for minimum standards of practice in conducting child custody and visitation evaluations. *Journal of Child Custody, 1*(1), 61–75. Binghamton, NY: The Haworth Press.

Kuehnle, K. F. (1996). *Assessing allegations of child sexual abuse*. Sarasota, FL: Professional Resource Press.

Kuehnle, K. (2003). Child sexual abuse evaluations. In A. M. Goldstein & I. B. Weiner (Eds.), *Handbook of psychology, Vol. 11: Forensic psychology* (pp. 437–460). New York: Wiley & Sons.

Kuehnle, K., & Connell, M. (in press). Child sexual abuse evaluations. In R. Otto & I. B. Weiner (Eds.), *Comprehensive handbook of psychology, Vol. 11: Forensic psychology* (2nd ed.). New York: Wiley & Sons.

Kuehnle, K. & Connell, M. (2009, Eds.). *The evaluation of child sexual abuse allegations: A comprehensive guide to assessment and testimony*. Hoboken, NJ: John Wiley & Sons.

Kuehnle, K., Coulter, M., & Firestone, G. (2000). Child protection evaluations: The forensic stepchild. *Family & Conciliation Courts Review, 38*, 368–391. *Kumho Tire Co. v. Carmichael*, 526 U.S. 137 (1999).

Lamb, M. E., Orbach, Y., Sternberg, K. J., Hershkowitz, I., & Horowitz, D. (2000). Accuracy of investigators' verbatim notes of their forensic interviews with alleged child abuse victims. *Law and Human Behavior, 24*, 699–708.

Lamb, M., Sternberg, K., & Esplin, P. (1998). Conducting investigative interviews of alleged sexual abuse victims. *Child Abuse & Neglect, 22*, 813–823.

Malloy, L. C., & Quas, J. A. (2009). Children's suggestibility: Areas of consensus and controversy. In K. Kuehnle & M. Connell (Eds.), *The evaluation of child sexual abuse allegations: A comprehensive guide to assessment and testimony* (pp. 267–297). Hoboken, NJ: Wiley & Sons.

Mayzer, R., Bradley, A. R., Rusinko, H., & Ertelt (2009). Juvenile competency to stand trial in criminal court and brain function. *Journal of Forensic Psychiatry & Psychology, 20*(6), 785–800.

McGaha, A., Otto, R. K., McClaren, M. D., & Petrila, J. (2001). Juveniles adjudicated incompetent to proceed: A descriptive study of Florida's competence restoration program. *Journal of the American Academy of Psychiatry & Law, 29*, 427–437.

Melton, G. B., Petrila, J., Poythress, N. G., & Slobogin, C. (2007). *Psychological evaluations for the courts: A handbook for mental health professionals and lawyers* (3rd ed.). New York: Guilford Press.

Murray, D., Martindale, D., & Epstein, M. (2009). Unsupported assessment techniques in child sexual abuse evaluations. In K. F. Kuehnle & M. Connell (Eds.), *The evaluation of child sexual abuse allegations: A comprehensive guide to assessment and testimony*. Hoboken, N.J.: Wiley & Sons.

Myers, J. E. B. (1997). *Evidence in child abuse and neglect cases* (3rd ed). New York: John Wiley.

Myers, J. E. B. (1998). *Legal issues in child abuse and neglect practice* (2nd ed.). Thousand Oaks, CA: Sage.

Otto, R. (2006). Competency to stand trial. *Applied Psychology in Criminal Justice, 2*(3), 82–113.

Poythress, N. P., Lexcen, F. J., Grisso, T., & Steinberg, L. (2006). The competence-related abilities of adolescent defendants in criminal court. *Law & Human Behavior, 30*(1), 75–91.

Quas, J.A, & Schaaf, J. M. (2002). Children's memories of experienced and non-experienced events following repeated interviews. *Journal of Experimental Child Psychology, 83,* 304–338.

Rohrbaugh, J. B. (2008). *A comprehensive guide to child custody evaluations: Mental health and legal perspectives.* New York: Springer.

Sawaya, T. D. (2010–2011 ed.). *Florida personal injury law and practice with wrongful death actions,* §3:12. Eagan, MN: Westlaw.

Sedlak, A. J., & Broadhurst, D. D. (1996). *The third national incidence study of child abuse and neglect.* Washington, DC: U.S. Department of Health and Human Services.

Shuman, D. W. (2003). Persistent reexperiences in psychiatry and the law. In R. I. Simon (Ed.), *Post-traumatic stress disorder in litigation: Guidelines of forensic assessment* (2nd ed.; pp. 1–18). Washington, DC: American Psychiatric Publishing, Inc.

Sparta, S. (1998) Evaluating children's expressed preferences in divorce proceedings. *Family Law News, Official Publication of the State Bar of California Family Law Section,* Vol. *21,* No. 3.

Sparta, S. N. (2003). Assessment of childhood trauma. In A. M. Goldstein (Ed.), *Handbook of psychology, Vol. 11: Forensic psychology* (pp. 209–231). New York: Wiley.

Sparta, S. N., & Koocher, G. P. (Eds.). (2006). *Forensic mental health assessment of children and adolescents.* New York: Oxford Press.

Trawick, H. P. (2010 ed.). *Trawick's Florida practice and procedure.* §13:7, 19:2, 19:3, 3:12. Eagan, MN: Westlaw.

Uniform Marriage and Divorce Act (UMDA). (1979). §402 (National Conference of Commissioners on Uniform State Laws, 1979).

Weiner, I., & Kuehnle, K. (1998). Projective assessment of children and adolescents. In M. Hersen & A. Bellack (Eds.), *Comprehensive clinical psychology* (Vol. 4, pp. 431–458). Tarrytown, NY: Elsevier Science.

Assessing Non-Cognitive Constructs in Education: A Review of Traditional and Innovative Approaches

Anastasiya A. Lipnevich, Carolyn MacCann, *and* Richard D. Roberts

Abstract

This chapter provides a broad overview of both conventional and novel approaches for assessing non-cognitive skills, specifically focusing on their application in educational contexts. Conventional approaches include self-assessments, other-ratings, letters of recommendation, biodata, and interviews. We outline the current uses and validity evidence for these methods, and discuss the theory of planned behavior as a useful heuristic for assessment development. Novel approaches to non-cognitive assessment include the situational judgement test, day-reconstruction method, and use of writing samples. After reviewing these new approaches, we discuss the issue of response distortion in non-cognitive assessment, outlining some assessment techniques thought to be less susceptible to faking. Suggested fake-resistant assessments include the implicit association test and conditional reasoning test, as well as forced-choice tests and the Bayesian truth serum. We conclude with a series of summary statements concerning uses of non-cognitive testing in education.

Key Words: non-cognitive assessment, self-report, other-reports, situational judgement test, biodata

Introduction

It is increasingly obvious that succeeding in education requires much more than just "book smarts." To succeed, students need to be not just intelligent, they need to work hard, believe in themselves, cope with the stress of academic evaluations, develop and maintain networks of social and academic support, and organize their homework, projects, and study. That is, students' non-cognitive qualities can be as influential as their cognitive skills in influencing their academic achievement and educational aspirations (e.g., Burrus, MacCann, Kyllonen, & Roberts, 2011). Moreover, these non-cognitive qualities do not just predict the grades awarded by teachers or schools, but the hard data collected by large-scale testing programs. For example, research demonstrates that children and adolescent's levels of self-efficacy, self-concept, and self-confidence predict their mathematics, science, and reading scores

(Campbell, Voelkl, & Donahue, 1997; Connell, Spencer, & Aber, 1994). Non-cognitive constructs are important predictors of academic achievement and behavioral adjustment from early childhood, with Abe's (2005) research demonstrating that personality at age three predicted academic achievement in later schooling.

Perhaps even more importantly, these non-cognitive constructs are not simply proxies for a privileged background or for student ability variables. Duckworth and Seligman (2005) demonstrate that non-cognitive variables still predict academic achievement even after controlling for key socioeconomic variables such as demographics, school attendance, and home educational materials. Meta-analyses testify that non-cognitive constructs such as conscientiousness, self-efficacy, achievement motivation, and test anxiety predict academic achievement and attrition rates over and above the effects of cognitive ability and socioeconomic status (Poropat, 2009; Robbins, Lauver, Le, Davis, Langley, & Carlstrom, 2004; Seipp, 1991). It seems that students' non-cognitive qualities are important in their own right, and play a vital role in whether students are able to profit from their experience of school.

Given the importance of non-cognitive factors for school success, the goal of the current chapter is to provide a broad overview of the different ways that these non-cognitive constructs can be conceptualized and measured. We begin with a brief explanation of the different types of non-cognitive qualities that have been examined in the literature, focusing primarily on an education context. We then discuss both traditional and innovative measurement methods for indexing these kinds of constructs, and evaluate the strengths and weaknesses of each psychometric approach. Traditional approaches include self- and other-report rating scales and interviews. Novel approaches include situational judgement tests (SJTs), day reconstruction, implicit association tests (IATs), and conditional reasoning tests (CRTs). One commonly stated disadvantage of non-cognitive compared to cognitive assessment is the concern that test-takers are able to distort their responses to create an erroneous impression. We therefore discuss faking in non-cognitive assessment, devoting special attention to whether innovative assessment methodologies can mitigate the effects of faking. In a concluding section, we discuss the existing and potential applications of non-cognitive measurement in educational research, policy, and practice.

What Are Non-cognitive Factors?

"Non-cognitive constructs" is a broad umbrella term in the education literature that refers to a range of student characteristics thought to be distinct from students' intellectual competence and their capacity for mastering the "three Rs" of schoolwork. The extensive research on non-cognitive constructs crosses many different disciplines, including education, educational psychology, social psychology, developmental psychology, personnel psychology, and individual differences (to name just a few). This breadth of research can sometimes result in inconsistent use of construct labels across studies from different disciplines, thus leading to both the "jingle fallacy" (assuming that two constructs are the same because they share the same label) and the "jangle fallacy" (assuming that two constructs differ because they have different labels; e.g., Block, 1995). For

example, the meta-cognition literature uses the term *confidence* to refer to an evaluation of correctness (e.g., "I am confident my answer is right") whereas the positive psychology literature uses the term *confidence* to refer to a positive emotional state (e.g., "I am feeling happy and confident today"). Conversely, the term *integrity* may vary widely in meaning from *intellectual integrity* to through to *absenteeism*. While we acknowledge that terminology is currently not set in stone and may vary slightly from discipline to discipline, we provide a rough taxonomy of some of the most commonly researched non-cognitive constructs, grouped into four domains: (1) attitudes and beliefs, (2) social and emotional qualities, (3) habits and processes, and (4) personality traits.

Attitudes and Beliefs

The first broad group of non-cognitive constructs includes the beliefs that students hold about themselves as learners, the nature of learning, the fairness or supportiveness of the school environment, and their attitudes towards different disciplinary areas and towards school in general. One prominent self-belief system is Dweck and Leggett's (1988) "implicit theories of intelligence." This model proposes that students may hold different types of beliefs about the malleability of intelligence. Entity theorists believe that ability is preset, and cannot be changed through training or practice. In contrast, incremental theorists believe that ability is malleable. As might be expected, entity theorists tend to perform worse at school (Blackwell, Trzesniewski, & Dweck, 2007). This beliefs-and-attitudes grouping of non-cognitive constructs also includes the conscious or unconscious attitudes that students may hold about particular disciplines (e.g., beliefs that mathematics is difficult or that science is fun). Such attitudes may strongly influence students' subsequent behavior and thus their academic success (e.g., Lipnevich, MacCann, Krumm, Burrus, & Roberts, 2011). Students may also hold particular beliefs relating to their self-concept, self-confidence, or self-efficacy, which predict their achievement in various academic and life domains (e.g., Marsh, Byrne, & Shavelson, 1988).

Social and Emotional Qualities

There is a range of non-cognitive constructs that relate to students dealing with their emotions and the emotions of others. Perhaps the most salient and most frequently studied of these constructs is test anxiety (e.g., Sarason, 1984; Zeidner, 1998).

Students who suffer from test anxiety become overwhelmed by the thoughts and physiological sensations of anxiety during assessment situations and thus will be distracted from the task at hand, impairing their performance (e.g., Wine, 1971). Other non-cognitive constructs relating to students' emotions include self-regulation, emotion management, emotional control, coping with stress, and students' emotional states (e.g., MacCann, Fogarty, & Roberts, 2012; MacCann, Wang, Matthews, & Roberts, 2010; Pekrun, Elliot, & Maier, 2006). Research has demonstrated plausible causal pathways that relate greater emotional skills to higher levels of achievement. For example, students with better emotion management tend to use more effective coping strategies in response to academic stressors, which relates to higher levels of academic achievement (MacCann et al., 2011). Social and interpersonal constructs such as teamwork and leadership might also be considered under this broad banner (e.g., Wang, MacCann, Zhuang, Liu, & Roberts, 2009).

Habits and Processes

A further category of non-cognitive constructs relates to particular classes of habits or processes that students engage in when completing academic tasks. For example, students differ in the extent to which they engage in time management practices such as list-making, using time management aids (e.g., a planner or a system of electronic reminders), allocating time to particular tasks, or carefully noting deadlines for assignment due dates. Liu, Rijmen, MacCann and Roberts (2009) demonstrate that time management predicts academic achievement at middle school, and that girls at this age tend to have better time management habits than boys. Similarly, some students may routinely set particular kinds of learning goals, whereas others may not set goals at all, or may set goals that relate to publicly proving their ability rather than learning new things (Grant & Dweck, 2003). Other constructs in this category include organizational skills, study habits, learning strategies, and test-taking strategies (e.g., Crede, & Kuncel, 2008; Liu, 2009). Students' meta-cognitive skills such as self-monitoring and self-evaluation might also be considered part of this broad group of constructs (e.g., Flavell, 1979; Stankov & Lee, 2008).

Personality Traits

Finally, the broad personality domains and narrow personality facets have a long research history within psychology and education (e.g., Fiske, 1949; Norman, 1963). Personality traits are thought to be relatively stable and long-lasting, and describe an individual's consistent patterns of thoughts, behaviors, and emotions across different situations. Although there are several competing personality models, there is a rough consensus that five broad domains are the best starting points for describing differences between individuals' personalities (e.g., Digman & Inouye, 1986; Tupes & Christal, 1992). These five factors are:

(1) Extraversion (the tendency to be social, positive, and energetic);
(2) Agreeableness (the tendency to be kind, truthful and trusting);
(3) Conscientiousness (the tendency to be detail-oriented, achievement striving, and work-focused);
(4) Neuroticism (the tendency to experience negative emotions easily, often, and strongly) and
(5) Openness to Experience (the tendency to be open to new feelings, thoughts, and experiences).

Both conscientiousness and openness to experience show a robust relationship with academic achievement, although only conscientiousness predicts achievement independently of cognitive ability (Poropat, 2009; Trapmann, Hell, Hirn, & Schuler, 2007). In addition to the five broad personality domains, most contemporary models of personality also acknowledge more specific facets of personality that underlie each domain (e.g., Costa & McCrae, 1995; MacCann, Duckworth, & Roberts, 2009). For instance, Costa and McCrae propose six relatively distinct facets of conscientiousness: competence, order, dutifulness, achievement striving, self-discipline, and deliberation. Some research indicates that the narrow facets of personality may be more predictive than the broad domains (e.g., Paunonen & Ashton, 2001).

Each of these different types of non-cognitive factors can be assessed in a variety of ways, and each method of assessment has different strengths and weaknesses. The method of assessment can affect a large variety of test characteristics. These include (but are not limited to):

(a) the nature of what is measured,
(b) the potential for response distortion,
(c) the accuracy of measurement in different groups (e.g., some methods may be more appropriate for young children or test-takers with developing English-language literacy);

(d) the type and variety of feedback that can be given;

(e) the feasibility of large-scale testing and group assessment, compared to individual assessment;

(f) the cost of testing in terms of time, money, required equipment, assessor-training, and assessment development expenses;

(g) the reliability of the tests;

(h) the ease of building interventions or development plans targeting the measured construct;

(i) the sensitivity of the measure to changes over time;

(j) the potential for adverse impact, particularly if the assessment is used for high-stakes purposes such as selection; and

(k) test-taker reactions and engagement with the testing process.

In the paragraphs below, we describe and evaluate some of the most commonly used assessment methodologies, as well as some of the innovative and emerging methods that may be used in future assessments.

Traditional Non-cognitive Assessment Techniques
Self-Assessments

Self-assessments are undoubtedly the most widely used approach for gauging students' non-cognitive characteristics. These uses include: evaluating the effects of training; program evaluation; outcomes assessment; research; and large-scale, group-level national and international comparisons, to name a few. Indeed, most insights concerning the relationship between non-cognitive qualities and educational (or for that matter, work-related) outcomes come from research, practice, and policy conducted with self-report questionnaires.

GENERAL APPROACH

Self-assessments usually ask individuals to describe themselves by answering a series of standardized questions. The answer format is generally a Likert-type rating scale, but other formats may also be used (such as Yes/No or constructed response). Typically, questions assessing the same construct are aggregated; this aggregate score serves as an indicator of the relevant non-cognitive domain. The variety of constructs that can plausibly be assessed with self-reports are myriad. At a broad or abstract level these include personality, values, beliefs, and affect. Examples of specific

constructs that may be assessed with self-reports include communication skills, time management, teamwork, leadership, self-regulation, self-efficacy, and altruism. (Table 33.1 in this chapter includes a selection of sample items indicative of this approach.)

Self-assessments are a relatively pragmatic, cost-effective, and efficient way of gathering information about the individual. However, many issues must be taken into account when one is developing a psychometrically sound questionnaire, and there is a large literature on a wide variety of such topics. The optimal number of points on a scale, scale point labels, the inclusion of a neutral point, alternative ordering, and other test characteristics have been widely analyzed and examined in the literature (e.g., Krosnick, Judd, & Wittenbrink, 2005). For instance, studies reveal that response scale format influences individuals' responses (Rammstedt & Krebs, 2007), while the inclusion of negatively keyed questions (to avoid acquiescence) is considered controversial, especially with younger children (e.g. Barnette, 2000; DiStefano & Motl, 2006). Respondents vary in their use of the scale—for example, young males tend to use extreme answer categories (Austin, Deary, & Egan, 2006), as do Hispanics (Marin, Gamba, & Marin, 1992); and in general, there are large cultural effects in response style (Harzing, 2006; Lipnevich et al., 2011).

Respondents can fake their responses on self-assessments to appear more attractive to a prospective educational institution or employer, or to avoid remedial programs (e.g., Griffith, Chmielowski & Yoshita, 2007; Viswesvaran & Ones, 1999; Zickar, Gibby & Robie, 2004). Researchers have identified several promising methods for collecting data through self-reports while reducing fakeability. These include giving real-time warnings (Sackett, 2006), using a forced-choice format (Stark, Chernyshenko, & Drasgow, 2005), and using one's estimates of how others will respond to help control for faking (Prelec, 2004; Prelec & Weaver, 2006). However, evidence for the effectiveness of these procedures in controlling for faking remains to be demonstrated unequivocally (Converse, Oswald, Imus, Hedricks, Roy, & Butera, 2008; Heggestad, Morrison, Reeve, & McCloy, 2006). We consider the issue of fakeability in greater detail in a later section of this chapter.

THEORY OF PLANNED BEHAVIOR (TPB) AS A FRAMEWORK FOR DEVELOPING SELF-ASSESSMENTS

Self-assessments are based on a number of different conceptual frameworks, including those based

Table 33.1 Self-Report: Examples of Constructs, Items, and Response Scales

	Construct	Sample Items	Response Scale
1	Achievement Striving	1. I detect mistakes. 2. I do just enough work to get by (R).	Five-point Likert scale: "Not At All Like Me" (1) to "Very Much Like Me" (5).
2	Conscientiousness	1. I am always prepared. 2. I work hard.	Five-point Likert Scale: "Very Inaccurate of Me" (1) to "Accurate" (5).
3	Goals	1. I focus on the happy ending. 2. I fully focus on the obstacles (R).	Seven-point Likert scale: "Never" (1) to "Always" (7).
4	Grit	1. I am diligent 2. Failures double my motivation to succeed.	Five-point Likert scale: "Not at all like me" (1) to "Very much like me" (5).
5	Learning Strategies	1. When I study, I try to figure out which parts of the material I need to study most. 2. When I do my homework, I check to see whether I understand the material.	A four-point Likert-type scale: Never or Hardly Ever (1), Sometimes (2), Often (3), Always or Almost Always (4).
6	Self-Efficacy	1. I am certain that I can accomplish my goals. 2. I can handle whatever comes my way.	A four-point Likert-type scale: Hardly Ever (1), Sometimes (2), Often (3), or Almost Always (4).
7	Academic Motivation	1. I do only as much work as I have to for the grade I want. 2. I put little effort into my classes (R).	A four-point Likert-type scale: Strongly Agree (4), Agree (3), Disagree (2), Strongly Disagree (1).
8	Feelings About School Life	1. When doing after-school activities, I have felt nervous (R). 2. When doing homework, I have felt confident.	A four-point Likert-type scale: Never or Rarely (1), Sometimes (2), Often (3), Usually or Always (4).
9	Anxiety	1. I worry about things. 2. Fear for the worst.	Yes/No
10	Leadership	1. Can talk others into doing things. 2. Wait for others to lead the way.	Five-point Likert scale: "Not at all like me" (1) to "Very much like me" (5).

Notes: (R) refers to items that are reverse-keyed for respective scales of the instruments.

on clinical criteria, lexical analysis, and psychological theory. TpB has been particularly effective in serving as a framework for the development of assessments of individuals' attitudes (see Table 33.2 in this chapter for examples of items measuring TpB components). Only recently has the theory of planned behavior been applied in educational contexts (see Davis, Ajzen, Saunders, & Williams, 2002; Lipnevich et al., 2011). The initial findings appear promising. Hence, a brief overview follows.

The TpB is based on the psychological theory of reasoned behavior (Ajzen, 1991, 2002). The TpB posits that the central determinant of volitional behavior is one's intention to engage in that behavior. The theoretical model of the TpB is shown in Figure 33.1. Ajzen (1991) further proposes three independent determinants of behavior that exert

their effects through intentions. These are: (1) attitudes, (2) subjective norms, and (3) perceived behavioral control. *Attitudes* are defined as the overall positive or negative evaluation of the behavior. In general, the more favorable the attitude towards the behavior, the stronger the individual's intention is to perform it. Subjective norms assess the social pressures on the individual to perform or not to perform a particular behavior. Finally, perceived behavioral control provides information about the potential constraints on action as perceived by the individual (Armitage & Conner, 2001).

Several meta-analyses and literature reviews show support for the general principles underlying the TpB model (see Ajzen, 1991; Armitage & Conner, 2001). Studies reveal that the TpB accounts for 27 percent and 39 percent of the variance in behavior

Table 33.2 Self-Report: Theory of Planned Behavior–Based Assessment of Attitudes Toward Mathematics (after Lipnevich et al., 2011).

	TpB Component	Sample Item	Response Scale
1.	Attitudes	I enjoy studying math.	(1) Strongly Disagree
2.	Subjective Norm	My friends think that math is an important subject.	(2) Disagree (3) Neither Agree nor Disagree
3.	Perceived Behavioral Control	If I invest enough effort, I can succeed in math.	(4) Agree (5) Strongly Agree
4.	Intentions	I will try to work hard to make sure I learn math.	

and intention, respectively (Armitage & Conner, 2001; Sheeran, 2002). Davis et al. (2002) used the TpB to successfully predict high school completion (Davis, Ajzen, Saunders, & Williams, 2002). Results revealed that the TpB questionnaire significantly predicted high school completion. The model was a good fit to the data, and attitudes, subjective norms, and perceived control accounted for 51 percent of the variance in the intention to complete the present school year. Furthermore, attitudes, subjective norms, and perceived control all significantly predicted intention.

Another study that applied TpB to an educational context was conducted by Lipnevich et al. (2011). The researchers examined the effectiveness of the TpB in predicting students' mathematics performance. They found that between 25 percent and 32 percent of the variance in mathematics grades could be explained by TpB components. Moreover, 17 percent of the variation in test grades can be

explained by the TpB over and above the effects of mathematics ability test scores. So, development and implementation of TpB-based self-assessments may be instrumental in predicting a number of meaningful educational outcomes. Additionally, researchers suggest that the TpB has tremendous potential to inform the development of behavior-change interventions (see e.g. Armitage & Conner, 2001; Hardeman, Johnston, Johnston, Bonetti, Wareham, & Kinmonth, 2002; Rutter, 2000).

Other-Ratings

Other-ratings are assessments in which others (e.g., supervisors, trainers, colleagues, friends, faculty advisors, coaches, etc.) rate individuals on various non-cognitive skills. This method has a long history, and numerous studies have been conducted that employed this methodology to gather information (e.g., Tupes & Christal, 1961/1992). Other-ratings have an advantage over self-assessments in that they

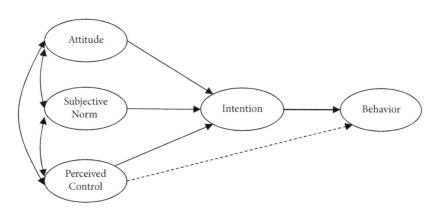

Figure 33.1 Representation of the Components of the TpB model.

Key: *Attitudes*—the overall evaluation of whether a behavior is positive or negative (based on prior behavioral contingencies). *Subjective Norms*—the perceived social pressure to perform the behavior. *Perceived Control*—the person's estimate of his or her capacity to perform the behavior. *Intentions*—the readiness or willingness to perform the behavior.

preclude socially desirable responding, although they are prone to rating biases. Self- and other-ratings do not always converge (Oltmanns & Terkheimer, 2006), but other-ratings have been demonstrated to often be more effective in predicting a range of educational outcomes, compared to self-ratings (Kenny, 1994; Wagerman & Funder, 2006).

TEACHER- AND PARENT-RATINGS

Teacher- or parent-ratings of personality have been widely used for gauging younger students' non-cognitive characteristics due to concerns that children lack the cognitive ability and/or psychology-mindedness to self-rate on personality instruments (e.g., Hendriks, Kuyper, Offringa, & VanderWerf, 2008). Other-ratings are also most appropriate when used to evaluate individuals with low verbal ability. For instance, the Child Behavior Check List (CBCL; Achenbach, 1991)—completed by teachers and/or parents—has been successfully employed to assess behavioral and emotional competencies (e.g., Anxious/Depressed, Rule-breaking Behavior) of children aged 6 to 18 years. Similarly, the Parent Rating Scale of the Behavioral Assessment System for Children (currently in its second edition—BASC-2) has been widely used to gauge adaptive and behavior problems of children between the ages of two and 21 (Reynolds & Kamphaus, 2004). Both CBCL and BASC-2 has been shown to capture a range of problems and competencies that would be difficult—if not impossible—to capture through self-reports.

MacCann, Lipnevich, and Roberts (2013) conducted a series of studies to compare parent judgements of personality with sixth to eighth-grade students' self-assessments. The results from three studies suggested that parent-ratings were both more reliable and more useful in predicting academic achievement than students' self-reports. This large difference in utility between self- and parent-reports of personality is noteworthy: Parent-reported Conscientiousness explained over twice as much variation in grades as students' self-reported Conscientiousness. Although such results might be used to justify the idea that younger children (in their preteens and early teens) might lack the psychology-mindedness or cognitive ability to accurately self-rate on personality questionnaires, it is worth comparing current results to studies of self- versus other-reports in older teenagers and adults. Thus, research studies demonstrate that peer-, co-worker-, supervisor-, and customer-ratings may be more reliable and more predictive of

valued outcomes than self-ratings, particularly for Conscientiousness (e.g., Mount, Barrick, & Strauss, 1994; Small & Diefendorff, 2006).

There are several possible reasons that parent-reports might differ from self-reports. John and Robins (1993) speculate that self-reporting differs from other-reporting in three main ways: (1) ego involvement is implicated in self-reports but not other-reports; (2) perspectives are different (the other-report is from an external observer, whereas the self is actively involved in the phenomena that personality items ask about); and (3) the self has access to privileged information such as previous experiences, internal thoughts, values, and intentions that are not available to others. If point (1) is responsible for the greater prediction by parent-reports, response bias in self-reports might attenuate correlations with grades. However, large-scale results from personnel psychology demonstrate that response bias does not actually affect the predictive power of personality tests (Barrick, & Mount, 1996; Ones, Viswesvaran, & Reiss, 1996). Moreover, when comparing mean differences in self- versus parent-reports, MacCann et al. (2013) demonstrated the opposite effect—parent-ratings resulted in higher means (i.e., were more flattering) than self-ratings. MacCann et al.'s study showed that score inflation in parent- versus child-reports might relate to different processes, with parent-reports prone to self-deceptive denial, whereas inflation of self-reports appears due to self-deceptive enhancement. Newspapers are full of illustrative examples of parents who deny that their children could possibly have behaved in such an immoral or unrestrained fashion as to commit crimes, for example, despite all the evidence to the contrary. When the other-rater shares a close emotional bond with the individual being assessed, the general rule that score inflation will be greater for self- than other-reports appears controvertible.

Point (3) might also account for differences in parent and self-report prediction. Given that parents do not have access to privileged internal information, they may need to use cues from the child's academic outcomes (which they know) to answer questions about the child's personality. That is, parents may make estimates on available information (which may be drawn from other constructs) when answering questionnaire items that refer to this privileged or internalized information. The implication of this finding for test development is that parent-reports (and other-reports more generally) should refer to observable information or facts to avoid the risk of criterion contamination.

However, parent-reports do have the advantage over self-reports in terms of point (2). A more external perspective might be viewed as a more objective reporting of the facts and so might result in more accurate measurement of the construct. Overall, parent- and teacher- reports are indispensable when assessing non-cognitive characteristics of younger students or students with limited verbal abilities.

LETTERS OF RECOMMENDATION

Letters of recommendation represent a specific form of other-rating and have been extensively used in a broad range of educational (e.g., Vannelli, Kuncel, & Ones, 2007) and workplace contexts (e.g., Arvey, 1979). Letters of recommendation provide stakeholders with detailed information about applicants' past performance, with the writers' opinion about the applicant being presented in the form of an essay. One major drawback of letters of recommendation is that they are not in a standardized format: different letter-writers may include or exclude qualitatively different types of information, so it is difficult to judge one letter against another. Walters, Kyllonen, and Plante (2003, 2006) developed a standardized format for such letters to counter this perceived problem (see Table 33.3 in this chapter for sample items). Initially termed the Standardized Letter of Recommendation, and now the Educational Testing Service (ETS)® Personal Potential Index (ETS, 2009), this assessment system prompts faculty members to respond to specific items using a Likert scale, in addition to eliciting their open-ended comments. It has been used operationally at ETS for selecting summer interns and fellows (Kyllonen & Kim, 2004; Kim & Kyllonen, 2008), through Project 1000 for the selection of graduate student applicants (Liu, Minsky, Ling, & Kyllonen, 2007), and since 2009, it has supplemented the Graduate Record Examination (GRE; see ETS, 2009; Kyllonen, 2008). Several research teams are currently collecting and analyzing data to address questions of validity and predictive power of letters of recommendation, but preliminary results provide some evidence for the reliability and validity of this method of measurement.

Biodata

Biographical data (biodata) have been explored for college admissions in the United States (Oswald, Schmitt, Kim, Ramsay, & Gillespie, 2004), Chile (Delgalarrando, 2008), and other countries. Biodata has also been a standard methodology for assessing constructs such as opportunity to learn

Table 33.3 The ETS® Personal Potential Index: Sample Items

Construct and Sample Items	Response Scale
1 Knowledge and Creativity Has a broad perspective on the field Produces novel ideas	(1) Below average (2) Average (3) Above average
2 Ethics and Integrity Is among the most honest persons I know Maintains high ethical standards	(4) Outstanding (5) Truly exceptional (7) Insufficient opportunity to evaluate
3 Planning and Organization Sets realistic goals Meets deadlines	
4 Resilience Accepts feedback without getting defensive Works well under stress	
5 Teamwork Supports the efforts of others Works well in group settings	
6 Communication Skills Speaks in a clear, organized, and logical manner Writes with precision and style	

and socioeconomic status in large-scale national and international group-level comparative studies (e.g., the National Assessment of Educational Progress, Programme for International Student Assessment, and Trends in International Mathematics and Science Study) (Chapter 6, this volume). Biodata are typically obtained by asking standardized questions about individuals' past behaviors, activities, or experiences. Respondents are typically offered multiple-choice answer options or are requested to answer questions in an open format (e.g., "state frequency of behavior"). Baird and Knapp (1981; see also Stricker, Rock, & Bennett, 2001) developed a biodata (documented accomplishments) measure that produced scores for six scales: Academic Achievement, Leadership, Practical Language, Aesthetic Expression, Science, and Mechanical.

Jackson, Wood, Bogg, Walton, Harms, & Roberts (2010) demonstrated that biodata approach can be effective when assessing individuals' personality. The researchers attempted to identify the behavioral component of conscientiousness and to specify a relatively large pool of behaviors that represent this personality facet. They developed and validated the Behavioral Indicators of Conscientiousness (BIC) and showed that the lower-order structure of conscientious behaviors (as assessed by BIC) is nearly identical to the lower-order structure obtained from extant self-report measures. Furthermore, the researchers used a daily-diary method to validate the BIC against frequency counts of conscientious behavior and found that behaviors assessed with BIC were strongly related to behaviors assessed daily through a diary method. The findings of Jackson et al. (2010) allow for a conclusion that may be extended to the biodata method in general: "Reports of past behavior are at least partially valid, mitigating a criticism often applied to self-reports of behavior" (p. 7).

Measures of biodata show incremental validity beyond SAT scores and the Big Five personality scores in predicting students' performance in college (Oswald, et al., 2004). Biodata may offer a less fakeable method of assessment than standard self-report scales, as there are several test characteristics that can be implemented to minimize faking (e.g., Dwight & Donovan, 2003; Schmitt, Oswald, Kim, Gillespie, & Ramsay, 2003). These include asking students to elaborate on the biodata details (e.g., "What was the name of the last foreign movie you saw?") or triangulating results obtained with alternative measurement approaches (e.g., other-reports). A sample biodata item is presented in Table 33.4 in this chapter.

Interviews

Interviews are the most frequently used method of personnel-selection in industry (Ryan, McFarland, Baron, & Page, 1999) and in clinical practice (Meyer et al., 2001), but they are also used for admissions, promotions, scholarships, and other awards in educational contexts (Goho & Blackman, 2006; Hell, Trapmann, Weigand, & Schuler, 2007). Interviews vary in their content and structure. In a

Table 33.4 Sample Biodata Item (from the Leadership scale of Oswald et al., 2004, p. 204).

Item	Response
How many times in the past year have you tried to get someone to join an activity in which you were involved or leading?	(A) never (B) once (C) twice (D) three or four times (E) five times or more

structured interview, questions are prepared before the interview starts. An unstructured interview simply is a free conversation between an interviewer and interviewee giving the interviewer the freedom to adaptively or intuitively switch topics. Research has shown that unstructured interviews lack predictive validity (Arvey & Campion, 1982) or show lower predictive validity than structured interviews (Schmidt & Hunter, 1998).

Structured interviews can be divided into three types: the behavioral description interview (BDI; Janz, Hellervik, & Gilmore, 1986), situational interview (SI; Latham, Saari, Pursell & Campion, 1980), and multi-modal interview (MMI; Schuler, 2002). The behavioral description interview involves questions that refer to the candidate's past behavior in real situations. The situational interview uses questions that require that interviewees imagine hypothetical situations (derived from critical incidents) and state how they would act in such situations. The multi-modal interview combines the two approaches and adds unstructured parts to ensure high respondent acceptance.

Meta-analyses of the predictive validity of interviews for job performance (Huffcutt, Conway, Roth, & Klehe, 2004; Marchese & Muchinski, 1993; McDaniel, Whetzel, Schmidt, & Maurer, 1994; Schmidt & Hunter, 1998) show that structured interviews: (a) are good predictors of job performance (corrected correlation coefficients range from 0.45 to 0.55); (b) they add incremental validity above and beyond general mental ability; and that (c) behavior description interviews show a higher validity than situational interviews.

Similarly, in educational contexts, interviews have been deemed moderately effective for the prediction of meaningful outcomes. For example, Goho and Blackman (2006) investigated the effectiveness of using selection interviews for admissions into medical schools, conducting meta-analyses to predict academic achievement and clinical performance. The mean effect size for studies examining the predictive power of interviews for academic success was 0.06 (95% confidence intervals 0.03–0.08), indicating a very small effect, whereas the sample of studies for predicting clinical success had a mean effect size of 0.17 (95% confidence intervals 0.11–0.22), indicating modest positive predictive power.

Wilkinson et al. (2008) report similar findings. Their study examined how well prior academic performance, admission tests, and interviews predicted academic performance in a graduate medical school. The researchers found that medical school grade point average (GPA) was most strongly correlated with prior academic performance (e.g., for overall score, partial $r = 0.47$; $p < 0.001$), followed by interviews (partial $r = 0.12$). Interestingly, whereas the relationship between GPA and performance weakened from Year 1 to Year 4, the association between interview score and performance increased from Year 1 to Year 4. Considering that the admissions interviews mostly focus on assessing candidates' non-cognitive characteristics (i.e., their motivation to become doctors, interest, drive, etc.), these findings attest to the effectiveness of interviews as methods for gauging students' non-cognitive skills. Thus, interviews were found to be better predictors of both medical school GPA and clinical practice than the Graduate Australian Medical School Admissions Test (Wilkinson et al., 2008), a finding reminiscent of the Swedish enlistment study conducted by Lindqvist and Vestman (2011).

Innovative Non-cognitive Assessment Techniques
Situational Judgement Tests (SJTs)

SJTs are a type of test where individuals are presented with a situation and then select either the most appropriate response or their typical response out of a list of possible choices (see Table 33.5, this chapter, for sample items). SJTs can be text-based or presented through multimedia, and responses can be multiple-choice (i.e., pick the best response), constructed response (i.e., provide a response to this situation), or ratings (i.e., rate each response for its effectiveness, on a Likert-type scale) (see, e.g., McDaniel, Morgesen, Finnegan, Campion, & Braverman, 2001). SJTs represent fairly simple, economical simulations of relevant academic- (or job-) related tasks (Kyllonen & Lee, 2005).

SELF-RATED SJTS

SJTs have several advantages over traditional self-assessment instruments. First, SJTs may be developed to reflect more subtle and complex judgement processes than are possible with conventional tests. Carefully constructed, the methodology of the SJT enables the measurement of many relevant attributes of applicants, including social competence, communication skills, critical thinking, and leadership, to name a few (e.g., Oswald et al., 2004; Waugh & Russell, 2003). By getting at these hard-to-measure constructs, SJTs carry the possibility of overcoming the validity ceiling found for conventional cognitive assessments in personnel selection and college admissions. Second, SJTs appear to be associated

Table 33.5 Situational Judgement Test Item: Teamwork Assessment

Item stem	You are part of a study group that has been assigned a large presentation for class. As you are all dividing up the workload, it becomes clear that both you and another member of the group are interested in researching the same aspect of the topic. Your colleague already has a great deal of experience in this area, but you have been extremely excited about working on this part of the project for several months. Which of the following is the best approach to dealing with this situation?
Responses	(A) Flip a coin to determine who gets to work on that particular aspect of the project. (B) Insist that, for the good of the group, you should work on that aspect of the project because your interest in the area means you will do a particularly good job. (C) Compromise your preferences for the good of the group and allow the other person to work on that aspect of the project.* (D) Choose a different group member to work on that aspect of the project so that no one person is privileged over another.

with less adverse impact on (ethnic) minorities. Of relevance in this context, reduced subgroup differences have indeed been found with SJTs (e.g., McDaniel et al., 2001). Third, SJTs can be used in training sessions to provide a student or prospective employee with feedback on his or her competencies in the domain of interest. Finally, SJTs appear to be less susceptible to faking than are self-assessments, where the improvement due to incentives can be up to a full standard deviation.

SJTs have been shown to predict a range of important outcomes such as college success (Lievens & Coestsier, 2002; Oswald et al., 2004) and leadership (Krokos, Meade, Cantwell, Pond, & Wilson, 2004). Although applications in education have been relatively limited, using SJTs in educational domains is certainly on the rise (Lievens, Buyse, & Sackett, 2005; MacCann et al., 2010; Oswald et al., 2004; Wang et al., 2009). This trend is partly due to the fact that there is more and more evidence that SJTs have high construct validity, both of predictive and consequential nature (e.g., Etienne & Julian, 2005; Sternberg et al., 2000). A recent study of high school students compared showed that an SJT of teamwork showed a higher correlation with GPA than a self-report rating scale of teamwork (Wang et al., 2009).

Depending on the information delivery mode, SJTs are typically dichotomized into text-based and multimedia-based types. Text-based SJTs fall into the category of traditional SJTs in the sense that they are presented in a paper-and-pencil format where scenarios and response options are in written form. Quite differently, multimedia SJTs use multimedia technology to present scenarios and sometimes also response options in video format (Lievens et al., 2005; McHenry & Schmitt, 1994; Olson-Buchanan & Drasgow, 2006; Weekley & Jones, 1997). Recent meta-analytic results demonstrate that multimedia SJTs show stronger criterion-related validity than written SJTs for predicting interpersonal skills (Christian, Edwards, & Bradley, 2010), and appear most effective when used to assess students' affective characteristics. A figural representation of a multimedia SJT item is presented in Table 33.6 in this chapter.

Table 33.6 Figural Representation of a Typical Multimedia SJTEA Item

Scenario

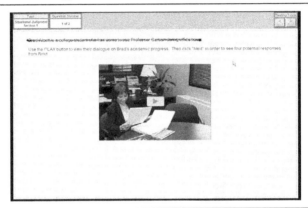

Response scale

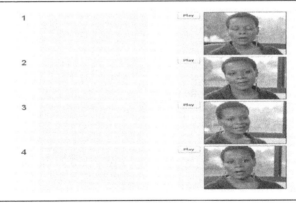

Response justification

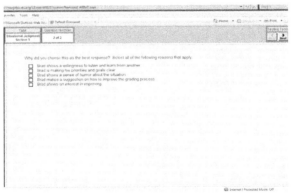

There are several reasons for the above-mentioned finding. First, multimedia SJTs enable the assessment of certain emotional abilities that cannot easily be assessed with other methodologies that are limited by the delivery medium. For instance, written SJTs can only provide verbal content, but multimedia SJTs represent a richer medium because they can present many more social cues, including verbal, nonverbal, and paralinguistic information.

Secondly, the use of multimedia technology enhances the degree to which the test mirrors the real environment, also referred to as *stimulus fidelity* (i.e., the extent to which the assessment task and context mirror those actually present in real life, Callinan & Robertson, 2000). Higher stimulus fidelity of multimedia SJTs is related to (a) enhanced ecological validity of the test (Chan & Schmitt, 1997), (b) more favorable test-taker reactions (Richman-Hirsch, Olson-Buchanan, & Drasgow, 2000), and (c) better prediction of meaningful outcome variables (Christian et al., 2010; Lievens & Sackett, 2006).

Thirdly, the use of multimedia technology does not rely excessively on verbal ability, a problem that has characterized the field to date. For example, written SJTs require the understanding and interpretation of text, making them dependent on text comprehension. The fact that text-based SJTs assume fairly advanced levels of reading comprehension may constitute a source of construct-irrelevant variance and may lead to higher correlations with cognitive ability. Contrary to text-based SJTs, multimedia SJTs do not require as much reading comprehension, instead more clearly targeting focal processes such as perceiving emotions and understanding the causes of these emotions. Indeed, recent studies confirm that multimedia SJTs have lower correlations with cognitive ability than do text-based SJTs (Lievens & Sackett, 2006).

In sum, SJTs represent a promising method for assessment of students' non-cognitive characteristics, with multimedia SJTs offering something that text-based assessments do not. Despite relatively high cost associated with their production (e.g., hiring actors and videotaping) and special requirements for administration (e.g., computers), we predict that multimedia SJTs will become an increasingly popular tool for measuring students' affective characteristics in a range of educational contexts (e.g., as supplements to college or graduate school admission interviews). An example of an SJT item is presented in Table 33.5.

OTHER-RATED SJTS

It is possible to administer SJTs in other-report format. That is, an observer such as a parent or teacher would be presented with a particular situation, and would judge what the target student would do in that situation. An example of the other-rated SJT item is presented in Table 33.7. MacCann, Wang, Matthews, and Roberts (2010) demonstrated that SJTs can be reliably administered in other-report format. This study used both self-report and parent-report SJTs to assess middle schools students' emotion-management skills. They found that although self- and parent-judgements were only weakly related, they both independently predicted valued criteria such as school grades, life satisfaction, and emotional reactions (both positive and negative) to the school environment. These findings support the idea that the non-shared variation between self- and parent-judgements is not random error, but represents different aspects of the phenomenon under investigation (in this case, emotion management). The researchers suggest that self- and parent-evaluations may index the frequency of different types of emotion management strategies. Parent-evaluations might relate to strategies involving interaction with others (e.g., seeking social support, talking through the issues), whereas self-evaluations might relate to strategies involving kind and sympathetic feelings towards others (e.g., expressing sympathy to diffuse tension, complimenting others). Other-rated SJTs represent a very promising approach for assessing non-cognitive characteristics, as they combine the benefits of SJTs

Table 33.7 Situational Judgement Test Item: Parent-Report of Teamwork Assessment (after MacCann et al., 2010).

Item stem	Your child and a classmate, James, sometimes help each other with homework. After your child helps James on a difficult project, the teacher is very critical of this work. James blames your child for his bad grade. Your child responds that James should be grateful, because helping him was a favor. What would your child do in this situation?
Responses	(A) Tell James that from now on he has to do his own homework. (B) Apologize to James. (C) Tell James "I am happy to help, but you are responsible for what you turn in." (D) Don't talk to James.

(e.g., high ecological validity of situations) and other-reports (e.g., suitable for younger kids and those with limited verbal abilities).

Time Use: Day-Reconstruction Method

A relatively new behavioral science domain concerns how people use their time. An assessment technique is the Day-Reconstruction Method (DRM; Kahneman, Krueger, Schkade, Schwarz, & Stone, 2004). The DRM assesses how people spend their time and how they experience the various activities and settings of their lives. It combines features of two other time-use techniques, time-budget measurement (the respondent estimates how much time is spent on various categories of activities) and experience sampling (the respondent records his or her current activities when prompted to do so at random intervals throughout the day). The DRM requires that participants systematically reconstruct their activities and experiences of the preceding day with procedures designed to reduce recall biases.

When using the DRM, a respondent first recreates the previous day by producing a confidential diary of events. Confidentiality encourages respondents to include details they may not want to share through any other assessment approach (such as an interview). Next, respondents receive a standardized response form and use their confidential diary to answer a series of questions about each event, including (1) when the event began and ended, (2) what they were doing, (3) where they were, (4) whom they were interacting with, and (5) how they felt on multiple affect dimensions. The response form is returned to the researcher for analysis. In addition, respondents answer a number of demographic questions.

Respondents complete the diary before they are informed about the content of the standardized response form, so as to minimize biases. A study of 909 employed women showed that the DRM closely corresponds with experience sampling methods (Kahneman et al., 2004). The DRM is a time-consuming and intrusive form of assessment that requires a significant effort from respondents. More research is needed to capture psychometric qualities of the method. However, initial evidence suggests that this method is effective in assessing characteristics otherwise difficult to capture (Belli, 1998; Kahneman et al., 2004). Moreover, the method appears generalizable to high school and college populations. For example, Roberts et al. (2011) report similar findings with the DRM for 131 college freshman as found for employee samples. In particular, participants reported significantly greater positive affect while engaging in hobbies or socializing than attending class or completing homework. In this study, the DRM was also substantially correlated (i.e., r's exceeding 0.40 for each activity) with a self-assessment of psychological well-being and a situational judgement test of emotional management.

Writing Samples

Chung and Pennebaker's (2007) analysis of writing samples as a gateway to personality is based on the idea that what we write and say, as well as how we write and say it, reflects our personality. This stream of research involves correlating words and word types from open-ended writing (e.g., emails) with personality and behavioral measures. Research suggests that the use of particular function words (e.g., pronouns, adjectives, articles) is related to individuals' affective states, reactions to stressful life events, social stressors, demographic factors, and biological conditions (Chung & Pennebaker, 2007; Mehl & Pennebaker, 2003). For example, the use of "I" is associated with depression, and speaking to a superior, based on email correspondence. Moreover, word choices can be used to detect deception (Hancock, Curry, Goorha, & Woodworth, 2004; Newman, Pennebaker, Berry, & Richards, 2003).

Vast volumes of materials are available to explore this research program further (especially given the preponderance of social networks and the archival capabilities that are part of the Internet), while the availability of inexpensive automated classification tools provides noteworthy research opportunities to continue to identify relationships between written communication and non-cognitive skills. The magnitude of correlations found tends to be quite low, but the method's low cost and unobtrusiveness suggests that it may lead to future applications in psychological testing. Although most of this research has focused on adult behaviors, the amount of writing that needs to be completed in secondary and tertiary education poses some intriguing possibilities for the assessment of non-cognitive skills during childhood and adolescence.

The Thorny Issue of Response Distortion

A potential problem with using non-cognitive assessments for high-stakes purposes such as educational selection is that test-takers may try to "fake" high scores in order to get into the course. Even an exceptionally lazy person is unlikely to agree with the statement "I am lazy" if they are answering this item as part of a college admissions process. Meta-analytic research from personnel psychology supports this intuitive idea with hard empirical data. Viswesvaran and Ones' (1999) meta-analysis demonstrates that people can fake personality tests when asked to do so, raising their personality test scores by the equivalent of 7 to 14 IQ points. Furthermore, research suggests that between 20 percent and 40 percent of people actually do fake when taking personality tests for selection purposes (Birkeland, Manson, Kisamore, Brannick, & Smith, 2006).

Psychologists have long realized that people are prone to exaggerate on rating-scale tests in order to get a better score and so get into the school of their choice or procure a better job. The predominant approach to dealing with faking has been to detect fakers with lie scales, also known as *response distortion scales* (e.g., Crowne & Marlowe, 1960; Paulhus, 1998). Lie scales intermix items such as "I never swear," or "I always pick up my litter" with focal personality items. Fakers are identified by their high scores on lie scales. Although lie scales are immensely popular and commonly used, there is a growing consensus that that they do not work (Dilchert, Ones, Viswesvaran, & Deller, 2006; Ellingson, Sackett, & Hough, 1999; MacCann, Zeigler, & Roberts, 2011). Both logic and empirical evidence suggest that people scoring high on lie scales might actually be exemplary individuals who always pick up their litter and never swear. Correlations of lie scores with substantive personality traits like conscientiousness and agreeableness suggest that it is not liars, but nice, kind, hard-working people who are caught out by lie scales (e.g., Li & Bagger, 2006).

Given that lie scales do not seem to catch the liars, there are two broad strategies for dealing with response distortion when assessing non-cognitive constructs. First, non-cognitive constructs, particularly as measured with self-reported rating scales, simply cannot be used as selection criteria for high-stakes purposes. For example, it may be reasonable for medical schools to exclude applicants with very low scores on empathy, given that these applicants might make poor healthcare professionals. However, it would be unreasonable to select only the top applicants based on empathy, as the very top scores on a rating-scale measure of empathy might be fakers who displace genuinely empathetic applicants. That is, using non-cognitive scores to screen out wildly inappropriate applicants is still a useful exercise, even if some people fake.

The second strategy to combat faking in non-cognitive assessments is to use a range of innovative assessment methods that show greater resistance to faking than standard rating scales. Implicit measurement techniques are chief among these new methods. In implicit measurement, the measurement objective is not obvious to the participants, such that these measures may be less susceptible to faking (e.g. Ziegler, Schmidt-Atzert, Buehner, & Krumm, 2008). Implicit measurement techniques include the implicit association test (IAT) paradigm, as well as the conditional reasoning test (CRT) paradigm, which we describe below. Other testing methods that may reduce faking include forced-choice assessment and the Bayesian truth serum. Many of these measurement techniques are still in their infancy, with limited empirical data to provide evidence of their validity and their non-fakeability. In the paragraphs below, we describe each of these techniques in turn and outline the empirical evidence for these techniques as viable methods to measure non-cognitive constructs.

Implicit Assessments: Implicit Association Tests (IATs)

The implicit association test (Greenwald, McGhee, & Schwartz, 1998) has become an incredibly popular method for researching non-cognitive factors, particularly attitudes, having been examined in many hundreds of empirical studies (see Greenwald, Nosek, & Sriram, 2006). IATs record the reaction time it takes to classify stimulus pairs (e.g., word, picture), which is then treated as an indirect measure of whether a participant sees the stimuli as naturally associated. IATs thus measure the strength of implicit associations to gauge attitudes, stereotypes, self-concepts, and self-esteem (Greenwald, Banaji, Rudman, Farnham, Nosek, & Mellot, 2002; Greenwald & Farnham, 2000).

IATs generally exhibit reasonably good psychometric properties. Meta-analyses have revealed high internal consistencies (0.80 to 0.90) (Hofmann et al., 2005), although somewhat lower test-retest reliabilities (0.50 and 0.70), which is a common finding in reaction time research. IATs predict a wide variety of criteria, particularly spontaneous (as opposed to controlled) behavior (Bosson, Swann, & Pennebaker, 2000; Gawronski & Bodenhausen, 2006; McConnel & Leibold, 2001). However, to our knowledge, they have not been used in studies of educational outcomes, although there is an emerging literature using this method to explore the attitudes of children and adolescents to health-related behaviors (e.g., smoking; see Andrews, Hampson, Greenwald, Gordon, &

Widdop, 2010). The Hofmann et al. meta-analysis estimated the correlation between implicit (IATs) and explicit (self-reports) measures of personality to be 0.24, with about half of variability being due to moderating variables.

The promise of the IAT is that it should be less susceptible to faking. However, preliminary findings demonstrate the IAT is to a certain extent fakeable (Fiedler, Messner, & Bluemke, 2006). Given that there is still controversy about what the IAT measures (Rothermund & Wentura, 2004), and that there is a lot of method-specific (construct-irrelevant) variance associated with IATs (Mierke & Klauer, 2003), it is clear that more research is needed before IATs (and the related Go–No Go Association Test, Nosek & Banaji, 2001) can be regarded as viable tools in various applied educational contexts.

Implicit Assessments: Conditional Reasoning Tests (CRTs)

Conditional reasoning tests are multiple-choice tests consisting of items that look like reading comprehension or logical reasoning items, but are used to measure world-view, personality, biases, and motives (James, 1998; LeBreton, Barksdale, & Robin, 2007). Following a passage and a question, the CRT presents two or three logically incorrect alternatives, and two logically correct alternatives, which reflect different (often opposing) worldviews. Participants are asked to state which of the alternatives seems to be most reasonable, based on the information given in the text. Thus, respondents assume that they can solve a problem by reasoning about it, not realizing that there are two correct answers, and that their selection is guided by implicit assumptions underlying answer alternatives.

Participants are prompted to select one of the logically correct alternatives, presumably according to his or her underlying beliefs, rationalizing the selection through the use of justification mechanisms. For example, the examinee might select an aggressive response to a situation, justifying it as an act of self-defense or as retaliation (LeBreton et al., 2007). These justification mechanisms serve to reveal hidden or implicit elements of the personality. To see an illustration of this idea, consider the example from LeBreton et al. (2007) presented in Tables 33.1–33.4.

The CRT for aggression has been shown to be unrelated to cognitive ability, yet reliable and valid for predicting different behavioral manifestations of aggression in the workplace (average r over 10 studies = 0.44) (James, McIntyre, & Glisson, 2004). Most of the research on CRTs has been in measuring aggression or achievement motivation (James, 1998). However, the method has proven difficult to replicate (Gustafson, 2004), and so far there is a paucity of research with children and adolescents (indeed, the cognitive difficulty of the items is currently such that applications would need to be restricted to high school populations and above). Also, as with IATs, the promise of resistance to faking has not been established (LeBreton et al., 2007). Thus, it seems that CRTs may need further work before being used in high-stakes academic situations. A sample CRT item is presented in Table 33.8.

Forced Choice

Peabody's (1967) early musings on personality assessments proposed a distinction between descriptive and evaluative judgements of personality. In any personality item, there is both a descriptive element and an evaluative element. For example, the descriptive element of the item "I am lazy" is that it measures conscientiousness (reverse-coded). The evaluative element is that "I am lazy" sounds like a bad thing. The basis for forced-choice testing is that test-takers are forced to choose between two or more statements that are equal in evaluative content (i.e., are equally socially desirable) but differ in terms of their descriptive content (i.e., measure different personality traits). Test-takers cannot then

Table 33.8 Conditional Reasoning Item (after James et al., 2004)

Item	Response
Half of all marriages end in divorce. One reason for the large number of divorces is that getting a divorce is quick and easy. If a couple can agree on how to split their property fairly, then they can get a divorce simply by filling out forms and taking them to court. They do not need lawyers. Which of the following is the most reasonable conclusion, based on the above?	(A) People are getting older when they get married. (B) If one's spouse hires a lawyer, then he or she is not planning to play fair. (C) Couples might get back together if getting a divorce took longer. (D) More men than women get divorced.

grade themselves highly on all positive statements, but must choose between them. Thus, faking-related variation in scores should be minimized.

There are several methods for forced-choice measurement, including pair comparisons, rank-ordering, and multidimensional forced-choice. In pair comparisons, the test-taker must choose between two equally desirable statements (e.g., "Which is more like you: 'I work hard' or 'I think up new ideas?'"). In rank-ordering, test-takers must rank a series of equally desirable statements in order from "most like me" to "least like me." Both these methods require that statements included in any one item be carefully matched for social desirability so that test-takers cannot use the evaluative aspects of the statements in their responses. In multidimensional forced-choice assessments, test-takers are presented with a dichotomous quartet of four different traits in which two socially desirable statements are paired with two socially undesirable statements (Jackson, Wroblewski, & Ashton, 2000). For example, a test-taker would be asked to select which is "most like you" and which is "least like you" from the following four statements: (1) "I work hard," (2) "I lose my temper," (3) "I love to help others," and (4) "I cannot deal with change." The statement selected as "most like you" would be scored +1; the statement selected as "least like you" would be scored –1, and the statements that were not endorsed at all would be scored zero.

There is some evidence to suggest that forced-choice tests are less fakeable than standard rating scales, and show stronger relationships with performance (e.g., Jackson et al., 2000; Martin, Bowen, & Hunt, 2002). However, forced-choice measures may have ipsative or partly ipsative properties. That is, scores on forced-choice measures may be appropriate for comparing the relative level of different traits within an individual, but inappropriate for comparing the relative levels of a trait across different people. Essentially, personality dimensions are not independent: one cannot be high on them all. This poses a problem for test-takers who really are high on multiple personality dimensions, or for test users who want to select individuals based on high scores on more than one personality dimension.

However, Stark, Chernyshenko, and Dragow (2011) propose a number of IRT-based processes for constructing forced-choice items that ameliorate these issues of ipsativity. For example, in the sequential approach to developing a multi-dimensional pair-wise preference (MDPP) measure, one first determines both social desirability and item parameters of a large number of items presented in conventional format. Social desirability ratings and item parameters may then be used to develop pairs of statements that act as a pair-comparison judgement (e.g., "I work hard" versus "I think up new ideas"). An important feature is that within most pair comparisons, items are drawn from two different personality domains (e.g., a Conscientiousness item is compared to an Agreeableness item). However, at least for some pairs, the items belong to the same domain. That way, it is possible to compute scores that also have a normative value; that is, can be used to differentiate between people. Empirical evidence to date suggests that tests constructed and scored using the MDPP method appear resistant to faking, and that normative rather than ipsative information can be recovered from this process. In this way, an empirically based procedure for item selection and test development combined with new statistical modeling techniques seems to produce the best of both worlds: fake-proof tests that also lack the ipsativity that plagued earlier operationalizations of forced-choice measurement. For this reason, we contend the approach will be explored much more in educational contexts in the years ahead. For example, an upcoming Program for International Student Assessment (PISA) field trial uses several variants of this approach to assess learning strategies. Table 33.9 contains a sample multidimensional forced-choice item.

Bayesian Truth Serum

The Bayesian Truth Serum (BTS) calculates how often people endorse item content they perceive as unusual and therefore possibly undesirable (Prelec, 2004). A person who rarely agrees with unpopular attitudes or behaviors is assumed to be adjusting their answers based on conformity to group opinion or expectations, rather than giving an honest appraisal of the item content. The extent of agreement with self-perceived "unpopular" items can be taken as an index of truth-telling. The method requires the test-taker to provide two pieces of

Table 33.9 Multi-dimensional Forced-Choice Item

Item	Response
Consider the four statements at right.	I work hard.
	I lose my temper.
Which is most like you, and which is least like you?	I love to help others.
	I cannot deal with change.

information for every item: their own response, and the proportion of people they estimate would respond the same way on that item. For example, a test-taker might have to choose which statement described them better: "I think up new ideas" or "I work hard." The test-taker would also have to estimate the preference of the wider population (e.g., guessing that perhaps 75% of the overall population would choose "I think up new ideas" over "I work hard" to describe themselves). Prelec argues that respondents who answer questions honestly will tend to overestimate the percentage of other people who agree with them. In this way, an index of truth telling can be calculated.

However, estimating the beliefs of other people is both meta-cognitively complex, and may be subject to frame-of-reference effects as to who these "others" are considered to be (other college applicants, other people the test-taker personally knows, other people of similar SES and demographics to the test-taker, or all other people in the world). For these reasons, the BTS may not function accurately for test-takers with poor meta-cognitive skills or test-takers using an unusual frame of reference. In addition, collecting additional information doubles the test-taking time, since twice as many questions are asked. Like the conditional reasoning test, the complexity of the Bayesian truth serum suggests that the method might only be accurately applied after the mid-teens, and then only among cognitively normal populations. Young children may not have the meta-cognitive skill to answer such questions, nor the concentration to sit through tests of double the normal length.

Future Directions: Potential Uses of Non-cognitive Assessments

In the final section of this chapter, we consider the findings from the literature analysis, and synthesize them in a way to suggest several ways in which comprehensive non-cognitive assessments might be used (or are currently used) in education.

High-Stakes Assessment

High-stakes applications of non-cognitive tests in education include diagnosis and selection. For diagnosis, non-cognitive assessments have an important role to play in augmenting traditional cognitive assessments aimed at diagnosing learning disorders and difficulties. For example, test anxiety shows frequent comorbidity with learning difficulties, as students who struggle with scholastic material develop an aversion to and fear of evaluative

situations (e.g., Bryan, Sonnefeld, & Grabowski, 1983; Sena, Lowe, & Lee, 2007). Test anxiety can function as both a symptom of learning difficulties and an exacerbation of learning difficulties, and may even affect scores on cognitive assessments designed to diagnose learning difficulties. Thus, this particular non-cognitive factor may be a pertinent factor to consider when diagnosing a student with a particular learning disorder.

The second major high-stakes application of non-cognitive assessments is selection for college, graduate school, preparatory school, gifted classes, or the honors or advanced placement track. Large-scale, high-stakes non-cognitive assessment, based on faculty ratings, has been implemented recently for graduate school admissions (Kyllonen, 2008). If this is successful, it is reasonable to expect that a similar application for undergraduate admissions could follow. Recent meta-analytic evidence shows that non-cognitive assessments are just as predictive of academic achievement as traditional intelligence testing (Poropat, 2009). Moreover, this prediction is separate from intelligence, that such non-cognitive assessments retain their strong relationship to achievement even after controlling for ability. Such results imply that accuracy in selection decisions could be improved drastically with the addition of non-cognitive assessments. For example, two students of equal intelligence might have very different chances of success in advanced placement classes if one of them is willing to work hard, seek help, and extend effort to maintain a supportive social network, whereas the other believes that success is due to lucky breaks and chance factors. Using appropriate non-cognitive tests to augment selection decision could feasibly result in better outcomes. Moreover, there is some evidence to suggest that including non-cognitive factors in selection decisions would result in less adverse impact on ethnic minorities and women (e.g., McDaniel et al., 2001)

A diagnosis or selection decision may be vastly influential for children and adolescents, with long-term consequences. Therefore, the potential for motivated individuals to try to gain a particular outcome should be not ignored: it is quite possible that even young children will give a socially correct answer rather than one that describes their actual tendencies. For this reason, several safeguards against response distortion should be considered when tests are used for high-stakes purposes. First, a non-cognitive assessment should never be the sole basis for a high-stakes decision, but should be considered in conjunction with other key factors (e.g., cognitive test scores, teacher and parent interviews, and record of achievement relative to ability for learning disorder diagnosis). Second, in most selection scenarios, it may be more beneficial to exclude those with unacceptably low non-cognitive skills, rather than select the top few with exceptionally high non-cognitive skills. Third, an aggregate of multiple other-reports should be preferred over self-reports, as in the case of the Personal Potentiality Index assessment for post-graduate admissions (Kyllonen, 2008). With these appropriate safeguards in mind, non-cognitive assessments have the potential to drastically improve selection and diagnosis decisions.

Developmental Scales

Another possible application of non-cognitive assessments is to track students' development over time (Roberts, 2009; Roberts & Wood, 2006). At the individual level, a "report card" each year could show the students' development of non-cognitive skills such as impulse control, social skills, coping strategies, and attitudes towards school and schoolwork. Particularly in the early grades, this sort of feedback could feasibly be used for early identification of individuals or cohorts at risk for learning disorders, conduct disorders, or other academic or social problems. At the institutional level, schools that provide programs for social and emotional learning, peer support, or the development of academic skills such as time management or learning strategies could monitor the progress of their student body in developing and maintaining these skills. Schools would also be able to track trends at specific levels (e.g., the adjustment to a new environment by students beginning kindergarten or high school; or the stress experienced by students undertaking college preparations in the last two years of secondary school). At the wider level, district, state or national comparisons of students' non-cognitive tests scores would allow a strong evidence base for policy development in education.

Interventions

One of the strengths of using non-cognitive tests as developmental scales is the potential for interventions or training. There are several ways that assessments can form the backbone of intervention and training development. First, as mentioned above, large-scale developmental assessments can be used to guide policy change, as well as to evaluate the effectiveness of policy implementation. Second, scores on specific assessments may serve as the basis for particular suggestions in the form of tailored feedback and action plans. For example, a high-school student might complete a three-component measure of time management, and score much lower on the *planning* component than the other two parts. Such a student would receive the information that they are (for example) good at coping with change, and tend to refrain from procrastination, but that planning is their weak point. Such information should increase their self-knowledge (and potentially their meta-cognitive skills). The student could also receive a series of suggestions about how to improve their planning skills, some helpful tools such as a weekly or monthly time-and-task calculator, or a referral to existing school- or district-based programs for assisting with academic-readiness skills. As we mentioned in earlier sections of this chapter, the TpB is a particularly powerful technique for linking assessments with interventions, as its theoretical basis focuses on behavior and behavior change (Ajzen, 2011).

Educational applications of non-cognitive testing might also borrow from personnel psychology, applying ideas such as the development assessment center, which directly links assessment with development activities (e.g., Thornton & Rupp, 2005). In developmental assessment centers, the test-taker:

(a) learns about the non-cognitive dimensions the test measures (e.g., learns about the underlying components of time management);

(b) learns their own strengths and weaknesses;

(c) learns how to set goals to improve;

(d) learns how to monitor their progress in improvement;

(e) is provided with exercises, feedback, and experiential learning activities.

These programs are currently being implemented by several research teams, and the initial results are promising (Elias & Clubby, 1992). This paradigm holds great promise for improving non-cognitive skills for education.

Concluding Comments

In this chapter we presented an overview of a rather wide variety of both conventional and novel methods for assessing non-cognitive skills in an educational context. Self-assessments are the most common and are likely to be useful in any kind of non-cognitive assessment system, particularly when the stakes are not high. Other-ratings, such as teacher ratings, parent reports, letters of recommendation, and interviews, are also quite useful, and as discussed in corresponding sections of this chapter, they are currently the most viable for high-stakes selection applications. A range of non-traditional assessments hereby reviewed—such as the implicit association test, day reconstruction method, and conditional reasoning tests—are intriguing and may potentially be quite useful for assessing students' non-cognitive characteristics. Situational judgement tests are an increasingly popular way to measure non-cognitive characteristics. They have been used in so many studies over the past 10 years that the methodology for developing them is now fairly affordable, and the measures are becoming increasingly reliable and valid. All of these methods are constantly evolving, so more information attesting to their validity and applicability for educational contexts will be accrued in the upcoming years.

Overall, our understanding of non-cognitive factors influencing academic achievement and possible approaches toward the measurement and assessment of these factors allows us to identify students who are more or less likely to do well in a specific academic program. Additionally, our knowledge of the relationships among a range of non-cognitive constructs and educational outcomes can be used to develop effective interventions. These interventions can be successful in enhancing students' non-cognitive characteristics, and, consequently, their achievement. In sum, these constructs can be successfully assessed and modified, and it is our hope that more and more researchers will start designing studies investigating the quality of such assessments and the effectiveness of such interventions.

Authors' Note

We thank Anthony Betancourt, Jeremy Burrus, Daniel Howard, Teresa Jackson, Stefan Krumm, Mary Lucas, Bobby Naemi, Jen Minsky, and Patrick Kyllonen for supporting the preparation of this manuscript. All statements expressed in this chapter are the authors' and do not reflect the official opinions or policies of the authors' host affiliations. Correspondence concerning this article should be directed to Anastasiya A. Lipnevich via email: a.lipnevich@gmail.com.

References

Abe, J. A. A. (2005). The predictive value of the Five-Factor Model of personality with preschool-age children: A nine year follow-up study. *Journal of Research in Personality, 39,* 423–442.

Achenbach, T. M. (1991). *Manual for the Child Behavior Checklist/ 4–18 and 1991 profile.* Burlington: University of Vermont, Department of Psychiatry.

Ajzen, I. (1991). The theory of planned behavior. *Organizational Behavior & Human Decision Processes, 50,* 179–211.

Ajzen, I. (2002). Perceived behavioral control, self-efficacy, locus of control, and the theory of planned behavior. *Journal of Applied Social Psychology, 32,* 665–683.

Ajzen, I. (2011). Behavioral interventions: Design and evaluation guided by the theory of planned behavior. In M. M. Mark, S. I. Donaldson, & B. C. Campbell (Eds.), *Social psychology for program and policy evaluation* (pp. 74–100). New York: Guilford.

Andrews, J. A., Hampson, S. E., Greenwald, A. G., Gordon, J., & Widdop, C. (2010). Using the Implicit Association Test to assess children's implicit attitudes toward smoking. *Journal of Applied Social Psychology, 40,* 2387–2406.

Armitage, C., & Conner, M. (2001). Efficacy of the theory of planned behaviour: A meta-analytic review. *British Journal of Social Psychology, 40,* 471–499.

Arvey, R. D. (1979). Unfair discrimination in the employment interview: Legal and psychological aspects. *Psychological Bulletin, 86,* 736–765.

Arvey, R. D., & Campion, J. E. (1982). The employment interview: A summary and review of recent research. *Personnel Psychology, 35,* 281–322.

Austin, E. J., Deary, I. J., & Egan, V. (2006). Individual differences in response scale use: Mixed Rasch modelling of responses to NEO-FFI items. *Personality & Individual Differences, 40,* 1235–1245.

Baird, L. L., & Knapp, J. E. (1981). *The inventory of documented accomplishments for graduate admissions: Results of a field trial study and its reliability, short-term correlates, and evaluation.* (ETS Research Rep. No. 81–18, GRE Board Research Rep. No. 78–3R). Princeton, NJ: Educational Testing Service.

Barnette, J. J. (2000). Effects of stem and Likert response option reversals on survey internal consistency: If you feel the need, there is a better alternative to using those negatively worded stems. *Educational & Psychological Measurement, 60,* 361–370.

Barrick, M. R., & Mount, M. K. (1996). Effects of impression management and self-deception on the predictive validity of personality constructs. *Journal of Applied Psychology, 81,* 261–272.

Belli, R. (1998). The structure of autobiographical memory and the event history calendar: Potential improvements in the quality of retrospective reports in surveys, *Memory, 6,* 383–406.

Birkeland, S. A., Manson, T. M., Kisamore, J. L., Brannick, M. T., & Smith, M. A. (2006). A meta-analytic investigation of job applicant faking on personality measures. *International Journal of Selection & Assessment, 14,* 317–335.

Blackwell, L. S., Trzesniewski, K. H., & Dweck, C. S. (2007). Implicit theories of intelligence predict achievement across an adolescent transition: A longitudinal study and an intervention. *Child Development, 78,* 246–263.

Block, J. (1995). A contrarian view of the five-factor approach to personality description. *Psychological Bulletin, 117,* 187–215.

Bosson, J. K., Swann, W. B., & Pennebaker, J. W. (2000). Stalking the perfect measure of implicit self-esteem: The blind men and the elephant revisited? *Journal of Personality & Social Psychology, 79,* 631–643.

Bryan, J. H., Sonnefeld, J. L., & Grabowski, B. (1983). The relationship between fear of failure and learning disabilities. *Learning Disability Quarterly, 6,* 217–222.

Burrus, J., MacCann, C., Kyllonen, P., & Roberts, R. D. (2011). Non-cognitive constructs in K–16: Assessments, interventions, educational and policy implications. In P. J. Bowman & E. P. St John (Eds.), *Diversity, merit, and higher education: Toward a comprehensive agenda for the twenty-first century* (pp. 233–274). Ann Arbor, MI: AMS Press.

Callinan, M., & Robertson, I. T. (2000). Work sample testing. *International Journal of Selection & Assessment, 8,* 248–260.

Campbell, J. R., Voelkl, K. E., & Donahue, P. L. (1997). *NAEP 1996 trends in academic progress.* (NCES Publication No. 97985r). Washington, DC: U.S. Department of Education.

Chan, D., & Schmitt, N. (1997). Video-based versus paper-and-pencil method of assessment in situational judgement tests: Subgroup differences in test performance and face validity perceptions. *Journal of Applied Psychology, 82,* 143–159.

Christian, M. S., Edwards, B. D., & Bradley, J. C. (2010). Situational judgement tests: Constructs assessed and a meta-analysis of their criterion-related validities. *Personnel Psychology, 63,* 83–117.

Chung, C. K., & Pennebaker, J. W. (2007). The psychological function of function words. In K. Fiedler (Ed.), *Social communication: Frontiers of social psychology* (pp. 343–359). Mahwah, NJ: Erlbaum.

Connell, J. P., Spencer, M. B., & Aber, J. L. (1994). Educational risk and resilience in African-American youth: Context, self, action, and outcomes in school. *Child Development, 65,* 493–506.

Converse, P. D., Oswald, F. L., Imus, A., Hedricks, C., Roy, R., & Butera, H. (2008). Comparing personality test formats and warnings: Effects on criterion-related validity and test-taker reactions. *International Journal of Selection & Assessment, 16,* 155–169.

Costa, P. T. Jr., & McCrae, R. R. (1995). Domains and facets: Hierarchical personality assessment using the Revised NEO Personality Inventory. *Journal of Personality Assessment, 64,* 21–50.

Crede, M., & Kuncel, N. R. (2008). Study habits, skills, and attitudes: The third pillar supporting collegiate academic performance. *Perspectives on Psychological Science, 3,* 425–453.

Crowne, D. P., & Marlowe, D. (1960). A new scale of social desirability independent of psychopathology. *Journal of Consulting Psychology, 24,* 349–354.

Davis, L. E., Ajzen, I., Saunders, J., & Williams, T. (2002). The decision of African American students to complete high school: An application of the theory of planned behavior. *Journal of Educational Psychology, 94,* 810–819.

Delgalarrando, M. G. (July 9, 2008). *Validan plan de admisión complementaria a la UC. (p. 9),* El Mercurio, Santiago Chile.

Digman, J. M., & Inouye, J. (1986). Further specification of the five robust factors of personality. *Journal of Personality & Social Psychology, 50,* 116–123.

Dilchert, S., Ones, D. S., Viswesvaran, C., & Deller, J. (2006). Response distortion in personality measurement: Born to deceive, yet capable of providing valid self-assessments? *Psychology Science, 48,* 209–225.

DiStefano, C., & Motl, R. W. (2006). Further investigating method effects associated with negatively worded items on self-report surveys. *Structural Equation Modeling: A Multidisciplinary Journal, 13,* 440–484.

Duckworth, A., & Seligman, M. (2005). Self-discipline outdoes IQ in predicting academic performance of adolescents. *Psychological Science, 16,* 939–944.

Dweck, C. S., & Leggett, E. L. (1988). A social-cognitive approach to motivation and personality. *Psychological Review, 95,* 256–273.

Dwight, S. A., & Donovan, J. J. (2003). Do warnings not to fake reduce faking? *Human Performance, 16,* 1–23.

Elias, M. J., & Clabby, J. (1992). *Building social problem solving skills: Guidelines from a school-based program.* San Francisco: Jossey-Bass.

Ellingson, J. E., Sackett, P. R., & Hough, L. M. (1999). Social desirability corrections in personality measurement: Issues of applicant comparison and construct validity. *Journal of Applied Psychology, 84,* 155–166.

Etienne, P. M., & Julian, E. R. (2005). Assessing the personal characteristics of premedical students. In W. J. Camara & E. W. Kimmel (Eds.), *Choosing students: Higher education admissions tools for the 21st century* (pp. 215–230). Mahwah, NJ: Erlbaum.

Fiedler, K., Messner, C., & Bluemke, M. (2006). Unresolved problems with the "I," the "A," and the "T": A logical and psychometric critique of the Implicit Association Test. (IAT). *European Review of Social Psychology, 17,* 74–147.

Fiske, D. W. (1949). Consistency of the factorial structures of personality ratings from different sources. *Journal of Abnormal & Social Psychology, 44,* 329–344.

Flavell, J. H. (1979). Metacognition and cognitive monitoring: A new area of cognitive-developmental inquiry. *American Psychologist, 34,* 906–911.

Gawronski, B., & Bodenhausen, G. V. (2006). Associative and propositional processes in evaluation: An integrative review of implicit and explicit attitude change. *Psychological Bulletin, 132,* 692–731.

Goho, J., & Blackman, A. (2006). The effectiveness of academic admission interviews: an exploratory meta-analysis. *Medical Teacher, 28,* 335–340.

Grant, H., & Dweck, C. S. (2003). Clarifying achievement goals and their impact. *Journal of Personality & Social Psychology, 85,* 541–553.

Greenwald, A. G., McGhee, D. E., & Schwartz, J. L. K. (1998). Measuring individual differences in implicit cognition: The Implicit Association Test. *Journal of Personality and Social Psychology, 74,* 1464–1480.

Greenwald, A. G., & Farnham, S. D. (2000). Using the Implicit Association Test to measure self-esteem and self-concept. *Journal of Personality & Social Psychology, 79,* 1022–1038.

Greenwald, A. G., Banaji, M. R., Rudman, L. A., Farnham, S. D., Nosek, B. A., & Mellott, D. S. (2002). A unified theory of implicit attitudes, stereotypes, self-esteem, and self-concept. *Psychological Review, 109,* 3–25.

Greenwald, A. G., Nosek, B. A., & Sriram, N. (2006). Consequential validity of the Implicit Association Test: Comment on Blanton and Jaccard (2006). *American Psychologist, 61,* 56–61.

Griffith, R. L., Chmielowski, T., & Yoshita, Y. (2007). Do applicants fake? An examination of the frequency of applicant faking behavior. *Personnel Review, 36,* 341–357.

Gustafson, S. (Chair). (2004). *Making conditional reasoning test work: Reports from the frontier.* Symposium conducted at the 19th Annual Conference of the Society for Industrial and Organizational Psychology Conference, Chicago, IL.

Hancock, J. T., Curry, L., Goorha, S., & Woodworth, M. T. (2004). Lies in conversation: An examination of deception using automated linguistic analysis. *Proceedings, Annual Conference of the Cognitive Science Society, 26,* 534–540.

Hardeman, W., Johnston, M., Johnston, D. W., Bonetti, B., Wareham, N. J., & Kinmonth, A. L. (2002). Application of the Theory of Planned Behaviour in behaviour change interventions: a systematic review. *Psychology & Health, 17*, 123–158.

Harzing, A-W . (2006). Response styles in cross-national survey research. *International Journal of Cross-Cultural Management, 6*, 243–266.

Heggestad, E. D., Morrison, M., Reeve, C. L., & McCloy, R. A. (2006). Forced-choice assessments of personality for selection: Evaluating issues of normative assessment and faking resistance. *Journal of Applied Psychology, 91*, 9–24.

Hell, B., Trapmann, S., Weigand, S., & Schuler, H. (2007). Die Validität von Auswahlgesprächen im Rahmen der Hochschulzulassung—eine Metaanalyse. *Psychologische Rundschau, 58*, 93–102.

Hendriks, A. A. J., Kuyper, H., Offringa J. G., & Van der Werf, M. P. (2008). Assessing young adolescents' personality with the five-factor personality inventory. *Assessment, 15*, 304–316.

Hofmann, W., Gawronski, B., Gschwendner, T., Le, H., & Schmitt, M. (2005). A meta-analysis on the correlation between the Implicit Association Test and explicit self-report measures. *Personality & Social Psychology Bulletin, 31*, 1369–1385.

Huffcutt, A. I., Conway, J. M., Roth, P. L., & Klehe, U. C. (2004). The impact of job complexity and study design on situational and behavior description interview validity. *International Journal of Selection & Assessment, 12*, 262–273.

Jackson, D. N., Wroblewski, V. R., & Ashton, M. C. (2000). The impact of faking on employment tests: Does forced-choice offer a solution? *Human Performance, 13*, 371–388.

Jackson, J. J., Wood, D., Bogg, T., Walton, K. E., Harms, P. D., & Roberts, B. W. (2010). What do conscientious people do? Development and validation of the Behavioral Indicators of Conscientiousness (BIC). *Journal of Research in Personality, 44*, 501–511.

James, L. R. (1998). Measurement of personality via conditional reasoning. *Organizational Research Methods, 1*, 131–163.

James, L. R., McIntyre, M. D., & Glisson, C. A. (2004). The Conditional Reasoning Measurement System for aggression: An overview. *Human Performance, 17*, 271–295.

Janz, T., Hellervik, L., & Gillmore, D. C. (1986). *Behavior description interview.* Boston, MA: Allyn & Bacon.

John, O. P., & Robins, R. W. (1993). Determinants of inter-judge agreement on personality traits: The big five domains, observability, evaluativeness, and the unique perspective of the self. *Journal of Personality, 61*, 521–551.

Kahneman, D., Krueger, A. B., Schkade, D. A., Schwarz, N., & Stone, A. A. (2004). A survey method for characterizing daily life experience: The Day Reconstruction Method. *Science, 306*, 1776–1780.

Kenny, D. A. (1994). *Interpersonal perception: A social relations analysis.* New York: Guilford Press.

Kim, S., & Kyllonen, P. C. (2008). Rasch measurement in developing faculty ratings of students applying to graduate school. *Journal of Applied Measurement, 9*, 168–181.

Krokos, K. J., Meade, A. W., Cantwell, A. R., Pond, S. B., & Wilson, M. A. (2004). Empirical keying of situational judgment tests: Rationale and some examples. Paper presented at the annual conference of the Society for Industrial and Organizational Psychology, Chicago, IL.

Krosnick, J. A., Judd, C. M., & Wittenbrink, B. (2005). Attitude measurement. In D. Albarracin, B. T. Johnson, & M. P. Zanna (Eds.), *Handbook of attitudes and attitude change.* Mahwah, NJ: Erlbaum.

Kyllonen, P. C. (2008). *The research behind the ETS Personal Potential Index.* Princeton, NJ: Educational Testing Service. Retrieved from http://www.ets.org/Media/Products/PPI/10411_PPI_bkgrd_report_RD4.pdf on January 15, 2009.

Kyllonen, P. C., & Kim, S. (2004). Personal qualities in higher education: Dimensionality of faculty ratings of graduate school applicants. Paper presented at the Annual Meeting of the American Educational Research Association, Montreal, Canada.

Kyllonen, P. C., & Lee, S. (2005). Assessing problem solving in context. In O. Wilhelm & R. Engle (Eds.), *Handbook of understanding and measuring intelligence.* Thousand Oaks, CA: Sage Publications, Inc.

Latham, G. P., Saari, L. M., Pursell, E. D., & Campion, M. A. (1980). The situational interview. *Journal of Applied Psychology, 65*, 422–427.

LeBreton, J. M., Barksdale, C. D., & Robin, J. (2007). Measurement issues associated with Conditional Reasoning Tests: Indirect measurement and test faking. *Journal of Applied Psychology, 92*, 1–16.

Li, A., & Bagger, J. (2006). Using the BID-R to distinguish the effects of impression management and self-deception on the criterion validity of personality measures: A meta-analysis. *International Journal of Selection & Assessment, 14*, 131–141.

Lievens, F., & Coestsier, P. (2002). Situational tests in student selection: An examination of predictive validity, adverse impact, and construct validity. *International Journal of Selection & Assessment, 10*, 245–257.

Lievens, F., & Sackett, P. R. (2006). Video-based versus written situational judgement tests: A comparison in terms of predictive validity. *Journal of Applied Psychology, 91*, 1181–1188.

Lievens, F., Buyse, T., & Sackett, P. R. (2005). The operational validity of a video-based situational judgement test for medical college admissions: Illustrating the importance of matching predictor and criterion construct domains. *Journal of Applied Psychology, 90*, 442–452.

Lindqvist, E., & Vestman, R. (2011). The labor market returns to cognitive and non-cognitive ability: Evidence from the Swedish Enlistment. *American Economic Journal: Applied Economics, 3*, 101–128.

Lipnevich, A. A., MacCann, C., Krumm, S., & Roberts, R. D. (2011). Mathematics attitudes in Belarusian and U.S. middle school students. *Journal of Educational Psychology, 103*, 105–118.

Liu, O. L. (2009). Evaluation of a learning strategies scale for middle school students. *Journal of Psychoeducational Assessment, 27*, 213–322.

Liu, O. L., Minsky, J., Ling, G., & Kyllonen, P. (2007). *The standardized letter of recommendation: Implications for selection.* ETS Research Report RR-07-38. Princeton, NJ: ETS.

Liu, O. L., Rijmen, F., MacCann, C., & Roberts, R. D. (2009). The assessment of time management in middle-school students. *Personality & Individual Differences, 47*, 174–179.

MacCann, C., Duckworth, A., & Roberts, R. D. (2009). Empirical identification of the major facets of conscientiousness. *Learning & Individual Differences, 19*, 451–458.

MacCann, C., Fogarty, G. J., & Roberts, R. D. (2012). Strategies for success in vocational education: Time management is more important for part-time than full-time students. *Learning & Individual Differences, 22*, 518–623.

MacCann, C., Lipnevich, A. A., & Roberts, R. D. (2013). Parents know best! Comparing self- and parent-reported personality in predicting academic achievement. Submitted to the ETS Research Report Series. Princeton, NJ: ETS.

MacCann, C., Matthews, G., Wang, L., & Roberts, R. D. (2010). Emotional intelligence and the eye of the beholder: Comparing self- and parent-rated situational judgements in adolescents. *Journal of Research in Personality, 44*, 673–676.

MacCann, C., Ziegler, M., & Roberts, R. D. (2011). Faking in personality assessment: Reflections and recommendations. In M. Ziegler, C. MacCann, & R. D. Roberts (Eds.), *New perspectives on faking in personality assessment* (pp. 309–329). New York: Oxford University Press.

Marchese, M. C., & Muchinski, P. M. (1993). The validity of the employment interview: A meta-analysis. *International Journal of Selection & Assessment, 1*, 18–26.

Marin, G., Gamba, R. J., & Marin, B. V. (1992). Extreme response style and acquiescence among Hispanics. *Journal of Cross-Cultural Psychology, 23*, 498–509.

Marsh, H. W., Byrne, B. M., & Shavelson, R. J. (1988). A multifaceted academic self-concept: Its hierarchical structure and its relation to academic achievement. *Journal of Educational Psychology, 80*, 366–380.

Martin, B. A., Bowen, C. C., & Hunt, S. T. (2002). How effective are people at faking on personality questionnaires? *Personality & Individual Differences, 32*, 247–256.

McDaniel, M. A., Morgesen, F. P., Finnegan, E. B., Campion, M. A., & Braverman, E. P. (2001). Use of situational judgement tests to predict job performance: A clarification of the literature. *Journal of Applied Psychology, 86*, 730–740.

McDaniel, M. A., Whetzel, D. L., Schmidt, F. L., & Maurer, S. D. (1994). The validity of employment interviews: A comprehensive review and meta-analysis. *Journal of Applied Psychology, 79*, 599–616.

McHenry, J. J., & Schmitt, N. (1994). Multimedia testing. In M. J. Rumsey, C. D. Walker, & J. Harris (Eds.), *Personnel selection and classification research* (pp. 193–232). Mahwah, NJ: Lawrence Erlbaum.

Mehl, M. R., & Pennebaker, J. W. (2003). The sounds of social life: A psychometric analysis of students' daily social environments and natural conversations. *Journal of Personality & Social Psychology, 84*, 857–870.

Meyer, G. J., Finn, S. E., Eyde, L. D., Kay, G. G., Moreland, K. L., Dies, R. R., et al. (2001). Psychological testing and psychological assessment: A review of evidence and issues. *American Psychologist, 56*, 128–165.

Mierke, J., & Klauer, K. C. (2003). Method-specific variance in the Implicit Association Test. *Journal of Personality & Social Psychology, 85*, 1180–1192.

Mount, M. K., Barrick, M. R., & Strauss, J. P. (1994). Validity of observer ratings of the Big Five personality factors. *Journal of Applied Psychology, 79*, 272–280.

Newman, M. L., Pennebaker, J. W., Berry, D. S., & Richards, J. M. (2003). Lying words: Predicting deception from linguistic style. *Personality & Social Psychology Bulletin, 29*, 665–675.

Norman, W. T. (1963). Personality measurement, faking, and detection: An assessment method for use in personnel selection. *Journal of Applied Psychology, 47*, 225–241.

Nosek, B. A., & Banaji, M. R. (2001). The go/no-go association task. *Social Cognition, 19*, 161–176.

Olson-Buchanan, J. B., & Drasgow, F. (2006). Multimedia situational judgment tests: The medium creates the message. In J. A. Weekley & R. E. Ployhart (Eds.), *Situational judgment tests* (pp. 253–278). San Francisco: Jossey-Bass.

Olson-Buchanan, J. B., Drasgow, F., Moberg, P. J., Mead, A. D., Keenan, P. A., & Donovan, M. A. (1998). Interactive video assessment of conflict resolution skills. *Personnel Psychology, 51*, 1–24.

Oltmanns, T. F., & Turkheimer, E. (2006). Perceptions of self and others regarding pathological personality traits. In R. Krueger & J. Tackett (Eds.), *Personality and psychopathology: Building bridges*. New York: Guilford.

Ones, D. S., Viswesvaran, C., & Reiss, A. D. (1996). The role of social desirability in personality testing in personnel selection: The red herring. *Journal of Applied Psychology, 81*, 660–679.

Oswald, F. L., Schmitt, N., Kim, B. H., Ramsay, L. J., & Gillespie, M. A. (2004). Developing a biodata measure and situational judgement inventory as predictors of college student performance. *Journal of Applied Psychology, 89*, 187–207.

Paulhus, D. L. (1998). *The Balanced Inventory of Desirable Responding (BIDR-7)*. Toronto/Buffalo: Multi-Health Systems.

Paunonen, S. V., & Ashton, M. C. (2001). Big five predictors of academic achievement. *Journal of Research in Personality, 35*, 78–90.

Peabody, D. (1967). Trait inferences: Evaluative and descriptive aspects. *Journal of Personality & Social Psychology, 7*, 1–13.

Pekrun, R., Elliot, A. J., & Maier, M. A. (2006). Achievement goals and discrete achievement emotions: A theoretical model and prospective test. *Journal of Educational Psychology, 98*, 583–597.

Poropat, A. E. (2009). A meta-analysis of the Five-Factor Model of personality and academic performance. *Psychological Bulletin, 135*, 322–338.

Prelec, D. (2004). A Bayesian truth serum for subjective data. *Science, 306*, 462–466.

Prelec, D., & Weaver, R. G. (2006). Truthful answers are surprisingly common: Experimental tests of Bayesian truth serum. Paper presented at the ETS Mini-conference on Faking in Non-cognitive Assessments. Princeton, NJ: Educational Testing Service

Rammstedt, B., & Krebs, D. (2007). Does response scale format affect the answering of personality scales? Assessing the big five dimensions of personality with different response scales in a dependent sample. *European Journal of Psychological Assessment, 23*, 32–38.

Reynolds, C. R., & Kamphaus, R. W. (2004). *BASC-2: Behavior Assessment System for Children, second edition manual*. Circle Pines, MN: American Guidance Service.

Richman-Hirsch, W. L., Olson-Buchanan, J. B., & Drasgow, F. (2000). Examining the impact of administration medium on examinee perceptions and attitudes. *Journal of Applied Psychology, 85*, 880–887.

Robbins, S., Lauver, K. J., Le, H., Davis, D., Langley, R., & Carlstrom, A. (2004). Do psychosocial and study skill factors predict college outcomes? A meta-analysis. *Psychological Bulletin, 130*, 261–288.

Roberts, B. W. (2009). Back to the future: Personality and assessment and personality development. *Journal of Research in Personality, 43*, 137–145.

Roberts, B. W., & Wood, D. (2006). Personality development in the context of the Neo-socioanalytic model of personality.

In D. Mroczek & T. Little (Eds.), *Handbook of personality development* (pp. 11–39). Mahwah, NJ: Lawrence Erlbaum Associates.

Roberts, R. D., Betancourt, A. C., Burrus, J., Holtzman, S., Libbrecht, N., MacCann, C., et al. (2011). *Multimedia assessment of emotional abilities: Development and validation*. Army Research Institute Report Series. Arlington, VA: ARI.

Rothermund, K., & Wentura, D. (2004). Underlying processes in the Implicit Association Test: Dissociating salience from associations. *Journal of Experimental Psychology: General, 133,* 139–165.

Rutter, D. (2000). Attendance and reattendance for breast cancer screening: a prospective 3-year test of the Theory of Planned Behaviour. *British Journal of Health Psychology, 5,* 1–13.

Ryan, A. M., McFarland, L., Baron, H., & Page, R. (1999). An international look at selection practices: Nation and culture as explanations for variability in practice. *Personnel Psychology, 52,* 359–391.

Sackett, P. R. (2006). *Faking and coaching effects on non-cognitive predictors*. Paper presented at the ETS Mini-conference on Faking in Non-cognitive Assessments. Princeton, NJ: Educational Testing Service.

Sarason, I. G. (1984). Stress, anxiety, and cognitive interference: Reactions to tests. *Journal of Personality & Social Psychology, 46,* 929–938.

Schmidt, F. L., & Hunter, J. E. (1998). The validity and utility of selection methods in personnel psychology: Practical and theoretical implications of 85 years of research findings. *Psychological Bulletin, 124,* 262–274.

Schuler, H. (2002). *Das Einstellungsinterview.* Göttingen, Germany: Hogrefe.

Seipp, B. (1991). Anxiety and academic performance: A meta-analysis of findings. *Anxiety Research, 4,* 27–41.

Sena, J. D. W., Lowe, P. A., & Lee, S. W. (2007). Significant predictors of test anxiety among students with and without learning disabilities. *Journal of Learning Disabilities, 40,* 360–376

Sheeran, P. (2002). Intention-behavior relations: A conceptual and empirical review. *European Review of Social Psychology, 12,* 1–36.

Small, E. E., & Diefendorff, J. M. (2006). The impact of contextual self-ratings and observer ratings of personality on the personality-performance relationship. *Journal of Applied Social Psychology, 36,* 297–320.

Stankov, L., & Lee, J. (2008). Confidence and cognitive test performance. *Journal of Educational Psychology, 100,* 961–976.

Stark, S., Chernyshenko, O. S., & Drasgow, F. (2005). An IRT approach to constructing and scoring pairwise preference items involving stimuli on different dimensions: An application to the problem of faking in personality assessment. *Applied Psychological Measurement, 29,* 184–201.

Stark, S., Chernyshenko, O. S., & Drasgow, F. (2011). Constructing fake-resistant personality tests using Item Response Theory: High stakes personality testing with Multidimensional Pairwise Preferences. In M. Zeigler, C. MacCann, & R. D. Roberts (Eds.), *New perspectives on faking in personality assessment* (pp. 214–239). New York: Oxford University Press.

Sternberg, R. J., Forsythe, G. B., Hedlund, J., Horvath, J. A., Wagner, R. K., & Williams, W. M . (2000). *Practical intelligence in everyday life.* New York: Cambridge University Press.

Stricker, L. J., Rock, D. A., & Bennett, R. E. (2001). Sex and ethnic-group differences on accomplishment measures. *Applied Measurement in Education, 14,* 205–218.

Thornton, G. C. III, & Rupp, D. E. (2005). *Assessment centers in human resource management: Strategies for prediction, diagnosis, and development.* Mahwah, NJ: Lawrence Erlbaum.

Trapmann, S., Hell, B., Hirn, J. W., & Schuler, H. (2007). Meta-analysis of the relationship between the Big Five and academic success at university. *Journal of Psychology, 215,* 132–151.

Tupes, E. C., & Christal, R. E. (1961/1992). Recurrent personality factors based on trait ratings. *Journal of Personality, 60,* 225–251.

Vannelli, J., Kuncel, N. R., & Ones, D. S. (2007, April). A mixed recommendation for letters of recommendation. In N. R. Kuncel (Chair), Alternative Predictors of Academic Performance: The Glass is Half Empty. Symposium conducted at the annual meeting of the National Council on Measurement in Education, Chicago, IL.

Viswesvaran, C., & Ones, D. S. (1999). Meta-analyses of fakeability estimates: Implications for personality measurement. *Educational & Psychological Measurement, 59,* 197–210.

Wagerman, S. A., & Funder, D. C. (2006). Acquaintance reports of personality and academic achievement: A case for conscientiousness. *Journal of Research in Personality, 41,* 221–229.

Walters, A., Kyllonen, P. C., & Plante, J. W. (2006). Developing a standardized letter of recommendation. *The Journal of College Admission, 191,* 8–17.

Walters, A. M., Kyllonen, P. C., & Plante, J. W. (2003). Preliminary research to develop a standardized letter of recommendation. Paper presented at the Annual Meeting of the American Educational Research Association, San Diego, CA.

Wang, L., MacCann, C., Zhuang, X., Liu, O. L., & Roberts, R. D. (2009). Assessing teamwork and collaboration in high school students: A multi-method approach. *Canadian Journal of School Psychology, 24,* 108–124.

Waugh, G. W., & Russell, T. L. (2003). Scoring both judgement and personality in a situational judgement test. Paper presented at the 45th Annual Conference of the International Military Testing Association. Pensacola, Florida.

Weekley, J. A., & Jones, C. (1997). Video-based situational testing. *Personnel Psychology, 50,* 25–49.

Wilkinson, D., Zhang, J., Byrne, G. J., Luke, H., Ozolins, I. Z., Parker, M. H., et al. (2008). Medical school selection criteria and the prediction of academic performance: Evidence leading to change in policy and practice at the University of Queensland. *Medical Education, 188,* 349–354.

Wine, J. (1971). Test anxiety and the direction of attention. *Psychological Bulletin, 76,* 92–104.

Zeidner, M. (1998). *Test anxiety: The state of the art.* New York: Plenum Press.

Zickar, M. J., Gibby, R. E., & Robie, C. (2004). Uncovering faking samples in applicant, incumbent, and experimental data sets: An application of mixed-model item response theory. *Organizational Research Methods, 7,* 168–190.

Ziegler, M., Schmidt-Atzert, L., Bühner, M., & Krumm, S. (2008). Motivated, unmotivated, or faking? Susceptibility of three achievement motivation tests measures to faking: Questionnaire, semi-projective, and objective. *Psychology Science, 49,* 291–307.

Assessment of Subjective Well-Being in Children and Adolescents

E. Scott Huebner *and* Kimberly J. Hills

Abstract

Research has suggested that measures of positive subjective well-being add incremental validity in relation to traditional measures of psychopathological symptoms in predicting child and adolescent psychsocial adaptation. Measures of subjective well-being, including measures of life satisfaction and positive affect, have been constructed that are appropriate for children and/or adolescents. Several measures are reviewed and recommendations for future research are provided. A case study is employed to illustrate the usefulness of subjective well-being instruments in school-based psychological assessments.

Key Words: subjective well-being, life satisfaction, positive affect, assessment, children

Research on the subjective well-being or happiness of adults and children has increased significantly in the last decade. Prominent scholars (e.g., Seligman & Csikszentmihalyi, 2000) have proposed that psychologists study positive constructs of well-being to provide a more comprehensive understanding of human development, including optimal development. In doing so, measures of subjective well-being and other positive psychology constructs have been developed to advance a science and practice of "positive psychology" to complement the field's traditional emphasis on psychopathology (Frisch, 2000; Lopez & Snyder, 2003).

Although numerous alternative conceptual models of positive mental health or well-being have been put forth, most models include subjective well-being (SWB) as a central component. The most widely accepted definition of SWB has been offered by Diener (1984, 2000). In his tripartite model, SWB comprises the three major components of *positive affect*, *negative affect*, and *life satisfaction*. Positive affect involves the experience of frequent positive

emotions (e.g., joy, enthusiasm, interest) over time, whereas negative affect involves the experience of frequent negative emotions (e.g., sadness, anxiety, anger) over time. Life satisfaction is conceptualized as a cognitive judgment of the degree of positivity of one's life as a whole or with specific domains (e.g., family, school, work). Taken together, an individual is thought to have high SWB if s/he reports relatively frequent positive emotions, infrequent negative emotions, and a high degree of satisfaction with her or his life (Diener, 2000).

Research has supported the differentiability of the three domains of SWB among adults and children, as early as third grade (Huebner, 1991a). Research has also supported the differentiability of the SWB constructs from related constructs. For example, global life satisfaction has been shown to be distinct from such constructs as self-esteem (Huebner, Gilman & Laughlin, 1999; Lucas, Diener, & Suh, 1996), depression (Lewinsohn, Redner & Seeley, 1991), and optimism (Lucas, Diener, & Suh, 1996). Furthermore, it is important to note that when measured across relatively lengthy periods of time (e.g., several months), respondents' reports of positive and negative emotions are not strongly inversely related as might be expected, but rather are somewhat independent. Although the reasons for this relative independence are complex, they involve the particular emotions sampled, the time period sampled, and distinctions and interrelationships between affect intensity and frequency of affect (Diener, Larsen, Levine, & Emmons, 1985; Pavot, 2008). The general conclusions emerging from the body of research support the need to measure positive affect and negative affect separately to adequately understand persons' SWB.

Fredrickson's Broaden-and-Build Theory of positive emotions and the associated research provide further distinctions between positive affect and negative affect (see Cohen & Fredrickson, 2009; and Fredrickson, 2001, for reviews). The Broaden-and-Build Theory hypothesizes that negative and positive emotions serve different purposes, resulting in different long-term outcomes. On the one hand, negative emotions, such as fear or anger, elicit narrowed perceptions and cognitions and specific action tendencies, such as "fight or flight" responses. On the other hand, positive emotions, such as joy or interest, are thought to elicit broadened perceptions and an associated wider range of behavioral response options. Both positive and negative emotions are crucial for survival. Fredrickson and colleagues have produced considerable evidence that in the long run, the experience of frequent positive emotions is associated with broader thought-action repertoires, resulting in greater resilience and physical and intellectual resources, and increased positive affect in the future (Fredrickson, 2001).

The benefits of frequent positive affect have been further supported by a large meta-analysis of cross-sectional, longitudinal, and experimental studies of positive affect (Lyubormirsky, King, & Diener, 2005. The findings of the meta-analysis revealed that frequent positive emotions precede a wide variety of indicators of individuals' success, including a higher likelihood of satisfying interpersonal relationships, high incomes, high productivity at work, good health, and a long life. Thus, frequent positive emotions are more than a simple byproduct of positive life circumstances. Rather, frequent positive emotions appear to facilitate more positive life experiences in many important arenas of life.

Such research findings are not inconsistent with evolutionary theory, which postulates that the mechanisms and processes associated with SWB maintenance have been shaped by evolution through natural selection to address fundamental problems of survival and reproduction. According to Hill and Buss (2008), SWB reflects "an internal signaling device that tells an organism than an adaptive problem has been solved successfully or is in the process of being solved successfully" (p. 71). In other words, SWB can be construed as a process as well as an outcome. As a process associated with evolutionary fitness, SWB serves as both an internal reward and motivator, increasing the probability that an individual will continue to approach and move toward attaining important goals related to universal needs, such as personal safety, financial resources, professional success, intimate relationships, and physical health (Hill & Buss, 2008). Thus, again, the monitoring and maintenance of relatively high levels of SWB over the long term is crucial to the adaptation of humans.

The tripartite model of SWB implies that positive mental health and psychopathology are distinguishable psychological constructs, not simply opposite ends of a single continuum of mental health. Thus, positive mental health is not equivalent to the absence of psychopathology. That is, a child who is not depressed or anxious does not necessarily demonstrate an optimal level of mental health functioning. Thus, comprehensive assessments of children's well-being are thought to require measures of positive functioning as well as psychopathological functioning to capture the full range of children's developmental possibilities.

The notion that students who are not depressed or anxious may not have high SWB has been investigated through variable-centered and person-centered research approaches. Using variable-centered approaches, Wilkinson and Walford (1998) administered measures of subjective well-being (e.g., life satisfaction, positive affect) and distress (e.g., anxiety, depression) to 345 adolescents. Although correlated, two distinguishable factors emerged. In a study of the differentiability of adolescents' reports of positive and negative affect, Lewis, Huebner, Reschly, and Valois (2009) evaluated the independent contribution of positive affect data (e.g., frequency of joy, interest) relative to negative affect data (e.g., anxiety, sadness) in predicting adaptive school functioning with a sample of middle and high school students. Their results indicated that measures of positive affect demonstrated significant incremental validity in explaining individual differences in school satisfaction, adaptive coping, and student engagement. Taken together, such studies support the differentiability of SWB and psycho-pathological symptoms.

Person-centered approaches have also been used to investigate the distinction between positive psychological health, such as SWB and psychopathology. Such a distinction is manifested in the Dual-Factor Model of Mental Health (Greenspoon & Saklofske, 2001), in which positive indicators of SWB are included with traditional negative indicators of psychopathology (i.e., internalizing and externalizing behavior problems) in a comprehensive assessment of child well-being. Results indicated that among the students with low psychopathology, those who had higher SWB showed significantly higher global self-esteem, academic self-efficacy, internal locus of control, and overall social support. Among students with significant psychopathological symptoms, children with higher SWB also showed higher global self-esteem, locus of control, sociability, and social support from fathers. The group of students with high psychopathology and low SWB demonstrated the lowest psychological functioning. Greenspoon and Saklofske underscored the fact that if only the presence of psychopathological symptoms had been investigated, then important group differences could not have been identified, indicating that both SWB and psychopathology need to be assessed to develop the most comprehensive portrait of a child's mental health.

In another critical demonstration of the importance of differentiating SWB and pathology, Suldo and Shaffer (2008) demonstrated the existence of four distinct groups of middle school students: 57 % of the sample who had "positive mental health" (i.e., high SWB and low pathology), 13% who were "vulnerable" (low SWB and low pathology), 13% who were "symptomatic but content" (high SWB and high pathology), and 17% who were "troubled" (low SWB and high psychopathology). Although the means of all four groups differed significantly on a variety of variables, most importantly, the "vulnerable" group had lower standardized test scores, academic self-concepts, valuing of school, and social support from classmates and parents, as well as more school absences, self-perceived physical health problems, and social problems, compared to the students with positive mental health. The identification of a group of students who were non-symptomatic, but relatively low in SWB, and who were clearly distinctive in terms of academic, physical, and interpersonal functioning, provides strong support for the additional utility of the inclusion of positive psychology measures (e.g., SWB) in comprehensive child and youth assessments.

Antaramian, Huebner, Hills, and Valois (2010) also identified four groups of adolescents based on the Dual-Factor Model. Their findings extended beyond those of Suldo and Shaffer by showing significant differences on behavioral, cognitive, and emotional engagement as well as academic achievement measures (i.e., GPA). The results of their analyses showed that the positive mental health youth had behavioral, cognitive, and emotional engagement scores significantly greater than all other groups. Additionally, Antaramian and colleagues reported that the symptomatic, but content, youth had significantly higher engagement scores than did troubled youth. In terms of academic achievement, the authors found the positive mental health youth had significantly higher GPA scores compared to the other three groups, including vulnerable youth.

Taken together, the variable- and person-centered studies support the assumption that measures of positive SWB provide important, incremental information in comprehensive assessments of child and youth functioning. Greenspoon and Saklofske (2001) note that the Dual-Factor Model of Mental Health is "surely a crude representation of reality," but they further note that it represents a "doubling of the current taxonomy" and " a step forward" (p. 100).

Review of SWB Measures for Children and Adolescents

In line with the tripartite conceptual foundation of SWB described above (Diener, 1984), the measures described in this section will be limited to measures of life satisfaction and generic measures of positive and negative affect (versus measures of specific emotions, such as curiosity or anxiety). Self-reported assessments of SWB, developed primarily for students of about grades three to 12, have received the most attention to date (Huebner, Gilman, & Suldo, 2006; Proctor, Linley, & Maltby, 2009).

Life satisfaction measures have been based on three distinct theoretical models: general, global, and domain-specific life satisfaction. Instruments based on general models of life satisfaction assume that overall or "general" life satisfaction comprises bottom-up judgments of specific life domains (e.g., family, peers, and school domains). Thus, a general or total life satisfaction score on such instruments reflects a simple (or weighted) sum of scores on items tapping life satisfaction across specific domains. Some instruments that attempt to assess life satisfaction "as a whole" or overall life satisfaction are based on a global model.

A global model assumes that overall life satisfaction is best assessed by an exclusive emphasis on items that are domain free (e.g., "My life is going well") versus domain-specific (e.g., "My *school* life is going well"). In contrast to general life satisfaction scores, in which the number and nature of the domains are predetermined by the instrument developer, global life satisfaction scales allow individual respondents to formulate their overall judgments based on their own criteria. Multidimensional measures have been developed with the intent of eliciting respondents' judgments across multiple domains of life that are considered to be important to most, if not all, individuals of the particular age group. In this manner, such measures yield profiles of individuals' reports of life satisfaction, providing more differentiated, contextualized satisfaction reports. Hence, a student who has average global life satisfaction, along with high family and low school satisfaction, can be differentiated from one who has average global life satisfaction, along with low family and high school satisfaction. The resulting context-specific profiles may provide targeted information relevant to the design of more healthy environments for individual students or groups of students.

Examples of global and domain-specific measures of life satisfaction and general measures of positive and negative affect are discussed below. These instruments include the Students' Life Satisfaction Scale (Huebner, 1991b), Multidimensional Students' Life Satisfaction Scale (Huebner, 1994), Brief Multidimensional Students' Life Satisfaction Scale (Seligson, Huebner, & Valois, 2003), and Positive and Negative Affect Schedule—Child Version (Laurent et al., 1999). Strengths and limitations of each scale are highlighted.

Students' Life Satisfaction Scale

The rationale for the construction of the Students' Life Satisfaction Scale (SLSS: Huebner, 1991b) was the previously mentioned increased interest in the promotion of positive psychological well-being in children and adolescents. Prior to the 1990s, research and practice had been hindered by the lack of psychometrically sound SWB instruments for children and adolescents (Bender, 1997).

In contrast to models that infer well-being from the absence of psychopathological symptoms, as early as 1964, the World Health Organization defined health as a state of complete physical, mental, and social well-being. The SLSS was thus designed to differentiate levels of life satisfaction above a neutral point of well-being. In this fashion,

"high" levels of life satisfaction would not be defined simply as the absence of dissatisfaction. For example, students who were "mildly satisfied" could be differentiated from students who were "moderately" and "strongly" satisfied.

The SLSS is a seven-item self-report measure that has been used with children ages eight to 18. The items require respondents to rate their satisfaction with respect to items that are context free (see above). The original version of the SLSS consisted of 10 items, but was subsequently reduced to seven items based on item analysis and internal consistency data (Huebner, 1991b). Supplemental positive and negative affect items were analyzed along with the SLSS items to clarify the boundaries of the construct tapped by the SLSS in relation to other SWB variables (Huebner, 1991a & c).

Early work with the SLSS used a four-point frequency response format, with 1 = never, 2 = sometimes, 3 = often, and 4 = always. Recent studies have used a six-point extent format, with 1 = strongly disagree, 2 = moderately disagree, 3 = mildly disagree, 4 = mildly agree, 5 = moderately agree, and 6 = strongly agree. One study raised issues regarding the comparability of scores across the extent and frequency response formats, thus the extent format is generally recommended (Gilman & Huebner, 1997).

SLSS studies of non-clinical samples of students aged eight to 18 in the US began in the 1990s (e.g., Dew & Huebner, 1994; Huebner, 1991b) and have continued to the present (e.g., Lewis, Huebner, Malone, & Valois, 2011). Additional samples from clinical and other special populations have included at-risk students (Huebner & Alderman, 1993), adjudicated adolescents (Crenshaw, 1998), gifted students (Ash & Huebner, 1998), students with learning disabilities (McCullough & Huebner, 2003), emotional disturbance (Huebner & Alderman, 1993), hearing impairments (Gilman, Easterbrooks, & Frey, 2004), and chronic health conditions (Hexdall & Huebner, 2007). The SLSS has also been used in studies of children and youth from other nations, for example, Portugal (Marques, Lopez, & Pais-Ribeiro, 2011) and South Korea (Park & Huebner, 2005).

Psychometric Properties

Studies of internal consistency have consistently revealed coefficient alphas in the .70–.80 range across all age groups. For example, Huebner (1991b) reported an alpha of .82 in a sample of students in grades four to eight in an American Midwestern state, and Dew and Huebner (1994) reported an alpha of

.86 in a sample of students in grades nine through twelve in a Southeastern state. Comparisons of alpha coefficients for African-American and Caucasian adolescents have demonstrated comparability across groups (Huebner & Dew, 1993). Studies of test-retest reliability with school- age students have yielded correlations of .76, .64, and .53 across 1- to 2-week (Terry & Huebner, 1995), 1-month (Gilman & Huebner, 1997), and 1-year (Huebner, Funk, & Gilman, 2000) time intervals, respectively.

Studies of the validity of SLSS scores have supported its meaningfulness. Factor analytic studies have consistently demonstrated a unidimensional factor structure (Dew & Huebner, 1994; Gilman & Huebner, 1997; Huebner, 1991b). Convergent validity has been supported by strong correlations between SLSS scores and a variety of other self-report life satisfaction measures (e.g., Huebner 1991b & c; Seligson, Huebner, & Valois, 2003) as well as parent reports of their children's life satisfaction (Dew & Huebner, 1994; Gilman & Huebner, 1997).

The validity of SLSS reports has been further supported by the wide-ranging nomological network of variables related to SLSS scores (see Huebner, 2004 and Proctor, Linley, & Maltby, 2009, for reviews). For example, as expected, SLSS reports of children and youth are significantly positively related to theoretical antecedents of positive life satisfaction, such as temperament (extraversion), positive family and peer relationships, and adaptive cognitions (e.g., self-efficacy and self-esteem). Additionally, SLSS scores are related in expected ways to a variety of positive outcomes, including positive mental health and school behavior and performance.

Evidence of discriminant validity is also available. SLSS reports have been distinguished from several constructs with which life satisfaction is not expected to relate. First, SLSS scores display weak correlations with social desirability responding (Huebner, 1991b) and IQ scores (Huebner & Alderman, 1993). Also, using conjoint factor analysis procedures, SLSS scores have been differentiated from measures of positive and negative affect (Huebner, 1991a; Huebner & Dew, 1996) and self-concept (Huebner, 1995; Huebner, Gilman, & Laughlin, 1999; Terry & Huebner, 1995). Finally, consistent with many studies of adults within countries, SLSS scores are modestly related to demographic variables (e.g., gender, socioeconomic status) at best (Huebner, 1991b & c).

Discriminative validity studies have also been conducted, with SLSS scores distinguishing appropriately among various known groups. On the one hand, compared to normal students, SLSS scores were lower for students with emotional disorders (Huebner & Alderman, 1993) and adjudicated adolescents (Crenshaw, 1998). On the other hand, consistent with studies in which SLSS scores were unrelated to IQ scores, SLSS scores did not distinguish between normal students and gifted students (Ash & Huebner, 1998).

Lastly, predictive validity studies have been supportive of the SLSS. For example, Huebner, Funk, and Gilman (2000) reported that SLSS scores significantly predicted depression and anxiety scores one year later. Similar results were obtained by Haranin, Huebner, and Suldo (2007) using a two-year time frame. Studies have also shown that low SLSS scores predict peer relational victimization (Martin, Huebner, & Valois, 2008) and student disengagement from school, especially cognitive disengagement (Lewis, Huebner, Malone, & Valois, 2011).

Summary of the SLSS

Two decades of research supports the SLSS as a brief, psychometrically sound measure of global life satisfaction for students from grades three to 12. Predictive validity studies suggest that the SLSS predicts important mental health outcomes. The SLSS has been used effectively with a variety of student populations, including students with emotional disabilities, students with learning disabilities, and gifted students. However, difficulties have been encountered in using the SLSS with adolescents with mild mental disabilities (Brantley, Huebner, & Nagle, 2002), despite the fact that the students were able to reliably respond to other, specific domain-based life satisfaction items. Major limitations of the SLSS include: (a) a lack of nationally representative samples, and (b) a need for additional research with students with cognitive impairments (e.g., children with mental disabilities).

The most important limitation of the SLSS may be that it measures only *global* life satisfaction. The SLSS does not allow for the evaluation of satisfaction across various, important domains of interest to children and youth, such as satisfaction with family, school, community, and so forth. Multidimensional measures, which assess satisfaction with multiple life domains, would offer more differentiated assessments of life satisfaction. For one example, although a large statewide sample of more than 5,000 high school students in a US southeastern state revealed generally positive global life satisfaction scores, scores across five specific domains (family, friends, school, self, living environment) were more variable, with substantial dissatisfaction observed among students' reports of satisfaction with their school experiences in particular (Huebner, Drane, & Valois, 2000). Furthermore, Antaramian, Huebner, and Valois (2008) found that family structure (intact vs. non-intact families) was related to satisfaction with family experiences, but not to general life satisfaction. Such differences in levels of life satisfaction illustrate the usefulness of considering overall and domain-based measures of life satisfaction separately. Thus, in the next sections, research findings for two multidimensional measures of life satisfaction for children and youth will be reviewed.

Multidimensional Students' Life Satisfaction Scale

As noted above, early research on children's life satisfaction instruments was limited to the development of unidimensional measures of global or general life satisfaction, which yielded only a single overall score (e.g., Perceived Life Satisfaction Scale: Adelman, Taylor, & Nelson, 1989; Students' Life Satisfaction Scale: Huebner, 1991b). In contrast, the MSLSS was designed to provide a multidimensional profile of children's life satisfaction judgments. Such differentiated assessments enable more focused diagnostic, prevention, and intervention efforts. For example, students who indicate relatively high levels of satisfaction with their families along with low levels of satisfaction with school experiences should necessitate different academic and health promotion strategies than students who indicate dissatisfaction with their families and school experiences. Contextualized life satisfaction assessments may also yield more revealing comparisons with traditional objective indicators used to assess the quality of life of children and adolescents (e.g., divorce rates, family income levels, per-pupil expenditures on schooling).

Specifically, the MSLSS was therefore developed in an effort to:

(a) provide a profile of children's satisfaction with important, specific domains (e.g., school, family, friends) in their lives;

(b) assess their general overall life satisfaction;

(c) demonstrate acceptable psychometric properties (e.g., acceptable subscale reliability);

(d) reveal a replicable factor structure indicating the meaningfulness of the five dimensions; and

(e) use effectively with children across a wide range of age (grades three to 12) and ability levels (e.g., children with mild developmental disabilities through gifted children).

The 40-item MSLSS can be administered to individuals or groups of children. Similar to the development of the SLSS, the original version of the MSLSS used a four-point frequency response option scale (e.g., Huebner, 1994). However, more recent work with the MSLSS has used a six-point extent scale, with 1 = strongly disagree; 2 = moderately disagree, 3 = mildly disagree; 4 = mildly agree; 5 = moderately agree; and 6 = strongly agree (Huebner, Laughlin, Ash, & Gilman, 1998). Higher scores thus indicate higher levels of life satisfaction throughout the scale. Because the domains consist of unequal number of items, the domain and total scores can be made comparable by summing the item responses and dividing by the number of domain (or total) items.

Like the SLSS, the MSLSS has been used in a variety of studies with samples of students ranging in age from eight to 18. For some examples, data are available for elementary (grades three to five) (Huebner, 1994), middle (Huebner, Laughlin, Ash, & Gilman, 1998), and high school students (Gilman, Huebner, & Laughlin, 2000). The MSLSS has also been used in studies in other nations, for example, South Korea and Ireland (e.g., see Gilman et al. 2008).

Psychometric Properties

Internal consistency (alpha) coefficients for subscales have been reported in various publications (Greenspoon & Saklofske, 1997; Huebner, 1994; Huebner, Laughlin, Ash, & Gilman, 1998), with reliabilities ranging from .70s to low .90s. Test-retest coefficients for two- and four-week time periods have also been reported (Huebner, 1994; Huebner, Laughlin, Ash, & Gilman, 1998; Terry & Huebner, 1995) falling mostly in the .70 to .90 range, providing further support for the reliability of the scale.

The results of exploratory factor analyses have supported the dimensionality of the MSLSS (Huebner, 1994). Confirmatory factor analyses have provided further support for the multidimensionality of the instrument (Gilman, Huebner, & Laughlin, 2000; Huebner, Laughlin, Ash, & Gilman, 1998; Irmak & Kuruuzum, 2009), including a study spanning individualistic and collectivistic nations (Gilman et al., 2008).

Convergent and discriminant validity have also been demonstrated through predicted correlations with other self-report well-being indexes (Gilman et al., 2000; Greenspoon & Saklofske, 1997; Huebner, 1994; Huebner et al., 1998), parent reports (Gilman & Huebner, 1997; Huebner, Brantley,

Nagle, & Valois, 2002), teacher reports (Huebner & Alderman, 1993), and social desirability scales (Huebner et al., 1998). Findings of weak relationships with demographic variables (e.g., age, gender) also fit with theoretical expectations (Huebner, 1994; Huebner, Laughlin, Ash, & Gilman, 1998).

Summary of the MSLSS

As with the SLSS, the major limitations of the MSLSS involve: (a) the lack of representative national standardization data and (b) a need for further research with students with cognitive limitations. For example, Griffin and Huebner (2000) reported that four items from MSLSS needed to be omitted in order to achieve acceptable reliability coefficients for the assessment of middle school students with emotional disorders. Similarly, Brantley, Huebner, and Nagle (2002) had to delete several items to achieve acceptable internal consistency coefficients for use with adolescents with mental disabilities. Another drawback of the MSLSS is the relative length of the scale, which is prohibitive with respect to purposes such as large-scale survey research or clinical screening.

Brief Multidimensional Students' Life Satisfaction Scale

The Brief Multidimensional Students' Life Satisfaction Scale (BMSLSS: Seligson, Huebner, & Valois, 2003) was designed to fill the need for a reliable and valid measure of life satisfaction that was relevant, developmentally appropriate, and sufficiently brief to be useful in screening contexts or in large-scale surveys of children and adolescents, such as national and cross-national surveys. Specifically, it was designed to reflect the conceptual model underlying the MSLSS. The BMSLSS is thus a five-item self-report measure that assesses satisfaction with respect to each of the five domains included on the MSLSS (see above). That is, students rate their satisfaction on a single item for each of the five domains of family life, friendships, school experiences, self, and living environment. Response options are on a seven-point scale (Andrews & Withey, 1976) that ranges from 1 = terrible to 7 = delighted. An additional item, measuring students' satisfaction with their overall life, has been included in the BMSLSS in some studies.

Like the SLSS and MSLSS, the BMSLSS has been used in studies of children from ages eight to 18. In particular it has been used in two large-scale studies in the US. The BMLSS was included in the 1997 South Carolina Youth Risk Behavior Survey

of the Center for Disease Control and administered to over 5,500 public school students from 63 high schools (Huebner, Drane, & Valois, 2000). It was also used in a study of 2,502 students from grades six to eight in South Carolina (Huebner, Valois, Paxton, & Drane, 2005). The BMLSS has also been employed in studies of children and youth from other nations, such as China (Kwan, 2009) and Turkey (Siyez & Kaya, 2008).

Psychometric Properties

Coefficient alphas for the total score (i.e., the sum of respondents' ratings across the five items) have been reported ranging from .68 (elementary school students) to .75 (middle and high school students (Funk, Huebner, & Valois, 2006; Seligson, Huebner, & Valois, 2003; 2005). Inclusion of the additional global life satisfaction item in the total score raised the alpha coefficients to .76 for elementary students and .85 for secondary level students. Test-retest coefficients for a two-week interval were .91 (five-item total score), .85 (family), .80 (living environment), .79 (self), .75 (school), and .62 (friends) (Funk, Huebner, & Valois, 2006). A one-year test-retest reliability coefficient of .52 has been reported for the total score (Huebner, Antaramian, Hills, Lewis, & Saha, 2011).

Studies of construct validity have been undertaken. As noted above, the BMSLSS was designed to tap the same dimensions of life measured by the MSLSS (Huebner, 1994). The MSLSS is based on a hierarchical model of life satisfaction with general life satisfaction at the apex, along with the five lower-order domains (i.e., family, friends, school, etc.). Confirmatory factor analyses have supported the hierarchical model underlying the MSLSS (see Huebner, Laughlin, Ash, & Gilman, 1998).

Construct validity of the BMSLSS has been supported in several other ways. First, the meaningfulness of the general or total life satisfaction score has been assessed. Specifically, BMSLSS reports of 221 middle school students were subjected to principal axis factor analysis. Based on an eigenvalue greater than 1 criterion, and the results of a scree test, a single higher-order factor solution was supported (Funk, Huebner, & Valois, 2006; Seligson, Huebner, & Valois, 2005). Additionally, item-total correlations, ranging from .65 to .73, were observed with a middle school sample (Seligson, Huebner, & Valois, 2003).

The construct validity of the five single-item domain scores for the BMSLSS has been supported by multitrait-multimethod correlation matrix comparisons of the multi-item domain scores from the MSLSS with the single items on the BMSLSS using Campbell and Fiske's (1959) recommendations (see Seligson, Huebner, & Valois, 2003). In all cases, intercorrelations among the measures' corresponding domains were substantially higher than intercorrelations among the BMSLSS domains, as well as between different domains of the BMSLSS and MSLSS (e.g., MSLSS family domain score, BMSLSS friend item score). This pattern was demonstrated in separate analyses of middle and high school samples, with higher convergent validity coefficients observed in the high school students. Acceptable convergent validity correlations have also been obtained between the BMSLSS Total score and other validated measures of life satisfaction, such as the MSLSS Total score ($r = .66$) and the SLSS ($r = .62$) (Seligson, Huebner, & Valois, 2003).

The BMSLSS has demonstrated criterion-related validity through expected relationships with various adolescent problem behaviors. For example, adolescents' BMSLSS reports have shown concurrent, negative relationships with their alcohol, tobacco, and other drug use (Zullig, Valois, Huebner, Oeltmann, & Drane, 2001); violent and aggressive risk behaviors, such as physical fighting and carrying a weapon (Valois, Zullig, Huebner, Oeltmann, & Drane, 2001); sexual risk-taking behaviors (Valois, Zullig, Huebner, Kammermann, & Drane, 2002); inappropriate dieting behaviors (Valois, Zullig, Huebner, & Drane, 2003); suicidal ideation and behavior (Valois, Zullig, Huebner, & Drane, 2004); and lack of physical activity (Valois, Zullig, Huebner, & Drane, 2003). Evidence of predictive validity has been demonstrated by significant one-year correlations in the expected directions with measures of school engagement and grades (Huebner, Antaramian, Hills, Lewis, & Saha, 2011).

Finally, evidence of discriminant validity has been reported. BMSLSS scores yield a low correlation with indicators of social desirability (Seligson, Huebner, & Valois, 2003). In addition, the BMSLSS demonstrated relatively weak relationships with physical health-related quality of life measures (Zullig, Valois, Huebner, & Drane, 2005). Similar to other measures of general life satisfaction, BMLSS scores show modest relationships at best with a variety of demographic variables, such as gender, ethnicity, and so forth (Huebner, Suldo, Valois, Drane, & Zullig, 2004).

Summary of the BMSLSS

Research has supported the usefulness of the BMSLSS with students from grades –three to 12. The BMSLSS may be most useful in large national and international databases evaluating students' overall subjective well-being as well as pinpointing specific areas of life that may serve as protective or risk factors. In addition, the straightforward, concrete wording of the items lends itself well to large-scale surveys in which data are often analyzed at the item level. It may also be useful in clinical screening contexts, where brevity is also a virtue. For example, Huebner, Nagle, and Suldo (2003) provide examples of interview questions that could be used to follow up on responses of individuals, to provide more comprehensive understanding of students' responses. Nevertheless, as with the previous SLSS and MSLSS, major limitations of the BMSLSS include (1) the lack of nationally representative normative samples, and (b) the need for additional research with children with special needs.

Subjective Well-Being—Positive and Negative Affect

The Positive and Negative Affect Schedule for Children (PANAS-C; Laurent et al., 1999) assesses students' positive and negative affect. The PANAS-C is the child version of the PANAS designed by Watson, Clark, and Tellegen (1988). The scale includes 27 items that comprise two subscales (Positive Affect and Negative Affect) and is based on the conceptualization that both PA and NA reflect dispositional activations of positive and negatively valenced emotions and are conceptually somewhat independent constructs. The Positive Affect subscale consists of 12 items, such as energetic, interested, excited, cheerful, and proud. The Negative Affect subscale includes 15 items, such as sad, nervous, ashamed, lonely, and frightened. Respondents rate the extent to which they have felt each emotion during the past few weeks on a five-point Likert scale ranging from "very little or not at all" to "extremely or all of the time."

The PANAS-C has been used in studies of children from ages eight to 14. One study involved children with a diagnosed anxiety disorder (Hughes & Kendall, 2009). The PANAS-C has been also been translated and used in a study of Japanese children (Katsuma, Risa, & Akiko, 2006).

Psychometric Properties

Prior studies investigating the psychometric properties of the PANAS-C suggest preliminary support. Alpha coefficients reported in the literature range from .87 to .90 for the Positive Affect subscale and from .87 to .94 for the Negative Affect subscale (Antaramian, Huebner, Hills, & Valois, 2010; Laurent et al., 1999). Test-retest reliability coefficients for a 20-item version have been reported as in the lower .70 range (negative emotions) and upper .60 range (positive emotions) across two-week intervals, suggesting adequate stability (Crook, Beaver, & Bell, 1998). Research investigating the construct validity of the PANAS-C has supported a two-factor model of affect in samples of children and adolescents, using exploratory factor analysis procedures with the 27-item version (Laurent et al., 1999) and the earlier 20-item version (Crook, Beaver, & Bell, 1998).

Evidence also provides some support for the convergent and discriminant validity of the PANAS-C. The Negative Affect subscale was strongly, positively correlated with measures of trait anxiety and depression while the Positive Affect subscale was strongly, negatively correlated with the depression measure, but less strongly correlated with the anxiety measure (Laurent et al., 1999). However, concerns have been expressed over the PANAS-C's ability to discriminate social anxiety and depression in a sample of children diagnosed with a principal anxiety disorder (Hughes & Kendall, 2009).

Summary of the PANAS-C

As mentioned earlier, a significant body of research supports the need to measure positive affect and negative affect to adequately understand persons' SWB. Research has supported the usefulness of the PANAS-C with children and adolescents as one such measure. The relative length of the PANAS-C may be prohibitive with respect to purposes such as large-scale survey research; however, it may be useful in clinical screening and targeted samples to gather important data regarding emotional status and engagement-disengagement. Major limitations of the PANAS-C include (a) the lack of nationally representative normative samples, and (b) the need for additional research further investigating its construct validity, especially its discriminant validity.

Needed Future Research on SWB Measures

Gilman and Huebner (2000) identified a number of issues and associated directions for future research in the assessment of children's SWB. The issues continue to need attention.

First, most SWB measures lack good standardization samples. Most samples are geographically, ethnically, and socioeconomically limited.

Differences in definitions of "a good life" and "positive emotions" necessitate the availability of norms that are representative of the individuals or groups under consideration. Given that norm-referenced interpretations may be desired for some purposes, the development of additional SWB measures with nationally representative samples would be a critical next step.

Second, although preliminary research findings have been positive, additional research on the psychometric properties of SWB scales would be useful. With respect to reliability, investigations of test-retest reliability have been particularly sparse. Studies of test-retest reliabilities across differing time periods are needed for many measures. Investigations of predictive validity have also been quite sparse, thus longitudinal studies using SWB are critical for the future of SWB research. More cross-group construct validity studies are also needed to ensure the comparability of the meaning of various measures across different groups. For example, the equivalence of the factor structure of a multidimensional SWB measure across various groups of students (e.g., age groups, gender, ethnicity) should be evaluated empirically, not assumed.

Third, the use of SWB measures with different age groups and abilities has been understudied. The possibility of important developmental differences in the nature and determinants of SWB reports has received little research attention. The ability of students below the age of eight to respond meaningfully to SWB items remains unclear. The nature and number of relevant domains included in multidimensional measures also remains unclear. Although recognizing that some domains of life satisfaction may be important at some ages but not others (e.g., romantic relationships in adolescence), some instruments (e.g., the MSLSS) have been based on the notion that there are some broad domains that are important across a wide age range. The benefits and limitations of developing scales that attempt to assess multidimensional SWB across a wide age range have not been addressed thoroughly. Furthermore, as noted above, some research has suggested that measures may need to be modified for use with special populations. For example, Griffin and Huebner (2000) demonstrated that five reverse-keyed items on the MSLSS had to be eliminated when used with adolescents with serious emotional difficulties. For another example, global ratings of life satisfaction proved to be difficult to interpret for students with mental disabilities (Brantley, Huebner, & Nagle, 2002), but not for students with learning disabilities

(McCullough & Huebner, 2003). Thus, the SWB reports of students with special needs should be interpreted very cautiously.

Finally, the relationships between SWB measures and other methods needs further study. Although findings overall support the use of self-report techniques to measure *subjective* well-being of students, multi-method, multi-occasion assessments are generally recommended (Diener, 1994). Although little research has been conducted with children and adolescents, research with adults reveals that various situational factors (e.g., current mood, specific previous and current events, memory) can influence SWB reports (Pavot, 2008). Although such effects can be modest, they reflect the complex cognitive processing associated with making SWB judgments and highlight the need to consider alternative methods of assessing SWB. The reports of knowledgeable others (e.g., parent reports) may serve as a useful alternative method in some cases, although some scholars (e.g., Cummins, 2002) have noted the shortcomings of such methods. Other methods showing some promise include physiological and non-verbal indices (e.g., facial expression, vocal tones), experience sampling methodology, in-depth interview, and memories of good and bad events) (Diener, 1994). Studies of the convergence and divergence of responding across different methods would be particularly useful to understand the strength and limitations of the various alternatives.

Overall, scores on a variety of self-report measures of SWB, such as those above, demonstrate reasonable reliability and validity for various purposes (Diener, 1994; Gilman & Huebner, 2000; Proctor, Linley, & Maltby, 2009). Within the context of multi-method, multi-occasion assessments, SWB measures should prove useful in developing more comprehensive pictures of the adaptation of children and youth. Supported by data from other sources (e.g., observations, interview, other tests), SWB instruments should be able to provide incremental validity to the traditional testing armamentarium available to school psychologists, especially when the evaluation of students' psychosocial strengths and optimal functioning are under consideration. Given the lack of large national standardization samples, the use of criterion-referenced interpretation is more appropriate than norm-referenced interpretations. The use of absolute interpretations (e.g., Maggie rates her life satisfaction as "terrible" versus "delighted") is likely to be more meaningful than norm-referenced comparisons (e.g., Maggie is happier than 95 out of 100 children her age) for many purposes. Teachers, parents, and other caregivers may be as interested in a given child's level of SWB relative to the various response options as much as in a comparison to normative data.

Case Study

The following is a brief case study of "E.S.," a 13-year-old male who was referred for evaluation due to poor response to intervention and limited academic progress. The school multidisciplinary team recommended an evaluation for E.S. due to a lack of academic progress and behavioral concerns that were emerging in the classroom. E.S. had attended Tier II reading intervention services for 45 minutes each school day combined with after-school tutoring a few days a week for the past year with minimal progress. He had not been evaluated previously. Cognitive and achievement norm-referenced test results obtained during this evaluation process indicated average to above-average cognitive skills and below-average reading skills; however, his performance on academic measures during the evaluation was higher than expected given his poor academic performance in the classroom.

As part of this evaluation, E.S. was administered two measures of SWB: the MSLSS and the PANAS-C, in addition to a traditional, norm-referenced measure of mental health, which focused on symptoms of psychopathology (i.e., internalizing and externalizing behavior problems). Results of teacher, parent, and self-reports on the norm-referenced measure indicated minimal to no concerns with social and emotional functioning (i.e., symptoms). However, E.S.' total score on the MSLSS (M = 3.0) suggested that his perceived satisfaction with life was in the negative range. An examination of the MSLSS individual subscale scores (see Figure 34.1) suggested that E.S. is happy with his family and his living situation; for example, he responded "Strongly Agree" to items like "I like where I live" and "My family gets along well together."

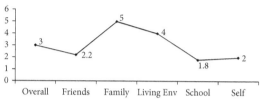

Figure 34.1 MSLSS Scores for E.S.

In contrast to his life satisfaction scores in family and living environment domains, his perceived satisfaction with friends, school, and self was of significant concern. Despite noting existing friendships during the parent, teacher, and individual interview and adequate social skills/relations on the norm-referenced social/emotional measure, E.S. rated his satisfaction with these relationships in the low range. For example, he responded "Strongly Disagree" to items "I have enough friends" and "My friends treat me well." In response to follow-up questions, he noted that he didn't see his friends as much as he used to and they didn't seem to be as interested in hanging out with him, further noting his friends were all in the Honors-level classes and had a different lunch schedule than his. Although during the initial interview E.S. simply reported "none" to a question about participation in extracurricular activities, during the follow-up interview using the MSLSS results to guide questioning, E.S. noted that he used to play sports for the school, but couldn't this year because of having to attend tutoring after school.

Upon follow-up, it became evident that given the salience of peers throughout adolescence and the positive impact of social relationships on well-being, his peer satisfaction was likely negatively impacting another important area of life satisfaction: self. E.S.' scores in the self-domain were also low (M = 2.0), with responses of "Agree" to statements like "I wish I had a different kind of life" and "Disagree" to many statements like "I like myself." His level of satisfaction with his school experiences was also of concern, with responses of "Disagree" to statements like "I enjoy school activities" and "I like being in school." He noted that although he complies with requests to attend tutoring and completing homework, he often remains disengaged throughout these activities, just completing them based on "what it takes to pass."

Ratings on the PANAS-C indicated that E.S. experiences only moderate levels of positive emotions (M = 3.1) and moderate levels of negative emotions (M = 3.9). For example, most of his ratings on positive emotion items ranged from 2 (A little) to 3 (moderately), with only a few ratings of 4 (quite a bit). His ratings of negative emotion items suggested that he experiences feelings of sadness (4—quite a bit) and upset (5—all of the time) on a regular basis. When questioned further about these ratings, E.S. indicated that he often felt sad at school, given that he never sees his friends, and is upset with how things are going academically at school, which can lead to his parents' being upset with him at home. Throughout this follow-up interview, he made several references to the fact that, given his isolation from his identified friends and his minimal academic progress, he has grown to "not care as much about school... because what's the point?"

Information collected from the MSLSS and PANAS-C was instrumental in the evaluation process to form data-based recommendations for appropriate interventions. Despite average ratings on teacher, parent, and self-report norm-referenced social-emotional measures, suggesting adequate mental health, and few psychological symptoms, results of the SWB scales (MSLSS and PANAS-C) provided information that was key to understanding E.S.' perceptions of his overall satisfaction with different areas of his life and the type of emotions he regularly experiences. This provides a context to help understand the factors that may be negatively affecting his academic progress. The results within this case study support the notion that gathering information about well-being enhances the information collected with more traditional, routine assessment measures, reflected in the previously mentioned Dual-Factor Model of Mental Health (Greenspoon & Saklofske, 2001). The results of SWB measures provided a more comprehensive context that allowed the psychologist to elicit information based on the SWB data provided by E.S. These results suggested that his peer isolation and discontinuation of sports participation may be negatively affecting his achievement motivation and causing him to engage in subtle, yet impactful, withdrawal behaviors at school.

As a result of this evaluation, the multidisciplinary team, which included his parents, determined that E.S. was not eligible for special education services; however, they implemented a number of interventions. Many of these interventions capitalized on E.S.' strengths indicated through this assessment. Measures of SWB indicated that his overall perception and satisfaction with his family life and living environment were positive and could be relied upon to provide support and progress monitoring. Throughout this process, it was revealed that his family was friendly with many of his close friends' families and could help with arranging social gatherings to give E.S. time to maintain and strengthen his current, but dwindling (as he perceives) friendships. In the school setting, the nature and time of tutoring was restructured to allow him to continue to participate in activities he values and activities that provide him time to engage socially with peers. Strong neighborhood support made it possible for this restructuring to occur, given the need for assistance with transportation to/from tutoring. The school team worked with the family to help set up neighborhood transportation networks for E.S. and other students in the area to get to/from important events (e.g., tutoring, extracurricular activities).

Although this restructuring did not allow him to participate in the school sports team (due to timing; it was midseason), it did allow him to participate in a recreational sports team in the community until the next sport season arrived. Six months later, he easily transferred to the school sports team, given the new season, his restructured schedule, and the athletic conditioning level he maintained through his participation on a recreational sports team. Combined with this change in his extracurricular activity participation, his trajectory of academic progress had significantly improved, which suggests that E.S.' school engagement and overall achievement motivation increased as well.

Concluding Comments

Extending beyond the Dual-Factor Theory of Mental Health (Greenspoon & Saklofske, 2001), the value of differentiating levels among average and higher levels of SWB has been suggested by a study by Suldo and Huebner (2006). Based on their life satisfaction scores, they divided secondary-level students into three groups: low (lowest 10%), average (middle 25%), and very high levels (top 10%) of life satisfaction. Not only were the high and low groups different, but the high and average groups differed on a variety of important adolescent variables. More specifically, although rates of clinical levels of behavior problems (e.g., internalizing and externalizing behaviors) did not differ significantly between the very high and average groups, significant differences were observed on measures of adaptive psychosocial functioning, and on academic, social, and emotional self-efficacy, as well as parent, teacher, close friend and classmate social support. A similar study by Gilman and Huebner (2006) revealed comparable findings, including significant differences between high and average groups of adolescents on measures of global self-esteem, hope, and internal locus of control. Taken together, the findings support the notion that the highest levels of well-being are not captured by the absence of psychopathological behaviors. Rather, assessing mental health requires measures of constructs, such as SWB constructs, that reflect experiences above a neutral point or the absence of indicators of psychopathology. Measures of life satisfaction and positive affect may thus provide a useful complement to the more traditional measures that focus on the presence of psychopathology in comprehensive assessments of child and adolescent mental health. As observed by Beaver (2008), families of children with behavior problems do not simply seek reductions in their behavior problems when they seek psychological assessments and counseling. They want their children to "be happy and to fully engage in the academic and social experiences of childhood" (Beaver, 2008, p. 134). Such a broadened focus, encompassing positive SWB, should aid in the accomplishment of such goals.

Author Note

Address correspondence to: Scott Huebner, Ph.D., Dept. of Psychology, University of South Carolina, Columbia, SC 29208; phone: 803.777.3591; fax: 803.777.9558; e-mail: huebner@sc.edu.

References

Adelman, H. S., Taylor, L., & Nelson, P. (1989). Minors' dissatisfaction with their life circumstances. *Child Psychiatry & Human Development, 20*, 135–147.

Andrews, F. M., & Withey, S. B. (1976). *Social indicators of well-being: Americans' perceptions of life quality*. New York: Plenum.

Antaramian, S. P., Huebner, E. S., Hills, K. J., & Valois, R. F. (2010). A dual-factor model of mental health: Toward a more comprehensive understanding of youth functioning. *American Journal of Orthopsychiatry, 80*, 462–472.

Antaramian, S. P., Huebner, E. S., & Valois, R. F. (2008). Adolescent life satisfaction. *Applied Psychology: Health & Well-Being, 57*, 705–714.

Ash, C., & Huebner, E. S. (1998). Life satisfaction reports of gifted middle-school children. *School Psychology Quarterly, 13*, 310–321.

Beaver, B. R. (2008). A positive approach to children's internalizing problems. *Professional Psychology: Research & Practice, 39*, 129–136.

Bender, T. A. (1997). Assessment of subjective well-being during childhood and adolescence. In G. D. Phye (Ed.), *Handbook of classroom assessment: Learning, achievement, and adjustment* (pp. 199–225). San Diego, CA: Academic Press.

Brantley, A., Huebner, E. S., & Nagle, R. J. (2002). Multidimensional life satisfaction reports of adolescents with mild mental disabilities. *Mental Retardation, 40*, 321–329.

Campbell, D. T., & Fiske, D. W. (1959). Convergent and discriminant validation by the multitrait-multimethod matrix. *Psychological Bulletin, 56*, 81–105.

Cohen, M. A., & Fredrickson, B. L. (2009). Positive emotions. In C. R. Snyder & S. J. Lopez (Eds.), *Oxford handbook of positive psychology* (pp. 13–24). Oxford: Oxford University Press.

Crenshaw, M. (1998). *Adjudicated violent youth, adjudicated non-violent youth vs. non-adjudicated, non-violent youth on selected psychological measures*. Unpublished Masters thesis, University of South Carolina.

Crook, K., Beaver, B. R., & Bell, M. (1998). Anxiety and depression in children: A preliminary examination of the utility of the PANAS-C. *Journal of Psychopathology & Behavioral Assessment, 20*, 333–350.

Cummins, R. A. (2002). Proxy responding for subjective well-being: A review. In L. Masters (Ed.), *International review of research in mental retardation* (Vol. 25: pp. 183–207), San Diego, CA: Academic Press.

Dew, T., & Huebner, E. S. (1994). Adolescents' perceived quality of life: An exploratory investigation. *Journal of School Psychology, 33*, 185–199.

Diener, E. (1984). Subjective well-being. *Psychological Bulletin, 95*, 542–575.

Diener, E. (1994). Assessing subjective well-being: Progress and opportunities. *Social Indicators Research, 31*, 103–157.

Diener, E. (2000). Science of well-being: The science of happiness and a proposal for a national index. *American Psychologist, 55*, 34–43.

Diener, E., Larsen, R. J., Levine, S., & Emmons, R. A. (1985). Intensity and frequency: Dimensions underlying positive and negative affect. *Journal of Personality & Social Psychology, 48*, 1253–1265.

Funk, B. A., Huebner, E. S., & Valois, R. F. (2006). Reliability and validity of a life satisfaction scale with a high school sample. *Journal of Happiness Studies, 7*, 41–54.

Fredrickson, B. (2001). The role of positive emotions in positive psychology: The broaden-and-build theory of positive emotions. *American Psychologist, 56*, 218–226.

Frisch, M. B. (2000). Improving mental and physical health care through quality of life therapy and assessment. In E. Diener & D. R. Rahtz (Eds.), *Advances in quality of life theory and research* (pp. 207–241). Great Britain: Kluwer Academic Publishers.

Gilman, R., Easterbrooks, S. R., & Frey, M. (2004). A preliminary study of multidimensional youth life satisfaction among deaf/hard of hearing youth across environmental settings. *Social Indicators Research, 66*, 143–164.

Gilman, R., & Huebner, E. S. (1997). Children's reports of their life satisfaction. *School Psychology International, 18*, 229–243.

Gilman, R., & Huebner, E. S. (2000). Review of life satisfaction measures for adolescents. *Behaviour Change, 17*, 178–195.

Gilman, R., & Huebner, E. S. (2006). Characteristics of adolescents who report very high life satisfaction. *Journal of Youth & Adolescence, 35*, 311–319.

Gilman, R., Huebner, E. S., & Laughlin, J. (2000). A first study of the Multidimensional Students' Life Scale with adolescents. *Social Indicators Research, 52*, 135–160.

Gilman, R., Huebner, E. S., Tian, L., Park, N., O'Byrne, J., Schiff, M., & Sverko, et al. (2008). Cross-national adolescent multidimensional life satisfaction reports: Analyses of mean scores and response style differences. *Journal of Youth & Adolescence, 37*, 142–154.

Griffin, M., & Huebner, E. S. (2000). Multidimensional life satisfaction reports of students with serious emotional disturbance. *Journal of Psychoeducational Assessment, 18*, 111–124.

Greenspoon, P. J., & Saklofske, D. H. (1997). Validity and reliability of the Multidimensional Students' Life Satisfaction Scale with Canadian children. *Journal of Psychoeducational Assessment, 15*, 138–155.

Greenspoon, P. J., & Saklofske, D. H. (2001). Toward an integration of subjective well-being and psychopathology. *Social Indicators Research, 54*, 81–108.

Haranin, E. C., Huebner, E. S., & Suldo, S. M. (2007). Predictive and incremental validity of global and domain-based adolescent life satisfaction reports. *Journal of Psychoeducational Assessment, 25*, 127–138.

Hexdall, C. M., & Huebner, E. S. (2007). Subjective well-being in pediatric oncology patients. *Applied Research in Quality of Life, 2*, 189–208.

Hill, S. E., & Buss, D. M. (2008). Evolution and subjective well-being. In M. Eid & R. J. Larsen (Eds.), *The science of subjective well-being* (pp. 62–79). New York: Guilford.

Huebner, E. S. (1991a). Further validation of the Student's Life Satisfaction Scale: Independence of satisfaction and affect ratings. *Journal of Psychoeducational Assessment, 9*, 363–368.

Huebner, E. S. (1991b). Initial development of the Students' Life Satisfaction Scale. *School Psychology International, 12*, 231–240.

Huebner, E. S. (1991c). Correlates of life satisfaction in children. *School Psychology Quarterly, 6*, 103–111.

Huebner, E. S. (1994). Preliminary development and validation of a multidimensional life satisfaction scale for children. *Psychological Assessment, 6*, 149–158.

Huebner, E. S. (1995). The Students' Life Satisfaction Scale: An assessment of psychometric properties with black and white elementary school students. *Social Indicators Research, 34,* 315–323.

Huebner, E. S. (2004). Research on assessment of life satisfaction in children and adolescents. *Social Indicators Research, 66,* 3–33.

Huebner E. S., & Alderman, G. L. (1993). Convergent and discriminant validation of a children's life satisfaction scale: Its relationship to self- and teacher-reported psychological problems and school functioning. *Social Indicators Research, 30,* 71–82.

Huebner, E. S., Brantley, A., Nagle, R. J., & Valois, R. F. (2002). Correspondence between parent and adolescent ratings of life satisfaction for adolescents with and without learning disabilities. *Journal of Psychoeducational Assessment, 20,* 20–29.

Huebner, E. S., & Dew, T. (1993). An evaluation of racial bias in a life satisfaction scale. *Psychology in the Schools, 30,* 305–309.

Huebner, E. S., & Dew, T. (1996). The interrelationships of positive affect, negative affect and life satisfaction in an adolescent sample. *Social Indicators Research, 38,* 129–137.

Huebner, E. S., Drane, J. W., & Valois, R. F. (2000). Levels and demographic correlates of adolescent life satisfaction reports. *School Psychology International, 21,* 281–292.

Huebner, E. S., Gilman, R., & Laughlin, J. E. (1999). A multimethod investigation of the multidimensionality of children's well-being reports: Discriminant validity of life satisfaction and self-esteem. *Social Indicators Research, 46,* 1–22.

Huebner, E. S., Funk, B. A., & Gilman, R. (2000). Cross-sectional and longitudinal psychosocial correlates of adolescent life satisfaction reports. *Canadian Journal of School Psychology, 16,* 53–64.

Huebner, E. S., Antaramian, S. J., Hills, K. J., Lewis, A. D., & Saha, R. (2011). Stability and predictive validity of the Brief Multidimensional Students' Life Satisfaction Scale. *Child Indicators Research, 4,* 161–168.

Huebner, E. S., Gilman, R., & Suldo, S. M. (2006). Assessing perceived quality of life in children and youth. In S. R. Smith & L. Handler (Eds.), *The clinical assessment of children and adolescents: A practitioners' guide* (pp. 349–366). Mahwah, NJ: Erlbaum.

Huebner, E. S., Laughlin, J. F., Ash, C., & Gilman, R. (1998). Further validation of the Multidimensional Students' Life Satisfaction Scale. *Journal of Psychoeducational Assessment, 16,* 118–134.

Huebner, E. S., Nagle, R. J., & Suldo, S. M. (2003). Quality of life assessment in child and adolescent health care: The use of the Multidimensional Students' Life Satisfaction Scale. In M. J. Sirgy, D. Rahtz, & A. C. Samlii (Eds.), *Advances in quality of life theory and research* (pp. 179–190). Dordrecht, Netherlands: Kluwer Academic Press.

Huebner, E. S., Valois, R. F., Paxton, R., & Drane, J. W. (2005). Middle school students' perceptions of quality of life. *Journal of Happiness Studies, 6,* 15–24.

Huebner, E. S., Suldo, S. M., Valois, R. F., Drane, J. W., & Zullig, K. (2004). Brief Multidimensional Students' Life Satisfaction Scale: Gender, race, and grade effects in a high school sample. *Psychological Reports, 94,* 351–356.

Hughes, A. A., & Kendall, P. C. (2009). Psychometric properties of the Positive and Negative Affect Scale for Children (PANAS-C) in children with anxiety disorders. *Child Psychiatry & Human Development, 40,* 343–352.

Irmak, S., & Kuruuzun, A. (2009). Turkish validity examination of the Multidimensional Students' Life Satisfaction Scale. *Social Indicators Research, 92,* 13–23.

Katsuma, Y., Risa, K., & Akiko, S. (2006). Development of a Japanese version of the Positive and Negative Affect Schedule for children. *Psychological Reports, 99,* 535–546.

Kwan, Y. K. (2009). Life satisfaction and self-assessed health among adolescents in Hong Kong. *Journal of Happiness Studies, 11,* 383–393.

Laurent, J., Catanzaro, S. J., Joiner, T. E., Rudolph, K. D., Potter, K. I., Lambert, S., et al. (1999). A measure of positive and negative affect for children: Scale development and preliminary validation. *Psychological Assessment, 11,* 326–338.

Lewinsohn, P. M., Redner, J. E., & Seeley, J. R. (1991). The relationship between life satisfaction and psychosocial variables: New perspectives. In F. Strack, M. Argyle, & N. Schwartz (Eds.), *Subjective well-being* (pp. 193–212). New York: Plenum.

Lewis, A., Huebner, E. S., Malone, P., & Valois, R. F. (2011). Life satisfaction and student engagement in adolescence. *Journal of Youth & Adolescence, 40,* 249–262.

Lewis, A., Huebner, E. S., Reschly, A., & Valois, R. F. (2009). The incremental validity of positive emotions in predicting school satisfaction, engagement, and academic success. *Journal of Psychoeducational Assessment, 27,* 397–408.

Lopez, S. J., & Snyder, C. R. (2003). *Positive psychological assessment: A handbook of models and measures.* Washington, DC: American Psychological Association.

Lucas, R. E., Diener, E., & Suh, E. (1996). Discriminant validity of well-being measures. *Journal of Personality & Social Psychology, 71,* 616–628.

Lyubormirsky, S., King, L. A., & Diener, E. (2005). The benefits of frequent positive affect: Does happiness lead to success? *Psychological Bulletin, 131,* 803–855.

Marques, S. C., Lopez, S. J., & Pais-Ribeiro, J. L. (2011). "Building hope for the future": A program to foster strengths in middle school students. *Journal of Happiness Studies, 12,* 129–152.

Martin, K. M., Huebner, E. S., & Valois, R. F. (2008). Does life satisfaction predict adolescent victimization experiences? *Psychology in the Schools, 45,* 419–431.

McCullough, G., & Huebner, E. S. (2003). Life satisfaction of adolescents with learning disabilities. *Journal of Psychoeducational Assessment, 21,* 311–324.

Park, N., & Huebner, E. S. (2005). A cross-cultural study of the levels and correlates of life satisfaction of adolescents. *Journal of Cross-Cultural Psychology, 36,* 444–456.

Pavot, W. (2008). The assessment of subjective well-being: Successes and shortfall. In M. Eid & R. J. Larsen (Eds.), *The science of subjective well-being* (pp. 124–140). New York: Guilford.

Proctor, C. L., Linley, P. A., & Maltby, J. (2009). Youth life satisfaction measures: A review. *The Journal of Positive Psychology, 4,* 128–144.

Proctor, C. L., Linley, P. A., & Malby, J. (2009). Youth life satisfaction: A review of the literature. *Journal of Happiness Studies, 10,* 583–603.

Seligman, M. E., & Csikszentmihalyi, M. (2000). Positive psychology: An introduction. *American Psychologist, 55,* 5–14.

Seligson, J. L., Huebner, E. S., & Valois, R. F. (2003). Preliminary validation of the Brief Multidimensional Students' Life Satisfaction Scale (BMSLSS). *Social Indicators Research, 61,* 121–145.

Seligson, J. L., Huebner, E. S., & Valois, R. F. (2005). An investigation of a brief life satisfaction scale with elementary school students. *Social Indicators Research*, *73*, 355–374.

Siyez, D. M., & Kaya, A. (2008). Validity and reliability of the Brief Multidimensional Students' Life Satisfaction Scale with Turkish children. *Journal of Psychoeducational Assessment*, *26*, 139–147.

Suldo, S. M., & Huebner, E. S. (2006). Is extremely high life satisfaction during adolescence advantageous? *Social Indicators Research*, *78*, 179–203.

Suldo, S. M., & Shaffer, E. J. (2008). Looking beyond psychopathology: The dual-factor model of mental health in youth. *School Psychology Review*, *37*, 52–68.

Terry, T., & Huebner, E. S. (1995). The relationship between self-concept and life satisfaction in children. *Social Indicators Research*, *35*, 39–52.

Valois, R. F., Zullig, K. J., Huebner, E. S., Drane, J. W. (2001). Relationship between life satisfaction and violent behaviors among adolescents. *American Journal of Health Behavior*, *25*, 353–366.

Valois, R. F., Zullig, K. J., Huebner, E. S., & Drane, J. W. (2003). Relationship between perceived life satisfaction and dieting behavior among public high school adolescents. *Eating Disorders: The Journal of Treatment & Prevention*, *11*, 271–288.

Valois, R. F., Zullig, K. J., Huebner, E. S., & Drane, J. W. (2004). Physical activity behaviors and life satisfaction among public high school adolescents, *Journal of School Health*, *74*, 59–65.

Valois, R. F., Zullig, K. J., Huebner, E. S., & Drane, J. W. (2004). Relationship between life satisfaction and suicidal ideation and behaviors among adolescents. *Social Indicators Research*, *66*, 81–105.

Valois, R. F., Zullig, K. J., Huebner, E. S., Kammermann, S. K., & Drane, J. W. (2002). Relationship between life satisfaction and sexual risk-taking behaviors among public high school adolescents. *Journal of Child & Family Studies*, *11*, 437–440.

Watson, D., Clark, L. A., & Tellegen, A. (1988). Development and validation of brief measures of positive and negative affect: the PANAS scales. *Journal of Personality & Social Psychology*, *54*, 1063–1070.

Wilkinson, R. B., & Walford, W. A. (1998). The measurement of adolescent psychological health: One or two dimensions? *Journal of Youth & Adolescence*, *22*, 443–455.

Zullig, K. J., Valois, R. F., Huebner, E. S., & Drane, J. W. (2005). The relationship between health-related quality of life and life satisfaction in adolescents. *Quality of Life Research*, *14*, 1573–1584.

Zullig, K. J., Valois, R. F., Huebner, E. S., Oeltmann, J. E., & Drane, W. J. (2001). Relationship between perceived life satisfaction and adolescent substance use. *Journal of Adolescent Health*, *29*, 279–288.

Assessment of Parenting Behaviors and Style, Parenting Relationships, and Other Parent Variables in Child Assessment

Laura G. McKee, Deborah J. Jones, Rex Forehand, *and* Jessica Cuellar

Abstract

This chapter provides an historical and theoretical context for the assessment of parenting, including the ways in which the concept of parenting has morphed over time, the ways in which assessment tools have been constructed to capture the complexities of the parent–child relationship, and the ways in which parenting assessment has contributed to basic developmental science and applied intervention/prevention science. The chapter also highlights integral cultural considerations of assessment design, validation, and application by focusing, primarily, on ethnicity. Three questionnaire tools and three observational coding schemes are explored in detail. The impact of parenting relationships and parental physical and mental illness are addressed, with implications for assessment noted. Finally, a summary of the literature provides potential avenues for future research.

Key Words: parenting practices, parenting behaviors, parenting style, child behavior, coparenting, culture, socioeconomic status, parental illness

Overview

Any theoretical model or empirical research designed to explain the development of child psychosocial adjustment must account for the influence of parenting, either directly or indirectly. Borrowing Baumrind's words, "there is no way in which parents can evade having a determining effect upon their children's personality, character, and competence" (1978, p. 239). Consistent with Baumrind's assertion, social, clinical, and developmental psychologists have spent the past half century seeking to answer the questions, "Does parenting contribute to child psychological well-being or psychopathology, and if so, how might parenting best be conceptualized and measured?" Given the now robust empirical evidence indicating "yes," parents do contribute to child psychosocial adjustment, researchers have more recently amended the question to capture the dynamic and reciprocal genetic, behavioral, and environmental interplay that unfolds over time between the parent–child dyad in the family, neighborhood, and cultural and economic contexts (Belsky & Jaffee, 2006).

Several theoretical models of human development, including ecological systems theory originally proposed by Bronfenbrenner (1979) and updated by others (Cummings, Davies, & Campbell, 2000), as well as Super and Harkness's (1999) concept of the "developmental niche," recognize the influence of caregivers as agents of emotional, cognitive, and relational socialization for their offspring. Bronfenbrenner's model, often presented graphically, consists of a series of concentric circles, with the individual child situated in the innermost circle, surrounded by the microsystem (e.g., parents and siblings, neighborhood, peers, schools), the mesosystem (representing the relations between aspects of the microsystem), the exosystem (e.g., extended family, mass media, community health services, parental workplace), and finally the macrosystem (e.g. cultural, subcultural, and social and economic class regulations). One of the more proximal forces, the caregiver, exerts influence on the child's development directly via shared genetics, parenting style, and parenting behaviors and, indirectly, as a filter and interpreter of more distal forces. For example, in the case of child aggressive behavior, McLoyd (1990) has argued that the relation between poverty (component of the macrosystem) and child externalizing symptoms is mediated by parental disciplinary strategies (microsystem), and several empirical studies have garnered support for this perspective (Dodge, Pettit, & Bates, 1994; Sampson & Laub, 1994). Super and Harkness's concept of the "developmental niche" emerged from a tradition that has conceptualized the child's *cultural* environment as a set of *proximal* sources of influence, providing an alternative to Bronfenbrenner's hierarchical schematic; nonetheless, caretakers are considered to be powerful direct and indirect regulators of the three subsystems surrounding the child (Super & Harkness, 1999). In sum, both frameworks, representing different lenses through which to examine the influence of the child's environment on development, highlight the central role of caretakers, most often biological parents, but increasingly other caregivers as well, including non-marital coparents (e.g., grandmothers assisting single mothers with childrearing), in the lives of youth.

As will be discussed in more depth in the pages that follow, the construct and assessment of "parenting" has morphed over time; thus, a number of different conceptual perspectives have been presented in the literature and will be reviewed and synthesized here. Parenting variables have also occupied a prominent place in a wide array of empirical studies, with foci ranging from youth academic achievement (e.g., Burchinal, Roberts, Zeisel, & Rowley, 2008; Glasgow, Dornbusch, Troyer, & Steinberg, 1997; Prelow, Bowman, & Weaver, 2007) to perpetration of violent crime (Bradshaw, Glaser, Calhoun, & Bates, 2006; Caspi et al., 2002; Widom, 1989) and diagnosis of major depressive disorder in offspring (Fendrich, Warner, & Weissman, 1990; Hammen, Shih, & Brennan, 2004). Despite the variation in parent predictors and developmental outcomes, researchers studying parenting have focused on remarkably similar underlying parenting dimensions—warmth/acceptance, harshness/hostility, strictness/behavioral control, permissiveness/lax control, involvement, and monitoring (e.g., Barber, Stolz, & Olsen, 2005; Patterson & Fisher, 2002). As a result of the consistency across studies

of parenting, as well as the sheer number of studies, significant empirical support has emerged for the robust association between parenting practices typified by warmth and affection, positive reinforcement, firm and consistent discipline, and active involvement in and monitoring of child and adolescent activities and child psychosocial well-being (Baumrind, 1978; Brody & Flor, 1998; Gray & Steinberg, 1999), including reduced externalizing (e.g., Barber & Olsen, 1997; Pettit, Laird, Dodge, Bates, & Criss, 2001) and internalizing (e.g., Barber & Olsen, 1997; Gray & Steinberg, 1999) symptoms. The converse—that negative parenting, including high levels of hostility, low levels of warmth and involvement, coercive disciplinary tactics, and inconsistent monitoring, is associated with youth psychosocial maladjustment—also has a broad base of empirical support (e.g., Baumrind, 1978; Ge, Conger, Lorenz, & Simons, 1994; Teicher, Samson, Polcari, & McGreenery, 2006).

Although the unidirectional, deterministic view of parents' influence on the etiology of child and adolescent psychopathology has been overstated at times, either by failing to consider the child evocative effects (e.g., Lytton, 2000; Scarr, 1992) or passive gene-environment correlations (e.g., Foley et al., 2004; Kim-Cohen et al., 2006), sophisticated contemporary research continues to assert that "parenting matters," albeit in complex interactions with heredity, nonfamilial influences, and the broader contexts (e.g., Collins, Maccoby, Steinberg, Hetherington, & Bornstein, 2000; Galambos, Barker, & Almeida, 2003). In fact, a number of causal theories of child and adolescent problems implicate parenting behaviors and parent–child interactions. Researchers at the Oregon Social Learning Center, for example, developed a social learning model and have studied extensively the coercive processes at play in families with aggressive or conduct-disordered children (e.g., Patterson et al., 1992; Snyder & Patterson, 1995). According to the theory and empirical tests of it, the irritable, hostile exchanges between parents and children often contain a negative reinforcement mechanism that perpetuates parental harshness and child externalizing problems (see Granic & Patterson, 2006). Consistent with this body of research, the intervention of choice for treating and preventing child and adolescent disruptive behavior problems is Parent Management Training, in which maladaptive parenting practices are replaced with a repertoire of skills to more effectively manage the child's behavior while improving the broader parent–child relationship quality (e.g., Forehand, Kotchick, Shaffer, & McKee, 2010; McMahon & Forehand, 2003; McMahon, Wells, & Kotler, 2006).

Of note, although interventions for internalizing symptoms have largely grown out of an individual-focused tradition with less emphasis on the parent–child relationship (Clarke, Lewinsohn, & Hops, 1990; Stark & Kendall, 1996), a special issue on evidence-based psychosocial treatments for children and adolescents published by the *Journal of Clinical Child & Adolescent Psychology* admonishes researchers to consider the impact of parental involvement in interventions targeting youth with anxiety and depressive disorders (David-Ferdon & Kaslow, 2008; Silverman, Pina, & Viswesvaran, 2008). In an example of such a program, Webster-Stratton and Herman (2008) recently examined the efficacy of *Incredible Years*, a parent training program with an established history of reducing externalizing problems in young children, for reducing internalizing problems. Importantly, the authors highlight that many of the same mechanisms that contribute to externalizing problems in youth also likely contribute to internalizing problems, including parenting, and that comorbidity between internalizing and externalizing problems in youth makes disentangling specific effects difficult. Findings revealed that the *Incredible Years* program was associated with a significant reduction in internalizing symptoms in youth relative to a wait-list control, particularly for youth who scored in the clinical range on internalizing symptoms at baseline. Moreover, perceived changes in parenting mediated the effect of treatment on children's internalizing symptoms. In sum, the assessment of parenting style and parenting behaviors is an integral component in the pursuit of causal theories of child and adolescent psychopathology, and, thus, in the development and testing of targeted prevention and intervention programs for externalizing, as well as internalizing, symptoms.

Ethnicity, Culture, and Parenting Constructs

While a vast body of research on parenting style and parenting behavior has produced, replicated, and extended a robust core of findings, and although the treatment literature has been informed and innovated by these consistent outcomes, important questions remain regarding the influence of ethnic, cultural, and socioeconomic contexts on the relations between parenting behaviors and child outcomes. For example, some research on low-income African American parents and their children, particularly those living in high-risk communities or exposed to high-risk peer groups, suggests that parents who adjust their approach to parenting in response to environmental risk factors (e.g., "no-nonsense parenting"—a term adopted to describe a parenting approach consisting of high levels of behavioral control combined with affectionate behaviors) have children who evidence fewer adjustment difficulties (Brody & Flor, 1998; see also Mason, Cauce, Gonzales, & Hiraga, 1996). Importantly, however, this work does not suggest that heightened monitoring in response to risk is beneficial in the absence of or at the expense of warmth. On the contrary, some work suggests that warmth is an important, if not the most important parenting behavior for children raised in high-risk contexts (Masten & Coatsworth, 1998).

Another example of the importance of considering the cultural ecology when ascertaining the effects of specific parenting behaviors on youth comes from the study of Hispanic American families. A "hierarchical/autocratic" parenting approach, typified by strong parental authority and rules/consequences *not* based on consensus, may more accurately characterize Hispanic American families whose practices are influenced by the values of *familism* and *respeto* (Arcia, Reyes-Blanes, & Vazquez-Montilla, 2000; Harwood, Leyendecker, Carlson, Asencio, & Miller, 2002). As such, some research has shown that a hierarchical or autocratic style is associated with positive outcomes among Hispanic children (Lindahl & Malik, 1999); however, other research has indicated that autonomy granting and democracy is related to adaptive offspring outcomes regardless of ethnicity, class, or family structure (Steinberg, Mounts, Lamborn, & Dornbusch, 1991). In sum, there is a growing body of evidence suggesting that socialization goals and cultural norms within a particular racial, ethnic, or socioeconomic group may determine the effect of a specific parenting style on child outcomes (e.g., Forehand & Kotchick, 1996; Lindahl & Malik, 1999); however, additional fine-tuned analysis is warranted.

Although much of the research focused on minority groups has utilized parenting assessment tools originally designed for use with majority families and may not reflect equivalent constructs/processes (Garcia Coll, & Pachter, 2002; Guerra & Jagers, 1999; Knight & Hill, 1998; Knight, Tein, Shell, & Roosa, 1992), the validation of tools with different populations and culturally informed measure development is gaining empirical ground (see Taylor, Barnett, Longest, & Raver, 2009; and Smetana, Abernethy, & Harris, 2004, for examples). Given that minorities, who now constitute roughly one-third of the US population, are expected to become the majority by mid-century (U.S. Census Bureau News, 2008), attention to the accurate assessment of diverse parenting practices is of paramount importance. Accordingly, we include examples, when available, not only of Caucasian families, which have been the primary focus of parenting research, but also of empirical data representing ethnic minority families. Although still paling in comparison to the depth and breadth of research on parenting in Caucasian families, the ethnic minority group that has received the most attention in the literature and has been a primary focus of the work by the authors is African American families; however, we make an effort to include studies of other ethnic minority groups as well, including some work on Hispanic families.

Assessing Correlates of Parenting Style and Behavior

Beyond the more direct effects of parenting style and behaviors on child psychosocial, emotional, and cognitive development, both Bronfenbrenner's (1979) and Super & Harkness's (1999) theoretical models recognize additional factors that may influence the relations between caregiver behavior and child outcomes, including but not limited to marital and coparenting relationships, parental psychopathology, and chronic illness. Each of these broad areas of study has important implications for adaptive and pathological child and adolescent development and will be addressed, in turn, in the chapter.

Parenting Measures: Overview of Content, Administration, and Feasibility

Just as the theories informing parenting research represent alternative perspectives, the assessment tools designed to assess the constructs of interest vary widely in terms of content, administration, and feasibility. As discussed further in this and the following section, a number of factors contribute to the content, administration, and feasibility, including the age and developmental stage of the child; the racial, ethnic, and class characteristics of the family; and the purpose of the assessment and its intended audience. All of these factors influence, in concert with the guiding theory, the variables included and the format imposed. For example, investigators and clinicians focused on adolescents

living in single-mother–headed families or urban families of low socioeconomic status may consider monitoring and limit setting as the most salient parenting issues (Bank, Forgatch, Patterson, & Fetrow, 1993; Elder, Eccles, Ardelt, & Lord, 1995; Jones, Forehand, O'Connell, Armistead, & Brody, 2005), while intrusiveness and disengagement may be more prominent for researchers working with depressed caregivers (Lovejoy, Graczyk, O'Hare, & Neuman, 2000). Given the wide range of parenting assessment tools available, this chapter will serve not as a comprehensive list but rather will highlight exemplars in each of two broad categories. The reader is referred to the *Handbook of Family Measurement Techniques*, Volumes 1–3 (Touliatos, Perlmutter, & Straus, 2001) for abstracts describing nearly 1,000 instruments utilized in the measurement of the family as well as selected examples of actual instruments. Other resources of interest are provided in subsequent sections.

With regard to administration, parenting assessment techniques fall into two broad categories: questionnaire data (parents reporting on their own practices and children/adolescents reporting on their caregiver's behaviors) and structured observations of dyadic (parent–child) or triadic (parent-parent–child) family interactions. The two general approaches provide different perspectives on parenting behavior and function (Fiske, 1987) and have distinct strengths and weaknesses, which, in turn, have implications for content and feasibility. Questionnaire data are generally less costly (Fiske, 1987; Ramey, 2002), often require little to no training to administer, are easily scored, and may elicit, depending upon the measure employed, response sets that take into account parenting behaviors across time and context (Zaslow et al., 2006). However, as with all questionnaire data, particularly self-reports, threats to validity are inherent, including a social desirability response bias, among others (Schwarz, 1999). While structured observational data are more burdensome to collect and score (more costly in terms of observer time or video equipment, require highly trained coders), advantages include the provision of a standard context and task, reduced likelihood of bias by independent raters, and the opportunity to assess characteristics of parenting not accessible by questionnaires (e.g., tone of voice, physical proximity of parent to child, child's response to particular parenting behaviors). Finally, in addition to issues of cost and ease of administration and scoring, transportability of the assessment tool also affects feasibility. While questionnaire data can be mailed to parents and children, utilized in telephone interviews, or completed online without a researcher or clinician present and, thus, ostensibly reach a larger and wider audience, observational data must be gathered in a clinical or research setting or in the field.

Parenting Behaviors and Parenting Style

Parenting, both positive and negative, has been explored from a variety of perspectives, ranging from a focus on (1) the effects of broad typologies of parenting to (2) the main effects of particular parenting behaviors (e.g., Baumrind, 1966; Schaefer, 1965; see also McKee, Colletti, Rakow, & Forehand, 2008). One approach to a review of this vast literature is to document the progression and development of concepts and theories from an historical perspective. Such an approach reveals the increasing sophistication of theory, methodology, and analytic strategies over the decades, and also allows for the identification of those concepts that have stood the test of time and empirical inquiry. In one of the earlier conceptualizations of parenting, many researchers suggested that it was particular, fixed constellations of parenting behaviors, as opposed to the unique impact of any single parenting behavior, that contributed to child and adolescent competency or psychopathology. This idea originated in Baumrind's traditional paradigm, which conceptualized parenting as a combination of varying levels of behavioral control and affection (Maccoby & Martin, 1983) (see Figure 35.1). *Authoritative parenting*, for example, was initially conceptualized as high levels of parental affection combined with high levels of behavioral control or supervision (Baumrind, 1966). Over time, the authoritative parenting approach was modified by Steinberg and colleagues to include psychological autonomy, or democracy, to more fully account for adolescent healthy psychological development and school success (Steinberg, 1990; Steinberg, Lamborn, Dornbusch, & Darling, 1992). Importantly, authoritative parenting has been shown to be positively related to healthy adjustment in children and adolescents (Baumrind, 1966; 1967; 1989; Maccoby & Martin, 1983; Steinberg et al., 1992). Conversely, *authoritarian parenting*, which was defined as low levels of affection and high levels of behavioral control or harsh discipline, *permissive parenting*, which consisted of high levels of warmth and caring but low levels of behavioral control, and *neglecting parenting*, which was characterized by a combination of low levels of both warmth and control, have all been associated with child and

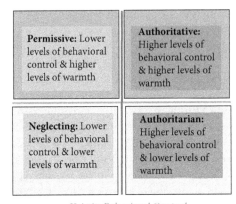

Permissive: Lower levels of behavioral control & higher levels of warmth	**Authoritative:** Higher levels of behavioral control & higher levels of warmth
Neglecting: Lower levels of behavioral control & lower levels of warmth	**Authoritarian:** Higher levels of behavioral control & lower levels of warmth

X Axis: Behavioral Control
Y Axis: Warmth and Responsiveness

Figure 35.1 Representation of parenting styles, based on Baumrind, 1966, and Maccoby & Martin, 1983.

adolescent internalizing and externalizing behaviors (Baumrind, 1989; Heller, Baker, Henker, & Hinshaw, 1996; Jewell & Stark, 2003).

It is worth noting, however, that much of the research using Baumrind's paradigm has focused on Caucasian families. When the paradigm is applied to ethnic minorities, some evidence emerges suggesting that *authoritarian* parenting may not have the same negative consequences demonstrated with Caucasian samples and may, in fact, be related to more positive outcomes (Garcia Coll, Meyer, & Brillon, 1995; Jambunathan, Burts, & Pierce, 2000). Although the findings are mixed, authoritarian parenting has been found to have positive associations with independence in African American children (Baumrind, 1972), mastery orientation in African American college students (Gonzalez, Greenwood, & Hsu, 2001), and school success in first-generation Chinese youth (Chao, 2001). Is it possible, then, that the negative connotation of authoritarian parenting in much of the literature is not accurate when applied to other cultural groups because of the various meaning attached to high levels of control. For example, the concepts of *chiao shun* (Chao, 1994) and *guan* (Tobin, Wu, & Davidson, 1989) in Chinese families, as well as no-nonsense parenting (Brody & Flor, 1998) in African American families, cast monitoring or control as indicative of parental love and concern. To overstate between-group differences at the expense of within-group variability, however, would be a mistake, as few of these studies actually examine the cultural meanings of parenting dimensions across racial/ethnic/cultural groups (Markus, Steele, & Steele, 2002; Takahashi, Ohara, Antonucci, &

Akiyama, 2002). Careful consideration of the ecological context of the parent–child dynamic (e.g., income, child peer group, acculturation status, immigrant status) often highlights important moderators of what may appear to be a "universal" association (see Steinberg, Dornbush, & Brown, 1992; Ang & Goh, 2006).

Although research based on Baumrind's typological approach to parenting has yielded an impressive body of findings linking parenting behavior to child outcome, this approach does not allow us to examine the impact of specific components (e.g., warmth) of the constellation on child adjustment (e.g., Bean, Bush, McKenry, & Wilson, 2003; Darling & Steinberg, 1993; Davidov & Grusec, 2006). In other words, the focus on the parenting composite (e.g., warmth plus firm control in authoritative parenting) and its relation to child outcome impedes the dismantling of the typology, by which it might be determined that an individual parenting behavior (e.g., warmth) is primarily associated with a specific child outcome (e.g., decreased levels of child externalizing symptoms) (Jones et al., 2008; McKee et al., 2008; McKee, Colletti, Rakow, & Forehand, 2008). As a result, some researchers have advocated for a more differentiated approach to examining the relation of specific parenting behaviors and specific child outcomes (e.g., Barber, 1997; Herman, Dornbusch, Herron, & Herting, 1997).

Consistent with this line of thinking, three behavioral dimensions, based on Schaefer's (1965) earlier work, have emerged as key elements of parenting: warmth (e.g., affection, involvement, supportiveness, attentiveness, acceptance); hostility (e.g., criticism, aggression, withdrawal); and behavioral control (e.g., monitoring, limit setting). Some of the behavioral indicators used to operationalize each of these constructs are presented in Table 35.1. Although some investigators have conceptualized warmth and hostility as opposite endpoints of the same spectrum (e.g., Child's Report of Parental Behavior Inventory; Schludermann & Schludermann, 1970), others have considered them to be distinct categories of behaviors (e.g., INTERACT Coding System; Dumas, 1984; 1986). With the latter approach, withdrawal, or the absence of warmth, and warmth are the opposing poles on the warmth continuum, and the absence of hostility and hostility are the opposing poles of the hostility continuum. Conceptualizing warmth and hostility as separate constructs provides richer information about parenting; it becomes possible, for example, to derive information about warmth, the absence of

Table 35.1 Behaviors Representative of Parental Warmth, Control, and Hostility

Warmth	Behavioral Control	Hostile Behavior
Acceptance	Behavioral directives	Aggression
Caring	Firm control	Anger
Involvement	Monitoring	Aversiveness
Positive affect	Rules	Criticism
Positive behavior	Supervision	Disapproval
Positive support	(Laxness)[2]	Intrusiveness
Praise		Irritability
(Withdrawal)[1]		Negative affect
		Overreactivity
		Verbal punishment

[1] Low levels indicate positive behavior
[2] Low levels indicate behavioral control

Reprinted from *Aggression & Violent Behavior*, Vol. 13, L. McKee, C. Colletti, A. Rakow, and R. Forehand, "Do parenting behaviors have specific or diffuse associations with externalizing and internalizing childhood problem behaviors?" pp. 201–215 (2008), with permission from Elsevier.

warmth—which is not necessarily the presence of aversive (i.e., hostile) parenting—*and* hostility.

Comparable to the body of research inspired by Baumrind's typologies, there are numerous empirical investigations linking specific parenting behaviors to child outcome. First, in terms of warmth, a number of studies have documented a link between relatively lower levels of parental warmth and negative child outcomes, particularly externalizing symptomatology (e.g., Jones, Forehand, Rakow, Colletti, McKee, & Zalot, 2008; Masten & Coatsworth, 1998; Shaw et al., 1998) and also the protective effects of relatively higher levels of warmth against the development of internalizing symptoms (e.g., Hammen, Shih, & Brennan, 2004; Muris, Meesters, & Van den Berg, 2003). In the case of parental behavioral control, lower levels have been associated with both child and adolescent externalizing symptoms, including conduct disorder, drug use, delinquency, and sexual risk behaviors (Chilcoat, Breslau, & Anthony, 1996; Dishion, Patterson, Stoolmiller, & Skinner, 1991; Li, Feigelman, & Stanton, 2000; Miller, Forehand, & Kotchick, 1999; Gray & Steinberg, 1999), and internalizing symptoms (e.g., Barber, 1996; Galambos et al., 2003; Kurdek & Fine, 1994). Finally, relatively higher levels of parental hostility have been associated with offspring externalizing behaviors (Conger, Ge, Elder, Lorenz, & Simons, 1994; O'Leary, Slep, & Reid, 1999; Patterson et al., 1992) and identified as a significant correlate of adolescent depressive symptoms (Buehler, Benson, & Gerard, 2006; see also Cole & McPherson, 1993).

In addition to the three well-studied parenting behaviors (i.e., warmth, hostility, and behavioral control), a number of other constructs, including parental overprotectiveness (Lieb, Wittchen, Hofler, Fuetsch, Stein, & Merikangas, 2000; Moore, Whaley, & Sigman, 2004) and psychological control (e.g., Barber & Harmon, 2002; Pettit et al., 2001; Rakow et al., 2011), have more recently been the subject of examination and merit further attention. Psychological control, for example, has been conceptualized as an intrusive and limiting form of control in which the child's autonomy is violated by manipulative guilt inducing and love withdrawal tactics (Barber, 2002). Despite the fact that psychological control has received relatively less attention in the literature, it has recently been linked with a broad array of adjustment problems in both the internalizing (depressed mood, anxiety, low self-confidence and low self-reliance) (Barber, 1996; Conger, Conger, & Scaramella, 1997; Pettit, Laird, Dodge, Bates, & Criss, 2001) and externalizing (delinquency, aggressive behaviors, and risky sexual behaviors) (Barber 1996, Barber & Harmon, 2002, Gray & Steinberg, 1999) clusters of behavior.

Furthermore, researchers studying minority families are increasingly focused on identifying and measuring constructs that are salient for particular cultural groups. For example, Smetana and colleagues (2004) used a conceptual and empirical approach to derive a family interaction scale for middle-income African American families. Principal component analyses revealed two types of composite variables. The first, pertaining to positive communication ability and style, consisted of items almost identical to the composite positive communication factors in Caucasian middle-class families (Smetana, Yau, Restrepo, & Braeges, 1991, as cited in Smetana, Abernethy, & Harris, 2000) while the second, reflecting "relational and reflected parents' supportiveness of their adolescents and adolescents' receptivity to their parents" (Smetana, Abernethy, & Harris, 2000, p. 469), emerged as unique from previous analyses of their Caucasian counterparts. Others have also suggested that the concepts of

respectfulness and obedience toward elders within African American families and "proper demeanor" or respect toward adults in Hispanic families is highly valued (e.g., Harwood, Miller, & Irizarry, 1995). In their examination of parent-adolescent conflict, for example, Dixon and colleagues (2008) created a measure of adolescent respect. Findings revealed that both African American and Hispanic mothers exerted more restrictive discipline (i.e., behavioral control) than the Caucasian mothers and that both African American and Latino adolescents showed higher levels of respect for authority than did their Caucasian counterparts.

In an effort to address the tension in the literature between the two primary theoretical and measurement approaches to understanding parenting and child socialization (i.e., broader parenting styles versus more specific parenting behaviors), Darling and Steinberg (1993) proposed an integrative model that incorporates both distinct but overlapping parenting attributes. Parenting practices are "behaviors defined by specific content and socialization goals" (p. 492). In the domain of academic achievement, for example, germane parenting practices may include attendance at parent-teacher conferences, establishing a specific homework routine with the child, and discussing assignments. Parenting *style*, alternatively, is distinguished as the "emotional climate in which the parents' behaviors are expressed" (p. 492) and includes tone of voice, body language, and temper outbursts as well as actual parenting practices through which children infer the parent's emotional attitude. Darling and Steinberg assert that both practices and style are influenced by parent socialization goals and values and that both influence child development but through different processes. Specifically, they theorize that parenting practices directly impact child outcomes while parenting style acts as a moderator of the relation between specific parenting practices and specific outcomes. Although the widespread adoption of such a model would increase the conceptual uniformity of the vast body of parenting research and allow for comparisons across studies, the current literature continues to represent a variety of orientations and numerous different operational definitions of parenting dimensions.

Tools for the Assessment of Parenting Behavior and Style
Questionnaires
Because an exhaustive review of all parenting assessment tools in questionnaire format is beyond

the scope of this chapter, we have chosen to focus on three representative measures. The choice of these three was guided by an attempt to include tools representing a range of developmental periods (toddlerhood, middle childhood, and adolescence) and reporters (parent versus child). The following assessment instruments are presented in detail and include a discussion of psychometric properties as well as the samples of parents and children with which the tools have been used: The Children's Report of Parental Behavior Inventory (CRPBI; Schaefer, 1965), The Alabama Parenting Questionnaire (APQ; Frick, 1991), and the Parenting Scale (Arnold, O'Leary, Wolff, & Acker, 1993). Because we realize that readers may be interested in a broader representation of parenting assessment tools than we can adequately review here, we refer them to two comprehensive resources. The first represents a review of 76 questionnaires, 27 interviews, and 33 observational systems all designed to assess discipline, nurturance, or both (Locke & Prinz, 2002). The second useful reference, mentioned in the previous section, is *The Handbook of Family Measurement Techniques* (Touliatos, Perlmutter, & Straus, 2001), which abstracts and provides examples of family measurement tools reported in the literature from 1929 through 1996.

Children's Report of Parental Behavior Inventory

In his initial publication describing the construction and psychometric properties of the Children's Report of Parental Behavior Inventory (CRPBI; Schaefer, 1965), Schaefer began by establishing one of the hypotheses motivating the development of a then-novel set of scales: "A child's perception of his parents' behavior," he wrote, "may be more related to his adjustment than is the actual behavior of his parents" (p. 413). Although the child-focused orientation had, by 1965, already produced volumes of research, and measurement of children's perceptions of parental behavior had proliferated, Schaefer criticized existing methodology for its inattention to "discrete components of parental behavior" (p. 414), its failure to differentiate maternal from paternal behavior, and its inability to discriminate the parent–child interaction from marital conflict and parental psychopathology. In an attempt to address these shortcomings, Schaefer factor analyzed psychologists' ratings of parental behavior. The two orthogonal dimensions revealed by the analyses—love versus hostility and autonomy versus control—were conceptualized as the

molar concepts in the guiding conceptual scheme (Schaefer, 1959). These higher-order factors were then defined by concepts such as ignoring, possessiveness, and lax discipline at an intermediate level of abstraction, and finally, 26 of these concepts were each described by 10 specific, observable parental behaviors. Inventory psychometrics were based on a sample of 165 12- to 14-year-old Caucasian girls and boys and a comparison group of 81 institutionalized delinquent Caucasian and African American boys aged 12 to 18 years. Analyses indicated sufficient internal-consistency reliability for each of the three groups (Caucasian boys, Caucasian girls, and institutionalized Caucasian and African American boys). Furthermore, discriminant validity was indicated by the following findings: 1) when the total scale score distributions for Caucasian boys and institutionalized Caucasian and African-American boys were compared, significant differences emerged for the majority of the 26 scales, and 2) when total scale score distributions for mothers and fathers as reported by the institutionalized sample were compared, significant differences again emerged for the majority of scales.

As stated, the original version of the CRPBI consists of 260 questions, 10 for each of 26 concepts, in which children and adolescents indicate whether each parent is "like," "somewhat like," or "not like" such statements as "Enjoys talking things over with me" and "Acts as though I am in the way." Since its inception, several shorter forms have been developed to decrease the administration time (Margolies & Weintraub, 1977; Raskin, Boothe, Reatig, Schulterbrand, & Odle, 1971; Schludermann & Schludermann, 1970). Although a recent review of the literature by Safford and colleagues (Safford, Alloy, & Pieracci, 2007) suggested that the 108-item version developed by Schludermann and Schludermann (1970) is the most commonly used revision, its 18 conceptually overlapping factors renders interpretation difficult. Alternatively, the 90-item scale (Raskin, Boothe, Reatig, Schulterbrand, & Odle, 1971) derived using a factor analysis of the original CRPBI resulted in 48 items that loaded onto three factors—Positive Involvement (Acceptance versus Rejection), Negative Control (Psychological Autonomy versus Psychological Control), and Lax Discipline (Firm Control versus Lax Control)—with adequate psychometrics including internal consistency ranging from .81 to .94. As with the original, children and adolescents rate scale items to indicate how similar the sample of parental behavior is to their perceptions of mother and father behavior. Finally, the 56-item CRPBI (Margolies & Weintraub, 1977) also appears to be an acceptable substitute for the original, as it yielded a factor structure approximating the Positive Involvement, Negative Control, and Lax Discipline dimensions with high test-retest reliability at one and five weeks, although the Lax Discipline evidenced less stability.

The CRPBI and its short-form revisions have been utilized widely with a range of child and adolescent respondents to examine the associations between parenting behaviors and myriad child outcomes. For example, the 108-item scale was administered to young adolescents (aged 11 through 14) from intact and recently divorced families to test a model positing parenting behaviors as mediators of the relation between inter-parental conflict and child adjustment (Fauber, Forehand, Thomas, & Wierson, 1990). It has also recently been utilized with African American adolescents from single mother-headed households to examine the impact of maternal behavior and coparent involvement on youth internalizing and externalizing behaviors (e.g., Sterrett, Jones, & Kincaid, 2009). Specific subscales of the original full-length version have also been employed in studies examining the relation between parenting behaviors and self-esteem (Ruiz, Roosa, & Gonzales, 2002) and internalizing and externalizing symptoms, broadly, and depression and conduct disorder, specifically (Dumka, Roosa, & Jackson, 1997; Manongdo & Ramirez Garcia, 2007) among Mexican American and Mexican immigrant children and families. The factor structure of the CRPBI and its revisions has been examined with a variety of samples, including children living with married and divorced parents (Teleki, Powell, & Dodder, 1982), Catholic school children in grades four through eight (Armentrout & Burger, 1972), French-speaking Belgian high school students (Renson, Schaefer, & Levy, 1968), Mexican American middle school children (Knight, Tein, Shell, & Roosa, 1992), and Canadian elementary and high school students (Kawash & Clewes, 1988).

In addition to the adolescent and child report forms of the CRPBI, some researchers have adapted the measure to be utilized by adults, both to gather retrospective reports of parent behavior and to assess parent self-report. Schwartz and colleagues (1985) examined the reliability and validity of the scales from the 108-item short form with a sample of college students, their siblings, and their mothers and fathers reporting on their own and each other's parenting behaviors; results revealed moderate internal consistency on all 18 subscales for all reporters and replicated the Schludermann and Schludermann (1970) factor structure for all raters. In another example, Fauber et al. (1990) examined both adolescent-report and parent-report on the Schludermann and Schluderman short form of the CRBPI. Both sources were utilized as indicators for the latent variable parenting constructs in a structural equation model testing the direct and indirect effects (via parenting behaviors) of marital conflict on adolescent adjustment in divorced and intact families.

Alabama Parenting Questionnaire

Like the CRPBI, the Alabama Parenting Questionnaire (APQ; Frick, 1991) was developed to address limitations of standardized questionnaires and observational assessments. Specifically noted in the rationale for constructing the measure was the limitation that a number of questionnaire tools in the research literature measure the emotional climate of the family (i.e., parenting style) as opposed to parent behaviors or practices. Although Schaefer's (1965) CRPBI is an exception, as it assesses distinct parenting behaviors, it does not include items tapping corporal punishment or monitoring and supervision, both of which have consistently been linked to child conduct problems (Frick, 1994). The APQ, a 42-item measure of parenting behaviors, yields five parenting constructs that have been associated with disruptive behaviors and delinquency in children and adolescents (Frick, Christian, & Wootton, 1999; Shelton, Frick, & Wootton, 1996):parental involvement, positive parenting, poor monitoring/supervision, inconsistent discipline, and corporal punishment. The APQ is available in parent- and child- "Global Report" forms and can also be administered to both parents and children via telephone interviews. Items on the Global Report forms are rated on a five-point scale to indicate how often the specific parenting behavior is performed in the home context, ranging from 1 (never) to 5 (always). During the telephone interviews, respondents are asked to respond to each item with his/her best estimate of the frequency (e.g., number of times) that behavior has occurred over the previous three-day period; item frequencies are collected over four telephone interview periods and averaged to compute scale scores.

Because the two positive parenting scales (i.e., involvement, positive parenting) have been found to be highly correlated across informant and assessment formats (e.g., $r = .45–.85$; Shelton et al., 1996) and because the three-item corporal punishment construct has been found to have low internal consistency ($\alpha = .49$) (Shelton et al., 1996), a three-factor model has been adopted and utilized by some researchers. Indeed, Hinshaw et al. (2000) reported that a first-order principal component analysis (PCA) of the APQ parent report with a middle childhood ADHD sample revealed a three-factor structure: positive involvement (16 items; e.g., praise, attends school meetings, helps with homework; $\alpha = .85$), negative/ineffective discipline (11 items; e.g., threatens to punish but doesn't, spanks child, lets child out of punishment early; $\alpha = .70$), and deficient monitoring (8 items; e.g., child out with friends unknown to you, child comes home one or more hours late; $\alpha = .72$). However, most recently, exploratory and confirmatory factor analyses of the Child Global Report version of the APQ with 1,219 10- to 14-year-old urban and rural German school children supported a five-factor solution consistent with the findings of Shelton et al. (1996), with only minor revisions to scale content (Essau, Sasagawa, & Frick, 2006). The findings thus far suggest that both the three-factor and five-factor solutions are acceptable, albeit with different samples in terms of child age and clinical versus community status.

In addition to explorations of the factor structure with distinct samples, several modifications to the original APQ have been suggested and tested. First, Clerkin et al. (2007) put forth a revision for use with preschool-aged children and examined the factor structure and psychometrics with a sample of 160 ethnically diverse children in urban public pre-kindergarten programs ($M_{age} = 4.47$; $SD = 0.62$). From the original version of the scale, the Alabama Parenting Questionnaire—Preschool Revision (APQ-PR) retained 32 items which loaded on three factors: positive parenting (12 items; $\alpha = .82$), negative/inconsistent parenting (7 items; $\alpha = .74$) and punitive parenting (5 items; $\alpha = .80$). Second, a nine-item parent report short form of the APQ was developed and validated with an Australian community sample of families with children ages four to nine years old (APQ-9; Elgar, Waschbusch, Dadds, & Sigvaldason, 2007). Principal components analysis of the original 42-item version of the scale supported a three-factor solution; the first factor was labeled positive involvement, the second, ineffective discipline, and the third, poor supervision; the remaining two domains that emerged, labeled involvement and punishment, were not supported.

The nine-item scale was constructed by drawing the three highest loading items from each of three factors. Internal consistency reliability of the APQ-9 was adequate, with the poor supervision factor evidencing the lowest internal consistency ($\alpha = .59$ in mothers; $\alpha = .63$ in fathers). The APQ-9 distinguished between parents of children with ODD or CD, who evidenced less consistent discipline and lower levels of supervision, and parents of children without a behavior disorder—but did not distinguish between parents of ADHD children and parents of non-ADHD children, suggesting the need for research to further explore the stand-alone validity of the shortened form (Elgar et al., 2007).

With regard to validity of the original APQ, data from several investigations suggest APQ scales are sensitive to interventions designed to modify parenting behaviors (e.g., August, Lee, Bloomquist, Realmuto, & Hektner, 2003; Feinfield & Baker, 2004; Lochman & Wells, 2002). Furthermore, a body of evidence supports the relation between problematic parenting practices as indexed by the APQ and conduct problems in clinic-referred children and adolescents (e.g. Chi & Hinshaw, 2002; Hinshaw, 2002; Frick, Christian, & Wootton, 1999) and non-referred children (e.g., Frick, Kimonis, Dandreaux, & Farell, 2003; Oxford, Cavell, & Hughes, 2003). While the use of child-report on the APQ, particularly in the telephone interview format, has raised some concern in the literature when used with younger samples (Shelton et al., 1996) Frick et al. (1999) reported increasing validity of child report in later childhood and adolescence.

The APQ has been used in research primarily as a measure of parenting practices associated with child and adolescent delinquent behavior in community and clinic-referred samples ranging in age from six to 17 years old; however, it has also been used with children as young as three (Brubaker & Szakowski, 2000) and as old as 18 (Stanger, Dumenci, Kamon, & Burstein, 2004). Furthermore, it has also been used to examine the relation between caregivers' self ratings of their parenting behavior and a) treatment outcome for children with Combined-type ADHD (Hinshaw et al., 2000), b) behavior problems in hearing-impaired children (Brubaker & Szakowski, 2000), and c) kindergartners' internalizing symptoms and peer relations (Cummings, Keller, & Davies, 2005).

The APQ was originally developed with clinical and community samples representative of some racial/ethnic and economic diversity (Shelton, Frick, & Wootton, 1996). Beyond the original study, the

APQ has been utilized in research with samples including ethnic minority families and representing a range of family income (e.g., Cummings et al., 2005; Hinshaw et al., 2000; McCoy, Frick, Loney, & Ellis, 1999; Stanger et al., 2004). Furthermore, August and colleagues (2003) examined the APQ factor structure with a culturally diverse urban sample: approximately 81 percent of the children were African American, 42 percent lived in single-parent households, and the mean family socioeconomic status fell in the low to middle-lower range. Similar to Hinshaw et al. (2000), factor analysis using principal components extraction revealed a three-factor structure (positive involvement, deficient monitoring, and harsh/ineffective discipline) as the best fit to the sample's data.

Parenting Scale

Consistent with the impetus behind the development of the CRPBI and APQ, the Parenting Scale (PS; Arnold, O'Leary, Wolff, & Acker, 1993) was developed by Arnold and colleagues as a brief measure of problematic discipline strategies for parents of young children (ages 18 to 48 months). Explicitly stated goals for the measure indicated that it should 1) build upon current empirical knowledge, 2) offer quick and easy administration, and 3) identify dysfunctional discipline strategies with the clinical goal of assisting in treatment and prevention of child externalizing problems. While the PS measures specific parenting behaviors, the format of the tool is distinct from the others reviewed in that its 30 items are rated on a seven-point scale, with each item anchored on one end with a parenting "mistake" and on the other end with its more adaptive counterpoint. For example, parents rate how closely their disciplinary strategy is linked to the mistake anchor (e.g., I coax or beg my child to stop) or the alternative effective strategy anchor (e.g., I firmly tell my child to stop). In this way, all parenting mistakes can be identified regardless of how often they occur, which would not be possible using a format based on frequency of encounters (e.g., How often do beg your child to stop?).

Principal components factor analysis with a sample of 168 mothers (65 of whom had presented for clinical services because of "extreme parenting difficulties") and their preschool-aged children yielded the following three factors: Laxness (11 items reflecting permissive discipline; $\alpha = .83$), Overreactivity (10 items related to irritability, anger, hostility; $\alpha = .82$), and Verbosity (7 items indicating use of lengthy, ineffective verbal strategies;

$\alpha = .63$) (Arnold et al., 1993). A Parenting Total Score was also computed by averaging the ratings of all items, including the four items that did not load on any factor, as a global index of parenting dysfunction ($\alpha = .84$). In addition to adequate internal consistency, reliability was further demonstrated with test-retest stability over a two-week period ($r = .79–.83$). PS scores also discriminated between clinic and non-clinic families, correlated strongly with Child Behavior Checklist scores, and related to observational measures of mother and child behavior. Despite the sound psychometrics of the PS in the Arnold et al. (1993) study, three subsequent studies of parents and their children ranging from two to 12 years old yielded a two-factor structure (Laxness and Overreactivity) as the best fit for the data (Collett, Gimpel, Greenson, & Gunderson, 2001; Harvey, Danforth, Ulazek, & Eberhardt, 2001; Irvine, Biglan, Smolkowski, & Ary, 1999).

While the original scale development and validation were performed with a relatively homogenous sample (middle income, well educated), the PS has subsequently been subjected to confirmatory and exploratory factor analyses with ethnically and socioeconomically diverse samples. First, Reitman and colleagues (2001) administered the PS to two primarily African American samples of mothers of 3.5–4.5-year-old children who attended a Head Start program. Confirmatory factor analysis with the first sample indicated that neither the original three-factor solution, nor a two-factor solution, consisting of the original Laxness and Overreactivity factors, fit the data. Exploratory factor analysis revealed a modified two-factor structure (also labeled Laxness and Overreactivity) with five items retained on each scale. The revised scales demonstrated adequate internal consistency ($\alpha = .70–.74$) and were highly correlated with the Arnold et al. (1993) Laxness and Overreactivity factors ($r = .91$ and .89) and Parenting Total Score ($r = .87$). The modified PS was then confirmed with a second sample of Head Start families and evidenced concurrent validity via significant correlations with measures of parenting stress and maternal depression. Second, Steele et al. (2005) examined the goodness of fit indices for both the original three-factor model (Arnold et al., 1993) and the two-factor model proposed by Reitman et al. (2001) with a sample of rural and urban low-income African American children ($M_{age} = 11.34$; SD = 1.82) from single-parent households. Results were consistent with the Reitman et al. (2001) two-factor model (Laxness and Overreactivity), which yielded a better fit to the data than the original model proposed by Arnold and colleagues (1993). Correlational data provided evidence of convergent validity for the Laxness dimension (when compared with Firm/Lax Control scale of the CRPBI), and also revealed an unexpected positive relation between the Overreactivity dimension and two measures of parental warmth (i.e., CRPBI Acceptance/Rejection subscale and Interaction Behavior Questionnaire total score), lending indirect support to Brody and Flor's (1998) concept of "no nonsense" parenting. Third, Karazsia and colleagues (2008) conducted a series of confirmatory factor analyses to test five different factor solutions presented in the literature with a community sample of 408 children ranging in age from two to 12 years old and their parents recruited from pediatric medical practices. The two-factor model proposed by Reitman et al. (2001) once again provided the best fit, and multi-group confirmatory factor analysis results suggested the factor structure was reliable and valid across ethnicity (Caucasian and African American), child gender, and child age.

The Parenting Scale and its multiple revisions have been utilized as a measure of parenting practices with parents and their children ranging from preschool (Arnold et al., 1993; Reitman et al., 2001) to elementary school (Harvey et al., 2001) and middle school (Irvine et al., 1999) age. Furthermore, the factor structure of the scale has been explored with economically, ethnically, and behaviorally diverse samples (Reitman et al., 1999; Karazsia et al., 2008; Steele et al., 2005) with various foci: 1) to test theoretical models linking disciplinary tactics and child psychopathology (e.g., Del Vecchio & O'Leary, 2006), 2) to identify determinants of parenting behaviors (e.g., Dorsey, Forehand, & Brody, 2007; Gerdes et al., 2007; Morawska & Sanders, 2007), and 3) to measure the impact of clinical interventions (e.g., Conners, Edwards, & Grant, 2007; Sanders, Turner, & Markie-Dadds, 2002).

In sum, all three of the measures reviewed—the CRPBI, the APQ, and the PS—share a similar guiding theoretical orientation and common goal of quantifying specific parenting behaviors (as opposed to a focus on a more global parenting style) in order to examine their relation to child adjustment. In addition, the factor structure of all three measures has been subjected to analysis in multiple studies subsequent to original scale development, and the psychometric qualities of each assessment tool are sound. Finally, the three questionnaires have been employed with minority as well as majority samples, reliably predict child/adolescent problem behavior,

and show sensitivity to changes in parenting as a result of intervention programs.

Although the measures reviewed share a number of qualities, each is also rendered distinct by relative strengths and limitations. For example, each scale was designed to target different age groups and, thus, utilizes different reporters. Because the CRPBI was developed with the intention of capturing the child's perception of parenting behaviors, its administration is limited to those children and adolescents with the cognitive capacity to read, comprehend, and respond to the item prompts. In contrast, the PS was designed explicitly to assess parenting of preschool children with the caregiving adult required to read and respond to the scale items. Straddling the two approaches, the APQ was developed to assess parenting from both the caregiver and child perspectives and targets a wide age range of children and adolescents (six to 17 years old). Although this approach increases the scale's applicability, it also implies that the same parenting behaviors are important across all age ranges.

Observational Measures

Because this section is not intended to represent an exhaustive review of all observational systems that include an assessment of parenting constructs, we refer the reader to several resources. First, Kerig and Lindahl's (2001) edited volume provides resources for clinicians and researchers interested in family observational coding systems: fourteen independent laboratories describe the theoretical bases for their systems, provide psychometric data, detail the content of the measure codes, and discuss the process for coder training. Second, as mentioned in the previous section, Locke and Prinz (2002) review 33 observational systems, all of which assess parental discipline, nurturance, or both in a variety of formats (e.g., structured versus unstructured tasks) and age-group referents. The choice of the three systems reviewed here was guided by an attempt to include tools that represent a range of developmental periods (toddlerhood, middle childhood, and adolescence), vary in terms of level of analysis (e.g., micro- versus macro-analytic) and content of the focal interactions, and are more or less suited to applied clinical work, research, or both. The following assessment instruments are presented in detail and include a discussion of psychometric properties as well as the samples of parents and children with which the tools have been used: The Behavioral Coding System (BCS; Forehand & McMahon, 1981), The Iowa Family Interaction Rating Scales (IFIRS; Melby et al., 1998), and The Family Interaction Coding System (FICS; Patterson, 1982; Reid, 1967; Reid, 1978) and its successor, the Family Process Code (Dishion, Gardner, Patterson, Reid, Spyrou, & Thibodeaux, 1987).

As will be evident from the review of the aforementioned instruments, relatively less attention has been focused on tool validation with ethnic minority groups. Just as with the questionnaire instruments, it is equally important, if not more so, that an interest in construct validity necessitates the determination that "... the meanings and interpretations associated with an inventory developed in one culture can validly accompany its use in another" (Ben-Porath, 1990, p. 28). When information was extant with regard to a coding system's applicability to an understudied group, it is noted. However, there are also a number of observational systems that either represent modifications of existing systems or novel contributions to the assessment repertoire that evidence increased sensitivity of code content and coder training to salient cultural nuances. Lindahl and Malik (2001), for example, developed the System for Coding Interactions and Family Functioning (SCIFF) explicitly to assess behavioral family functioning across Caucasian, Hispanic American, and African American ethnic groups. Alternatively, Smetana and colleagues (2000) modified the Global Coding System (Smetana, Yau, Restrepo, & Braeges, 1991), which was originally developed for use with divorced and intact middle-class Caucasian parents and their adolescents, to increase its sensitivity and relevance to middle-class African American families. Although both of these systems and others (e.g., Lefkowitz, Romo, Corona, Au, & Sigman, 2000; Taylor, Barnett, Longest, & Raver, 2009) represent progress, the validity of otherwise well-established coding systems across ethnic groups has yet to be empirically established.

Behavioral Coding System

The Behavioral Coding System (BCS; Forehand & McMahon, 1981) was developed for trained therapists and researchers to utilize in their assessment of parent–child interactions and specific parent and child behaviors, particularly as an integral component in delivering and testing the empirically supported parent training program for caregivers and their two- to six-year-olds, *Helping the Noncompliant Child* (*HNC*; Forehand & McMahon, 1981; McMahon & Forehand, 2003). The BCS may be used in both the clinic and home settings and, when utilized as a part of *HNC*, is administered as a pre-and post-treatment assessment, as well as throughout the intervention, both to measure parent mastery of skills and child compliance and non-compliance and to determine the timing of progression from one skill to the next (i.e., achievement of predetermined behavioral criteria). In the clinic setting, parents are provided with setting instructions to engage in two five-minute play sessions with their child while a trained coder observes from behind a one-way mirror. The first coding session, the "Child's Game," is essentially a free-play task in which parents are instructed to follow the child's lead and to refrain from imposing rules. The second coding session, the "Parent's Game," is a command situation during which the parent is advised to lead the child in activities of the parent's choosing. Six parent behaviors (i.e., verbal rewards, attends, questions, clear and unclear instructions, warnings, and time outs) and three child behaviors (i.e., compliance, noncompliance, and appropriateness of child behavior) are the primary targets of each observational period and are recorded in 30-second increments. The format of the score sheet permits the recording of the parent–child interaction or sequence of behaviors such that for any one interaction, a parent antecedent (e.g., parent issues command), child response (e.g., child complies with command), and parental consequence (e.g., parent provides verbal reward for compliance) may be documented. The BCS also includes an interval sampling component in which inappropriate child behavior is recorded if the child has a tantrum, aggresses, or uses deviant verbalizations at any point during each 30-second time period. At the conclusion of the clinic observation, data are summarized in the following ways: 1) for the Child's Game, rates per minute of each parent behavior and percentage of child inappropriate behavior are calculated, and 2) for the Parent's Game, the number of clear and unclear instructions coupled with the percentage child compliance to instructions, the percentage of parental attention (attends plus verbal rewards) following child compliance, and the total number of time-outs are calculated. As stated, the BCS may also be utilized to code parent and child interactions and behaviors during a naturalistic home observation (for additional information regarding the parental instructions, see McMahon and Forehand, 2003); however, because home observations are not always feasible and because observation sessions in the clinic and in the home have produced similar results (Peed, Roberts, & Forehand, 1977), clinic sessions may be sufficient.

A number of studies utilizing the BCS have established its sound psychometric qualities. First, an average inter-observer agreement of .75 or higher has been obtained for each of the coded parent and child behaviors (e.g., Forehand, Wells, & Griest, 1980; McMahon, Forehand, & Griest, 1981). Second, with regard to test-retest reliability, at least one investigation noted the stability and consistency of parent–child interactions in dyads assigned to a non-intervention condition (Peed, Roberts, & Forehand, 1977). Third, with respect to validity, the BCS discriminates between clinic-referred and non-referred children (Forehand, King, Peed, & Yoder, 1975; Forehand, Sturgis, et al., 1979; Griest, Forehand, Wells, & McMahon, 1980), and is sensitive to acute intervention effects and maintenance effects with clinical samples (e.g., Forehand, Griest, & Wells, 1979; Forehand, Sturgis, et al., 1979; Peed et al., 1977).

Iowa Family Interaction Rating Scales

The Iowa Family Interaction Rating Scales (IFIRS; Melby et al., 1998) were originally developed at Iowa State's Institute for Social and Behavioral Research as a global observation tool to assess individual-level qualities and behavior displays as well as relationship processes at the individual, dyadic, and group levels (Conger & Elder, 1994). Since its original conceptualization and implementation, the IFIRS has been utilized in myriad longitudinal research studies with diverse age groups (e.g., early adulthood, young adulthood, middle age) to study individuals and relationship processes in multiple contexts (e.g., interactions between parent–child, marital partners, siblings, friend pairs). The theoretical underpinnings of the system, drawn from social interactional, social contextual, and behavioral approaches, posit that relatively brief observations (15 to 30 minutes) of behavior and reciprocal interactions provide a window into dynamic systems that develop and unfold over time. In addition to providing information about the adjustment of the individual and the relationship observed, the snapshots are also purported to capture interaction styles and individual dispositions thought to be relatively stable, even "traitlike" (Melby & Conger, 2001, p. 34).

The IFIRS was initially intended for use in coding interactions during discussion-based tasks. In that case, interviewers provide instructions to the family regarding the content of the discussion, set up videotaping equipment, provide cue cards for the family highlighting the discussion topics, and then leave the room for the conversation to occur without the intrusion of the interviewer's presence. Although the topics range from project to project (see Melby & Conger, 2001, for additional information), the *parent–child discussion task* and the *family problem solving task* both involve a triadic interaction (two parents and one child or one parent and two children). The foci of the *parent–child discussion task* include enjoyable shared activities, parental expectations and rules, and recent child disappointments or accomplishments. During the *problem-solving task*, family participants are instructed to discuss and work toward resolution of a problem that causes family conflict (e.g., chores, sibling fighting) (Melby & Conger, 2001).

Recently, however, the system has been adapted to capture interactions between parents and their young children (ages two to eight) during a *parent–child teaching* task and/or *clean-up task*. In both five- to 10-minute activity-based tasks, the interviewer provides materials and instructions for the parent–child dyad, and a camera operator tapes the interaction to ensure that movement out of a still-camera range is captured. In the *teaching task,* the parent is instructed to help the child with a puzzle or other activity too difficult for the child to complete independently. In the *clean-up task*, the interviewer instructs the child to put away the toys in provided containers, and the parent is told to offer whatever assistance he or she deems necessary.

Highly trained observers who review and code the videotaped interactions are taught to document behavior without making inferences about motivation or intent on the part of the focal subject(s). Ratings are influenced by the frequency and intensity of behaviors; additional considerations when determining how to categorize a behavior or relationship process include affect, context, and proportion. However, given the macro-level focus of the IFIRS, the scoring of the interaction does not produce actual frequencies of behaviors or exchanges (e.g., in the form of rates per minute) or duration of observed behaviors.

The fifth edition of the IFIRS manual describes 60 behavioral scales, most of which are rated from one to nine, with the odd-numbered points as anchors. For example, many of the scales are scored as: *1= not at all characteristic, 3 = mainly uncharacteristic, 5 = somewhat characteristic, 7 = moderately characteristic,* and *9 = mainly characteristic* of the individual, dyad, or group observed. The scales are designed to rate behaviors and interaction processes at four levels (individual characteristics, dyadic interactions, dyadic relationships, and group interactions) and are divided into three categories encompassing items from one or more of the four levels. The General Interaction Rating Scales category is the largest and contains 35 scales that rate observed behaviors in all types of interaction tasks at the individual, dyadic, and group levels. Most pertinent to the assessment of parenting behaviors, however, are the two specialty scales: The Parenting Scales (15 scales) and the Problem-Solving Scales (10 scales). The Parenting Scales are all assessed at the dyadic interaction level and are used to rate childrearing behaviors as observed and reported by parents and children. For example, the Child Monitoring scale rates the parent's demonstration of knowledge regarding the child's activities and whereabouts. The Problem-Solving Scales utilize individual and group level ratings to assess problem-solving behaviors during a family or group task. Agreement on Solution, for example, rates the resolution and satisfaction with the resolution of a problem discussed. The number and type of scales employed varies depending upon the observation task and number of participants. In the case of the activity-based tasks with parents and young children, 31 scales are appropriate for use in coding observations of the clean-up task, and 35 scales can be applied to the puzzle task.

Numerous studies have employed the IFIRS to examine the relation between parenting behaviors and child/adolescent healthy adaptation and psychopathology: depending upon the focus of the investigation, researchers have employed single scales and/or composite observational measures (e.g., Conger, Ge, Elder, Lorenz, & Simons, 1994) and have utilized ratings as indicators of latent constructs (e.g., Melby, Conger, Ge, & Warner, 1995). A wide range of relations have been explored with the IFIRS, from the impact of economic stress on parenting and adolescent adjustment (Conger et al., 1992; 1993) to family processes and characteristics related to adolescent alcohol use (Conger, Rueter, & Conger, 1994), academic performance (Melby & Conger, 1996), and problem-solving (Rueter & Conger, 1995; Rueter & Conger, 1998). More recently, parent behaviors in a free-play interaction task with their preschool-aged male children were demonstrated to be significantly related to teacher ratings of boys' problem behaviors (Davenport, Hegland, & Melby, 2008). As with the BCS (Forehand & McMahon, 1981), the IFIRS has also been used to document change in parenting behaviors and affect targeted by interventions (Spoth, Redmond, Haggerty, & Ward, 1995; Spoth, Redmond, & Shin, 1998).

The psychometric properties of the system have been shown to be acceptable. A technical report summarizing over 50 published works that utilize the IFPRS (Franck & Anderson, 2004) documented inter-rater reliability (as measured by ICCs) ranging from .33 (father's warmth toward youth summed across two tasks; Fletcher, Elder, & Mekos, 2000) to .97 (solution quality; Rueter & Conger, 1995). Additionally, evidence presented for convergent validity in the form of positive correlations between observational scales and self report (see Ge et al., 1996, for an example) and discriminant validity in the form of negative correlations between scales that theoretically should be inversely related (e.g., see Simons, Lorenz, Wu, & Conger, 1993) further attest to the scale's sound properties.

Although the IFIRS scales were originally developed for use with primarily lower- to middle-class intact Caucasian families living in rural communities, they have also been used by trained African American coders to characterize caregiver relationship quality and nurturant-involved parenting among African American families in rural and suburban Iowa and Georgia (Conger, Wallace, Sun, Simons, McLoyd, & Brody, 2002). Furthermore, in an attempt to investigate the relations between coder training and rater bias, Melby and colleagues (2003) examined observations by African American and Caucasian coders on 30 IFIRS scales when characterizing two videotaped interactions, one of an African American mother–child dyad and the second of a Caucasian mother–child dyad. Although the majority of scales showed a reduction in rater bias as training progressed, race-related bias did not seem to decrease with training; in particular, main effects for coder race were evident for scales assessing emotional state (i.e., positive mood, sadness, anxiety, avoidant). Accordingly, although more research on the role of race in observational coding using the IFIRS, as well as other observational coding systems, is necessary before the nuances detailed in the Melby et al. study can be fully understood, the findings suggest that conventional training techniques may not be adequate to reach reliable consensus on what may be more culturally mediated interpretations of behavior and affect.

Family Interaction Coding System and Family Process Code

The Family Interaction Coding System (FICS; Patterson, 1982; Reid, 1967; Reid, 1978) is a microanalytic coding system developed by researchers at the Oregon Social Learning Center (OSLC) as a portable observational tool designed to characterize the aggressive behaviors, as well as their antecedents and consequences, of children with conduct disorder (Patterson, 1982). Patterson, Reid, and colleagues revised the system six times over three years, yielding a coding system that captures the unfolding processes of family aggression, measures change in interaction styles, and identifies entry points for intervention.

The FICS is composed of 29 code categories, approximately half of which identify aversive behaviors (e.g., destructiveness, noncompliance, humiliate) and half that recognize pro-social or neutral actions (e.g., play, laugh, physical positive). Originally, the system developers intended to observe family members in the natural home setting without formal rules for structuring the session; however, in order to maximize actual interactions (e.g., all family members in the same room) and limit interruptions (e.g., telephone calls, visitors), several boundaries were established. During the session, which varies in length depending upon number of family members present, each member is identified as the "target" and coded during two separate five-minute periods. For each 30-second period, approximately five interaction units can be recorded to document the behavior of the target as well as the precipitant or response behaviors of another family member. Although data are coded continuously, each 30-second period is divided into six-second intervals, which precludes differentiating recurrence of a behavior from duration. For example, a child crying for 24 seconds is coded as three instances of "Cry" (Patterson, 1982). Behaviors then are summed over the coding period and expressed as rate per minute. A Total Aversive Behavior (TAB) score may also be calculated by summing 14 of the 29 code categories.

Because of the limitations of the FICS, particularly with regard to its inability to denote duration of behaviors, modifications to the system were made by a group of researchers at the OSLC to capture interactions in real time. Research and modification yielded a new coding system called the Interaction Coding System (ICS; Moore, Forgatch, Mukai, Toobert, & Patterson, 1978), which included 26 behaviors (14 aversive, seven neutral, and five positive). Observers used voice recorders to capture onset and sequencing of behaviors as well as frequency and duration, and transcriptions of recordings were then transferred to coding sheets divided

into 30-second increments. Despite the improvements of the ICS, several deficiencies in both the FICS and ICS remained. Specifically, neither system was sufficiently sensitive to pro-social behavior or changes in affect. As a result, an additional iteration of the system called the MOSAIC was developed, which culminated, finally, in the Family Process Code (Dishion, Gardner, Patterson, Reid, Spyrou, & Thibodeaux, 1987).

The Family Process Code, like its predecessors, is designed to code interactions between the targets of the observation period and their family members. Two features of the FPC, however, distinguish it from prior systems. First, a unique coding device, referred to as the OC-3, is utilized by the observers to record data. Second, each interaction is coded with regard to the following five factors. First, the initiator of the behavior is denoted. Second, an activity code is designated to characterize the general context of the interaction as Work, Play, Read, Eat, Attend, or Unspecified. Third, 25 content codes, divided among five independent categories (Verbal, Vocal, Nonverbal, Physical and Compliance Behavior), are available to document the actual behavior. Fourth, the recipient of the behavior is denoted. Finally, the valence or emotional flavor of the exchange is rated based upon observations of body language and other nonverbal gestures, tone of voice, and inflection (Dishion, Gardner, Patterson, Reid, Spyrou, & Thibodeaux, 1987).

The psychometric properties of the FICS have been extensively evaluated. First, Patterson and colleagues have considered several factors that may influence the reliability and validity of data collected over a number of observational sessions. The first is the possibility that family members would display less pro-social and more deviant behavior in later versus earlier sessions (i.e., the habituation hypothesis), which would result in smaller correlations of behavior over time. Several attempts to examine possible habituation effects, however, revealed no significant changes in mean levels of parent or child behavior across sessions for any of the coded behaviors (Johnson & Bolstad, 1973; Patterson & Cobb, 1971; Patterson & Cobb, 1973). The second consideration was how many samplings of behavior would be necessary to produce a stable estimate of behavior, particularly given that the contextual variables may change substantially across coding sessions. Several sets of findings suggest that behavioral scores based on 60 to 120 minutes of data provide stable estimates (Jones et al., 1975; Patterson, 1982). Utilizing these findings, Patterson (1974a) demonstrated adequate reliability of the Total Aversive Behavior (TAB) score based on at least 60 minutes of observational data per subject from at least six sessions conducted over two weeks. With regard to validity, the FICS significantly differentiates families with an antisocial child, characterized by higher levels of a coercive interaction style, from control families (Burgess & Conger, 1978; Patterson, 1976; 1981b; Reid, Taplin, & Lorber, 1981). It also shows convergent validity with a parent-report questionnaire measure of child deviant behavior both before and after intervention (Patterson, 1974b).

The FICS was used from 1968 until 1977 as a data collection tool for families treated at the OSLC. The sample is characterized by target children and adolescents (median age seven to eight years old, largely male), referred primarily for antisocial behavior, approximately 80 percent of whom were from working-class families. The modified FPC has been utilized in research, again primarily with male children and adolescents identified as engaging in delinquent behaviors. Dishion and colleagues (1991), for example, used the FPC to examine longitudinal relations among poor disciplinary practices (i.e., nattering and punishment density, or the proportion of negative relative to positive parent–child interactions), parental monitoring, youth antisocial behavior, and deviant peer affiliation in a sample of predominantly Caucasian preadolescent boys. In fact, the group of scientists employing the FPC has provided the field with a body of research documenting the trajectories of young antisocial males (Patterson, Forgatch, Yoerger, & Stoolmiller, 1998; Vuchinich, Bank, & Patterson, 1992), detailing both the temperamental, familial and peer antecedents (Capaldi, Peers, Patterson, & Owen, 2003; Dishion, Patterson, Stoolmiller, & Skinner, 1991; Patterson, DeGarmo, & Knutson, 2000) and the effects of clinical intervention on that trajectory (Patterson & Forgatch, 1995).

As with the questionnaire measures reviewed, each of the observational systems has relative strengths and challenges, depending upon the purpose of the assessment. One perhaps obvious advantage of all the observational tools reviewed is that they provide a window into dynamic relationship systems and thus reach beyond what may be captured at an individual-focused level of analysis. Furthermore, some have argued that the observational methodology aids in the identification of mechanisms linking parenting behaviors and a host of child outcomes and may, in fact, capture behaviors that would otherwise be outside the researchers' purview (Brody & Stoneman, 1990; Cowan & Cowan, 1990). The BCS, for example, is designed to assess the contingency of child compliance / noncompliance to parental directives, and in turn, the parental response to child compliance / noncompliance in a structured parent-directed analog task, which produces both frequency and sequencing data that may be difficult to measure with a questionnaire-based tool. Similarly, both the IFIRS and the FPC are sensitive to the emotional valence or flavor of the parent–child exchanges; this component of parenting style, again, may be more difficult to access with other tools.

Despite the advantages afforded by the observational methodology, there are also significant challenges to the validity and integrity of the data collected. Patterson (1982), for example, warns against systematic observer bias and observer presence effects, the latter which he characterizes as nonspecific reactivity (e.g., "orienting" behaviors that typically habituate over the observation period(s)) and impression management (e.g., attempts to perform in socially desirable ways that are less likely to habituate). Explicit coder training procedures and reliability checks to prevent "coder drift" combined with coder "blindness" to research hypotheses may address observer bias. With regard to observer presence effects, Patterson suggests that "habitual models of interaction provide powerful constraints for familial interactions" (1982, p. 56) such that even mothers aware that they were being observed because of reports of child abuse hit their children during sessions at 10 times the rate of comparison mothers (Reid et al., 1981). In sum, the decision to employ an observational approach to the measurement of parenting style and behaviors must be driven by a cost-benefit analysis of the time and resource investment required by the methodology relative to the type and quality of the data, the choice of the appropriate unit of analysis (e.g., the individual versus the family unit; macro versus micro level codes), and the practicality of the tool for repeated measurement in longitudinal research and clinical work.

Focus on Parenting Relationships

Thus far, we have focused almost exclusively on the "what" and "how" in our discussion of the assessment of parenting without much regard for the "who" and "why." If we return briefly to our starting point and the theoretical framework on which our discussion of parenting has been built, we are reminded by an ecological systems perspective that parents (and parenting behaviors and style) are influenced by a host of inter- and intra-personal, social, economic, and cultural factors. The three sections that follow, then, serve to highlight three such factors—marital relationships, coparenting relationships, and parent psychological and physical health—that are integral considerations in the assessment of parenting.

With regard to the "who" of parenting, it may be concluded by research presented herein that the constructs examined, such as warmth and responsiveness, and the methodologies employed may have been informed by the implicit assumption, borne out by decades of research privileging the mother–child relationship, that the child's primary caregiver is the mother. Only one of the questionnaire measures discussed extensively here, the CRPBI, explicitly denotes the father's contribution by requiring the child or adolescent reporter to consider the behaviors of mothers *and* fathers separately. Needless to say, even when the mother is the primary or sole caregiver, other adults with whom she is in relationship (e.g., child's biological father and/or stepfather, mother's parents and other kin, mother's residential and non-residential romantic partners, mother's friends and coworkers) make contributions to the child's caregiving environment, directly and/or indirectly.

We begin with a brief description of research linking the quality of the marital relationship, typically characterized in the literature by the mother's relationship with the child's biological father (i.e., intact families), to parenting behavior and the quality of the parent–child relationship. Then, we proceed to a brief discussion of coparenting—a construct related to marital relationship quality in intact families—that is also of relevance to divorced and single parents, as it captures how well two caregivers coordinate their childrearing efforts. Finally, we turn to a brief discussion of the role of parental mental and physical health in parenting. Building upon our own research, we review the research on maternal depression as an example of the link between parental mental health and parenting, and on maternal HIV/AIDS as an example of the link between parental physical health and parenting.

Marital Relationship Quality

As with the bulk of work on parenting, research on the link between the quality of the marital relationship between two parents and parenting behavior has focused almost entirely on Caucasian, middle-class families and the mother–child (rather than the father–child) relationship. Thus, it must be clarified up front that the generalizability of much of this work to families that are separated/divorced, headed by a single parent, lower income, or ethnically diverse is questionable. With this caveat in mind, the interrelatedness of marital quality, parenting, and parent–child relationship quality has been well established, and several seminal reviews highlight advancements in this literature (e.g., Erel & Burman, 1995; Fincham, 1998). Collectively, this work suggests that the link between marital and parent–child relationship quality may best be characterized by a "spillover" of negative mood, affect, and behavior between the two individuals in a marital relationship to the parent–child relationship (Erel & Burman, 1995). Numerous mechanisms by which such spillover is posited to occur have been detailed elsewhere, but range from more family systems–oriented processes such as "scapegoating," or the process by which parents distract themselves from their own problems by focusing on the problems of their child (e.g., Minuchin, Rosman, & Baker, 1978; Vogel & Bell, 1960), to more behavioral processes such as modeling, by which children model the maladaptive patterns of their parents' marital conflict in the parent–child relationship (e.g., Easterbrooks & Emde, 1988). In addition, marital conflict is thought to directly influence the quality of both maternal and paternal parenting behaviors, such that more discordant parents are more likely to evidence disrupted and less consistent parenting behaviors (e.g., Frosch & Mangelsdorf, 2001; Kitzmann, 2000). Regardless of the specific mechanism by which marital conflict spills over into compromises in parenting, most agree that the interrelationship of the marital discord, parenting disruptions, and parent–child conflict is cyclical: namely, the strain of marital discord may compromise the extent to which a parent can be available to a child, which negatively impacts the parent–child relationship, which, in turn, likely exacerbates the strain on the marital relationship (e.g., Emde & Easterbrooks, 1985; Kerig, Cowan, & Cowan, 1993).

Although much more work has focused on marital quality in intact families, the quality of the relationship between ex-marital partners has also been implicated in parenting behavior and, in turn, child adjustment (e.g., Fauber, Forehand, Thomas, & Wierson, 1990; also see Kelly, 2000, for a review). Of note, although it was once believed that divorce in and of itself was harmful for children, evidence now more clearly suggests that it is not divorce that necessarily compromises children's outcomes. Rather, it is more likely that parents continue to experience conflict after their divorce, which compromises their parenting relationship and the quality of parenting behaviors as well (Fauber et al., 1990).

Building upon the well-established link between marital quality, parenting behavior, and parent–child relationship quality, a thorough assessment of parenting behavior should also consider the quality of the parents' marital relationship. Although a comprehensive review of potential measures is beyond the scope of the current chapter, others (e.g., Fincham, 1998) have provided detailed guidelines for researchers and clinicians interested in the assessment of various domains of the marital relationship as they may relate to child development. Like parenting, the assessment of marital quality is nuanced and includes measures of different domains of the marital relationship (e.g., satisfaction, conflict, communication), as well as different methods to assess these domains (e.g., self-report, observational) (Fincham, 1998).

Next, we turn to the literature on the interrelationship of coparenting, or the process by which two individuals coordinate childrearing efforts, and parenting behavior. The following section highlights a rich body of research examining a range of parenting relationships, from coparenting in traditional marital relationships to coparenting after divorce and, finally, to coparenting dyads that characterize a growing number of ethnic minority families in the United States, including single mothers coparenting with the child's biological father, grandmothers, and other extended family members.

Coparenting

As previously noted, one focus of many married couples is childrearing. Although the quality of the marital relationship is associated with how well two individuals work together in their role as parents to coordinate their childrearing responsibilities (i.e., coparenting), coparenting has been shown to be a unique construct of relevance to a broader sample of families than only those which are intact. Interest in the study of "coparenting" can be traced to the advent of family systems theory and the subsequent increase in attention to triadic (e.g., mother, father, child) interactions, rather than dyadic (e.g., mother–child) interactions alone (Minuchin, 1974; 1985). Coparenting is conceptualized as a triadic, or whole family, level of analysis within the family system (Belsky et al., 1996). Thus, the construct of coparenting is typically characterized along varying dimensions of supportive interactions, or the extent to which two parents support and reinforce one another's parenting activities, as well as unsupportive interactions, or the level of inconsistent parenting, amount of conflict, and extent to which parents undermine one another's parenting efforts.

Initially, coparenting research focused on Caucasian parents who were divorced or in the process of divorcing (e.g., Ahrons, 1981; 1983). Prevention and intervention researchers were interested in identifying the processes that characterized the parenting efforts of divorcing parents who potentially had very negative feelings for one another, but managed to successfully parent together. Not surprisingly, divorcing parents who were more supportive of one another's parenting efforts and goals, despite their feelings for one another, had children who adjusted more favorably to the divorce (e.g., Coiro & Emery, 1998). Subsequently, researchers turned their attention to intact or two-parent Caucasian families and the processes by which married parents successfully parented together (e.g., McHale, 1995; 1997). Again, children whose parents evidenced more support for one another's parenting efforts, and less conflict regarding parenting goals and values, evidenced fewer difficulties.

Given the importance of coparenting for predicting child and adolescent adjustment, research on Caucasian families has also focused on predictors of successful coparenting relations (e.g., Stright & Bales, 2003). With regard to sociodemographic factors, a higher level of education has been associated with more stable levels of coparenting support than lower levels of education (e.g., Stright & Bales, 2003). Parental psychosocial variables are predictive of the quality of the coparenting relationship as well. Parents with fewer psychological problems are more likely to have coparenting relationships that are initially more positive and stay more positive over time compared to parents with more severe psychological problems (e.g., Stright & Bales, 2003; Moore, Florsheim, & Butner, 2007). Finally, parents who experience lower levels of stress enjoy more positive coparenting relations (e.g., Belsky, Crnic, & Gable, 1995).

Although leaders in the coparenting field have highlighted that coparenting is a construct of relevance to diverse (Feinberg, 2002) and single-parent (Van Egeren & Hawkins, 2004) families, far less attention has been devoted to the role of coparenting in ethnic minority or single-parent families (see Jones, Zalot, Foster, Sterrett, & Chester, 2007, for a review). In our own work, young adult and adult (age range = 28 to 40 years old) African American single mothers of preadolescent children were asked whether another adult or family member assisted them with childrearing and, if so, were asked to identify the most important person. Only 3 percent of mothers failed to identify another adult or family member who assisted with childrearing; the majority identified the child's maternal grandmother (31%) or biological father (26%). Others identified a maternal aunt (11%), the child's older sister (11%), and a diverse group of other relatives and non-relatives, such as friends and neighbors (Jones, Shaffer, Forehand, Brody, & Armistead, 2003).

Building upon the coparenting literature more broadly, the quality of the relationships that these single mothers evidenced with their nontraditional coparents was associated with both maternal and child adjustment (Jones et al., 2003; Jones et al., 2005a). African American single mothers who reported experiencing greater conflict regarding childrearing issues with their nontraditional coparents had children who reported greater internalizing and externalizing difficulties than mothers who reported less conflict. The link between mother-coparent childrearing conflict and child adjustment was shown to be mediated, in part, by parenting behavior, as well as maternal mental health (Dorsey et al., 2007; Jones, et al., 2003). Mothers who experienced more conflict with their coparents experienced more compromises in parenting, as well as more depressive symptoms which, in turn, negatively affected child outcomes. Finally, research to date also suggests that the quality of the coparenting relationship may affect other contextual factors that influence the parenting behaviors of African American single mothers, including neighborhood risk. For example, African American single mothers who reside in riskier neighborhoods are more likely to appropriately heighten their monitoring behavior in the context of better relationships with their nontraditional coparents than in the context of poorer ones (Jones et al., 2005b).

With regard to the assessment of coparenting, it is important to note here that the methods utilized to assess coparenting in ethnic minority families lag behind the methods generally considered to be gold standard in the broader coparenting literature. For example, the research on the role of nontraditional coparents in African American single mother families has focused almost exclusively on mother-report of the quality of her relationship with her nontraditional coparent (e.g., Forehand & Jones, 2003;

Jones et al, 2005a; Jones et al., 2005b). In contrast to the broader coparenting literature with Caucasian two-parent families, the other adults or family members identified by mothers as coparents have not been included in the previously mentioned work. Rather, all data have been based on the mother's report of the coparent and the coparenting relationship. Moreover, while children have been included, the bulk of prior research has not considered their reports of the quality of the mother-coparent relationship or their perception of the nontraditional coparents' involvement (see Sterrett, Jones, & Kincaid, 2009, for a notable exception). Given the triadic nature of the coparenting construct, assessment of the single mother alone ignores two important contributors to the coparenting relationship, namely, the coparent and the child.

In extant coparenting research focused on ethnic minorities, young adult and adult African American single mothers in prior research have been asked about two relatively broad domains of the coparenting relationship: support and conflict regarding childrearing activities. State-of-the-field coparenting measures, however, include much richer assessments of the coparenting relationship, including division of childrearing labor and parental relationship quality (e.g., Belsky & Hsieh, 1998). Coparenting is now considered a multidimensional (rather than two-dimensional) construct, including more nuanced aspects of communication between parents, such as verbal sparring (e.g., hostility), conflict (e.g., arguing), and disparagement (e.g., undermining) (e.g., McHale, Kuersten-Hogan, Lauretti, & Rasmussen, 2000).

Finally, in addition to self-report methods, the broader coparenting literature includes observation and coding of interactions between married parents and children, which we did not include in our work on adult African American single mothers parenting with their nontraditional coparents. Observational methods have been notably underutilized in research on African American families in general (McLoyd et al., 2000), and the research on coparenting in African American families headed by a young adult or adult single mother is not an exception.

We cannot leave a review of the interrelationship of coparenting and parenting behavior without mentioning the dearth of research in this area on families with gay and lesbian parents. Such families have not been the focus of much empirical research; therefore, we know relatively little about their coparenting relationships or the links between coparenting and parenting in same-sex parents (see Patterson & Farr, 2011, for a recent review). That said, the literature that has begun to accumulate suggests that the experiences of these families may be more similar than different from families with opposite-sex parents (see Tasker, 2005, for a review). In part, this may be due to the growing number of "diverse" family structures in the United States, including some we have already discussed (e.g., parents coparenting after divorce, single mothers coparenting with grandmothers, etc.). More research is needed, however, to determine how the unique factors facing same-sex parents may influence their coparenting efforts and, in turn, parenting behavior and the quality of the parent–child relationship. Among these unique factors are the extent to which children are aware of lesbian and gay relationships and homophobia (Tasker, 2005).

Focus on Other Parent Variables in Child Assessment

Returning to the "why" of parenting—why parents utilize particular strategies and/or create specific caregiving environments—entails consideration of a vast number of influences, including, but not limited to, parental beliefs and values, parent knowledge of and expectations for child development, economic and social pressures, cultural norms and the prevailing folk psychological theories, child and parent temperament and the relative fit between the two, and siblings. However, no discussion of factors shaping parental behavior would be complete without mention of several key intrapersonal variables, namely, parental psychological and physical health or, alternatively, psychopathology, disease, and disability.

Scientific interest in parental psychopathology as it relates to parenting behaviors and offspring outcomes has burgeoned in the last two decades from its origins in developmental and clinical science in the 1950s and 1960s (Zahn-Waxler, Duggal, & Gruber, 2002). The nature of the questions and the sophistication of the models and methodologies utilized have evolved from simple correlational relations (assumed to be unidirectional) to include the gene x environment interactions and correlations that typify the intergenerational transmission of mental illness. The general pattern detected for any number of psychiatric diagnoses fits the following oversimplified formula: parental psychological symptoms and/or clinical disorders affect parenting behaviors and the family environment and are reflected in the quality of the parent–child relationship, which, in turn,

has bearing on concurrent and long-term offspring outcomes (Zahn-Waxler, Duggal, & Gruber, 2002). Specificity of the formula, however, is required to delineate which domains of parenting are affected by the particular psychiatric symptoms or disorders under study and to highlight the relative influence of specific parenting deficits or excesses on domains of child development. Important considerations in the specificity of the model include the timing, chronicity, and severity of the parental mental illness, the age and developmental stage of the child, and the availability and quality of additional coparenting relationships.

Major Depressive Disorder and HIV/AIDS: Two Cases in Point

Given that depression is 1) one of the leading causes of disease-related disability worldwide (Murray & Lopez, 1997), 2) estimated to be twice as common in women than in men (see Nolen-Hoeksema, 1987, for a review), and 3) related to childbirth and childrearing (Zahn-Wexler, Duggal, & Gruber, 2002), the likelihood of exposure to parental depression in a child's lifetime is relatively high (Zahn-Wexler et al., 2002). Data amassed over the past half century indicate that children and adolescents living with depressed caregivers are at substantial risk for a variety of developmental and adjustment difficulties across the lifespan (Goodman & Gotlib, 1999). Such difficulties include, but are not limited to, an increased risk for psychiatric disorders, increased guilt, problems with attachment, and sub-optimal interpersonal functioning (Beardslee, Versage, & Gladstone, 1998)

The detrimental effects of parental depression on their offspring are apparent in infancy. Some work suggests that newborns of mothers with significant depressive symptoms exhibit a profile or symptom cluster of dysregulation in their behavior, physiology, and biochemistry; these infants are typified by elevated norepinephrine and cortisol levels, lower vagal tone, and disrupted sleep patterns (Field, 1995). Additionally, newborns of clinically depressed mothers have shown poorer performance on a measure of motor tone and activity levels and increased irritability when compared to newborns of non-depressed mothers (Abrams, Field, Scafidi, & Prodromidis, 1995). Finally, infants of depressed caregivers evidence atypical frontal lobe activity (reduced left versus right activity) during interactions with mothers and non-depressed familiar adults (Dawson, Frey, Panagiotides, Yamada, Hessl, & Osterling, 1999).

Research on offspring at the preschool age suggests that attachment security is compromised when a caregiver suffers from depressive symptoms: toddlers born to mothers with both intermittent and chronic depressive symptoms and decreased sensitivity were more likely to be classified as having insecure attachments (Campbell et al., 2004). Additionally, research focused on behavioral and cognitive indices of dysfunction indicate that preschool offspring of mothers with severe or chronic depressive symptoms evidence higher levels of child behavior problems of both a hostile/aggressive and anxious/withdrawn nature, as well as lower vocabulary test scores (Alpern & Lyons-Ruth, 1993; Brennan, Hammen, Andersen, Bor, Najman, & Williams, 2000).

School-aged children and adolescents of depressed parents evidence more physical and psychological problems, including greater depression and anxiety, than do controls. They also exhibit significantly more difficulty with academics, school discipline, and social interactions than same-age peers with never-depressed caregivers (Anderson & Hammen, 1993; Billings & Moos, 1983). In terms of actual diagnostic outcomes, children and adolescents of depressed parents are three times more likely to qualify for any affective disorder, six times more likely to be diagnosed with Major Depressive Disorder (Downey & Coyne, 1990), and at least two to five times more likely to experience externalizing disorders than are controls (Billings & Moos, 1983; Cummings & Davies, 1994).

The literature reviewed here, which is reflective of the literature at large, has focused primarily on depressed mothers. Relatively recently, however, investigators have begun to include depressed fathers in their explorations of the effects of parental depression on child psychological health. A recent meta-analysis by Kane and Garber (2004), for example, suggests that outcomes for preschool, middle childhood, and adolescent-aged offspring of depressed fathers are very similar to those reported for children of depressed mothers.

Over the past ten to twenty years, empirical attention has shifted from establishing the risk of parental depression to exploring potential pathways or mechanisms of risk. What factors are responsible for predisposing children of depressed parents to abnormal development? In a developmentally sensitive, integrative theoretical model of the transmission of depression from parent to offspring, Goodman and Gotlib (1999) suggest four mechanisms: (1) heritability of depression; (2) innate dysfunctional neuroregulatory mechanisms; (3) exposure to negative maternal cognitions, behaviors, and affect; and (4) the stressful context of the child's life. The first two proposed mechanisms are primarily genetic in nature, while the latter two focus on interpersonal and environmental contributions.

The third transmission pathway highlighted by Goodman and Gotlib (1999) concerns the offspring's exposure to maternal maladaptive cognitions, behaviors, and affect. Several distinct but interrelated lines of research suggest that two parallel processes inflate the offspring's risk: (1) depressed mothers are unable to parent effectively because of their distorted cognitions, behaviors, and affect and, thus, are unable to meet their children's social and emotional needs; and (2) a social learning dynamic unfolds, by which children acquire the cognitions, behaviors, and affect exhibited by their depressed mothers. Both the inadequate parenting and the depressogenic style characteristic of depressed caregivers negatively impact the development of the offspring's cognitive and social skills and restrict the child's range of affect and behavior, placing the youth at a heightened risk for the development of depression and other psychopathology.

Each piece of the proposed process constituting the third mechanism has garnered convincing empirical support. First, it is well established that depressed adults demonstrate more negative self-perceptions and cognitions (e.g., Beck, 1967, 1987; Ingram, Miranda, & Segal, 1998), including negative views of themselves as parents (Gelfand & Teti, 1990), more negative behaviors in interactions with others (Jacobson & Anderson, 1982), and more sad and irritable affect (Hops, Biglan, Sherman, Arthur, Friedman, & Osteen, 1987). This cognitive, behavioral, and affective symptomatology makes it difficult for depressed mothers to provide the requisite sensitivity, stimulation, and affectionate contact with their infants (e.g., Egeland & Farber, 1984; Fleming, Ruble, Flett, & Shaul, 1988; Livingood, Daen, & Smith, 1983), adequate scaffolding to support the social and cognitive developmental transitions of their toddlers and preschool-aged children (e.g., Breznitz & Friedman, 1988; Goldsmith & Rogoff, 1997), or the general emotional support and consistent discipline integral to the social and academic success of their school-aged children and adolescents (e.g., Hops et al., 1987; Sheeber, Hops, & Davis, 2001; Patterson, 1982).

In a meta-analytic review of 46 observational studies, Lovejoy, Graczyk, O'Hare, and Neuman (2000) highlight specific deficits and excesses typical of depressed mothers. Namely, the authors report a positive association between maternal depression and both of these parenting behaviors: (1) negative or coercive parenting (i.e., threatening gestures, negative facial expressions, criticism, and negative commands) and (2) disengaged parenting (i.e., decreased vocalization, responsiveness, positive affect, and participation in play). In addition, some support emerged for a negative association between maternal depression and positive parenting behaviors (i.e., positive tone of voice, affectionate gestures, expression of pleasure and enthusiasm, and praise). Research suggests that offspring are not only negatively affected by the parenting deficiencies and emotional unavailability of their caretakers, but that they also are at a higher risk for dysfunction because they model or internalize their caretakers' negative cognitions, behaviors, and affect. As an illustrative example, school-aged children and adolescents of depressed parents are more likely to be self-critical, have lower self-concepts, and report more negative cognitive styles when compared to children of well mothers (Garber & Robinson, 1997); they are, in effect, potentially modeling their mothers' negative cognitions.

Given the research suggesting that caregiver depression affects the quality of the parent–child relationship and is associated with particular problematic parenting behaviors and patterns, which in turn impact offspring cognitive, emotional and, social health, and well-being, clinicians and developmental scientists may wish to explore parental depression as one of many contributors to individual differences in parenting beliefs, style, and behaviors. A number of self-report screening tools, structured and semi-structured interviews, and clinician-rated measures are available (see Nezu, Nezu, McClure, & Zwick, 2002, for a review of depression assessment tools). Both the Beck Depression Inventory—II (BDI-II; Beck, Steer, & Brown, 1996) and the Center for Epidemiological Studies Depression Scale (CES-D; Radloff, 1977) are psychometrically sound self-report questionnaires that provide an assessment of depressive symptoms with suggested clinical cut-offs. Often cited as the gold standard for clinical diagnosis of Major Depressive Disorder in research are standardized clinical interviews, such as the Structured Clinical Interview for *DSM-IV* Axis I Disorders (SCID-I; First, Spitzer, Gibbon, & Williams, 1997) and the Diagnostic Schedule for Affective Disorders and Schizophrenia (SADS; Endicott & Spitzer, 1978). Clinician-rated measures, such as the Hamilton Rating Scale for Depression (HRSD, Hamilton, 1960), have also been utilized widely in psychiatric and primary care settings as well as in research protocols.

In addition to psychological illness, many parents face physical health problems as well, and a review of procedures for assessing parenting would not be complete without a discussion of how parenting behavior may be influenced by parental physical illness. Although there are literatures on a range of parental illnesses (see Armistead, Klein, & Forehand, 1995, for a review), our focus here will be on HIV/AIDS, since it is a primary focus of our own work and an illness confronting more families, particularly ethnic minority families, in the United States than many realize.

Early in the HIV/AIDS epidemic, women were rarely diagnosed with the disease; however, today women account for more than 25 percent of all new HIV/AIDS diagnoses, and African American women are especially affected by the disease (Corea, 1992; Centers for Disease Control and Prevention [CDC], 2005). Sixty-four percent of the women currently living with HIV/AIDS are African American, a rate that is more than three times that of the percentage (19%) of Caucasian women living with the illness (CDC, 2005). Moreover, HIV/AIDS is the leading cause of death for African American women aged 25 to 34 years and the third-leading cause of death for African American women aged 35 to 44 years (CDC, 2005). Both of these time periods represent prime childbearing and childrearing years for women.

Given that many African American women with HIV/AIDS are also mothers, the extent to which the illness influences maternal parenting behavior and the quality of the mother–child relationship is of critical public health importance for understanding the psychosocial adjustment of the growing number of African American youth being raised by mothers infected with the disease (e.g., Forehand et al., 2002; Stein, Rotheraum-Borus, & Lester, 2007; Tompkins & Wyatt, 2008). Collectively, the findings of research to date suggest that maternal HIV/AIDS may disrupt both maternal parenting behaviors and the quality of the relationship that the infected mother has with her child. For example, infected mothers have been shown to evidence compromises on both the warmth/support and monitoring/control domains of parenting behaviors (e.g., Forehand et al., 2002; Tompkins & Wyatt, 2008).

Importantly, the extent to which HIV compromises maternal parenting and mother–child relationship quality depends on several factors related to parenting in general, but also on factors specific to HIV/AIDS in particular, including whether or not mothers disclose their illness to their children (e.g., Antle et al., 2001; Armistead, Tannenbaum, Forehand, Morse, & Morse, 2001; Shaffer et al., 2001). A mother's disclosure of any chronic or life-threatening illness to her child is often accompanied by some level of hesitation or worry regarding the child's reaction (Semple et al., 1993; Tompkins, Henker, Whalen, Axelrod, & Comer, 1999). Mothers with HIV/AIDS may be particularly worried about their children learning of their illness given the stigma associated with the disease, as well as the methods of transmission (Armistead et al., 2001; DeMatteo et al., 2002; Kirshenbaum & Nevid, 2002). Perhaps for these reasons, maternal disclosure of HIV/AIDS has not been associated with the same sense of relief experienced by mothers who disclose other life-threatening, but less stigmatized diseases, such as cancer (Armistead, Morse, Forehand, Morse, & Clark, 1999; Levy et al., 1999). It is not surprising then that only about one-third of mothers with HIV/AIDS disclose their disease to their children, even as the disease progresses and death becomes more imminent (Armistead et al., 2001; Murphy, Koranyi, Crim, & Whited, 1999; Murphy, Steers, & Stritto, 2001).

Although initial work suggested that maternal HIV/AIDS had negative effects on parenting and, in turn, on child adjustment, more recent work suggests that the impact of maternal HIV/AIDS is more heavily dependent on whether the child is aware of the mother's illness and the extent to which the mother–child relationship has been compromised by the illness. For example, in our own work we have found that children who knew of their mothers' diagnosis, but who viewed their relationships with their mother as more warm and supportive, evidenced fewer adjustment difficulties than children who viewed their relationships with their mother as less warm and supportive (Jones et al., 2007). In contrast, mother–child relationship quality was not associated with the psychosocial adjustment of children who were not aware of their mothers' diagnosis.

In addition to the direct effects of HIV/AIDS on parenting behaviors, we have already noted that maternal depressive symptoms are associated with a range of compromises in parenting behaviors (e.g., Lovejoy et al., 2000). Of note, mothers with HIV/AIDS evidence higher levels of depressive symptoms than demographically matched non-infected women (e.g., Jones, Beach, Forehand, & the Family Health Project Research Group, 2001; Miles, Gillespie, & Holditch-Davis, 2001), Accordingly, more attention needs to be devoted to understanding whether parenting behavior may be particularly compromised in mothers who are both HIV positive and depressed; however, research to date is mixed (e.g., Cho, Holditch-Davis, & Miles, 2008; Jones et al., 2008; McKee et al., 2007).

Before concluding our discussion of maternal HIV/AIDS, it should be noted that far less attention has been devoted to paternal than maternal illness in general and the area of HIV/AIDS is no exception. As previously noted, the focus on mothers in the HIV/AIDS literature is likely due in large part to increased awareness of HIV/AIDS as a disease affecting women over the past two decades. In addition, the focus on mothers has come from the increased rates of HIV/AIDS among African American women of childbearing age, drawing attention to the disproportionate number of African American youth in this country being raised by an infected mother. Of course, as with the parenting literature more generally, our understanding of the impact of HIV/AIDS on parenting depends on greater attention to infected fathers and paternal parenting as well.

Our review of the associations of parental depression and parental HIV/AIDS with parenting, and, in turn, child adjustment provides evidence for the role that parental psychiatric and physical health can play in parenting. Any assessment or intervention focused on parenting behaviors should, therefore, consider these and other intrapersonal variables (e.g., personality) and their impact on parenting behaviors, coparenting relationships, and offspring development.

Conclusions and Future Directions

Throughout this chapter, a number of theoretical and methodological contributors to the assessment of parenting style and behaviors have been articulated, accompanied by an in-depth exploration of three questionnaire-based measures and three observational tools. Despite the surprising similarity in the molar constructs that have been the focus of parenting research and assessment both over time and across theoretical orientations, decisions regarding which of several hundred assessment tools to employ require thoughtful consideration. Nezu and colleagues (2009) highlight key issues and relevant questions to guide those decisions, including: (1) the goals of the assessment (e.g., case formulation versus outcome evaluation), (2) the intended target of the assessment (e.g., considerations of age and ethnicity), (3) the value assigned to a given assessment strategy (i.e., the likelihood that the tool will yield the desired information in the context of a cost-benefit analysis), and (4) the source of the information (e.g., the parent or the child versus a neutral observer). From the vast collection of assessment tools available, both a behavioral scientist seeking to explore the relation between parental monitoring and adolescent alcohol use and a clinician evaluating the outcome of a behavioral parent training intervention can be served well.

Despite advances in the assessment of parenting over the last five decades, a number of challenges in the field remain. First, as we have highlighted throughout the chapter, the cultural relevance and sensitivity of assessment tools initially designed for use with a specific segment of the population (e.g., Caucasian middle class parents) may or may not yield meaningful or valid data when utilized with subjects outside that population segment. This issue, of course, is particularly relevant to research and clinical assessments targeting historically understudied groups (e.g., working-class African and Hispanic Americans, same-sex parents). Although advances in the modification, creation, and validation of culturally appropriate parenting assessment tools have bolstered the confidence with which claims about the relation between parenting behaviors and child development can be made, a host of questions remain unanswered and beg continued study. For example, how have class and ethnicity been confounded in the study of parenting? Furthermore, how might within-group factors, such as acculturation status and racial socialization, impact the validity of a tool designed for an ethnic minority group?

Second, there are distinct advantages and disadvantages to the sheer number of assessment tools available and the disparate ways in which parenting behaviors have been defined. Although there is considerable overlap in the broad underlying parenting dimensions measured by different tools, the ways different research groups have operationalized these dimensions vary greatly. For example, warmth may be defined in one measure by displays of positive affect and in a different measure by an index of involvement in the child's life (see Table 35.1). As a result, drawing conclusions across studies regarding the effects of parental warmth on child disruptive behavior, for example, can prove difficult. Some might argue, then, that the field would benefit from widespread adoption of a model (such as the one proposed by Darling and Steinberg [1993]) that may serve to increase both the conceptual uniformity and operational definitions of parenting constructs. In a related vein, the situational specificity of particular parent–child exchanges could be further refined. Warmth, for example, may be appropriate in some contexts (e.g., dinnertime conversation) but counter-indicated (depending upon the definition) if a child has just engaged in an aggressive act at which time limit setting or a combination of warmth and behavioral control may be a more appropriate response. A similar argument is made by Caron et al. (2006) in that the "effects of at least some parenting behaviors may differ as a function of the interaction task or larger context in which the behavior occurs" (p. 35). Although observational assessment tools may have a relative advantage over questionnaire-based tools in this regard, a number of studies have averaged across different tasks, perhaps masking subtleties, or examined only one task; as a result, cross-study comparisons examining the same parenting behavior but during different tasks render interpretation difficult.

Because parenting is a complex, multifaceted, and dynamic process, the assessment tools designed to capture such a wide range of nuanced behaviors must be sophisticated and sensitive to micro- and macro-level interactions. And because no one tool can meet the demands of every researcher and practitioner, the assessment pendulum swings between generality and specificity, and the field, as a whole, balances the advantage of a grand, unifying theory with the allure of methods and measures that can address the needs of increasingly specialized interest groups.

References

Abrams, S. M., Field, T., Scafidi, F., & Prodromidis, M. (1995). Newborns of depressed mothers. *Infant Mental Health Journal, 16*(3), 233–239.

Ahrons, C. (1981). The continuing coparental relationship between divorced spouses. *American Journal of Orthopsychiatry, 51*, 415–428.

Ahrons, C. (1983). Predictors of paternal involvement post-divorce: Mothers' and fathers perceptions. *Journal of Divorce, 6*, 55–69.

Alpern, L., & Lyons-Ruth, K. (1993). Preschool children at social risk: Chronicity and timing of maternal depressive symptoms and child behavior problems at school and at home. *Development and Psychopathology, 5*, 371–387.

Anderson, C. A., & Hammen, C. L. (1993). Psychosocial outcomes of children of unipolar depressed, bipolar, medically ill, and normal women: a longitudinal study. *Journal of Consulting and Clinical Psychology, 61*, 448–454.

Ang, R. P., & Goh, D. H. (2006). Authoritarian parenting style in Asian societies: A cluster-analytic investigation.

Contemporary Family Therapy: An International Journal, 28, 131–151.

Antle, B. J., Wells, L. M., Goldie, R. S., DeMatteo, D., & King, S. M., (2001). Challenges of parenting for families living with HIV/AIDS. *Social Work, 46,* 159–169.

Arcia, E., Reyes-Blanes, M. E., & Vazquez-Montilla, E. (2000). Constructions and reconstructions: Latino parents' values for children. *Journal of Child and Family Studies, 9,* 333–350.

Armentrout, J. A., & Burger, G. K. (1972). Children's reports of parental child-rearing behavior at five grade levels. *Developmental Psychology, 7,* 44–48.

Armistead, L. P., Klein, K., & Forehand, R. (1995). Parent physical illness and child functioning. *Clinical Psychology Review, 15,* 409–422.

Armistead, L. P., Morse, E., Forehand, R., Morse, P. S., & Clark, L. (1999). African American women and self-disclosure of HIV infection: Rates, predictors, and relationship to depressive symptomatology. *AIDS & Behavior, 3,* 195–204.

Armistead, L. P., Tannenbaum, L., Forehand, R., Morse, E., & Morse, P. S. (2001). Disclosing HIV status: Are mothers telling their children? *Journal of Pediatric Psychology, 26,* 11–20.

Arnold, D. S., O'Leary, S. G., Wolff, L. S., & Acker, M. M. (1993). The Parenting Scale: A measure of dysfunctional parenting in discipline situations. *Psychological Assessment, 5,* 137–144.

August, G. J., Lee, S. S., Bloomquist, M. L., Realmuto, G. M., & Hektner, J. M. (2003). Dissemination of an evidence-based prevention innovation for aggressive children living in culturally diverse, urban neighborhoods: The Early Risers effectiveness study. *Prevention Science, 4,* 271–286.

Bank, L., Forgatch, M. S., Patterson, G. R., & Fetrow, R. A. (1993). Parenting practices of single mothers: Mediators of negative contextual factors. *Journal of Marriage & the Family, 55,* 371–384.

Barber, B. K. (1996). Parental psychological control: Revisiting a neglected construct. *Child Development, 67,* 3296–3319.

Barber, B. K. (1997). Introduction: Adolescent socialization in context—the role of connection, regulation, and autonomy in the family. *Journal of Adolescent Research, 12,* 5–11.

Barber, B. K. (2002). Violating the self: Parental psychological control of children and adolescents. In B. K. Barber (Ed.), *Reintroducing parental psychological control* (pp. 3–13). Washington, DC: American Psychological Association.

Barber, B. K., & Harmon, E. L. (2002). Violating the self: Parental psychological control of children and adolescents. In B. K. Barber (Ed.), *Intrusive parenting: How psychological control affects children and adolescents* (pp. 15–52). Washington, DC: American Psychological Association.

Barber, B. K., & Olsen, J. A. (1997). Socialization in context: Connection, regulation, and autonomy in the family, school, and neighborhood, and with peers. *Journal of Adolescent Research, 12,* 287–315.

Barber, B. K., Olsen, J. E., & Shagle, S. C. (1994). Associations between parental psychological and behavioral control and youth internalized and externalized behaviors. *Child Development, 65,* 1120–1136.

Barber, B. K., Stolz, H. E., & Olsen, J. A. (2005). Parental support, psychological control, and behavioral control: Assessing relevance across time, method, and culture. *Monographs of the Society for Research in Child Development, 70*(4), 1–137.

Baumrind, D. (1966). Effects of authoritative control on child behavior. *Child Development, 37,* 887–907.

Baumrind, D. (1972). An exploratory study of socialization effects on black children: Some black-white comparisons. *Child Development, 43,* 261–267.

Baumrind, D. (1978). Parental disciplinary patterns and social competence in children. *Youth & Society, 9,* 239–251.

Baumrind, D. (1989). Rearing competent children. In W. Damon (Ed.), *Child development today and tomorrow* (pp. 349–378). San Francisco: Jossey-Bass.

Bean, R. A., Bush, K. R., McKenry, P. C., & Wilson, S. M. (2003). The impact of parental support, behavioral control, and psychological control on the academic achievement and self-esteem of African American and European American adolescents. *Journal of Adolescent Research, 18,* 523–541.

Beardslee, W. R., Versage, E. M., & Gladstone, T. R. (1998). Children of affectively ill parents: A review of the past 10 years. *Journal of the American Academy of Child & Adolescent Psychiatry, 37,* 1134–1141.

Beck, A. T. (1967). *Depression: Causes and treatment.* Philadelphia, PA: University of Pennsylvania Press.

Beck, A. T. (1987). Cognitive models of depression. *Journal of Cognitive Psychotherapy, 1,* 5–37.

Beck, A. T., Steer, R. A., & Brown, G. (1996). *Beck Depression Inventory—II manual.* San Antonio, TX: The Psychological Corporation.

Belsky, J., Crnic, K., & Gable, S. (1995). The determinants of coparenting in families with toddler boys: Spousal differences and daily hassles. *Child Development, 66,* 629–642.

Belsky, J., & Hsieh, K. H. (1998). Patterns of marital change during the early childhood years: Parent personality, coparenting, and division-of-labor correlates. *Journal of Family Psychology, 12,* 511–528.

Belsky, J., Putnam, S., & Crnic, K. (1996). Coparenting, parenting, and early emotional development. *New Directions in Child Development, 74,* 45–55.

Belsky, J., & Jaffee, S., R. (2006). The multiple determinants of parenting. In D. Cicchetti & D. J. Cohen (Eds.), *Developmental psychopathology, 3: Risk, disorder, and adaptation* (2nd ed.; pp. 38–85). Hoboken: John Wiley & Sons Inc.

Ben-Porath, Y. (1990). Cross-cultural assessment of personality: The case for replicatory factor analysis. In J. N. Butcher & C. D. Spielberger (Eds.), *Advances in personality assessment, vol. 8.* (pp. 27–48). Hillsdale, NJ: Lawrence Erlbaum Associates, Inc.

Billings, A. G., & Moos, R. H. (1983). Comparisons of children of depressed and nondepressed parents: A social-environmental perspective. *Journal of Abnormal Child Psychology, 11,* 463–485.

Bradshaw, C. P., Glaser, B. A., Calhoun, G. B., & Bates, J. M. (2006). Beliefs and practices of the parents of violent and oppositional adolescents: An ecological perspective. *The Journal of Primary Prevention, 27,* 245–263.

Brennan, P. A., Hammen, C., Andersen, M. J., Bor, W., Najman, J. M., & Williams, G. M. (2000). Chronicity, severity, and timing of maternal depressive symptoms: Relationships with child outcomes at age 5. *Developmental Psychology, 36,* 759–766.

Breznitz, Z., & Friedman, S. L. (1988). Toddler's concentration: Does maternal depression make a difference? *Journal of Child Psychology and Psychiatry, 29,* 267–279.

Brody, G. H., & Flor, D. L. (1998). Maternal resources, parenting practices, and child competence in rural, single-parent African American families. *Child Development, 69,* 803–816.

Brody, G. H., & Stoneman, Z. (1990). Sibling relationships. In I. E. Sigel & G. H. Brody (Eds.), *Methods of family research:*

Biographies of research projects: Vol. 1. Normal families (pp. 182–212). Hillsdale, NJ: Erlbaum.

Bronfenbrenner, U. (1979). Contexts of child rearing: Problems and prospects. *American Psychologist, 34,* 844–850.

Brubaker, R. G., & Szakowski, A. (2000). Parenting practices and behavior problems among deaf children. *Child & Family Behavior Therapy, 22,* 13–28.

Buehler, C., Benson, M. J., & Gerard, J. M. (2006). Interparental hostility and early adolescent problem behavior: The mediating role of specific aspects of parenting. *Journal of Research on Adolescence, 16,* 265–292.

Burchinal, M. R., Roberts, J. E., Zeisel, S. A., & Rowley, S. J. (2008). Social risk and protective factors for African American children's academic achievement and adjustment during the transition to middle school. *Developmental Psychology, 44,* 286–292.

Burgess, R. L., & Conger, R. D. (1978). Family interaction in abusive, neglectful, and normal families. *Child Development, 49,* 1163–1173.

Campbell, S. B., Brownell, C. A., Hungerford, A., Spieker, S. J., Mohan, R., & Blessing, J. S. (2004). The course of maternal depressive symptoms and maternal sensitivity as predictors of attachment security at 36 months. *Development And Psychopathology, 16,* 231–252.

Capaldi, D. M., Pears, K. C., Patterson, G. R., & Owen, L. D. (2003). Continuity of parenting practices across generations in an at-risk sample: A prospective comparison of direct and mediated associations. *Journal of Abnormal Child Psychology, 31,* 127–142.

Caron, A., Weiss, B., Harris, V., & Catron, T. (2006). Parenting behavior dimensions and child psychopathology: Specificity, task dependency, and interactive relations. *Journal of Clinical Child & Adolescent Psychology, 35,* 34–45.

Caspi, A., McClay, J., Moffitt, T., Mill, J., Martin, J., Craig, I. W., et al. (2002). Role of genotype in the cycle of violence in maltreated children. *Science, 297*(5582), 851–854.]

Centers for Disease Control and Prevention (2005). *HIV/AIDS Surveillance Report, 2005. Vol. 17.* Atlanta: US Department of Health and Human Services, CDC; 2006:1–46.

Chao, R. K. (1994). Beyond parental control and authoritarian parenting style: Understanding Chinese parenting through the cultural notion of training. *Child Development, 65,* 1111–1119.

Chao, R. K. (2001). Extending research on the consequences of parenting style for Chinese Americans and European Americans. *Child Development, 72,* 1832–1843.

Chi, T. C., Hinshaw, S. P. (2002). Mother–child relationships of children with ADHD: The role of maternal depressive symptoms and depression-related distortions. *Journal of Abnormal Child Psychology, 30,* 387–400.

Chilcoat, H. D., Breslau, N., & Anthony, J. C. (1996). Potential barriers to parent monitoring: Social disadvantage, marital status, and maternal psychiatric disorder. *Journal of the American Academy of Child & Adolescent Psychiatry, 35,* 1673–1682.

Cho, J., Holditch-Davies, D., & Miles, M. (2008). Effects of maternal depressive symptoms and infant gender on the interactions between mothers and their medically at-risk infants. *Journal of Obstetric, Gynecologic, & Neonatal Nursing: Clinical Scholarship for the Care of Women, Childbearing Families, & Newborns, 37,* 58–70.

Clarke, G. N., Lewinsohn, P. M., & Hops, H. (1990). *Adolescent coping with depression course.* Eugene, OR: Castalia Publishing.

Clerkin, S. M., Marks, D. J., Policaro, K. L., & Halperin, J. M. (2007). Psychometric Properties of the Alabama Parenting Questionnaire-Preschool Revision. *Journal of Clinical Child & Adolescent Psychology, 36,*19–28.

Coiro, M., & Emery, R. (1998). Do marriage problems affect fathering more than mothering? A quantitative and qualitative review. *Clinical Child & Family Psychology Review, 1,* 23–40.

Cole, D. A., & McPherson, A. E. (1993). Relation of family subsystems to adolescent depression: Implementing a new family assessment strategy. *Journal of Family Psychology, 7,* 119–133.

Coll, C., & Pachter, L. M. (2002). Ethnic and minority parenting. In M. H. Bornstein (Ed.), *Handbook of parenting: Vol. 4: Social conditions and applied parenting* (2nd ed., pp. 1–20). Mahwah, NJ: Lawrence Erlbaum Associates Publishers.

Collett, B. R., Gimpel, G. A., Greenson, J. N., & Gunderson, T. L. (2001). Assessment of discipline styles among parents of preschool through school-age children. *Journal of Psychopathology & Behavioral Assessment, 23,* 163–170.

Collins, W. A., Maccoby, E. E., Steinberg, L., Hetherington, E. M., & Bornstein, M. H. (2000). Contemporary research on parenting: The case for nature and nurture. *American Psychologist, 55,* 218–232.

Conger, R., & Elder, G. (1994). *Families in troubled times: Adapting to change in rural America.* New York: Aldine De Gruyter.

Conger, R. D., Ge, X., Elder, G. H., Lorenz, F. O. & Simons, R. L. (1994). Economic stress, coercive family process, and developmental problems of adolescents. *Child Development, 65,* 541–561.

Conger, R. D., Wallace, L. E., Sun, Y., Simons, R. L., McLoyd, V. C., & Brody, G. H. (2002).Economic pressure in African American families: A replication and extension of the family stress model. *Developmental Psychology, 38,* 179–193.

Conger, R. D., Conger, K. J., Elder, G. H., Lorenz, F. O., Simons, R. L., & Whitbeck, L. B. (1992). A family process model of economic hardship and adjustment of early adolescent boys. *Child Development, 63,* 526–541.

Conger, R. D., Conger, K. J., Elder, G. H., Lorenz, F. O., Simons, R. L., & Whitbeck, L. B. (1993). Family economic stress and adjustment of early adolescent girls. *Developmental Psychology, 29,* 206–219.

Conger, K. J., Conger, R. D., & Scaramella, L. V. (1997). Parents, siblings, psychological control, and adolescent adjustment. *Journal of Adolescent Research, 12,* 113–138.

Conger, R. D., Rueter, M. R., & Conger, K. J. (1994). The family context of adolescent vulnerability and resilience to alcohol use and abuse. *Sociological Studies of Children, 6,* 55–86.

Conners, N. A., Edwards, M. C., & Grant, A. S. (2007). An evaluation of a parenting class curriculum for parents of young children: Parenting the strong-willed child. *Journal of Child & Family Studies, 16,* 321–330.

Corea, G. (1992). *The invisible epidemic: The story of women and AIDS.* New York: Harper Collins.

Cowan, C. P., & Cowan, P. A. (1990). Who does what? In J. Touliatos, B. F. Perlmutter, & M. A. Straus (Eds.), *Handbook of family measurement techniques* (pp. 447–448). Beverly Hills, CA: Sage.

Cummings, E., & Davies, P. T. (1994). Maternal depression and child development. *Journal of Child Psychology and Psychiatry, 35,* 73–112.

Cummings, E. M., Davies, P. T., & Campbell, S. B. (2000). *Developmental psychopathology and family process: Theory, research, and clinical implications.* New York: Guilford Press.

Cummings, E. M., Keller, P. S., & Davies, P. T. (2005). Towards a family process model of maternal and paternal depressive symptoms: Exploring multiple relations with child and family functioning. *Journal of Child Psychology & Psychiatry, 46,* 479–489.

Darling, N., & Steinberg, L. (1993). Parenting style as context: An integrative model. *Psychological Bulletin, 113,* 487–496.

Davenport, B. R., Hegland, S., & Melby, J. N. (2008). Parent behaviors in free-play and problem-solving interactions in relation to problem behaviors in preschool boys. *Early Child Development & Care, 178,* 589–607.

Dawson, G., Frey, K., Panagiotides, H., Yamada, E., Hessel, D. & Osterling, J. (1999). Infants of depressed mothers exhibit atypical frontal electrical brain activity during interactions with mother and with a familiar, nondepressed adult. *Child Development, 70,* 1058–1066.

David-Ferdon, C., & Kaslow, N. J. (2008). Evidence-based psychosocial treatments for child and adolescent depression. *Journal of Clinical Child & Adolescent Psychology, 37,* 62–104.

Davidov, M., & Grusec, J. E. (2006). Multiple pathways to compliance: Mothers' willingness to cooperate and knowledge of their children's reactions to discipline. *Journal of Family Psychology, 20,* 705–708.

Del Vecchio, T., O'Leary, S. G. (2006). Antecedents of toddler aggression: Dysfunctional parenting in mother-toddler dyads. *Journal of Clinical Child & Adolescent Psychology, 35,* 194–202.

DeMatteo, D., Harrison, C. C., Arneson, C. C., Goldie, R., Lefebvre, A. A., Read, S. E., & King, S. M. (2002). Disclosing HIV/AIDS to children: The paths families take to truthtelling. *Psychology, Health & Medicine, 7,* 339–356.

Dishion, T. J., Gardner, K., Patterson, G. R., Reid, J. B., Spyrou, S., & Thibodeaux, S. (1987). *The family process code: A multidimensional system for observing family interactions* (Rev. ed.). Unpublished technical manual.

Dishion, T. J., Patterson, G. R., Stoolmiller, M., & Skinner, M. L. (1991). Family, school, and behavioral antecedents to early adolescent involvement with antisocial peers. *Developmental Psychology, 27,* 172–180.

Dixon, S. V., Graber, M. A., & Brooks-Gunn, J. (2008). The roles of respect for parental authority and parenting practices in parent–child conflict among African American, Latino, and European American families. *Journal of Family Psychology, 22,* 1–10.

Dodge, K. A., Pettit, G. S., & Bates, J. E. (1994). Socialization mediators of the relation between socioeconomic status and child conduct problems. *Child Development, 65,* 649–665.

Dorsey, S., Forehand, R., & Brody, G. (2007). Coparenting conflict and parenting behavior in economically disadvantaged single parent African American families: The role of maternal psychological distress. *Journal of Family Violence, 22,* 621–630.

Downey, G., & Coyne, J. C. (1990). Children of depressed parents: An integrative review. *Psychological Bulletin, 108,* 50–76.

Dumas, J. E. (1984). *INTERACT—A computer-based coding system for family interaction. Manual.* Unpublished manuscript available from the author.

Dumas, J. E. (1986). Parental perception and treatment outcome in families of aggressive children: A causal model. *Behavior Therapy, 17,* 420–432.

Dumka, L. E., Roosa, M. W., & Jackson, K. M. (1997). Risk, conflict, mothers' parenting, and children's adjustment in low-income, Mexican immigrant, and Mexican American families. *Journal of Marriage and the Family, 59,* 309–323.

Easterbrooks, M. A., & Emde, R. N. (1988). Marital and parent–child relationships: The role of affect in the family system. In R. A. Hinde & J. S. Hinde (Eds.), *Relationships within families: Mutual influences* (pp. 83–103). New York: Oxford University Press.

Egeland, B., & Farber, E. A. (1984). Infant-mother attachment: Factors related to its development and changes over time. *Child Development, 55,* 753–771.

Elder, G. H. Jr., Eccles, J. S., Ardelt, M., & Lord, S. (1995). Inner-city parents under economic pressure: Perspective on the strategies of parenting. *Journal of Marriage & the Family, 57,* 771–784.

Elgar, F. J., Waschbusch, D. A., Dadds, M. R., & Sigvaldason, N. (2007). Development and validation of a short form of the Alabama Parenting Questionnaire. *Journal of Child & Family Studies, 16,* 243–259.

Emde, R. N., & Easterbrooks, M. A. (1985). Assessing emotional availability in early development. In W. K. Frankenburg, R. N. Emde, & J. Sullivan (Eds.), *Early identification of the at-risk child: An international perspective* (pp. 79–102). New York: Plenum.

Endicott, J., & Spitzer, R. L. (1978). A diagnostic interview: the Schedule for Affective Disorders and Schizophrenia. *Archives of General Psychiatry, 35,* 837–844.

Erel, O., & Burman, B. (1995). Interrelatedness of marital relations and parent–child relations: A meta-analytic review. *Psychological Bulletin, 118,* 108–132.

Essau, C. A., Sasagawa, S., Frick, P. J. (2006). Psychometric properties of the Alabama Parenting Questionnaire. *Journal of Child & Family Studies, 15,* 597–616.

Fauber, R., Forehand, R., Thomas, A. M., & Wierson, M. (1990). A mediational model of the impact of marital conflict on adolescent adjustment in intact and divorced families: The role of disrupted parenting. *Child Development, 61,* 1112–1123.

Feinberg, M. (2002). Coparenting and the transition to parenthood: A framework for prevention. *Clinical Child & Family Psychology Review, 5,* 173–195.

Feinfield, K. A., & Baker, B. L. (2004). Empirical support for a treatment program for families of young children with externalizing problems. *Journal of Clinical Child & Adolescent Psychology, 33,* 182–195.

Fendrich, M., Warner, V., & Weissman, M. M. (1990). Family risk factors, parental depression, and psychopathology in offspring. *Developmental Psychology, 26,* 40–50.

Field, T. (1995). Infants of depressed mothers. *Infant Behavior & Development, 18,* 1–13.

Fincham, F. (19988). Child development and marital relations. *Child Development, 69,* 543–574.

First, M. B., Spitzer, R. L., Gibbon, M., & Williams, J. B. W. (1997). *User's guide for the Structured Clinical Interview for DSM-IV Axis I Disorders: Clinical version.* Washington, DC: American Psychiatric Press.

Fleming, A. S., Ruble, D. N., Flett, G. L., & Shaul, D. L. (1988). Postpartum adjustment in first-time mothers: Relations between mood, maternal attitudes, and mother-infant interactions. *Developmental Psychology, 24,* 71–81.

Fletcher, A. C., Elder, G. H. J., & Mekos, D. (2000). Parental influences on adolescent involvement in community activities. *Journal of Research on Adolescence, 10,* 29–48.

Fiske, Donald W. (1987). Construct invalidity comes from method effects. *Educational & Psychological Measurement, 47,* 285–307.

Foley, D. L. Eaves, L. J., Wormley, B., Silberg, J., L., Maes, H. H., Kuhn, J., et al. (2004). Childhood adversity, monoamine oxidase a genotype, and risk for conduct disorder. *Archives of General Psychiatry, 61,* 738–744.

Forehand, R., Griest, D. L., & Wells, K. C. (1979). Parent behavioral training: An analysis of the relationship among multiple outcome measures. *Journal of Abnormal Child Psychology, 7,* 229–242.

Forehand, R., Jones, D. J., Kotchick, B. A., Armistead, L., Morse, E., Morse, P. S., & Stock, M. (2002). Non-infected children of HIV-infected mothers: A four year longitudinal study of child psychosocial adjustment and parenting. *Behavior Therapy, 33,* 579–600.

Forehand, R., King, E., Peed, S., & Yoder, P. (1975). Mother–child interaction: Comparison of a noncompliant clinic group and a nonclinic group. *Behaviour Research & Therapy, 1975, 13,* 79–84.

Forehand, R., & Kotchick, B. A. (1996). Cultural diversity: A wake-up call for parent training. *Behavior Therapy, 27,* 187–206.

Forehand, R., Kotchick, B. A., Shaffer, A., & McKee, L. (2010). Parent management training. In I. Weiner & W.E. Craighead (Eds.), *Concise encyclopedia of psychology* (4th ed.). New York: John Wiley & Sons.

Forehand, R. & McMahon, R. J. (1981). *Helping the non-compliant child.* New York: Guilford Press.

Forehand, R., Sturgis, E. T., McMahon, R. J., Aguar, D., Green, K., Wells, K. D., et al. (1979). Parent behavioral training to modify child noncompliance: Treatment generalization across time and from home to school. *Behavior Modification, 3,* 3–25.

Forehand, R., Wells, K. C., & Griest, D. L. (1980). An examination of the social validity of a parent training program. *Behavior Therapy, 11,* 488–502.

Franck, K., & Anderson, O. (2004). *Summary of published works that include the observational measures from the Iowa Family Project Rating Scales* (Tech. Rep. No. 2). The University of Tennessee at Knoxville, Family Life Project.

Frick, P. J. (1991). *The Alabama Parenting Questionnaire.* Tuscaloosa, AL: University of Alabama.

Frick, P. J. (1994). Family dysfunction and the disruptive behavior disorders: A review of recent empirical findings. *Advances in Clinical Child Psychology, 16,* 203–226.

Frick, P. J., Christian, R. E., & Wootton, J. M. (1999). Age trends in association between parenting practices and conduct problems. *Behavior Modification, 23,* 106–128.

Frick, P. J., Kimonis, E. R., Dandreaux, D. M., & Farell, J. M. (2003). The 4 Year Stability of Psychopathic Traits in Non-Referred Youth. *Behavioral Sciences & the Law, 21,* 713–736.

Frosch, C. A., & Mangelsdorf, S. C. (2001). Marital behavior, parenting behavior, and multiple reports of preschoolers' problem behavior. *Developmental Psychology, 37,* 502–519.

Galambos, N. L., Barker, E. T., & Almeida, D. M. (2003). Parents do matter: Trajectories of change in externalizing and internalizing problems in early adolescence. *Child Development, 74,* 578–594.

Garber, J., & Robinson, N. S. (1997). Cognitive vulnerability in children at risk for depression. *Cognition and Emotion, 11*(5–6), 619–635.

Garcia Coll, C. T., Meyer, E. C., Brillon, L. (1995). Ethnic and minority parenting. In M. H. Bornstein (Ed.), *Handbook of parenting, 2: Biology and ecology of parenting.* (pp. 189–209). Mahwah, NJ: Lawrence Erlbaum Associates, Inc.

Garcia Coll, C. T., & Pachter, L. M. (2002). Ethnic and minority parenting. In M. H. Bornstein (Ed.), *Handbook of parenting: 4: Social conditions and applied parenting* (2nd ed.; pp. 1–20). Mahwah, NJ: Lawrence Erlbaum Associates Publishers.

Ge, X., Conger, R. D., Lorenz, F. O., & Simons, R. L. (1994). Parents' stressful life events and adolescent depressed mood. *Journal of Health & Social Behavior, 35,* 28–44.

Ge, X., Conger, R. D., Cadoret, R. J., Neiderhiser, J. M., Yates, W., Troughton, E., et al. (1996). The developmental interface between nature and nurture: A mutual influence model of child antisocial behavior and parent behaviors. *Developmental Psychology, 32,* 574–589.

Gelfand, D. M., & Teti, D. M. (1990). The effects of maternal depression on children. *Clinical Psychology Review, 10,* 329–353.

Gerdes, A. C., Hoza, B., Arnold, L. E., Pelham, W. E., Swanson, J. M., Wigal, T., et al. (2007). Maternal depressive symptomatology and parenting behavior: Exploration of possible mediators. *Journal of Abnormal Child Psychology, 35,* 705–714.

Glasgow, K. L., Dornbusch, S. M., Troyer, L., & Steinberg, L. (1997). Parenting styles, adolescents' attributions, and educational outcomes in nine heterogeneous high schools. *Child Development, 68,* 507–529.

Goldsmith, D. F., & Rogoff, B. (1997). Mothers' and toddlers' coordinated joint focus of attention: Variations with maternal dysphoric symptoms. *Developmental Psychology, 33,* 113–119.

Goodman, S. H., & Gotlib, I. H. (1999). Risk for psychopathology in the children of depressed mothers: A developmental model for understanding mechanisms of transmission. *Psychological Review, 106,* 458–490.

Granic, I., & Patterson, G. R. (2006). Toward a comprehensive model of antisocial development: A dynamic systems approach. *Psychological Review, 113,* 101–131.

Gray, M. R., & Steinberg, L. (1999). Unpacking authoritative parenting: Reassessing a multidimensional construct. *Journal of Marriage & the Family, 61,* 574–587.

Griest, D. L., Forehand, R., Wells, K. C., & McMahon, R. J. (1980). An examination of differences between non clinic and behavior problem clinic-referred children and their mothers. *Journal of Abnormal Psychology, 24,* 33–41.

Guerra, N. G., & Jagers, R. (1998). The importance of culture in the assessment of children and youth. In V. C. McLoyd & L. Steinberg (Eds.), *Studying minority adolescents: Conceptual, methodological, and theoretical issues* (pp. 167–181). Mahwah, NJ: Lawrence Erlbaum Associates Publishers.

Hamilton, M. (1960). A rating scale for depression. *Journal of neurology, neurosurgery, and psychiatry, 23,* 56–61.

Hammen, C., Shih, J. H., & Brennan, P. A. (2004). Intergenerational transmission of depression: Test of an interpersonal stress model in a community sample. *Journal of Consulting & Clinical Psychology, 72,* 511–522.

Harvey, E. Danforth, J. S., Ulaszek, W. R., Eberhardt, T. L. (2001). Validity of the parenting scale for parents of children with attention-deficit/hyperactivity disorder. *Behaviour Research & Therapy, 39,* 731–743.

Harwood, R., Leyendecker, B., Carlson, V., Asencio, M., & Miller, A. (2002). Parenting among Latino families in the U.S. In M. H. Bornstein (Ed.) *Handbook of parenting, Vol. 4: Social conditions and applied parenting* (2nd ed., 21–46). Mahwah, NJ: Lawrence Erlbaum.

Harwood, R. L., Miller, J. G., & Irizarry, N. L. (1995). *Culture and attachment: Perceptions of the child in context.* New York: Guilford Press.

Heller, T. L., Baker, B. L., Henker, B., & Hinshaw, S. P. (1996). Externalizing behavior and cognitive functioning from preschool to first grade: Stability and predictors. *Journal of Clinical Child Psychology, 25*, 376–387.

Herman, M. R., Dornbusch, S. M., Herron, M. C., & Herting, J. R. (1997). The influence of family regulation, connection, and psychological autonomy on six measures of adolescent functioning. *Journal of Adolescent Research, 12*, 34–67.

Hinshaw, S. P. (2002). Intervention research, theoretical mechanisms and causal processes related to externalizing behavior patterns. *Development & Psychopathology, 14*, 789–818.

Hinshaw, S. P., Owens, E. B., Wells, K. C., Kraemer, H. C., Abikoff, H. B., Arnold, L. E., et al. (2000). Family processes and treatment outcome in the MTA: Negative/ineffective parenting practices in relation to multimodal treatment. *Journal of Abnormal Child Psychology, 28*, 555–568.

Hops, H., Biglan, A., Sherman, L., Arthur, J., Friedman, L., & Osteen, V. (1987). Home observations of family interactions of depressed women. *Journal of Consulting and Clinical Psychology, 55*, 341–346.

Ingram, R. E., Miranda, J., & Segal, Z. V. (1998). *Cognitive vulnerability to depression.* New York: Guilford Press.

Irvine, A. B., Biglan, A., Smolkowski, K., & Ary, D. V. (1999). The value of the Parenting Scale for measuring the discipline practices of parents of middle school children. *Behaviour Research & Therapy, 37*, 127–142.

Jacobson, N. S., & Anderson, E. A. (1982). Interpersonal skill and depression in college students: An analysis of the timing of self-disclosures. *Behavior Therapy, 13*, 271–282.

Jambunathan, S., Burts, D. C., & Pierce, S. (2000). Comparisons of parenting attitudes among five ethnic groups in the United States. *Journal of Comparative Family Studies, 31*, 395–406.

Jewell, J. D., & Stark, K. D. (2003). Comparing the family environments of adolescents with conduct disorder or depression. *Journal of Child & Family Studies, 12*, 77–89.

Johnson, S. M., & Bolstad, O. D. (1973). Methodological issues in naturalistic observation: Some problems and solutions for field research. In L. A. Hamerlynck, L. C. Handy, E. J. Mash, L. A. Hamerlynck, L. C. Handy & E. J. Mash (Eds.), *Behavioral change: Methodology, concepts, and practice.* Champaign, IL: Research Press.

Jones, D., Dorsey, S., Forehand, R., Foster, S., Armistead, L., & Brody, G. (2005a). Co-parent support and conflict in African American single mother-headed families: Associations with mother and child adjustment. *Journal of Family Violence, 20*, 141–150.

Jones, D. J., Forehand, R., O'Connell, C., Armistead, L., & Brody, G. (2005). Mothers' perceptions of neighborhood violence and mother-reported monitoring of African American children: An examination of the moderating role of perceived support. *Behavior Therapy, 36*, 25–34.

Jones, D., Forehand, R., O'Connell, C., Brody, G., & Armistead, L. (2005b). Neighborhood violence and maternal monitoring in African American single mother-headed families: An examination of the moderating role of social support. *Behavior Therapy, 36*, 25–34.

Jones, D. J., Forehand, R., Rakow, A., Colletti, C. J. M., McKee, L., & Zalot, A. (2008). The specificity of maternal parenting behavior and child adjustment difficulties: A study of inner-city African American families. *Journal of Family Psychology, 22*, 181–192.

Jones, D. J., Shaffer, A. Forehand, R., Brody, G., & Armistead, L. P. (2003). Coparent conflict in singlemother headed African American families: Do parenting skills serve as a mediator or moderator of children's psychosocial adjustment? *Behavior Therapy, 34*, 259–272.

Jones, D. J., Zalot, A. A., Foster, S. E., Sterrett, E., & Chester, C. (2007). A review of childrearing in African American single mother families: The relevance of a coparenting framework. *Journal of Child and Family Studies, 16*, 671–683.

Jones, R. R., Reid, J. B., & Patterson, G. R. (1975). Naturalistic observation in clinical assessment. In P. McReynolds (Ed.), *Advances in psychological assessment* (Vol. 3). San Francisco: Jossey-Bass, 1975. pp. 42–95.

Kane, P., & Garber, J. (2004). The relations among depression in fathers, children's psychopathology, and father–child conflict: A meta-analysis. *Clinical Psychology Review, 24*, 339–360.

Karazsia, B. T., van Dulmen, M. H. M., Wildman, B. G. (2008). Confirmatory factor analysis of Arnold et al.'s Parenting Scale across race, age, and sex. *Journal of Child & Family Studies, 17*, 500–516.

Kawash, G. F., Clewes, J. L. (1988). A factor analysis of a short form of the CRPBI: Are children's perceptions of control and discipline multidimensional? *Journal of Psychology: Interdisciplinary & Applied, 122*, 57–67.

Kelly, J. B. (2000). Children's adjustment in conflicted marriage and divorce: A decade review of research. *Journal of the Academy of Child & Adolescent Psychiatry, 39*, 963–973.

Kerig, P. K., & Lindahl, K. M. (Eds.). (2001). *Family observational coding systems: Resources for systemic research.* Mahwah, NJ: Lawrence Erlbaum Associates Publishers.

Kerig, P. A., Cowan, P. A., & Cowan, C. P. (1993). Marital quality and gender differences in parent–child interaction. *Developmental Psychology, 29*, 931–939.

Kim-Cohen, J., Caspi, A., Taylor, A., Williams, B., Newcombe, R., Craig, I. W., & Moffitt, T. E. (2006). MAOA, maltreatment, and gene-environment interaction predicting children's mental health: New evidence and a meta-analysis. *Molecular Psychiatry, 11*, 903–913.

Kirshenbaum, S. B., & Nevid, J. S. (2002). The specificity of maternal disclosure of HIV/AIDS in relation to children's adjustment. *AIDS Education & Prevention, 14*, 1–16.

Kitzmann, K. (2000). Effects of marital conflict on subsequent triadic family interactions and parenting. *Developmental Psychology, 36*, 3–13.

Knight, G. P., & Hill, N. E. (1998). Measurement equivalence in research involving minority adolescents. In V. C. McLoyd, & L. Steinberg (Eds.), *Studying minority adolescents: Conceptual, methodological, and theoretical issues* (pp. 183–210). Mahwah, NJ: Lawrence Erlbaum Associates Publishers.

Kurdek, L. A., & Fine, M. A. (1994). Family acceptance and family control as predictors of adjustment in young adolescents: Linear, curvilinear, or interactive effects? *Child Development, 65*, 1137–1146).

Lee, C. M., & Gotlib, I. H. (1991). Adjustment of children of depressed mothers: A 10-month follow-up. *Journal of Abnormal Psychology, 100*, 473–477.

Lefkowitz, E. S., Romo, L. F., Corona, R., Au, T. K., & Sigman, M. (2000). How Latino American and European American adolescents discuss conflicts, sexuality, and AIDS with their mothers. *Developmental Psychology, 36*, 315–325.

Levy, A., Laska, F., Abelhauser, A., Delfraissy, J., Goujard, C., Boue, F. et al. (1999). Disclosure of HIV seropositivity. *Journal of Clinical Psychology, 55*, 1041–1049.

Li, X., Feigelman, S., & Stanton, B. (2000). Perceived parental monitoring and health risk behaviors among urban low-income African-American children and adolescents. *Journal of Adolescent Health, 27*, 43–48.

Lieb, R., Wittchen, H., Höfler, M., Fuetsch, M., Stein, M. B., & Merikangas, K. R. (2000). Parental psychopathology, parenting styles, and the risk of social phobia in offspring: A prospective-longitudinal community study. *Archives of General Psychiatry, 57*, 859–866.

Lindahl, K. M., & Malik, N. M. (1999). Marital conflict, family processes, and boys' externalizing behavior in Hispanic American and European American families. *Journal of Clinical Child Psychology, 28*, 12–24.

Lindahl, K. M., & Malik, N. M. (2001). The System for Coding Interactions and Family Functioning. In K. P. Kerig, & K. M. Lindahl (Eds.), *Family observational coding systems: Resources for systemic research* (pp. 77–91). Mahwah, NJ: Lawrence Erlbaum Associates Publishers.

Lochman, J. E., & Wells, K. C. (2002). The Coping Power program at the middle-school transition: Universal and indicated prevention effects. *Psychology of Addictive Behaviors, 16*, S40–S54.

Locke, L. M., & Prinz, R. J. (2002). Measurement of parental discipline and nurturance. *Clinical Psychology Review, 22*, 895–930.

Lovejoy, M. C., Graczyk, P. A., O'Hare, E., & Neuman, G. (2000). Maternal depression and parenting behavior: A meta-analytic review. *Clinical Psychology Review, 20*, 561–592.

Lytton, H. (2000). Toward a model of family-environmental and child-biological influences on development. *Developmental Review, 20*(1), 150–179.

Manongdo, J. A., & Ramirez Garcia, J. I. (2007). Mothers' parenting dimensions and adolescent externalizing and internalizing behaviors in a low-income, urban Mexican American sample. *Journal of Clinical Child and Adolescent Psychology, 36*(4), 593–604.

Margolies, P. J., & Weintraub, S. (1977). The revised 56-item CRPBI as a research instrument: Reliability and factor structure. *Journal of Clinical Psychology, 33*(2), 472–476.

Markus, H. R., Steele, C. M., & Steele, D. M. (2002). Color blindness as a barrier to inclusion: Assimilation and nonimmigrant minorities. In R. A. Shweder, M. Minow, & H. R. Markus (Eds.), *Engaging cultural differences: The multicultural challenge in liberal democracies* (pp. 453–472). New York: Russell Sage Foundation.

Mason, C. A., Cauce, A. M., Gonzales, N., & Hiraga, Y. (1996). Neither too sweet nor too sour: Problem peers, maternal control, and problem behavior in African American adolescents. *Child Development, 67*, 2115–2130.

Masten, A. S., & Coatsworth, J. D. (1998). The development of competence in favorable and unfavorable environments: Lessons from research on successful children. *American Psychologist, 53*, 205–220.

McCoy, M. G., Frick, P. J., Loney, B. R., & Ellis, M. L. (1999). The potential mediating role of parenting practices in the development of conduct problems in a clinic-referred sample. *Journal of Child & Family Studies, 8*, 477–494.

McHale, J. (1995). Coparenting and triadic interactions during infancy: The roles of marital distress and gender. *Developmental Psychology, 31*, 985–996.

McHale, J. (1997). Overt and covert parenting processes in the family. *Family Process, 36*, 183–201.

McHale, J., Kuersten-Hogan, R., Lauretti, A., & Rasmussen, J. (2000). Parental reports of coparenting and observed coparenting behavior during the toddler period. *Journal of Family Psychology, 14*, 220–236.

McKee, L., Colletti, C., Rakow, A., Jones, D. J., & Forehand, R. (2008). Parenting and child externalizing behaviors: Are the associations specific or diffuse? *Aggression & Violent Behavior, 13*, 201–215.

McKee, L., Forehand, R., Rakow, A., Reeslund, K., Roland, E., Hardcastle, E., et al. (2008). Parenting specificity: An examination of the relation between three parenting behaviors and child problem behaviors in the context of a history of caregiver depression. *Behavior Modification, 32*, 638–658.

McKee, L., Jones, D. J., Roland, E., Coffelt, N., Rakow, A., & Forehand, R. (2007). Maternal HIV/AIDS and depressive symptoms among inner-city African American youth: The role of maternal depressive symptoms, mother–child relationship quality, and child coping. *American Journal of Orthopsychiatry, 77*, 259–266.

McLoyd, V. C. (1990). The impact of economic hardship on Black families and children: Psychological distress, parenting, and socioemotional development. *Child Development, 61*, 311–346.

McLoyd, V. C., Cauce, A. M., Takeuchi, D., & Wilson, L. (2000). Marital processes and parental socialization in families of color: A decade review of research. *Journal of Marriage & the Family, 62*, 1070–1093.

McMahon, R. J., & Forehand, R. L. (2003). *Helping the noncompliant child: Family-based treatment for oppositional behavior* (2nd ed.). New York: Guilford Press.

McMahon, R. J., Forehand, R., & Griest, D. L. (1981). Effects of knowledge of social learning principles on enhancing treatment outcome and generalization in a parent training program. *Journal of Consulting & Clinical Psychology, 49*, 526–532.

McMahon, R. J., Wells, K. C., & Kotler, M. S. (2006). Conduct problems. In E. J. Mash, & R. A. Barkley (Eds.), *Treatment of childhood disorders* (3rd ed.; pp. 137–268). New York: Guilford Press.

Melby, J. N., & Conger, R. D. (1996). Parental behaviors and adolescent academic performance: A longitudinal analysis. *Journal of Research on Adolescence, 6*, 113–137.

Melby, J., & Conger, R. D. (2001). The Iowa Family Interaction Rating Scales: Instrument summary. In P. K. Kerig & K. M. Lindahl (Eds.), *Family observational coding systems: Resources for systemic research* (pp. 33–58). Mahwah, NJ: Erlbaum.

Melby, J. N., Hoyt, W. T., & Bryant, C. M. (2003). A generalizability approach to assessing the effects of ethnicity and training on observer ratings of family interactions. *Journal of Social & Personal Relationships, 20*, 171–189.

Melby, J. N., Conger, R. D., Ge, X., & Warner, T. D. (1995). The use of structural equation modeling in assessing the quality of marital observations. *Journal of Family Psychology, 9*, 280–293.

Melby, J. N., Conger, R. D., Book, R., Rueter, M., Lucy, L., Repinski, D., et al. (1998). The Iowa Family Interaction Rating Scales (5th ed.). Unpublished manuscript. Institute for Social & Behavioral Research, Iowa State University, Ames, IA.

Miles, M. S., Gillespie, J. V., & Holditch-Davis, D. (2001). Physical and mental health in African American mothers with HIV. *Journal of the Association of Nurses in AIDS Care, 12*, 42–50.

Miller, K. S., Forehand, R., & Kotchick, B. A. (1999). Adolescent sexual behavior in two ethnic minority samples: The role of family variables. *Journal of Marriage and the Family, 61*, 85–98.

Minuchin, S. (1974). *Families and family therapy*. Cambridge, MA: Harvard University.

Minuchin, S. (1985). Families and individual development: Provocations from the field of family therapy. *Child Development, 56*, 289–302.

Minuchin, S., Rosman, B. L., & Baker, L. (1978). Psychosomatic families: Anorexia nervosa in context. Cambridge, MA: Harvard University Press.

Moore, D. R., Florsheim, P., & Butner, J. (2007). Interpersonal behavior, psychopathology, and relationship outcomes among adolescent mothers and their partners. *Journal of Clinical Child & Adolescent Psychology, 36*, 541–556.

Moore, D., Forgatch, M., Mukai, L., Toobert, D., & Patterson, G. (1978). *Interactional Coding System*. Unpublished manuscript, Oregon Social Learning Center, Eugene, OR.

Moore, P. S., Whaley, S. E., & Sigman, M. (2004). Interactions between mothers and children: Impacts of maternal and child anxiety. *Journal of Abnormal Psychology,113*, 471–476.

Morawska, A., Sanders, M. R. (2007). Concurrent predictors of dysfunctional parenting and maternal confidence: Implications for parenting interventions. *Child: Care, Health & Development, 33*, 757–767.

Muris, P., Meesters, C., & van den Berg, S. (2003). Internalizing and externalizing problems as correlates of self-reported attachment style and perceived parental rearing in normal adolescents. *Journal of Child & Family Studies, 12*, 171–183.

Murphy, L. M. B., Koranyi, K., Crim, L., & Whited, S. (1999). Disclosure, stress, and psychological adjustment among mothers affected by HIV. *AIDS Patient Care & STDs, 13*, 111–118.

Murphy, D. A., Steers, W. N., & Stritto, M. E. D. (2001). Maternal disclosure of mothers' HIV serostatus to their young children. *Journal of Family Psychology, 15*, 441–450.

Murray, C. J., & Lopez, A. D. (1997). Mortality by cause for eight regions of the world: Global Burden of Disease Study. *The Lancet, 349*(9061), 1269–1276.

Nezu, A. M., Nezu, C. M., Friedman, J., & Lee, M. (2009). Assessment of depression. In I. H. Gotlib & C. L. Hammen (Eds.), *Handbook of depression*. (2nd ed., pp. 44–68). New York: Guilford Press.

Nolen-Hoeksema, S. (1987). Sex differences in unipolar depression: Evidence and theory. *Psychological Bulletin, 101*, 259–282.

O'Leary, S. G., Slep, A. M. S., & Reid, M. J. (1999). A longitudinal study of mothers' overreactive discipline and toddlers' externalizing behavior. *Journal of Abnormal Child Psychology, 27*, 331–341.

Oxford, M., Cavell, T. A., & Hughes, N. (2003). Callous/unemotional traits moderate the relation between ineffective parenting and child externalizing problems: A partial replication and extension. *Journal of Clinical Child & Adolescent Psychology, 32*, 577–585.

Patterson, G. R. (1974a). Intervention for boys with conduct problems: Multiple settings, treatments, and criteria. *Journal of Consulting & Clinical Psychology, 42*, 471–481.

Patterson, G. R. (1974b). Retraining of aggressive boys by their parents: Review of recent literature and follow-up evaluation. *Canadian Psychiatric Association Journal, 19*, 142–161.

Patterson, G. R. (1976). The aggressive child: Victim and architect of a coercive system. In E. J. Mash, L. A. Hamerlynck, & L. C. Handy (Eds.), *Behavior modification and families* (pp. 267–316). New York: Brunner/Mazel.

Patterson, G. R. (1982). *Coercive family processes*. Eugene, Oregon: Castalia Publishing Company.

Patterson, G. R., & Cobb, J. A. (1971). A dyadic analysis of "aggressive" behaviors. In J. P. Hill (Ed.), *Minnesota symposia on child psychology* (Vol. 5, pp. 72–129). Minneapolis: University of Minnesota.

Patterson, G. R., & Cobb, J. A. (1973). Stimulus control for classes of noxious behaviors. In J. F. Knutson (Ed.), *The control of aggression: Implications from basic research* (pp. 144–199). Chicago: Aldine.

Patterson, G. R., DeGarmo, D. S., & Knutson, N. (2000). Hyperactive and antisocial behaviors: Comorbid or two points in the same process? *Development and Psychopathology, 12*, 91–106.

Patterson, C. J., & Farr, R. H. (2011). Coparenting among lesbian and gay couples. In J. P. McHale, K. M. Lindahl (Eds.), *Coparenting: A conceptual and clinical examination of family systems* (pp. 127–146). Washington, DC: American Psychological Association.

Patterson, G. R., & Fisher, P. A. (2002). Recent developments in our understanding of parenting: Bidirectional effects, causal models, and the search for parsimony. In M. H. Bornstein (Ed.), *Handbook of parenting: Vol. 5: Practical issues in parenting* (2nd ed.; pp. 59–88). Mahwah, NJ: Lawrence Erlbaum Associates Publishers.\

Patterson, G. R., & Forgatch, M. S. (1995). Predicting future clinical adjustment from treatment outcome and process variables. *Psychological Assessment, 7*, 275–285.

Patterson, G. R., Forgatch, M. S., Yoerger, K. L., & Stoolmiller, M. (1998). Variables that initiate and maintain an early-onset trajectory for juvenile offending. *Development and psychopathology, 10*, 531–547.

Patterson, C. J., Griesler, P. C., Vaden, N. A., & Kupersmidt, M. B. (1992). Family economic circumstances, life transitions, and children's peer relations. In R. D. Parke, & G. W. Ladd (Eds.), *Family-peer relationships: Modes of linkage* (pp. 385–424). Hillsdale, NJ: Lawrence Erlbaum Associates, Inc.

Peed, S., Roberts, M., & Forehand, R. (1977). Evaluation of the effectiveness of a standardized parent training program in altering the interaction of mothers and their noncompliant children. *Behavior Modification, 1*, 323–350.

Pettit, G. S., Laird, R. D., Dodge, K. A., Bates, J. E., & Criss, M. M. (2001). Antecedents and behavior-problem outcomes of parental monitoring and psychological control in early adolescence. *Child Development, 72*, 583–598.

Prelow, H. M., Bowman, M. A., & Weaver, S. R. (2007). Predictors of psychosocial well-being in urban African American and European American youth: The role of ecological factors. *Journal of Youth & Adolescence, 36*, 543–553.

Radloff, L. S. (1977). The CES-D scale: A self-report depression scale for research in the general population. *Applied Psychological Measurement, 1*(3), 385–401.

Rakow, A., Forehand, R., Haker, K., McKee, L. G., Champion, J. E., Potts, J., et al. (2011). Use of parental guilt induction among depressed parents. *Journal of Family Psychology, 25*, 147–151.

Ramey, S. L. (2002). The science and art of parenting. In J. G. Borkowski, S. L. Ramey, & M. Bristol-Power (Eds.), *Parenting and the child's world: Influences on academic, intellectual, and social-emotional development* (pp. 47–71). Mahwah, NJ: Lawrence Erlbaum Associates Publishers.

Raskin, A., Booth, H. H., Reatig, N. A., Schulterbrandt, J. G., & Odle, D. (1971). Factor analyses of normal and depressed patients' memories of parental behavior. *Psychological Reports, 29*, 871–879.

Reid, J. B. (Ed.). (1978). *A social learning approach to family interaction, II: Observation in home settings.* Eugene, OR: Castalia Publishing Company.

Reid, J. B. (1967). Reciprocity in family interaction. Unpublished doctoral dissertation, University of Oregon.

Reid, J. B., Taplin, P. S., & Lorber, R. (1981). A social interactional approach to the treatment of abusive families. In R. Stuart (Ed.), *Violent behavior: Social learning approaches to prediction, management, and treatment* (pp. 83–101). New York: Brunner/Mazel.

Reitman, D., Currier, R. O., Hupp, S. D., Rhode, P. C., Murphy, M. A., & O'Callaghan, P. M. (2001). Psychometric characteristics of the Parenting Scale in a Head Start population. *Journal of Clinical Child Psychology, 30*, 514–524.

Renson, G. J., Schaefer, E. S., & Levy, B. I. (1968). Cross-national validity of a spherical conceptual model for parent behavior. *Child Development, 39*, 1229–1235.

Rueter, M. A., & Conger, R. D. (1995). Interaction style, problem-solving behavior, and family problem-solving effectiveness. *Child Development, 66*, 98–115.

Rueter, M. A., & Conger, R. D. (1998). Reciprocal influences between parenting and adolescent problem-solving behavior. *Developmental Psychology, 34*, 1470–1482.

Ruiz, S. Y., Roosa, M. W., & Gonzales, N. A. (2002). Predictors of self-esteem for Mexican American and European American youths: A reexamination of the influence of parenting. *Journal of Family Psychology, 16*, 70–80.

Safford, S. M., Alloy, L. B., & Pieracci, A. (2007). A comparison of two measures of parental behavior. *Journal of Child & Family Studies,16*, 375–384.

Sampson, R. J., & Laub, J. H. (1994). Urban poverty and the family context of delinquency: A new look at structure and process in a classic study. *Child Development, 65*, 523–540.

Sanders, M. R., Turner, K. M. T., & Markie-Dadds, C. (2002). The development and dissemination of the triple P-positive parenting program: A multilevel, evidence-based system of parenting and family support. *Prevention Science, 3*, 173–189.

Scarr, S. (1992). Developmental theories for the 1990s: Development and individual differences. *Child Development, 63*, 1–19.

Schaefer, E. S. (1959). A circumplex model for maternal behavior. *The Journal of Abnormal & Social Psychology, 59*, 226–235.

Schaefer, E. S. (1965). Children's reports of parental behavior: An inventory. *Child Development, 36*, 413–424.

Schludermann, E., & Schludermann, S. (1970). Replicability of factors in children's report of parent behavior (CRPBI). *Journal of Psychology: Interdisciplinary & Applied, 76*, 239–249.

Schwarz, N. (1999). Self-reports: How the questions shape the answers. *American Psychologist, 54*(2), 93–105.

Semple, S. J., Patterson, T. L., Temoshok, L. R., McCutchan, J. A., Straits-Tröster, K. A., Chandler, J. L., et al. (1993). Identification of psychobiological stressors among HIV positive women. *Women & Health, 20*, 15–36.

Shaffer, A., Jones, D. J., Kotchick, B. A., Forehand, R., & the Family Health Project Research Group (2001). Telling the children: Disclosure of maternal HIV infection and its effects on child psychosocial adjustment. *Journal of Child & Family Studies, 10*, 301–313.

Shaw, D. S., Winslow, E. B., Owens, E. B., Vondra, J. I., Cohn, J. F., & Bell, R. Q. (1998). The development of early externalizing problems among children from low-income families: A transformational perspective. *Journal of Abnormal Child Psychology, 26*, 95–107.

Sheeber, L., Hops, H., & Davis, B. (2001). Family processes in adolescent depression. *Clinical Child and Family Psychology Review, 4*, 19–35.

Shelton, K. K., Frick, P. J., & Wootton, J. (1996). Assessment of parenting practices in families of elementary school-age children. *Journal of Clinical Child Psychology, 25*, 317–329.

Silverman, W. K., Pina, A. A., & Viswesvaran, C. (2008). Evidence-based psychosocial treatments for phobic and anxiety disorders in children and adolescents. *Journal of Clinical Child & Adolescent Psychology, 37*, 105–130.

Simons, R. L., Lorenz, F. O., Wu, C., & Conger, R. D. (1993). Social network and marital support as mediators and moderators of the impact of stress and depression on parental behavior. *Developmental Psychology, 29*, 368–381.

Smetana, J. G., Abernethy, A., & Harris, A. (2000). Adolescent-parent interactions in middle-class African American families: Longitudinal change and contextual variations. *Journal of Family Psychology, 14*, 458–474.

Smetana, J. G., Metzger, A., & Campione-Barr, N. (2004). African American late adolescents' relationships with parents: Developmental transitions and longitudinal patterns. *Child Development, 75*, 932–947.

Smetana, J. G., Yau, J., Restrepo, A., & Braeges, J. L. (1991). Adolescent-parent conflict in married and divorced families. *Developmental Psychology, 27*, 1000–1010.

Snyder, J. J., & Patterson, G. R. (1995). Individual differences in social aggression: A test of a reinforcement model of socialization in the natural environment. *Behavior Therapy, 26*, 371–391.

Spoth, R., Redmond, C., Haggerty, K., & Ward, T. (1995). A controlled parenting skills outcome study examining individual difference and attendance effects. *Journal of Marriage & the Family, 57*, 449–464.

Spoth, R., Redmond, C., & Shin, C. (1998). Direct and indirect latent-variable parenting outcomes of two universal family-focused preventive interventions: Extending a public health-oriented research base. *Journal of Consulting & Clinical Psychology, 66*, 385–399.

Stanger, C., Dumenci, L., Kamon, J., & Burstein, M. (2004). Parenting and children's externalizing problems in substance-abusing families. *Journal of Clinical Child & Adolescent Psychology, 33*, 590–600.

Stark, K. D., & Kendall, P. C. (1996). *Treating depressed children: Therapist manual for "Taking Action".* Ardmore, PA: Workbook Publishing, Inc.

Steele, R. G., Nesbitt-Daly, J. S., Daniel, R. C., & Forehand, R. (2005). Factor structure of the Parenting Scale in a low-income African American sample. *Journal of Child & Family Studies, 14*, 535–549.

Stein, J. A., Rotheram-Borus, M. J., & Lester, P. (2007). Impact of parentification on long-term outcomes among children of parents with HIV/AIDS. *Family Process, 46*, 317–333.

Steinberg, L. (1990). Autonomy, conflict, and harmony in the family relationship. In S. S. Feldman, G. R. Elliott (Eds.), *At the threshold: The developing adolescent.* (pp. 255–276). Cambridge: Harvard University Press.

Steinberg, L., Lamborn, S. D., Dornbusch, S. M., & Darling, N. (1992). Impact of parenting practices on adolescent achievement: Authoritative parenting, school involvement, and encouragement to succeed. *Child Development, 63,* 1266–1281.

Steinberg, L., Dornbusch, S.M., Brown, B. B. (1992). Ethnic differences in adolescent achievement: An ecological perspective. *American Psychologist, 47,* 723–729.

Steinberg, L., Mounts, N. S., Lamborn, S. D., & Dornbusch, S. M. (1991). Authoritative parenting and adolescent adjustment across varied ecological niches. *Journal of Research on Adolescence, 1,* 19–36.

Sterrett, E., Jones, D. J., & Kincaid, C. (2009). Psychosocial adjustment of low-income African American youth from single mother homes: The role of youth coparent relationship quality. *Journal of Clinical Child & Adolescent Psychology, 38,* 427–438.

Stright, A., & Bales, S. (2003). Coparenting quality: Contributions of child and parent characteristics. *Family Relations, 52,* 232–240.

Super, C. M., & Harkness, S. (1999). The environment as culture in developmental research. In S. L. Friedman, & Wachs, T. D. Theodore (Eds.), *Measuring environment across the life span: Emerging methods and concepts* (pp. 279–323). Washington, DC: American Psychological Association.

Takahashi, K., Ohara, N., Antonucci, T. C., & Akiyama, H. (2002). Commonalities and differences in close relationships among the Americans and Japanese: A comparison by the individualism/collectivism concept. *International Journal of Behavioral Development, 26,* 453–465.

Tasker, F. (2005). Lesbian mothers, gay fathers, and their children: A review. *Developmental & Behavioral Pediatrics, 26,* 224–240.

Taylor, L. C., Barnett, M. A., Longest, K., & Raver, C. (2009). Observational methods and diversity in parenting for African American and European American low-income families with young children. Unpublished manuscript.

Teicher, M. H., Samson, J. A., Polcari, A., & McGreenery, C. E. (2006). Sticks, stones, and hurtful words: Relative effects of various forms of childhood maltreatment. *American Journal of Psychiatry, 163,* 993–1000.

Teleki, J. K., Powell, J. A., & Dodder, R. A. (1982). Factor analysis of reports of parental behavior by children living in divorced and married families. *Journal of Psychology: Interdisciplinary & Applied, 112,* 295–302.

Tobin, J. J., Wu, D. Y. H., & Davidson, D. H. (1989). *Preschool in three cultures: Japan, China, and the United States.* New Haven: Yale University Press.

Tompkins, T. L., Henker, B., Whalen, C. K., Axelrod, J., & Comer, L. K. (1999). Motherhood in the context of HIV infection: Reading between the numbers. *Cultural Diversity and Ethnic Minority Psychology, 5,* 197–208.

Tompkins, T. L., & Wyatt, G. E. (2008). Child psychosocial adjustment and parenting in families affected by maternal HIV/AIDS. *Journal of Child & Family Studies, 17,* 823–838.

Touliatos, J., Perlmutter, B. F., & Straus, M. A. (2001). *Handbook of family measurement techniques* (Vols. 1–3). Thousand Oaks, CA: Sage Publications, Inc.

U. S. Census Bureau News, U. S. Department of Commerce (2008). An older and more diverse nation by mid-century. Retrieved October 16, 2008, from http://www.census.gov/Press-Release/www/releases/archives/population/012496.html

Van Egeren, L., & Hawkins, D. (2004). Coming to terms with coparenting: Implications of definition and measurement. *Journal of Adult Development, 11,* 165–178.

Vogel, E. F., & Bell, N. W. (1960). The emotionally-disturbed child as the family scapegoat. In N. W. Bell & E. F. Vogel (Eds.), *A modern introduction to the family* (pp. 382–397). New York: Free Press.

Vuchinich, S., Bank, L., & Patterson, G. R. (1992). Parenting, peers, and the stability of antisocial behavior in preadolescent boys. *Developmental Psychology, 28,* 510–521.

Webster-Stratton, C., & Herman, K. C. (2008). The impact of parent behavior-management training on child depressive symptoms. *Journal of Counseling Psychology, 55,* 473–484.

Widom, Cathy S. (1989). Does violence beget violence? A critical examination of the literature. *Psychological Bulletin, 106,* 3–28.

Zahn-Waxler, C., Duggal, S., & Gruber, R. (2002). Parental psychopathology. In M. H. Bornstein (Ed.), *Handbook of parenting: Vol. 4: Social conditions and applied parenting* (2nd ed., pp. 295–328). Mahwah: NJ: Lawrence Erlbaum.

Zaslow, M. J., Weinfield, N. S., Gallagher, M., Hair, E. C., Ogawa, J. R., Egeland, B., et al. (2006). Longitudinal prediction of child outcomes from differing measures of parenting in a low-income sample. *Developmental Psychology, 42,* 27–37.

Linking Children and Adolescent Assessment to Effective Instruction: An Evidence-based Perspective from the Experimental Literature

H. Lee Swanson

Abstract

This chapter reviews the outcomes of meta-analysis studies that provide potential links between assessment and instruction. The review covers three areas: (1) dynamic assessment, (2) general models of instruction that combine the components of direct and strategy instruction, and (3) treatment outcomes related to definition x treatment interactions. The implications of the review were (a) when dynamic assessment procedures are coupled with static assessment, they provide important differential weights in predicting learning outcomes, (b) effective instruction is neither a bottom-up nor top-down approach in isolation, and (c) variations in IQ and reading cannot be ignored when predicting treatment outcomes.

Key Words: Dynamic assessment, meta-analysis, evidence-based intervention, direct instruction, and strategy instruction

The purpose of this chapter is to link effective assessment practices to effective instruction for children and adolescents at risk for learning problems. No doubt, this first sentence begs the question as to what is effective assessment and what is effective instruction. We will attempt to answer these questions by considering outcomes related to quantitative syntheses (meta-analyses) of the intervention and assessment literature. Prior to reviewing this research, however, some of the goals of assessment and effective instruction need to be stated. The goal of assessment in the educational and/or instructional context is to determine those underlying cognitive, social, and environmental variables that contribute to a student's academic performance. Effective instruction, on the other hand, complements assessment by monitoring the intensity of instruction and making systematic changes in the instructional context as a function of a student's overt performance. These two activities are complementary. One focuses on systematic manipulation of the environmental

context (e.g., instruction, classroom, school) to determine procedures that maximize learning, whereas the other focuses on mapping the internal and social dynamics of learning for the purposes of informing instruction. Given these assumptions, we now review our meta-analyses that attempt to link assessment with instruction (also see Swanson, 2011, for further discussion). Prior to our review we define meta-analysis.

Meta-analysis

Meta-analysis refers to a statistical technique used to synthesize data from separate comparable studies in order to obtain a quantitative summary of research that addresses a common question. Prior to conducting a meta-analysis, the researcher defines the problem (i.e., determining interventions that work), collects the research relevant to the problem (i.e., evidence-based reading interventions), and evaluates the quality of the data (i.e., experimental designs). The procedures for conducting a meta-analysis are described in detail in Cooper and Hedges (1994), Lipsey and Wilson (2001), and Rosenthal and DiMatteo (2001). There are at least two advantages of meta-analysis over traditional narrative techniques for synthesizing research. First, when discussing research linking assessment to instruction, the structured methodology of meta-analysis requires careful review and analysis of all contributing methodologically sound research. As such, meta-analysis overcomes biases associated with the reliance on single assessment or intervention studies, or on subsets of studies that inevitably occur in narrative reviews of a literature. Second, meta-analysis can address questions about variables that moderate effects. For example, questions such as whether key assessment information (e.g., variations in intelligence and reading in samples at risk for learning problems) plays a significant role in moderating treatment outcomes can be addressed. Specifically, meta-analysis provides a formal means for testing whether different features of studies explain variation in their outcomes (e.g., see Gersten, Chard, Jayanthi, Baker, Morphy, & Flojo, 2009).

Although there are many different metrics to describe an effect size, in this chapter we use the *d-index* by Cohen (1988). The d-index is a scale-free measure of the separation between two means that is used when one variable is dichotomous (e.g., children at risk for learning problems versus children not at risk; control vs. treatment group) and the other is continuous (e.g., dependent measures related to cognitive processes, reading, and/ or math). Calculating the *d*-index for any study involves dividing the difference between the two group means by either their average standard deviation or the standard deviation of the control group. To make *d*'s interpretable, statisticians have usually adopted Cohen's (1988) system for classifying *d*'s in terms of their size (i.e., .00–.19 is described as TRIVIAL; .20–.49, SMALL; .50–.79, MODERATE; .80 or higher, LARGE). Cohen's *d* (1988) is further weighted by the reciprocal in the sampling variance (Hedges & Olkin, 1985). The dependent measure for the estimate of effect size (ES) can be defined as ES = d/(1/v), where **d** [(Mean of treatment group – Mean of comparison group)/ average of standard deviation for both groups)], and **v** is the inverse of the sampling variance, $v = (N_{rd} + N_{nrd})/(N_{rd} \times N_{nrd}) + d^2/[2(N_{rd} + N_{nrd})]$ (Hedges & Olkin, 1985). Thus, ESs are computed with each ES weighted by the reciprocal of its variance, a procedure that gives more weight to ESs that are more reliably estimated. As suggested by Hedges and Olkin (1985), the majority of syntheses remove outliers from the analysis of main effects. Outliers are defined as ESs lying beyond the first gap of at least one standard deviation between adjacent ES values in a positive direction (Bollen, 1989).

Dynamic Testing

One of the clearest links between assessment and instruction are procedures referred to as dynamic assessment (e.g., Caffrey, Fuchs, & Fuchs, 2008; Fuchs, Compton, Fuchs, Hollenbeck, Craddock, & Hamlett, 2008; Hasson & Joffe, 2007; Jeltova, Birney, Fredine, Jarvin, Sternberg, & Grigorenko, 2007; Macrine & Sabatino, 2008; Sternberg & Grigorenko, 2002; Swanson & Lussier, 2001; Tzuriel & Flor-Maduel, 2010). Dynamic assessment has long been argued as a direct means to integrate assessment with instruction. For example, several authors (e.g., Campione & Brown, 1987; Feuerstein, 1980; Haywood, Brown, & Wingenfeld, 1990; Lidz, 1996) suggest that traditional testing procedures that rely on intelligence or aptitude tests underestimate general ability. That is, traditional or static approaches to assessment of aptitude typically provide little feedback or practice prior to testing, and therefore performance on such measures often reflects the child's misunderstanding of instructions more than his ability to perform the task (e.g., Brown & Ferrara, 1999; Campbell & Carlson, 1995). A supplement to traditional assessment is to measure a child's performance when given examiner assistance. This procedure that attempts to modify performance, via examiner assistance, in an effort to understand learning potential, captures the essence of dynamic assessment (DA). Thus, DA is defined as a procedure that determines whether substantive changes occur in examinee behavior if feedback is provided across an array of increasingly complex or challenging tasks. This procedure contrasts with traditional models of assessment in which there is no feedback on student performance from the examiner.

Traditional DA Approaches

Traditional approaches of DA include learning potential assessment (e.g., Budoff, 1987), testing-the-limits (Carlson & Wiedl, 1979; Swanson, 1995b), mediated assessment (e.g., Feuerstein, 1980; Tzuriel & Flor-Maduel, 2010), and assisted learning and transfer (e.g., Bransford, Delclos, Vye, Burns, & Hasselbring, 1987; Campione, Brown, Ferrara, Jones, & Steinberg, 1985). Although DA is a term used to characterize a number of distinct approaches (see Sternberg & Grigorenko, 2002, for a review), two common features of this approach are to determine the learner's potential for change when given assistance, and to provide a prospective measure of performance change independent of assistance (e.g., Embretson, 1987; 1992). Unlike traditional testing procedures, score changes due to examiner intervention are not viewed as threatening task validity. In fact, some authors argue that construct validity increases (e.g., Carlson & Wiedl, 1979; Lidz, 1996; Swanson, 1995; also see Sternberg & Grigorenko, 2002, for a review). To obtain information about a child's responsiveness to hints or probes, DA approaches require the interaction of an examiner and the examinee. When a student is having difficulty, the examiner attempts to move the student from failure to success by modifying the format, providing more trials, providing information on successful strategies, or offering increasingly more direct cues, hints, or prompts. The intensity of the intervention ranges from several sessions to brief intensive prompts in one session. Thus, "potential" for learning new information (or accessing previously presented information) is measured in terms of the distance, difference between, and/or change from unassisted performance to a performance level with assistance.

Although DA has been suggested as an alternative and/or supplement to traditional assessment, only a few critical reviews of such procedures have been published (e.g., Caffrey et al., 2008; Elliott & Lauchlan, 1997; Grigorenko & Sternberg, 1998; Jitendra & Kameenui, 1993; Laughon, 1990). The most comprehensive qualitative review of DA procedures to date was conducted by Grigorenko and Sternberg (1998; also see Sternberg & Grigorenko, 2002). Their study reviewed the strengths and weaknesses of five different dynamic testing models: Feuerstein and colleague's model of structural cognitive modifiability (e.g., Feuerstein, Miller, Hoffman, Rand, Mintzker, & Jensen, 1981; Feuerstein & Schur, 1997), Budoff's (1987) learning potential testing model, Campione and Brown's (Campione & Brown, 1987) transfer model, Carlson's (Carlson & Wiedl, 1978, 1979) testing-the-limits model, and an information-processing framework as conceptualized by the Swanson Cognitive Processing Test (S-CPT, Swanson, 1994, 1995a, 1995b; Swanson & Howard, 2005). In general, after reviewing these different approaches, Grigorenko and Sternberg (1998) concluded "that it is difficult to argue that this approach (DA) has proved its usefulness and

has shown a distinct advantage over traditional static testing relative to the resources that need to be extended ..." (p. 105).

Goals of DA

More specifically, Grigorenko and Sternberg (1998) questioned whether the experimental literature supports the goals of DA. These goals are related to (a) providing a better estimate of ability, (b) measuring new abilities, and (c) improving mental efficiency when compared to static testing procedures (see Embretson, 1987; then see Grigorenko & Sternberg, 1998, p. 103). For example, Grigorenko & Sternberg review questioned whether DA increased the comparability of performance among students from differing backgrounds and handicapping conditions when compared to static conditions. That is, when compared to static measures, DA has not been shown to equate the performance among children with differing learning abilities (i.e., level the playing field). In addition, Grigorenko and Sternberg (1998) suggested that cognitive modifiability (a psychological construct frequently referred to in the DA literature) has not been shown to be independent of initial learning ability. Likewise, their review questioned whether changes in mental processing come about because of DA or merely reflect artifacts related to retesting. That is, they argue that approximately 30 percent of children improve to a statistically significant extent simply because of retesting (see Grigorenko & Sternberg, 1998, p. 104). Thus, changes in performance may be unrelated to intervention instructions.

DA Outcomes

So, what's the data on dynamic testing? Swanson and Lussier (2001) addressed this question with meta-analytic techniques. Their synthesis included those studies cited in the comprehensive review by Grigorenko and Sternberg (1998) (N = 229 articles), but was also expanded by a review of the PSYCINFO database over a 35-year period. The search resulted in a list of 303 potential articles for analysis. Most of these articles were eliminated because ESs could not be computed. Thirty articles were included for the final analysis. Each of these articles contained at least a pretest/post-test situation and appropriate statistical information (means, standard deviations, or F tests) to calculate ESs. Each article was coded for: sample size, type of ability group, assessment instruments, mean age of participants, IQ range of participants, gender ratio, length of treatment sessions, amount of time per session, and type of experimental design.

The majority of information coded is shown in Table 36.1. For example, studies were coded on whether participants were average achievers or reflected special education categories. This resulted in five classification categories: Average Achievers, Mentally Retarded, Learning Disabled, Under Achieving, and Hearing Impaired. Participants were classified as Average Achieving if the article stated participants were of "average ability" or served as "age matched" participants when compared to a special education group, or if the study stated that the sample was considered a normal representation of the population. Participants were coded as Mentally Retarded if IQs were 71 or lower on a standardized intelligence test (e.g., Wechsler Intelligence Scale for Children). Participants were

Table 36.1 Weighted Effect Size as a Function of Moderator Variables

Participant Ages				95% Confidence Interval	
1. Young (< 10)	N	K	ES	Low	High
2. Middle (10–13)	4,480	55	0.65	0.62	0.7
3. Older (> 13)	4,906	78	0.36	0.31	0.4
	2,558	31	0.38	0.32	0.44
Sample Size					
1. < 40	2,033	74	0.47	0.41	0.54
2. > 39 AND < 80	2,613	44	1.11	1.05	1.18
3. > 79	7,270	46	0.29	0.26	0.32
Domain					
Verbal	368	11	0.31	0.16	0.47
Visual-Spatial	11,548	153	0.48	0.45	0.51
Participants					
Average Ach.	7,523	98	0.41	0.38	0.45
Ment. Retard.	2,645	23	0.49	0.43	0.55
Learning Dis.	633	20	0.1	-0.01	0.22
Under Ach.	419	8	0.98	0.81	1.14
Hearing Imp.	350	9	0.75	0.58	0.91
Number of Sessions					
Single	9,154	127	0.48	0.45	0.52
Multiple	2,762	37	0.43	0.37	0.49
Type of Instruction					
1. Test Limits	8,221	128	0.48	0.45	0.52
2. Training	1,695	14	0.21	0.15	0.28
3. General-Feedback (strategy)	2,000	22	0.85	0.58	0.71

K = Number of Dependent Measures, Ach = Achievers, Inst = Instruction, Imp = Impaired, Test. Limits = Testing the Limits, Train = Test-Train-Test Model labeled Learning Disabled if so designated by the primary author and/or if IQ scores were in the normal range (85 – 115) and achievement scores in one or more domains (e.g., reading) were below the 25th percentile. Participants were coded Under Achieving if samples were labeled by the primary author as "under achieving," "slow learning," or participants in a Head Start program. The final category, Hearing Impaired or Deaf, included participants who were identified as pre-lingually deaf or classified as "deaf."

Dependent measures were also coded as reflecting primarily visual-spatial or verbal assessment measures. Tasks coded as visual-spatial measures included: the Test of Early Math Ability, the Kohs Block Design, Piagetian Matrices Task, The Order of Appearance Test, The Representational Stencil Design Test, Number Finding Task, Visual Search Test, Child's Analogical Thinking Modifiability Test, The Differential Ability Test, The Raven's Colored Progressive Matrices Test and its sub-tests (including the picture booklet and puzzle forms), the Wechsler Preschool and Primary Scale of Intelligence-the Block Design subtest, the Picture Analogy Test, the Leiter International Performance Scale, and the "balance-scale strategy using moving pegs" (Day & Cordon, 1993). Tasks labeled as primarily verbal were verbal subtests from the Swanson-Cognitive Process Test (e.g., Story Retelling, Semantic Association, Rhyming, Semantic Classification, Phrase Sequencing, Digit-Sentence), verbal subtests from the Wechsler Preschool and Primary Scale of Intelligence (e.g., Similarities subtest), the Yopp-Singer Test (phoneme segmentation task), the Picture Vocabulary Test, and the Electricity Knowledge Test.

In terms of design, studies were classified as "between comparisons" if two *independent* samples in two treatment conditions (i.e., static vs. dynamic) were compared or "within design comparisons," if the *same* participants were compared on both the static and dynamic measures. The later condition reflects pretest–post-test only situations (i.e., the pre-test reflects the static measure, usually, followed by a scaffolded/mediated learning period, and then a post-test). If a study was classified as a "Within Design Comparison," then the pre-test was considered the static test and the post-test (i.e., after interaction) was considered a measure of dynamic testing.

Studies were also divided into three general models. One set of studies tested the limits by using systematic scaffolding, via verbal mediation or probes, to push performance to *upper* limits (e.g., Carlson & Wiedl, 1979; Swanson, 1992). These studies compared various cuing procedures but had the goal of maximizing performance at an upper or asymptotic level. A second set of studies used techniques that trained participants to solve problems or intervened on performance in order to instruct (e.g., Budoff, 1987). This set of studies used a test-train-test format usually involving coaching and/or mediated training. The final set of studies relied on structured strategy training, modeling, and/or general feedback (e.g., Larson et al., 1991). The terms "scaffolding" (pushing the limits), "mediated learning" (training), and "general feedback" are used to reflect, respectively, the three models.. Clearly these overlapped in some areas (cues, instruction, and practice), but the primary form of assessment in each study was assessed.

All together, 170 effect sizes (ESs) were generated. Table 36.1 provides a summary of the mean ESs and standard deviations across studies as a function of the categories of variables. Column one reports the sample size (N); column 2, the number of dependent measures (K); column 3, ES; and columns 4 and 5, the confidence intervals. As shown in Table 36.1, the magnitude of the ESs varied significantly ($ps < .05$) as a function of age (ages 10 to 13 = samples less than 10 years > samples with ages > 13), sample size (samples < 80 but larger than 39 yield larger ES than samples > 79 or < 40), and type of dynamic assessment (scaffolding and general feedback yields higher ESs than explicit training). Comparisons were made between studies that only included pretest/post-test designs (within or repeated design) and those that made between-conditions comparisons. When a correction was made related to pretest–post-test correlations, a significant difference in ESs emerged in favor of between-comparison designs (M = .91) when compared to within designs (.17).

The most important findings were related to ability group. When compared with the other ability groups, the highest mean ES (M = .98) emerged for underachieving participants, whereas the lowest ES emerged for learning-disabled participants (M = .10). These findings on children with learning disabilities (LD) will also be discussed later when we discuss evidence-based practices below.

Links to Instruction

How does DA inform us about child performance? First, DA procedures positively influence the magnitude of ES. The overall magnitude of

ES was found to be 1.69 for between-comparison studies (samples are assigned to either static or DA testing condition) and 1.40 for studies that use the same sample in a pretest–post-test only design. Thus, based on Cohen's criterion of .80 as a large ES, DA procedures substantially improved testing performance over static testing conditions. However, the magnitude of the ES was substantially reduced for between-comparison design studies when weighted for sample size (ES = .91) and when pretest–post-test only designs were corrected for upward biases and artifacts-related retesting (ES = .16). The positive ES does suggest, however, that dynamic testing does make positive changes in performance.

Second, the magnitude of ES was directly influenced by the type of assessment used. ESs were higher for studies that included strategy training, general feedback, and modeling (ES = .85), followed by those that allowed for testing the limits (e.g., scaffolding, ES = .48), followed by those conditions that focused on coaching and/or mediated training (ES = .21). Further, these effects were not an artifact of ability group, number of assessment sessions, or the age of the sample.

Third, the conditions under which ability-group differences across diverse dependent measures are reduced or maximized were identified. Through various regression modeling Swanson and Lussier (2001) found that ability group differences in responsiveness to DA procedures were non-significant. However, advantages were found for underachievers when variables related to age, number of sessions, and types of assessment were left to co-vary. Their synthesis suggested that DA equated ability groups in terms of *responsiveness* to dynamic test conditions when variables related to instruction, type of measure, age, and type of design were held constant in the analysis. This finding supports the contention that changes in performance as a function of DA procedures reflected abilities independent of measures of traditional classification and procedures. That is, in reference to the goals of DA discussed earlier (providing better estimates of ability and providing a measure independent of ability), comparability of ES as a function of ability group was supported. However, the playing field was only equalized when all variables are entered into the regression model. Given the common finding that normal and handicapped groups differ on a host of verbal and visual-spatial measures, finding no significant differences in the magnitude of ESs related to ability group suggests that some new abilities are being tapped.

Fourth, the results support the notion that the magnitudes of ESs are not merely an artifact of length of intervention. No differences in ES emerged related to the number of treatment sessions. Rather, the results clearly supported the notion that treatment effects, particularly those studies that emphasized general feedback or scaffolding, contributed independent variance to the magnitude of the ES. These findings suggested that changes in mental efficiency are related to DA conditions and not merely to re-testing conditions.

Finally, the synthesis complemented the findings of Grigorenko and Sternberg (1998) and others more recently (Caffrey et al., 2008; Fuchs et al., 2008; Swanson & Howard, 2005; Yeomans, 2008), but also suggested that DA procedures may provide an estimate of processing potential not necessarily tapped by traditional assessment approaches. DA training resulted in better performance than traditional (referred to as static testing), even when studies under different conditions were considered (multiple sessions versus single, between groups versus within groups) and ESs were corrected for pretest sensitivity and upward biases. In terms of new abilities, a relationship was found between ES and responsiveness to the type of DA procedures used; this pattern holds true in the full regression model (with all variables present). It is important to note, however, that the results did not hold up when only main effects were considered in isolation from the influence of other variables. When the categories of studies were considered in isolation, underachievers clearly yield higher ESs, and LD children lower ESs than other ability groups. Further, there is a trend to find higher ESs in younger age groups (younger participants yield higher ESs than the older ages).

Qualifications in Using DA

Although the analyses by Swanson and Lussier (2001) suggested some positive benefits to using DA techniques when linking assessment and instruction, there are at least three qualifications to their findings when linking the results of DA to practice. First, most DA procedures in the studies we reviewed have been validated primarily on tasks that may have weak contextual validity within the classroom. For example, some of the tasks in which changes in performance have been shown (e.g., Raven Progressive Matrices, and Block Designs) may have very little relevance to areas in which high-risk children experience difficulties—such as reading (reading comprehension and writing) or math (calculation, problem solving).

Second, there is some question about the "level" or "meaning of" the dependent measures used in DA procedures. Some DA approaches focus on change scores (products), rather than the processes that are changing. Although the assessment of children at risk can certainly focus on "how much change can occur in a score," of greater interest to the educator are the cognitive processes or strategies that may have been influenced by such changes. For example, in some of the DA approaches reviewed by Swanson and Lussier, it is was uncertain whether changes in performance reflected information that is available or accessible in the "mind" of the child tested or merely reflected changes in testing format. That is, in some DA procedures changes in performance may be related to increasing task familiarity, instructions, expectations, and/or individual attention. Thus, changes are not necessarily influencing any deep cognitive structures, as much as they are directing the child's attention to important task parameters.

Finally, it is uncertain in some studies whether examiner feedback to the child suspected of being at risk for learning activates the information that is already in the child's mind or reintroduces the concept again to a poorly stored original memory trace. The differences between learners on these later issues are important if gains in scores are to be attributed to changes in environment or changes in cognition, or both.

Summary

A meta-analysis of the literature shows that DA procedures improve testing performance of children and adolescents over traditional (static) conditions. Other important findings were that the influence of ability-group classification, except for learning disabilities, was mitigated with DA procedures when a full array of contextual variables was considered. Clear advantages were found for DA procedures that use general feedback and modeling during testing. We now review a meta-analysis related to evidence-based instruction for children and adolescents with learning disabilities (LD). A focus is placed on children and adolescents with LD because this group reflects the largest incidence of children in special education.

Effective Instruction and Role of Psychometric Information

Children with LD are a heterogeneous group and, therefore, no general instructional effective model can be recommended for all of them. However, we think some common general principles from the experimental intervention literature have emerged, and effective instructional programs capitalize on these principles. We summarize findings related to our meta-analysis of the literature (Swanson, Hoskyn, & Lee, 1999; Swanson & Deshler, 2003). There have been several excellent meta-analyses on instructional research in LD (Gersten et al., 2009), but none to our knowledge have considered intervention research across a broad array of academic domains and/or controlled for variations in methodology. In addition, none of these syntheses have attempted to link instructional outcomes with variations in definitions of LD.

The primary meta-analysis referred to (Swanson et al., 1999) was funded by the U.S. Department of Education. This research synthesized experimental intervention research conducted on children with LD over a 35-year period. Swanson and several colleagues (e.g., Swanson, 1999a; 2000, Swanson & Deshler, 2003; Swanson & Hoskyn, 1998; Swanson & Sachse-Lee, 2000) synthesized articles, technical reports, and doctoral dissertations that reported on group design and single design studies published between the years of 1963 and 2000. Condensing over 3,000 ESs, they found a mean ES of .79 for LD treatment versus LD control conditions for group design studies (Swanson & Hoskyn, 1998) and 1.03 for single-subject design studies (Swanson & Sachse-Lee, 2000). According to Cohen's (1988) classification system, the magnitude of the ES was large. Thus, on the surface, the results are consistent with the notion that children with LD are highly responsive to intense intervention. However, when children with LD were compared to non-disabled children of the same grade or age who also were receiving the same best evidence intervention procedure, ESs (ES M = .97, SD = .52) were substantially in favor of non-disabled children (see Swanson et al., 1999, pp. 162–169).

There were two other important findings from this synthesis as applied to effective instruction. First, the analysis showed that combined direct and explicit strategy instruction (explicit practice, elaboration, strategy cuing) and small group interactive settings best predicted the size of treatment outcomes across various academic domains. The implication of this finding is that a combination of direct instruction (DI) and cognitive strategy (SI) instruction provided the best evidence-based instructional heuristic for improving academic performance (effect sizes >.80) in children with LD. However, these components accounted for less that

15 percent of the variance in predicting outcomes (Swanson, 1999b). This finding held when controls were made in the analysis for methodology, age, and type of academic domain (e.g., reading, math, and writing).

A further analysis of the data divided the studies up in terms of their emphasis on key activities or components of instruction. Swanson (2000) divided studies into eight models based on key instructional tactics: direct instruction (a focus on sequencing and segmentation of skills), explicit strategy training, monitoring (teaching children strategies), individualized and remedial tutoring, small interactive group instruction, teacher-indirect instruction (teacher makes use of homework and peers' help for instruction), verbal questioning/attribution instruction (asking children key questions during the learning phase and whether they thought what they were learning would transfer), and technology (using computers to present concepts). The results indicated that explicit strategy instruction (explicit practice, elaboration, strategy cuing) and small group interactive settings best improved the magnitude of treatment outcomes.

In terms of presentation format, Swanson (1999b) found that effective instructional models follow a *sequence of events*:

1. State the learning objectives and orient the students to what they will be learning and what performance will be expected of them.

2. Review the skills necessary to understand the concept.

3. Present the information, give examples, and demonstrate the concepts/ materials.

4. Pose questions (probes) to students and assess their level of understanding and correct misconceptions.

5. Provide group instruction and independent practice. Give students an opportunity to demonstrate new skills and learn the new information on their own.

6. Assess performance and provide feedback. Review the independent work and give a quiz. Give feedback for correct answers and reteach skills if answers are incorrect.

7. Provide distributed practice and review.

Swanson also found that some instructional components were far more important than others in various instructional domains. For example in the domain of reading comprehension (Swanson, 1999b), those key instructional components that contributed in significantly (as shown in regression analyses) improving the magnitude of outcomes (ES) were:

1. *Directed Response/Questioning.* Treatments related to dialectic or Socratic teaching, the teacher directing students to ask questions, the teacher and a student or students engaging in reciprocal dialogue.

2. *Control Difficulty or Processing Demands of Task.* Treatments that included short activities, level of difficulty controlled, teacher providing necessary assistance, teacher providing simplified demonstration, tasks sequenced from easy to difficult, and/or task analysis.

3. *Elaboration.* Treatments that included additional information or explanation provided about concepts, procedures, or steps, and/or redundant text or repetition within text.

4. *Modeling by the Teacher of Steps.* Treatments that included modeling by the teacher in terms of demonstration of processes and/or steps the students are to follow to solve the problem.

5. *Small Group Instruction.* Treatments that included descriptions about instruction in a small group, and/or verbal interaction occurring in a small group with students and/or teacher.

6. *Strategy Cues.* Treatments that included reminders to use strategies or multi-steps, use of "think aloud models," and/or teacher presenting the benefits of strategy use or procedures.

In contrast, the important instructional components that significantly increased the ESs for word recognition were:

1. *Sequencing.* Treatments included a focus on breaking down the task, fading of prompts or cues, sequencing short activities, and/or using step-by-step prompts.

2. *Segmentation.* Treatments included a focus on breaking down the targeted skill into smaller units, breaking into component parts, segmenting and/or synthesizing components parts.

3. *Advanced Organizers.* Treatments included a focus on directing children to look over material prior to instruction, directing children to focus on particular information, providing prior information about task ahead, and/or the teacher stating objectives of instruction prior to commencing.

The importance of these findings is that only a few components from a broad array of activities were found to moderate treatment outcomes. Regardless of the instructional focus (math, writing, reading), two instructional components emerged in Swanson et al.'s analysis of treatments for children with LD. One component was explicit practice, which included activities related to distributed review and practice, repeated practice, sequenced reviews, daily feedback, and/or weekly reviews. The other component was advanced organizers, which included: (a) directing children to focus on specific material or information prior to instruction, (b) directing children about task concepts or events before beginning, and/or (c) the teacher stating objectives of the instruction.

There is a note of caution when interpreting best evidence studies. This is because the results of "best evidence studies" (or in this case, studies reporting on effective instruction) are influenced by a host of moderating variables. For example, in the Swanson and colleagues' meta-analysis (Swanson & Hoskyn, 1998; Swanson et al., 1999), all studies for comparative purposes had well-defined control groups and treatments and/or baseline conditions before their inclusion in the synthesis. The synthesis eliminated the analysis of all studies of poor methodological quality (see Valentine & Cooper, 2005, for a rationale). Simmerman and Swanson (2001) analyzed these best evidence studies and found that slight variations in the internal and external validity significantly moderated the magnitude of treatment outcomes.

More specifically, Simmerman and Swanson (2001) analyzed studies in the Swanson et al. (1999) synthesis and found that slight variations in the internal and external validity moderated that magnitude of treatment outcomes for students with LD. Violations that were significantly related to treatment outcomes included the following:

- teacher effects (studies that used the very same experimenter for treatment and control in administrating treatments yield smaller ESs than those studies that used different experimenters in administering treatments);
- establishment of a criterion level of instructional performance before moving to the next level (studies that specified performance criteria yield significantly larger weighted ESs than those that did not);
- reliance on experimental measures (studies that did not use standardized measures had much larger ESs than those that reported using standardized measures), using different measures between pretest and post-test (larger ESs emerge for studies that used alternative forms when compared to those that used the same test);

- use of a heterogeneous sample in age (studies that included both elementary and secondary students yielded larger ESs than the other age level conditions);
- and use of the correct unit of analysis (those studies that applied the appropriate unit of analysis [i.e., when small groups were presented, the interventions and the unit of analysis was groups instead of individuals], yield smaller ESs than those that used the incorrect unit of analysis).

Furthermore, studies that left out critical information inflated treatment outcomes in a positive direction. The under-reporting of information related to the following yielded larger ESs than those that positively inflated the magnitude of treatment outcomes:

- ethnicity (studies that reported ethnicity yielded smaller ESs than those that did not report ethnicity);
- locale of the study (larger ESs occurred when no information was provided about the locale of the study);
- psychometric data (larger ESs occurred when no psychometric information was reported when compared to the other conditions); and
- teacher application (studies that provide minimal information in terms of teacher implications and recommendations yielded larger ESs than those that provide more information).

The magnitude of ESs was also influenced by whether studies relied on federal definitions (studies that did not report using the federal definition yielded a larger weighted effect score than those that did) or reported using multiple definitional criteria (studies that included multiple criteria in defining their sample yielded smaller ESs than those that did not report using multiple criteria) in selecting their sample. In addition, they found that some methodological variables that influenced the magnitude of ESs were not violations of internal or external validity, but rather were moderating variables that appear to maximize the effects of treatment. These variables relate to the instructional setting (small instructional groups yield larger ESs than individual or large group instruction), direct teaching of transfer (studies that trained for transfer to different abstract skills yield larger ESs than those that do not), and the degree to which treatments were implemented as intended (studies that indicated the specific sessions in which treatment integrity was assessed yielded larger ESs than those that did not). In sum, studies considered as "best evidence" for intervention effects must be carefully scrutinized.

More importantly, when applied to the issues of assessment, studies that left out critical information commonly used in most assessment test batteries (e.g., IQ and achievement scores) greatly inflated treatment outcomes. More specifically, the analysis addressed the question, "Does it matter, in terms of treatment outcomes, whether samples with LD have high or low IQ scores or have large or minimal discrepancies between IQ and achievement or if such children are merely defined by cut-off scores?" Quite simply, do variations in how samples with LD are defined interact with treatment outcomes? No doubt, research efforts in search of definition x treatment interactions may suffer the same fate as research that has focused on aptitude x treatment interactions. These latter interactions among children (either with or without LD) have been equivocal, and few studies have shown that children are differentially responsive to teaching methods. However, this may be because, among other things, aptitude and treatment are multivariate variables. One means of evaluating whether aptitude variations in the LD sample interact with treatment is to compare the relationship between treatment outcomes with multivariate data that include different configurations of how samples with LD are defined. This can be accomplished by placing studies on the same metric (effect size) and comparing the magnitude of these outcomes as a function of variations in the sample definition (e.g., on measures of intelligence and reading).

Thus, we briefly review some of the results of Swanson et al. (1999) testing whether variations in how the samples of students with LD are defined interact with treatment outcomes. Specifically, we review whether (a) those studies that include samples with large differences in intelligence and reading (defined by discrepancy criteria) and/or (b) those studies defined by cut-off score criteria (children and adolescents with LD suffer a discrepancy between their actual achievement and their expected level of achievement based upon IQ scores) yield quantitatively different outcomes as a function of the type of treatment (e.g., strategy or direct instruction) when compared to competing conditions.

The two aptitude measures (intelligence and reading) were isolated because they are the most frequently reported psychometric measures across all studies. Thus, aptitude in this context is defined narrowly by focusing only on variations in reported intelligence and reading scores across studies. Various treatments in the synthesis were categorized as reflecting a critical threshold of instructional components related to strategy instruction (SI), direct instruction (DI), and/or both instructional models (SI + DI). The models of instruction were operationally defined as the occurrence or nonoccurrence of specific instructional components (to be described in the methods section) reflected in the treatment description (see Swanson et al. 1999, for a detailed description). Based upon a set number of activities, studies were classified as a Combined SI and DI model (referred to as the combined model), DI-alone (DI), SI-alone (SI) and a model (non SI & non DI) that failed to reach a critical threshold of "reported" information. We drew upon the literature to operationalize direct instruction and strategy instruction approaches. Several reviews suggested that direct instruction emphasizes fast-paced, well-sequenced, highly focused lessons. The lessons are delivered usually in small groups to students who are given several opportunities to respond and receive feedback about accuracy and responses (see Kaméenui, Jitendra, & Darsch, 1995, for a review of model variations). Those activities coded that reflect direct instruction in the present synthesis include breaking down a task into small steps, administering probes, administering feedback repeatedly, providing a pictorial or diagram presentation, allowing for independent practice and individually paced instruction, breaking the instruction down into simpler phases, instructing in a small group, teacher modeling a skill, providing set materials at a rapid pace, providing individual child instruction, teacher asking questions, and teacher presenting the new (novel) materials. A second instructional variable coded was strategy instruction. Components related to effective strategy instructional programs are reviewed elsewhere (see Wong, Harris, Graham, & Butler, 2003, for review). Based upon these reviews, we categorized studies as reflecting strategy instruction if they include at least three of the following instructional components: elaborate explanations (i.e., systematic explanations, elaborations, and/or plans to direct task performance), modeling from teachers (i.e., verbal modeling, questioning, and demonstration from teachers), reminders to use certain strategies or procedures (i.e., cued to use taught strategies, tactics, or procedures), step-by step prompts or multi-process instructions, dialogue (i.e., the teacher and student talk back and forth), teacher asks questions, and teacher provides only necessary assistance. Based upon these criteria, studies were classified into one of the four aforementioned models: (SI + DI, SI-alone, DI-alone, or non SI and non DI). As a validity check on our classifications, we compared our classification of the treatment conditions with that of the primary author's general theoretical model and/or the label attached to the treatment condition. There was substantial overlap (approximately 70 percent of the studies) between those studies we classified as DI and strategy instruction models with the primary authors' titles or descriptions of the independent variables. For example, frequent terms provided by the author were strategy, cognitive intervention, monitoring, metacognition, self-instruction, and cognitive-behavior modification for the strategy model. Those that were classified as DI by our criteria used such labels as directed instruction, advanced organizers, adapting materials, corrective feedback, or direct computation.

Although the majority of studies had samples identified as LD, studies varied tremendously on the criteria and detail for participant selection. In terms of reporting group mean scores on psychometric information, only 104 studies reported group mean scores for intelligence, 84 studies reported group mean scores on achievement scores in reading, and 22 studies reported group mean scores in mathematics. Beyond IQ, reading, and mathematics scores, psychometric information on other characteristics of the sample was infrequently reported (< 3% of the studies). In terms of those studies that reported scores, 83.7 percent of the studies that reported IQ scores used tests from the Wechsler series (e.g., WISC-III) as the measure of intelligence, and 80 percent of the studies that reported achievement scores used the Wide Range Achievement Test, Peabody Individual Achievement Test, Woodcock-Johnson Reading Mastery Test, or the reading section (cluster) from Woodcock-Johnson Psycho-educational Inventory as the measure of reading achievement. The mean reported treatment IQ for the LD sample was 93.51 (SD = 16.51, range of 85 to 115). Of those studies reporting standardized reading scores (42%), the mean reported standard score was 71.44 (SD = 25.38). For the studies that report descriptive criteria for selecting subjects identified as LD, 73 percent mention the concept of a discrepancy between achievement and IQ, and differences in IQ and achievement scores, and/or that children with LD were presently placed in a special education class (e.g., pull-out classroom).

Table 36.2 shows the variations in ES as a function of the reported sample psychometric characteristics.

The table shows the total sample of students with LD, number of studies in each category, unweighted ES, standard deviation, and weighted ES, averaged within each study. The general pattern was that studies that fail to report psychometric information on participants with LD yield significantly higher ESs than those studies that report psychometric information. For example, as shown in Table 36.2, studies were categorized by the amount of psychometric information reported. Four categories were developed for comparisons (no information, standardized intelligence test scores, standardized intelligence scores + standardized reading test scores, and standardized intelligence test scores + reading scores + mathematics scores). The results indicated that those studies providing no psychometric information on the LD sample produced significantly larger ESs than those studies that reported intelligence, reading, and/or mathematics scores. No significant differences (all ps >.05) were found between those studies that reported intelligence scores and those that reported standardized intelligence scores and reading and/or mathematics scores. Our best explanation for this pattern is that samples that are poorly defined in the assessment process inflate treatment outcomes by introducing greater heterogeneity into the sample when compared to studies that select samples based upon psychometric criteria.

Given that psychometric information is related to ES, the reported sample characteristics were further categorized by the reported range in intelligence scores and the reported range of reading scores. As shown in Table 36.2, three categories for comparison were created for intelligence: those studies that reported mean standard scores between 85 and 92, those that reported mean standardized intelligence scores greater than 91, and those that did not report standardized information. If studies provided multiple IQ scores (verbal, performance, nonverbal, etc.), these scores were averaged within studies. As shown in Table 36.2, the results indicated that the highest ESs occurred when no information about IQ was presented (.77) when compared to conditions that reported IQ (.60 range). No significant differences in ES emerged between studies that report high-average or low-average IQs.

The next category considered in our sample analysis was reading severity. The majority of studies that reported reading scores included measures of word recognition. If multiple standardized reading measures were provided in the study, reading scores were averaged across word recognition and reading comprehension. Four categories of reading

Table 36.2 Effect Size Estimates as a Function of Reported Psychometric Information

I. All Studies	Sample Size	N	Mean	SD	Weighted Mean
All Studies with Outliers Removed	4,871	180	0.79	0.52	0.61
1. No Information					
	2,560	73	0.83	0.5	0.82
2. Intelligence					
	1,111	55	0.8	0.58	0.62
3. Intelligence + Reading					
	849	39	0.76	0.54	0.63
4. Intelligence + Reading + Math					
	349	13	0.66	0.28	0.6
II. Intelligence					
1. > 84 & < 92[a]					
	1,464	69	0.77	0.57	0.63
2. No Reported information					
	2,822	86	0.82	0.5	0.77
3. > 91					
	584	25	0.79	0.48	0.66
III. Reading Severity					
1. < 85					
	771	35	0.86	0.52	0.71
2. > 84 & < 91					
	127	9	0.57	0.39	0.51
3. No Score					
	3,629	122	0.8	0.54	0.73
4. > 90					
	293	14	0.69	0.44	0.55

[a]Standard Score Range

level were created for comparisons: scores below 85, scores above 84 and less than 91, scores greater than 90, and no standardized scores reported. The results indicated that ESs for studies that reported scores below 85 were comparable to those studies that reported no scores. The lowest ESs occurred between studies that reported reading scores between 84 and less than 91 when compared to other conditions (ps <.05).

In summary, our analysis shows that reported intelligence and reading level in isolation had minimal influence on the magnitude of ES (see Table 36.2).

This was not the case, however, when the simultaneous impact of *both* aptitude variables on treatment outcome was taken into consideration. The important findings were that samples that would be considered as reflecting slow learners (IQ and reading scores in the same low range, < 90 standard score), yielded larger ESs (Mean ES = .95) in terms of treatment outcomes than did children with the same low level of reading but higher IQ scores (> 90) (Mean ES = .52). The results also indicated a depressed pattern of performance for studies that reported intelligence scores above 90. For this IQ range, ESs were significantly lower when reading scores were in the 85 to 90 range (M = .52) when compared to studies that included severe readers (< 85, M = .78) and readers in the average range (reading score > 90, M = .68, ps <.05).

Definition x Treatment

As previously stated, a combination of direct instruction and cognitive strategy instruction (SI + DI) provided the best evidence-based instructional heuristic for improving academic performance (effect sizes >.80) in children with LD across various academic domains. An investigation was conducted to investigate whether various configurations of IQ and reading scores were related to the magnitude of ES as a function of the type of treatment (Swanson & Hoskyn, 1999). The Swanson and Hoskyn analysis found that the level of cut-off scores (study meets a cut-off score criteria vs. study does not meet cut-off score) significantly interacted with the instructional contrast variables of orientation (SI-alone vs. DI-alone) and Combination (Combined vs. DI-alone & SI-alone). This finding was important because reading scores at or below the 25th percentile in reading recognition and standardized intelligence performance above 84 have been considered as critical cut-off scores for defining LD (e.g., Francis, Fletcher, Stuebing, Lyon, Shaywitz, & Shaywitz, 2005).

Table 36.3 shows the comparison of the studies reflecting the four models that meet or do not meet "cut-off score criteria." Also shown are the mean IQ and reading scores as a function of the four models. As shown, the ES means for studies that meet cut-off score criterion vs. those that do not were .81 vs. .72, .77 vs. 59, .67 vs. .52, .58 vs. .57 for the Combined model, DI-only, SI-only model, and non DI & non SI models, respectively. The post hoc tests indicated that significant differences emerged in favor of the Combined model (Combined > DI-only = SI-only = non DI & non SI). Except for studies that did not reflect either strategy or direct instruction, the remaining models yielded higher ESs when studies met cut-off score criteria when compared to studies that do not meet criteria.

Table 36.3 Effect Sizes as a Function of Instruction and Definition (Cut-off Scores)

	Sample N	Study N	Effect Size	IQ Scores	Reading Scores
Strategy Instruction–Alone					
	544	15	0.67	93.5	73.94
	1,514	42	0.52	100	92.00
Direction Instruction–Alone					
	535	23	0.77	92.42	77.85
	1,527	74	0.59	98.93	99.88
Combined Strategy and Direct					
	367	14	0.81	97.84	82.58
	2,212	82	0.72	97.08	90.28
No Direct or Strategy Instruction					
	706	23	0.58	97.75	79.25
	3,271	104	0.57	100.56	90.04

Sample N = Total Sample Size, Study N = Number of Independent Studies,
Effect Size = Mean Weighted Effect Size

Summary and Implications

The obvious implication is that variations in IQ and reading have relevance to the magnitude of instructional outcomes. On this issue there are two important findings: First, studies that produced the highest ESs reported both intelligence and reading scores in same low average range (intelligence scores between 84 and 91 and reading scores between 84 and 91) when compared to other studies reporting higher IQ (intelligence scores > 91) but low reading scores (scores between 84 and 91). Although these findings are not related to a particular type of treatment, they support the notion that greater changes emerge in studies whose samples have mean intelligence and reading scores in the same low range (we refer to this sample as a nondiscrepancy or low-discrepancy group).

Second, outcomes related to an instructional approach (e.g., SI, DI) vary across studies that can be separated into those that meet operational definitions (meet cut-off score criteria) and those that do not meet operational definitions. ESs were higher for strategy instruction and/or direct instruction for studies that meet cut-off score criteria when compared to studies that do not meet cut-off score criteria. Thus, the magnitude of outcomes for both direct instruction and strategy instruction models are moderated by sample variations in IQ and reading.

What are the implications of our findings for assessment? There are two clear applications: First, groups of students at risk for LD who have aptitude profiles similar to generally poor achievers or slow learners (low IQ and low reading), produced higher ESs than those samples whose level of IQ is higher than the level of reading. Second, we identified a general approach to instruction (strategies + direct instruction) that remains robust across a diversity of studies.

Traditional Assessment in the Context of RTI

We would be remiss in discussing the link between assessment and effective instruction if we did not discuss links to current procedures referred to as response to intervention (RTI). RTI models are partially based on intervention programs that have distinguished children experiencing academic difficulty due to instructional deficits from those with disability-related deficits (Al Otaiba & Fuchs, 2002; Fuchs & Fuchs, 2006; Vellutino, Scanlon, Sipay, Small, Pratt, Chen, et al., 1996). The RTI model identifies whether a student's current skill level is substantially lower than the instructional level (based on predetermined criteria: e.g., below the 25th percentile in reading achievement). Low academic performance is established using standardized, norm-referenced and/or curriculum-based measurements (Compton, Fuchs, Fuchs & Bryant, 2006; Fuchs, Fuchs, & Compton, 2004). After establishing low performance, empirically based interventions are implemented to determine if a disability is present. Student progress is monitored during the intervention. The impetus for using RTI models for identifying children at risk for learning problems has been partly in response to validity issues related to using discrepancy criteria in defining LD. The controversial question has been whether IQ is a relevant construct in the assessment process. Some research has argued that IQ has little relevance in the assessment process when groups are defined at low levels of reading (e.g., Francis, Fletcher, Stuebing, Lyon, Shaywitz, & Shaywitz, 2005). This question is important since the Individuals with Disabilities Education Improvement Act (IDEA, 2004) and the final regulations published August 14, 2006, by the federal government recognized potential problems with the IQ-discrepancy method for the diagnosis of children with LD. Three criteria were included in IDEA (2004) to better identify children with LD:

1. States are not required to use a severe discrepancy between intellectual ability and achievement.

2. The procedure must include a process where the children's response to scientifically based research interventions is considered in the assessment process.

3. States are permitted to use alternative research-based procedures to determine a specific learning disability.

This law has spurred an intense interest in RTI procedures. We have provided some evidence above that high IQ levels in context of low reading are related to variations in the magnitude of instructional outcomes. However, are variations in IQ important in the assessment process in separating children at risk for RD and those children who are generally poor achievers?

Three meta-analyses addressed this issue prior to the passage of IDEA (2004; Fuchs, Fuchs, Mathes, & Lipsey, 2000; Stuebing, Fletcher, LeDoux, Lyon, Shaywitz, & Shaywitz, 2002; Hoskyn & Swanson, 2000). The contradictions in the three meta-analyses are reviewed in Stuebing et al. (2002). Stuebing et al. considered the Hoskyn and Swanson (2000) selection process of studies most conservative of the three, and therefore I want to highlight the findings related to the relevance of IQ. Hoskyn and Swanson (2000) analyzed only published literature comparing children who were poor readers but either had higher IQ scores than reading scores or had IQ scores commiserate with their reading scores. The findings of the synthesis were consistent with previous studies outside the domain of reading that report on the weak discriminative power of discrepancy scores. Although the outcomes of Hoskyn and Swanson's synthesis generally supported current notions about comparable outcomes on various measures among the discrepancy and non-discrepancy groups, verbal IQ significantly moderated ESs between the two groups. That is, although the degree of discrepancy between IQ and reading was irrelevant in predicting ESs, the magnitude of differences in performance (effect sizes) between the two groups was related to verbal IQ. Hoskyn and Swanson (2000) also found that when the ES differences between discrepancy (reading disabled group) and non-discrepancy groups (low achievers in this case) on verbal IQ measures were greater than 1.00 (the mean verbal IQ of the reading disabled [RD] group was approximately 1.00 and the verbal IQ mean of the low achieving [LA] group was approximately 85) the approximate mean ES on various cognitive measures was 0.29. In contrast, when the ES for verbal IQ was less than 1.00 (the mean verbal IQ for the RD group was approximately 95 and the verbal IQ mean for the LA group was at approximately 90), estimates of ES on various cognitive measures was close to 0 (M = -0.06). Thus, the further the RD group moved from IQs in the 80 range (the cut-off score used to select RD samples), the greater the chances their overall performance on cognitive measures would differ from the low achiever. In short, although the Hoskyn and Swanson's (2000) synthesis supports the notion that "differences in IQ and achievement" are unimportant in predictions of ES differences on various cognitive variables, the magnitude of differences in verbal IQ between these two ability groups did significantly moderate general cognitive outcomes as measured by ESs. Moreover, robust differences on measures between the two groups were found by Fuchs, Fuchs, Mathes, and Lipsey (2000). For example, Fuchs et al. (2000), comparing low-achieving students with and without LD, found moderate ESs (ES = .61, see p. 94) in favor of low achievers without LD. My point in reviewing these major syntheses of the literature is to suggest that removing IQ from the assessment battery in classifying children as LD, especially verbal IQ, is not uniformly supported by the literature.

Summary

The results of these syntheses have enhanced understanding of the potential links between effective assessment and effective instruction in three ways:. First, measuring responsiveness of an individual's performance to feedback has long been viewed as an alternative (or complement) to traditional (static) ability assessment (e.g., Dearborn, 1921; see Embretson, 1992, for a review). Dynamic assessment has been suggested to teachers as a means to enhance children's performance and tap potential that might otherwise be undiscovered by traditional testing approaches. For example, children with identical performance on psychoeducational tests may profit differentially from feedback.

Furthermore, DA provides information necessary to design intervention programs. For example, Day and Cordon (1993) provided third-graders with either scaffolding or complete explanations to solve balance scale problems. As children worked on the problems, scaffolding was provided only if someone experienced difficulties. Thus, the procedures determined what children had already learned (pretest or static measure), as well as how easily they learned (the number of hints needed, the number of explanations required, or DA measure). The application of DA also appears practical to most testing situations. That is, increased validity (changes in ES) in the Swanson and Lussier (2001) synthesis was not due to the labor-intensive time spent with children, but was derived from variations in the type of DA model used. Thus, an assessment of the effects of feedback does not require multiple sessions to assess responsiveness (or too much time to be practically feasible). Further, it could be argued that when DA procedures are coupled with static assessment, they may each provide differential weights in predicting learning criteria. Thus, under some circumstances, static measures may have equal or greater weight in predicting response to instruction than DA measures in some children (children with LD), but not others (underachievers).

Second, an effective general model of instruction that combines the components of direct and strategy instruction supersedes other models for children with LD. There has been some lively debate over the years in the literature about whether instruction should be top-down, via emphasizing the knowledge base, heuristics, and explicit strategies; or a bottom-up emphasis that entails hierarchical instruction at the skill level (e.g., Adams & Carnine, 2003). Based on previous meta-analyses, we conclude that effective instruction is neither a bottom-up nor top-down approach in isolation. Lower-order and higher-order skills interact to influence treatment outcomes. What is clear from the aforementioned syntheses, however, is that varying degrees of success across treatment domains draw from treatments that focus on both high- and low-order instruction (i.e., strategy and direct instruction).

A final application is that the extant literature suggests that significant definition x treatment interactions exist across evidence-based studies (see Swanson & Hoskyn, 1999, for review). Individual variations in IQ and reading level are important moderators of instructional outcomes in group design studies (Swanson & Hoskyn, 1998, 1999). Although not reviewed here, IQ and reading level also serve as significant moderators for single-subject design studies (Swanson & Sachse-Lee, 2000). We find in our meta-analysis of intervention studies that variations in standardized IQ and reading influenced the magnitude of treatment effects (Swanson & Hoskyn, 1998). The general pattern in our data is that poorly defined samples (i.e., minimal information on IQ and achievement) inflated treatment outcomes by introducing greater heterogeneity into the sample when compared to studies that selected samples based on psychometric criteria. The influence of IQ scores on the magnitude of the treatment outcomes became especially relevant when reading scores were below the 25th percentile. Thus, the implication of these findings is that variations in IQ and reading cannot be ignored when predicting treatment outcomes and therefore are a critical ingredient to the identification process.

References

Adams, G., & Carnine, D. (2003). Direct instruction. In H. L. Swanson, K. Harris, & S. Graham (Eds.), *Handbook of learning disabilities* (pp. 323–344). New York: Guilford.

Al Otaiba, S., & Fuchs, D. (2002). Characteristics of children who are unresponsive to early literacy intervention: A review of the literature. *Remedial and Special Education*, 23(5), 300–316.

Bollen, K. A. (1989). *Structural equations with latent variables.* New York: Wiley Interscience.

Bransford, J. C., Delclos, J. R., Vye, N. J., Burns, M., & Hasselbring, T. S. (1987). State of the art and future directions. In C. S. Lidz (Ed.), *Dynamic assessment: An interactional approach to evaluating learning potential* (pp. 479–496). New York: Guilford Press.

Brown, A. L., & Ferrara, R. A. (1999). Diagnosing zones of proximal development. In P. Lloyd & L. Vygotsky (Eds.), *Critical assessments: The zones of proximal development*, Vol. III, (pp. 225–256). New York: Routledge.

Budoff, M. (1987). Measures for assessing learning potential. In C. S. Lidz (Ed.), *Dynamic testing* (pp. 173–195). New York: Guilford Press.

Caffrey, E., Fuchs, D., & Fuchs, L. S. (2008). The predictive validity of dynamic assessment: A review. *The Journal of Special Education*, 41, 254–270.

Campbell, C., & Carlson, J. S. (1995). The dynamic assessment of mental abilities. In J. S. Carlson (Ed.), *Advances in cognition and educational practice: Vol. 3, European contributions to dynamic assessment.* London: JAI Press.

Campione, J. C., & Brown, A. L. (1987). Linking dynamic testing with school achievement. In C. S. Lidz (Ed.), *Dynamic testing* (pp. 82–115). New York: Guilford Press.

Campione, J. C., Brown, A. L., Ferrara, R. A., Jones, R. S., & Steinberg, E. (1985). Breakdowns in the flexible use of information: Intelligence-related differences in transfer following equivalent learning performance. *Intelligence*, 9, 297–315.

Carlson, J. S., & Wiedl, K. H. (1978). Use of testing-the-limits procedures in the assessment of intellectual capabilities in children with learning difficulties. *American Journal of Mental Deficiency*, 82, 559–564.

Carlson, J. S., & Wiedl, K. H. (1979). Toward a differential testing approach: Testing the limits employing the Raven Matrices. *Intelligence*, 3, 323–344.

Cohen, J. (1988). *Statistical power analysis in the behavioral sciences.* Hillsdale, NJ: Erlbaum.

Compton, D. L., Fuchs, D., Fuchs, L. S., & Bryant, J. D. (2006). Selecting at-risk readers in first grade for early intervention: A two-year longitudinal study of decision rules and procedures. *Journal of Educational Psychology*, 98(2), 394–409.

Cooper, H. & Hedges, L. V. (Eds.) (1994). *Handbook of research synthesis.* New York: Russell Sage.

Day, J. D., & Cordon, L. A. (1993). Static and dynamic measures of ability: An experimental comparison. *Journal of Educational Psychology*, 85, 75–82.

Della Toffalo, D. A., & Milke, R. M. (2008). Test reviews: Dynamic assessment of test accommodations. *Journal of Psychoeducational Assessment*, 26, 83–91.

Dearborn, D. F. (1921). Intelligence and its measurement: A symposium. *Journal of Educational Psychology*, 12, 123–147.

Elliott, J. & Lauchlan, F. (1997). Assessing potential—the search for the philosopher's stone? *Education & Child Psychology*, 14, 6–16.

Embretson, S. E. (1987). Improving the measurement of spatial aptitude by dynamic testing. *Intelligence*, 11, 333–358.

Embretson, S. E. (1992). Measuring and validating cognitive modifiability as an ability: A study in the spatial domain. *Journal of Educational Measurement*, 29, 25–50.

Francis, D. J., Fletcher, J. M., Stuebing, K. K., Lyon, G. R., Shaywitz, B. A., & Shaywitz, S. E. (2005). Psychometric approaches to the identification of LD: IQ and achievement scores are not sufficient. *Journal of Learning Disabilities*, 38(2), 98–108.

Fuchs, D., & Fuchs, L. S. (2006). Introduction to response to intervention: What, why, and how valid is it? *Reading Research Quarterly*, 41(1), 93–99.

Fuchs, L. S., Compton, D. L., Fuchs, D., Hollenbeck, K. N., Craddock, C. F., & Hamlett, C. L. (2008). Dynamic assessment of algebraic learning in predicting third graders' development of mathematical problem solving. *Journal of Educational Psychology*, 100(4), 829–850.

Fuchs, D., Fuchs, L. S., & Compton, D. L. (2004). Identifying reading disabilities by responsiveness-to-instruction:

Specifying measures and criteria. *Learning Disability Quarterly, 27*(4), 216–227.

Fuchs, D., Fuchs, L., Mathes, P. G., & Lipsey, M. (2000). Reading differences between low achieving students with and without learning disabilities. In R. Gersten, E. P. Schiller, & S. Vaughn (Eds.), *Contemporary special education research: Synthesis of knowledge base of critical issues* (pp. 81–104). Mahwah, NJ: Erlbaum.

Feuerstein, R. (1980). *Instrumental enrichment: An intervention program for cognitive modifiability*. Baltimore, MD: University Park Press.

Feuerstein, R., Miller, R., Hoffman, M. B., Rand, Y., Mintzker, Y., & Jensen, M. R. (1981). Cognitive modifiability in adolescence: Cognitive structure and the effects of intervention. *The Journal of Special Education, 15*, 269–287.

Feuerstein, R., & Schur, Y. (1997). Process as content in regular education and in particular in education of low functioning retarded performer. In A. L., Costa & R. M. Liebmann (Eds.), *Envisioning process as content: Toward a renaissance curriculum*. Thousand Oaks, CA: Corwin Press.

Gersten, R., Chard, D. J., Jayanthi, M., Baker, S. K., Morphy, P., & Flojo, J. (2009). Mathematics instruction for students with learning disabilities: A meta-analysis of instructional components. *Review of Educational Research, 79*(3), 1202–1242.

Grigorenko, E. L., & Sternberg, R. J. (1998). Dynamic testing. *Psychological Bulletin, 124*, 75–111.

Grigorenko, E. L., Sternberg, R. J., Jukes, M., Alcock, K., Lambo, J., Ngorosho, D., et al. (2006). Effects of antiparasitic treatment on dynamically and statically tested cognitive skills over time. *Journal of Applied Developmental Psychology, 27*, 499–526.

Hasson, N., & Joffe, V. (2007). The case for dynamic assessment in speech and language therapy. *Child Language Teaching & Therapy, 23*(1), 9–25.

Haywood, H. C., Brown, A. L., & Wingenfeld, S. (1990). Dynamic approaches to psychoeducational assessment. *School Psychology Review, 19*, 411–422.

Hedges, L. V., & Olkin, I. (1985). *Statistical methods for meta-analysis*. Orlando, FL: Academic Press.

Hoskyn, M., & Swanson, H. L. (2000). Cognitive processing of low achievers and children with reading disabilities: A selective meta-analytic review of the published literature. *School Psychology Review, 29*, 102–119.

Jeltova, I., Birney, D., Fredine, N., Jarvin, L., Sternberg, R. J., & Grigorenko, E. L. (2007). Dynamic assessment as a process-oriented assessment in educational settings. *Advances in Speech Language Pathology, 9*, 273–285.

Individuals with Disabilities Education Improvement Act of 2004 (IDEA), Pub. L. No. 108-446,118 Stat. 2647 (2004). [Amending 20 U.S.C. §§ 1400 et. seq.].

Jitendra, A. K., & Kameenui, E. J. (1993). Dynamic testing as a compensatory testing approach: A description and analysis. *RASE: Remedial and Special Education, 14*, 6–18.

Kaméenui, E. J., Jitendra, A. K., & Darch, C. B. (1995). Direct instruction reading as contronym and eonomine. *Reading & Writing Quarterly: Overcoming Learning Difficulties, 11*, 3–17.

Laughon, P. (1990). The dynamic assessment of intelligence: A review of three approaches. *School Psychology Review, 19*, 459–470.

Larson, G. E., Alderton, D. L., & Kaupp, M. A. (1991). Dynamic administration of a general intelligence test. *Learning and Individual Differences, 3*, 123–134.

Lipsey, M. W., & Wilson, D. B. (2001). *Practical meta-analysis*. Thousand Oaks, CA: Sage.

Lidz, C. S. (1996). Dynamic assessment approaches. In D. P. Flanagan, J. L. Genshaft, & P. L. Harrison (Eds.), *Contemporary intellectual assessment: Theories, tests, and issues* (pp. 281–296). New York: Guilford Press.

Macrine, S. L., & Sabatino, E. D. (2008). Dynamic assessment and remediation approach: Using the DARA approach to assist struggling readers. *Reading & Writing Quarterly: Overcoming Learning Difficulties, 24*(1), 52–76.

Palinscar, A., Brown, A., & Campione, J. (1991). Dynamic assessment. In H. L. Swanson (Ed.), *Handbook on the assessment of learning disabilities: Theory, research, and practice* (pp. 79–95). Austin, TX: Pro-ed.

Rosenthal, R. & DiMatteo, M. R. (2001). Meta-analysis: Recent developments in quantitative methods for literature reviews. *Annual Review of Psychology, 52*, 59–82.

Simmerman, S., & Swanson, H. L. (2001). Treatment outcomes for students with learning disabilities: How important are internal and external validity? *Journal of Learning Disabilities, 34*, 221–236.

Sternberg, R. J., Grigorenko, E. L., Ngorosho, D., Tantufuye, E., Mbise, A., Nokes, C., et al. (2002). Assessing intellectual potential in rural Tanzanian school children. *Intelligence, 30*(2), 141–162.

Sternberg, R. J., & Grigorenko, E. L. (2002). *Dynamic testing: The nature and measurement of learning potential*. New York: Cambridge University Press.

Stuebing, K. K., Fletcher, J. M., LeDoux, J. M., Lyon, G. R., Shaywitz, S. E., & Shaywitz, B. A. (2002). Validity of IQ-discrepancy classifications of reading disabilities: A meta-analysis. *American Educational Research Journal, 39*, 469–518.

Swanson, H. L. (1992). Generality and modifiability of working memory among skilled and less skilled readers. *Journal of Educational Psychology, 84*, 473–488.

Swanson, H. L. (1994). The role of working memory and dynamic assessment in the classification of children with learning disabilities. *Learning Disabilities Research & Practice, 9*(4), 190–202.

Swanson, H. L. (1995a). Effects of dynamic testing on the classification of learning disabilities: The predictive and discriminant validity of the Swanson-cognitive processing test. *Journal of Psychoeducational Assessment, 13*(3), 204–229.

Swanson, H. L. (1995b). Using the cognitive processing test to assess ability: Development of a dynamic assessment measure. *School Psychology Review, 24*, 672–693.

Swanson, H. L. (1999a). Instructional components that predict treatment outcomes for students with learning disabilities: Support for a combined strategy and direct instruction model. *Learning Disabilities Research & Practice, 14*(3), 129–140.

Swanson, H. L. (1999b). Reading research for students with LD: A meta-analysis in intervention outcomes. *Journal of Learning Disabilities, 32*, 504–532.

Swanson, H. L. (2000). Searching for the best cognitive model for instructing students with learning disabilities: A component and composite analysis. *Educational and Child Psychology, 17*, 101–121.

Swanson, H. L. (2001). Research on interventions for adolescents with learning disabilities: A meta-analysis of outcomes related to higher-order processing. *The Elementary School Journal, 101*, 331–348.

Swanson, H. L. (2011). Meta-analysis of research on children with reading disabilities. In A. McGill-Franzen & R. Allington (Eds.), *Handbook of reading disability research* (pp. 477–487). New York: Routledge.

Swanson, H. L., & Deshler, D. (2003). Instructing adolescents with learning disabilities: Converting a meta-analysis to practice. *Journal of Learning Disabilities, 36,* 124–135.

Swanson, H. L., & Hoskyn, M. (1998). Experimental intervention research on students with learning disabilities: A meta-analysis of treatment outcomes. *Review of Educational Research, 68,* 277–321.

Swanson, H. L., & Hoskyn, M. (1999). Definition × treatment interactions for students with learning disabilities. *School Psychology Review, 28,* 644–658.

Swanson, H. L., & Hoskyn, M. (2001). Instructing adolescents with learning disabilities: A component and composite analysis. *Learning Disabilities Research & Practice, 16,* 109–119.

Swanson, H. L., Hoskyn, M., & Lee, C. M. (1999). *Interventions for students with learning disabilities: A meta-analysis of treatment outcomes.* New York: Guilford.

Swanson, H. L., & Howard, C. B. (2005). Children with reading disabilities: Does dynamic assessment help in the classification? *Learning Disability Quarterly, 28,* 17–34.

Swanson, H. L., & Lussier, C. M. (2001). A selective synthesis of the experimental literature on dynamic assessment. *Review of Educational Research, 71*(2), 321–363.

Swanson, H. L., & Sachse-Lee, C. (2000). A meta-analysis of single-subject-design intervention research for students with LD. *Journal of Learning Disabilities, 33,* 114–136.

Tzuriel, D., & Flor-Maduel, H. (2010). Prediction of early literacy by analogical thinking modifiability. *Journal of Cognitive Education & Psychology, 9,* 107–227.

Valentine, J. C., Cooper, H. M. (2005).Can we measure the quality of causal research in education. In G. Phye, D. Robinson, & J. Levin (Eds.), *Empirical methods for evaluating interventions* (pp. 85–112). San Diego: Elsevier Academic Press.

Vellutino, F. R.; Scanlon, D. M.; Sipay, E. R.; Small, S. G.; Pratt, A.; Chen, R.; et al. (1996). Cognitive profiles of difficult-to-remediate and readily remediated poor readers: Early intervention as a vehicle for distinguishing between cognitive and experimental deficits as basic causes of specific reading disability. *Journal of Educational Psychology, 88,* 601–638.

Wong, B., Harris, K., Graham, S., & Butler, D. (2003). Cognitive strategies instruction research in learning disabilities. In H. L. Swanson, K. Harris, & S. Graham (Eds.), *Handbook of learning disabilities* (pp. 383–402). New York: Guilford.

Yeomans, J. (2008). Dynamic assessment practice: Some suggestions for ensuring follow up. *Educational Psychology in Practice, 24*(2), 105–114.

INDEX

Note: Page numbers followed by "*f*" and "*t*" denote figures and tables, respectively.

CPSIA information can be obtained
at www.ICGtesting.com
Printed in the USA
LVHW061327220119
604800LV00026B/422/P